GERIATRIC EMERGENCY MEDICINE

GERIATRIC EMERGENCY MEDICINE

American College

of Emergency

Physicians

Edited by

Stephen W. Meldon, MD
Associate Professor
Case Western Reserve University
Department of Emergency Medicine
MetroHealth Medical Center
Cleveland, OH

O. John Ma, MD
Associate Professor and Vice Chairman
University of Missouri-Kansas City School of Medicine
Department of Emergency Medicine
Truman Medical Center
Kansas City, MO

Robert H. Woolard, MD
Department of Emergency Medicine
Rhode Island Hospital
Providence, RI

McGraw-Hill
Medical Publishing Division

*New York   Chicago   San Francisco   Lisbon
London   Madrid   Mexico City
Milan   New Delhi   San Juan   Seoul
Singapore   Sydney   Toronto*

Geriatric Emergency Medicine

Copyright © 2004 by **The McGraw-Hill Companies, Inc.** All rights reserved. Printed in the United States of America. Except as permitted under the United States Copyright Act of 1976, no part of this publication may be reproduced or distributed in any form or by any means, or stored in a data base or retrieval system, without the prior written permission of the publisher.

1234567890 DOC DOC 09876543

ISBN 0-07-138385-9

This book was set in Times Roman by Binghamton Valley Composition.
The editors were Andrea Seils and Regina Y. Brown.
The production supervisor was Richard Ruzycka.
The index was prepared by Robert Swanson.
RR Donnelly was the printer and binder.

This book was printed on acid-free paper.

Library of Congress Cataloging-in-Publication Data

Geriatric emergency medicine / edited by Stephen Meldon, O. John Ma, Robert Woolard.–
    1st ed.
        p. ; cm.
    Includes bibliographical references and index.
    ISBN 0-07-138385-9
    1. Geriatrics. 2. Emergency medicine.   I. Meldon, Stephen.   II. Ma, O. John. III.
Woolard, Robert.
    [DNLM: 1. Geriatrics—methods. 2. Emergencies—Aged. 3. Emergency
Medicine—methods. WT 100 G36616 2004]
RC952.5.G3482 2004
618.97—dc21
                                                                    2003051182

To my sons, William and Michael;
to Stephanie, on behalf of dedicated and caring emergency nurses everywhere;
and to our elders who inspire us with their life experience, wisdom, and grace.

Stephen W. Meldon

To my parents, Mark and Simone,
whose love, support, and sacrifice allowed me to enter the field of medicine;
and to Joseph C. Darin, M.D., who provided me the opportunity to practice
emergency medicine and has demonstrated enduring character and leadership.

O. John Ma

To my residents and faculty who will create a better practice of emergency medicine;
to Caroline, Cyrus, and Nancy who have helped me get this far;
and to Alana Ducharme who assisted with editing many of these chapters.

Robert H. Woolard

CONTENTS

Foreword   *xvii*
Preface   *xix*

SECTION I   **Special Considerations**

1   Geriatric Emergency Department Use and Care
     Samuel M. Keim and Arthur B. Sanders   *1*
2   The Physiology of Aging   *Rajeshwar Peddi and John Morley*   *4*
3   Pharmacotherapy and Adverse Drug-Related Events in Elders
     Treated in the Emergency Department
     Laura Snyder, Shannon Connolly, and Bruce Becker   *13*
4   Functional Assessment and Decline   *David J. Peter and Lowell W. Gerson*   *22*
5   Falls   *Manish N. Shah*   *28*
6   Elder Abuse and Neglect   *Elizabeth deLahunta Edwardsen*   *32*
7   Ethical Issues in Geriatric Emergency Medicine   *Catherine A. Marco*   *40*
8   Nursing Home Transfers   *Martin A. Docherty*   *51*
9   Fever and Immune Function in the Elderly
     Eric Daniel Katz and Christopher R. Carpenter   *55*

SECTION II   **Cardiovascular Emergencies**

10   Acute Coronary Syndromes   *Brian F. Erling and William J. Brady*   *71*
11   Syncope   *Jeffrey N. Glaspy*   *78*
12   Heart Failure   *Benjamin J. Freda and W. Franklin Peacock, IV*   *86*
13   Dysrhythmias   *Thomas Lemke*   *99*
14   Valvular Heart Disease   *Stefanie R. Ellison*   *111*
15   Hypertensive Emergencies   *Timothy D. Babbitt and Matthew C. Gratton* *121*
16   Sudden Cardiac Death and Resuscitation   *Stefanie R. Ellison*   *131*

SECTION III   **Pulmonary Emergencies**

17   Acute Dyspnea   *T. Paul Tran*   *137*
18   Geriatric Pneumonia   *Scott T. Wilber*   *144*
19   Chronic Obstructive Pulmonary Disease (COPD)   *T. Paul Tran*   *154*
20   Pulmonary Embolism   *Janet Poponick*   *165*

SECTION IV   **Gastrointestinal Emergencies**

21   Abdominal Pain
      Jeffrey N. Glaspy, O. John Ma, Robert A. Schwab, and Stephen W. Meldon   *173*
22   Peptic Ulcer Disease and Gastrointestinal Bleeding   *Mark E. Hoffmann*   *179*
23   Esophageal Emergencies   *Mark E. Hoffmann*   *185*
24   Diverticular Disease   *Robert A. Schwab and Kary Kaltenbronn*   *191*
25   Bowel Obstruction   *Walter N. Simmons and Gavin J. Putzer*   *198*

26 Volvulus *Walter N. Simmons and Anika Parab* *202*
27 Constipation *Walter N. Simmons and Gavin J. Putzer* *208*
28 Biliary Emergencies *Matthew A. Bridges and O. John Ma* *214*
29 Acute Appendicitis *Robert D. Sidman, Colleen N. Roche, and Stephen W. Meldon* *220*
30 Mesenteric Ischemia *Jeffrey A. Manko and Phillip D. Levy* *227*

SECTION V   Genitourinary Emergencies

31 Renal Emergencies *Jeffrey Cox* *237*
32 Urologic Emergencies *Charles F. Pattavina* *245*
33 Gynecologic Emergencies *Marc R. Toglia* *251*
34 Urinary Tract Infections *Michelle Blanda* *259*

SECTION VI   Vascular Emergencies

35 Abdominal Aortic Aneurysm *Robert L. Rogers and Amal Mattu* *267*
36 Aortic Dissection *Andrew K. Chang* *275*
37 Arterial Insufficiency *Chris J. Richter* *280*
38 Venous Disorders *Natalie A. Kayani* *285*

SECTION VII   Neurologic Emergencies

39 Altered Mental Status *Fredric M. Hustey and Joseph LaMantia* *291*
40 Headache in the Elderly *Richard A. Walker and Michael C. Wadman* *304*
41 Stroke *Melissa Ann Eirich* *316*
42 Seizures and Status Epilepticus in the Elderly *Gary Bubly* *326*
43 Dizziness, Weakness, and Vertigo *Melissa Ann Eirich* *333*

SECTION VIII   Trauma

44 Geriatric Trauma Overview *O. John Ma and Stephen W. Meldon* *337*
45 Head Trauma *David F.E. Stuhlmiller* *343*
46 Chest and Abdominal Trauma *Liudvikas Jagminas and Jeremiah Schuur* *349*
47 Orthopedic and Spinal Injuries *Jason Wilkins* *358*

SECTION IX   Metabolic and Endocrine Emergencies

48 Dehydration and Electrolyte Disorders *Ethan Heit and Stephen W. Meldon* *369*
49 Hypothermia and Hyperthermia *Alexander Rachmiel and Mark D. Levine* *386*
50 Diabetes and Diabetic Emergencies *Micheal D. Rush* *394*
51 Thyroid Emergencies *Jonathan Glauser* *402*
52 Nutritional Issues *David C. Lee and Christopher C. Raio* *416*

SECTION X   Dermatologic Emergencies

53 Toxic Epidermal Necrolysis and Stevens-Johnson Syndrome *Victor A. Pinkes* *427*
54 Autoimmune Bullous Diseases *Paula F. Moskowitz* *432*
55 Zoster *Matthew A. Kopp* *438*
56 Wound Care Issues *Jonathan H. Valente and Mark C. Muetterties* *444*

SECTION XI **Ophthalmologic Emergencies**

57 Approach to Ocular Complaints *Steven Go and Anne L. Clevenger*   455
58 Narrow-Angle-Closure Glaucoma *MaryAnn E. Smith*   462
59 Retinal Vascular Occlusions and Ischemic Optic Neuropathy *MaryAnn E. Smith*   466
60 Eye Infections *Steven Go and Craig T. Florea*   469

SECTION XII **ENT Emergencies**

61 Epistaxis *Thomas K. Swoboda*   475
62 ENT Infections *Jason Graham and Michael Polka*   479
63 Tracheostomy Issues *Robert J. Vissers*   485

SECTION XIII **Hematologic and Oncologic Emergencies**

64 Bleeding and Coagulation *Lance C. Hoffman*   491
65 Anemia *Ryan Davis and Alex Garza*   502
66 Emergency Complications of Malignancy *John P. Sverha and O. John Ma*   506

SECTION XIV **Musculoskeletal and Rheumatologic Emergencies**

67 Back Pain *Andrew D. Perron and Brian F. Erling*   517
68 Acute Arthritis *Harriet Young*   526
69 Giant Cell Arteritis (Temporal Arteritis) and Polymyalgia Rheumatica *Mark Levine*   534
70 Ankylosing Spondylitis *John R. Lindbergh and Andrew D. Perron*   539

SECTION XV **Psychiatric Emergencies**

71 Depression and Suicide *Stephen W. Meldon and Sarah Delaney-Rowland*   545
72 Psychosis *Stephen W. Meldon and Sarah Delaney-Rowland*   550
73 Alcoholism in the Elderly *James W. Campbell*   553

Index *559*

CONTRIBUTORS

Tim Babbitt, MD
Department of Emergency Medicine
Truman Medical Center
University of Missouri-Kansas City School of Medicine
Kansas City, MO

Bruce Becker, MD, MPH, FACEP
Rhode Island Hospital
Department of Emergency Medicine
Providence, RI

Michelle Blanda, MD
Summa Health System
Professor of Emergency Medicine
Northeastern Ohio Universities College of Medicine
Akron, OH

William Brady, MD
Associate Professor and Vice Chair
Department of Emergency Medicine
University of Virginia School of Medicine
Charlottesville, VA

Matthew Bridges, MD
Assistant Professor
University of Missouri-Kansas City School of Medicine
Department of Emergency Medicine
Truman Medical Center
Kansas City, MO

Gary Bubly, MD, FACEP
Clinical Assistant Professor of Medicine
Brown University School of Medicine
Providence, RI
Associate Director
Department of Emergency Medicine
The Miriam Hospital
Providence, RI

James W. Campbell, MD, MS
Chairman, Department of Family Practice and
   Geriatrics
Case Western Reserve University School of Medicine

MetroHealth System
Cleveland, OH

Christopher R. Carpenter, MD
Allegheny General Hospital
Pittsburgh, PA

Andrew K. Chang, MD
Assistant Clinical Professor
Department of Emergency Medicine
University of California, Irvine
Irvine, CA
UCI Medical Center
Department of Emergency Medicine
Orange, CA

Anne L. Clevenger, DO
Truman Medical Center
University of Missouri-Kansas City
Kansas City, MO

Shannon Connolly, MD, MPH, FACEP
Rhode Island Hospital
Department of Emergency Medicine
Providence, RI

Jeffrey Cox, MD
Assistant Clinical Professor of Surgery
Brown University Emergency Medicine Foundation
Providence, RI
Rhode Island Hospital
Department of Emergency Medicine
Providence, RI

Ryan Davis, MD
Department of Emergency Medicine
Truman Medical Center
Kansas City, MO

Martin A. Docherty, MD, FAAEM
Assistant Professor
Division of Emergency Medicine
Washington University School of Medicine
St. Louis, MO

Elizabeth deLahunta Edwardsen, MD
Associate Professor
Department of Emergency Medicine
University of Rochester
Rochester, NY

Melissa Ann Eirich, MD
Assistant Professor
Department of Emergency Medicine
Medical Director for Prehospital Education
Strong Memorial Hospital
University of Rochester
Rochester, NY

Stefanie R. Ellison, M.D.
Department of Emergency Medicine
Truman Medical Center
Kansas City, MO

Brian F. Erling, MD
Clinical Instructor
Department of Emergency Medicine
University of Virginia
Charlottesville, Virginia

Craig T. Florea, MD
Truman Medical Center
Hospital Hill
University of Missouri-Kansas City School of Medicine
Kansas City, Missouri

Benjamin J. Freda, DO
Department of Emergency Medicine
The Cleveland Clinic Foundation
Cleveland, OH

Alex Garza, M.D.
Department of Emergency Medicine
Truman Medical Center
Kansas City, MO

Lowell W. Gerson, PhD
Professor of Epidemiology
Northeastern Ohio Universities
College of Medicine
Rootstown, OH

Jeff Glaspy, MD
Department of Emergency Medicine
Truman Medical Center
Kansas City, MO

Jonathan Glauser, MD, FACEP
Cleveland Clinic Foundation
Cleveland, OH

Steven Go, MD
Director of Emergency Medicine Student Education
Truman Medical Center
Hospital Hill Department of Emergency Medicine
Kansas City, MO
Assistant Professor of Emergency Medicine
University of Missouri-Kansas City School of Medicine
Kansas City, MO

Jason Graham, MD
Department of Emergency Medicine
Truman Medical Center
Kansas City, MO

Matthew Gratton, MD
Department of Emergency Medicine
Truman Medical Center
Kansas City, MO

Ethan Heit, MD
Senior Clinical Instructor
University of Rochester
Rochester, NY

Lance H. Hoffman MD
Assistant Professor
Section of Emergency Medicine
University of Nebraska College of Medicine
Omaha, NE

Mark E. Hoffmann, M.D
Department of Emergency Medicine
St. Cloud Hospital
St. Cloud, MN

Fredric M. Hustey, MD
Assistant Clinical Professor
Emergency Medicine
The Ohio State University
Associate Staff Physician
Department of Emergency Medicine
The Cleveland Clinic Foundation
Cleveland, OH

Liudvikas J. Jagminas, MD
Assistant Professor
Brown Medical School

Department of Emergency Medicine
Rhode Island Hospital

Kary Kaltenbronn, MD
Department of Emergency Medicine
Northwestern University School of Medicine
Chicago, Illinois

Eric Daniel Katz, MD
Washington University School of Medicine
St. Louis, MO

Natalie A. Kayani, MD
Division of Geriatrics
The Cleveland Clinic Foundation
Cleveland, OH

Samuel M. Keim, MD
Associate Professor and Residency Director
Department of Emergency Medicine
University of Arizona College of Medicine
Tucson, Arizona

Matthew A. Kopp, MD
Miriam Hospital
Brown University Department of Emergency
    Medicine
Providence, RI

Joseph LaMantia, MD
Program Director, Emergency Medicine
North Shore University Hospital
Manhasset, NY
Assistant Professor, Clinical Emergency Medicine
New York University School of Medicine
New York, NY

David C. Lee, MD
North Shore University Hospital
Manhasset, New York

Thomas Lemke, MD
Assistant Professor
Brown Medical School
Department of Emergency Medicine
Rhode Island Hospital
Providence, RI

Mark D. Levine, MD
Attending Physician
Division of Emergency Medicine
Washington University School of Medicine
St. Louis, MO

Phillip D. Levy, MD
Assistant Professor of Emergency Medicine
Wayne State University
Detroit Receiving Hospital
Emergency Department
Detroit, MI

John R. Lindbergh, MD
Department of Emergency Medicine
University of Virginia Health Sciences Center
Charlottesville, VA

O. John Ma, MD
Associate Professor and Vice Chair
University of Missouri-Kansas City School of
    Medicine
Department of Emergency Medicine
Truman Medical Center
Kansas City, MO

Jeffrey Manko, MD
Associate Program Director
Department of Emergency Medicine
NYU/Bellevue Medical Center
New York, NY

Catherine A. Marco, MD
Associate Professor, The Medical College of Ohio
Attending Physician, St. Vincent's Mercy Medical
    Center
Acute Care Services
Toledo, OH

Amal Mattu, MD
Director of Academic Development
Department of Surgery, Division of Emergency
    Medicine
Co-Director, Emergency Medicine/Internal Medicine
Combined Residency Training Program
University of Maryland School of Medicine
Baltimore, MD

Stephen W. Meldon, MD
Associate Professor
Case Western Reserve University
Department of Emergency Medicine
MetroHealth Medical Center
Cleveland, OH

John Morley, MD
Dammert Professor of Gerontology
Division of Geriatric Medicine

St. Louis University Health Sciences Center
The Geriatric Research, Education, and Clinical Center
Veterans Administration Hospital
Saint Louis, MO

Paula F. Moskowitz, MD, PhD
Assistant Professor, Department of Dermatology and
    Skin Surgery
Roger Williams Medical Center
Providence, RI
Instructor in Dermatology, Department of Dermatology
Boston University Medical Center
Boston, MA

Mark C. Muetterties, MD
Rhode Island Hospital
Department of Emergency Medicine
Brown University Medical School
Providence, RI

Anika Parab
Department of Emergency Medicine
Rhode Island Hospital
Providence, RI
University of Massachusetts School of Medicine
Amherst, MA

Charles F. Pattavina, MD, FACEP
Assistant Professor of Medicine (Emergency
    Medicine)
Brown University School of Medicine
Providence, RI
Member, Board of Directors
American College of Emergency Physicians
Dallas, TX
Miriam Hospital
Providence, RI

W. Frank Peacock, MD
Associate Professor
The Ohio State University
Director of Clinical Operations
Emergency Department
The Cleveland Clinic
Cleveland, OH

Rajeshwar Peddi, MD
Fellow in Geriatric Medicine
Division of Geriatric Medicine
St. Louis University Health Sciences Center
The Geriatric Research, Education, and Clinical Center

Veterans Administration Hospital
Saint Louis, MO

Andrew D. Perron, MD
Assistant Professor of Emergency Medicine &
    Orthopedic Surgery
Associate Program Director
Department of Emergency Medicine
University of Virginia
Charlottesville, Virginia

David J. Peter, MD
Associate Professor of Clinical Emergency Medicine
Akron General Medical Center
Akron, OH

Victor A. Pinkes, MD
Clinical Assistant Professor of Emergency Medicine
    Brown University
Rhode Island Hospital Department of Emergency
    Medicine
Providence, RI

Michael Polka, MD
Department of Emergency Medicine
SwedishAmerican Health System
Rockford, IL
Truman Medical Center
Kansas City, MO

Janet Poponick, MD
Assistant Professor of Emergency Medicine
Case Western Reserve University
MetroHealth Medical Center
Department of Emergency Medicine
Cleveland, OH

Gavin J. Putzer, MD, MPH
Department of Emergency Medicine
Rhode Island Hospital
Providence, RI
Harvard University, Graduate School of Public
    Health
Boston, MA

Alexander Rachmiel, MD
Resident, Emergency Medicine
Barnes Jewish Hospital
St. Louis, MO

Christopher C. Raio, MD
North Shore University Hospital
Manhasset, New York

Chris J. Richter, MD
Department of Emergency Medicine
St. Johns Mercy Medical Center
Crevecouer, MO

Colleen N. Roche, MD
Associate Residency Director
George Washington University
Washington, DC

Robert L. Rogers, MD
Clinical Instructor
Department of Surgery
Division of Emergency Medicine and Department of
    Medicine
University of Maryland School of Medicine

Sarah Delaney-Rowland, MD
Emergency Medicine Consulting Staff
University of Nebraska Medical Center
Omaha, NE

Mike Rush, MD, FACEP, FAAEM
Department of Emergency Medicine
Truman Medical Center
Kansas City, MO

Arthur B. Sanders, MD
Professor
Department of Emergency Medicine
University of Arizona College of Medicine
Tucson, Arizona

Jeremiah Schuur, MD
Department of Emergency Medicine
Rhode Island Hospital
Providence, RI

Robert A. Schwab, MD
Professor and Chair
University of Missouri-Kansas City School of
    Medicine
Department of Emergency Medicine
Truman Medical Center
Kansas City, MO

Manish N. Shah, MD
Assistant Professor
Department of Emergency Medicine
Department of Community and Preventive Medicine
University of Rochester School of Medicine and
    Dentistry
Rochester, NY

Robert D. Sidman, MD
Residency Director
Department of Emergency Medicine
Rhode Island Hospital
Providence, RI

Walter Simmons, MD
Department of Emergency Medicine
Rhode Island Hospital
Providence, RI

MaryAnn E. Smith, MD
Emergency Physician
Emergency Department
William W. Backus Hospital
Norwich, CT

Laura Snyder, MD
Rhode Island Hospital
Department of Emergency Medicine
Providence, RI

David F Stuhlmiller, MD
Senior Instructor
Case Western Reserve University
Department of Emergency Medicine
MetroHealth Medical Center
Cleveland, OH

John P. Sverha, MD
Assistant Director, Emergency Department
Virginia Hospital Center—Arlington
Arlington, VA

Thomas K. Swoboda, MD, MS
Assistant Professor of Emergency Medicine and
    Pediatrics
Department of Emergency Medicine
Medical College of Wisconsin
Milwaukee, WI

Marc R. Toglia, MD, FACOG
Director, Division of Gynecology
Riddle Memorial Hospital
Media, PA
Assistant Clinical Professor
Department of Obstetrics and Gynecology
Thomas Jefferson University
Philadelphia, PA

T. Paul Tran, MD
Assistant Professor

Section of Emergency Medicine
Department of Surgery
University of Nebraska Medical Center
Omaha, Nebraska

Jonathan H. Valente, MD
Department of Emergency Medicine
Rhode Island Hospital
Assistant Professor, Department of Community
  Health
Brown University Medical School
Providence, RI

Robert J. Vissers, MD
Department of Emergency Medicine
UNC Hospitals
Chapel Hill, NC

Michael C. Wadman, MD
Assistant Professor
Section of Emergency Medicine
Department of Surgery
University of Nebraska College of Medicine
Omaha, NE

Richard A. Walker, MD
Associate Professor
Section of Emergency Medicine

Department of Surgery
University of Nebraska College of Medicine
Omaha, NE

Scott T. Wilber, MD
Summa Health System
Associate Research Director
Department of Emergency Medicine
Akron, OH
Assistant Professor of Emergency Medicine
College of Medicine
Northeastern Ohio Universities
Akron, OH

Jason Wilkins, MD
Department of Emergency Medicine
Cox Medical Center
Springfield, MO

Robert H. Woolard, MD
Department of Emergency Medicine
Rhode Island Hospital
Providence, RI

Harriet Young, MD
University of Rochester Medical Center
Department of Emergency Medicine
Rochester, NY

Foreword

WHILE MOST EMERGENCY PHYSICIANS (EP) readily understand that diseases in infants and children are age related, and have very different presentations and courses that are distinctly dependant upon age, they either don't know that this applies equally to the elderly, of they forget this in the heat of multiple problems. There isn't much in the Emergency Medicine (EM) literature that is specific to geriatrics, and certainly the normal aging changes in physiology are not recognized, remembered or understood.

It has been enormously educational for me to read this book. Not only does it reinforce many of the hard learned lessons that I have had to acquire over the past thirty years, but introduced me to many topics that I had never before been exposed to. I would certainly advise that this book become a compulsory reading for every EM residency, and would also advise a copy be available in every Emergency Department (ED).

The overview chapter is a very effective way to start; there are many physiologic changes of aging that need to be as well remembered and understood as are the physiologic changes of vital signs in infancy. For example, while the infant has a normal tachycardia, the geriatric patient often has a normal bradycardia, even without such a common medication as a beta blocking agent such as Popranolol.

There are many chapters in the book that provide excellent reviews of uncommon diseases that we think we understand, such as endocrine problems involving the thyroid. Nevertheless as the population ages, we see the ravages of many diseases that started much earlier in the patients life, such as treatment for hyperthyroidism with radioactive iodine that is now presenting as hypothyroidism in the elderly. The telltale neck surgical scar is not there to help, and the chapter describes very well the subtle and non classical presentation that is frequent in the elderly.

There are some very strong chapters that have a very common theme, such as dementia, trauma, and pneumonia and other sepsis in the elderly. The theme (and if the practicing physician learns nothing else from this book than this, there will be a markedly improved EM practice): elderly patients do not, and often cannot manifest the classical signs and symptoms that we have learned to appreciate with specific diseases. This means that we don't think of those diagnoses, don't search for evidence of their presence, and frequently underestimate the seriousness of the patient's problems. This leads to inappropriate workups, inappropriate failures in disposition, and mistakes in management that causes significant increases in morbidity and mortality. The repeated message in most if not all of these topics is that the EP must be quick to order diagnostic studies, must not fall into the trap of thinking it safe to treat as an outpatient, because it is safe in a younger patient, and must not underestimate the impending catastrophic decline in the elderly patient who "looks pretty good" on presentation. This is especially true of the septic elder who doesn't have a fever, despite a major infection; who can't manufacture an elevated white blood count, even though there might be a multi-lobar pneumonia present; and whose slight confusion is ascribed to an advanced age rather than a disease process. As well pointed out in the trauma chapter, advanced age alone invalidates many of the schemes for prediction of trauma seriousness, and is enough to warrant evaluation of the patient, thought to have sustained a minor mechanism of injury, in a trauma center. If there is one lesson I have personally learned from prior error in the geriatric patient, it is that they must be expected to do badly, not well, with a new onset trauma or illness.

In part this is because of the many comorbidities that will be present in virtually every elderly patient. In part, this is due to the polypharmacy with a bewildering complex series of interactions. These are often misses, as is well pointed out by many of the authors because of the patient's poor memory for the multiple medications being consumed, poor communication from the custodian of the elder, and lack of knowledge of the EP who cannot be expected to know every new oncology drug that is being used.

In part this is because the elder simply doesn't have the physiologic ability to show the result of the injury or disease. Perhaps the diminished pain perception of the geriatric patient is a blessing, but it certainly doesn't assist the EP to recognize impending failure of an organ.

The chapter on back pain is an excellent place to learn that the elder probably has a greater chance for significant pathology than an otherwise healthy young adult. This must translate to earlier use of diagnostic imaging that will be unfruitful in the young adult, but may reveal a spontaneous vertebral compression fracture, or a bony metastasis in the geriatric patient.

There are a number of chapters that represent material that ordinarily isn't part of the EP cognizance, but represent important parameters of observation for the elderly. One that I particularly enjoyed since it was a first for me, was the chapter on nutrition. In the past, this is a subject that is covered rarely, if ever, other than perhaps for the alcoholic patient, but is definitely not part of a standard curriculum for the care of the adult patient.

There are also a number of serious ethical concerns in the management of the geriatric patient, that I suspect often lead to incomplete workups and assumptions that management won't make any difference. For example, the chapter on alcoholism reminds the EP that this disease hasn't disappeared just because the patient has aged. Moreover I suspect many EPs don't look for this problem because they feel the elderly patient is entitled to drink since there are so few other pleasures still available to them. As a result, they assume that an alcohol induced dementia is irreversible and represents Alzheimer's or some other chronic aging dementia; that atrial fibrillation is chronic rather than an example of "holiday heart" and that alcohol is "salutary" rather than causing a deterioration in otherwise stable chronic diseases.

There are of course many other chapters that I haven't referred to that are filled with useful and thoughtful recommendations for diagnosis, management, and will surely improve the knowledge of the reader; but even if you don't wish to read the book from cover to cover, and I heartily enjoyed my journey through the book, you should consult it often. This book is a tremendous addition to the literature of Emergency Medicine, and I hope it will see many editions because it can only improve with time.

Peter Rosen, M.D.
Associate Professor Harvard University
Professor Emeritus
University of California San Diego
Visiting Professor University of Arizona
Attending Physician Beth Israel/Deaconess Hospital
Teaching Attending Massachusetts General Hospital
Attending Physician
St. John's Hospital, Jackson, Wyoming

PREFACE

THE FAMILIAR ADAGE IN PEDIATRICS—"children are not just small adults"—applies as well to the care of geriatric patients. While elders may technically be "just older adults," overwhelming evidence demonstrates that they possess unique pathophysiologic and clinical concerns, which require the application of special management principles. This specialized understanding is particularly important within the confines of a busy emergency department.

This textbook was developed as a resource for clinicians who provide emergency care for older persons. Older patients who present to the emergency department may have baseline functional impairment and multiple comorbidities that may make them vulnerable to mismanagement. For frail or impaired elders an emergency department visit is often a sentinel event, one that may mark the beginning of significant functional decline and loss of independence.

Most physicians are aware of the demographic changes that are occurring as our society ages. Elders currently make up approximately 13% (or more than 35 million people) of the United States population. The Census Bureau estimates that the number of older individuals will reach almost 68 million by 2024. Furthermore, the elder population is becoming increasing older, with the number of persons older than age 85 increasing at 3 to 4 times the rate of the general population. This unprecedented increase in the elder population will have a significant impact on healthcare in general and emergency medicine in particular.

Older patients represent a unique and heterogeneous population. Aging physiology, differences in presentation for common illnesses, and the accumulation of illness in this population highlight this observation. Emergency physicians usually view older patients with trepidation since their care requires more complex medical management and decision making. These tasks are made more difficult in the patient with cognitive impairment or if the patient is transferred from a nursing home setting. The result is often a prolonged evaluation that may still conclude with diagnostic uncertainty. Surveys have indicated that more than half of emergency physicians believe they have received insufficient training in geriatric emergency medicine and the majority note very few continuing medical education hours on this subject.

This textbook was written by and for health care workers who are engaged in the practice of emergency medicine. The breadth of the topics reflects the large number of important issues in geriatric emergency medicine. We have included key clinical concerns ranging from cardiovascular and pulmonary disease to falls, functional assessment, and nursing home issues. Emergency physicians certainly will find this textbook applicable to their daily practice. Physicians who practice in family medicine, internal medicine, and geriatrics should also find this book to be of value for specific clinical scenarios.

In each chapter, the epidemiology and pathophysiology are first reviewed. The clinical features, diagnosis and differential, and emergency department management of each clinical topic are then discussed. Each chapter emphasizes the key aspects as they pertain to geriatric emergency medicine; this textbook does not attempt to cover every element of emergency or geriatric medicine, but only those that relate to the acute care of the older patient.

A number of experts from a variety of specialties have contributed to this textbook. We would like to express our deep appreciation to the *Geriatric Emergency Medicine* chapter contributors for their commitment and hard work in helping to produce this textbook. We are indebted to several individuals who assisted us with this project; in particular, we would like to thank Andrea Seils, Jennifer Cosgrove, Martin Wonsiewicz, Regina Brown, and Richard Ruzycka at McGraw-Hill Medical Publishing.

Dr. Stephen Meldon has been supported in part by an American Geriatrics Society/John A. Hartford Foundation Dennis W. Jahnigen Career Development Scholars Award.

Stephen W. Meldon
O. John Ma
Robert H. Woolard

GERIATRIC EMERGENCY MEDICINE

1

Geriatric Emergency Department Use and Care

Samuel M. Keim
Arthur B. Sanders

HIGH-YIELD FACTS

- By 2030, 20 percent of us population will be 65 years of age and older, almost 9 million people will be over age 85.
- Both healthy individuals and some with chronic diseases such as hypertension, diabetes, and heart disease are surviving into older age.
- People over age 75 visit the emergency department (ED) almost twice as often as the younger population.
- Elders visiting the ED are more likely to arrive by ambulance and more likely to be admitted to hospital (46 percent) and to intensive care.
- Elder ED visits involve more comprehensive, longer evaluations with more testing and more cost.
- A more comprehensive evaluation is required when managing an elder patient. Emergency physicians must be alert to more subtle atypical presentations of disease, construct a broader differential diagnosis, account for underlying diseases and medication effects, assess cognitive and functional deficits, and talk with a caregiver to get an adequate history and plan an appropriate disposition.

DEMOGRAPHICS OF THE AGING POPULATION IN THE UNITED STATES

The overall aging of the United States and the unprecedented expansion of the 65 years and older age group create an imperative for the specialty of emergency medicine. Older adults will create the greatest future challenge and consume the most emergency department resources of any segment of our population. While people over age 65 currently represent 13 percent of the U.S. population, this segment consumes one-third of the health care spending and occupies one-half of all physician time. As the population ages, more health resources will be required, and an even greater proportion of resources will be consumed by elders.[1–4]

Three major factors contribute to our nation's evolving age structure: changing mortality patterns, decreased fertility, and aging of the baby-boom cohort born between 1946 and 1964 (75 million persons). These factors and, specifically, the aging of the baby-boom generation, will have far-reaching effects on the future overall health status and ED use of Americans. By 2030, 20 percent of the U.S. population will be 65 years of age and older. Demographic changes within the older segment of the population will increase the proportion of persons 85 years of age and older, from our current 4.3 million to 8.9 million individuals during the next three decades. This oldest segment is also the group with the greatest need for health care services.[1–5]

It is important for the clinician to distinguish physiologic age from biologic age. Physiologic age of the older person is highly variable. Although many of the oldest elderly have chronic diseases, some are quite healthy and have better physiologic reserve than younger individuals. During the period from 1994 to 1996, 72 percent of older Americans reported that their health was good, very good, or excellent. Women and men reported comparable levels of health status. While the prevalence of hypertension remained fairly constant, the prevalence of stroke, diabetes, heart disease, and cancer all increased in Americans over age 70, between 1984 and 1995. This increase in prevalence of disease, may reflect decreasing mortality rates for these diseases. The aging of the population in the United States includes the healthy as well as some segments with chronic diseases.[6]

DEMOGRAPHICS OF ED USE BY OLDER PATIENTS

The 2000 National Hospital Ambulatory Medical Care Survey (NHAMCS) reveals that ED use continues to increase in this country. Between 1997 and 2001, ED use increased by 14 percent, whereas the number of EDs decreased from 4,005 to 3,934. Persons 75 years of age and older had an estimated 64.8 visits per 100 persons per year, compared with an overall rate in the population of 39.4 visits. In the latest NHAMCS report, 43.1 percent, of older patients arrived by ambulance, whereas the ambulance arrival rate for all ages was 14 percent. Ambulance use by the elderly increased significantly, between 1990 and 2000. Finally, despite revealingly significant differences between Caucasian and African-American ED use in the general population, the NHAMCS reported no such racial use disparity in the older segment.[7-10]

In 1998, Strange and Chen reported results from a 5-year review of ED visits by older patients to 88 EDs in 21 states. The rate of admission among older patients increased from 1990 to 1995. In 1995, patients 65 years of age and older were admitted to hospitals on 46 percent of their ED visits. There was an 11 percent admission rate for younger patients. The higher and increasing admission rate is the result of several factors. The American health system increasingly has moved more care to the outpatient setting. Older patients are likely to be more ill when they visit the ED.

The increase in the oldest segment of the population is also an important factor.[10] Older patients arrive at the ED with higher levels of acuity and, therefore, require more immediate and more comprehensive care. They are also more likely to require prolonged stays in the ED, secondary to the complexity of their evaluations and therapeutic interventions. Prolonged patient stays in the ED may have consequences on hospital and departmental finances. When EDs are operating at full capacity, an increasing percentage of long patient stays can result in the loss of potential revenue. Strange and Chen reported that the elder ED patient was five times more likely to be admitted to an intensive care unit (ICU) than the nonelder patient. Their acuity and propensity to vague presentation of common, critical illness clearly require extensive laboratory and radiologic evaluations. There is no evidence that these expensive evaluations are the result of either inefficient or under-educated physicians. They are simply necessary for adequate evaluation of the older patient in the ED. Older patients require more nursing and ancillary staff time. These resources are limited when EDs are at full capacity. Since there is no reason to expect the trend

of increased ED use among older patients to flatten out or subside, the aging of the baby-boom generation easily could overwhelm our ED resources, especially staff and space, which are experiencing shortages now.[10-12]

Independent of the aging of America is the larger issue of ED overcrowding. Hospital restructurings and closures, government regulations on teaching and non-teaching hospitals, managed care, increased numbers of uninsured, the nursing shortage, and decreases in reimbursement all have contributed significantly to the current state of chaos that exists in many of the nations EDs. A recent national survey reported that EDs in this country are "overcrowded" about 35 percent of the time.[13] A need certainly exists in most EDs to better distribute resources. Increasing numbers of elders with more severe illness, more prolonged evaluations, and higher admission rates will further highlight the need to address ED overcrowding problems. These must be addressed by developing strategies involving the entire hospital. These might include increasing flexibility of inpatient resources, improving information systems for notifying physicians and obtaining laboratory and radiology results, floating nurses to assume care of admitted patients in the ED, implementing community-wide diversion protocols, and employing multidisciplinary administrative teams to better distribute patients from the ED to clinical areas.[13-19]

PRINCIPLES OF GERIATRIC EMERGENCY MEDICINE[20]

Older individuals have unique physiologic, medical, and social requirements that must be considered during their ED evaluation. Studies of ED personnel have reported a lack of education regarding this segment of our population. In one study, 69 percent of practicing emergency physicians reported insufficient availability of continuing medical education courses in geriatric emergency medicine. In the same study, 53 percent of residency—trained emergency physicians and 40 percent of residency directors reported that geriatric emergency medicine training was inadequate.[12] Considering the unique evaluation and treatment issues related to older emergency patients, an educational initiative for this expanding patient group is necessary. This educational initiative should include undergraduate, medical school, and graduate medical programs, as well as continuing medical education strategies.

The Society for Academic Emergency Medicine Geriatric Task Force has recommended that a more comprehensive model of care be used for older patients in the ED. The model includes an assessment of the patient's presentation in the context of his or her social, psychological, and emotional setting. A simple medical problem such as a sprained ankle can be devastating for an older person without a social support system. Further, multiple studies have demonstrated that emergency physicians may miss key conditions, such as delirium or elder abuse. Emergency staff must be trained to become aware of these problems. As part of this expanded model of care, the following principles of geriatric emergency medicine have been defined:

1. The patient's presentation is frequently complex.

2. Common diseases present atypically in this group.

3. The confounding effects of comorbid diseases must be considered.

4. Polypharmacy is common and may be a factor in presentation, diagnosis, and management.

5. Recognition of the possibility of cognitive impairment is important.

6. Some diagnostic tests may have normal values.

7. The likelihood of decreased functional reserve must be anticipated.

8. Social support systems may not be adequate, and patients may need to rely on caregivers.

9. A knowledge of baseline functional status is essential in evaluating new complaints.

10. Health problems must be evaluated for associated psychosocial adjustment.

11. The emergency department encounter is an opportunity to assess important conditions in the patients personal life.

In the ideal ED environment, care for older patients would be optimized by an emergency health care team of physicians, nurses, medics, pharmacists, and allied health care professionals who are aware of these principles.

REFERENCES

1. Administration on Aging: *A Profile of Older Americans—2001;* available at *http://www.aoa.dhhs.gov.*

2. Census 2000, *http://www.census.gov/.*

3. Perry D: Testimony to Senate Special Committee on Aging, Feb. 27, 2002. Alliance for Aging Research, *http://www.agingresearch.org/news.*

4. Cefalu C: Testimony to Senate Special Committee on Aging, Feb. 27, 2002. American Geriatrics Society, *http://www.americangeriatrics.org/news.*

5. *Trends in Causes of Death—2001,* National Center for Health Statistics, *http://www.cdc.gov/nchs/.*

6. *Older Americans 2000: Key indicators of Well-Being.* Federal Interagency Forum on Aging-Related Statistics, *http://www.agingstats.gov/.*

7. McCaig LF, Ly N: *National Hospital Ambulatory Medical Care Survey: 2000 Emergency Department Summary.* Washington, National Center for Health Statistics, Centers for Disease Control and Prevention, Department of Health and Human Services, 2002.

8. McCaig LF: *National Hospital Ambulatory Medical Care Survey: 1998 Emergency Department Summary.* Washington, National Center for Health Statistics, Centers for Disease Control and Prevention, Department of Health and Human Services, 2000.

9. McCaig, LF: *National Hospital Ambulatory Medical Care Survey: 1992 Emergency Department Summary.* Washington, National Center for Health Statistics, Centers for Disease Control and Prevention, Department of Health and Human Services, 1994.

10. Strange GR, Chen EH: Use of emergency departments by elder patients: A five-year follow-up study. *Acad Emerg Med* 5(12):1157, 1998.

11. Evans R, Ireland G, Morley JE, et al: Pharmacology and aging, in Sanders AB (ed): *Emergency Care of the Elder Person.* St. Louis, Beverly Cracom, 1996, pp 29–42.

12. Gerson LW, Rousseau E, Hogan J, et al: A multicenter study of case findings in elderly emergency department patients. *Acad Emerg Med* 2:729, 1995.

13. Derlet RW, Weiss SL, Ernst AA, et al: Development of an emergency department overcrowding scale: Results of the National ED Overcrowding Study (NEDOCS). *Acad Emerg Med* 9:366a, 2002.

14. Bayley MD, Schwartz S, Shofer FS, et al: The financial burden of ED congestion and hospital overcrowding for chest pain patients awaiting admission. *Acad Emerg Med* 9:367a, 2002.

15. Spaite DW, Bartholomeaux F, Guisto J, et al: Rapid process redesign in a university-based emergency department: decreasing waiting time intervals and improving patient satisfaction. *Ann Emerg Med* 39(2):168, 2002.

16. Schneider S, Zwemer F, Doniger A, et al: Rochester, New York: A decade of emergency department overcrowding. *Acad Emerg Med* 8(11):1044, 2001.

17. Schull MJ, Szalai JP, Schwartz B, Redelmeier DA: Emergency department overcrowding following systematic hospital restructuring: Trends at twenty hospitals over ten years. *Acad Emerg Med* 8(11):1037, 2001.

18. McCabe JB: Emergency department overcrowding: A national crisis. *Acad Med* 76(7):672, 2001.

19. Grimace K, Keane D, Bondman A: Primary care and public emergency department overcrowding. *Am J Public Health* 83(3):372, 1993.

20. Sanders AB. *Emergency Care of the Elder Person.* St. Louis, Beverly Cracom, 1996.

2

The Physiology of Aging

Rajeshwar Peddi
John Morley

HIGH-YIELD FACTS

- Aging itself is not a disease process, but with aging, reserve capacity is lost, hemostatic mechanisms become less robust, and the ability to effectively meet challenges such as infection or injury is lost.
- Older individuals are physiologically heterogeneous, any organ or system within the individual can loose more reserve than other organs, and the individual at any age may be more or less healthy.
- With age, systolic blood pressure rises, cardiac output falls, and heart rate slows.
- With age, the work of breathing is greater, alveolar surface area is lost, and arterial oxygenation is less.
- With age, renal blood flow and glomerular filtration rate drop, but the serum creatinine level remains constant due to decreased muscle mass.
- With age, lean body weigh decreases, fat increases, and bone mass decreases.
- With age, hearing and vision losses are common but easily correctable; however, changes in cognition are pathologic and not expected.
- Elder patients have an impaired ability to prevent temperature fluctuations due to lower metabolic rate, problems with vasoconstriction, decreased skin temperature receptors, and diminished shivering and sweating.
- Aging is associated with a steady loss of reserve that does not cause problems with daily activities until disease occurs.
- As more Americans adjust to healthy lifestyles, the majority will live to age 85 in good health.

DEFINITION OF AGING

"Aging is characterized by a decline in the ability to maintain homeostasis under conditions of physiologic stress, a failure of which is associated with a decrease in the viability and an increase in the vulnerability of the individual."[1] Evolution and nature have endowed the body with abundant reserve capacity. What aging represents is an attrition of this reserve capacity. As the individual grows older, "he or she is less capable of adapting to challenges from the external environment such as injury and infection and to challenges from the internal environment such as arterial occlusion and malignant cell clones. As homeostatic mechanisms become less sensitive, less accurate, slower and less well sustained, sooner or later, individuals encounter challenges that they are unable to deal with effectively,"[2] and death is the result of this ultimate failure of reserve capacity.

Aging is a complex phenomenon that results from the interaction between extrinsic (environmental) and intrinsic (genetic) factors. At the physiologic level, the most prominent characteristic of human aging is its variability.[3] There is tremendous variation among individuals, as well as within the same individual, among their bodily systems. Aging also has been refined into chronologic, psychological, and biologic aging. Chronologic aging, or the number of birthdays celebrated by an individual, is mainly used for statistical and demographic purposes. Psychological aging mainly deals with the attitudes of the individual toward aging as well as that of society. Biologic aging has been defined as "the sum of all changes that occur in an organism with the passage of time."[4] Such a definition makes no distinction between changes related to different stages in human development, maturation, disease, or degenerative processes. It acknowledges the difficulty of deciding whether an age-related change is attributable to true aging or to some other process.

Characteristics of Aging

Physiologic or biologic aging has the following characteristic features:

1. Aging is universal; it affects all living organisms.
2. Aging is progressive; the aging process is continuous.
3. The changes associated with aging are detrimental.
4. Aging by itself is not a disease.
5. Aging makes the individual more vulnerable to disease.[5]

Clinical Significance of Aging

The changes attributable to aging may be viewed as a spectrum, with changes associated with aging alone at one end and those associated with disease at the other end. Realistically, what happens in individuals are changes that are between the two ends of this spectrum. The morbidity and longevity of any particular individual depend on the spectrum from which his or her aging changes eminate.

Although some changes associated with aging are seen with increasing frequency in elders and may be considered as "normal," it is important to realize that normal aging changes are not necessarily harmless. "If healthy old individuals perform less well on glucose tolerance tests compared to younger individuals, it does not mean that carbohydrate intolerance, insulin resistance and elevated insulin levels which might be normal for their age are harmless."[6] Emergency physicians must realize that "aging is not synonymous with disease."[7] Clinically, they must distinguish changes of normal aging from those which occur as a result of disease. At the same time, they should be aware that the physiologic changes associated with aging alter the presenting symptoms of disease, make the onset of serious illnesses more insidious, and increase the difficulty of diagnosis.[8]

PHYSIOLOGIC CHANGES OF AGING (TABLE 2-1)

Cardiovascular System

The heart is a muscular organ that pumps blood to the various organs and to the tissues of the body. The heart and blood vessels are highly dependent for their normal function on their physical properties of distensibility, contractility, and elasticity, all of which may be affected by the changes associated with aging. The degree to which the efficiency of the heart and blood vessels are affected could be determined by looking at the following three clinical functions: blood pressure, cardiac output, and heart rate.

Blood Pressure

Blood pressure depends on cardiac output and peripheral resistance.[9] Peripheral resistance is increased in the elderly because of damage to the elastic fibers in the arteries. Aging causes the blood vessels to become more rigid and less compliant. Blood pressure is therefore increased in the elderly. "Diastolic pressure rises with age but stabilizes after age 60, whereas systolic pressure continues to increase, rising steeply after age 55 in both sexes but to a greater degree in women."[10] An increase in peripheral resistance and diastolic blood pressure results in left ventricular hypertrophy (LVH).

Cardiac Output

Cardiac output is dependent on the contractility of the heart muscle, end-diastolic volume, and heart rate. One of the factors determining stroke volume and cardiac output is the strength of the heart muscle. Studies have suggested that the capacity to develop force is not compromised in the senescent heart. Another factor that determines cardiac output is the end-diastolic volume, the volume of blood in the left ventricle prior to the contraction. A number of studies have shown that diastolic filling in the early diastolic period (passive diastolic filling) is reduced by about half between the ages of 20 and 80. This is due to an increase in left ventricular stiffness and a reduction in its compliance. Most of the ventricular filling in the elderly takes place in the late diastolic period, which is facilitated by active atrial contraction ("atrial kick"). In fact, about 40 percent of ventricular filling takes place in the late diastolic period, as opposed to 15 percent in younger individuals. In the elderly this increased ventricular filling in the late diastolic phase has two important clinical consequences. It can result in an additional heart sound, such as a fourth heart sound, which can be normal in the elderly. Since about 40 percent of the ventricular filling takes place in the late diastolic period and filling is facilitated by active atrial contraction, with new onset or rapid atrial fibrillation patients may develop heart failure.

Elderly individuals are predisposed to diastolic dysfunction. A number of studies have indicated that heart failure in the elderly is mainly a result of diastolic dysfunction. Dougherty and Soufer (1984) demonstrated that a subset of elderly patients with clinical heart failure had normal contracting hearts. The problem was ventricular diastolic dysfunction; not systolic dysfunction.[11] In Olmstead County, Minnesota, 43 percent of patients with congestive heart failure had a left ventricular ejection fraction of greater than or equal to 50 percent.[12] Similarly, investigators from the Framingham study found that 51 percent of their cohort with heart failure had a left ventricular ejection fraction of greater than or equal to 50 percent.[13] It is believed that heart failure secondary to diastolic dysfunction is mainly a disorder of elderly patients.[11] Wong[14] found that only 6 percent of patients aged 60 years and younger had normal systolic function as

Table 2-1. The Physiology of Aging

Organ/System	Physiologic Changes of Aging	Clinical and Functional Implications
Cardiovascular system	Increased peripheral resistance; increased left ventricular stiffness and decreased compliance; increase in ventricular filling during the late diastolic period facilitated by atrial contraction; decreased response in heart rate to catecholamines; atherosclerosis	Elevated BP; left ventricular hypertrophy; reduction in cardiac output; increased susceptibility to diastolic heart failure; presence of a fourth heart sound; reduced response in heart rate to exercise; reduced blood supply to organs
Respiratory system	Decreased elastic recoil; overall decrease in compliance of the respiratory system; increasing number of alveoli do not participate in gas exchange; decreased alveolar surface area; decreased lung defenses	Decrease in FEV_1, FVC, CO diffusion factor; increased residual volume; decreased Pao_2; decreased effectiveness of mucociliary reflex; increased susceptibility to aspirations and respiratory infections
Renal system	Progressive loss of one-third of renal mass; reduction in renovascular bed; narrowing of renal arteries; reduction in renal blood flow	Reduction in GFR not reflected by elevation of serum creatinine; dose adjustments of drugs to be done based on creatinine clearance
Musculoskeletal system	Loss of muscle mass; reduction in lean body mass; progressive loss of bone mass and osteoporosis.	Impaired mobility; increased likelihood of falls; increased susceptibility to fractures
Glucose regulation	Reduction in insulin sensitivity; elderly achieve normal levels of blood glucose at expense of a higher rate of insulin secretion; glucose tolerance test shows a significant rise in 2-hour blood glucose level with age	Impairment of glucose regulation
Thyroid function	Total T_4, T_3, and free T4 index may give false results in elderly patients with acute nonthyroid illnesses	TSH and free T_4 are the most reliable tests of thyroid function in the elderly; thyroid hormone production is reduced; normal values maintained by a reduction in metabolic clearance
Sexual function	Testosterone, free testosterone, and bioavailable testosterone all decline with age; atherosclerotic vascular disease	Gradual slowing of sexual function; more time needed for sexual arousal and climax; erectile dysfunction
Gastrointestinal system	Decreased esophageal contractions; lower esophageal sphincter pressure; slowing in gastric emptying; decrease in fundal compliance	Minimal changes in GI function; increase in gastric acid production; varying degrees of lactase deficiency; constipation
Immune system	Decrease of cell-mediated immunity; reduced basal and stimulated interleukin-2 levels; diminished proliferative response of lymphocytes to antigens	Increased incidence of infections like tuberculosis and herpes zoster
	Levels of IgG and IgA increased; IgM decreased; response to antigen delayed	Diminished and delayed antibody response to antigens; increase in autoantibodies
	Decrease in number or effectiveness of killer cells	Increase in incidence of cancer

(continues)

Table 2-1. The Physiology of Aging (continued)

Organ/System	Physiologic Changes of Aging	Clinical and Functional Implications
Nervous system	Reduction in number of nerve cells; compensatory increase in length and dendritic connections of remaining nerve cells	Cognition and behavior essentially remain normal in healthy elderly
Vision	Increase in size of lens; decreased flexibility of the lens; smaller pupil; increased lens permeability	Presbyopia; impaired dark adaptation; reduced visual acuity; cataract
Hearing	Loss of elasticity of tympanum; impaired articulation of ossicles; loss of neurons in auditory cortex	High-frequency hearing loss; impaired functional capacity
Skin	Reduced contact between epidermis and dermis; reduction in melanocytes; decrease in number of cutaneous nerves; reduction in subcutaneous fat; decrease in sweat glands; reduction in sebum	Impaired thermal regulation; graying of hair; reduced sensitivity to touch and pain; predisposition to burns, pressure sores, hypothermia, heat strokes; dry skin or xerosis
Body temperature	Diminished sweating responses; decreased generation of heat; impaired conservation of heat; diminished ability to discriminate differences in temperature	Heat strokes; hypothermia; burns

compared with 21 percent of patients aged 61 to 70 years and 41 percent of patients older than 70 years. In nursing home residents (mean age 84 years) with heart failure, Aronow and colleagues[15] reported normal systolic function in 47 percent.

Heart Rate

Heart rate is the third factor on which cardiac output is dependent. Although the resting heart rate is not greatly affected by aging, there is a striking decrease in heart rate response to exercise. This decrease occurs because of a reduced sensitivity to circulating catecholamines. The reduced sensitivity is not caused by a reduction in the number of receptors. Rather, it is due to a defect in the uncoupling of the beta receptor from the adenylyl cyclase system, which is essential to the catecholamine cascade mechanism.[16] This reduced sensitivity results in increased levels of circulating catecholamines. With aging, a small decrease in resting cardiac output is expected. However, with exercise, there is a marked lack of increase in cardiac output.

Atherosclerosis

The main change in blood vessels occurs as atherosclerosis develops, especially in coronary arteries. "Athero-

sclerosis (also known as arteriosclerosis or atheroma) is a patchy focal disease of the arterial intima"[17] that causes damage to the blood vessels through the accumulation of lipid-filled smooth-muscle cells, macrophages, and fibrous tissue. The process is unique in that some arteries, such as the radial artery and the internal mammary artery, are frequently spared, whereas others, such as the coronary arteries, are at high risk and are frequently affected.[17] The consequences of atherosclerosis can be devastating when atheromatous plaques block blood vessels, resulting in myocardial infarction or stroke. It is now accepted that atherosclerosis begins at a young age, possibly infancy. Fatty streaks, the earliest change associated with atherosclerosis, are seen in the ascending aorta of infants a few months old, in the coronary arteries of adolescents, and in the cerebral arteries of young adults.[18]

Respiratory System

Aging is associated with a gradual loss of elastic lung recoil, resulting in an increase in compliance. Age-related increase in lung compliance is due to damage or loss of the elastic fibers in the alveolar walls attached to small airways.[19] This results in an increase in the proportion of collapsible airways so that an increasing number of alveoli do not participate in gas exchange. This results in a ventilation-perfusion imbalance that partly explains the reduced arterial oxygen tension in the elderly. The increased compliance leads to thinning and disruption of alveolar walls, resulting in a decreased alveolar surface (decreasing from 70 m^2 in a 20-year-old to 60 m^2 by age 70), which also contributes to a reduction in arterial oxygen tension.

Aging changes also occur in the chest wall. The rib cartilages become calcified, and there is increased curvature of the spine. The decreased compliance of the chest wall exceeds the increased compliance of the lungs. Total compliance of the entire respiratory system, therefore, decreases. Hence more muscular work is required to move air in and out of the lungs. A 60-year-old does an estimated 20 percent more work at any given ventilatory rate than a 20-year-old. All measures of respiratory function are decreased in the elderly except residual volume, which is increased. Forced expiratory volume in 1 second (FEV$_1$), forced vital capacity (FVC), and carbon monoxide diffusion are all decreased. Age-related reduction in diffusing capacity is due primarily to increased thickness of the alveolar-capillary membrane. Cross-sectional studies of pulmonary function have identified a constant decline in FEV$_1$ of 32 mL/y and FVC of 25 mL/y in males, whereas reductions in FEV$_1$ of 25 mL/y and FVC of 24 mL/y have been observed in females.[19]

Aging causes a gradual decline in Pa$_{O_2}$. The reasons for this decline are loss of elastic recoil, maldistribution of ventilation and a ventilation-perfusion imbalance, and reductions in cardiac output.[19] Smoking further accelerates the decline in pulmonary function. Even asymptomatic smokers have a significantly greater decrease in FEV$_1$ with age than do nonsmokers.

In elderly individuals, lung defenses are decreased against inhaled matter (predisposing elderly to aspiration pneumonia). The mucociliary reflex in the elderly is not as effective as in younger individuals. Cilia are lost from the airways, and the vigor of the remaining cilia is reduced. Their mucus becomes less effective in removing material from the lungs. The macrophages that form the last line of defense at the alveolar level also become less efficient.

Renal System

Aging is associated with a progressive loss of renal mass. Kidney weight decreases from an average of 300 g in young adults to 200 g at age 80. Most of the reduction in this weight is because of a loss of the renal cortex, with a relative sparing of the renal medulla. The glomeruli and Bowman's capsule are located in the cortex, whereas the tubules and the collecting ducts are located in the medulla. The renal cortex contains about 85 percent of the nephrons. There is a decrease in the number of glomeruli with age.

Renal blood flow decreases from 1200 mL/min in young adulthood to 600 mL/min by age 80 because of a reduction in the renovascular bed and a narrowing of the renal arteries secondary to atherosclerosis. This results in a linear reduction in glomerular filtration rate (GFR) from the middle of the fourth decade at about 8 mL/min/1.73 m^2 per decade.[19] The decline in GFR is not reflected by an elevation of serum creatinine. Creatinine is derived from the breakdown of muscle. Because a concomitant reduction in muscle mass parallels the decline in GFR, serum creatinine levels are unchanged. On average, a healthy 80-year-old has a creatinine clearance of 32 mL/min less than that of his or her 30-year-old counterpart with the same serum creatinine levels.[19]

Therefore, dose adjustments based on creatinine clearance need to be made when drugs are prescribed to elders. (See Chap. 32 for the formula to calculate creatinine clearance.)

Muscular System

Aging brings a loss of muscle strength. The lean body mass falls from about 80 percent of total-body weight (TBW) at age 20 to 60 percent of TBW by age 80. At the same time, total-body fat increases from 20 to 40 percent of TBW. Muscle weakness increases from the sixth decade onward, and much of this deterioration is due to a loss of muscle mass because of a decrease in the number of muscle fibers. Muscle strength is maintained by hypertrophy of the remaining muscle fibers. Exercise, therefore, becomes vital in preventing or slowing the progression of functional loss in the elderly.[20] Numerous scientific studies provide evidence that physical activity leads to better physical health for elders.[21]

The extent to which muscle strength is reduced is such that a healthy 20-year-old requires only 50 to 70 percent of maximum quadriceps contraction to rise from a low armless chair, whereas a healthy 80-year-old must make a maximal quadriceps contraction to perform the same activity. One important consequence of muscle weakness is falls.

Skeletal System

Loss of skeletal mass is a universal accompaniment to aging. One of the consequences of a declining bone mass is osteoporosis. Factors that determine development of osteoporosis include peak bone mass, sex, race, and body weight. Peak bone mass is achieved in the fourth decade. Thereafter, 3 to 5 percent of bone density is lost per decade, increasing to as much as 10 to 20 percent per decade in women in the perimenopausal and immediate postmenopausal periods.[19] While postmenopausal endocrinal changes are thought to be responsible for most osteoporosis, aging-related changes in the synthesis of vitamin D may be responsible for some osteoporosis.

Primary osteoporosis is essentially of two types: type 1, postmenopausal osteoporosis, and type 2, senile osteoporosis. Type 1 occurs predominantly in women (female-to-male ratio of 6:1) between the ages of 50 and 75 years. The type of bone loss involved is primarily trabecular. The rate of bone loss typically is accelerated and of short duration, with vertebral fractures and Colles' fractures being the most common fractures with type 1 osteoporosis. Type 2 osteoporosis occurs equally among both sexes (female-to-male ratio of 1:1), usually past age 70 years. The type of bone loss includes both trabecular and cortical. The rate of bone loss is gradual and of long duration, with vertebral and hip fractures being the most common fractures. One study indicates that despite the availability of various therapeutic agents, recognition and appropriate treatment of this condition are less than ideal, leading to serious, debilitating consequences.[22] Exercise may have an important role as therapy both for prevention and for treatment of osteoporosis.[23]

Endocrine System

Glucose Regulation

Aging is associated with progressive impairment of glucose tolerance. Due to a reduction in insulin sensitivity, elderly individuals achieve normal levels of blood glucose at the expense of a higher rate of insulin secretion. Under resting conditions, blood sugar levels remain essentially unchanged throughout life. However, when a person is put under stress by a glucose load, the 2-hour blood glucose level shows a significant rise with age. The reasons for impairment of glucose tolerance in the elderly are physical inactivity, the decrease in the amount of lean body mass, impairment of insulin secretion, and most important, insulin antagonism due to either a reduction in the number of receptors or decreased insulin binding.

Thyroid Function

Thyroid function is essentially normal with aging. The values of triiodothyroxine (T_4), free T_4, free T_4 index, triiodothyronine (T_3), and thyroid-stimulating hormone (TSH) remain normal. The two most reliable tests to evaluate thyroid function in the elderly are determinations of TSH and free T_4. Tests of total T_4, T_3, and free T_4 index may yield false results in patients because of changes in thyroid-binding globulin caused by nonthyroid illnesses.

Thyroid hormone production is decreased in the elderly, but normal hormone levels are maintained by a reduced metabolic clearance and increased half-life.[10] TSH response to thyrotropin-releasing hormone (TRH) is reduced, especially in elderly males.[10]

Aging and Sexual Function

"Sexual change in old age is a process of gradual slowing; more time is needed to become sexually aroused and to reach sexual climax."[19] "The circulating levels of male hormone, testosterone, decline with aging in all males. This is due predominantly to a failure of the hypothalamic-pituitary component of the hypothalamic-pituitary-testicular axis. This results in a defined syndrome of androgen deficiency in aging males (ADAM) which is similar to that seen in females at menopause, but less dramatic. Testosterone, free testosterone, and bioavailable testosterone all decline with age. The reason for this decline seems to be multifactorial and includes failure at both the testicular and hypothalamic-pituitary level, particularly the latter. Androgen deficiency is related to the decline in muscle strength, some age-related cognitive dysfunction, and decreased libido. While there are clear age-related changes in erectile function with aging, true erectile dysfunction (impotence) is usually associated with disease. The most common cause of erectile dysfunction is atherosclerotic vascular disease."[16]

Gastrointestinal System

Aging causes clinically insignificant changes in gastrointestinal function. Some older individuals seem to have decreased esophageal contractions and a lower esophageal sphincter pressure, but this is relatively rare. There is a small slowing in gastric emptying and a decrease in fundal compliance. Atrophic gastritis appears in 20 percent of elderly individuals. In the rest, an increase in gastric acid secretion occurs secondary to decreased prostaglandin production. Small intestinal transit remains stable over the lifespan. There are minimal changes in nutrient absorption. Increased absorption of fat-soluble vitamins and decreased calcium absorption are notable exceptions.

Varying degrees of lactase deficiency occur in all geriatric patients. For elderly individuals with lactase deficiency, diarrhea may develop when milk products not enriched with lactose are consumed. Colonic transit time decreases slightly with aging. Only small changes in anorectal function have been found.

Constipation

Constipation is a major problem in the elderly. Colonic motility is of two types. Shuttling peristalsis is continuous and facilitates absorption of water, and mass peristalsis occurs two to three times a day, propeling the fecal bolus toward the rectum. Mass peristalsis is stimulated by the gastrocolic reflex initiated by the entry of food into the upper gastrointestinal tract. Physical activity also stimulates the gastrocolic reflex, whereas sedentary habits inhibit the reflex. Thus exercise may relieve constipation.

Immune System

Aging is associated with alterations in the immune system. (For a full account, see Chap. 9.)

Nervous System

One of the changes associated with aging is a reduction in the number of nerve cells because of their inability to regenerate. Certain compensatory mechanisms occur to overcome this reduction. One is an increase in the length and another is an increase in the number of dendritic connections of the remaining nerve cells. The deposition of the pigment lipofuscin in the nerve cells is another change seen with aging. Amyloid plaques and neurofibrillary tangles, pathognomonic of Alzheimer's disease, are also seen in the brains of normal elderly individuals without dementia but in much fewer numbers. Regardless of these changes in the nervous system, most healthy elderly individuals have normal cognition and behavior.

Sensory Systems

"Because vision and hearing losses are so common in the elderly, both elderly individuals and health professionals tend to overlook them. This can lead to passive acceptance of the disability rather than seeking appropriate correction through prescription lenses or provision of amplification to overcome hearing loss. Both visual and hearing losses in elderly individuals can severely affect their physical and psychological functioning."[24] The emergency visit may provide an opportunity to screen for these problems.

Vision

Visual changes associated with aging include presbyopia (impaired accommodation), impaired dark adaptation, and reduced visual acuity. Laxity of elastic tissue causes the eyelid to fall outwards (ectropion), whereas loss of periorbital fat can lead to a curling in of the lower eyelid (entropion). Both these conditions are seen more frequently in the elderly. Loss of accommodation is due to decreased flexibility of the lens and to an increase in the size of the lens (there is a 50 percent increase in the size of the lens from age 20 to 80 years). Impaired dark adaptation and reduced visual acuity are caused by the pupil becoming smaller. The range of dilatation and constriction of the pupil to changes in ambient light is decreased. This is the result of atrophic changes of aging to muscles in the iris. At age 60, the amount of light that falls on the retina is only 33 percent of that occuring at age 20. Reduced visual activity can be explained by the smaller pupil that allows less light to fall on the retina, light scattering in the lens, vitreous and lens opacities, and cataracts. Most cataracts are age-related due to increased lens permeability. Genetic (people of India and Egypt) and environmental differences (high levels of ultraviolet light exposure) may be significant in the development of cataracts.

Hearing

Speech ranges from 25 dB (whisper) to above 80 dB (shouting). Loss of hearing becomes obvious when 30 to 40 dB of acuity is lost. Speech frequencies range from 500 to 6000 Hz, with consonants having higher frequencies than vowels. Much of the sense of speech is embodied in consonants. Aging is associated with high-frequency hearing loss that affects the ability to comprehend speech. Changes associated with aging of the ear include loss of elasticity of the tympanum, impaired articulation of the ossicles, and loss of neurones in the auditory cortex.

Body Temperature

Aging is associated with an impairment in the body's ability to prevent fluctuations in core body temperature. The problem is both generation and conservation of heat. Decreased generation of heat results from reduced basal metabolic rate (BMR), reduced cellular mass, and decreased activity. The shivering response is not as effective as in the young. Elderly people have problems with vasoconstriction in the skin. Thus they cannot easily reduce the loss of heat or conserve heat. The ability to discriminate differences in temperature is reduced in the elderly secondary to a decrease in the number of functioning nerve cells and receptors in the skin. Added to this, diminished sweating predisposes the elderly to heat strokes, and decreased subcutaneous fat makes them more susceptible to hypothermia.

Skin

The thickness and resistance of the stratum corneum are unchanged. The barrier function is preserved. Reduced contact between epidermis and dermis results in an epidermis that separates easily from dermis by simple trauma (epidermis can be easily peeled off by simple trauma). A decrease in dermal vasculature results in impaired thermal regulation. Reduction in melanocytes results in graying of the hair, which is one of the earliest signs of aging. The decrease in the number of cutaneous nerves reduces sensitivity to touch and pain, making the elderly more susceptible to burns. Reduction in subcutaneous fat predisposes elderly individuals to pressure sores and hypothermia (subcutaneous fat limits heat loss). A decrease in sweat glands predisposes the elderly to heat strokes, and a reduction in the production of sebum causes increased prevalence of dry skin or xerosis (see Chap. 56).

ADDITIONAL ASPECTS

Although aging is associated with a steady loss of body reserve, healthy elderly individuals have no problem being fully functional and carrying out their normal daily activities. "It is believed [that] the vast majority of individuals have genes that allow them to live to at least 85 years old."[25] Lifestyle behaviors influence healthy aging, especially nutrition, exercise, smoking, and stress. Prevention of heart and lung disease and treatment of diabetes and hypertension are associated with increased healthy lifespan. Obesity is an important risk factor for heart disease, diabetes, and cancer. "High-fat diets and sedentary behavior have led to increased obesity throughout the developed world."[25] Regular physical activity may increase longevity in middle-aged and older men and women.[26,27] Thus a majority of people can greatly compress the period of morbidity or ill-health in their lives by adopting healthy lifestyles and taking preventive steps to maximize good health.[25]

CONCLUSION

"Aging is not a disease." It is clinically important to distinguish changes of normal aging from those which occur as a result of disease. The physiologic changes of aging alter the presenting symptoms of disease, make the onset of serious illnesses more insidious, and increase the difficulty of accurate diagnosis. Aging is associated with a number of significant physiologic changes, including elevated blood pressure, left ventricular hypertrophy, more diastolic heart failure, reduced sensitivity to catecholamines, reduced respiratory function, decreased renal blood flow and glomerular filtration rate, reduced muscle strength and bone mass, impaired glucose tolerance, decreased immunity, and diminished visual and hearing capabilities. Despite these changes, it needs to be emphasized that normal aging in the absence of disease is benign. Aging is associated with a steady erosion of body reserve that usually does not cause problems with normal daily activities until disease occurs.

REFERENCES

1. Comfort A: *The Biology of Senescence.* New York, Elsevier, 1979.
2. Evans JG: Introduction, in Evans JG, Williams TF, Beattie BL, et al (eds): *Oxford Textbook of Geriatric Medicine,* 2d ed. Oxford, England, Oxford University Press, 2000, pp 1–4.
3. Horan MA: Introduction : Presentation of disease in old age, in Brocklehurst JC, Tallis RC, Fillit HM (eds): *Textbook of Geriatric Medicine and Gerontology,* 4th ed. London, Churchill Livingston, 1992, pp 145–149.
4. Sharma R: Definitions: Demographic, comparative and differential aging, in Timiras PS (ed): *Physiological Basis of Geriatrics,* 1st ed. New York, Macmillan, 1988, pp 7–26.
5. Strehler BL: *Time, Cells and Aging.* New York, Academic Press, 1977.
6. Elahi D, Muller DC, Rowe JW: Design, conduct and analysis of human aging research, in Schneider EL, Rowe JW (eds): *Handbook of the Biology of Aging,* 4th ed. New York, Academic Press, 1996, pp 24–36.

7. Austad SN: Concepts and theories of aging, in Masoro EJ, Austad SN (eds): *Handbook of the Biology of Aging,* 5th ed. New York, Academic Press, 2001, pp 3–22.

8. Anderson F: An historical overview of geriatric medicine, in Pathy MSJ (ed): *Principles and Practice of Geriatric Medicine,* 1st ed. New York, Wiley, 1986, pp 7–16.

9. Braunwald E, Williams GH: Alterations in arterial pressure and the shock syndrome, in Braunwald E, Isselbacher KJ, Petersdorf RG, et al (eds): *Harrison's Principles of Internal Medicine,* 11th ed. New York, McGraw-Hill, 1987, p 153.

10. Kane RL, Ouslander JG, Abrass IB: *Essentials of Clinical Geriatrics.* New York, McGraw-Hill, 1999.

11. Abdel Hafiz AH: Heart Failure in older people: Causes, diagnosis and treatment. *Age and Ageing* 31(1):29, 2002.

12. Senni M, Tribouilloy CM, Rodeheffer RJ: Congestive heart failure in the community: A study of all incident cases in Olmstead County, Minnesota in 1991. *Circulation* 98:2282, 1998.

13. Vasan RS, Larson MG, Benjamin EJ, et al: Congestive heart failure in subjects with normal versus reduced left ventricular ejection fraction: Prevalence and mortality in a population based cohort. *J Am Coll Cardiol* 33:1948, 1999.

14. Wong WF, Gold S, Fukuyama O, et al: Diastolic dysfunction in elderly patients with Congestive heart failure. *Am J Cardiol* 63:1526, 1989.

15. Aronow WS, Ahn C, Kronszon I: Prognosis of congestive heart failure in elderly patients with normal versus abnormal left ventricular systolic function associated with coronary artery disease. *Am J Cardiol* 66:1257, 1990.

16. Morley JE, Armbrecht HJ, Coe RM, Vellas B (eds): *The Science of Geriatrics*, 1st ed. New York, Springer, 2000.

17. Boon NA, Fox KAA: Diseases of the cardiovascular system, in Edwards CRW, Bouchier IAD, Haslett C (eds): *Davidson's Principles and Practice of Medicine,* 17th ed. Edinburgh, Churchill Livingstone, 1996, pp 245–256.

18. Ritchie AC (ed): *Boyd's Textbook of Pathology.* Philadelphia, Lea and Febiger, 1990.

19. Abrass IB, Besdine RW, Butler RN, et al: *The Merck Manual of Geriatrics.* Whitehouse Station, NJ, Merck, Sharp & Dohme Laboratories, 1990.

20. Whitehead JB: Exercise for older patients, in Gallo JJ, Whitehead JB, Rabins PV, et al (eds): *Reichel's Care of the Elderly: Clinical Aspects of Aging,* 5th ed. Baltimore, Williams & Wilkins, 1999, pp 141–146.

21. Blair SN, Kohn LW III, Gordon NF: How much physical activity is good for health? *Annu Rev Public Health* 13:99, 1992.

22. Gehlbach SH, Fournier M, Bigelow C: Recognition of osteoporosis by primary care physicians. *Am J Public Health* 92:271, 2002.

23. Harris SS, Caspersen CJ, DeFriese GH, et al: Physical activity counseling for healthy adults as a primary preventive intervention in the clinical setting. *JAMA* 261:3590, 1989.

24. Teshuva K, Stanislavsky Y, Kendig H: *Towards Healthy Ageing.* Victoria, Australia, Collins Dove, 1994.

25. Perls TT, Silver MH: *Living to 100.* New York, Basic Books, 1999.

26. Paffenbarger RS Jr, Hyde RT, Wing AL, et al: Physical activity, all-cause mortality and longevity of college alumni. *New Engl J Med* 314:605, 1986.

27. Sherman SE, D'Agostino RB, Cobb JL, et al: Does exercise reduce mortality rates in the elderly? Experience from the Framingham heart study. *Am Heart J* 128:965, 1994.

3

Pharmacotherapy and Adverse Drug-Related Events in Elders Treated in the Emergency Department

Laura Snyder
Shannon Connolly
Bruce Becker

HIGH-YIELD FACTS

- Elders use three times the number of prescription drugs and four times the number of of over-the-counter (OTC) drugs than younger patients use.

- Adverse drug-related effects (ADREs) account for 10 percent of emergency department (ED) visits and up to 25 percent of hospital admissions for elders.

- Taking two medications instead of one increases the risk of ADREs from 0 to 13 percent; with three medications, 30 percent; with five medications, 58 percent; and with seven medications, 82 percent.

- Herbal remedies, ginko biloba, St. Johns wort, and OTC medications such as Tylenol, nonsteroidal anti-inflammatory drugs (NSAIDs), and antihistamines can cause significant drug-drug interactions.

- Several factors, including loss of renal function (not reflected by serum creatine levels), lean body weight, and total-body water, can alter the response of elders to medications.

- Common ED presentations, such as change in mental status, weakness, dizziness, and syncope, can be the result from ADREs.

- Emergency physicians should prescribe medicines for the elderly with a full knowledge of ADREs, drug-drug interactions (DDIs), and changes in physiology with age.

People over age 65 represent 12 percent of the population;[1-4] they consume 30 percent of all prescription medications and 50 percent of all over-the-counter (OTC) medications.[1,3,5] More than 80 percent of this population takes at least one medication daily.[1,5,6] They have an increased risk of suffering adverse drug events (ADEs), including adverse drug reactions (ADRs) and drug-drug interactions (DDIs) because of impaired drug metabolism and clearance, poor compliance, and intentional or accidental polypharmacy. In addition, ADEs in this population tend to have more severe consequences because of the physiologic changes associated with aging and unrelentingly chronic diseases. This chapter reviews the etiology and consequences of ADEs in elders, examining specific medication problems and strategies for improved medication administration and tracking.

DEFINITION OF THE PROBLEM

An ADR is defined as any adverse change in a patient's condition that requires treatment or decrease or cessation of medicine use.[6] ADRs are the most common cause of iatrogenic illness in elders.[1] The term *adverse drug-related events* (ADREs) is more encompassing because ADRs exclude medication errors, an increasing concern as a cause of drug-related morbidity and mortality.[7] ADREs account for 2 to 27 percent of all hospital admissions.[1,3,6,8] Not surprisingly, the incidence of ADREs in hospitalized patients increases from approximately 10 percent in patients 40 to 50 years to 25 percent in patients older than 80.[1,3] For elders being treated in an emergency department (ED), a recent study showed that over 10 percent of ED visits were prompted by ADREs, 31 percent of patients had a potential adverse drug interaction (PADI) in their medication list, and 50 percent of those with ADREs had at least one unrecognized PADI that was unrelated to their current problem.[6]

There is a strong correlation between the number of prescribed medicines and an increased risk of ADREs. While this correlation was found to be independent of the patient's age, elders take more prescribed and nonprescribed medications per patient than any other demographic group.[1,3,5] Elders have more ADREs and a more severe morbidity from each event. In 1986, 51 percent of deaths from ADREs occurred in elders.[1,3,5]

Clearly, ADREs, and DDIs in particular pose, a significant problem for elder patients. The scope of this problem is broad, and the etiologies are complex. Nevertheless, seeking an understanding of the root causes can lead to the development of strategies and solutions. The following section delineates the factors supporting the increased prevalence and morbidity of ADREs in elders.

THE ETIOLOGY OF ADRE'S IN ELDERS

Polypharmacy

Although the benefits of modern pharmacotherapy often outweigh the risks to patients, in elders the balance is quite precarious, with risks frequently predominating. Many elders take at least one prescription medication daily as well as a number of documented and undocumented OTC drugs. Many potent medications that were available previously only by prescription and thus were prescribed with a physician's guidance and monitoring have become available as OTC medications. Elders also ingest other substances that have the potential to interact with both their physician-prescribed and self-prescribed personal pharmacy, including herbal medications, caffeine, nicotine, and alcohol. The probability of an ADRE increases dramatically with each additional ingested medication: Taking two drugs instead of one increases the risk of an ADRE from 0 to 13 percent. The risk increases exponentially with each additional medication. With three medications, the probability increases to almost 30 percent. It increases to 58 percent with five medications and 82 percent with seven or more medications. [3,9–11] The relationship of ADREs to the number of medications ingested clarifies the dangers of DDI in elders, for whom polypharmacy is common. Elders may have a number of specialists as well as a primary care provider (PCP), among whom communication is not always ideal. Medications are added; doses are changed. An elder who is not medically sophisticated and who may suffer from cognitive impairment may not keep track of these medication changes.

When that elder presents to an ED with an acute exacerbation of a chronic problem or with a new acute problem, it may be difficult or impossible for the ED physician to garner an accurate list of all the medications taken by the patient. When the visits occur at night or on weekends, the PCP's coverage is rarely aware of the patient's medications. Even if the elder's PCP is available, he or she may not have an up-to-date record of the drugs and doses, especially if the elder has visited a specialist recently, takes OTC medications, or "borrows" medications

from a spouse or friend to self-treat perceived problems (particularly pain or common acute illnesses such as an acute respiratory illness).

It is not surprising that the ED is the source of many ADREs in elders. Administering medications during an ED visit and adding or changing medications or doses on discharge from the ED are worrisome. If the patient is taking three or more prescribed medications, a 30 percent probability of a DDI can be expected when a medication is introduced in the ED.[4,12] Between 47 and 61 percent of patients, independent of age, receive a new drug prescription upon being discharged from an ED.[3,12]

OTC Medications

OTC medications are widely ingested for analgesia, sleep aids, and mood enhancement.[5] Even supposed "benign" OTC medications have effects on drug metabolism (Table 3-1). For example, acetominiphen can interfere with liver function, decreasing the metabolism of many medications. As few as four regular-strength tablets (325 mg) of acetaminophen a day can significantly affect the hepatic clearance of warfarin, increasing the patient's risk of bleeding complications.[13] NSAIDs decrease renal clearance and prolong the plasma half-life of other medications, as well as increase the risk of azotemia and gastrointestinal bleeds.[1,5,11,13] Antacids and H_2 blockers may reduce absorption of many medications by increasing gastric pH. Even in therapeutic doses, antihistamines commonly used as sleep aids can have deleterious anticholinergic side effects in elders, such as urinary retention, tachycardia, worsening of glaucoma, and delirium.[1,5,11,13]

Alternative remedies are often ingested by elders, adding to the risk of ADREs; the rising cost of prescription drugs and the wide variety and availability of alternative remedies have increased the probability that the elder patient may be taking one or more of them. Because of embarrassment, ignorance, or forgetfulness, an elder may omit these drugs from the medication list he or she reports. Ginkgo biloba can enhance the anticoagulant properties of aspirin and warfarin.[3,5] St. John's wort, marketed as a mood enhancer, may precipitate serotonin syndrome if taken with another serotonin-enhancing agent (SSRI). Serotonin syndrome classically presents as a disturbance in the central nervous system (CNS), with delirium, seizures or coma, autonomic instability, or neuromuscular hyperactivity. However, these findings may be masked in elders with chronic diseases who often take medications and add an herbal remedy, leading to delays in diagnosis and extensive evaluations for causes of symptoms related to DDI. Since psychotropic drugs are

Table 3-1. Effect of Over-the-Counter Medications on Metabolism of Selected Medications

Medication (Trade Name)	Clinical Actions Affecting Drug Metabolism	Potential Adverse Reaction
Antihistamines (Benadryl)	Decreased GI motility	Delirium, tachycardia, worsening of glaucoma, urinary retention, tardive dyskinesias, fatigue, ataxia
Cimetidine (Tagamet)	Increased gastric pH	Decreased absorption of medications
Aspirin and NSAIDs	Decreased gastric pH	Increased degradation of medications
Acetaminophen (Tylenol)	Decreased P450 activity	Increased activity of hepatically cleared medications
Ginkgo boloba	Antiplatelet function	Enhanced anticoagulation
St. John's wort	Serotoninergic activity	Serotonin syndrome
Vitamin E	Unknown method	Enhanced anticoagulation
Grapefruit juice	P450 activation	Increased absorption of certain medications
Caffeine	P450 activation	Decreased serum levels of hepatically cleared medications
Tobacco	P450 activation	Increased metabolism of medications
Ethanol	Decreased liver function	Inhibits drug metabolism in acute intoxication; enhances in chronic
Laxatives	Decreased GI absorption	Decreased absorption and increased clearance of medications and nutrients
Mineral oil	Decreased GI absorption	Decreased absorption and increased clearance of medications and fat soluble vitamins
Aluminum antacids	Decreased gastric absorption, increased gastric pH	Increased retention of aluminum, malabsorption of calcium

Sources: Adapted from Podrazik and Schwartz[5]; Beyth and Schorr.[1]

prescribed commonly for the elderly, serotonin syndrome may be more prevalent in this population than previously thought and should be considered in the evaluation of delirium and syncope.

Elder Medications

Elders face a variety of challenges when trying to understand and control their medication regimens. Poor eyesight and hearing, multiple caretakers and physicians, and decreased memory and cognition all may contribute to mistakes and confusion. Additionally, medication names can be misread or substituted because of similar trade or generic names of unrelated medications, e.g., Inderal and Adderal or Celebrex and Cerebrex.[1] Pharmacy and third-party-payer drives toward drug substitutions of generic equivalents for brand-name drugs can be a factor. Based on Food and Drug Administration (FDA) regulations,

generic substitutions may vary up to 20 percent in dosage from their trade-name equivalents.[9] The ED physician should review the elder's medication list carefully for errors and sources of DDIs. Prescriptions always should be written in a thoughtful and legible manner. Also, discharge instructions for elders should include prescription instructions in large type and clear language.

In the ED, patient recall of medications may not be accurate. Elders omitted an average of 1.3 medications; only 15 percent could correctly name all medications, dosages, frequencies, and indications.[4]

Elders' use of multiple pharmacies and mail-order pharmacies further complicates obtaining an accurate list of their medications. Additionally, they frequently omit or adjust medications themselves because of cost, inconvenience, forgetfulness, or side effects. As many as 70 percent of elders intentionally alter their intake of prescribed medication, and 90 percent of elder noncompliance is manifested by decreasing the dose of a prescribed medication.[1,10,11] Elder compliance can be improved significantly with a few simple strategies and guidelines.

Pharmacokinetics in Elders

Both the pharmacokinetics (drug absorption distribution, metabolism, and excretion) and pharmacodynamics (physiologic response) of drugs are altered in the elderly patient. Age-related changes can lead to high initial peak concentrations, increased bioavailablity, and prolonged clearance of lipid-soluble medications. While drug absorption can be impaired by achlorhydria, bacterial overgrowth, and surgical resection of digestive organs, this impairment is rarely clinically significant. Drug distribution, however, may be altered significantly due to decreased lean body mass, decreased total-body water, and increased adipose tissue. Drugs that are soluble in water or hydrophilic (e.g., coumadin, digoxin, propranolol, procainamide, and theophylline) have higher plasma concentrations at a given dose in the elderly. Hepatic clearance of certain drugs declines because of decreased liver volume and blood flow. Congestive heart failure, chronic renal disease, rheumatoid arthritis, cirrhosis, protein-calorie malnutrition, and malignancy may result in hypoalbuminemia and increase the free fraction of drugs that are usually protein-bound (e.g., coumadin, phenytoin, tolbutamide, indomethacin, and furosemide). Because laboratory assays generally report only the total drug concentration, an increase in pharmacologically active free drug will not be measured.

Metabolic Changes

Changes in drug metabolism and clearance are common in elders. Once introduced, a medication may require activation by gastric acids, multiple-pass metabolism by the liver, and clearance by the liver or kidney, with circulation of active products. Current scientific understanding of medication metabolism in elders is hampered by a paucity of pharmacologic research and data that are specific to this age group. Although medications are evaluated by the FDA on subjects prior to approval, they are rarely tested in elders. Elders with a multitude of medical problems taking a variety of medications often are ineligible for drug trials.[1,5,11] ADREs are reported and catalogued post hoc after the distribution and widespread prescription of a medication once they are recognized. The FDA then issues warnings or withdrawals. Recognition and reporting delays, as well as delays in distribu-

tion of information about ADREs and DDIs, contribute to the increasing number of these events. On average, patients over 65 years of age have five coexisting medical conditions.[3] Understanding the specific changes of drug action, metabolism, excretion, and toxicity in this population poses an almost insurmountable challenge for medical researchers.

Renal Function

There is an age-related decrease in renal function related to decreased GFR and tubular efficency. These changes are independent of renal disease, develop as the kidney ages, and remain unreflected by serum creatinine levels. Serum creatinine overestimates the actual rate of renal clearance in elders because production decreases with decreasing lean body mass. The average creatinine clearance decreases by 50 percent between the ages of 25 and 85.[1,3,5,11,13] To correct the creatinine clearance for age and weight, the following formula, by Cockroft and Gault, can be used [5,11]:

$$\text{Creatinine clearance} = \frac{[(140 - \text{age}) \times \text{weight (kg)}]}{[72 \times \text{serum creatinine (mg/dL)}]}$$
(Multiply by 0.85 in females)

This formula may assist in the proper renal dosing of medications in elders; however, it may not be accurate when applied to frail elders with severe loss of muscle mass.[11]

Decreased renal function affects drug clearance by prolonging the half-life of renally cleared medications, increasing the serum level, and prolonging the clinical effect. In medications with narrow therapeutic windows, such as digoxin and gentamycin, this decreased clearance may result in toxicity and harmful clinical manifestations. Table 3-2 lists some common medications that rely primarily on renal clearance.

Hepatic Function

Hepatic metabolic enzyme function and hepatic blood flow decline significantly with age (up to a 50 percent reduction).[1,3,5,11,13] Specifically, the cytochrome P450 system is responsible for clearance as well as oxidation and activation of many drugs. Certain medications and active substances can either induce or inhibit the cytochrome P450 system, thus changing the serum levels and clinical activity of other medications. Common inhibitors of the cytochrome P450 system include cimetidine (now available OTC), amiodarone, ciprofloxacin, diltiazem, fluoxe-

Table 3-2. Common Drugs with Decreased Renal Clearance in the Elderly

Class	Medication
Cardiovascular	Atenolol
	Digoxin
	Furosemide
	Hydrochlorothiazide
	Procainamide
	Sotalol
Antibiotics	Ampicillin
	Ceftriaxone
	Gentamycin
	Penicillin
Gastrointestinal	Cimetidine
	Rantitidine
Neurologic	Amantadine
	Lithium
	Pancuronium
	Phenobarbital

Source: Adapted from Beyth and Schorr.[1]

Table 3-3. Common Drugs with Decreased Hepatic Clearance in the Elderly

Class	Medication
Cardiovascular	Labetalol
	Lidocaine
	Prazosin
	Propranolol
	Quinidine
	Salicylates
	Warfarin
Analgesics	Acetaminophen
	Ibuprofen
	Merperidine
Neurologic	Amytriptyline
	Barbituates
	Benzodiazepines
	Nortriptyline
	Phenytoin
Pulmonary	Theophylline

Source: Adapted from Beyth and Schorr.[1]

tine, omeprazole, sulfonamides, and verapamil. These medications, as well as many others that induce cytochrome P450, can severely impair hepatic clearance of drugs (Table 3-3). Common inducers of cytochrome P450 that can decrease the serum concentrations of medications metabolized by the liver include barbiturates, antiepileptic agents such as carbamazepine and phenytoin, caffeine, nicotine, and chronic ethanol intake.[1,3,5,11] Special care must be taken to account for these effects on the medication regimen of any elder patient.

Other Changes Affecting Drug Metabolism

Total-body water and body fat decrease steadily with aging, decreasing the volume of distribution of medications and increasing their serum concentration. Changes in total-body water, lean tissue, and fat also affect the bioavailability of medications. Serum protein, especially albumen, declines with age, decreasing the available binding sites for protein-bound medications. Unbound drug is present in a higher serum concentration at any given dose and will be cleared and excreted (assuming normal renal and hepatic function) more rapidly than protein-bound drug. Malnutrition and dehydration occur more commonly in elders, especially those in nursing homes. Predicting drug serum concentrations and drug metabolism is complex in these patients. At least 5 per-

cent of community-dwelling elders and at least 33 percent of institutionalized elders are malnourished.[5]

Cardiovascular function also decreases in elders; cardiac output declines 1 percent per year after age 30. The heart also manifests a decreasing responsiveness to parasympathetic blockade.[3,5,11] Commonly, there is increased sensitivity to chronotropic and ionotropic drugs; elders may require lower bolus and maintenance doses of antiarrhythmic and antihypertensive agents in order to avoid adverse effects. Guidelines are not readily available. The clinician must use care and close clinical observation to titrate these medications in elder patients. The usual rule is to "start low and go slow." Start at half the usual bolus and half the usual drip dosage.

Decreased gastrointestinal motility and gastric pH in elders may inhibit gastric uptake or metabolism and clearance of certain medications. Also, the increasing resistance of elders to insulin may result in a higher tolerance for diabetic medications. Cognitive and CNS functional deficits in elders may lead to increased sensitivity and adverse effects from many medications. Patients presenting to the ED with confusion, ataxia, delirium, and falls should be evaluated for ADREs. ADREs must be considered as potential causes of ED presentations, and ADREs must be avoided when selecting new medications. Be aware of the physiologic changes of aging when prescribing for elderly patients in the ED.

Specific Medication Problems

Although almost any medication can lead to ADREs in an elder patient, some drugs are implicated more frequently and thus pose a higher risk. Some drugs have been associated with ADREs so frequently in elders that they should be prescribed only in clearly defined clinical situations and with an understanding of the risks (Tables 3-4 and 3-5).

Warfarin poses a large risk of ADREs and DDIs, most significantly intracranial hemorrhage, which occurs in 2 percent of patients.[5,13] Falls, DDIs, medication errors, poor compliance, and hepatic dysfunction all increase the risk of bleeding while taking warfarin. Its affects can be potentiated by a long list of drugs, including most antibiotics and analgesics.[13]

Angiotensin-converting enzyme (ACE) inhibitors can cause hyperkalemia and angioedema. Calcium channel blockers (CCBs), which are broadly prescribed for a number of clinical indications, pose a considerable risk for DDIs. Through a magnification of their clinical effects, they can precipitate bradycardia and hypotension. They also inhibit the cytochrome P450 system, decreasing the metabolism of other hepatically cleared medications.[3,5,11,13] Beta blockers have been associated with frequent ADREs in elders, precipitating hypotension, brady-dysrhythmia, bronchospasm, decreased cardiac output, and congestive heart failure and masking hypoglycemia.

Digitalis, although one of the oldest cardiovascular drugs, is particularly dangerous for elders because of its narrow therapeutic range. Excreted mainly by the kidneys, serum concentrations of digitalis can vary in the face of renal insufficiency, diuretic coingestion, alteration of gastrointestinal flora by antibiotics, and displacement from its receptors on albumin (already limited in elders) by quinidine and amiodarone. In one study, almost 50 percent of ADREs in hospitalized patients were related to digoxin. Presentation of symptoms may be subtle and difficult to differentiate from other conditions; clinical suspicion is key in making the correct and often lifesaving diagnosis.

Careful consideration should be given to anticholinergics such as diphenhydramine hydrochloride (Benadryl), which can increase the risk of delirium and cognitive decline. Many side effects of anticholinergics mimic symptoms traditionally associated with old age, such as dry mouth, constipation, and urinary problems, and these side effects increase when multiple anticholinergics are prescribed.

NSAIDs, commonly used as analgesics, can potentiate anticoagulation, gastrointestinal bleeding, nephritis, hypertension, and renal failure. They also interact with coumadin, digoxin, diuretics, and antihypertensives.

Psychotropic medicines are prescribed widely for elders. Benzodiazepines are given for anxiety and sleeplessness and have been linked to an increased risk of falls and hip fractures in this population.[1] All antidepressants are metabolized by the cytochrome P450 system and thus are

Table 3-4. High-Risk Medications in the Elderly

Class	Medication	Potential ADRE
Diuretic	ACE inhibitors	Hypotension, hypokalemia, renal failure
Antiarrhymics	Beta blockers	Hypotension, heart failure, bronchospasm, bradycardia, depression
	Calcium channel blockers	Decreased P450 metabolism, hypotension, bradycardia, heart failure
	Digitalis	Syncope, arrhythmia
Psychiatrics and hypnotics	Benzodiazepines	Falls, delirium, depression
	Lithium	SIADH, renal failure, CNS toxicity
	SSRIs	Serotonin syndrome
Analgesics	NSAIDs	Gastric irritation, bleeding
Anticoagulants	Warfarin	Bleeding
Pulmonary	Theophylline	Increases P450 metabolism
Metabolic	Insulin	Hypoglycemia
Anti-Seizure medication	Carbamazepine	Increases P450 metabolism

Sources: Adapted and compiled from Prybys et al.[3]; Harwood-Nuss 2001; Byeth and Schorr[1]; Podrazik and Schwartz.[5]

Table 3-5. Inappropriate Medication in the Elderly and Suggested Dosage Adjustments

Class	Agent (Example Trade Name)	Reason/Dosage Adjustment*
Analgesics	Pentazocine (Talwin)	Seizures, cardiotoxicity
	Propoxyphene (Darvon)	Relatively poor pain relief, CNS, and cardiotoxicity
	Merperidine (Demerol)	Seizures, cardiotoxicity, sedation
	Ergot mesyloids	Cardiotoxicity and hypertension
Antidepressants	Amitriptyline (Elavil)	Anticholinergic effects and orthostatic
	Doxepin (Sinequan)	hypotension higher than with other TCAs
Antiemetic	Trimethobenzamide (Tigan)	Less effective, drowsiness, diarrhea,
	Promethazine (Phenergan)	rash, dystonia
Antihypertensives	Methyldopa (Aldomet)	CNS side effects
	Resperpine	
	Propranolol (Inderal)	
	Disopyramide (Norpace)	Hypotension, bradycardia
Cardiac	Digoxin	Arrhythmia, CNS toxicity 0.125 mg
Muscle Relaxants	Carisprodol (Soma)	CNS toxicity (far greater than drug
	Cyclobenzaprine (Flexeril)	benefits)
	Methocarbamol (Robaxin)	
	Orphenadrine (Norflex)	
NSAIDs	Indomethacin	CNS toxicity
	Phenylbutazone	Bone marrow toxicity
Oral hypoglycemic	Chlorpropamide (Diabinese)	Prolonged half-life, risk of SIADH
Platelet inhibitor	Dipyridamole (Aggrenox, Persantine)	CNS side effects
Sedative-hypnotics	Chlordiazepoxide (Librium)	Prolonged clearance, active metabo-
	Diazepam (Valium)	lites
	Flurazepam (Dalmane)	
	Meprobamate (Miltown)	
	All barbiturates except phenobarbital	
	Aprazolam (Xanax)	2 mg
	Lorazepam (Ativan)	3 mg
	Oxazepam	60 mg
	Temazepam (Restoril)	15 mg
	Triazolam (Serax)	0.25 mg
	Zolpidem (Ambien)	5 mg
Other	Iron supplements > 325 mg	GI toxicity
	Dicyclomine	Anticholenergic side effects, drowsi-
	Hyoscyamine	ness

Abbreviations: TCAs = tricyclic antidepressants; CNS = central nervous system; NSAIDs = non-steroidal anti-inflammatory drugs.
*Recommended daily dosage limit.

Sources: Adapted and compiled from Beers M: *Arch Intern Med,* 1997; Prybys et al.[13]; Golden et al.[2];
Becker B: Geriatric considerations: drug toxicity, in Harwood-Nuss 2001.

prone to interfere with other drugs that are metabolized by the liver. Up to 50 percent of nursing home residents receive some form of antipsychotic medication.[1,9] These drugs can precipitate serious ADREs, including disorientation, change in mental status, extrapyramidal effects, and neuroleptic malignant syndrome (NMS).

Diagnosis

The most common manifestations of drug toxicity in the elderly are cardiovascular and neurologic.[1,7,13,14] ADREs always should be considered in any elder patient who is evaluated in the ED with a change in mental status, motor vehicle accident, fall, or syncopal episode. Worsening of preexisting clinical conditions may be linked to a change in the elder patient's medication or the dosage of a preexisting medication. ADREs often mimics another medical condition and are diagnosed only by the careful clinician who obtains and confirms the elder's medication history. ADREs are a diagnosis of exclusion, made when other conditions such as myocardial infarction or cerebrovascular accident have been ruled out or the patient improves with drug withdrawal.

ADDITIONAL ASPECTS

Successful pharmacotherapy for the elder patient who is treated in the ED should not result in ADREs. There are simple strategies to improve ED drug treatment of elder patients, avoiding nearly all iatrogenically induced medication-related problems. Physician awareness may address the problem because 22 percent of ADREs were caused by a lack of physician understanding of the prescribed drug effects.[13] Fortunately, technology can have a significant impact on improving physician ignorance. The Internet and personal digital assistants (PDAs) with pharmaceutical databases provide the clinician with easy access to drug information. Nearly all pharmacies now have DDI and proper-dosing programs, as well as 24-hour access to patients' medication information. Giving clear, legible, written or typed medication instructions to elder patients about their prescriptions increases medication compliance up to 80 to 90 percent.[1]

Other suggestions include

- Inquire about *all* OTC medications that the patient may be taking, including antacids, pain relievers, sleep aids, and alternative therapies.
- Obtain the patient's current medication list—call the pharmacy, primary physician, *and* specialist. Ask a family member or the prehospital health care worker to bring in all the medication bottles from home.
- Attach a list of medications to the patient's chart, and provide a wallet-sized copy for the patient.
- Calculate creatinine clearance for each patient, and adjust medication doses as needed.
- Limit the number of prescriptions. Use the "rule of five": no more than five drugs at a time and in the lowest dose possible for clinical efficacy.[9]
- Avoid starting or continuing high-risk drugs in the ED. If absolutely necessary, communicate verbally and in writing with the PCP or his or her coverage.
- Prescribe a limited number of medications; understand and be comfortable with these drugs, including their potential for DDIs.
- Recommend stool softeners when prescribing narcotic pain relievers
- Prescribe NSAIDs for a limited amount of time at the lowest effective dosage. Consider COX-1 inhibitors.
- "Start low and go slow" on dosages of new medications.[9] Avoid starting any new medications.
- Give written instructions to the patient detailing the diagnosis, medications, instructions on administration, and possible side effects.
- Consider computer-generated discharge instructions and prescriptions. Initiate a drug alert system as part of the discharge process that highlights DDIs.
- Inform family members and caretakers about the type of drugs being prescribed and the possible side effects
- Call in the prescriptions to the pharmacy directly to decrease the paper trail and the possibility of introducing errors.
- Consider home nursing compliance checks and home safety assessment.
- Ensure appropriate follow up. Some elders seen in the ED lack any regular health care provider.[13]

REFERENCES

1. Beyth RJ, Schorr RI: Medication use, in Duthie EH Jr, Katz PR (eds): *Duthie: Practice of Geriatrics,* 3d ed. St. Louis, Saunders, 1998, Chap 5, p 38.
2. Golden AG, Preston RA, Barnett SD: Inappropriate medication prescribing in homebound older adults. *J Am Geriatr Soc* 47:8: 1999.

3. Prybys KM, Melville KA, Hanna JR: Polypharmacy in the elderly: Clinical challenges in emergency practice. I. Overview, etiology, and drug interactions. *Emer Med Rep* 23:11, 2002.

4. Chung MK, Bartfield JM: Knowledge of prescription medications among elderly emergency department patients. *Ann Emerg Med* 39:605, 2002.

5. Podrazik PM, Schwartz JB: Cardiovascular disease in the elderly: Cardiovascular pharmacology of aging. Cardial Clin 17:1, 1999.

6. Hohl CM, Dankoff, J, Calacone, A: Polypharmacy, adverse drug-related events, and potential adverse drug interactions in elderly patients presenting to an emergency department. *Ann Emerg Med* 83:666, 2002.

7. Hafner JW Jr, Belknap, SM, Squillante, MD: Adverse drug events in emergency department patients. *Ann Emerg Med* 39:258, 2002.

8. Johnson JA, Bootman JL: Drug-related morbidity and mortality: A cost-of-illness model. *Arch Intern Med* 155:1949–56, 1995.

9. Cadieux RJ: Geriatric psychopharmacology, a primary care challenge. *Postgrad Med* 93:4, 1993.

10. Nolan L, O'Malley K: Prescribing for the elderly: I. Sensitivity of the elderly to adverse drug reactions. *J Am Geriatr Soc* 36:142, 1988.

11. Montamat SC, Cusack BJ, Vestal RE: Medical intelligence: Management of drug therapy in the elderly. *New Engl J Med* 321:5, 1989.

12. Beers MH, Storrie M, Lee G: Potential adverse drug interactions in the emergency room: An issue of quality of care. *Ann Intern Med* 112:61, 1990.

13. Prybys KM, Melville KA, Hanna JR: Polypharmacy in the elderly: Clinical challenges in emergency practice: II. High-risk drugs, diagnosis, and the role of the emergency physician. *Emerg Med Rep* 23:12, 2002.

14. Romac DR: Drug interactions in the intensive care unit. *Clin Chest Med* 20(2):385, 1999.

15. Grymonpre RE, Mitenko, PA, Sitar, DS: Drug-associated hospital admissions in older patients. *J Am Geriatr Soc* 36:1092, 1988.

4

Functional Assessment and Decline

David J. Peter
Lowell W. Gerson

HIGH-YIELD FACTS

- Functional impairment is common, varies widely in severity, and frequently is not identified in elder emergency department (ED) patients.
- Interview the patient and adjunct historians to determine the time and degree of functional limitations.
- Functional impairment is often due to acute illness, cognitive impairment (delirium or dementia), depression medications, environmental factors, pain, and/or chronic disease.
- Consider baseline and current functional status in patient evaluation and disposition.
- Link functional assessment with and evaluation of caregiver and other support availability and capability.
- Functional assessment as a part of geriatric case finding may reduce emergency department visits and decrease functional decline.

Elder patients presenting to the ED routinely require more time and resources than do younger patients. Their chief complaints are associated with an expanded differential diagnosis and greater medical complexity. Functional, cognitive, and social factors affect the management of elder patients, especially those who are frail. The usual emergency medicine model of care—chief complaint, evaluation, diagnosis, and disposition—may not be best for elders.[1]

Routine assessment of the patient's baseline status and change from baseline represents part of a better model for geriatric emergency care. Collecting evidence of decline in functional performance is important in the initial eval-

uation and final disposition planning. Perhaps the simplest example of this is a patient with a proximal humeral fracture for whom a sling will not provide assistance in performing basic activities of daily living. Functional evaluation includes evaluation of activities necessary for self-care and independent living. Informal questions as a part of the patient history can provide clues to the patient's baseline and any new decline. Formal tests of function include the Katz Activities of Daily Living (ADLs)[2] and the Lawton and Brody Instrumental Activities of Daily Living (IADLs).[3]

An acute decline in functional performance may be caused by new acute disease or exacerbation of chronic illness. Slower decline can indicate more chronic processes (such as dementia, arthritis, or congestive heart failure) that may still be amenable to timely diagnosis and management. Because of illness bringing patients to the ED, functional status deteriorates significantly at the time of an ED visit.[4] Decline in functional status affects the morbidity and mortality of the patient.[5,6] Predictors of poor outcomes in elder ED patients include deficiencies in ADLs, needing more help with everyday tasks, comorbid disease, polypharmacy, recent ED visits, hospitalizations, and a need for a proxy to complete the initial history.[4,7–9] Denman and colleagues[6] found that functional impairment at baseline is an independent predictor of poor medical outcome.

The ED is a useful site for identification of elders at risk for adverse health outcomes, including nursing home admission, death, or future hospitalization. Functional screening of elder patients in the ED is feasible and identifies many problems.[10,11] Screening or case-finding programs attempt to identify high-risk elders who need more comprehensive assessment. Screening in the ED requires tools that are brief, efficient, easily administered, and sensitive to identify elders at risk for poor outcomes. A more complete assessment of those with positive screens may focus on functional impairment, cognitive status, elder abuse, depression, alcohol, malnutrition, or social and environmental factors. Patients identified as at high risk in the ED can be linked to appropriate medical and community services. These ED case-finding programs require additional resources and time but potentially may lead to improved outcomes for elder patients.[7–9]

EPIDEMIOLOGY

Elder ED patients have a high rate of functional problems. The inability to perform one or more ADLs is found in more than three-quarters of elder patients presenting to the ED.[10,11] Gerson and colleagues[11] report finding problems with vision (55 percent), mental status (46 percent), falls (40 percent), and depression (36 percent). Aminzadeh and Dalziel,[12] as part of a systematic review, concluded that "10 to 45 percent of older patients experience functional decline in the 3 months following an ED visit." Chin and colleagues[4] found that physical function declines at the time of the ED visit and then improves over the next 3 months, but not to where the patient was 1 month prior to the visit. Minor trauma may be followed by functional decline. Shapiro and colleagues[13] found that 7 percent of elder patients had a decline in ADLs and that 23 percent had a decline in IADLs 3 months following an ED visit for minor trauma.

CLINICAL FEATURES

Acute and decompensated chronic illness in the elder ED patient often presents as change in cognitive and functional status. Examples include urosepsis, pneumonia, acute coronary syndrome, congestive heart failure, subdural hematoma, stroke, medication effects, electrolyte abnormalities, thyroid disease, and vitamin B_{12} and thiamine deficiency. Falls may be the result of either or both cognitive and functional decline. Worsening dementia, delirium, or depression can result in functional decline, too. An extensive search for medical causes is required when the elder patient presents with unexplained cognitive or functional status changes.

MEASURES OF FUNCTIONAL DECLINE

The Medical History

In general, a cognitive assessment for delirium or dementia should precede the assessment of functional status and should occur early in the patient evaluation to give the physician some assurance of the validity of the patient's self-reported history. Hustey and Meldon[14] recently emphasized the importance of specific screening for delirium and dementia when they found that 26 percent of screened elder patients had a cognitive deficit, 72 percent of which were not documented. They found that 82 percent of patients who were discharged to home with cognitive deficits had no plan for addressing the impairment. Additionally, 37 percent of patients with delirium were discharged to home. The cognitive assessment can include questions and observations (e.g., asking the caretaker or accompanying person about confusion and not-

ing the use of a proxy to answer questions) and formal testing using one of the cognitive assessment tools discussed in Chap. 39.

The medical history should establish the patient's functional baseline and any recent declines in functional ability. When available, the patient and family or other caregivers should be interviewed. It is noteworthy that patients usually will rate their physical abilities higher than do their caretakers.[15] Any changes should be defined in terms of the approximate time of onset, severity, and chronology in relation to other patient factors. These factors can include illness, social factors such as loss of a spouse or caregiver, environmental factors such as a move from the home, the start of a new medication or a change of medication dose, pain, and cognitive decline. The goal is to establish the patient's capabilities at baseline, define the degree and time course of any new impairment, and determine the effect new functional impairment may have on patient disposition.

Activities of Daily Living

Functional status assessment tends to look for hierarchical losses from the highest functions, personal and social fulfillment, to the most basic functions described by the ADLs.

The Activities of Daily Living Scale, as described by Katz (Table 4-1), is used most frequently for assessing the basic functions necessary for self-care. The Katz ADLs consist of bathing, dressing, toileting, transferring, continence, and feeding. Katz rated each item on a three-point scale based on the amount of assistance required: none (1), some (2), or substantial (3).[2]

The ADLs are supposed to be hierarchical. In other

Table 4-1. Activities of Daily Living

Each item is rated (1) no assistance required, (2) needs some assistance, or (3) needs substantial assistance or unable to perform
Bathing
Dressing
Toileting
Transfer
Continence
Feeding

Source: Adapted from Katz S, Ford AB, Moskowitz RW, et al: Studies of illness in the aged. The index of ADL: A standardized measure of biological and psychosocial function. *JAMA* 185:914, 1963. Used with permission.

words, functions usually are lost in order, with bathing the first to go and feeding last. Toileting requires that the patient first transfer. Dressing represents a more difficult task than those that follow. Thus, the person who is able to bathe independently probably can perform the other ADLs satisfactorily. Lazarides and colleagues[16] reported that while the Katz proposed hierarchy does exist, there are other patterns of ADLs loss. Emergency physicians may choose to focus their questions on the need for assistance in performing the ADLs associated with the patient's illness or injury. It may be sufficient in the ED to start with the most complex tasks associated with the patient's condition and ask if the patient has been able to perform them and will be able to continue to perform them. For brevity, the emergency physician could ask about the ADLs in order and stop ADLs questions whenever an impairment is reported, since lower levels of ADLs functioning also will be impaired. We believe that the easiest approach to remembering ADLs in order is to think about what you do when you wake up. You get out of bed, walk to the toilet, wash up, bathe, get dressed, and eat a meal, performing the six ADLs in hierarchical order.

The emergency physician should assess whether the ADLs deficits exceed available resources. If so, the patient is at risk, and discharge without support may lead to readmission. The degree of assistance required by the patient can be determined, in part, by ADLs deficits. Those with deficits in bathing or dressing only may require assistance at predictable times of the day. When greater disability is present, the patient will require more frequent monitoring and assistance throughout the day.[2]

Nearly all studies evaluating function in the ED have incorporated some version of the Katz ADLs.[4,6–11,13] They can be fully assessed in about 2 minutes.[10] ADLs are combined with IADLs when assessing more functional elders.

Instrumental Activities of Daily Living

The IADLs described by Lawton and Brody (Table 4-2) attempt to define the patient's ability to live independently within the community.[3,5] The components include telephone use, shopping, food preparation, housekeeping, transportation, medications, and ability to handle finances. Each is rated from completely or mostly independent (1) to completely or mostly dependent (0). As with the ADLs, the baseline in comparison with available support and changes in level of functioning are important. Screening of IADLs takes less than 2 minutes to complete; when combined with ADLs, the assessment requires about 3 minutes to complete.[10] Sloan[17] offers a use-

Table 4-2. Instrumental Activities of Daily Living

Each item is rated (1) no assistance required, (2) needs some assistance, or (3) needs substantial assistance or unable to perform

Telephone use
Shopping
Food preparation
Housekeeping
Transportation
Medications
Ability to handle finances

Source: Adapted from Lawton WP, Brody EM: Assessment of older people: Self-maintaining and instrumental activities of daily living. *Gerontology* 9:179, 1969. Used with permission.

ful mnemonic, SHAFT, for remembering the IADLs: *s*hopping, *h*ousework, *a*ccounting, *f*ood preparation, and *t*ransportation.

A positive screen for IADLs deficits should trigger an assessment of available support and needed services. Referral options in response to a positive screen include home health care referral and assessment, physical therapy, occupational therapy, home health aids, meals on wheels, and others. The patient may need more urgent intervention or social admission. When deficits exceed the support that is readily available, IADLs predict mortality. For patients 65 years of age and older, Fillenbaum[5] found the yearly mortality rate to be 27 percent for patients unable to perform any of the IADLs unaided and 2 percent for patients able to independently perform all IADLs.

Performance-based screening of functional status has been shown to be superior to question-based assessment. This approach is not practical under the time constraints of the ED. However, an easily performed performance measure that may be suited to the ED is the timed "up and go" test.

Timed "Up and Go" Test

The timed "up and go" test correlates with balance, gait speed, and functional capacity. The patient is asked to rise from an armchair, walk 3 m, turn, return to the chair, and sit. For screening, the authors suggest 10 seconds as the cutoff for patients to be described as "freely mobile," which appears to predict the patient's ability to go outside safely.[18] Moore and Siu[19] used 15 seconds for the screening cutoff.

Lachs and colleagues[20] preferred an untimed approach, simply observing the patient and assessing the ability to complete the task. Many emergency physicians routinely perform untimed "up and go" tests, observing the patient rise from the stretcher, walk, turn, and then return to the stretcher with or without assistance. Qualitative assessments such as this may be helpful as part of functional screening in the ED. When impairments are found, more formal testing and appropriate disposition planning are required.

Functional Screening

Lachs and colleagues[20] developed a brief functional assessment for use in ambulatory settings. They recommend testing vision with a Jaeger card; hearing using the whisper test; proximal and distal arm mobility, leg strength, and mobility with an untimed "up and go" test; urinary continence via question; nutrition by weight and height; mental status by three-item recall; depression by question; home environment by questions; and social support by asking, "Who would be able to help you in case of illness or emergency?" ADLs and IADLs were assessed by asking about four items: ability to get out of bed, dress, prepare meals, and shop by oneself. All positive responses on the screen were linked to a further evaluation or referral.[20] Gerson and colleagues[11] used the Lachs and colleagues screen in combination with questions on general health, polypharmacy, influenza vaccination, and alcohol and elder abuse in order to determine the frequency of problems in older ED patients and to identify which questions and tests would be useful in the ED setting. Patients with problems were referred to their personal physician.[11] The screen found 281 conditions in 242 patients, with difficulty in performing ADLs being the most common finding. The screen required about 18 minutes to complete. Often patients did not have glasses or hearing aids available, which limits ED evaluation.

Moore and Sui[21] have developed a 10-minute test for geriatric conditions. The items include questions about vision, urinary incontinence, weight loss, memory, depression, and physical ability. It also includes an "up and go" test, audiometry, and a Snellen chart for those who, because of their eyesight, answer that they have trouble with driving, television, or reading. The question items could be obtained while taking a history. To what extent these screening tests would add time to the ED encounter or require additional personnel is unknown.

ED Case Finding

Teams of emergency physicians, geriatricians, and nurses in Montreal, Canada,[7,8] and Cleveland, Ohio,[9] have developed and implemented a two-stage screening process to identify patients at risk for poor health outcomes. Each group developed a brief screening instrument. Patients with a positive brief screen received a comprehensive geriatric assessment performed by a geriatric nurse specialist. The screening tests were derived empirically from studies identifying predictors of poor outcome, such as hospitalization. Each screen has unique questions, but there are questions that are common to both. The Canadian screen, Identification of Seniors at Risk (ISAR), is displayed in Table 4-3.[7,8] The Cleveland project is known as the Systematic Intervention for a Geriatric Network of Evaluation and Treatment (SIGNET), and its screen, Triage Risk Screening Tool (TRST), is displayed in Table 4-4.[9]

The Canadian team demonstrated a significant decrease in functional decline in the 4 months following the ED visit for patients identified by the screen and referred to their family physician. The ISAR screen is also predictive of increased risk for return to the ED. This screen

Table 4-3. Identification of Seniors at Risk (ISAR)

1. Before the illness or injury that brought you to the emergency department, did you need someone to help you on a regular basis?	Yes	No
2. Since the illness of injury brought you to the emergency department, have you needed more help than usual to care for yourself?	Yes	No
3. Have you been hospitalized for one or more nights during the past 6 months (excluding a stay in the emergency department)?	Yes	No
4. In general, do you see well?	Yes	No
5. In general, do you have serious problems with your memory?	Yes	No
6. Do you take more than three different medications every day?	Yes	No

Two or more positive (yes) answers—high risk elder patient.

Source: Adapted from McCusker J, Cardin S, Bellavance F, et al.: Return to the emergency department among elders: Patterns and predictors. *Acad Emerg Med* 7:249, 2000. Used with permission.

Table 4-4. Triage Risk Screening Tool (TRST) Used in the SIGNET Program

1. Presence of cognitive impairment. Example: disorientation, unable to follow directions, diagnosis of delirium or dementia.	(Yes, no)
2. Lives alone or no caregiver available, willing, or able.	(Yes, no, unable to determine)
3. Difficulty with walking or transfers, history of recent falls.	(Yes, no)
4. ED use (past 30 days) or hospitalization (last 3 months)	(Yes, no, unable to determine)
5. Five or more medications.	(Yes, no, unable to determine)

6. Professional recommendations: Nurse believes this patient requires
   further follow-up at home for any of the following:
   a. Suspected abuse, neglect, self-neglect, or exploitation.
   b. Noncompliant patient with less than five medications who keeps coming back to the ED.
   c. Suspected substance abuse (alcohol or drug).
   d. Problems with meeting IADLs, such as getting prescriptions filled, problems with transportation, problems
      with getting food or meals, etc.
   e. Other (please specify).

Any patient with cognitive impairment (1) or two or more of the remaining risk factors is considered at risk and should be followed up by the geriatric nurse specialist.

Source: Adapted from Mion LC, Palmer RM, Anetzberger GJ, et al: Establishing a case-finding and referral system for at-risk older individuals in the emergency department setting: The SIGNET model. *J Am Geriatr Soc* 49:1379, 2001. Used with permission.

is rapid and can be initiated by nursing or physician staff during the patient's evaluation in the ED.[7,8]

The initial evaluation with the TRST, followed by the comprehensive geriatric assessment, resulted in a significant increase in referrals to community agencies. The estimated annual cost of this case finding is $8.99 to $17.08 per elder screened in the ED.

CONCLUSION

A new model of care for elder patients emphasizes that emergency physicians must consider the patients' biologic, social, and cognitive function. Some simple tests for assessment of functional status are presented (see Chap. 38 for cognitive assessment). These functional and cognitive assessments are best administered as part of the history and physical examination. The information they yield is crucial in patient evaluation and decisions about disposition.

More comprehensive programs of screening for geriatric problems and functional status in the ED were discussed. These experimental programs have shown that ED case finding is feasible and has a high yield, identifying significant problems. Case finding involves universal initial screening, comprehensive geriatric assessment for patients who screen positive, and the potential for improved outcomes.

Without the benefit of ancillary personnel to perform these screens and provide the needed links to community and medical services, emergency physicians need to target only those issues directly affecting patient disposition. This includes assessing the need for home health care referral, durable medical equipment, transportation services, and assistance with procuring medications or arranging follow-up appointments. If any of these cannot be accomplished by the patient and caregiver and the patient cannot get additional support, "social" admission may be necessary. Involvement of case managers or a geriatric assessment team may mobilize outpatient resources and obviate the need for admission.

Since avoidable admissions are undesirable, the ED will become a place where elder patients with functional, cognitive, and social impairments should be identified and linked to appropriate services prior to discharge. Addressing these deficits constitutes secondary prevention, which should be an important aspect of ED care for elders.

ADDITIONAL ASPECTS

The following are pitfalls to be avoided in the assessment of elder patients. Do not fail to assess the patient's need for resources during the course of an injury or illness. Do not fail to appreciate that illness treated in the ED may affect the patient's ability to perform ADLs and IADLS. Do not fail to recognize impaired functional status as a comorbidity and consider it in management decisions.

REFERENCES

1. Sanders AB: Older persons in the emergency medical care system (editorial). *J Am Geriatr Soc* 49:1390, 2001.
2. Katz S, Ford AB, Moskowitz RW, et al: Studies of illness in the aged. The index of ADL: A standardized measure of biological and psychosocial function. *JAMA* 185:914, 1963.
3. Lawton WP, Brody EM: Assessment of older people: Self-maintaining and instrumental activities of daily living. *Gerontology* 9:179, 1969.
4. Chin MH, Ma LJ, Karrison TG, et al: Older patients' health-related quality of life around an episode of emergency illness. *Ann Emerg Med* 34:595, 1999.
5. Fillenbaum GG: Screening the elderly: A brief instrumental activities of daily living measure. *J Am Geriatric Soc* 33:698, 1985.
6. Denman SJ, Ettinger WH, Zarkin BA, et al: Short-term outcomes of elderly patients discharged from an emergency department. *J Am Geriatr Soc* 37:937, 1989.
7. McCusker J, Cardin S, Bellavance F, et al: Return to the emergency department among elders: Patterns and predictors. *Acad Emerg Med* 7:249, 2000.
8. McCusker J, Verdon J, Tousignant P, et al: Rapid emergency department intervention for older people reduces risk of functional decline: Results of a multicenter randomized trial. *J Am Geriatr Soc* 49:1272, 2001.
9. Mion LC, Palmer RM, Anetzberger GJ, et al: Establishing a case-finding and referral system for at-risk older individuals in the emergency department setting: The SIGNET model. *J Am Geriatr Soc* 49:1379, 2001.
10. Miller DK, Lewis LM, Nork MJ, et al: Controlled trial of a geriatric case-finding and liaison service in an emergency department. *J Am Geriatr Soc* 44:513, 1996.
11. Gerson LW, Rousseau EW, Hogan TM, et al: Multicenter study of case finding in elderly emergency department patients. *Acad Emerg Med* 2:729, 1995.
12. Aminzadeh F, Dalziel WB: Older adults in the emergency department: A systematic review of patterns of use, adverse outcomes, and effectiveness of interventions. *Ann Emerg Med* 39:238, 2002.
13. Shapiro MJ, Partridge RA, Jenouri I, et al: Functional decline in independent elders after minor traumatic injury. *Acad Emerg Med* 8:78, 2001.
14. Hustey FM, Meldon SW: The prevalence and documentation of impaired mental status in elderly emergency department patients. *Ann Emerg Med* 39:248, 2002.
15. Gerson LW, Blanda M, Dhingra P, et al: Do elder emergency department patients and their informants agree about the elder's functioning? *Acad Emerg Med* 8:721, 2001.
16. Lazaridis EN, Rudberg MA, Furner SE, et al: Do activities of daily living have a hierarchical structure? An analysis using the Longitudinal Study of Aging. *J Gerontol* 49:M47, 1994.
17. Sloan JP: *http://www.mayo.edu/geriatrics-rst, ADLs.html.*
18. Podsiadlo D, Richardson S: The times "up and go": A test of basic functional mobility for frail elderly persons. *J Am Geriatr Soc* 39:142, 1991.
19. Moore AA, Siu AL: Screening for common problems in ambulatory elderly: Clinical confirmation of a screening instrument. *Am J Med* 100:438, 1996.
20. Lachs MS, Feinstein AR, Cooney LM, et al: A simple procedure for general screening for functional disability in elderly patients. *Ann Intern Med* 112:699, 1990.
21. Moore AA, Siu AL, Partridge JM, et al: A randomized trial of office-based screening for common problems in older persons. *Am J Med* 102:371, 1997.

5

Falls

Manish N. Shah

HIGH-YIELD FACTS

- Falls among older adults are common, affecting 30 percent of all individuals each year.
- Falls are associated with significant physical and psychological morbidity, mortality, and cost.
- Treatment for falls requires assessment of injuries resulting from the fall and determination of the cause of the fall.
- Falls can be effectively prevented by modifying risk factors.

Falls are a leading and preventable cause of morbidity, mortality, and loss of quality of life among older adults.[1-4] The complete extent of the impact on patients from falling is difficult to assess but includes both physical and psychological trauma. The public health burden caused by falls is extensive but also difficult to estimate. Patients may modify lifestyle or require more assistance, but often they do not seek care after minor falls.

Emergency physicians frequently care for older adults who fall, particularly when they sustain injury. Falls in elders may be the result of underlying illness, and a careful history must be obtained from the patient and caregiver to ascertain the cause of any fall. When in doubt about the cause because of lack of witnesses and unreliable or contradicting history or findings on physical examination or laboratory results, the prudent emergency physician considers and carefully rules out the life-threatening diagnoses associated with syncope. In some patients, a fall is "just a fall." Then the emergency physician also needs to provide acute care for injury and promote secondary prevention by considering causes of falling.

EPIDEMIOLOGY

Community-Dwelling Adults

Falls are among the most common accidental injury in older persons. Approximately 30 percent of older adults fall annually, and of those who fall, 50 percent fall repeatedly.[5,6] Studies report an increasing incidence of falls with advancing age, with an average fall rate of 40 percent among those 80 years of age and older.[5] Falls may be more common among women, but results from studies are contradictory.[5,7-10]

Approximately 10 to 15 percent of falls result in serious physical injuries, and half result in minor injuries. Catastrophic injuries, such as subdural hemorrhage or vertebral fractures, occur only occasionally from falls. More common are hip, pelvis, and extremity fractures (as well as minor injuries such as contusions and sprains).

After falling, individuals may have difficulty getting up and, as a result, can spend significant time lying on the ground. These long ground times may result in rhabdomyolysis, dehydration, and pressure sores. These complications fortunately occur in less than 10 percent of cases.[11]

The emotional consequences of falling have been recognized as much more common than the physical consequences. One study reports that after an initial fall, 50 percent of community-dwelling older adults report being afraid of additional falls, and 25 percent of older adults who fall report limiting basic activities due to worries about falling again.[5]

The combined result of the physical and psychological injuries caused by falls has been shown to include functional limitations, skilled nursing facility admission, death, and a significant increase in both health care use and medical charges.[12,13] One study reports that the direct costs for fall-related injuries among both institutionalized and community-dwelling older adults was $20 billion in 1995 and is estimated to be $32 billion by 2020.[14] The total cost which would include indirect costs for disability, long-term consequences, and decreased productivity, and certainly is much higher but difficult to estimate.

Institutionalized Adults

Falls sustained by institutionalized individuals are slightly different from those sustained by community-dwelling older adults. Among institutionalized older adults, studies report that between 29 and 61 percent of patients fall each year. Approximately 15 percent of these falls result in serious injuries, including approximately 4 percent resulting in fractures.[10,15-17] A disproportionately high incidence of hip fractures occurs, but pelvic and extremity fractures, contusions, and sprains are also seen.[15-17]

PATHOPHYSIOLOGY

A number of studies have examined risk factors for falls among older adults. Table 5-1 shows the relative risk (for prospective studies) or odds ratio (for retrospective studies) associated with risk factors among institutionalized and community-dwelling adults. The risk factors for falls are separated into intrinsic and extrinsic causes, but many falls are felt to be a combination of both. Intrinsic causes of falls include factors such as lower extremity weakness, poor grip strength, balance disorders, cognitive impairment, and visual and auditory deficits. Extrinsic causes include the effects of medication and environmental factors such as a lack of hand rails in the home, dark walk-ways, improperly fitting shoes, and unsafe objects (e.g., throw rugs or cords) on which the patient can trip. While intrinsic and extrinsic factors can affect both institutionalized and community-dwelling older adults, published data show associations with intrinsic factors among institutionalized patients and associations with extrinsic factors among community-dwelling patients.[18]

Studies document an increased risk of falling as the number of risk factors experienced by an individual increases. Robbins and colleagues[19] examined three simple risk factors—hip weakness, unstable balance, and four or more medications. The 1-year risk of falling increased from 12 percent for an individual with no risk factors to 100 percent for an individual with all three risk factors. In another study, Tinetti and colleagues[20] showed that the risk of falling ranged from 0 percent for individuals with zero to three risk factors to 100 percent for individuals with seven or more risk factors.

Table 5-1. Statistically Significant Risk Factors for Falls

Factor	Community-Dwelling Adults[5] (Relative Risk)	Institutionalized Adults[17] (Average Risk)
Fall in previous 2 years	2.5	N/A
Balance deficit	1.7	4.6
Bedroom hazard	3.5	N/A
Cognitive impairment	2.3	1.5
Decreased functional status	1.8	3.1
Decreased vision	1.7	2.7
Depression	1.7	1.6
Gait deficit	1.8	3.6
Impaired mobility	1.7	3.3
Sedative use	3.1	2.0
Weakness (lower extremity)	2.4	6.2

Sources: Tinetti ME, Speechley M, Ginter SF: Risk factors for falls among elderly persons living in the community. *New Engl J Med* 319:1701, 1988; and Rubenstein LZ, Josephson KR, Robbins AS: Falls in the nursing home. *Ann Intern Med* 121:442, 1994.

PREHOSPITAL CONSIDERATIONS

Emergency medical technicians (EMTs) are often the first responders to patients who have fallen. EMTs should rapidly evaluate for injuries such as fractures, as well as processes that could have caused the fall, such as cardiac or neurologic dysfunction. Then the patient should be transported to an emergency department (ED).

EMTs have an important role to play in the overall care of the patient who has fallen. EMTs have entered the patient's home. Beyond the acute care delivery in the prehospital setting, they can gather information, aiding the emergency physician who must assess each patient's social needs and ultimately make a disposition. For example, the EMTs are uniquely able to describe the state of the home and evaluate patient safety in the home.[21] For this reason, it is important for the emergency staff and physician to elicit this type of history from the EMTs when receiving the patient in the ED.

CLINICAL FEATURES

History

Obtaining a history of the events surrounding a fall from an older patient may be challenging, depending on the medical conditions from which the patient suffers (e.g., dementia) and the effect of the fall (e.g., loss of consciousness). If the patient is unable to provide significant, clear information, speaking with family members, caregivers, and EMTs, reviewing medical records, and consulting the patient's primary care physician may be helpful. Information of particular value to the physician can include the patient's recent functional status and illnesses, as well as events surrounding the fall, including any loss of consciousness, time spent on the ground, injuries sustained, and previous medical conditions (e.g., arrhythmias or neurologic disorders).

DIAGNOSIS AND DIFFERENTIAL

Multiple health issues present a challenge to the evaluation of patients suffering falls. Emergency physicians must base their diagnostic workup and treatment of patients on (1) illnesses and injuries resulting from the actual fall and (2) illnesses or events causing the fall. While both levels of disease are important to consider, physicians must decide on a case-by-case basis which conditions require immediate intervention. A key point to remember is that older patients can deteriorate rapidly without any warning.

When evaluating and treating illnesses that could have caused a fall that remains unexplained, an evaluation for syncope is appropriate (see Chap. 11). Injuries resulting from a fall should be evaluated and treated following general trauma principles (see Chap. 44). Injuries are quite common, and the physician should expect to find contusions and fractures. The physician should first perform a rapid primary survey, followed by a thorough secondary survey. Common injuries include hip, wrist, femur, and ankle fractures; head and facial trauma; and lacerations. Adequate diagnostic imaging and laboratory testing must be performed, as discussed in Chaps. 45 through 47. Injuries that seem minor initially may be associated with more significant traumatic injuries, such as subdural hematomas and spinal fractures.

Because older persons often have difficulty getting up after falling and therefore are lying on the ground for prolonged periods of time, physicians should look for hypothermia or hyperthermia, dehydration, and rhabdomyolysis. Many medical illnesses can lead to falls (details about these illnesses are contained in other chapters in this book).

When evaluating the illnesses that may have caused the fall, the emergency physician may have limited success. For instance, if the patient provides a clear history of an environmental cause, such as tripping over an object, further workup may be limited because the cause is known and can be addressed. However, if the patient provides an unclear history or a history compatible with an intrinsic cause (e.g., weakness, dizziness, or syncope) of the fall, then a much broader workup will be necessary to identify and treat the actual cause. Central to any workup, even when the history appears to identify an external cause, should be thorough cardiac, neurologic, and musculoskeletal evaluations, as well as an analysis of medications that could cause falls.

ED CARE AND DISPOSITION

Treatment

The injuries and illnesses resulting from the fall should be treated immediately. Chapters 45 through 47 discuss the appropriate treatment in detail.

If the cause of the fall is identified, the treating physician should attempt to remedy the cause. An unsafe home may require that family, friends, or social workers intervene to ensure that obstacles are removed and that the patient can ambulate safely. Sedatives and narcotics may need to be altered or discontinued. Cardiac or neurologic problems require further workup as an inpatient. Consulting the primary care physician also can help when assessing causes of a fall, but the emergency physician must make an independent assessment of the patient's need for hospital admission.

If the patient is to be discharged to home, the emergency physician must ensure that the older adult will be safe and able to manage daily activities successfully. The potential impact on home safety of ED treatments, such as splints and medications, also must be considered. If available, a geriatric assessment team, case manager, or social worker can arrange a safe discharge by providing detailed patient evaluation, communicating with family members and friends to organize support, and organizing additional services such as home health aids or nursing services. The emergency physician must consider admitting the older patient until appropriate and safe disposition is obtained.

Prevention

While care in the ED must focus initially on acute medical therapy, emergency physicians have a tremendous opportunity to identify, educate, and refer older individuals who are at risk for falling. Unfortunately, only limited research has been performed to evaluate preventive efforts aimed at reducing falls. Only one study, published as an abstract, shows the benefit of an ED-based primary falls prevention program.[22] A second study, the PROFET study, shows that a structured interdisciplinary intervention program for ED patients who have fallen (tertiary prevention) decreases the number of falls, risk of recurrent falls, and number of hospitalizations.[23] The emergency physician must be aware of the risk of fall inherent in the prescription of narcotics and sedatives. With better prescription practices, emergency physicians will contribute less to their older patients' risk of falling.

ADDITIONAL ASPECTS

The following pitfalls should be avoided in the care of patients evaluated after falling: incomplete trauma and illness evaluation, discharging the patient to an unsafe environment, and initiating medications such as narcotics or sedatives that are unsafe in older populations.

REFERENCES

1. American Geriatrics Society: Guideline for the prevention of falls in older persons. *J Am Geriatr Soc* 49:664, 2001.
2. Tinetti ME, Baker DL, McAvay G, et al: A multifactorial intervention to reduce the risk of falling among elderly people living in the community. *New Engl J Med* 1(331):821, 1994.
3. Bell AJ, Talbot-Stern JK, Hennessy A: Characteristics and outcomes of older patients presenting to the emergency department after a fall: A retrospective analysis. *Med J Aust* 173:179, 2000.
4. Tynan C, Cardea JM: Home health hazard assessment. *J Gerontol Nurs* 13:25, 1987.
5. Tinetti ME, Speechley M, Ginter SF: Risk factors for falls among elderly persons living in the community. *New Engl J Med* 319:1701, 1988.
6. Tinetti ME, Speechley M: Prevention of falls among the elderly. *New Engl J Med* 320:1055, 1989.
7. Northridge ME, Nevitt MC, Kelsey JL, Link B: Home hazards and falls in the elderly: The role of health and functional status. *Am J Public Health* 85:509, 1995.
8. Sorock, GS: Falls among the elderly: Epidemiology and prevention. *Am J Prevent Med* 4:282, 1988.
9. Alexander BH, Rivara FP, Wolf ME: The cost and frequency of hospitalization for fall-related injuries in older adults. *Am J Public Health* 82(7):1020, 1992.
10. Sattin RW: Falls among older persons: A public health perspective. *Annu Rev Public Health* 13:489, 1992.
11. Nevitt MC, Cummings SR, Kidd S, Black D: Risk factors for recurrent nonsyncopal falls. *JAMA* 261:2663, 1989.
12. Tinetti ME, Williams CS: Falls, injuries due to falls, and the risk of admission to a nursing home. *New Engl J Med* 337:2379, 1997.
13. Kiel DP, O'Sullivan P, Teno JM, Mor V: Health care utilization and functional status in the aged following a fall. *Med Care* 29:221, 1991.
14. Englander F, Hodson TJ, Terregrossa RA: Economic dimensions of slip and fall injuries. *J Forens Sci* 41:733, 1996.
15. Tinetti ME: Factors associated with serious injury during falls by ambulatory nursing home residents. *J Am Geriatr Soc* 35:644, 1987.
16. Kiely DK, Kiel DP, Burrows AB, Lipsitz LA: Identifying nursing home residents at risk for falling. *J Am Geriatr Soc* 46:551, 1998.
17. Rubenstein LZ, Josephson KR, Robbins AS: Falls in the nursing home. *Ann Intern Med* 121:442, 1994.
18. Sehested P, Severin-Nielsen T: Falls by hospitalized elderly patients: Causes, prevention. *Geriatrics* 4:101, 1977.
19. Robbins AS, Rubenstein LZ, Josephson KR, et al: Predictors of falls among elderly people: Results of two population based studies. *Arch Intern Med* 149:1628, 1989.
20. Tinetti ME: Performance-oriented assessment of mobility problems in elderly patients. *J Am Geriatr Soc* 34:119, 1986.
21. Gerson LW, Schelble DT, Wilson, JE: Using paramedics to identify at-risk elderly. *Ann Emerg Med* 21:688, 1992.
22. Gerson LW, Blanda M, Janakiram M: A randomized trial of three strategies for primary prevention of falls in elders. *Acad Emerg Med* 8:530, 2001.
23. Close J, Ellis M, Hooper R, et al: Prevention of falls in the elderly trial (PROFET): A randomized control trial. *Lancet* 353:93, 1999.

6

Elder Abuse and Neglect

Elizabeth deLahunta Edwardsen

HIGH-YIELD FACTS

- Institutional issues regarding elder abuse, which may vary, should be addressed by individual institutions and made available in the clinical area for quick referral.

- Required interventions and legal considerations are under the jurisdiction of the states.

- Elderly patients have the right to choose their care if they are competent.

- Reporting requirements of suspected cases of elder abuse are determined by state law. A good-faith report is immune from liability.

- Exercising power to protect persons who choose not to protect themselves is considered ageist and is not legal. Restraining orders against perpetrators can be obtained by the victim.

- Emergency physicians should remember their duty to a victim to do what is medically best or most appropriate.

- Despite patient confidentiality, there is a general duty to warn a third party of a patients intent to harm that third party.

- Well-documented medical records can be important to court testimony.

- Interventional options and financial support vary by state. However, the ethical responsibility of society and especially emergency physicians is to strongly advocate for elderly patients who may be victims of abuse or neglect.

Elder abuse and neglect are increasingly recognized problems in our society that present commonly in clinical practice.[1,2] Physicians may be the only regular contact outside of the home or institution for patients who experience abuse. Therefore, physicians must assume the roll of patient advocate, ask appropriate questions, and authorize necessary social services.

Elder abuse exists in many forms, including physical, psychological, sexual, and financial. Neglect of daily needs and deprivation of personal rights are common forms of abuse. A commission of an act or an omission of appropriate care can result in harm or potential harm to an elder. The term *elder mistreatment* has been coined to indicate a violation of legal or human rights to self-respect, dignity, and liberty. If cognitive ability is sufficient, older persons should be allowed to maintain property, privacy, and free speech. Care providers may intentionally or unintentionally (inadvertently due to ignorance, inexperience, or inability) compromise the health or well-being of an elderly person.

Examples of abuse are diverse. A variety of actions of family members or caregivers can result in physical or mental harm to or neglect of an elder. A willful direct infliction of physical pain or injury—pushing, pinching, slapping, striking, burning, force feeding, improper use of physical restraints or medications, and sexual coercion and assault—are examples of physical abuse. Neglect may consist of the lack of attention, denial of the necessities of life, incorrect positioning, confinement, or abandonment. Psychological abuse includes the removal of decision-making power, arbitrary changes in care without patient input, withholding affection, denying privacy, or isolation from companionship, news, or information. Exploitation is the dishonest use of an elderly persons resources such as fraud, misuse of money, provision of substandard care to reallocate money for other purposes, stealing property or possessions, or supporting chemical dependency. Coercion regarding power of attorney or a will or ownership of a home and forcing an elderly person into home labor or child care are further examples. Verbal abuse may include constant shouting, harassment, humiliation, berating, insults, intimidation, or threats.

Historically, elder abuse and neglect were not recognized in the United States until the 1970s, when a few small case studies were published. Subsequently, the U.S. Senate created a Committee on Aging. In the 1980s, federal inquiries resulted in recommendations by the Institute of Medicine. The 1990s saw the creation of the Elder Abuse Task Force and the formation of the National Institute on Elder Abuse by the Department of Health and Human Services. Finally, the Joint Commission on Accreditation of Healthcare Organizations (JCAHO) has developed standards for improved identification and management of abuse, including elder abuse and neglect.

EPIDEMIOLOGY

An estimated 1.5 to 2.0 million elderly persons are victimized each year, or approximately 4 percent of the elder population. With the current rise in this population, emergency department (ED) detection of cases of abuse and neglect is expected to increase steadily in the years to come. Settings of abuse include the elderly individuals home, the home of relatives, institutions, and extended-care facilities. The ED may be an area for more intensive screening of patients for abuse.

There is a suspicion that many cases, unfortunately, are undetected and unreported. This is accentuated by the home-bound state of many elderly persons and their lack of access to medical or social service professionals. Abused individuals may be embarrassed, intimidated, and overwhelmed. They may fear and experience threats of reprisal. Some are unaware of the availability of help and may have suffered prior discrimination due to societal attitudes. Many professionals receive inadequate training with respect to geriatric abuse. Cognitive impairment of the elderly may limit their ability to report abuse. Social pressure may exist to overlook abuse, but EDs can provide a safety net for these patients.

PREDISPOSITION

Several theories exist about the causes of elder abuse. Some espouse a theory of learned behavior in which violence is used to deal with stress. Alternately, some believe that the psychopathology of the caregiver (due to alcoholism, drug addiction, or emotional problems) leads to the abuse of an older individual. Families and communities can be part of a cycle of violence that includes elder, child, and spousal violence. A history of abusive relationships may predispose individuals to abuse. Family problems often exacerbate and predispose individuals. Medical, functional, and cognitive disability of elderly persons increases their vulnerability, dependency, and isolation. Caregivers may experience ambivalence and resentment when they are dependent on an elderly individual, particularly for housing and financial resources. Finally, the stress of economic issues, care needs, and lack of societal support may surpass the coping abilities of some caregivers.[3]

All race, ethnic, socioeconomic, and educational groups are at risk for elder abuse from a perpetrator who is often a spouse, an adult child, or a caregiver. Within institutions, potential abusers include staff members, other patients, intruders, and visitors. The clinical course of an abusive relationship is toward escalation of severity and frequency of abuse over time if no correction of risk factors occurs.

CLINICAL FEATURES

Elder abuse and neglect can be diagnosed with a thorough history and physical examination.[4] Unfortunately, barriers to identification exist, including false beliefs that functional decline and frailty are inevitable, lack of training for professionals, and an overemphasis on the time-consuming nature of unraveling a potentially complex situation. A multidisciplinary approach involving psychiatric and social workers and all ED staff members as well as a geriatric consult team if available can limit the time and resources expended by any individual provider.

Interviewing

Interviewing must include routine screening for potential abuse if physicians are to discover and advocate for the abused elder (Fig. 6-1 and Table 6-1). Interviewing the patient alone (cognitive deficits often do not negate the elderly patients ability to describe mistreatment) and then with the caregiver will optimize the information obtained about the patients quality of life. Direct questions about potentially unmet needs and the patients feelings of safety (or lack thereof) are suggested. Inquiry as to whether the patient wishes to reside where he or she presently is living and observation of interactions with the caregiver may reveal fear or intimidation. Differing accounts of symptoms and injuries should prompt concern about abuse. Concern also should arise if a caregiver expresses indifference, hostility, or excessive concern with finances or hovers over the patient. Speaking with several family members, any patient advocates, and the primary care physician may lead to an understanding of any potentially unsafe situation. The social history should include any problems related to the caregiver (financial, stress, chemical dependency), demographic data, family composition, financial status, and the general sense of well-being of the patient.

Red flags for potential abuse include presentation of an elderly patient to the health care environment with a non-family member or noncaregiver, delays in presentation, noncompliance with medications or withholding care, missed appointments, physician or hospital hopping, and stress-related illnesses (somatic pain, poor sleep or appetite) (Table 6-2). Inconsistency between the history and

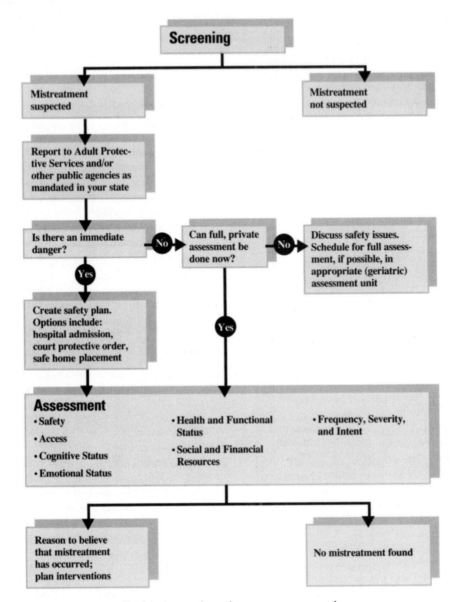

Fig. 6-1   Intervention and case management, part 1.

findings or contradictory explanations, repetitive injuries, and unexplained injuries are most consistent with abuse. Another cause for concern would be emergency medical technicians (EMTs) or others reporting a debilitated patient at home without supervision. Presenting symptoms may include injuries, worsening of chronic health conditions, vague pain syndromes, or mental decline. Key historical information to obtain in the interview includes

how an event happened or a symptom occurred, when and who was involved, how the patient feels about the present situation, and how the patient copes with daily issues, including the current chief complaint. Finally, how dangerous does the patient perceive the current situation to be? What does the patient want to be done? Ultimately, a competent patient is allowed to make autonomous decisions about any intervention.

Table 6-1. Interviewing Questions and Statements

1. Abuse and violence are epidemics in our society; therefore, we are asking all patients about the possibility for abuse in their lives in addition to other health problems.
2. Please be assured that whatever you say will be kept confidential. If you are or have been abused or neglected, we would like to give you a chance to talk about it. I will not push you to do anything you do not want to do.
3. Has anyone at home ever hurt you?
4. Has anyone ever touched you without your consent?
5. Has anyone ever made you do things you did not want to do?
6. Has anyone taken anything that was yours without asking?
7. Have you ever signed any document that you did not understand?
8. Are you alone a lot?
9. Has anyone ever failed to help you take care of yourself when you need help?
10. Are you (have you ever been) with someone who has ever verbally, emotionally, sexually, or physically harmed or threatened you?
11. We all fight or disagree sometimes with the people we live with. When you disagree at home, are you ever afraid of what your caregiver or family might do to you or your possessions?
12. Has your family or caregiver threatened to kill you?
13. Does your family or caregiver ever try to control what you do, where you go, your money, or relationships with your other family and friends?
14. Does your family or caregiver ever force you to engage in sex?
15. We see many patients who have been abused. Remember, help is available.

Physical Examination

The physical examination can reveal many clues to potential abuse (Table 6-3). The patient may appear unkempt or physically disabled, shivering, or cyanotic. Abnormal vital signs may point to poor hydration or hypothermia due to exposure. There may be unaddressed infections, lice-infested hair, or noncompliance with medications. The patient must be completely undressed. Specific findings and associated findings may involve any organ system, but the head and musculoskeletal systems

Table 6-2. High-Risk History for Family Violence

Incident

Mechanism described by patient does not fit injury
Delay in seeking care

Past medical history

"Accident-prone" patient
Frequent health care visits (review past medical history)
Drug/alcoholism (caregiver or patient)

Family circumstances

History of other family members being abused
High stress in family (e.g., financial concerns, chemical dependency)

Patient affect

Patient evasive or guarded, embarrassed, depressed
Patient denies abuses too strongly
Patient minimizes injury or demonstrates inappropriate responses (cries, laughs)

Interaction with caregiver

Patient has hypervigilant behavior with caregiver
Patient defers to caregiver
Caregiver hovers

should receive particular attention. Suspicious injuries include unusual fractures and dislocations; bruises, lacerations, and burns of unusual shapes, sizes, or locations; a closed head injury without a mechanism; contusions at various stages of healing; and unexplained abrasions, bruises, welts, grip marks, or rope marks. Additional concerning signs include unattended pressure sores; unexplained dehydration, genital complaints (including symptoms of sexually transmitted diseases), and bleeding in the perineum; and unexplained alopecia, bumps, pain, restricted movement, or immobility. Injuries or sores that have been left untreated or that are partially healed may indicate neglect or abuse (Tables 6-4 and 6-5).

Neglect often presents as poor hygiene; malnutrition or dehydration; lack of needed dentures, glasses, or hearing aids; poor skin integrity, rashes, or soiled linen; clothes inappropriate for the season; oversedation; or unexplained weakness, immobility, and contractures. Psychosocial symptoms may include shame, humiliation, low self-esteem, passivity, easy intimidation, fear, unjustified guilt, lack of self-determination, agitation, anxiety, withdrawn affect, depression, lack of privacy, or infantilization. The caregiver berating or threatening the pa-

Table 6-3. Typical Findings of Abuse

Central injuries

Black eyes
Front teeth injuries
Midface injury
Neck injury
Breast or abdomen injury
Vague gynecologic complaints

Hidden injuries

Injuries to hidden sites (covered by clothing)
Internal injuries

Defensive injuries

Midarm injuries

Inconsistent injuries

Injuries to areas not injury prone
Symmetric injuries
Old as well as new injuries
Injuries to multiple sites

Abusive mechanism of injury

Weapon injuries or marks
Strangulation marks
Bites or burns (scalds or cigarette burns)

Table 6-4. Physical Examination for Abuse

Patient must be completely undressed.

Clues to potential abuse revealed by examination include

Patient appears unkempt, physically disabled, shivering or cyanotic, or has lice-infected hair.
Abnormal vital signs that may point to poor hydration, hypothermia due to exposure, unaddressed infections, or noncompliance with medications.

Suspicious injuries include

Head and musculoskeletal systems should receive particular attention.
Unusual fractures and dislocations, bruises, lacerations, and burns of unusual shapes sizes or locations.
Closed head injury without a mechanism, contusions at various stages of healing; unexplained abrasions, bruises, welts, grip marks, or rope marks.
Injuries or sores left untreated or partially healed may indicate neglect or abuse.

Additional signs of concern are

Unattended pressure sores, unexplained dehydration, genital complaints (including symptoms of sexually transmitted diseases), bleeding in the perineum, and unexplained alopecia, bumps, pain, restricted movement, or immobility.

tient with isolation, abandonment, or institutionalization actually may be witnessed during the patient encounter[5] (Table 6-6).

DIAGNOSIS AND DIFFERENTIAL

A low threshold for considering abuse must be maintained. Any presenting complaint can bring an abused patient to the ED. Elder abuse should be considered in all elders, but it should be specifically added to the differential diagnosis of patients who have any of the "red flags" of abuse listed earlier, such as injuries of concern (Table 6-7). On initial presentation, assessment of medical problems and physical injuries should be pursued, as with any other patient. However, if abuse is identified, evaluation of psychosomatic complaints may be shortened in lieu of psychosocial evaluation and intervention as appropriate. In addition to pursuing the workup required for the patient's medical problems, laboratory data should be requested to document the patients status with regard to hydration, nutrition, and compliance with medications.

EMERGENCY DEPARTMENT CARE AND DISPOSITION

As with domestic violence and unlike child abuse, the physician can only hospitalize victims of elder abuse with their consent. Treatment must include both physical and emotional care. Referral to subspecialists may be indicated based on the extent of physical injuries or the degree of psychopathology. However, all physicians who see elderly patients need a basic level of knowledge and understanding of elder abuse and neglect.[6] The ED must have a policy that coordinates care for victims of abuse. Advice about future options and referral to counseling agencies must be available.

Immediate priorities are the future safety of the patient and protecting the patient from further injury. Confronting a potential perpetrator may escalate abuse and put the patient and hospital staff at risk.

ED management of potentially abused patients includes routine patient care. An objective, nonjudgmental,

Table 6-5. Signs of Neglect

Physical	Psychosocial
Poor hygiene	Shame/humiliation
Malnutrition or dehydration	Low self-esteem/passivity
Lack of needed dentures, glasses, or hearing aids	Easy intimidation/fear
Poor skin integrity	Unjustified guilt
Rashes, soiled linen	Lack of self-determination
Clothes inappropriate for the season	Agitation/anxiety
Oversedation	Withdrawn affect/depression
Unexplained weakness, immobility, and contractures	Lack of privacy/infantilization

Note: The caregiver berating or threatening the patient with isolation, abandonment, or institutionalization actually may be witnessed during the patient encounter.

and empathetic demeanor is essential. Do not blame the victim; demonstrate concern and respect at all times. The patient should be assured that confidentiality will be maintained. Consider admission if the patient is willing or incompetent when no alternative, safe disposition exists. Psychiatric assessment to address cognitive status and competence may be indicated. If the patient is mentally or physically impaired and cannot give a history or does not accept a plan for a safe environment, consult psychiatry for a competence evaluation.

Referral to hospital social workers to address patient safety, health care access, and resource (social and financial) management will be helpful. Even when social services are only available on call, they should be called to evaluate potential victims of abuse. Delays in patient disposition may save patients from continued and eventually escalated abuse. Multiple community resources such as respite care, visiting nurse, health aide, and legal and financial services can be recruited by social work after assessing the home environment, adequacy of support, and access to care, transportation, food, or other services. Relocation or admission to hospital ultimately may be necessary.

EDs can play a role in stopping the escalation and continuation of elder abuse. Early identification and action to increase patient safety will require time, training, and screening involving all ED staff. The ultimate goal is to decrease patient pain and suffering by eliminating elder abuse. Physicians must be proactive to recognize abuse and neglect in patients presenting with typical problems such as incontinence, confusion, impaired mobility, falling, and failure to thrive. As required by JCAHO, EDs must have established policies, but these policies must address ongoing care, resources to provide care, educational programs, and a mechanism to meet reporting requirements that follows state guidelines.

Nursing home residents with decubiti must be considered potential victims of neglect. Institutions also must guard against abuse. EDs may be community watch dogs when nursing homes are neglectful.

Elderly patients have a right to choose their care if they are competent. Reporting suspected cases of elder abuse is determined in accordance with local statutes because required interventious and legal considerations are under the jurisdiction of individual states. In many states, physicians may be required to report abuse and a patient allowed to refuse "help." The power to protect persons who cannot or will not protect themselves is, in some states, considered to be ageist. Local resources and requirements vary. They should be addressed by institutional policies that are made available in the clinical area for quick referral.

Table 6-6. Mnemonic to Identify and Treat Elder Abuse

	Identification		Treatment
S	Screen	S	Safety
C	Central injuries	C	Crime
R	Repetitive injuries	R	Referral
A	Abuse (physical + psychological)	A	Acknowledge abuse
P	Possessive caregiver	P	Protocols
E	Explanation inconsistent	E	Evidence collection
D	Direct questions	D	Documentation

Table 6-7. Approach to Patients Who Are Victims of Abuse

Screen all patients.
Identify abuse or neglect.
Validate experience.
Plan for safety.
Maintain confidentiality.
Report only with patient's knowledge.
Document objectively.
Empower patients to make their own informed decisions.

Restraining orders against perpetrators may be indicated. Access should be easily available to the patient and hospital staff. Cooperation with police and local courts will better inform elder abuse policies and procedures. Institutional abuse and elder neglect are a growing concern. Photographs of injuries when taken with legally acceptable equipment may help victims of abuse in court. Equipment should be available in the ED, and staff should be trained to use it. A patient must consent to photographs, and all photographs should be included in the patients medical record with the history and physical examination. Photographs can be persuasive in court and add to the weight of evidence that compels lawyers and patients to pursue legal action. Regulatory agencies, national standards for care, and statements of patient rights inform all citizens to expect care and compassion. ED staff must take care not to abuse or neglect elders and also not to "appear" to ignore their needs. Efforts to reduce chemical and physical restraints and monitor medication use are already required by JCAHO. Documentation should be meticulous whenever using these devices.

Similarly, documentation of patients with suspected abuse must be compulsive. Consents and refusals, along with a thorough history, physical examination, observations, services, and interventions, are even more important to track. Well-documented medical records can limit in-court testimony. A good-faith report is immune to liability. It is the duty of ED personnel to advise a victim as to what is medically best and most appropriate. Record at the time of any evaluation the chief complaint in the patients own words, preferably in quotes. A body chart and drawing, as well as photographs, are helpful to denote type, number, size, location, and stages of all injuries. A health care provider must collect appropriate evidence, including evidence for sexual assault, when needed, and retain evidence with a formal consent. Inform the assaulted patient of the legal right to file a report with law enforcement authorities. Documentation may be subpoenaed for potential legal proceedings. Discussion with the patient and any decisions made must be noted in the chart. Protocols and standardized forms can help with documentation (Fig. 6-2 and Table 6-8).

Table 6-8. Resources for Physicians

Adult protective services	This service agency has legal responsibility and authority to investigate reports of abuse and neglect in the home.
Facility abuse investigations	Every nursing care facility must have a process for investigating reports of abuse, neglect, and misappropriation of resident property.
Law enforcement	Local police and sheriffs are being given more power to intervene in family violence, and where state statutes define elder abuse as a crime, physicians may be required to report suspected abuse to law enforcement officials.
Long-term care ombudsmen	Every state has a long-term care ombudsman program established in 1978 by the Older Americans Act. Each program regularly visits nursing facilities. Information is generally available from local agencies on aging.
Medicaid fraud control units (MFCU)	Each MFCU, located in the state attorney general's office, is required by federal law to investigate and prosecute Medicaid provider fraud and patient abuse or neglect in health care facilities that participate in Medicaid.
State elder abuse and domestic violence hotline(s)	Most states have one or more 24-hour toll-free numbers for receiving reports of abuse and neglect. Calls are confidential.

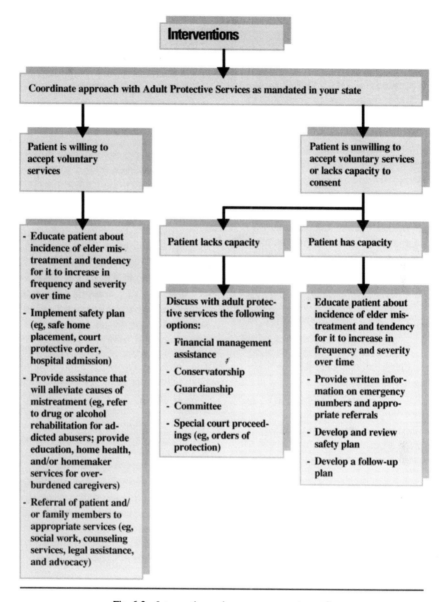

Fig. 6-2 Intervention and case management, part 2.

REFERENCES

1. AMA Council on Scientific Affairs: Elder abuse and neglect. *JAMA* 257:966, 1987.
2. Kleinschmidt KC: Elder abuse: A review. *Ann Emerg Med* 30(4):463, 1997.
3. Jones JS, Holstege C, Holstege H: Elder abuse and neglect: Understanding the causes and potential risk factors. *Am J Emerg Med* 15(6):579, 1997.
4. Bloom JS, Ansell P, Bloom MN: Detecting elder abuse: A guide for physicians. *Geriatrics* 44:40, 1989.
5. Marshall CE, Benton D, Brazier JM: Elder abuse: Using clinical tools to identify clues of mistreatment. *Geriatrics* 55(2):42, 2000.
6. Jones J, Doughery J, Schelble D, et al: Emergency department protocol for the diagnosis and evaluation of geriatric abuse. *Ann Emerg Med* 17:1006, 1988.

7

Ethical Issues in Geriatric Emergency Medicine

Catherine A. Marco

HIGH-YIELD FACTS

- Decision-making capacity may be lost due to cognitive impairment and severe illness. The emergency physician needs an organized approach to assess decision-making capacity and ensure consent or informed refusal of care.

- Decision-making communication that corrects temporary impediments is facilitated by discussing values and understanding consequences.

- Emergency physicians must employ effective communication techniques such as establishing eye contact, demonstrating empathy, and employing active listening when addressing ethical issues.

- Documentation of decision-making capacity is crucial when a patient accepts or refuses an intervention carrying significant risk.

- When decision-making capacity is impaired, the emergency physician should attempt to follow patient wishes by consulting family members, patient representatives, or legal documents such as advance directives.

- Rendering resuscitative care often includes discussing patient wishes with the patients loved ones and effectively communicating the death of the patient.

- Emergency physicians can follow legally documented advance directives and should not feel compelled to undertake ineffective resuscitation.

A number of ethical issues are relevant to geriatric emergency medicine. A basic understanding of com-monly accepted principles of bioethics can be valuable when confronted by ethical dilemmas. Determining a patients decision-making capacity is often important to obtaining informed consent or informed refusal of care. As patients increase in age, often in a diseased state, the importance of end-of-life issues becomes paramount. Communication regarding the end of life and resuscitation preferences will match the care provided with the desires of the patient.

GENERAL PRINCIPLES OF MEDICAL ETHICS

The study of ethics has been defined as the way of understanding and examining the moral life (T. I. Beauchamp and J. F. Childress, *Principles of Biomedical Ethics,* 4th ed. New York, Oxford University Press, 1994) and as the study of standards of conduct and moral judgment (*Webster's Dictionary*). The Hippocratic Oath has been revered as one of the oldest codes of medical ethics. More recently, the American Medical Association (AMA) Code of Ethics (earliest version from 1847) and American College of Emergency Physicians (ACEP) Code of Ethics (1997) have provided guidance to emergency physicians in the application of ethical principles to clinical practice. Most ethical codes address common features, such as beneficence (doing good), nonmaleficence (*primum non nocere,* or "do no harm"), respect for patient autonomy, confidentiality, honesty, distributive justice, and respect for the law. Ethical dilemmas may arise when there is a seeming conflict between two ethical principles or values. Ethical dilemmas may be resolved by various means, including individual judgment, additional information, and consensus meetings. In some circumstances, the involvement of the institutional ethics committee or the judicial system may be sought.

DETERMINATION OF DECISION-MAKING CAPACITY

The determination of decision-making capacity is an essential component of medical practice and is an important step in securing voluntary informed consent for medical treatment, as well as for refusal of care.[1–4] In most clinical situations, emergency physicians have little difficulty determining a patients implicit capacity or competency to participate in decision making. At times, this determination is more challenging, particularly when issues of underlying medical conditions,[5] dementia,[6,7] delirium, polypharmacy, substance abuse, psychiatric issues, and social issues commonly arise in the practice of geriatric emergency medicine. It is best to consider impairment of capacity on a sliding scale not as an absolute yes or no. Emergency physicians must make an individual assessment of the relative decision-making capacity relevant to the specific decision at hand.[8] Under the doctrine of informed consent, patients with adequate capacity are allowed to make autonomous choices about their own health and health care, even choices that may appear irrational to health care providers.[9]

The Code of Ethics of the American College of Emergency Physicians states that "patients with decision-making capacity must give their voluntary consent to treatment. . . . Emergency physicians should be able to determine whether a patient has decision-making capacity and who can act as a decision maker if the patient is unable to do so.[10] The Society for Academic Emergency Medicine (SAEM) Code of Conduct also underscores a promise of "Respect, securing the safety, privacy, and personal welfare of patients, and offering informed choice whenever possible."[11]

Definition of Decision-Making Capacity

This capacity reflects cognitive and affective functions, which manifest in intellect, memory, judgment, insight, language, attention, emotion, calculation, and communication skills. This capacity includes the ability to receive information, process and understand information, deliberate, and make articulate choices.

Unlike the more static entity of legal competency, decision-making capacity may be variable over time as a function of host and environmental factors. Often, impairment of capacity is situational; the same patient may have appropriate capacity for one decision and not another, depending on the gravity and consequences of the decision and the potential for harm. In emergency situations, physicians must promptly assess whether a patient is capable of making an often complex decision.

Determination of Decision-Making Capacity

In most patient encounters, a certain level of capacity is obvious by the patients ability to communicate rationally. In others, the emergency physician may need a more standardized approach to determine this capacity, particularly when the decisions involve potentially grave or serious consequences.[12] The elements of a stepwise approach to determine capacity are summarized in Table 7-1.

Table 7-1. The Determination of Capacity

1. Ensure that patient has the ability to communicate voluntarily (free from coercion).
2. Correct reversible environmental, metabolic, mental, and physical impediments to capacity.
3. Investigate affect and cognition using standardized tests of competency, when necessary.
4. Examine patient goals, values, and fears.
5. Assess patients understanding of alternatives and the foreseeable consequences.
6. Document the essential elements of capacity, or its impairment, in the medical record.

Step 1: Ensure the Patients Ability to Communicate Voluntarily

Patients should be free to make independent medical decisions without undue influence. All patient choices are, on some level, influenced by a multitude of factors that may include such elements as personal beliefs, religious beliefs, cultural practices, family wishes, finances, etc. Voluntary communication is best ensured by listening to the patient to understand the degree to which coercive forces enter into the patients decision. If certain visitors or consultants are found to exert undue coercion, the patient should be encouraged to make a personal and independent decision in their absence. At times, education and persuasion may be an appropriate and important part of decision making. It is legitimate for a physician, family member, or other interested party to use medical knowledge to persuade the patient to agree to an intervention or treatment. This communication must be nonthreatening and noncoercive. Undue influences, coercion, and manipulation are unethical. Coercion occurs when the patient experiences a credible threat of punishment or harm, such as the presence of police, when making decisions. Manipulation may occur when autonomous decision making is jeopardized, for example, by exaggerating, lying, withholding information, or threatening (such as abandoning the patient).

Step 2: Correct Reversible Environmental, Metabolic, Mental, and Physical Impediments to Capacity

Some medical, environmental, pharmacologic, and psychological conditions are potentially reversible. Reversing them may allow the patient full participation in the decision-making process.[13] Examples of reversible impediments to capacity include pain, narcotic overdose, benzodiazepine overdose, alcohol intoxication, hypothermia, hypotension, hypoxia, and hypoglycemia. Whenever the patients condition allows the time, reversible causes of incapacity should be addressed prior to making a final determination of decision-making capacity.

Step 3: Investigate Affect and Cognition Using Standardized Tests of Capacity When Indicated

Numerous standardized tests are available that may prove valuable adjuncts in the determination of capacity.[14–22] One example of a simple standardized assessment tool is the Mini-Mental Status Examination[23–25] (Table 7-2). Another easily administered test is the Quick Confusion Scale (QCS).[26] Regardless of the testing methodology used, it is important to recognize that many patients with some apparent cognitive deficits may still have sufficient capacity to participate in health care decisions. Cognitive testing is useful as an adjunct to and not a substitute for sound clinical judgment.

Step 4: Examine Patient Goals, Values, and Fears

Evaluation of the patients reasons for holding certain beliefs or fears can be an important step in the determination of capacity. The patient may refuse a given test or intervention based on his or her perceptions or misperceptions. Knowledge of patient concerns and values may facilitate the development of alternate, acceptable therapeutic directions. For example, a patient afraid of needlesticks and pain may not necessarily be averse to a recommended treatment. The use of topical or local anesthetics (e.g., EMLA, warmed, buffered lidocaine, etc.) or changing the route of administration (from intravenous to oral) may allay legitimate patient concerns of pain and allow treatment.

Step 5: Assess Patient Understanding of Alternatives and Their Foreseeable Consequences

Patients who can communicate an understanding of choices and consequences generally should be assumed

Table 7-2. Mini-Mental Status Examination

	Score	Maximum Score
Orientation		
What is the (year) (season) (date) (day) (month)?	—	5
Where are we? (state) (county) (town) (hospital) (floor)	—	5
Registration		
Name three objects, and ask patient to repeat.	—	3
Attention and calculation		
Serial 7s (one point for each correct up to 5)		
Option: Spell *world* backwards.	—	5
Recall		
Ask for the three objects repeated above.	—	3
Language		
Name a pencil and watch. (2 points)	—	9
Repeat "no ifs, ands, or buts." (1 point)		
Follow a three-stage command. (3 points)		
Read and follow the command "Close your eyes." (1 point)		
Write a sentence. (1 point)		
Copy a design. (1 point)		
TOTAL	—	30

to have decision-making capacity. This can be ascertained by asking patients to repeat the treatment plan and its expected consequences in their own words. Adequate informed consent or refusal can occur when the patient understands both the short- and long-term consequences of a decision. Clinicians must weigh the patients level of understanding against of the patients stated goals and values.

Step 6: Document the Essential Elements of Capacity or Its Impairment in the Medical Record

The medical and legal importance of documentation is especially crucial when an intervention or its forbearance carries a significant risk. Conversations with patients and their advocates should be documented to show that the process of determing decision-making capacity was fair and patient-centered. A signed copy of such conversations, outlining the likely risks and benefits of a proposed course of action, should be given to the patient whenever possible. Patients who refuse care always should be invited to return should they change their mind at any time, when appropriate alternative therapy should be offered.

When Capacity Is Impaired

When the physician determines that capacity is impaired, a surrogate decision maker should be identified. In some cases a patient may have executed a legal document identifying a surrogate as well as specific instructions. This document could be in the form of a living will, a health care power of attorney, or an advance directive. Where the patient has identified a surrogate, consent should involve that individual. In the absence of such identification, consent usually is sought from close family members or other interested parties. Most states have codified the next-of-kin hierarchy of decision makers. To the extent that the care needed is urgent, the physicians responsibility to seek out, inform, and get consent from a surrogate may be modified. In true emergency situations, implied consent is accepted practice. The emergency physician must treat the patient who has impaired capacity. However, a physician who knows that a patient would refuse treatment cannot wait until an emergency exists and then proceed without consent. Even when clinicians must act in an emergency situation, they should strive to involve patients and their representatives as much as possible.

ETHICAL ISSUES AT THE END OF LIFE

Resuscitation

During resuscitation, decisions must be made rapidly and often based on the suboptimal information available. Issues considered include positive aspects of resuscitation (restoring life to the patient, a sense of closure and resolution of guilt for the survivors) and negative aspects (resuscitation to a suboptimal quality of life, misuse of resources).

In the United States, sudden cardiac death occurs in an estimated 250,000 patients annually.[27] It has been estimated that $58 million in Medicare expenditures result from unsuccessful resuscitations in the United States annually.[28] Resuscitation is a high-cost, invasive, and labor-intensive endeavor that in most clinical settings carries a low likelihood of success. Traditionally, physicians routinely attempt cardiopulmonary resuscitation for most patients who present with cardiac arrest unless a legal advance directive is presented.[29,30] Since very few patients have completed legal advance directives and only a fraction of those have the document readily available in most cases, the default option is to attempt resuscitation.

Recent reviews report widely variable survival rates for victims of cardiac arrest depending on a number of factors. These include time elapsed since arrest (down time),[31–33] presenting rhythm,[34,35] underlying medical condition,[36] response to prehospital advanced life support (ALS) protocols,[37,38] age,[39] and long-term care.[40] Overall, survival to hospital discharge for victims of cardiac arrest has been estimated at between 0 and 16 percent.[41–47] Certain identifiable groups of patients have survival rates approaching 0 percent, such as residents of long-term care facilities with unwitnessed arrests. Despite this relatively low success rate, current American Heart Association guidelines and hospital policies typically suggest resuscitation for all patients except those with prior do-not-attempt-resuscitation (DNR) orders, clear signs of death such as rigor mortis or dependent lividity, or if no physiologic benefit can be expected after maximal therapy.[48–50] Many emergency physicians continue to attempt resuscitation on patients in cardiac arrest in situations considered nonbeneficial, often because of fears of litigation or criticism.[29]

Despite the apparent lack of communication through the use of advance directives, many individuals have strong personal preferences regarding cardiopulmonary resuscitation.[51] Depending on a variety of factors, including age, state of health, and clinical setting, such preferences regarding resuscitation attempts vary widely.[52–58] Recent reports suggest that full resuscitative efforts are not necessarily desired by patients and that trends toward societal consensus exist in a variety of hypothetical resuscitation scenarios.[59–62] Physician decisions regarding attempts at resuscitation often are influenced by such issues as perceived quality of life, age, down time, presenting rhythm, whether the arrest was witnessed, family preferences, fear of litigation, and other factors.[63,64]

ADVANCE DIRECTIVES

An *advance directive* refers to any proactive document stating the patients wishes should the patient be incapacitated. The *living will,* which was adopted by many states in 1990, is a document suitable for terminally ill individuals. Many living wills state that no life support should be used in cases where meaningful recovery will not occur. *Durable power of attorney* specifies a surrogate decision maker in the event the patient no longer has the capacity to make medical decisions. In 1991, the Federal Patient Self-Determination Act mandated the opportunity to sign an advance directive for all patients admitted to a hospital. In many cases, the existence of an advance directive can facilitate implementation of the patients specific wishes.

Unfortunately, despite widespread advocacy and legal mandates (such as the 1991 act) for the increased use of advance directives, only a minority of patients have taken advantage of the opportunity,[65–67] with an even smaller minority who present to the emergency department (ED) with the necessary documentation. Although some health care providers are reluctant to discuss issues such as end-of-life care and advance directives, many patients welcome the opportunity to discuss their wishes.[51,68–73] Most have definite opinions regarding resuscitation despite their lack of legal advance directives.[62,74] A recent study demonstrated the effective reduction of health care services used in nursing homes following a prospective advance directive implementation system.[75] There are many cases in which dying should be accepted as a natural process. Perhaps palliative care, judgment, communication, and counseling with the patient, family, and friends may be of greater benefit to all.[76–84]

Although studies conducted outside the ED have demonstrated variable compliance with advance directives,[85–89] recent studies indicate that emergency medical personnel usually comply with advance directives. Most emergency physicians (78 percent) withhold resuscitation attempts for patients with a legal advance directive, indicating a general willingness to honor patients' wishes.[29] Additionally, most prehospital providers (89 percent)

withhold resuscitation attempts for patients with a legal advance directive.[89] These studies show that advance directives are especially useful to emergency health care providers.

The Concept of *Futility*

The term *futility,* although used commonly, is fraught with difficulties in definition and interpretation. The word *futile* is derived from the Latin *futilis,* meaning "leaky." According to Greek myth, the daughters of King Danaus were condemned by the gods to carry water in sieves, a futile task. Scholars have proposed a variety of different standards for both the quantitative and qualitative aspects of futility. Some definitions include *quantitative futility* (the likelihood of benefit to the patient falls below a minimal threshold) and a *patient-centered* definition (failure to produce effects that the patient can appreciate).[90–92] Health care professionals may interpret "futile" interventions as those which carry an absolute impossibility of successful outcome, a low likelihood of success, a low likelihood of survival, a low likelihood of discharge from the hospital, or a low likelihood of restoration to a meaningful quality of life.

Many ethicists agree that physicians are under no obligation to render treatments that they deem of little or no benefit to the patient. The Hastings Center concluded: "If a treatment is clearly futile . . . there is no obligation to provide the treatment.[93] The AMA Council on Ethical and Judicial Affairs wrote that cardiopulmonary resuscitation (CPR) may be withheld, even if requested by the patient, "when efforts to resuscitate a patient are judged by the treating physician to be futile.[94–99]

An ACEP policy asserts that "physicians are under no ethical obligation to render treatments that they judge have no realistic likelihood of medical benefit to the patient."

The AMA Council on Ethical and Judicial Affairs recommends a process-based approach to the determination of futility,[100] including such actions as

1. Deliberation and resolution
2. Joint decision making with physician and patient or proxy
3. Assistance of a consultant or patient representative
4. Use of an institutional committee (i.e., ethics committee)

Decisions regarding emergency interventions and treatments and the likelihood of benefit to the patient and decisions to provide, limit, or withhold interventions should be made by the emergency physician in the context of well-established research results, patient and family wishes, and professional judgment.[101,102]

DNR Document

For the patient with an advance directive, it is also important to know if there is an order for CPR or an order for palliative care. The confusion of *do not resuscitate* with *do not treat* still exists for patients and physicians. It is important to differentiate wishes for CPR, defibrillation, medications, and mechanical ventilation as life support from palliative care, which can include tube feeds, intravenous fluids, surgery, and intravenous antibiotics. It is also important to verify the exact wishes of the patient and family member before the resuscitation. Identifying a legally binding advance directive is important. It should have the patient's signature, a clearly stated next of kin or durable power of attorney, and the signature of the physician who has prepared the directive. At the time of arrest wishes can change. If the patient is still competent and able to express his or her wishes, those are what should be carried out.

THE PHYSICIAN'S ROLE AT THE END OF LIFE

Death in many cases should be accepted as a natural part of life by the patient, loved ones, and health care providers.[76,77] When curative therapies do not exist, the role of the physician is to address the numerous emotional and social challenges facing patients and their loved ones.[133–136] Comfort care should be provided, including treatment of pain, shortness of breath, nausea, fatigue, depression, or other symptoms.[103]

Rituals at the End of Life

Rituals have been an essential component of all life (both human and animal) since the beginning of time. Rituals are commonly performed in many diverse cultures surrounding important events signifying change, such as birth, puberty, marriage, and death. The significance of ritual is complex and multifaceted, often using symbolism to demonstrate social structure or to interpret the meaning of daily life.[104] Certain rituals may provide a sense of comfort and constancy amid change or an emo-

tional guarantee of future well-being to the participants, possibly serving anxiolytic functions.[105] Rituals may serve to "animate life with a certain level of enchantment."[106] Particularly at the end of life for the dying patient, family, and friends, ritual functions in several capacities, including spiritually, religiously, emotionally, socially, and physically.

Family Presence During Resuscitation

Although, traditionally, family members have not been allowed to witness resuscitation attempts, several recent reports have demonstrated the positive results of this practice.[107–110] Family presence may serve to allay guilt or disappointment and may be a helpful part of the grieving process. Many families simply wish to have the option of being present.

Communication

Effective communication with patients and loved ones is an essential component of end-of-life care and may in fact serve some of the function of rituals. Even following the patient's death, when some physicians are guilty of the perception that their duty has been fulfilled, there exists an imperative duty to address the needs of surviving loved ones; including communication, comfort, empathy, and assistance with meeting other needs. Some examples of effective communication techniques in end-of-life care are shown in Table 7-3.

Table 7-3. Effective Communication Techniques[115–123]

Spend adequate time.
Use a private, quiet location for communications.
Use appropriate nonverbal communication.
Be seated, if possible.
Establish and maintain eye contact.
Demonstrate empathy.
Address patient and loved ones by name.
Use understandable language (avoid jargon).
Ask open-ended questions.
Employ active listening techniques.
Use reassurance to resolve feelings of guilt or blame.
Accept emotions of patients and loved ones.
Avoid condescending speech or behavior.
Use additional resources (nursing, psychiatry, pastoral care, social services, etc.).

ADDITIONAL ASPECTS

Procedures on Recently Deceased Patients

The practice of teaching and performing procedures on recently deceased patients is controversial. The most important benefit of these practices is in fulfilling the recognized need for hands-on practice for students, housestaff, and experienced physicians.[111] The recently deceased patient provides a unique opportunity to practice procedures with literally *no* risk to the patient. As a result of this training, physicians may be more able to competently perform procedures on living patients, producing an overall benefit to society. However, informed consent is rarely obtained in these settings. Some consider that performing procedures without informed consent often is disrespectful, deceptive, or unethical.[112] Several recent studies have shown that consent is often easily obtained for such procedures and should be considered, if not mandated.[113,114]

Communication with Families Following Death

A majority of emergency physicians find the notification of death to survivors emotionally difficult. In many cases, however, the communication, care, and counseling provided to survivors (family, friends, etc.) of victims of cardiac arrest will have more impact than the actual resuscitative efforts. Optimal care should be given to families and friends regardless of the level of treatment rendered or the outcome (see Table 7-4).

CONCLUSION

There are a great number of ethical issues involving the geriatric patient. The basic principles of bioethics can inform our understanding. The determination of decision-making capacity is important when obtaining informed consent or informed refusal of care. Educating patients with regard to end-of-life issues, including resuscitation and advance directives, is crucial to providing care in accordance with patients' wishes. Communication with patients and families is an essential medical skill. A number of ethical issues can be solved by using appropriate resources and improving communication among patients and their families, staff, primary care physicians, and consultants.

Table 7-4. Guideline for Delivering "Bad News"

1. Give advance warning, if possible. A member of the health care team should communicate the gravity of the patient's condition during the resuscitative efforts.
2. Provide a private, quiet location for communications.
3. Spend adequate time in counseling and answering questions.
4. Use clear and succinct language. Often medical jargon is not accurately understood. It is generally appropriate to use straightforward language, such as *died* and *death* rather than *didn't make it, passed on,* etc.
5. Use proper names of the deceased and family members.
6. Accept any reaction as normal. Even unexpected reactions, such as apathy, anger, and hysteria, may not be inappropriate.
7. Use appropriate nonverbal communication. Use of appropriate eye contact, sitting rather than standing, and maintaining appropriate concentration and listening skills can all improve the quality of the message received by the survivors.
8. Do not hesitate to show emotion. Families may benefit from sharing emotions.
9. Reassure loved ones that the patient likely did not suffer.
10. Attempt to absolve any guilt feelings. It is generally inappropriate to suggest that a different course of action (calling 911 sooner, different actions by prehospital personnel, etc.) may have changed the outcome.
11. When appropriate, discuss organ donation. Many families find organ donation a means to make a tragedy result in some measurable good.
12. Allow the family to view the body. This may provide some closure and aid in their acceptance of the death.
13. Use additional resources when appropriate. This may include social work, nursing, psychiatry, clergy, or other ancillary and support staff.
14. Invite further questioning. The emergency physician may serve as an important resource for future concerns or questions.

REFERENCES

1. Larkin GL, Marco CA, Abbott JT: Emergency determination of decision making capacity (DMC): Balancing autonomy and beneficence in the emergency department. *Acad Emerg Med* 8:282, 2001.
2. Melsel A, Roth L: What we do and do not know about informed consent. *JAMA* 246:2473, 1981.
3. Moskop JC: Informed consent in the emergency department. *Emerg Med Clin North Am* 17:327, 1999.
4. Borak J, Veilleux S: Informed consent in emergency settings. *Ann Emerg Med* 13:731, 1984.
5. Marson DC, Ingram KK, Cody HA, et al: Assessing the competency of patients with Alzheimer's disease under different legal standards. *Arch Neurol* 52:949, 1995.
6. Fellows LK: Competency and consent in dementia. *J Am Geriatr Soc* 46:922, 1998.
7. Rockwood K, Stadnyk J: The prevalence of dementia in the elderly: A review. *Can J Psychiatry* 39:253, 1994.
8. Beachamp TI, Childress JF: The sliding-scale strategy, in *Principles of Biomedical Ethics*, 4th ed. New York, Oxford University Press, 1994, pp 138–141.
9. Brock D, Wartman SA: When competent patients make irrational choices. *New Engl J Med* 322:1595, 1990.
10. American College of Emergency Physicians: Code of ethics for emergency physicians. *Ann Emerg Med* 30:365, 1997.
11. Larkin GL: A code of conduct for academic emergency medicine. *Acad Emerg Med* 6:45, 1999.
12. Drane J: Competency to give an informed consent: A model for making clinical assessments. *JAMA* 252:925, 1984.
13. Dresser R, Whitehouse PJ: The incompetent patient on the slippery slope. *Hastings Center Rep* 24:6, 1994.
14. Markson I, Kern D, Annas G, et al: Physician assessment of patient competence. *J Am Geriatr Soc* 42:1074, 1994.
15. Tomoda A, Yasumiya R, Sumiyama T, et al: Validity and reliability of structured interview for competency incompetency assessment testing and ranking inventory. *J Clin Psychol* 53:443, 1997.
16. Pohjasvaara T, Ylikoski R, Leskela M, et al: Evaluation of various methods of assessing symptoms of cognitive impairment and dementia. *Alzheimer Dis Assoc Disord* 15:184, 2001.
17. Kirby M, Denihan A, Bruce I, et al: The clock drawing test in primary care: Sensitivity in dementia detection and specificity against normal and depressed elderly. *Int J Geriatr Psychiatry* 16:935, 2001.
18. Bean G, Nishisato S, Rector NA, et al: The psychometric properties of the competency interview schedule. *Can J Psychiatry* 39:368, 1994.
19. Kaufman DM, Zun L: A quantifiable, brief mental status examination for emergency patients. *J Emerg Med* 13:449, 1995.
20. Grisso T, Appelbaum PS: Comparison of standards for assessing patients' capacities to make treatment decisions. *Am J Psychiatry* 152:1033, 1995.
21. Grisso T, Appelbaum PS: Thinking about competence, in *Assessing Competence to Consent to Treatment: A Guide for Physicians and Other Health Professionals.* New York, Oxford University Press, 1998, pp 17–30.
22. Litovitz GL, Hedberg M, Wise TN, et al: Recognition of psychological and cognitive impairments in the emergency department. *Am J Emerg Med* 3:400, 1985.
23. Folstein MF, Robins LN, Helzer JE. The Mini-Mental State Examination. *Arch Gen Psychiatry* 40:812, 1983.
24. Giordani B, Boivin MJ, Hall AL, et al: The utility and generality of Mini-Mental State Examination scores in Alzheimer's disease. *Neurology* 40:1894, 1990.
25. Heeren TJ, Lagaay AM, von Beek WC, et al: Reference values for the Mini-Mental State Examination (MMSE) in octo- and nonagenarians. *J Am Geriatr Soc* 38:1093, 1990.
26. Huff JS, Farace E, Brady WJ, et al: The Quick Confusion Scale in the ED: Comparison with the Mini-Mental State Examination. *Am J Emerg Med* 19:461, 2001.
27. American Heart Association: *2002 Heart and Stroke Statistical Update.* Dallas, American Heart Association, 2002.
28. Suchard JR, Fenton FR, Powers RD: Medicare expenditures on unsuccessful out-of-hospital resuscitations. *J Emerg Med* 17:801, 1999.
29. Marco CA, Bessman ES, Schoenfeld CN, et al: Ethical issues of cardiopulmonary resuscitation: Current practice among emergency physicians. *Acad Emerg Med* 4:898, 1997.
30. Swig L, Cooke M, Osmond D, et al: Physician responses to a hospital policy allowing them to not offer cardiopulmonary resuscitation. *J Am Geriatr Soc* 44:1215, 1996.
31. Weaver WD, Cobb LA, Hallstrom AP et al: Considerations for improving survival from out-of-hospital cardiac arrest. *Ann Emerg Med* 15:1181, 1986.
32. Eisenberg MS, Bergner L, Hallstrom A: Cardiac resuscitation in the community: Importance of rapid provision and implications for program planning. *JAMA* 241:1905, 1979.
33. De Maio VJ, Stiell IG, Wells GA, Spaite DW: Cardiac arrest witnessed by emergency medical services personnel: Descriptive epidemiology, prodromal symptoms, and predictors of survival. *Ann Emerg Med* 35:138, 2000.
34. Bonnin MJ, Pepe PE, Clark PS: Survival in the elderly after out-of-hospital cardiac arrest. *Crit Care Med* 21:1645, 1993.
35. Aprahamian C, Thompson CM, Gruchow HW, et al: Decision making in prehospital sudden cardiac arrest. *Ann Emerg Med* 15:445, 1986.
36. Bedell SE, Delbanco TL, Cook EF, et al: Survival after cardiopulmonary resuscitation in the hospital. *New Engl J Med* 309:569, 1983.
37. Schoenenberger RA, von Planta M, von Planta I: Survival after failed out-of-hospital resuscitation: Are further therapeutic efforts in the emergency department futile? *Arch Intern Med* 154:2433, 1994.
38. Bonnin MJ, Pepe PE, Kimball KT, et al: Distinct criteria for termination of resuscitation in the out-of-hospital setting. *JAMA* 270:1457, 1993.

39. Murphy DJ, Murray AM, Robinson BE, et al: Outcomes of cardiopulmonary resuscitation in the elderly. *Ann Intern Med* 111:199, 1989.

40. Awoke S, Mouton CP, Parrott M: Outcomes of skilled cardiopulmonary resuscitation in a long-term facility: Futile therapy? *J Am Geriatr Soc* 40:593, 1992.

41. Engdahl J, Bang A, Lindqvist J, Herlitz J: Factors affecting short- and long-term prognosis among 1069 patients with out-of-hospital cardiac arrest and pulseless electrical activity. *Resuscitation* 51:17, 2001.

42. Becker LB, Ostrander MP, Barrett J, et al: Outcome of CPR in a large metropolitan area: Where are the survivors? *Ann Emerg Med* 20:355, 1991.

43. Callaham M, Madsen CD: Relationship of timeliness of paramedic advanced life support interventions to outcome in out-of-hospital cardiac arrest treated by first responders with defibrillator. *Ann Emerg Med* 27:638, 1995.

44. Eisenberg MS, Horwood BT, Cummins RO, et al: Cardiac arrest and resuscitation: A tale of 29 cities. *Ann Emerg Med* 19:179, 1990.

45. Kellerman AL, Hackman BB, Somes G: Predicting the outcome of unsuccessful prehospital advanced cardiac life support. *JAMA* 270:1433, 1993.

46. Stratton SJ, Niemann JT: Outcome from out-of-hospital cardiac arrest caused by nonventricular arrhythmias: Contribution of successful resuscitation to overall survivorship supports the current practice of initiating out-of-hospital ACLs. *Ann Emerg Med* 32:448, 1998.

47. Varon J, Fromm RE: In-hospital resuscitation among the elderly: Substantial survival to hospital discharge. *Am J Emerg Med* 14:130, 1996.

48. American Heart Association: Ethical aspects of CPR and ECC. *Circulation* 102:1, 2000.

49. Johnson AL. Towards a modified cardiopulmonary resuscitation policy. *Can J Cardiol* 14:203, 1998.

50. Bruce-Jones PN: Resuscitation decisions in the elderly: a discussion of current thinking. *J Med Ethics* 22:286, 1996.

51. Hakim RB, Teno JM, Harrell FE, et al: Factors associated with do-not-resuscitate orders: Patients' preferences, prognoses, and physicians' judgments. *Ann Intern Med* 125:284, 1996.

52. Murphy DJ, Santilli S: Elderly patients' preferences for long-term life support. *Arch Fam Med* 7:484, 1998.

53. Heap MJ, Munglani R, Klunck JR, Males AG: Elderly patients' preferences concerning life-support treatment. *Anaesthesia* 48:1027, 1993.

54. Rosenfeld KE, Wenger NS, Phillips RS, et al: Factors associated with change in resuscitation preference of seriously ill patients. The SUPPORT Investigators. Study to understand prognoses and preferences for outcomes and risks of treatments. *Arch Intern Med* 156:1558, 1996.

55. Schonwetter RS, Teasdale TA, Taffet G, et al: Educating the elderly: Cardiopulmonary resuscitation decisions before and after intervention. *J Am Geriatr Soc* 39:372, 1991.

56. Miller DL, Jahnigen DW, Gorbien MJ, Simbartl L: Cardiopulmonary resuscitation: How useful? Attitudes and knowledge of an elderly population. *Arch Intern Med* 152:578, 1992.

57. Hansdottir H, Gruman C, Curry L, Judge JO: Preferences for CPR among the elderly: The influence of attitudes and values. *Conn Med* 64:625, 2000.

58. Mead GE, O'Keeffe ST, Jack CI, et al: What factors influence patient preferences regarding cardiopulmonary resuscitation? *J R Coll Phys Lond* 29:295, 1995.

59. Hamel MB, Lynn J, Teno JM, et al: Age-related differences in care preferences, treatment decisions, and clinical outcomes of seriously ill hospitalized adults: Lessons from SUPPORT. *J Am Geriatr Soc* 48(suppl 1):76, 2000.

60. Marco CA, Schears RM: Resuscitation preferences among the general public (abstract). *Acad Emerg Med* 7:532, 2000.

61. Marco CA, Schears RM: Resuscitation preferences: What do people really Want? (abstract). *Ann Emerg Med* 35:S62, 2000.

62. Marco CA, Schears RM: Societal preferences regarding cardiopulmonary resuscitation. *Am J Emerg Med* 40:347, 2002.

63. Goodlin SJ, Qhong Z, Lynn J, et al: Factors associated with use of cardiopulmonary resuscitation in seriously ill hospitalized adults. *JAMA* 282:2333, 1999.

64. Lockey AS, Hardern RD: Decision making by emergency physicians when assessing cardiac arrest patients on arrival at hospital. *Resuscitation* 50:51, 2001.

65. Teno J, Lynn J, Wenger N, et al: Advance directives for seriously ill hospitalized patients. *J Am Geriatr Soc* 45:508, 1997.

66. The SUPPORT Principle Investigators: A controlled trial to improve care for seriously ill hospitalized patients. *JAMA* 274:1591, 1995.

67. Stolman CJ, Gregory JJ, Dunn D, Levine JL: Evaluation of patient, physician, nurse, and family attitudes toward do not resuscitate orders. *Arch Intern Med* 150:653, 1990.

68. Hakim RB, Teno JM, Harrell FE, et al: Factors associated with do-not-resuscitate orders: Patients' preferences, prognoses, and physicians' judgments. *Ann Intern Med* 125:284, 1996.

69. Gunasekera NP, Tiller DJ, Clements LT, Bhattacharya BK: Elderly patients' views on cardiopulmonary resuscitation. *Age Ageing* 15:364, 1986.

70. Schonwetter RS, Walker RM, Solomon M, et al: Life values, resuscitation preferences, and the applicability of living wills in an older population. *J Am Geriatr Soc* 44:954, 1996.

71. Kerridge IH, Pearson SA, Rolfe IE, Lowe M: Decision making in CPR: Attitudes of hospital patients and health care professionals. *Med J Aust* 169:128, 1998.

72. Uhlmann RF, Pearlman RA: Perceived quality of life and preferences for life-sustaining treatment in older adults. *Arch Intern Med* 151:495, 1991.

73. Marco CA, Larkin GL: A time to die: Patient-centered priorities in cardiac resuscitation. *Acad Emerg Med* 8:475, 2001.

74. Molloy DW, Guyatt GH, Russo R, et al: Systematic implementation of an advance directive program in nursing homes: A randomized, controlled trial. *JAMA* 283:1437, 2000.

75. Eisenberg MS, Mengert TJ: Cardiac resuscitation. *New Engl J Med* 344:1304, 2001.
76. McCue JD. The naturalness of dying. *JAMA* 273:1039, 1995.
77. Jecker NS. Medical futility and care of dying patients. *West J Med* 163:287, 1995.
78. Layde PM, Beam CA, Broste SK, et al: Surrogates' predictions of seriously ill patients' resuscitation preferences. *Arch Fam Med* 4:518, 1995.
79. Wenger NS, Phillips RS, Teno JM, et al: Physician understanding of patient resuscitation preferences: Insights and clinical implications. *J Am Geriatr Soc* 48:S44, 2000.
80. Uhlmann RF, Pearlman RA, Cain KC: Physicians' and spouses' predictions of elderly patients' resuscitation preferences. *J Gerontol* 43:M115, 1988.
81. Golin CE, Wenger NS, Liu H, et al: A prospective study of patient-physician communication about resuscitation. *J Am Geriatr Soc* 48:S52, 2000.
82. Ebell MH, Doukas DJ, Smith MA: The do-not-resuscitate order: A comparison of physician and patient preferences and decision-making. *Am J Med* 91:255, 1991.
83. Fischer GS, Tulsky JA, Rose MR, et al: Patient knowledge and physician predictions of treatment preferences after discussion of advance directives. *J Gen Intern Med* 13:447, 1998.
84. Bedell SE, Pelle D, Maher PL, Cleary PD: Do-not-resuscitate orders for critically ill patients in the hospital: How are they used and what is their impact? *JAMA* 256:233, 1986.
85. Davidson KW, Hackler C, Caradine DR, McCord RS: Physicians' attitudes on advance directives. *JAMA* 266:402, 1991.
86. Ebell MH, Doukas DJ, Smith MA: The do-not-resuscitate order: A comparison of physician and patient preferences and decision making. *Am J Med* 91:255, 1991.
87. Seckler AB, Meier DE, Mulvihill M, Paris BE: Substituted judgment: How accurate are proxy predictions? *Ann Intern Med* 115:92, 1991.
88. Dull SM, Graves JR, Larsen MP, Cummins RO: Expected death and unwanted resuscitation in the prehospital setting. *Ann Emerg Med* 23:997, 1994.
89. Marco CA, Schears RM: Prehospital resuscitation practices: A survey of prehospital providers. *J Emerg Med* 24:101, 2003.
90. Jecker NS: Medical futility and care of dying patients. *West J Med* 163:287, 1995.
91. Jecker NS, Schneiderman LJ: An ethical analysis of the use of "futility" in the 1992 American Heart Association guidelines for cardiopulmonary resuscitation and emergency cardiac care. *Arch Intern Med* 153:2195, 1993.
92. Schneiderman LJ, Jecker NS, Jonsen AR: Medical futility: Its meaning and ethical implications. *Ann Intern Med* 112:949, 1990.
93. Hastings Center: *Guidelines on the Termination of Life-Sustaining Treatment and the Care of the Dying* Indianapolis Indiana University Press. Hastings Center, 1987.
94. American Medical Association, Council on Ethical and Judicial Affairs: *Guidelines for the appropriate use of do-not-resuscitate orders. JAMA* 265:1868, 1991.
95. Blackhall LJ: Must we always use CPR? *New Engl J Med* 317:1281, 1987.
96. Tomlinson B: Ethics and communication in do-not-resuscitate orders. *New Engl J Med* 318:43, 1988.
97. Hackler JC, Hiller FC: Family consent to orders not to resuscitate: Reconsidering hospital policy. *JAMA* 264:1281, 1990.
98. Jecker NS, Schneiderman LJ: Futility and rationing. *Am J Med* 92:189, 1992.
99. Paris JJ, Reardon FE: Physician refusal of requests for futile or ineffective interventions. Cambridge Q Healthcare Ethics 2:127, 1992.
100. American Medical Association, Council on Ethical and Judicial Affairs: Medical futility in end-of-life care. *JAMA* 281:937, 1999.
101. Marco CA, Larkin GL, Moskop JC, Derse AR: The determination of "futility" in emergency medicine. *Ann Emerg Med* 35:604, 2000.
102. Marco CA, Larkin GL: Case studies in futility. *Acad Emerg Med* 7:1147, 2000.
103. Schears RM: Emergency physicians' role in end-of-life care. *Emerg Med Clin North Am* 17:539, 1999.
104. Morris I: *Death-Ritual and Social Structure in Classical Antiquity.* Cambridge, England, Cambridge University Press, 1992.
105. Goldbloom RB. Prisoners of ritual. *JAMA* 161:528, 1999.
106. Moore T. *Care of the Soul: A Guide for Cultivating Depth and Sacredness in Everyday Life.* New York, Harper Perennial Library, 1994.
107. Barratt F, Wallis DN: Relatives in the resuscitation room: Their point of view. *J Accid Emerg Med* 15:109, 1998.
108. Boyd R: Witnessed resuscitation by relatives. *Resuscitation* 43:171, 2000.
109. Doyle CJ, Post H, Burney RE, et al: Family participation during resuscitation: An option. *Ann Emerg Med* 6:107, 1987.
110. Eichhorn DJ, Meyers TA, Mitchell TG, et al: Opening the doors: Family presence during resuscitation. *J Cardiovascular Nurs* 10:59, 1996.
111. Goldblatt AD: Don't ask, don't tell: Practicing minimally invasive resuscitative techniques on the newly dead. *Ann Emerg Med* 25:86, 1995.
112. McNamara RM, Monti S, Kelly JJ: Requesting consent for an invasive procedure in newly deceased adults. *JAMA* 273:310, 1995.
113. Manifold CA, Storrow A, Rodgers K: Patient and family attitudes regarding the practice of procedures on the newly deceased. *Acad Emerg Med* 6:110, 1999.
114. Alden AW, Ward KL, Moore GP: Should postmortem procedures be practiced on recently deceased patients? A survey of relatives' attitudes. *Acad Emerg Med* 6:749, 1999.
115. Olsen JC, Buenese ML, Falso W: Death in the emergency department. *Ann Emerg Med* 31:758, 1998.

116. Marco CA. Ethical issues of resuscitation. *Emerg Med Clin North Am* 17:527, 1999.

117. Greenberg LW, Ochsenschlager D, Cohel GJ, et al: Counseling parents of a child dead on arrival: A survey of emergency departments. *Am J Emerg Med* 11:225, 1993.

118. Delbanco T: Enriching the doctor-patient relationship by inviting the patient's perspective. *Ann Intern Med* 116:414, 1992.

119. Suchman A, Metthews D: What makes the patient-doctor relationship therapeutic? Exploring the connexial dimension of medical care. *Ann Intern Med* 108:125, 1988.

120. Quill T: Recognizing and adjusting to barriers in doctor-patient communication. *Ann Intern Med* 111:51, 1989.

121. Ong LM, de Haes JC, Hoos AM, et al: Doctor-patient communication: A review of the literature. *Soc Sci Med* 40:903, 1995.

122. Lipkin M Jr: Patient education and counseling in the context of modern patient-physician-family communication. *Patient Ed Counsel* 27:5, 1996.

123. O'Mara K: Communication and conflict resolution in emergency medicine. *Emerg Med Clin North Am* 17:451, 1999.

8

Nursing Home Transfers

Martin A. Docherty

HIGH-YIELD FACTS

- Five percent of people over age 65 live in nursing homes.
- Twenty-five percent of all nursing home residents go to the emergency department (ED) for care each year, and 40 percent of these patients are admitted to hospitals.
- Most patients will require a comprehensive evaluation. The history should be obtained from a nursing home caregiver as well as the patient because many problems may be chronic or partially treated.
- Use of a standard nursing home transfer form that includes data such as the patients underlying medical problems, medications, advance directives, and baseline mental and functional status facilitates evaluation in the ED.
- The ultimate disposition decision should be made after considering the options for care available at the nursing home.

The overwhelming majority of elders are living unassisted, independently. Approximately 5 percent of elderly people in the United States reside in nursing homes. It is estimated that 25 to 50 percent of elders will reside, for some part of their lives, in a nursing home or extended-care facility.[1] Nursing home residents often have multiple medical problems, and many will require acute medical care beyond the capabilities of the facility. Nursing home residents can be some of the sickest and most challenging patients any physician manages. The combination of acute on chronic disease adds a layer of complexity to their evaluation and treatment. Acute care intervention increasingly has become the responsibility of emergency physicians. Several studies also have shown use of EDs by nursing home patients with only minor problems.[2,3] Unfortunately, a mismatch between emergency medical practice and the patient's desires sometimes leads to unwanted evaluation, intervention, and hospitalization.[4]

This chapter highlights problem areas, potential pitfalls, and possible remedies in the emergency care of nursing home transfers.

EPIDEMIOLOGY

Annually in the United States more than one-quarter of all nursing home residents are transferred to an ED for care.[5] This accounts for approximately 1 to 2 percent of all adult ED visits in a given year. Of these patients, about 40 percent are admitted to the hospital.[6,7] Studies have revealed a variety of reasons that nursing homes transfer patients to the ED. However, altered mental status, falls, respiratory and gastrointestinal problems, fever, lacerations, and gastrostomy tube problems made up the majority of reasons in two large studies.[7,8] The most common ED diagnoses were fractures, urinary tract infections, chronic obstructive pulmonary disease and pneumonia, complications of diabetes, and open wounds.[7,8] For nursing home patients admitted to the hospital from the ED, principal diagnoses were cardiovascular (myocardial infarction, stroke, congestive heart failure), infection (urinary tract infection, pneumonia), trauma (fractures), and gastrointestinal (acute abdomen and gastrointestinal bleed).[6–8]

Despite the perception among emergency care providers that patients from nursing homes tend to be transferred more often at night or on weekends, this has not been borne out in several studies. Most patients present during afternoon and evening hours, and there is an even distribution of transfers throughout the week.[3,7,8]

The vast majority of nursing home transfers arrive at the ED in advanced life support (ALS) ambulances staffed by paramedics. They may require a high level of prehospital care, although some data indicate that many nursing home patients are sent for "routine" reasons. For these patients, less care-intensive modes of transport may be more appropriate.[1,6,8]

EMERGENCY DEPARTMENT CARE

While the medical and surgical treatment of elderly patients is covered in detail elsewhere in this book, nursing home patients present with their own unique set of problems. The most problematic is obtaining accurate information regarding the patients medical history and the reason for transfer. In most instances, family is not available to give background information. The caregiver at the nursing home should be contacted as soon as possible after patient arrival to obtain an accurate presenting history. It is often very difficult to contact the regular caregiver at the nursing home several hours after patient arrival. Physicians caring for nursing home patients may be unable to provide detailed information.

Nurses are the usual source of useful details. Almost 70 percent of transfer decisions by nursing home physicians are made by telephone, and in 12 percent of cases, the physician is never contacted prior to the transfer being made. In the study by Brooks and colleagues,[5,8] 5 hours was the average time for a physician call back to the nursing home. Because of the complexity of medical illness in these patients and difficulty obtaining historical information, greater reliance is placed on the nursing home transfer sheet, which should accompany the patient. Such forms vary from community to community. However, most are designed to contain the reason for transfer, demographics, vital signs, patient problem lists, medications and allergies, functional and cognitive status, and advance directives.[9] While helpful in many instances, transfer forms need to be complete in order to aid the ED physician. In one survey conducted by the Society of Academic Emergency Medicine (SAEM), approximately 75 percent of ED physicians reported problems in obtaining information regarding nursing home transfers.[4] Additionally, one large study noted that 10 percent of patient transfers from nursing homes arrived without transfer documentation. When such documentation was provided, it most commonly lacked information regarding advance directives, past medical history, and baseline functional and mental status.[8] Miscommunication has the potential to greatly affect patient care. Lack of information (or inaccurate information) regarding the reason for transfer may lead to undertreatment of the patient and missed diagnoses.[10] Lack of a knowledge of underlying chronic conditions and baseline status can lead to extensive and unnecessary ED workups. Given the potential for spread of nosocomial infections, EDs should be made aware of patients infected with resistant organisms, and steps should be taken to prevent further contamination.[11] A standard transfer form was developed by the geriatric task force of SAEM to address these issues. Other regional efforts to standardize transfer forms have been published.[8] EDs that receive patients from a group of nursing facilities would benefit from development of consensus concerning a standard transfer form. Other problems encountered by ED physicians in caring for nursing home patients include the unavailability of recent electrocardiograms (ECGs), x-rays, and medical reports. Without these, an adequate understanding of the patients chronic illnesses may be difficult to achieve. Nursing homes and ambulance services often transfer patients without appliances such as glasses and hearing aids. Without these, baseline assessment and communication can become impossible.

Most nursing home transfer patients will require ED interventions such as placement of an intravenous line, intravenous fluids and medications, bladder catheterization, or supplemental oxygen. Most also will require comprehensive testing, blood chemistries, cardiac enzymes, blood gases, ECGs, and chest x-rays. Computed tomography is obtained in approximately 10 percent of nursing home patients transferred to EDs.[7]

The dismal outcome for nursing home patients who arrive undergoing cardiopulmonary resuscitation (CPR) is well documented.[7,12] ALS measures should be performed promptly during the prehospital care. Unfortunately, underlying illness and delays to recognition of arrest and start of resuscitation are common.

PATIENT DISPOSITION

While nursing home residents use the ED at a higher rate than do elderly patients in the community,[13] more treatment may be available in nursing homes than at home. However, the majority of staff at nursing homes have little or no formal medical training; thus patients who require close medical monitoring may not be returned safely from the ED to the nursing home. Indeed, admission criteria for nursing home transfers depend on the capabilities of the nursing home. Knowledge of the levels of care available at nursing facilities may better inform planning transfer of patients back to the nursing home. If treatment consists primarily of intravenous fluids, parenteral medications, or ongoing respiratory therapy, some nursing homes can manage these treatment options, whereas others cannot. The decision to return a patient to the nursing home for treatment depends on the capability of that facility. When the safety of return to the nursing home is not clear, patients benefit from observation (<23 hours) and then return to the nursing home. Most nursing facilities will hold a bed for 23 hours for an observation patient.[2,14] Obviously, such decisions need to be made with the input of the nursing home staff, patient, cargiver(s), and physician.

The following approach is reasonable in taking care of nursing home transfers. On receiving notification from the nursing home of a transfer, call the nursing home to obtain accurate information regarding the reason for transfer and current and baseline cognitive and functional status. An agreed data set should be established and a standard form used whenever patients are transferred. Devices such as hearing aids and glasses should accompany the patient. Medication lists, problem lists, medical records, x-rays, and ECGs should be sent with patient. When the patient arrives in the ED, seek any other pertinent information from the paramedics. Scan the transfer paperwork for completeness. Contact the transferring caregiver to obtain missing information. A call should be placed to the patient's physician to delineate new from chronic problems. When doubt exists as to the acute or chronic nature of symptoms, especially vague symptoms, use structured questions about activities of daily living. If at all possible, make contact with a caregiver rather than evaluating the patient completely under the assumption that all symptoms are new. When patients must be transported without delays and without paperwork, arrangements should made to fax the needed information to the ED. When patients are being returned to the nursing home, again an agreed data set should be conveyed. Be meticulous in providing a summary of care given in the ED and recommended treatment as well as test results in order to facilitate the patient's ongoing care.

ADDITIONAL ASPECTS

The predominant theme in this chapter is one of communication. Clearly, a proactive approach to this problem benefits both the ED care provider and the patient transferred from a nursing home. Various forms have been proposed, and use of any standard form should become routine. Since most EDs receive transfers from only a handful of local nursing homes, development of a good working relationship between entities will enhance patient care. In addition, developing a rapport with the community geriatricians can ease the patient disposition process in the ED. As proposed by Sanders,[15] this requires meetings of ED directors, geriatricians, and nursing home administrators. These meetings should facilitate understanding the capabilities and limitations of the referring nursing homes and the role of the ED in the community. ED administrators should be expected to take a leading role in facilitating these meetings.

CONCLUSION

Elderly patients in nursing homes are using EDs at increasingly higher rates. They often have multiple medical problems that may be chronic, making the ED evaluation difficult. The information from the nursing home must be complete and accurate. Development of good communication between ED and nursing home care providers is the key to maximizing appropriate care for these patients. Both exchange of standardized forms and direct discussions between providers of care should be routine in all cases.

REFERENCES

1. Vicente L, Wiley J, Carrington R: The risk of institutionalization before death. *Gerontologist* 19:361, 1979.
2. Kerr HG, Byrd JC: Nursing home patients transferred by ambulance to a VA emergency department. *J Am Geriatr Soc* 39:132, 1991.
3. Gillick M, Steel K: Referral of patients from long term to acute care facilities. *J Am Geriatr Soc* 31:74, 1983.
4. McNamara RM, Rousseau E, Sanders AB: Geriatric emergency medicine: A survey of practicing emergency physicians. *Ann Emerg Med* 21:796, 1992.
5. Brooks S, Warshaw G, Hasse L, et al: The physician decision-making process in transferring nursing home patients to the hospital. *Arch Intern Med* 154:902, 1994.
6. Bergmann H, Clarfield AM: Appropriateness of patient transfer from a nursing home to an acute care hospital: A study of emergency room visits and hospital admissions. *J Am Geriatr Soc* 39:1164, 1991.
7. Ackermann RJ, Kemle KA, Vogel RL, et al: Emergency department use by nursing home residents. *Ann Emerg Med* 31:749, 1998.
8. Jones JS, Dwyer PR, White LJ, et al: Patient transfer from nursing home to emergency department: Outcomes and policy implications. *Acad Emerg Med* 4:908, 1997.
9. Madden C, Garrett J, Busby-Whitehead J: The interface between nursing homes and emergency departments: A community effort to improve transfer of information. *Acad Emerg Med* 5:1123, 1998.
10. Kalbfleisch N: Altered mental status, in Sanders AB (ed): *Emergency Care of the Elder Person.* St Louis, Beverly Cracom, 1996, pp 119–142.
11. Stein D: Managing pneumonia acquired in nursing homes: Special concerns. *Geriatrics* 45:39, 1990.

12. Murphy DJ, Murray AM, Robinson BE, et al: Outcomes of cardiopulmonary resuscitation in the elderly. *Ann Intern Med* 111:192, 1989.

13. Gabow PA, Hutt DM, Baker S, et al: Comparison of hospitalization between nursing home and community residents. *J Am Geriatr Soc* 33:524, 1985.

14. Gordon M, Klapecki KC, Wilson DB: Emergency care and the patient in the long-term care facility. *Can Med Assoc J* 145:19, 1991.

15. Sanders AB: Emergency care for patients in long-term care facilities: A need for better communication. *Acad Emerg Med* 4:854, 1997.

9

Fever and Immune Function in the Elderly

Eric Daniel Katz
Christopher R. Carpenter

HIGH-YIELD FACTS

- Atypical presentation of infection is typical in the elderly.
- The elderly may be considered immunocompromised hosts.
- Fever in the elderly is not well defined, and a blunted fever response is common. Current recommendations for defining fever include considering as elevated oral or tympanic temperatures over 37.6°C or a rectal temperature over 37.2°C.
- The 1-month mortality of a geriatric emergency department (ED) patient with fever is 7 to 10 percent.
- Chest x-ray and urinalysis will only identify half of bacteremic patients.
- Nursing home residents are more prone to infection and have different microbial pathogens than community-dwelling elderly.
- Thirty percent of bacteremic elderly patients are afebrile on presentation to the ED.

IMPORTANCE

As use of the ED by the elderly increases, emergency physicians are evaluating more geriatric patients with fever. Ten percent of the elderly who present to the ED will have a fever.[1] In the nursing home population, fever is a frequent cause for transfer to an ED for evaluation. Fever, with or without the presence of infection, is worrisome in the geriatric population for a number of reasons. Of those patients who present to the ED with fever, 70 to 90 percent will be admitted, and 7 to 10 percent of those will die within the first month after presentation.[2,3] In comparison, less than 1 percent of patients aged 17 to 59 years who present with fever will die within 1 month.[2,3] Part of the reason for this is that 40 percent of all bacteremia and sepsis occur in the elderly and cause up to 60 percent of geriatric mortality.[4] Sepsis is one of the top 5 causes of death and one of the top 10 causes of hospitalization in the elderly.

When evaluating the elderly for infection, it is important to remember that some are immunocompromised. There is evidence that immune function peaks during puberty and decreases from 5 to 30 percent over a patient's lifetime.[5] Waning immune function perhaps is due primarily to the effects of age or to the effects of comorbidities. The increased risk of infection with age is manifest in frequent urinary tract, respiratory tract, wound, gastrointestinal, and nosocomial infections. Less common diseases, such as tuberculosis, influenza, and varicella, are also seen disproportionately in the aged population. More important, the morbidity and mortality from infections are higher in the elderly than in younger patients.

For these reasons, it is vital to consider the elderly patient with fever or other evidence of infection as acutely ill and requiring emergent intervention.

BLUNTED FEVER RESPONSE AND DEFINITION OF FEVER IN THE ELDERLY

"The fevers of old men are less acute than others for the body is cold."

—Hippocrates

Twenty to thirty percent of the elderly with bacterial or viral infections will present to the ED with blunted or absent fever response.[6–8] The reason may be due in part to a lower basal body temperature. Other causes for a decreased fever response are changes in thermal homeostasis, such as central nervous system (CNS) and temperature perception regulation; decreased response to endogenous and exogenous pyrogens; and decreased production and conservation of body heat.[9–12] Comorbidities also may play a significant role in the loss of fever response. For example, diabetes and malignancy are both correlated with a decreased immune response to infection. Patients with hypothyroidism, hypopituitarism, or renal insufficiency may have a decreased fever response as well.

Patients with lower basal body temperatures have been known to have a blunted fever response to an infectious challenge. There may be some delay between infection and the onset of fever, often as much as 12 hours.[13]

Afebrile bacteremia in the elderly can originate from infections of numerous sources, including the lungs, urinary tract, heart valves, peritoneum, gall bladder, and skin. The presence of afebrile bacteremia, however, is far more common in the elderly patient than in the young.

This lack of fever is an important prognostic sign. A blunted fever response to serious bacterial, viral, or fungal illness portends a poorer prognosis. Afebrile elderly patients presenting with infection are harder to diagnose and treat in an efficient manner. When evaluating and treating elderly patients with subtle presentations, it is important to consider infectious causes both in the presence of low-grade elevations of temperature and in the absence of any temperature evaluations.

It is also important to know that elders with fever often do not have infectious causes. Impoverished or isolated elders may not be able to physically remove themselves from environmental overheating. Thus, hyperthermia develops from excessive ambient temperatures. They are also at risk of hyperthermia from behavioral changes, medications, and malnutrition. Elders' ability to vasodilate and sweat is often impaired in extremes of temperature, making them more susceptible to ambient temperatures, medication effects, infections, and other causes of hyperthermia.

An accurate temperature may be difficult to abtain in a elderly patient. An inaccurate oral temperature may be measured in patients who are emotionally distraught, demented, tremulous, or mouth breathing or who have eaten recently. False hypothermia can be the result of poor positioning of the thermometer, short duration of sampling, an uncooperative patient, or rapid respiratory rate. Antipyretic medications may have lowered an elevated temperature.

The type of thermometer used and where the temperature is measured may have some relevance to the ability to detect a fever. Some EDs use the tympanic infrared thermometer. While one study in the operating room found pulmonary artery catheters and typmanic probe temperatures to be closely correlated,[14] ED studies have yielded poor results from tympanic thermometry when compared with oral, and rectal thermometry. Mercury thermometers and electronic thermometers also have shown divergence of measurements. Most studies of electronic thermometry have shown it to be superior to mercury thermometers for geriatric patients.[13,15,16] In one study comparing oral and rectal temperatures, it was found that oral temperatures are, on average, 0.66 degrees lower than rectal temperatures.

In order to define fever in the elderly, the normal mean temperature of a healthy geriatric population must be known, but this has not been well studied. Most studies report on either nursing home inpatients or afebrile elderly hospital patients. Mean morning rectal temperatures are 37.3°C, and oral temperatures are 36.7°C. In a sample of afebrile elderly patients, the upper level of normal was 37.5°C (rectal) and 37.3°C (oral).[17]

In perhaps the best study to determine the threshold for defining fever in the elderly, Castle and colleagues[18] followed 50 geriatric inpatients and found that while healthy, they had a mean temperature of 36.3°C (oral). In these patients, when definitive infection was diagnosed, the mean maximal temperature was 38.5°C (oral), but half these patients had a temperature of less than 38.3°C. Using a definition of 1.3°C above a patient's established baseline was a far more sensitive indicator of fever in nursing home patients. Lowering the threshold for fever from 101°F (38.3°C) to 100°F (37.8°C) improved the sensitivity of detecting infection from 40 to 70 percent, with little change in the specificity (98 percent). Darowsky and colleagues[16] showed that patients with confirmed infections had tympanic or oral temperatures above 37.2°C or rectal temperatures above 37.5°C and yielded a sensitivity of 86 percent for rectal temperatures and 66 percent for oral temperatures.

While a higher temperature cut point is more specific for infection, a lower cut pont with a higher sensitivity is important to avoid missing potentially serious infections. Many studies have documented the sensitivity and specificity of oral or rectal temperatures for the presence of acute bacterial infection. We recommend using a temperature of 1.1°F (2.0°C) greater than baseline regardless of the technique of measurement. An oral temperature of 37.2°C (99.0°F) from a normal baseline or a rectal temperature of 37.5°C (99.5°F) would be a fever. Using these numbers, McAlpine and colleagues[13] showed a 95 percent sensitivity for diagnosing "definite infections" on a geriatric unit.

PRESENTATION OF PATIENTS WITH INFECTIONS

In younger patients, classic symptoms are more reliable in guiding diagnostic testing and treatment than in older patients. In the elderly, presentations are often atypical. For example, pneumonia patients may present without cough or sputum production, and patients with a urinary tract infection may present without dysuria or frequency. In addition, two studies have shown that approximately a third of geriatric patients with acute infections have no febrile response whatsoever.[6,7,19] Twenty-five of 192 elderly hospitalized patients with bacteremia were afebrile at the time of diagnosis. For patients under age 65, only 5 of 128 barteremic patients were a febrile.[20]

Delays in diagnosis and prompt initiation of appropriate antibiotic therapy in the elderly adversely affect the prognosis. These delays may be due to atypical presentations, confusion between acute and chronic conditions, and underreporting of symptoms. The presence of comorbidities may be the most important cause of delay in the recognition of infection in the elderly. Clinicians in the ED have not previously treated their patients and hence do not know their baseline status. The manifestations of a chronic disease may mask or be mistaken as an explanation for an acute disease. In addition, elders underreport symptoms. Patients, caregivers, and doctors often credit "old age" as being the cause of acute symptoms. Patients may underreport symptoms because of cognitive impairment, dysphasia, aphasia, or depression. Further mental status changes may occur due to acute infection. These problems make the recognition of infection a true challenge to the emergency physician.

The emergency physician must have a low threshold for considering occult infectious disease in the decompensating geriatric patient regardless of the presence or absence of fever.

EPIDEMIOLOGY

Limitations of Studies

One of the difficulties in studying infectious disease in the elderly is defining the physiologic age of the population studied. Studies of the elderly population routinely use chronologic age as a criterion for admission into a study, thereby enrolling a physiologically heterogeneous population. Stratifying patients on the basis of age alone neglects important factors such as functional independence and comorbidities. The newly retired independent elder is a significantly different host from the moribund, bed-bound preterminal elder. Not all studies use the same age cutoff. The most common is age over 65. Also, studies on animals use models whose bioequivalence to an elderly human is not obvious or proven. Lastly, the pathophysiologic affects of aging are often studied in vitro and not studied in vivo.[21]

Critical differences among elder patients' immune systems could produce conflicting study results. Patients in nursing homes have a higher rate of anergy than healthy patients of similar age.[21,22] Anergy itself is associated with a higher 2-year mortality rate in patients over 80

years of age[23] and has predictive value for postoperative sepsis and other complications of surgery.[24,25]

Age and Disease Prevalence

When emergency physicians see young patients with fever, the most common diagnoses are pharyngitis, otitis and viruses. In the elderly, 90 percent of febrile patients will have serious and potentially life-threatening infection, such as pneumonia, urinary tract infection (UTI), intraabdominal infection, or bacteremia.[1] A fever has a high positive predictive value for serious illness in elders.[20,26–29] In addition, the elderly have disproportionate numbers of positive blood cultures. At one hospital, 192 of 320 positive blood cultures (60 percent) over a 1½-year period were from older patients, far outweighing their proportion among hospitalized patients at that institution.[20]

Even among the elderly there are differences in disease prevalence. In men aged 65 to 70 years there is approximately a 3 percent rate of bacteriuria, but this increases to 20 percent among men over age 70. In women between the ages of 65 and 70 there is a 20 percent rate of bacteriuria, whereas after age 80 it can range from 23 to 50 percent. Institutionalized patients have bacteriuria approximately 50 percent of the time.[30] In hospitalized patients, elderly (>85 years of age) compared with young (age 16–25) patients have rates of UTI and bacteremia five times higher, pneumonia three times higher, wound infections twice as high, and herpes zoster ten times as high.[31]

As we age, our response to immunization becomes less effective. One-third of patients over age 65 will not have a protective response to an influenza vaccination.[32] Similarly, 30 percent of patients beyond age 55 with diagnosed tuberculosis will have negative purified protein derivative (PPD) tests as compared with 10 percent of those under age 55.[32] Because of these deficiencies in immune response, there is an increase in the mortality from both influenza and tuberculosis.[30] These are two examples of diseases that increase in frequency and mortality as we age.

The Nursing Home Resident

Approximately 5 percent of the elderly in the United States are nursing home residents. Infection rates increase in patients in chronic care facilities. The patients who live in these facilities are physiologically different from their community-dwelling counterparts. They typically have compromised immune function, mental status abnormalities, chronic diseases, indwelling catheters, and multiple medications. In addition, the institutionalized are exposed to outbreaks of many highly communicable diseases such as influenza, scabies, gastroenteritis, tuberculosis, and sexually transmitted diseases. Because of this, the average nursing home patient can expect approximately 1.5 infections each year he or she is in a chronic care facility.[3,33–35] In fact, over three-quarters of all "functional decline" in nursing home residents is due to infection.[36]

The increased rate of infection may relate to comorbidities and other factors in nursing home residents. The rate of infection increases with the level of care from 9 percent per year for the independent-living elderly to 60 percent per year for the hospitalized elderly.[37] This increase obviously parallels the degree of debility and severe illness found in those patients. The most common infections (in order of decreasing frequency) are UTI, respiratory tract infection, skin and soft tissue infection, and gastroenteritis.[38] In addition, tuberculosis is contracted or reactivated in nursing home residents four times as often as in the community-dwelling elderly. In chronic care facilities, the PPD conversion rate is 5 percent per year, as compared with 3.4 percent in the community.[39]

Malnutrition

Between 40 and 85 percent of the elderly suffer from protein malnutrition.[40] Malnutrition may contribute to lowering a patient's febrile response to infection. The mechanism for this may be a decrease in the release of endogenous pyrogens. In aged rodents, the ability to mount a febrile response was related to qualitative and quantitative changes in brown fat.[12] In rats, brown fat losses occur late in malnutrition. Malnutrition also may increase the propensity for infection by breaking down the mucosal barrier within the tracheobronchial tree. This causes enhanced adherence of bacteria, thus increasing susceptibility to infection. Patients who are on supplemental nutrition have improved lymphocyte function.[41]

PATHOPHYSIOLOGY

The immunocompromise that comes with age can be seen at the cellular, biochemical, and organ system level. The cells produce a lesser amount of and less active immune reactants. The organs and organ systems change, predisposing the elderly to infection as well. In addition, when infection does take hold, the elderly are poorly equipped to respond. By the time the impaired immune system

mounts a response, the infection's damage may be irreversible. At baseline, many elderly have decreased cardiac output, decreased creatine clearance, conduction disease, worsened homeostasis, and low catecholamine reserves. For these reasons, sepsis may overwhelm the physiologic reserve of the elderly patient. When the patient becomes hypotensive, there is no catecholamine reserve to maintain cerebral perfusion. The patient needs increased cardiac output but does not have the reserve cardiac output or is tachycardic. When sepsis mandates that a patient deliver oxygen to the tissues in a more efficient manner, the elderly have lower levels of 2,3-DPG and are unable to adequately deliver oxygen (Fig. 9-1).

Cellular and Biochemical Changes with Aging

T-Cell and Thalamic Function

It has been observed that while the doubling rate of T cells decreases with age, the total number of T cells does not change. However, the proportion of cells in each subset of T cells does show significant change with age. This may be responsible for the observed deficiencies in T-cell function. In addition, the elderly are prone to have a higher percentage of immature T cells both in the thymus and in the blood at any given time.

Specific subsets of T cells that are affected by the aging process include a lowering of the CD4, CD8, and cytotoxic T-lymphocytes. In addition, there is a decrease in "naive" T cells capable of responding to new antigens. The decrease in these four cell lines is offset by an increase in "memory" cells, which respond to previously encountered antigens. The only other T-cell line that is increased is autoreactive T cells recognizing self-antigens.

The total number of T cells available to respond to a new antigenic challenge decreases. Some biochemical causes of decreased T-cell function include a lower rate of interleukin 2 (IL-2) synthesis and release and a less impressive response to IL-2. Other mitogens also are less effective in stimulating T cells. Meanwhile, thymic involution begins as early as puberty, and thymopoietin, which is responsible for the production of mature T cells, becomes undetectable after age 60. Other thymic hormones decrease with age as well and disappear even earlier. The result of thymic involution is that a lower percentage of T cells are available to recognize new antigens. Most of the T cells that remain are memory cells. This produces an immune function that is analogous to memory in demented patients: They are capable of remembering the

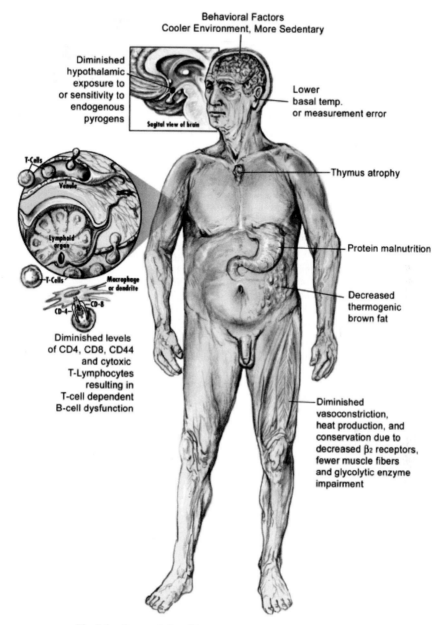

Fig. 9-1   Causes of altered immune and fever function in the elderly.

past but do not have the ability to incorporate new information. This involution of the thymus may represent the biologic clock of the immune system. However, early thymectomy has not been shown to change the life span or increase the risk of infection.

Other Cellular Components of the Immune System

While the change in T-cell function is clearly the dominant, age-associated, cellular dysfunction in the immune system, there is dysfunction associated with B-cell activity as well. Perhaps the most important component of B-cell dysfunction stems from their reliance on T-cell function for effect. There is controversy as to whether or not B-cell function that is independent of T cells decreases with age. Loss of B-cell function can best be seen in the poor response of the elderly to the influenza vaccine.

The effect of aging on neutrophil function remains controversial. While it appears that there is no difference in neutrophil function between sick and healthy elderly adults, it does appear that the elderly have a higher percentage of dysfunctional neutrophils. However, the functional ones appear to be equal to those of young adults. Deficits in opsonization and phagocytosis have been reported in geriatric neutrophils. There have been reports of loss of neutrophil chemotaxis (possibly due to a deficit in superoxide and ion production). Complement levels remain normal with age. It appears that there are no changes with aging in either antigen-presenting cells (APCs) or natural-killer (NK) cells.

Antibodies and Autoantibodies

Age-associated immune deficiencies are hallmarked by a decreased response to new foreign antigens and a relative preservation of response to previously encountered antigens. There is, however, ample evidence for a deficit in humoral immunity as well. For example, infections by encapsulated bacteria, such as *Streptococcus pneumoniae,* *Escherichia coli,* and *Klebsiella,* are more common in the elderly. In addition, serum antibodies generally lose the ability to recognize and bond to foreign antibodies with age. The relative deficits that are then found in the immune system's memory make the patient prone to new infections or relapses of latent diseases such as tuberculosis and herpes zoster infection.

Total levels of immunoglobulin do not change with age. However, like T-cell subsets, the proportions of the subsets do change. IgM may be decreased as much as 50 percent, whereas there is an overall increase in IgG and

IgA. There is increased autoantibody production, especially after age 80, with no higher risk of autoimmune disease. The increase in immune-complex formation and monoclonal gammopathies may represent impairment of suppressor T-cell function.

Biochemical Factors

Monokines are substances produced by macrocytes and macrophages. They mediate nonspecific host defenses to infection. These defenses include the development of fever as well as the production of acute-phase reactants. Examples of monokines include IL-1, IL-2, and tumor necrosis factor (TNF), and all are decreased in the elderly.

CLINICAL FEATURES

History

General Information

The history obtained from the febrile geriatric ED patient is of particular importance given the unfortunate reality that although less likely to have fevers, elderly people are more likely to develop infections. A detailed history should include recent hospitalizations, infections, antibiotics, indwelling devices (catheters, orthopedic plates, prosthetic valves, etc.), and a medication review (including identification of new medications, herbal supplements, and antipyretics). In addition, the ambient temperature should be considered, and when appropriate, inquiries should be made into the presence of heat or air-conditioning in the home (paramedics often can offer useful information in this regard). The duration of fever and any prior workup and treatment of infection should be ascertained. Most importantly, comorbities must be recognized and assessed. Although atypical presentation is expected, knowledge of the most common geriatric pathogens and a systematic history should guide diagnostic tests and empiric therapy. Of particular importance to emergency physicians is the fact that up to 10 percent of those over age 60 who present to the ED with fevers die within 1 month as compared with 1 to 5 percent of younger patients.[1,42] No studies have addressed the utility of history and physical examination in febrile residents of long-term care facilities. The American Geriatric Society has published guidelines for management of febrile nursing home residents. These guidelines reflect the frequent unavailability of subjective information from residents.[4]

The community-dwelling elderly often offer a more reliable and detailed history. Multiple studies, though, have demonstrated vague complaints as the most common presentation of serious bacteremia. A retrospective analysis by Fontanarosa and colleagues[43] identified only two independent predictors of bacteremia: altered level of consciousness and vomiting. Other nonspecific indicators of bacterial illness in the elderly include altered "general state," clinical evidence of infection, falls, functional decline, and new incontinence.[44] Not surprisingly, these vague presentations result in frequent misdiagnoses and delay the initiation of appropriate antimicrobial therapy, undoubtedly contributing to the increased mortality from infection in the elderly. Fontanarosa and colleagues[43] noted that emergency physicians correctly identified 66 percent of elderly bacteremic patients as septic. Unfortunately, they also incorrectly labeled 40 percent of nonbacteremic patients as septic. Others also have observed this inability to clinically identify serious bacterial illness in the elderly.[45]

If the patient is able to communicate, a thorough history should be obtained from the patient. A systematic history also should include a recent medical history from the patient's caregivers. A 5-minute phone call to the nursing home, physician's office, family, or a friend can differentiate the chronically debilitated patient from the acutely decompensating patient. Since 50 percent of geriatric emergency patients with serious bacterial illness lack any clinical features,[42] additional history may be crucial to prompt initiation of diagnostic testing and antibiotic therapy.

Marco and colleagues[42] identified the most common etiologies for fever in geriatric patients presenting to the ED (Table 9-1). Although each of these infections shares common presenting features, some signs or symptoms may help to direct diagnostic and therapeutic interventions (Table 9-2). Whereas pneumonia, UTI, soft tissue infection, intraabdominal abscess, and generalized bacteremia all can present with confusion, obtundation, functional decline, incontinence, falls, respiratory distress, vomiting, diarrhea, or abdominal pain, many patients will display localizing symptoms. Some of these localizing symptoms, however, can be misleading. One study demonstrated that less than 20 percent of elders with UTI had any urinary symptoms, but more than 33 percent had respiratory symptoms, leading to an initial misdiagnosis of respiratory infection.[46] In contrast, elderly ED patients with pneumonia are significantly less likely than younger patients to complain of cough, dyspnea, pleuritic chest pain, or hemoptysis.

Fever of Unknown Origin (FUO)

Geriatric patients may present to the ED complaining of prolonged fevers, sometimes with extensive nondiagnostic outpatient workups. Although these patients do not meet inpatient FUO criteria, they are often labeled as having an FUO. Elders with FUO presenting to the ED have not been studied systematically. The elderly patient who presents to the ED with an acute fever that remains unexplained after ED evaluation is not unusual, since 71 percent of fevers in those over age 50 remained unexplained after the initial evaluation.[45]

Twice as many elderly FUO patients have infection, tumors, or multisystem diseases as compared with younger groups. Drug-related fevers are six times as likely. Most impressive, however, is the eventual identification of a

Table 9-1. Infectious Etiologies of Fever in Geriatric ED Patients

Source	% Total	Common Associated Signs and Symptoms	Common Organisms
UTI	22–38%	ALOC, malaise, respiratory symptoms	*E. coli* (22–85%) *Klebsiella* (3–11%) Polymicrobial (12%)
Pneumonia	12–30%	Tachypnea	*S. pneumoniae* (69%)
Soft tissue	5–13%		
Biliary tract	20%	Anorexia, nausea, abdominal pain	*E. coli* (45%) *Klebsiella* (30%)
Unidentified	11–26%	Change in mental status, vomiting	*E. coli* (30%) *Bacteroides* (20%)

Source: Used with permission from Gallagher et al.[52]

Table 9-2. Differential Diagnosis and Relative Frequency of Various Etiologies of Fever in the Elderly

Infectious
  Respiratory
    Pneumonia (25%)
    Tuberculosis (13%)
    Bronchitis (6%)
    Viral syndrome (3%)
    Otitis media/externa
    Pharyngitis
    Sinusitis
  Genitourinary
    Urinary tract infection (22%)
    Epididymitis
    Prostatis
  Skin
  Musculoskeletal
    Osteomyelitis
    Septic arthritis (1%)
  Neurologic
    Meningitis
    Encephalitis
    CNS/epidural abscess
  Gastrointestinal
    Appendicitis
    Cholecystitis
    Diverticulitis
    Entertis/colitis
    Abscess
  Cardiovascular
Noninfectious
  Temporal arteritis (17%)
  Malignancy (12%)
    Colon cancer, Hodgkin's disease, leukemia
  Medication side effect (6%)
  Cerebral vascular accident (<2%)
  Intracranial hemorrhage (<2%)
  Myocardial infarction (<2%)
  Seizure disorder (<2%)
  Cirrhosis
  Crystaloid arthropathy
  Dehydration
  Environmental exposure
  Large hematoma
  Sarcoidosis
  Thyroid storm

source in 88 percent of elderly workups, as opposed to only 71 percent of younger cohorts.

Given the large number of comorbidities and the diminished ability to tolerate the side effects of extensive or repeated diagnostic testing, the febrile elderly patient's history and physical examination should be exceedingly thorough. The key to diagnosing the etiology of FUO may lie in the elaboration of nonspecific complaints or even trivial bits of history. For instance, a headache may represent temporal arteritis or a dental abscess, whereas abdominal pain can direct the evaluation away from the head.[47]

Physical Examination

In general, bacteremic elderly patients have fewer manifestations of infectious disease than do younger patients. Marco and colleagues[42] noted that several clinical features were independently associated with serious illnesses: initial temperature exceeding 103°F (39.4°C), respiratory rate greater than 30 breaths per minute, white blood cell count (WBC) greater than 11,000/ml, or pulse greater than 120 beats per minute. However, these factors are not good screening criteria because their negative predictive values did not exceed 36 percent. The presence of these factors may aid in identifying a high-risk population for admission, but their absence should not be reassuring enough to discharge patients to home.

Physical examination should begin with vital signs, including pulse oximetry. An assessment of respiratory effort, level of consciousness, and personal hygiene should be made. A complete examination should include otoscopic evaluation of the tympanic membrane and external auditory canal; palpation of the mastoid, sinuses, and temporal arteries; and visualization of oral structures with palpation as appropriate. The neck should be assessed for menigismus, adenopathy, and thyromegaly. Many elders have preexisting murmurs or rales related to chronic processes that are unrelated to the presenting problem. Any murmur, though, should be documented, and evaluation for the stigmata of bacterial endocarditis should be undertaken. A search of previous records for evidence of a murmur should be routine. Hearing rales on the examination of the chest should prompt radiographic evaluation.

A significant proportion of elderly patients with serious intraabdominal pathology lack pain or tenderness. When present, however, the localization of abdominal pain or tenderness can reliably point to the correct diagnosis. Right upper quadrant pain or tenderness is elicited in 74 to 84 percent of elderly cholecystitis patients, whereas two-thirds manifest left lower quadrant pain or tenderness with diverticulitis and right lower quadrant pain or tenderness with appendicitis.[39] In the absence of localizing complaints, a pelvic examination rarely will elucidate the fever source. Back pain or tenderness may indicate pyelonephritis or epidural abscess.

Two systems to include in the physical examination for fever are the neurologic and integumentary systems. An altered level of consciousness, ranging from confusion to coma, can occur with virtually any infectious process. Focal deficits should prompt evaluation for infectious etiologies such as cerebral abscess.[48] The preponderance of cellulitis as the source of elderly fever necessitates a complete evaluation of the skin. Common sources of infection include decubitus ulcers and diabetic ulcers, so all clothing and shoes must be removed, and the patient must be rolled to facilitate an evaluation of dependent areas.

Physical examination should reveal any indwelling devices. These may not be noted during the history. Sites of intravascular and bladder catheters, prosthetic valves, pacemakers, and defibrillators are worth checking on examination. Surgical scars should lead to queries about orthopedic hardware and vascular grafts.

DIFFERENTIAL DIAGNOSIS

When an emergency physician encounters a febrile or infected geriatric patient, he or she must keep a broad differential in mind. Table 9-2 summarizes an extensive list of infectious and noninfectious diagnoses that are encountered in febrile elders. The majority of patients presenting to EDs[42,45] with fever [49,50] have infectious etiologies. One study comparing four groups of adults, divided by age, noted that febrile patients aged 17 to 39 are diagnosed with viral syndrome, otitis media, or pharyngitis in 58 percent of cases: however, only 4 percent of those over age 60 and less than 1 percent of those over age 80 have these diagnoses.

Three diagnoses fairly unique to geriatric fevers have been identified: temporal arteritis, tuberculosis, and medication side effect. When history and physical examination are unclear, the emergency physician should consider adding an erythrocyte sedimentation rate (ESR) determination and a PPD test to the evaluation, and on admission or discharge, nonessential medications should be eliminated. Common sources of drug-induced fevers are listed in Table 9-3.

One review of drug-induced fever noted several fea-

Table 9-3. Drug-Induced Fever: Commonly Encountered ED Medications

Cardiovascular
Methyldopa
Quinidine
Procainamide
Hydralazine
Antimicrobials
Penicillin
Ampicillin
Vancomycin
Isoniazid
Amphotericin
Psychoactive agents
Carbamazepine
Haloperidol
LSD
Amphetamine
Others
Aspirin
Allopurinol
Interferon
Propylthiouracil

Source: Used with permission from Fry et al.[64]

tures of interest. First, fever onset is highly variable, with antimicrobial agents causing the most rapid onset (mean 8 days), whereas cardiac medications have both the longest lag time (mean 45 days) and the greatest variability (median 10 days) in onset. Second, contrary to classic teaching, drug-induced fever does not usually include additional manifestations such as rash or eosinophilia. Finally, the true incidence of drug-induced fever is currently unknown, and the diagnosis remains one of exclusion. Ruling out more immediate life-threatening causes of fever is the focus in the ED.[51]

DIAGNOSTIC TESTING

Given the limited clinical utility of the history and physical examination, diagnostic testing may play a key role in assessing the risk of serious bacterial illness and the need for antimicrobial therapy. The WBC and band percentage have both been demonstrated to predict bacteremia in the elderly. Marco and colleagues[42] showed that a WBC greater than 11,000 independently predicted serious illness, whereas Fontanarosa and colleagues,[43] in a retrospective review, indicated that bandemia of more than 6 percent predicted bacteremia. Others have used WBCs greater than 15,000/mm³[45,52] or less than 5,000/mm³[44] or an absolute band count of greater than 1500[53] as predictive of bacteremia. Wasserman and colleagues[54] analyzed the combination of fever, WBC, and differential count to predict bacterial infections. WBC less than 14,000/mm³, bands less than 500mm³, and the absence of fever, yielded a 6 percent likelihood of bacterial infection, whereas the presence of all three yielded a 100 percent likelihood.

Urinalysis is a high-yield study, but the results should be interpreted carefully. In general, though, negative test results are more useful in excluding UTI than positive tests results are in diagnosing UTI. The prevalence of pneumonia in adults with respiratory symptoms increases from 3 percent in the outpatient environment to 26 percent in the ED. Still, the majority of patients presenting to the ED with respiratory complaints do not have pneumonia. A chest radiograph (CXR) is necessary to establish the diagnosis.[55] The initial study should be a posteroanterior (PA) and lateral CXR when possible. A common myth is that infiltrates that are absent initially may "blossom" with rehydration when the patient presents dehydrated. Animal studies have demonstrated just the contrary.[56,57] However, disease progression may lead to the development of infiltrates after initial radiography. While the fever and leukocytosis may be lacking in pneumonia (and thereby predict increased mortality),[58] an infiltrate and/or effusion should be present. The radiographic appearance is not useful for distinguishing between viral or bacterial pneumonia.[59,60] The presence of fever and pulmonary symptoms without infiltrate may represent upper respiratory infection, bronchitis, or exacerbation of a chronic pulmonary condition.[46] Together urinalysis and CXR identify only 58 percent of occult bacterial infections.[45]

Blood cultures should be sent on all febrile elderly patients presenting to the ED for the initial work-up of fever. In addition, afebrile elderly patients with an unexplained acute functional decline, recent falls, incontinence, leukocytosis, bandemia, or pulmonary infiltrate should have blood cultures sent. The afebrile bacteremic geriatric patient usually is not recognized as septic.[51,61,62] Not surprisingly, studies demonstrate an inability to clinically distinguish the bacteremic from the nonbacteremic elderly patient.[43,46,52,63] Two sets of blood cultures should be obtained via two different venipuncture sites whenever bacteremia is suspected.[64] Urine cultures should be sent on all febrile elderly. Positive urine cultures in women over age 80 approach 20 percent in the community and 50 per-

cent in chronic care facilities.[65] Although debate exists, the prudent course dictates sending blood cultures even in the face of a suspicious urinalysis.

When diagnosis is not readily apparent, the differential diagnosis of acute fever or FUO is broad, and additional studies should be ordered as appropriate. An ESR determination may help distinguish temporal arteritis; a thyroid-stimulating hormone (TSH) determination, thyroid storm; a bone scan, osteomyelitis; a lumbar puncture, meningitis; and a computed tomographic (CT) scan, cerebral abscess, thoracoabdominal abscess, or sinusitis.[39] Figure 9-2 proposes one approach to the initial evaluation of the febrile elderly patient.

EMERGENCY CARE AND DISPOSITION

Early, appropriate antimicrobial therapy diminishes mortality. One study of bacteremic elderly patients revealed the highest survival with UTI and cellulitis and the lowest with pneumonia.[66] Often the diagnosis remains unclear after the ED workup. In such settings, empirical therapy and inpatient observation or close outpatient follow-up are often necessary.

Before choosing an antibiotic regimen, the emergency physician should take into consideration likely sources, clinical status, and potential complications. Table 9-4 summarizes treatment recommendations for common geriatric febrile illnesses, although local resistance patterns may alter any recommendations made.

The pharmacokinetics of many antibiotics are altered by an age-related decline in renal function. Since many of the drugs are eliminated via the renal system, the ED physician may need to check the frail elderly patient's creatinine level prior to discharge to home with antibiotics. Remember that the creatinine clearance decreases with age and smaller size, so a creatinine level within the "normal" range does not necessarily represent intact renal function (see Chap. 31). In general, the antibiotic dose should be decreased by 50 percent when the creatinine clearance is less than 30 mL/min (to approximate creatinine, see Chap. 31) for penicillins, aztreonam, quinolones, trimethoprim-sulfamethoxazole, and vancomycin.

Age does not appear to affect other aspects of pharmacokinetics, such as oral absorption or hepatic metabolism. Because the elderly use twice as many prescription medications and seven times as many nonprescription drugs as younger patients, drug interactions are another important consideration in determining optimal antimicrobial therapy for the geriatric ED patient.[67] Table 9-5

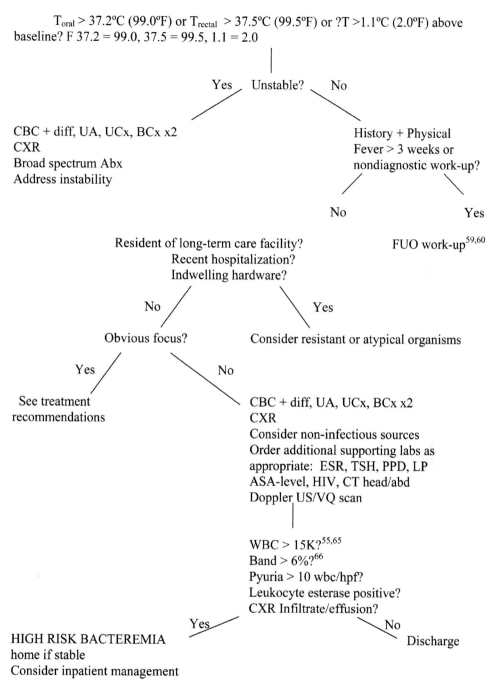

$T_{oral} > 37.2°C$ (99.0°F) or $T_{rectal} > 37.5°C$ (99.5°F) or ?T >1.1°C (2.0°F) above baseline? F 37.2 = 99.0, 37.5 = 99.5, 1.1 = 2.0

Yes   Unstable?   No

CBC + diff, UA, UCx, BCx x2
CXR
Broad spectrum Abx
Address instability

History + Physical
Fever > 3 weeks or
nondiagnostic work-up?

No   Yes

Resident of long-term care facility?
Recent hospitalization?
Indwelling hardware?

FUO work-up[59,60]

No   Yes

Obvious focus?   Consider resistant or atypical organisms

Yes   No

See treatment
recommendations

CBC + diff, UA, UCx, BCx x2
CXR
Consider non-infectious sources
Order additional supporting labs as
appropriate: ESR, TSH, PPD, LP
ASA-level, HIV, CT head/abd
Doppler US/VQ scan

WBC > 15K?[55,65]
Band > 6%?[66]
Pyuria > 10 wbc/hpf?
Leukocyte esterase positive?
CXR Infiltrate/effusion?

Yes   No

HIGH RISK BACTEREMIA
home if stable
Consider inpatient management

Discharge

Fig. 9-2   Proposed ED approach to the febrile elderly.[55,59,60,66]

Table 9-4. Empirical Treatment of Geriatric Fever Based on Suspected Source[116-119]

Infection	First-Line Therapy	Second-Line Therapy	Duration of Therapy (days)
Uncomplicated UTI	TMP-SMX	Ceph1 or Ceph2	7
	Fluroquinolone	Amoxicillin-clav	7
Pyelonephritis	Fluroquinolone PO/IV	Amox-clav	14
	Cefotaxime IV	Amp-sulb	14
		Ticarcillin-clav	14
In-dwelling catheter	Fluroquinolone	Aztreonam	14
	Piperacillin-tazobac	Ceph3	
	Imipenum	Aminoglycoside	
Community- acquired pneumonia	Macrolide	Doxycycline	5–14
	Fluroquinolone	Amox-clav	10–14
		Ceph2	
Hospital- or nursing home–Acquired pneumonia	β-Lactam ± Macrolide	Ceph3 + clindamycin	10–14
	Fluroquinolone	Amp-sulb	
		Amp + quinolone	
Bacterial meningitis	Amp + Ceph3	Substitute Aztreonam or aminoglycoside for Ceph3	14
Bacteremia NOS	Ceftizoxime ± aminoglycoside *or* Ampicillin + aminoglycoside + clindamycin	Aztreonam for aminoglycoside Metronidazole for clindamycin	Dependent on diagnosis
Cellulitis	Dicloxacillin Cephalexin	Erythromycin	14
Decubitus ulcer with systemic symptoms	Amox-clav Ceph3 Vancomycin	Pip-tazo Synercid	21+
Intraabdominal abscess/ infection	Ceph2 or Ceph3 Amp-sulb	Ampt + metronidazole + Quinolone	Diagnosis/ treatment -dependent
Diarrhea, *C. diff.*	Metronidazole oral	Vancomycin oral	14
Diarrhea, non *C. diff.* bacterial	Quinolone	TMP-SMX	3–5

lists some of the more common interactions. For example, before discharging an elderly patient with a quinolone prescription to home, be sure that no mineral-containing antacids (aluminum, magnesium) will be taken concurrently. These may significantly reduce oral absorption of quinolones.

The decision to admit or discharge, either to home or to a skilled care facility, is particularly relevant to the care of elders. While multiple studies have demonstrated an irreversible functional decline in elderly patients following admission for hip fractures and pneumonia despite optimal management of the admitting condition, no prospective, controlled data exist for the disposition of hemodynamically stable geriatric patients. In many cases the presentation dictates admission for hypotension, hypoxia, immobility, or unreliable social setting. A low

Table 9-5. Commonly Used Antibiotic Drug
Interactions and Side Effects

Antibiotic	Interaction/Side Effect
TMP-SMZ	Enhanced oral hypoglycemic effect
	Bone marrow toxicity
	Digoxin toxicity
	Coumadin attenuation
	Rash
	Megaloblastic anemia
Macrolides	Digoxin toxicity
	Nausea, diarrhea
Cipro	Theophylline toxicity
	Hypokalemia
	Seizure
	Tendon rupture
	Refractory hypoglycemia
Other quinolones	QT$_c$ prolongation
	Hepatitis
β-Lactams	Autoimmune hemolytic anemia
	Rash
Imipenum	Seizure

threshold for admission should be maintained. Advance directives, unless they preclude hospitalization, should have little influence on disposition decisions.

SUMMARY AND FUTURE RESEARCH QUESTIONS

The normal temperature range of community-dwelling elderly should be firmly established in order to allow a more accurate recognition of the febrile state. All such studies to date have focused on the hospitalized elderly or long-term care facility residents, not ED or community-dwelling patients. The better definition, incidence, and etiology of FUO in the ED elderly should be defined. The use of blood cultures in febrile and nonfebrile ED elderly patients should be explored. The efficacy of treatment of elders with infections outside the hospital setting should be determined. Finally, the ED length of stay, time to antimicrobial therapy, and effects of any delays on mortality should be studied.

Timely evaluation and appropriate disposition of the febrile elderly patient challenge even the most astute emergency physician. This chapter has summarized the current literature regarding the pathophysiology of im-

mune impairment and the breakdown of barriers to infection that often result in the atypical disease presentation seen in the elderly. The evaluation of a older patient with an infection, with or without fever, is difficult and time-consuming, but high mortality can be expected when treatable causes are missed.

REFERENCES

1. Keating HJ, Klimek JJ, Levine DS, et al: Effect of aging on the clinical significance of fever in the ambulatory adult patient. *Am Geriatr Soc* 32:282, 1984.
2. Ouslander JG, Osterweil D: Physician evaluation and management of nursing home residents. *Ann Intern Med* 121:584, 1994.
3. Smith PW, Rusnak PG: Infection prevention and control in the long-term-care facility. *Infect Control Hosp Epidemiol* 18:831, 1997.
4. Bentley DW, Bradley S, High K, et al: Practice guideline for evaluation of fever and infection in long-term care facilities. *Am Geriatr Soc* 49:210, 2001.
5. Walford RL: Henderson award lecture: Studies inimmunogerontology. *J Am Geriatr Soc* 30:617, 1982.
6. Jones SR: Fever in the elderly, in Machowiak P (ed): *Fever: Basic Mechanisms and Management.* New York, Raven Press, 1991, pp 233–241.
7. Norman DC, Grahn D, Yoshikawa TT: Fever and aging. *J Am Geriatr Soc* 33:859, 1985.
8. Norman DC, Yoshikawa TT: Fever in the elderly, in Cunha BA (ed): *Fever: Infectious Disease Clinics of North America.* Philadelphia, Saunders, 1991, pp 93–101.
9. Collins KJ, Exton-Smith AD: Thermal homeostasis in old age. *J Am Geriatr Soc* 31:519, 1983.
10. Jones PG, Kauffman CA, Bergman AG, et al: Fever in the elderly: Production of leukocytic pyrogen by monocytes from elderly persons. *Gerontology* 30:182, 1984.
11. Norman DC, Yokshikawa TT: Intraabdominal infections in the elderly. *J Am Geriatr Soc* 31:677, 1983.
12. Scarpace PJ, Bender BS, Burst SE: The febrile response of *E. coli* peritonitis in senescent rats. *Gerontologist* 30:215A, 1990.
13. McAlpine CH, Martin BJ, Lennox IM, et al: Pyrexia in infection in the elderly. *Age Ageing* 15:230, 1986.
14. Ferrara-Love R: A comparison of tympanic and pulmonary artery measures of core temperatures. *J Postop Anesth Nurs* 6:161, 1991.
15. Downton JH, Andrews K, Puxty JAH: Silent pyrexia in the elderly. *Age Ageing* 16:41, 1987.
16. Darowski A, Najim Z, Weinbrg JR, et al: The febrile response to mild infections in elderly hospital inpatients. *Age Aging* 20:193, 1991.
17. Darowski A, Weinberg JR, Guz A: Normal rectal, auditory canal, sublingual and axillary temperature in elderly afebrile patients in a warm environment. *Age Aging* 20:113, 1991.

18. Castle SC, Yeh M, Norman DC, et al: Fever response in the elderly: Are the older truly colder? *J Am Geriatr Soc* 39:853, 1991

19. Norman DC, Yoshikawa TT: Fever in the elderly. *Infect Dis Clin North Am* 10:93, 1996.

20. Gleckman RA, Hilbert D: Afebrile bacteremia: A phenomenon in geriatric patients. *JAMA* 248:1478, 1982.

21. Plewa MC: Altered host response and special infections in the elderly. *Emerg Med Clin North Am* 8:193, 1990.

22. Rodysill KJ, Hansen L, O'Leary JJ: Cutaneous-delayed hypersensitivity in nursing home and geriatric clinic patients: Implications for the tuberculin test. *J Am Geriatr Soc* 37:35, 1989.

23. Roberts-Thomson IC, Whittingham S, Youngchaiyud U, et al: Ageing, immune response and mortality. *Lancet* 13:358, 1974.

24. Powers DC, Nagel JE, Hoh J, et al: Immune function in the elderly. *Postgrad Med* 81:355, 1987.

25. Lewis RT, Klein H: Risk factors in postoperative sepsis: Significance of preoperative lymphocytopenia. *J Surg Res* 26:367, 1979.

26. Finklestein MS, Petkun WM, Freedman ML, et al: Pneumococcal bacteremia in adults: Age dependent differences in presentation and in outcome. *J Am Geriatr* Soc 31:19, 1983.

27. Gorse GJ, Thrupp LD, Nudleman KL, et al: Bacterial meningitis in the elderly. *Arch Intern Med* 144:1603, 1984.

28. Marrie TJ, Haldane EV, Faulkner RS, et al: Community-acquired pneumonia requiring hospitalization: Is it different in the elderly? *J Am Geriatr Soc* 33:671, 1985.

29. Terpenning MS, Buggy BP, Kauffman CA: Infective endocarditis: Clinical features in young and elderly patients. *Am J Med* 83:626, 1987.

30. Schneider EL: Infectious diseases in the elderly. *Ann Intern Med* 98:395, 1983.

31. Haley RW, Hooton TM, Culver DH, et al: Nosocomial infections in U.S hospitals 1975–1976: Estimated frequency by selected characteristics of patients. *Am J Med* 70:947, 1981.

32. Ben-Yehuda A, Weksler ME: Host resistance and the immune system. *Infect Dis* 8:701, 1992.

33. Nicolle LE, Garibaldi RA: Infection control in long-term-care facilities. *Infect Control Hosp Epidermiol* 16:348, 1995.

34. Yoshikawa TT, Nicolle LE, Norman DC: Management of complicated urinary tract infection in older patients. *J Am Geriatr Soc* 44:1235, 1996.

35. Muder RR: Pneumonia in residents of long-term care facility: Epidemiology, etiology, management and prevention. *Am J Med* 105:319, 1998.

36. Brody GM: Hyperthermia and hypothermia in the elderly. *Clin Geriatr Med* 10:213, 1994.

37. Valenti WM, Trudell RG, Bentley DW: Factors predisposing to oropharyngeal colonization with gram-negative bacilli in the aged. *New Engl J Med* 298:1108, 1978.

38. Leinicke T, Navitsky R, Cameron S, et al: Fever in the elderly: How to surmount the unique diagnostic and therapeutic challenges. *Emerg Med Pract* Newsletter 1999.

39. Stead WW, Lofgren JP, Warren E, et al: Tuberculosis as an endemic and nosocomial infection among the elderly in nursing homes. *New Engl J Med* 312:1483, 1983.

40. Linn BS, Jensen J: Malnutrition and immunocompetence in older and younger outpatients. *South Med J* 77:1098, 1984.

41. Chandra RK, Joshi P, Au B, et al: Nutrition and immunocompetence of the elderly: Effect of short-term nutritional supplementation on cell-mediated immunity and lymphocyte subsets. *Nutr Res* 2:223, 1982.

42. Marco CA, Schoenfeld CN, Hansen KN: Fever in geriatric emergency patients: Clinical features associated with serious illness. *Ann Emer Med* 26:18, 1995.

43. Fontanarosa PB, Kaeberlein FJ, Gerson LW: Difficulty in predicting bacteremia in elderly emergency patients. *Ann Emer Med* 21:99, 1992.

44. Chassagne P, Perol MB, Doucet J, et al: Is presentation of bacteremia in the elderly the same as in younger patients? *Am J Med* 100:65, 1996.

45. Mellors JW, Horwitz RI, Harvey MR, Horwitz SM: A simple index to identify occult bacterial infection in adults with acute unexplained fever. *Arch Intern Med* 147:666, 1987.

46. Barkham TMS, Martin FC, Eykey SJ: Delay in the diagnosis of bacteraemic urinary tract infection in elderly patients. *Age Ageing* 25:130, 1996.

47. Berland B, Gleckman RA: Fever of unknown origin in the elderly: A sequential approach to diagnosis. *Postgrad Med* 92:197, 1992.

48. Georgilis K, Plomaritoglou A, Dufni U, et al: Aetiology of fever in patients with acute stroke. *J Intern Med* 246:203, 1999.

49. Esposito AL, Gleckman RA: Fever of unknown origin in the elderly. *J Am Geriatr Soc* 26:498, 1978.

50. Knockaert DC, Vanneste LJ, Bobbaers HJ: Fever of unknown origin in elderly patients. *J Am Geriatr Soc* 41:1187, 1993.

51. Mackowiak PA, LeMaistre CF: Drug fever: A critical appraisal of conventional concepts. An analysis of 51 episodes diagnosed in two Dallas hospitals and 97 episodes reported in the English literature. *Ann Intern Med* 106:728, 1987.

52. Gallagher EJ, Brooks F, Gennis P: Identification of serious illness in febrile adults. *Am J Emeg Med* 12:129, 1994.

53. Pfitzenmeyer P, Decrey H, Auckenthaler R, Michel JP: Predicting bactermia in older patients. *J Am Geriatr Soc* 43:230, 1995.

54. Wasserman M, Levinstein M, Keller E, et al: Utility of fever, white blood cell count, and differential count in predicting bacterial infections in the elderly. *J Am Geriatr Soc* 37:537, 1989.

55. Bartlett JG, Breiman RF, Mandell LA, File TM: Community acquired pneumonia in adults: Guidelines for management *Clin Infect Dis* 26:811, 1998.

56. Caldwell A, Glauser FL, Smith WR, et al: The effects of dehydration on the radiologic and pathologic appearance of

experimental canine segmental pneumonia. *Am Rev Respir Dis* 112:651, 1975.

57. Cooligan TG, Light R, Duke K, et al: The effect of volume infusion in canine lobar pneumonia. *Am Rev Respir Dis* 121:122, 1980.

58. Ahkee S, Srinath L, Ramirez J: Community acquired pneumonia in the elderly: Association of mortality with lack of fever and leukocytosis. *South Med J* 90:296, 1997.

59. Tew J, Calenoff L, Berlin BS: Bacterial or nosocomial pneumonia: Accuracy of radiographic diagnosis. *Radiology* 124:607, 1977.

60. Farr BM, Kaiser DL, Harrison BDW, et al: Prediction of microbial etiology at admission to hospital for pneumonia from the presenting clinical features. *Thorax* 44:1031, 1989.

61. Sanders AB (ed): *Dermographics, Aging, and Emergency Medical Care: Emergency Care of the Elder Person.* St Louis, Beverly Cracom, 1996, pp 3–5.

62. Whitelaw DA, Rayner BL, Willcox PA: Community-acquired bacteremia in the elderly: A prospective study of 121 cases. *J Am Geriatr Soc* 40:996, 1992.

63. Bates DW, Cook EF, Goldman L, Lee TH: Predicting bacteremia in hospitalized patients: A prospectively validated model. *Ann Intern Med* 113:495, 1990.

64. Fry DE, Cox RA, Harbrecht PJ: Gangrene of the gallbladder: A complication of acute cholecystitis. *South Med J* 74:666, 1981.

65. Monane M, Gurwitz JH, Lipsitz LA, et al: Epidemiologic and diagnostic aspects of bacteriuria: A longitudinal study in older women. *J Am Geriatr Soc* 43:618, 1995.

66. Meyers BR, Sherman E, Mendelson MH, et al: Bloodstream infections in the elderly. *Am J Med* 86:379, 1989.

67. Colt HG, Shapiro AP: Drug-induced illness as a cause for admission to a community hospital. *J Am Geriatr Soc* 37:323, 1989.

10

Acute Coronary Syndromes

Brian F. Erling
William J. Brady

HIGH-YIELD FACTS

- The majority of patients with acute myocardial infarction are older than 65 years.
- Atypical presentations of unstable angina and acute myocardial infarction are much more common in the elderly.
- Elderly patients have a much higher risk of post-myocardial infarction complications, including congestive heart failure, atrial fibrillation, heart block, myocardial rupture, and cardiogenic shock.
- Elderly patients have a higher risk associated with pharmacologic and procedural intervention as compared with younger patients.
- While baseline risk is increased, failure to intervene in this population has been shown to have worse outcomes compared with similar groups who received appropriate intervention.

Among the cardiovascular ailments encountered in the elderly, acute coronary ischemic events are the most common. Coronary artery disease (CAD) is the underlying common "pathophysiologic denominator" in the older patient with such presentations. CAD is encountered commonly in the elderly; due to its prevalence in this age group, it is the number one cause of death in patients over age 60. Approximately 700,000 patients are hospitalized annually with CAD; the majority of these patients are elderly. Of those patients who succumb to CAD and its complications, more than 80 percent are 65 years of age or older.[1]

In the elderly patient the clinical presentations of CAD include stable angina, unstable angina, acute myocardial infarction (AMI), and sequelae of ischemic heart disease. The acute presentations of CAD—unstable angina and AMI—are best described collectively as *acute coronary syndrome* (ACS). These patients also may manifest the sequelae of ischemic heart disease, presenting with decompensated congestive heart failure (CHF) due to ischemic cardiomyopathy or malignant ventricular arrhythmia. Elderly patients present to the emergency department (ED) frequently with complaints related to the cardiovascular system. At times, these complaints include chest pain, shoulder pain, or jaw pain; such presentations are usually straightforward from a diagnostic perspective. Alternatively, anginal equivalent complaints and presentations are encountered, particularly in the very elderly; these presentations represent significant diagnostic challenges. Therapeutically, elderly patients are candidates for the range of therapies used in the ACS patient. Certain of these treatments, however, may demonstrate different risk-benefit analyses, thereby making treatment decisions more problematic.

EPIDEMIOLOGY

CAD is present in as many as 7 million Americans and is responsible for the death of more than 500,000 patients annually, with a significant percentage of these patients being elderly. In fact, a majority of patients aged greater than 70 years have CAD; for instance, approximately 70 percent of persons over age 70 will demonstrate coronary atherosclerosis at autopsy. In a large portion of these patients, CAD was clinically silent in life. At least 30 to 40 percent of persons over age 65, however, will demonstrate CAD clinically. These patients typically manifest CAD as stable angina; in fact, it is estimated that 10 percent of patients over age 65 have CAD that manifests as stable angina.[2] A large portion of these patients will manifest CAD as an acute coronary event, such as unstable angina or AMI; 60 percent of all AMIs occur in patients older than age 65. The long-term complications of the illness also account for many patients with CAD. Regardless of the presentation, a significant number of these patients are functionally impaired by this illness. CAD is found equally in geriatric men and women.

CAD, either in its acute form such as AMI or its chronic ischemic sequelae, is the leading cause of death in patients older than 65 years of age.[3] Ischemic heart disease is a frequent cause of death in the elderly, particularly in older men.[4] Geriatric patients experience a significantly higher mortality rate from AMI when compared with younger populations. For example, the GUSTO-I trial revealed that the mortality rate of the AMI patient who underwent thrombolysis was significantly higher in older individuals; patients over 75 years of age died at a much greater rate (10.3 percent) when compared with those individuals under age 65 (1.5 percent).[5] While the specific reasons responsible for this pronounced mortality rate are unclear, they likely involve a combination of factors, including more severe forms of the illness, decreased ability to tolerate physiologic dysfunction, and advanced comorbidity.

A significant disparity is found when one considers the elderly patient with ACS and the medical literature related to the topic in this population. Despite the widespread nature of this disease in the geriatric population and its significant medical impact, relatively fewer older patients are found in large, randomized studies investigating various treatment modalities.[6] In certain instances, the results of these studies are applicable to the elderly patient, whereas in other cases the possibility for an incomplete or incorrect description of the issue must be considered, and the literature must be interpreted from this perspective.

PATHOPHYSIOLOGY

Thrombus formation is considered an integral factor in all forms of ACS, including unstable angina, non-ST-segment-elevation AMI, and ST-segment-elevation AMI. All these syndromes are initiated by endothelial damage, usually by atherosclerotic plaque disruption, which leads to platelet aggregation and thrombus formation. The resulting thrombus can occlude more than 50 percent of the vessel lumen. Vessel occlusion can lead to myocardial ischemia, hypoxia, acidosis, and eventually, infarction. The consequences of the occlusion depend on the extent of the thrombotic process, the characteristics of the preexisting plaque, and the availability of collateral circulation.

Coronary arteries of patients with ACS tend to have eccentric, ragged, irregular walls and nearly occluded lumens. The wide variety of clinical presentations of patients with complete coronary artery occlusion suggests marked differences in the rate of development of total occlusion, the amount of collateral circulation, or both.

Another important aspect of ACS is vasospasm. After significant thrombotic occlusion, local mediators induce vasospasm, which further compromises blood flow. Central and sympathetic nervous system input increases as alpha receptors proliferate within minutes of the occlusion. Unopposed alpha-sympathetic stimulation can result in more coronary vasospasm. Coronary artery spasm with subsequent thrombus formation and without significant underlying CAD is involved in approximately 10 percent of AMIs and can precipitate sudden cardiac death; most elderly patients with vasospasm, however, have underlying CAD. This mechanism may be more prevalent during unstable angina and other coronary syndromes that do not result in infarction. Sympathetic stimulation by endogenous hormones such as epinephrine and serotonin also may result in increased platelet aggregation and neutrophil-mediated vasoconstriction.

Further myocardial injury at the cellular level occurs during the reperfusion phase, either by spontaneous or therapeutically induced fibrinolysis. In particular, the introduction of calcium, oxygen, and cellular elements into ischemic myocardium can lead to irreversible myocardial damage that causes reperfusion injury, prolonged ventricular dysfunction (known as *myocardial stunning*), or reperfusion dysrhythmias. Neutrophils probably play an important role in reperfusion injury, occluding capillary lumens, decreasing blood flow, accelerating the inflammatory response, and resulting in the production of chemoattractants, proteolytic enzymes, and reactive oxygen species.

CLINICAL FEATURES

Advanced age almost always has an impact on the emergency physician's ability to evaluate the patient and assess for the potential of AMI. In fact, the evaluation of acute chest pain with confirmation of the correct diagnosis is very difficult in geriatric patients. Numerous disease states, syndromes, and medications, as well as age-related changes in the cardiovascular and neurologic systems, contribute to make the elderly AMI presentation a significant diagnostic challenge. The increased rate of atypical presentation among the elderly translates into the not infrequent clinically unrecognized AMI. Based on autopsy information, the correct diagnosis of AMI is made in less than half the patients prior to death; the very elderly constitute a large portion of this group of patients with the postmortem diagnosis of AMI. As a patient ages, a multitude of factors—including autonomic neuropathy, injury to cardiac sensory afferent nerves due to past ischemic heart disease, cortical failure resulting from cerebrovascular or other central nervous system (CNS) disease, extensive comorbidity, higher pain thresholds, and preexisting mental status abnormalities—all contribute to a higher rate of atypical presentation and medically unrecognized AMI. These various factors combine and result clinically in an increased prevalence among the geriatric populace of anginal equivalent chief complaints, "silent" myocardial infarction, and a preponderance of neurologic symptom–based syndromes.

In contrast to the younger population, elderly patients are much less likely to present to the ED complaining of typical chest pain or pressure. In fact, the presentation of AMI in the elderly is frequently nonclassic; atypical presentations are encountered with increasing frequency in sequentially older populations.[7,8] Vague complaints are much more common, which can lead the clinician in the incorrect diagnostic direction. Presentations may be confounded by poor histories as a result of altered memory.[9]

The spectrum of presentation changes significantly with increasing age. In elderly patients younger than age 85 years, chest pain becomes less frequent, whereas equivalent complaints are noted more often; chest pain, however, still is found in the majority of patients. Stroke, weakness, and altered mentation became more common with increasing age and frequently are not accompanied by typical chest discomfort. While atypical presentations occur, they are still in the minority in this relatively younger geriatric population. Over the age of 85 years, atypical presentations are the norm and should be anticipated.[8] The incidence of "painless" AMI increases dramatically with age in that 60 to 70 percent of elderly infarct patients over age 85 will present with an anginal equivalent complaint or syndrome—most often with a change in the mental status. If one considers all elderly patients with altered mental status in an ED population, however, the diagnosis of AMI is found in only 1 percent of cases.[10] In most acutely ill patients over age 85, the clinician not only should consider the potential for AMI but also should actively exclude the diagnosis with appropriate investigations. The elderly frequently also present with complications of AMI rather than the actual symptoms of the acute ischemic event. For example, very elderly patients presenting with new-onset, unexplained CHF should be screened for acute ischemia. Similarly, the

elderly patient presenting with malignant bradycardia, atrioventricular block, or ventricular arrhythmia should be evaluated for cardiac ischemia while appropriate therapies and other evaluations are performed.[8,11]

The 12-lead electrocardiogram (ECG) of the elderly AMI patient is frequently nondiagnostic.[12] The ECG may be described as "nondiagnostic" if nonspecific ST-segment/T-wave changes are noted. These nonspecific changes are defined as ST-segment depression or ST-segment elevation of less than 1 mm with or without abnormal morphology and blunted, flattened, or biphasic T waves without obvious inversion or hyperacuity. Other electrocardiographic issues that may produce nondiagnostic changes are sinus tachycardia and bradycardia or artifactual issues such as a wandering or irregular baseline. Lee and colleagues[13] noted that adult chest pain patients with nonspecific or other nondiagnostic electrocardiographic features had a relatively low risk of AMI ranging from 3 to 4 percent but a significant risk of unstable angina that occurred in approximately one-fifth of all such patients and more often in older patients. Other investigators have found that approximately 6 percent of patients with AMI demonstrate a "nonspecifically abnormal" ECG on presentation. Alternatively, in a somewhat different application of the term, the nondiagnostic ECG is initially encountered in 50 to 75 percent of patients ultimately found to have experienced a myocardial infarction. With this use of the descriptor *nondiagnostic,* the clinician is referring to the lack of pathologic ST-segment elevation noted on the ECG. Significant ST-segment depression and/or T-wave changes may be seen in these situations, findings certainly suggestive of an active coronary ischemic event.

The classic ACS triad of chest pain, diagnostic ECG, and abnormal serum markers is seen in a minority of elderly patients ultimately diagnosed with AMI. In fact, these findings are present in only 25 percent of these patients.[14] The clinician must not expect the obvious abnormality in these three areas of evaluation—the patient's history, ECG, and serum markers. As noted, the rates of atypical presentation and nondiagnostic ECG increase with age. These altered patterns of presentation must be considered in the evaluation of the elderly patient.

DIAGNOSIS AND DIFFERENTIAL

The atypical presentation of ACS in the elderly sometimes can create a challenge in successful diagnosis. The heavy disease load common to this age group, with frequent gastroesophageal and musculoskeletal comorbidities, can further confuse the picture. The pain is commonly atypical or focused in the abdomen or back with vague associated symptoms. The chief complaint may be dyspnea, vomiting, dizziness, confusion, or the common "feels ill." Physicians must maintain a very low threshold to pursue a cardiac cause to vague complaints in the elderly, particularly if clinical deterioration becomes evident.

As in the younger population, the differential diagnosis of chest pain in the elderly includes diagnoses of cardiac, gastrointestinal, pulmonary, vascular, and musculoskeletal etiology (Table 10-1). Clinicians should consider this broad differential diagnosis when beginning their evaluation of the elderly patient who presents with chest pain.

The ECG is often confounded by chronic conduction or anatomic disease and must be interpreted with this in mind. Common masqueraders of ST-segment elevation, such as left bundle-branch block, left ventricular hypertrophy, and left ventricular aneurysm,[15,16] are much more common in the elderly. In addition, the usual pattern of Q-wave infarction and ST-segment-elevation AMI commonly seen in the young is much less common in the elderly. Myocardial infarction presenting with electrocardiographic ST-segment depression is much more common.[17,18] Additional confounders in ST-segment interpretation include drugs that may alter this signal. The most common drug associated with this is digoxin and its classic down-sloping ST segment.

Although ST-segment-elevation AMI is appropriately associated with a serious cardiac event, the more common ST-segment-depression AMI in the elderly is not benign. ST-segment depression is associated with a significant mortality, particularly in the elderly. Nevertheless, the standard indications for fibrinolysis pertain to all age groups—ST-segment elevation in two contiguous leads or new-onset left bundle-branch block. Although ST-segment-depression AMI may be serious, the ISIS-2 trial clearly demonstrates that fibrinolytics are not indicated with this electrocardiographic pattern regardless of age.[19]

Early differentiation between unstable angina and AMI is difficult in any age group but is particularly confounding in the elderly, where the history can be poor, the ECG can be misleading, and serum marker elevations (particularly CK-MB) can be minimal.[20] Unfortunately, even these small enzyme leaks can be of grave consequence in the elderly. Whether it is due to decreased proteins in the myocardium or diminished physiologic reserve, the level of CK-MB does not correlate well with outcome. Troponin I appears to have a higher sensitivity over CK-MB, particularly in the elderly, as an indication for myocardial

Table 10-1. Differential Diagnosis of Chest Pain in the Elderly

Cardiac
    Acute coronary syndrome—unstable angina or AMI
    Stable angina
Gastrointestinal
    Esophageal rupture
    Esophagitis
    Esophageal spasm
    Peptic ulcer disease
    Gastritis
    Cholelithiasis or cholecystitis
    Hepatitis
    Pancreatitis
Pulmonary
    Pulmonary embolism
    Pneumothorax
    Chronic obstructive pulmonary disease
    Pneumonia
Vascular
    Aortic dissection or aneurysm (thoracic)
Other
    Chest trauma
    Chest wall syndrome (musculoskeletal)
    Radicular (neurogenic) pain
    Herpes zoster infection
    Psychogenic

death. All these confounders can result in significant delays in diagnosis and suboptimal care in the elderly.

EMERGENCY DEPARTMENT CARE AND DISPOSITION

In general, elderly patients with an ACS should be approached using the same algorithms as younger patients. Aspirin, nitrates when appropriate, morphine, and beta blockers are the standard of care. Elderly patients' complex medical histories and potentially altered physiology can complicate therapeutic options. Since these patients have the highest mortality risk from coronary disease, they theoretically have the most to gain from aggressive treatment. It is this increased interventional risk that calls for caution and often leads to a candid discussion with the patient and family.

Interventions in elderly patients have been shown to have an increased morbidity and mortality as compared with younger patients.[21] When determining a patient's risk from a procedure, however, it is more important to consider the biologic age of the individual rather than the actual chronologic age. People do not age the same due to many factors, and the "young old" must be differentiated from the "old old" when determining risk. Healthy patients without comorbid disease will have procedural complication rates much closer to their younger counterparts.

While elderly patients have increased bleeding after fibrinolysis as compared with younger patients, the mortality benefits of giving the medication far outweigh the risks of withholding therapy in appropriate patients.[22,23] However, because of these higher rates of complications secondary to interventions, treatment should be very well thought out. The side effects and risk of complication must be well considered and weighed against the quality of life of the patient, especially in octogenarians, in whom the chance for an increase in life expectancy is minimal at best. Determining the patient's quality of life is a time-consuming process and can be difficult to accomplish in the ED. Factors that play into quality of life include social ties, physical activity, and independence. Most important, however, it involves a candid discussion with the patient as to his or her perceptions of quality of life and his or her wishes, as well as involving the family and primary care provider.

One theory of fibrinolytic risk relates the frequency of underweight elderly as a confounder in determining risk in the elderly. The ASSENT-2 trial demonstrated a reduction in intracranial hemorrhage in elderly and low-weight patients when using tenecteplase (TNK-tPA) as compared with alteplase (tPA), where the tPA was given in a standard non-weight-based dose.[24] In contrast, TNK-tPA is a one-time weight-based dose that may play a role in its improved safety profile. It is clear that when fibrinolytics must be used in the elderly, weight-optimized dosing has the highest efficacy and safety and is the standard of care at this time.

Elderly patients are also at increased risk of complications with primary angioplasty. However, when the risk of bleeding complications is high, it is the intervention of choice. The Primary Angioplasty in Myocardial Infarction (PAMI) trial has shown a significant decrease in mortality and stroke when compared with fibrinolysis in the 150 patients older than age 65.[25] As technical skill with this procedure has been refined over the last decade, it has become the standard of care when available in a timely fashion. The benefit is incontrovertible when performed at tertiary-care centers where interventions are performed with significant frequency.

The presence of baseline electrocardiographic abnormalities, the frequency of associated cardiac disease, and the common inability to exercise make the performance, interpretation, and prognostic value of noninvasive cardiac testing significantly less than in younger patients. If they are able to exercise, the resulting increase in heart rate commonly will fall short of predicted goals. Elderly patients do, however, have an appropriate increase in systolic blood pressure such that the heart rate pressure product, an indicator of myocardial oxygen demand, will reach adequate (but not ideal) levels. A negative or indeterminate exercise stress test does not exclude the disease, whereas a positive test is much more helpful.[26]

The data supporting exercise or pharmacologic stress tests in the elderly are limited. Electrocardiographic stress tests with nuclear augmentation seem to offer a greater sensitivity for the diagnosis of cardiac ischemia in the elderly. This was demonstrated during the Baltimore Longitudinal Study of Aging.[27] The presence of either ST-segment changes on electrocardiographic stress tests or thallium perfusion defects after exercise resulted in a 5-year cardiac event rate similar to that in patients with both tests negative. However, patients with both positive electrocardiographic and thallium stress tests had a high positive predictive yield for silent ischemia, with a 5-year cardiac event rate of 48 percent.

The data on echocardiographic stress tests are also limited in the elderly. These are technically difficult studies, however, because underlying anatomic and valvular disease is common. Determining wall-motion abnormalities either acutely in the ED or during functional testing can be a formidable task even to the specialized cardiologist. Baseline wall-motion abnormalities and reduced ejection fractions are common confounders to be considered in interpretation of the data.

Drug therapies for ACS in the elderly are similar to those agents used in younger patients; elderly patients, however, do not tolerate the cardiovascular effects of medications as well as younger patients. Their lack of physiologic reserve, one of the same reasons they have a poorer outcome after AMI, helps to explain this phenomenon. Drug selection should be performed thoughtfully, with dosages titrated carefully to avoid profound hypotension or bradycardia.

Low-molecular-weight heparin, particularly enoxaparin, has been shown to have a significant benefit over unfractionated heparin in treating ACS.[28,29] It is, however, contraindicated in patients with renal insufficiency. In elderly patients in whom decreased creatinine clearance may be expected, waiting for a chemistry panel would be prudent. Whether using unfractionated or low-molecular-weight heparin, careful prescreening to assess for bleeding risk must be undertaken. If the decision to start unfractionated heparin is made, special dosing considerations are important in the elderly. Age, comorbid states, and small body size will alter drug metabolism, and lower doses should be used with frequent assessments of the partial thromboplastin time (PTT).

Glycoprotein IIb/IIIa platelet inhibitors are increasing in popularity in EDs across the country. The most pertinent study to emergency medicine is the PURSUIT trial,[30] which demonstrated a weak reduction in overall mortality. There also was a reduction in adverse cardiac events while being treated with a glycoprotein IIb/IIIa inhibitor (and an increase in bleeding) that did not carry over after termination of the drug. Eptifibatide, the focus of the PURSUIT trial, is the drug of choice in the ED because it is the only one in this class that carries Food and Drug Administration (FDA) approval for both medical and interventional treatment of ACS. Abciximab is only approved for interventions, and tirofiban is only approved for medical management. While further studies of this drug class are ongoing, their exact role in the elderly population has yet to be defined. Knowing that they are associated with an increased bleeding risk, it is reasonable to use them with extreme caution in the elderly until further safety studies are available.

Understanding the complication rates and safety profiles of different drugs allows for use of the best drug for a particular patient. The ASSENT-3 trial demonstrated that TNK-tPA plus enoxaparin is associated with the lowest 30-day mortality of any clinical AMI study to date.[31] If the decision is made to use fibrinolytics, this is the current drug of choice. This study also demonstrated that abciximab plus TNK-tPA was associated with an unacceptable rate of bleeding. Abciximab should be reserved for use in the interventional laboratory by experienced cardiologists, particularly in the elderly.

ADDITIONAL ASPECTS

The following are pitfalls in the diagnosis and management of ACS in the elderly:

- Elderly patients commonly take numerous medications and may neglect timely prescription renewal. Chest pain not relieved by nitroglycerin may be due to an expired or deteriorated drug supply.
- The phosphodiesterase inhibitor sildenafil citrate (Viagra) is growing in popularity and has been associated with extreme hypotension and death when used in conjunction with nitrates.

- AMI in the elderly is more commonly associated with ST-segment depression rather than ST-segment elevation.
- Enzyme elevations are often less significant in elderly persons with AMI when compared with younger controls and do not predict severity of injury.
- Elderly patients deserve the same aggressive treatment as younger patients presenting with ACS. When the risk is high, involving the patient and family in decision making is prudent.

REFERENCES

1. Gillum RF: Trends in acute myocardial infarction and coronary heart disease death in the United States. *J Am Coll Cardiol* 23:1273, 1993.
2. Wei JR, Gersh BJ: Heart disease in the elderly. *Curr Probl Cardiol* 12:1, 1987.
3. Lerner DJ, Kannel WB: Patterns of coronary heart disease morbidity and mortality in the sexes: A 26-year follow-up of the Framingham population. *Am Heart J* 111:383, 1986.
4. Aronow WS, Ahn C: Risk factors for new coronary events in a large cohort of very elderly patients with and without coronary artery disease (abstract). *Am J Cardiol* 77:864, 1996.
5. The GUSTO Investigators: An international randomized trial comparing four thrombolytic strategies for acute myocardial infarction. *New Engl J Med* 329:673, 1993.
6. Prabhat JHA, Deboer D, Sykora K, et al: Characteristics and mortality outcomes of thrombolysis trial participants and nonparticipants: A population-based comparison. *J Am Coll Cardiol* 27:1335, 1996.
7. Aronow WS: Prevalence of presenting symptoms of recognized acute myocardial infarction and of unrecognized healed myocardial infarction in elderly patients. *Am J Cardiol* 60:1182, 1987.
8. Bayer AJ, Chadha JS, Farag RR, Pathy MSJ: Changing presentation of myocardial infarction with increasing old age. *J Am Geriatr Soc* 34:263, 1986.
9. Miller PF, Sheps DS, Bragdon EE, et al: Aging and pain perception in ischemic heart disease. *Am Heart J* 120:22, 1990.
10. Kanich W, Brady WJ, Huff JS, et al: Altered mental status: Evaluation and etiology in the emergency department. *Am J Emerg Med* 20:613, 2002.
11. Aronow WS: Prevalence of presenting symptoms of recognized acute myocardial infarction and of unrecognized healed myocardial infarction in elderly patients. *Am J Cardiol* 60:1182, 1987.
12. Brady WJ: The electrocardiographic diagnosis of AMI: Clinical features associated with an initial nondiagnostic electrocardiogram. Abstract presented at Society for Aca-

demic Emergency Medicine Mid-Atlantic Regional Meeting, Baltimore, April 1999.

13. Lee T, Cook F, Weisberg M, et al: Acute chest pain in the emergency room: Identification and examination of low risk patients. *Arch Intern Med* 145:65, 1985.

14. Brady WJ: Missing the diagnosis of acute MI: Challenging presentation, electrocardiographic pearls and outcome-effective management strategies. *Emerg Med Rep* 18:91, 1997.

15. Brady WJ, Perron A, Ullman E: Errors in emergency physician interpretation of ST segment elevation in ED chest pain patients. *Acad Emerg Med* 7:1256, 2000.

16. Brady WJ, Perron A, Chan T: Electrocardiographic ST segment elevation: Correct identification of AMI and non-AMI syndromes by emergency physicians. *Acad Emerg Med* 8:349, 2001.

17. Caird FL, Campbell A, Jackson TFM: Significance of abnormalities of the electrocardiogram in old people. *Br Heart J* 36:1012, 1974.

18. Campbell A, Caird FL, Jackson TFM: Prevalence of abnormalities of the electrocardiogram in old people. *Br Heart J* 36:1005, 1974.

19. ISIS-2 (Second International Study of Infarct Survival) Collaborative Group: Randomized trial of intravenous streptokinase, oral aspirin, both, or neither among 17,187 cases of suspected acute myocardial infarction. ISIS-2. *Lancet* 2:349, 1988.

20. Goldberg RJ, Gore JM, Gurwitz JH, et al: The impact of age on the incidence and prognosis of initial myocardial infarction: The Worcester Heart Attack Study. *Am Heart J* 117(3):543, 1989.

21. Peterson ED, Cowper PA, Jollis JG, et al: Outcomes of coronary artery bypass graft surgery in 24,461 patients aged 80 years or older. *Circulation* 92:85, 1995.

22. Fibrinolytic Therapy Trials (FTT) Collaborative Group: Indications for fibrinolytic therapy in suspected acute myocardial infarction: Collaborative overview of early mortality and major morbidity results from all randomized trials of more than 1000 patients. *Lancet* 343:311, 1994.

23. Ryan TJ, Antman EM, Brooks NH, et al: 1999 update: ACC/AHA guidelines for the management of patients with acute myocardial infarction: A report of the American College of Cardiology/American Heart Association Task Force on Practice Guidelines (Committee on Management of Acute Myocardial Infarction). *Circulation* 100:1016, 1999.

24. Assessment of the Safety and Efficacy of a New Thrombolytic (ASSENT-2) Investigators: Single-bolus tenecteplase compared with front loaded alteplase in acute myocardial infarction: The ASSENT-2 double-blind randomized trial. *Lancet* 354:716, 1999.

25. Grines CL, Brown KF, Marco J, et al: A comparison of immediate angioplasty with thrombolytic therapy for acute myocardial infarction: The Primary Angioplasty in Myocardial Infarction Study Group. *New Engl J Med* 328:673, 1993.

26. Glover DR, Robinson CS, Murray RG: Diagnostic exercise testing in 104 patients over 65 years of age. *Eur Heart J* 5:59, 1984.

27. Fleg FL, Gerstenblith G, Zonderman AB, et al: Prevalence and prognostic significance of exercise-induced silent myocardial ischemia detected by thallium scintigraphy and electrocardiography in asymptomatic volunteers. *Circulation* 81:428, 1990.

28. Cohen M, Demers C, Gurfinkel EP, et al: A comparison of low-molecular-weight heparin with unfractionated heparin for unstable coronary disease: Efficacy and Safety of Subcutaneous Enoxaparin in Non-Q-Wave Coronary Events Study Group. *New Engl J Med* 337(7):447, 1997.

29. Antman EM, and the TIMI 11B Trial Investigators: TIMI 11B: Enoxaparin versus unfractionated heparin for unstable angina or non-Q-wave myocardial infarction: A double-blind, placebo-controlled, parallel-group, multicenter trial: Rationale, study design and methods. *Am Heart J* 135:S353, 1998.

30. PURSUIT Trial Investigators: Inhibition of of platelet glycoprotein IIb/IIIa with eptifibatide in patients with acute coronary syndromes. The PURSUIT Trial Investigators. Platelet Glycoprotein IIb/IIIa in Unstable Angina: Receptor Suppression Using Integrilin Therapy. *New Engl J Med* 339(7):436, 1998.

31. Assessment of the Safety and Efficacy of a New Thrombolytic Regimen (ASSENT-3) Investigators: Efficacy and safety of tenecteplase in combination with enoxaparin, abciximab, or unfractionated heparin: The ASSENT-3 randomized trial in acute myocardial infarction. *Lancet* 358:605, 2001.

11

Syncope

Jeffrey N. Glaspy

HIGH-YIELD FACTS

- The history alone is responsible for diagnosing the cause of syncope in approximately 50 percent of cases in which a diagnosis is established. The physical examination is responsible for an additional 20 percent. Taken together, the history and physical examination are by far the most valuable diagnostic tools.

- A cardiac etiology is responsible for 34 percent of syncopal events in the elderly. Elderly patients with a cardiac cause of syncope have a 19 percent chance of death over the following year compared with a 6 percent chance in those with a noncardiac cause of syncope.

- Although common in the young, vasovagal syncope is rare in the elderly, with a reported incidence of only 2 percent.

- The cause of syncope in the elderly is often multifactorial; therefore, it is often difficult to implicate a single factor in the etiology.

Syncope is defined as a sudden loss of consciousness, with loss of postural tone, from which the patient recovers spontaneously without resuscitative intervention. Like congestive heart failure, syncope is not a disease but rather a symptom of an underlying condition or disease causing decreased cerebral perfusion. Although syncope occurs in all age groups, it is particularly concerning in the elderly. The human body undergoes considerable physiologic changes with aging. These changes make the elderly patient more prone to syncope along with the morbidity associated with the syncopal events. Furthermore, the underlying etiology is often multifactorial and therefore is difficult to diagnose.

EPIDEMIOLOGY

Syncope accounts for approximately 3 percent of emergency department (ED) visits, whereas 2 to 6 percent of hospital admissions are for syncope or syncope-related injuries.[1–3] In a study of elderly institutionalized patients, the 1-year incidence was 6 percent, with a recurrence rate of 30 percent over the following 2 years.[4] Lipsitz[5] reports that elderly patients with cardiac syncope have a 19 percent chance of death over the next year. In elderly patients with noncardiac syncope, the risk of death was 6 percent. As the proportion of elderly in our population increases, coupled with the ever-expanding technology of medical interventions and the increasing cost of health care, the diagnostic and therapeutic workup of patients admitted for syncope will become an even greater burden to the health care system.

PATHOPHYSIOLOGY

Age-Related Changes

Regardless of etiology, the underlying pathophysiologic mechanism of syncope is a decrease in cerebral blood flow to the reticular activating system. The human brain requires a constant supply of glucose and oxygen. If this supply is extinguished for 5 to 15 seconds, loss of consciousness occurs.[6] Under normal conditions, cerebral blood flow is approximately 55 mL of blood per 100 g of brain tissue per minute.[7] Syncope occurs if blood flow decreases below 20 mL/100 g/min.[7]

Several important age-related changes make elderly patients more prone to syncope. Cerebral blood flow decreases about 25 percent with aging, primarily due to vascular stiffening and decreased cardiac output.[8] Vascular compliance decreases as elastin within the blood vessel wall fragments and calcifies.[9] This poor compliance inhibits coronary vascular dilatation and prevents the necessary increase in coronary perfusion during times of stress, such as exercise or tachyarrythmias.[10] Furthermore, cardiac output is decreased as myocytes undergo age-related hypertrophy.[11] This hypertrophy causes a decrease in cardiac distensibility, leading to poor diastolic function. Under these circumstances, the preload volume becomes critical for maintaining adequate ventricular filling.[12,13] Therefore, any condition that decreases preload, such as vasodilating medications, dehydration, or atrial fibrillation, may lead to syncope in these patients.

Elderly patients also undergo changes in their autonomic nervous and endocrine systems that predispose them to syncope. Despite having increased plasma norepinephrine levels, the older patient's beta-adrenergic response is blunted.[14,15] This decrease in β_1 response results in impaired cardiac acceleration and contractility. The decrease in β_2 response results in unopposed α_1 vasoconstriction that increases afterload. These factors combine to cause a decrease in cardiac output that results in greater susceptibility to syncope. Furthermore, the elderly patient has lower plasma rennin and aldosterone levels and increased atrial natriuretic peptide levels, which result in sodium wasting.[16] Elderly patients also have impaired thirst mechanisms, which may make them prone to dehydration.[17] These factors make the elderly susceptible to syncope due to orthostatic hypotension, especially under conditions of decreased intravascular volume, such as fever or diuretic use.[11]

The key element to the successful treatment of syncope is identification of the underlying cause of decreased cerebral perfusion. The following are the most common causes of syncope (Table 11-1).

Cardiac

Cardiac syncope is two times more prevalent in the elderly compared with the general population and carries a much more serious prognosis.[18] Patients with a cardiac cause of syncope have a 21 to 30 percent mortality rate compared with a 6 to 12 percent mortality rate if the cause is noncardiac or undetermined.[19,20] Cardiac etiology is responsible for 34 percent of syncopal events in the elderly population.[18] There are many different etiologies of cardiac syncope. One classification system is to divide these causes up into electrical and mechanical causes.

Electrical causes include tachyarrhythmias, bradyarrhythmias, atrioventricular (AV) node blocks, and pacemaker malfunction. In patients with cardiac syncope, Kapoor and colleagues[18] reported the etiology to be 46 percent ventricular arrhythmia, 17 percent sick sinus syndrome, and 8 percent heart block. Patients with syncope related to cardiac conduction often had no preceding symptoms, although a brief episode of palpitation may be reported. It is therefore difficult to exclude electrical dysfunction by history and physical examination alone. Furthermore, the incidence of arrhythmia and sick sinus syn-

Table 11-1. Etiology of Syncope

Cardiac	Orthostatic hypotension
Electrical causes	Hypovolemia
Tachydysrhythmias	Hemorrhage
Bradydysrhythmias	Medication-induced
AV blocks	Neurologic
Pacer malfunction	Stroke/posterior cerebral ischemia
Mechanical causes	Subclavian steal
Valvular disease	Subarachnoid hemorrhage
Myocardial infarction	Medications (see Table 11-2)
Tumor	Other causes
Cardiomyopathy	Pulmonary embolus
Pulmonary hypertension	Aortic dissection
Reflex-mediated	Constrictive pericarditis
Vasovagal (neurocardiogenic)	Abdominal aortic aneurysm
Situational	Hyperventilation
Cough	Psychiatric
Micturition	
Defecation	
Swallow	
Postprandial	
Carotid sinus hypersensitivity	

drome is increased by certain medications that are frequently prescribed to elderly patients.

Mechanical causes of cardiac syncope include valvular disease, cardiomyopathy, myocardial infarction (MI), pulmonary hypertension, and tumor. In general, the mechanical causes of syncope share the common characteristic of obstructing the circulation at a cardiac valve or a major vascular level.[21] The most common structural cause of syncope in the elderly is aortic stenosis. In elderly patients with cardiac syncope, 11 percent was due to aortic stenosis and 6 percent to MI.[18] Furthermore, syncope occurs in about 25 percent of patients with symptomatic aortic stenosis.[11] Due to a fixed cardiac output, these patients do not tolerate vasodilatation. Therefore, any mechanism that causes vasodilatation, such as medication, exercise, or a hot environment, may predispose these patients to syncope.[11]

Reflex-Mediated

Vasovagal, or neurocardiogenic, syncope is a common cause of syncope in younger patients but is relatively rare in the elderly. It occurs in response to a noxious stimuli or intense sympathetic stimulation of the heart, most often in the standing position.[21,22] Forceful contraction of the heart occurs, causing a stimulation of cardiac C-fibers, which in turn inhibit sympathetic outflow and increase parasympathetic outflow.[7,23,24] This leads to two major phases.[21] The first phase is characterized by a drop in systolic blood pressure, most commonly due to peripheral vasodilatation. The second phase consists of a paradoxical bradycardia, known as a *cardioinhibitory response*. Elderly patients have impaired parasympathetic innervation of the heart and therefore are at decreased risk for vasovagal syncope.[11] Kapoor and colleagues[18] reported a 2 percent incidence of vasovagal syncope in the elderly.

Situational syncope includes cough, micturition, defecation, swallow, and postprandial syncope. These syndromes all have the common mechanism of decreased preload that triggers a cardioinhibitory or vasodepressor reflex similar to that of vasovagal syncope.[11] Cough, micturition, defecation, and swallow all induce this reflex by simulating a Valsalva maneuver. Micturition syncope is especially common in elderly men with benign prostatic hypertrophy who awaken during the night and strain to urinate. This change to an upright posture combines with the Valsalva maneuver to decrease preload, resulting in syncope. Postprandial syncope likely occurs as blood pools in the splanchnic system after a meal. This condition is very common in the elderly, accounting for 8 per-

cent of syncopal events in one population of nursing home patients.[25] In another study, 36 percent of nursing home patients developed postprandial hypotension, with 2 percent becoming symptomatic.[26] Situational syncope remains a frequent cause of syncope in the elderly.

The final type of reflex-mediated syncope is carotid sinus hypersensitivity (CSH). This syndrome is characterized by an overly sensitive carotid sinus complex, which induces a vagally mediated cardioinhibitory or vasodepressor response.[21] It is defined as sinus slowing of more than 50 percent or a systolic blood pressure drop of more than 50 mmHg or to an absolute systolic blood pressure of less than 90 mmHg.[11] This condition is present in approximately 10 percent of elderly adults, but only 5 to 20 percent of these patients experience syncope.[27–29] There are three types of CSH.[11] In the first and most common type, known as the *cardioinhibitory* type, patients experience asystole for 3 seconds or more with carotid sinus massage. This type accounts for approximately 50 percent of cases.[30] In the second type, a *vasodepressor* response is elicited by carotid sinus massage. It is defined as a systolic blood pressure drop of 50 mmHg or more without corresponding bradycardia.[11] This syndrome is responsible for about 5 to 20 percent of cases.[2,30] The last of these types is the *mixed* type. These patients experience asystole for 2 seconds or more with a greater than 50 percent drop in systolic blood pressure.[31] Risk factors for CSH include male sex, advanced age, hypertension, coronary heart disease, head and neck malignancy, and certain medications, such as digoxin, methyldopa, beta blockers, or calcium channel blockers.[21,32–35] Diagnosis of this condition usually is elicited by careful history of events leading to the syncopal event and a positive response to carotid sinus massage. Patients may experience syncope while shaving, head turning, or wearing tight-fitting clothes such as neck ties. It is important to exclude other more serious causes before attributing the cause of syncope to CSH.

Orthostatic Hypotension

Orthostatic hypotension is a common cause of syncope in the elderly. In one study, 30 percent of community-dwelling persons age 75 or older had orthostatic hypotension.[36] This condition is defined as a systolic blood pressure drop of more than 20 mmHg or a diastolic drop of more than 10 mmHg with standing. The etiology is likely due to blood pooling in the lower extremities. On standing, the decrease in preload causes a decrease in cardiac output leading to decreased cerebral perfusion. In normal patients, aortic, carotid, and cardiopulmonary baroreceptors cause an increase in sympathetic and a decrease in parasympathetic output.[11] This in turn causes an increase in heart rate and a decrease in cerebral vascular resistance. Elderly patients are at increased risk for this condition because baroreceptor responsiveness decreases with aging.[21] Elderly patients also frequently use medications such as beta blockers, vasodilators, diuretics, and digoxin that inhibit the increase in heart rate or cause a decrease in intravascular volume. Older adults also have impaired thirst mechanisms and comorbid conditions that predispose them to dehydration, leading to a decrease in intravascular volume.

Neurologic Causes

Posterior cerebral circulation ischemia is an infrequent cause of syncope, but it does occur occasionally in the elderly. These patients generally experience other symptoms, such as vertigo, nausea, diplopia, dysarthria, or hemiparesis, prior to and after their syncopal episode.[11,35] Patients with large strokes generally have a prolonged loss of consciousness and therefore do not fit the classic definition of syncope. Nevertheless, this diagnosis should be suspected in any elderly patient with syncope and symptoms of posterior circulation ischemia.

Subclavian steal syndrome occurs when the lumen of the subclavian artery is narrowed prior to the origin of the vertebral artery. This narrowing causes decreased blood flow through the vertebral artery and shunting of blood into the arm, more commonly on the left side of the body. Patients with this condition often give a history of passing out while doing any activity in which their arms are raised for a period of time.[7,35] These activities include shaving, combing hair, painting, etc.

Another rare but serious cause of neurologic syncope is subarachnoid hemorrhage (SAH). Syncope occurs secondary to a sudden rise in intracranial pressure, which, in turn, lowers cerebral perfusion pressure.[7] As the blood diffuses throughout the subarachnoid space, patients may regain consciousness. This diagnosis should be considered in patients with syncope and symptoms consistent with SAH.

Medications

Patients 65 years of age or older have an average of 3.5 chronic medical conditions.[37] Therefore, they commonly are prescribed medications that may increase their susceptibility to syncope. The most common of these medications are listed in Table 11-2. In one study of nursing home patients, 11 percent of syncopal episodes were at-

Table 11-2. Medications Associated with Syncope

Antidysrhythmics
Anticonvulsants
Antidepressants
Antiparkinsonian medications
Antipsychotics
Benzodiazepines
Beta blockers
Calcium channel blockers
Cardiac glycosides
Diuretics
Hypnotics
H_2 blockers
MAO inhibitors
Nitrates
Phenothiazines

tributed to medication-induced hypotension, of which 75 percent involved nitrates.[4]

Other Causes

Other less frequent etiologies of syncope include pulmonary embolus (PE), aortic dissection, cardiac tumors, constrictive pericarditis, leaking abdominal aortic aneurysm, and psychiatric conditions.[7,35] It is therefore necessary to keep a broad differential diagnosis in the management of elderly patients with syncope.

CLINICAL FEATURES
Prehospital Considerations

The history of events surrounding a patient's syncopal episode remains the most important indicator of etiology. It is therefore important for emergency medical service (EMS) providers to question witnesses carefully to aid in diagnosis. EMS personnel must balance the importance of rapid transport with the benefit for continued data gathering. Family members and friends who witnessed the event should be encouraged to find safe transport to the ED for further questioning.

Elderly patients with syncope have a higher morbidity and mortality when compared with younger individuals. These patients commonly experience trauma with syncope-related falls. These secondary injuries must be identified and managed accordingly. Cardiac and serious neurologic causes are also more common in these patients. Therefore, intravenous access should be established and continuous cardiac monitoring with supplemental oxygen provided during transport. If the EMS system has electrocardiographic capabilities, a 12-lead electrocardiogram (ECG) should be obtained, provided that it does not delay transport time significantly. If SAH is suspected, elevation of the head of the bed to 30 degrees may aid in lowering intracranial pressure.

History

The history of events surrounding the syncopal episode is often the most vital part of the evaluation. The history provides the diagnosis in 50 percent of the cases in which a cause can be determined.[11] What was the patient doing at the time he or she lost consciousness? A rapid rise after prolonged recumbence may point to orthostatic hypotension as the cause. Shaving, combing hair, or working with the arms above the head may indicate subclavian steal. Wearing a tight-fitting collar or turning of the head may indicate carotid sinus hypersensitivity. Urination, defecation, stress, pain, cough, swallow, and postprandial syncope are all recognized syndromes that may be elicited by careful history.

Associated symptoms and the patient's position at the time of syncope are also important factors. Chest pain, palpitations, dyspnea, and diaphoresis should increase suspicion for a cardiac cause or a PE. Headache, vertigo, dizziness, or nausea may indicate a neurologic cause. Lack of prodrome is indicative of a cardiac cause or a conduction system abnormality. It is important to note that many patients with syncope experience short episodes of myoclonic shaking or twitching.[7] These episodes usually last for less than 8 to 10 seconds and do not represent seizure. Witnesses, including EMS providers, should be questioned about the postictal phase to aid in differentiation from true seizure. Syncope in a recumbent position raises concern of cardiac etiology and essentially rules out orthostatic hypotension.

An attempt should be made to determine the duration of symptoms. A rapid resolution of symptoms with no residual may suggest a cardiac or conduction system cause.[11] Risk-factor assessment for coronary artery disease is also important. Approximately 6 percent of myocardial infarctions (MIs) have syncope as the presenting symptom, and ventricular arrhythmias are more likely to occur in patients with coronary artery disease.[11]

A list of current medications, including over-the-counter preparations, should be obtained. Recent addition, cessation, or alteration in dose may result in syncope. Any recent complaints or changes in health should be sought. Recent headache, chest pain, vomiting, diarrhea, bloody stools, or change in diet may suggest a potential cause for syncope.

Physical Examination

The physical examination is responsible for the diagnosis in approximately 20 percent of cases in which a cause for syncope can be found.[11] Taken together, the history and physical examination are by far the most valuable tools in establishing the etiology of syncope.

On initial inspection, patients with a chief complaint of syncope often have a completely normal general appearance. They often are totally asymptomatic and in no acute distress on presentation. They may be able to give an accurate account of events leading up to their syncope and everything that has occurred after they regained consciousness. The general appearance may be misleading because even patients with potentially life-threatening causes of syncope may look remarkably normal. Patients may, however, appear in acute distress, especially if a significant, life-threatening condition is ongoing, such as MI, arrhythmia, SAH, or PE.

Although a detailed physical examination is essential, particular attention should be given to the cardiovascular and neurologic systems. The cardiac examination should include palpation for apical impulse and regularity of rhythm and auscultation for intensity of the first and second heart sounds and presence of murmurs, gallops, or rubs. The vascular examination should include inspection of carotid upstroke, palpation of peripheral versus central pulse, and auscultation for carotid bruits. The neurologic examination should include assessment of mental status, cranial nerves, strength, sensation, visual fields, deep tendon reflexes, and cerebellar function. Identification of any acute deficit may indicate serious neurologic pathology.

Other components of the physical examination that deserve mention include the rectal examination for occult blood in stool, abdominal examination for a pulsatile mass, assessment of the skin and mucous membranes for hydration status, and examination for any evidence of trauma. Although carotid sinus massage may indicate an etiology for syncope, it remains somewhat controversial in elderly patients. Carotid sinus massage is absolutely contraindicated in patients with a carotid bruit or a history of stroke syndromes. In elderly patients, this maneuver is best left undone until plaques are excluded by carotid Doppler ultrasound. Although this is a conservative stance, the potential implications of a missed bruit and resulting plaque embolus are devastating.

Vital Signs

Evaluation of vital signs, including blood pressure determination in both arms, is essential. Frequent reassessment of vital signs is important, especially if the patient experiences any change in cardiac rhythm or frequency of ectopic foci. Orthostatic blood pressure determination may be helpful if an orthostatic cause is likely and serious cardiac or structural abnormality is unlikely. It is important to remember that many elderly patients have orthostatic hypotension and never experience syncope. Therefore, it is essential to search for and exclude other causes prior to making a diagnosis of orthostatic hypotension in an elderly patient.

DIAGNOSIS AND DIFFERENTIAL

Differential Diagnosis

Seizure remains in the differential diagnosis of syncope. Occasionally, differentiation between syncope and seizure is not possible. In these circumstances, a thorough workup for both conditions is essential. In most instances, however, the differentiation is possible with a detailed history. Any patient who fails to regain consciousness without intervention or has continued altered sensorium does not fit the classic definition of syncope. Conditions such as hypoglycemia, carbon monoxide poisoning, and narcotic overdose usually do not reverse without intervention and therefore do not fit the definition of syncope.

Laboratory Testing

If the history and physical examination point to a benign condition, such as situational or vasovagal syncope, laboratory testing is unnecessary. In general, laboratory testing is of little yield in any patient with syncope.[11] However, due to elderly patients' comorbidity, higher incidence of cardiac syncope, and often multifactorial etiology, laboratory testing in this population may be more useful. Basic laboratory workup includes a complete blood count and determinations of electrolytes (including calcium and magnesium) and cardiac enzymes (if MI remains in the differential).[38] Specific drug levels, such as digoxin, anticonvulsants, lithium, and antiarrhythmics, should be checked in patients taking them. A finger-stick glucose determination is warranted if hypoglycemia is suspected or if the patient has a neurologic abnormality or altered mental status. A urinalysis may be helpful because elderly patients are at increased risk for urinary tract infection and urosepsis. Other tests, such as plasma norepinephrine level, adrenal function tests, and autonomic function tests, should be reserved for the primary care and consulting services.

Ancillary Testing

All patients presenting to the ED with syncope should have a 12-lead ECG.[11,31] This is especially true in the elderly population. The ECG aids in diagnosis of MI, cardiac ischemia, and arrhythmia. Furthermore, elderly patients should be placed on continuous cardiac monitoring until a cardiac etiology of syncope has been excluded. A chest radiograph is warranted in patients with suspected cardiac etiology, new abnormalities on physical examination, or dyspnea and if the patient has not had a chest radiograph in the last 5 years.[21] A chest radiograph may aid in diagnosis of cardiomyopathy, aortic dissection, and rarely, in PE. Computed tomographic (CT) scanning of the head is almost never diagnostic and therefore should be obtained only if SAH or stroke is suspected.[31]

Echocardiogram is essential in the workup of patients with suspected structural cardiac abnormality, such as valvular disease, constrictive pericarditis, or cardiac tamponade.[11] Echocardiogram should be performed emergently in unstable patients with physical examination findings consistent with structural heart disease. This rapid bedside test yields valuable diagnostic information without subjecting these patients to the risk of leaving the ED.

Tilt-table testing may be helpful in establishing a vasovagal or neurally mediated cause of syncope.[11,21] Although helpful, such testing is not part of the immediate ED management and should be reserved for patients without structural cardiac abnormality.[21]

The electrophysiologic study (EPS) is an important tool for risk stratification and management of patients with unexplained syncope or in elderly patients with underlying organic heart disease, recurrent syncope, and a negative noninvasive workup.[11,39] In patients of all ages, the 3-year mortality with an abnormal EPS is approximately 60 percent, compared with a 15 percent mortality in patients with a normal EPS.[39] EPS testing, although not part of the ED workup, is a valuable tool for diagnosis and risk stratification in elderly patients with syncope of unexplained origin.

Ambulatory electrocardiography (Holter monitoring or loop recording) is indicated in elderly patients with an uncertain cause and a possible structural cardiac etiology of syncope.[21] Holter monitoring constantly records cardiac electrical activity, usually for a period of 24 hours. In contrast, loop recorders record over previous data unless activated by the patient to store data. For this reason, Holter monitors are useful if patients have no warning signs with their syncope or if symptoms occur very frequently.[40] Loop recorders are more useful in patients who experience prodromal symptoms, especially if these symptoms occur infrequently. The utility of prolonged outpatient ambulatory monitoring remains controversial.[40–42]

EMERGENCY DEPARTMENT CARE AND DISPOSITION

The elderly patient with syncope should be placed at high priority on presentation to the ED. Hemodynamic parameters, cardiac monitoring, intravenous access, and ECG should be obtained immediately. Any suspected unstable condition, such as arrhythmia, heart block, MI, PE, SAH, or stroke, should take precedence and be managed accordingly. Transcutaneous pacer pads should be placed if second- or third-degree heart block is diagnosed. In patients with an unstable cardiac rhythm, emergent electrical cardioversion must be performed.

In stable patients, a thorough history and physical examination should be undertaken, assessing for a specific etiology of syncope as well as resulting trauma. Appropriate laboratory and ancillary studies should be ordered. Hospital admission is required for any elderly patient with underlying cardiovascular disease or unknown cause of syncope.[11] It is important to remember that elderly patients often have a multifactorial cause of syncope; therefore, a low threshold for admission is warranted. Patients with a benign cause of syncope, such as situational syncope, may be discharged safely. It is important to educate these patients about ways to avoid future syncope. These precautions include sitting down to urinate, avoiding restrictive clothes, resting supine immediately after meals, and avoiding large carbohydrate meals and alcohol. It is essential to refer patients to their primary care physician for close follow-up.

ADDITIONAL ASPECTS

The following are common pitfalls in the management of syncope in geriatric patients:

- *Failure to recognize the often multifactorial nature of syncope in the elderly.* A thorough search for the etiology of syncope is necessary, even if the cause initially seems obvious.

- *Failure to complete a thorough history and physical examination.* Relying solely on laboratory data during the workup of a patient with syncope would be an error.

- *The belief that elderly patients who experience a syncopal episode should be automatically admitted into the hospital.* After a complete workup, if the etiology of syncope is obvious and benign, then the patient may be discharged with appropriate instructions and precautions.

REFERENCES

1. Day SC, Cook EF, Funkenstein H, et al: Evaluation and outcome of emergency room patients with transient loss of consciousness. *Am J Med.* 73:15, 1982.
2. Kapoor WN: Syncope in older persons. *J Am Geriat Soc.* 42:426, 1994.
3. Lipsitz LA: Syncope in the elderly patient. *Hosp Pract* 21:33, 1986.
4. Lipsitz L, Wei JY, Rowe JW: Syncope in an elderly, institutionalized population: Prevalence, incidence and associated risk. *Q J Med* 55:45, 1985.
5. Lipsitz LA: Syncope in the elderly. *Ann Intern Med.* 99(1):92, 1983.
6. Kapoor WN: Hypotension and syncope, in Braunwald E (ed): *Heart Disease: A Textbook of Cardiovascular Medicine,* 4th ed. Philadelphia, W.B. Saunders, 1992, p 875.
7. Hunt M: Syncope, in Rosen P, Barkin R (eds): *Emergency Medicine Concepts and Clinical Practice,* 4th ed. St Louis, Mosby–Year Book, 1998, p 1570.
8. Scheinberg P, Blackburn I, Saslaw RM: Effects of aging on cerebral circulation and metabolism. *Arch Neurol Psychiatry* 70:77, 1953.
9. Lakatta EG: Cardiovascular regulatory mechanisms in advanced age. *Physiol Rev* 73:413, 1993.
10. Wei JY: Age and the cardiovascular system. *New Engl J Med.* 327:1735, 1992.
11. Forman DE, Lipsitz LA: Syncope in the elderly. *Cardiol Clin* 15(2):295, 1997.
12. Bryg RJ, Williams GA, Labovitz AJ: Effect of aging on left ventricular function diastolic filling in normal subjects. *Am J Cardiol* 59:971, 1987.
13. Miyatake K, Okamoto M, Kinoshita N, et al: Augmentation of atrial contribution to left ventricular inflow with aging as assessed by intracardiac Doppler flowmetry. *Am J Cardiol* 53:586, 1984.
14. Morrow LA, Linares OA, Hill TJ, et al: Age differences in plasma clearance mechanisms for epinephrine and norepinephrine in humans. *J Clin Endocrinol Metab* 65:508, 1987.
15. Supiano MA, Linares OA, Smith MJ, et al: Age-related difference in norepinephrine kinetics: Effect of posture and sodium-restricted diet. *Am J Physiol* 259:E422, 1990.

16. Haller BG, Zust H, Shaw S, et al: Effects of posture and ageing on circulating atrial natriuretic peptide levels in man. *J Hypertens* 5:551, 1987.

17. Phillips PA, Phil D, Rolls BJ, el al: Reduced thirst after water deprivation in healthy elderly men. *New Engl J Med* 311:753, 1984.

18. Kapoor WN, Snustad D, Peterson J: Syncope in the elderly. *Am J Med* 80:419, 1986.

19. Kapoor WN, Karpf M, Wieand S, et al: A prospective evaluation and follow-up of patients with syncope. *New Engl J Med* 309:197, 1983.

20. Eagle KA, Black HR, Cook EF, et al: Evaluation of prognostic classifications for patients with syncope. *Am J Med* 79:455, 1985.

21. Farrehi PM, Santinga JT, Eagle KA: Syncope: Diagnosis of cardiac and noncardiac causes. *Geriatrics* 50(11):24, 1995.

22. Shalev Y, Gal R, Tchou P, et al: Echocardiographic demonstration of decreased left ventricular dimensions and vigorous myocardial contraction during syncope induced by head upright tilt. *J Am Coll Cardiol* 18:746, 1991.

23. Mark AL: The Bezold-Jarisch reflex revisited: Clinical implications of inhibitory reflexes originating in the heart. *J Am Coll Cardiol* 1:90, 1983.

24. Thoren P: Role of cardiac vagal C-fibers in cardiovascular control. *Rev Physiol Biochem Pharmacol* 86:1, 1979.

25. Lipsitz LA, Pluchino FC, Wei JY, et al: Syncope in institutionalized elderly: The impact of multiple pathologic conditions and situational stress. *J Chron Dis* 39:619, 1986.

26. Vaitkevicius PV, Esserwein DM, Maynard, AK, et al: Frequency and importance of postprandial blood pressure reduction in elderly nursing-home patients. *Ann Intern Med* 115:865, 1991.°

27. Morley CA, Sutton R: Carotid sinus syncope. *Int J Cardiol* 6:287, 1984.

28. Wenthick JRM, Jansen RWMM, Hoefnagels WHL: The influence of age on the response of blood pressure and heart rate to carotid sinus massage in healthy volunteers. *Cardiol Elderly* 1:453, 1993.

29. McIntosh SJ, de Costa D, Lawson J, et al: Heart rate and blood pressure responses to carotid sinus massage in healthy elderly subjects. *Age Aging* 23:57, 1994.

30. Schellack J, Fulenwider JT, Olson, RA, et al: The carotid sinus syndrome: A frequently overlooked cause of syncope in the elderly. *J Vasc Surg* 4(4):376, 1986.

31. Olsky M, Murray J: Dizziness and fainting in the elderly. *Emerg Med Clin North Am* 8(2):295, 1990.

32. Reyes AJ: Propranolol and the hyperactive carotid sinus reflexsyndrome. *Br Med J* 2:662, 1973.

33. Quest JA, Gillis RA: Effect of digitalis on carotid sinus baroreceptor activity. *Circ Res* 35:247, 1974.

34. Bauerfiend X, Hall d, Denes P, et al: Carotid sinus hypersensitivity with alpha methyldopa. *Ann Intern Med* 88:214, 1978.

35. Blok BA: Syncope, in Tintinalli JE (ed): *Emergency Medicine: A Comprehensive Study Guide,* 5th ed. New York, McGraw-Hill, 2000.

36. Caird FI, Andrews GR, Kennedy RD, et al: Effect of posture on blood pressure in the elderly. *Br Heart J* 35:527, 1973.

37. Besdine RW: Geriatric medicine: An overview. *Annu Rev Gerontol* 1:135, 1980.

38. Haddad RM, Sellers TD: Syncope as a symptom: A practical approach to etiologic diagnosis. *Psotgad Med* 79:48, 1986.

39. Bass, EB, Elson JJ, Fogoros RN, et al: Long-term prognosis of patients undergoing electrophysiologic studies for syncope of unknown origin. *Am J Cardiol* 62:1186, 1988.

40. Linzer M, Pritchett ELC, Pontinen M, et al: Incremental diagnostic yield of loop electrocardiographic recorders in unexplained syncope. *Am J Cardiol* 66:214, 1990.

41. Bass EB, Curtiss EI, Arena VC, et al: The duration of Holter monitoring in patients with syncope: Is 24 hours long enough? *Arch Intern Med* 150:1073, 1990.

42. Gibson TC, Heitzman MR: Diagnostic efficacy of 24-hour electrocardiographic monitoring for syncope. *Am J Cardiol* 53:1013, 1984.

12

Heart Failure

Benjamin J. Freda
W. Franklin Peacock, IV

HIGH-YIELD FACTS

- The prevalence of heart failure roughly doubles each decade, with nearly 10 percent of elderly persons affected by age 80.
- Natriuretic peptides have a beneficial hemodynamic profile of decreasing systemic vascular resistance, pulmonary capillary wedge pressure, right atrial pressure, and mean arterial pressure.
- Patients with diastolic dysfunction are preload-dependent, and the use of excessive diuresis or venodilatation may exacerbate the underlying deficit in ventricular filling, resulting in hypotension.
- The pharmacologic treatment of heart failure should be similar among the elderly and the general population.

Heart failure is a clinical syndrome characterized by an inability of the heart to meet the metabolic demands of the body. Cardiac filling pressures are increased in an attempt to augment cardiac output. In the absence of medical therapy, this increase in cardiac filling pressure often leads to respiratory symptoms and systemic fluid overload.

Heart failure may manifest as primarily systolic or diastolic dysfunction. A normal ejection fraction is defined as 60 percent. Some patients develop pure diastolic heart failure, in which they maintain a normal left ventricular ejection fraction. Diastolic heart failure may be the most common type of heart failure in elderly patients. Older age, female gender, and history of chronic hypertension are strongly associated with diastolic heart failure. Systolic heart failure is defined as an ejection fraction of less than 40 percent. Patients with systolic heart failure frequently have some degree of diastolic dysfunction. The distinction between pure diastolic and systolic heart failure has important therapeutic implications.

In the era of potent vasodilator and loop diuretic therapy, heart failure also can present without congestive manifestations of fluid overload. Therefore, it may be reasonable to avoid the term *congestive*. The terms *acute decompensated* or *chronic diastolic* or *systolic heart failure* should help clinicians tailor appropriate therapies to the different presentations of heart failure.

EPIDEMIOLOGY

With incidence and prevalence being age-dependent, heart failure is primarily a disorder of the elderly.[1] The prevalence of heart failure roughly doubles each decade, with nearly 10 percent of elderly persons affected by age 80,[2] and the number of people affected by this disorder will increase disproportionately as our population ages. Currently, heart failure is the most common reason for hospital admission among patients older than 65 years of age, and repeat hospitalization is common.[3,4]

Despite the use of pharmacotherapy known to target disease progression, the overall prognosis of heart failure is extremely poor. One-year mortality as high as 38 percent[5] makes this disorder as malignant as many oncologic disorders. Age is a powerful independent risk factor; 1-year mortality increases 2.8 percent per year of life.[5] Prognosis is also related to symptoms. Elderly New York Heart Association (NYHA) class IV heart failure (Table 12-1) patients have a 1-year mortality exceeding 50 percent.[6] Up to 85 percent of patients who present in cardiogenic shock die within 1 week.

PATHOPHYSIOLOGY

The development of heart failure is not a "normal" part of the aging process. Indeed, the ejection fraction is not reduced in otherwise healthy elderly subjects.[8] However, the aging cardiovascular system does undergo important changes in structure and function. How much of these changes are related to "normal aging" and how much result from concomitant diseases (e.g., atherosclerosis, diabetes, or hypertension) is controversial. Nevertheless, the aging heart is prone to changes that may leave it at a greater risk for the development of both systolic heart failure and heart failure with preserved systolic function (diastolic heart failure).

Normotensive patients experience a mild increase in left ventricular wall thickness with age,[9] but this is much

Table 12-1. New York Heart Association Class

Class	Limitations	Daily Living Symptoms	BNPL (pg/ml)
I	No limitation	Asymptomatic during usual daily activities	100
II	Slight limitation	Mild symptoms during ordinary daily activities	200
III	Moderate limitation	Symptoms noted with minimal activities	450
IV	Severe limitation	Symptoms present even at rest	>1000

more pronounced in the elderly with systemic hypertension. Although fibrous tissue may develop in the older heart, the primary mechanism for the increase in left ventricular thickness is myocyte hypertrophy.[10] Age-related changes also occur throughout the vascular tree. The arterial wall intima thickens, and more fibrous tissue appears in the tunica media.[11] Additionally, there is an age-related decrease in vascular compliance. These and other changes contribute to important functional changes in the geriatric heart, such as impaired ventricular relaxation and increased left ventricular wall stiffness. Most important, the aging heart has less functional reserve. Although the reason for this is multifactorial, attenuated intrinsic contractility plays a primary role. The elderly heart is particularly susceptible to "fail" during times of hemodynamic stress, such as ischemia, excess salt load, and the development of arrhythmias.

The most striking age-related change in cardiovascular function is a decrease in early diastolic filling.[9] Consequently, in order to maintain adequate ventricular filling (preload), the older heart becomes dependent on late diastolic filling. Late diastolic filling is provided by atrial contraction. Therefore, the elderly patient with a loss of atrial contraction is particularly sensitive to atrial fibrillation because the heart may not have adequate time to fill, and pulmonary congestion can develop.

Beyond the acute presentation, heart failure is predominately an endocrine disease. The driving force behind the pathophysiology of heart failure is the activation of a neurohormonal cascade resulting in further cardiac and vascular damage. While the initiating event is obvious in a patient with a large anterior myocardial infarction, in some patients, multiple subclinical insults are responsible for the myocardial injury. Specific to the elderly, heart failure may be accompanied by or partially the result of valvular diseases (e.g., calcific aortic stenosis or mitral regurgitation).[2] Regardless of the origin, once a critical portion of myocardium is injured or stressed, neurohormonal reflex activation occurs to counter the consequences of impaired myocardial func-

tion. Neurohormonal activation includes increases in the activity of the sympathetic nervous system and renin-angiotensin-aldosterone system and augmented release of endothelin (one of the most potent vasoconstrictors). These pathways are activated in an attempt to maintain circulatory integrity and adequate arterial pressure. They remain active during chronic heart failure and result in systemic vasoconstriction, increased afterload, fluid retention, cardiac interstitial fibrosis, and myocyte hypertrophy. Accordingly, the most effective therapies for chronic heart failure [e.g., beta blockers, angiotensin-converting enzyme (ACE) inhibitors, and spironolactone] are aimed at attenuating these neurohormonal pathways.

Natriuretic Peptides

The natriuretic peptides are a group of hormones released by the myocardium in response to increased chamber volumes and pressures. A-type natriuretic peptide is released predominately from the atria, B-type from the ventricle, and C-type from the vascular endothelium. Natriuretic peptides are the endogenous counterregulatory effectors that balance the consequences of increases in the sympathetic nervous and renin-angiotensin-aldosterone systems. Natriuretic peptides cause arterial, venous, and coronary artery vasodilatation and increase diuresis and urinary sodium losses. Natriuretic peptides have a beneficial hemodynamic profile of decreasing systemic vascular resistance, pulmonary capillary wedge pressure, right atrial pressure, and mean arterial pressure.

Diastolic Heart Failure

Diastolic dysfunction refers to a pathophysiologic process in which the left ventricle has difficulty receiving blood. The prevalence of diastolic dysfunction increases with age. Chronic systemic hypertension, with the development of left ventricular hypertrophy, is often responsible for this syndrome. Coronary artery disease also contributes because diastolic dysfunction is an early event in the ischemic cascade. In diastolic failure, systolic function is preserved such that the ejection fraction may be normal or higher but with an abnormal diastolic pressure-volume relationship. The primary pathologic abnormality is impaired ventricular relaxation. The decrease in left ventricular compliance from impaired myocardial relaxation necessitates higher atrial pressures to ensure adequate diastolic filling of the left ventricle.

As many as 30 to 50 percent of heart failure patients have circulatory congestion on the basis of diastolic dysfunction.[12] When congested, treatment for volume overload is the same as in systolic dysfunction. However, patients with diastolic dysfunction are preload-dependent, and the use of excessive diuresis or venodilation may exacerbate the underlying deficit in ventricular filling, resulting in hypotension. Ultimately, after the hemodynamic status has been stabilized and congestion resolved, treatment of diastolic dysfunction is directed at the underlying etiology.

Cardiogenic Shock

Cardiogenic shock is defined clinically as a state of decreased cardiac output with evidence of tissue hypoperfusion despite adequate intravascular volume.[13] The etiology of cardiogenic shock is usually a large myocardial infarction; other causes include septic shock with myocardial depression, pericardial tamponade, left ventricular outflow tract obstruction (e.g., aortic stenosis), myocarditis, the mechanical complications of myocardial infarction (e.g., ventricular septal defect, acute mitral regurgitation, myocardial free wall rupture), and end-stage cardiomyopathy.

The pathophysiology of cardiogenic shock is a result of progressive myocardial dysfunction from impaired myocardial perfusion.[13] In cardiogenic shock, a critical amount of functioning myocardial tissue is lost secondary to ischemia or infarction. As a result, cardiac output is decreased, and in an attempt to compensate for decreased stroke volume, tachycardia develops. The combination of hypotension and tachycardia drastically reduces coronary artery flow by decreasing perfusion pressure and diastolic filling time (when the majority of coronary flow takes place). This results in further ischemia and myocardial dysfunction.

Acute Pulmonary Edema

Acute pulmonary edema is characterized by pulmonary fluid overload. It may be cardiogenic in nature (i.e., secondary to increased left ventricular filling pressures) or noncardiogenic (i.e., secondary to renal failure). The development of acute pulmonary edema is best understood as a downward spiral of events resulting in progressive myocardial dysfunction that highlights the failing heart's exquisite sensitivity to increased afterload. The spiral starts when an individual with baseline left ventricular dysfunction (diastolic or systolic) experiences an additional myocardial stressor such as development of arrhythmia, uncontrolled hypertension, salt excess, ischemia, or a new or worsening valvular lesion. Filling pressures are increased, the myocardium is unable to compensate, and hence pulmonary congestion and dyspnea result. Catecholamine levels and vascular resistance are increased. This results in increases in blood pressure and afterload, further left ventricular dysfunction, and progressive increases in filling pressures with more pulmonary congestion. Diastolic dysfunction is present in the majority of patients presenting with hypertensive pulmonary edema.[14]

Heart failure is a heterogeneous syndrome with different etiologies, manifestations, and clinical presentations (Table 12-2). Some patients present to the emergency department (ED) in extremis with acute pulmonary edema or cardiogenic shock from a new myocardial infarction. Other patients present with a decompensation of known heart failure with symptoms of low cardiac output in the absence of systemic or pulmonary congestion. While cardiogenic shock and acute pulmonary edema can be more difficult to stabilize and treat, they are the more easily diagnosed of the heart failure presentations. The more protean types of heart failure presentations offer more diagnostic challenges, especially if a previous diagnosis of heart failure is not established. For example, the differential diagnosis is extensive in elderly patients presenting with symptoms of weakness, fatigue, dyspnea, or generalized failure to thrive, and the clinician must include heart failure in the differential diagnosis in such patients.

Table 12-2. Clinical Presentations of Heart Failure

Decompensation of known heart failure with congestive complaints

Low cardiac output complaints (i.e., fatigue) in the absence of congestion

Acute pulmonary edema with pure diastolic dysfunction

Acute pulmonary edema with mixed (systolic and diastolic) dysfunction

Cardiogenic shock (heart failure and systemic hypoperfusion)

CLINICAL FEATURES

A targeted history should be obtained from the patient, family, or emergenct medical services (EMS) provider. It should focus initially on the past medical history, signs or symptoms of myocardial ischemia, cardiac arrhythmia, infection, or thromboembolic disease. On stabilization of the patient, further questioning can be directed at salt intake, medicine compliance, alcohol or drug use, and recent changes in medical regimen. The patient also should be questioned regarding the use of negative inotropic agents, digitalis, and any over-the-counter or herbal medicines.

In the elderly, classic symptoms of heart failure (exertional dyspnea, fatigue, orthopnea) are neither sensitive nor specific.[2,6] Many patients may be sedentary and restricted by other conditions (arthritis, pulmonary or vascular disease) that limit the expression of exertional symptoms. The older patient with heart failure may complain mainly of nonspecific symptoms, such as generalized fatigue, nausea, anorexia, nocturia, or cough. Depression is also common among elderly patients with heart failure, and its presence is independently associated with a poor prognosis.[15] The emergency physician must have a high index of suspicion for the diagnosis of heart failure in older patients, especially in the presence of risk factors such as hypertension, coronary artery disease, or diabetes.

The emergency physician should perform an initial physical examination focused on the cardiopulmonary systems. Careful auscultation for murmurs of left ventricular outflow tract obstruction (aortic stenosis and hypertrophic cardiomyopathy) should be performed early in the evaluation. These cardiac lesions often require specialized care to avoid aggressive preload and afterload reduction with diuretics and vasodilators.

In elderly patients, there are significant limitations to the value of some physical examination findings commonly related to heart failure.[2,6] In the aged, the presence of lower extremity edema, pulmonary rales, or S_3/S_4 gallops is neither sensitive nor specific. Elderly patients frequently have ankle edema or pulmonary rales for reasons other than heart failure (e.g., venous insufficiency, atelectasis, chronic lung disease).[16] An S_4 gallop may be heard in clinically stable older patients with hypertension and is not helpful in the diagnosis of acute heart failure.[2] In patients with chronic heart failure, physical examination findings suggestive of congestion are poorly predictive of high pulmonary capillary wedge pressure.[17] Examination of respiration may reveal a Cheyne-Stokes pattern with alternating periods of apnea and hyperventi-

lation. However, such a pattern also may be seen in other disorders such as respiratory infections and cerebral vascular disorders.

Regardless of the concern for inaccuracy of the physical examination for findings of congestion, the emergency physician should use this information as part of the overall assessment. Indeed, a patient with hypotension, dyspnea, pulmonary rales, tachycardia, decreased mental status, and cool extremities has cardiogenic shock until proven otherwise. Examination of the lower extremities for calf tenderness, venous cords, or size asymmetry is important. Asymmetric adventitious breath sounds may point to a diagnosis of pneumonia or pneumothorax.

Once the patient is stabilized, the emergency physician must answer two important questions: (1) Is the patient presenting with signs and symptoms that can be attributed to heart failure? and (2) If heart failure is responsible for the patient's clinical syndrome, then what factor(s) are responsible for its development or recurrence?

DIAGNOSIS AND DIFFERENTIAL

There is no single radiographic, clinical, or laboratory test that always establishes the diagnosis of heart failure. It is therefore incumbent on the emergency physician to use information taken from the patient's risk factors, physical examination, and radiographic or laboratory results to establish the diagnosis of heart failure.

Electrocardiogram

In the acute setting of possible decompensated heart failure, obtaining an electrocardiogram (ECG) is needed to help exclude acute myocardial infarction. In the nonacute patient, the ECG is a useful tool to suggest the presence of underlying structural heart disease, such as left ventricular hypertrophy, atrial enlargement, or previous myocardial infarction. Arrhythmias and conduction abnormalities also may be found, and the ECG may suggest other underlying noncardiac disorders, such as emphysema (right-axis deviation, right bundle-branch block, low voltage) or pulmonary embolism (right-sided heart strain). However, neither the presence nor the absence of electrocardiographic abnormalities proves or excludes the diagnosis of heart failure. In patients with systolic dysfunction, the resting ECG is insensitive and nonspecific for identifying severe underlying coronary artery disease.

Chest Radiograph

Chest radiographs should be performed on all patients presenting with possible heart failure. This radiographic test is useful in identifying pulmonary congestion, pleural effusion, and cardiomegaly and may suggest the presence of other pulmonary (e.g., emphysema, pneumothorax, and pneumonia) or vascular diseases (e.g., aortic aneurysm or dissection). However, it is not a useful tool for excluding heart failure. Chest radiograph findings may lag as long as 6 hours, and patients with an acute presentation may have no evidence of cardiomegaly. In one study, the chest radiograph failed to detect pulmonary congestion in 53 percent of patients with chronic heart failure and a pulmonary capillary wedge pressure of 16 to 29 mmHg.[17] Although a large cardiothoracic ratio on the chest radiograph is predictive of a higher 5-year mortality rate,[12] the chest radiograph may miss as much as 20 percent of echocardiographically proven cardiomegaly.[18] Finally, although portable chest radiographs are convenient and used commonly in the ED, this technique worsens the sensitivity and specificity for the detection of pleural effusion and infiltrates.

Laboratory Studies

Underlying coronary artery disease is one of the most common comorbidities in elderly heart failure patients. Consequently, determinations of cardiac markers of ischemia (troponin I or T, CK-MB) are needed in all patients presenting to the ED with suspected decompensated heart failure. As many as 14 percent of patients with decompensated heart failure will have diagnostic cardiac markers,[19] and when these markers are elevated, these patients suffer acute adverse outcomes statistically identical to the non-heart failure cohort.[20] Consequently, patients with these markers represent a subgroup with increased risk of morbidity and mortality.

Arterial blood gase determinations are useful if the patient is at risk for CO_2 retention. They are not usually required unless there is acute pulmonary edema or cardiogenic shock. Metabolic acidosis also may suggest early or occult cardiogenic shock on the basis of inadequate peripheral perfusion. Patients with hypercarbia and heart failure should be observed closely (preferably in the intensive care unit) for impending respiratory failure.

Determination of brain natriuretic peptide (BNP) is currently available as a bedside test that takes 15 minutes to perform on whole blood. It is used to assist in the determination of elevated intracardiac pressures and can be considered a serum approximation of the pulmonary capillary wedge pressure. Physiologic levels may be as high as 3500 pg/mL; however, abnormal is defined as exceeding 100 pg/mL. BNP levels correlate with NYHA class (see Table 12-1). Aging does increase endogenous BNP levels, possibly due to increased ventricular stiffness resulting in increased left ventricular pressures, but this has not been reported to exceed the recommended cutoff of the test. Because increased left ventricular stretch or pressure results in increased BNP levels, conditions associated with this hemodynamic finding result in non-heart failure elevations of BNP. Elevated pressures occur in fluid overload states (e.g., renal failure requiring dialysis or liver failure with ascites), cardiac flow impairment conditions (e.g., a large pulmonary embolus), and other etiologies where elevated intracardiac pressure occurs secondarily to another pathology (e.g., primary pulmonary hypertension or left ventricular hypertrophy from chronic hypertension). The currently available BNP assay has a negative predictive value of 95 to 99 percent and a positive predictive value of 85 to 95 percent.[21] Therefore, if the BNP is negative, the patient is extremely unlikely to have heart failure. However, if the BNP is positive, heart failure is likely but must be confirmed by other testing.

Electrolytes need to checked because treatment with diuretics may produce hypokalemia and hypomagnesemia. Although rare, hypophosphatemia and hypocalcemia are potentially reversible causes of heart failure. Creatinine and blood urea nitrogen (BUN) levels can be abnormal because heart failure therapies (e.g., diuretics and ACE inhibitors) can have a potentially negative effect on renal function and blood flow. A complete blood count (CBC) helps to evaluate for anemia, leukocytosis, or thrombocytopenia (especially if antithrombotic agents may be used). If hepatomegaly is present, liver function studies may be obtained to evaluate for hepatic congestion or other liver disorders. If the diagnosis is unclear, albumin levels evaluate for the presence of a hypoproteinemic states mimicking heart failure. Thyroid function studies may need to be checked, especially if patients present with new-onset atrial fibrillation or if they are on thyroid-replacement therapy. Determination of digoxin levels is needed if there is suspicion for toxicity or worsening renal function. Urine or serum toxicology screens are performed when indicated.

Echocardiogram

The history, physical examination, and presence of risk factors provide the clinician with enough information to decide whether the diagnosis of heart failure is a clinical possibility. While echocardiography is not obtained routinely in the ED, it is considered in the critically ill patient with a suspected acute cardiac anatomic abnormality (e.g., valvular catastrophe). It is also useful in the observation unit for patients without a previous diagnosis of systolic dysfunction, unless it is performed within 1 year.

In elderly patients presenting with an exacerbation of previously documented heart failure, the emergency physician must search for likely reasons for the decompensation and consider the differential diagnosis (Table 12-3). The older cohort of patients is more likely than a younger group to exhibit the less obvious manifestations of myocardial ischemia. With increasing age, the "classic" symptoms of myocardial infarction are less common; consequently, the emergency physician must maintain a high index of suspicion for cardiac ischemia precipitating a presentation of decompensated heart failure. Other heart failure precipitants include atrial fibrillation, myocardial ischemia, and concomitant infection (e.g., pneumonia), especially in the elderly. Older patients have a higher incidence of valvular disease, and calcific aortic stenosis may complicate heart failure exacerbations in this patient population.

The most common reasons for heart failure readmissions in the elderly are noncompliance with medication (24 percent) or dietary restrictions (24 percent), inappropriate medication (16 percent), and failure to seek medical treatment (16 percent).[22] Since noncompliance is common, the elderly should be asked about their method of taking medications, and the clinician must search for signs of dementia via patient interview and family questioning. Financial constraints and inability to prepare meals also may limit the implementation of an adequately sodium-restricted diet. Some elderly patients may rely on institutionalized meal plans or preprepared (often high in

Table 12-3. Differential Diagnosis

Pulmonary embolism
Emphysema exacerbation
Acute myocardial infarction
Aortic dissection
Acute pericardial effusion
Tension pneumothorax
Superior vena cava syndrome
Pneumonia
Hypoproteinemias (nephrotic syndrome, liver failure)
Renal failure (acute on chronic)
Thyroid disease
Renal artery stenosis (hypertensive pulmonary edema)

sodium) foods. Identification of dietary or medicine noncompliance may avoid the addition of further drugs or other costly therapies in an effort to treat presumably "refractory" symptoms.

EMERGENCY DEPARTMENT CARE AND DISPOSITION

Initial management of a patient presenting with cardiopulmonary symptoms (dyspnea, chest pain) consists of evaluation of airway, breathing, and circulation. When the patient is hemodynamically unstable, therapy and diagnosis occur simultaneously. Endotracheal intubation should be considered early if the patient has an unstable airway or has mental status changes resulting from poor cardiac output or significant hypoxia. Oxygen should be administered to improve hypoxia. Intravenous access is indicated, and a cardiac monitor will determine if underlying arrhythmia is present. An ECG is needed early in the presentation of the unstable patient to identify acute cardiac injury requiring early reperfusion management.

The pharmacologic treatment of heart failure should be similar among the elderly and the general population.[23] This is especially true in the setting of acute heart failure syndromes such as acute pulmonary edema and cardiogenic shock. However, the elderly patient may have more comorbidity, polypharmacy, medicine-related side effects, and noncompliance with therapies. For example, in a study of almost 35,000 heart failure patients older than age 65, 33 percent had emphysema, 40 percent had diabetes, and greater than 50 percent had coronary artery disease and hypertension.[24] Elderly patients also were more likely to have renal insufficiency. Patients with hemodynamic instability or evidence of acute myocardial ischemia should be considered for urgent cardiology consultation (Table 12-4).

Table 12-4. Indications for Urgent Cardiology Consult

Positive troponin T or I
Unstable arrhythmias
ST-segment-elevation myocardial infarction or new left bundle-branch block
New ischemic changes on ECG
Concomitant severe valvular disease or left ventricular outflow tract obstruction
Hypoxemia despite supplemental oxygen
Hypercarbia
Cardiogenic shock

Cardiogenic Shock

The most severe acute presentation of heart failure is cardiogenic shock. Patients with cardiogenic shock are likely to be older and have a history of heart failure or prior myocardial infarction.[14] Medical therapy should be considered a temporizing measure while arranging for definitive treatment to reestablish coronary patency. Since some with cardiogenic shock will have relatively inadequate preload, those patients without evidence of severe pulmonary congestion may receive a small fluid bolus. Vasodilators cannot be used in most cases where hypotension is present. Pure vasoconstrictors such as phenylephrine generally are contraindicated because they increase cardiac afterload without augmenting cardiac inotropy. Dopamine is used if there is hypotension, but it may increase cardiac work by increasing heart rate. It also may increase the pulmonary capillary wedge pressure via its alpha-agonist effect. Dobutamine may be effective in increasing cardiac inotropy, but it generally should be used when blood pressure is greater than 90 mmHg because of its vasodilator potential. Phosphodiesterase inhibitors such as milrinone augment inotropy but have significant vasodilatory properties and can decrease blood pressure even greater then dobutamine. Combination therapy with a vasopressor (dopamine) and an inotropic agent (dobutamine) may be more effective than use of either agent alone.[25]

The only temporizing therapeutic modality that improves coronary perfusion without potentially increasing cardiac work is the intraaortic balloon pump. An intraaortic balloon pump may function as a bridge to definitive therapy aimed at myocardial reperfusion. Definitive therapy for cardiogenic shock associated with mechanical complications or myocardial infarction requires urgent repair or revascularization. Emergency invasive reperfusion therapy, accompanied by intraaortic balloon pump, is the treatment of choice.[26,27] In one study, however, treatment benefit was only apparent for patients younger than 75 years of age.[27] If an experienced center is not immediately available for invasive reperfusion therapy, fibrinolytic therapy and intraaortic balloon pump can be used.[28] Tissue plasminogen activator (tPA) may be more effective than reteplase.[29]

Acute Pulmonary Edema

The failing heart is sensitive to any afterload increase. Most patients with acute pulmonary edema present with elevated systemic arterial blood pressure, and therapy to achieve prompt blood pressure reduction often will break the downward spiral of pulmonary edema and avoid the need for intubation. Initial therapy includes serial administration of sublingual nitroglycerin (every 1 minute), which can be initiated while establishing stabilization procedures. Onset of action is within 2 to 3 minutes, and the effect of sublingual nitroglycerin usually lasts 15 to 20 minutes. Patients with hypertrophic obstructive cardiomyopathy (HOCM) or severe aortic stenosis may not tolerate such reductions in preload and afterload with nitrates.

After intravenous access is established, conversion to intravenous nitroglycerin is usually needed. The endpoint should be lowering of the mean arterial pressure. Nitroglycerin is rapidly titrated upward to obtain this effect (it should be increased at 20- to 40-μg increments every 1 to 5 minutes based on clinical status). If nitroglycerin reaches levels of 200 μg, further increases give little hemodynamic benefit, and a change to nitroprusside, a more potent agent, is required. Nitroprusside is rapidly titrated upward until blood pressure begins to decline or symptoms resolve.

Diuretic therapy with intravenous furosemide or bumetanide is also recommended. Ethacrynic acid is useful if the patient has a serious sulfa allergy. Loop diuretics have a quick onset, with diuresis expected to begin 10 to 15 minutes after their use. If urine output is inadequate after 30 to 60 minutes, the diuretic dose is doubled and repeated, not to exceed 360 mg. Diuretics also may have an earlier effect as weak venodilators. In addition, intravenous morphine may be used to help decrease respiratory distress, venodilate, and decrease circulating catecholamine levels.

Acute Pulmonary Edema and Hypertrophic Obstructive Cardiomyopathy

Patients with HOCM and acute pulmonary edema require special attention. They have a dynamic outflow obstruction that is exacerbated by increases in either heart rate or cardiac contractility or decreases in either preload or afterload. Therapy is aimed at decreasing heart rate with intravenous beta blockers. These patients do not tolerate atrial fibrillation, and every effort should be made to convert them to sinus rhythm. Urgent cardiology consultation is recommended. If shock is present, the vasopressor of choice is phenylephrine because of its action as a circulatory vasopressor and lack of effect on cardiac contractility.

Acute Decompensated Heart Failure

Patients in this group have stable vital signs, oxygenation, and ventilation without signs of hypoperfusion. These patients should be excluded for occult myocardial ischemia, assessed for cardiac rhythm changes, and evaluated for other causes of dyspnea (i.e., anemia, emphysema, pulmonary embolism, etc.). They require diuresis with an intravenous loop diuretic, supplemental oxygen, and therapy aimed at bringing the blood pressure down to acceptable levels. Nesiritide should be considered for use in this cohort. It is synergistic with standard therapy and results in superior dyspnea improvement at the acute presentation.[30]

Most patients with decompensated heart failure are fluid overloaded, and intravenous diuretics remain a cornerstone of therapy. In a study of elderly patients presenting to the hospital with NYHA class IV symptoms and elevated central venous pressure (>16 mmHg), aggressive diuresis was safe, efficacious, and cost-effective. Patients were given a 100-mg intravenous bolus of furosemide, followed by a 24-hour continuous infusion titrated to maintain a diuresis of more than 100 mL/h. Patients experienced a 9- to 20-L diuresis in an average of 3.5 days. They had shorter stays and a Medicare-calculated cost savings of $5000 compared with patients undergoing standard intravenous bolus therapy.[31]

Medications that are used commonly in the management of acute heart failure include the following.

Diuretics

Diuretics are the fastest agent for relief of fluid overload; however, compared with the young, the elderly are less responsive.[32,33] Diuretics are used in all patients with congestion, regardless of heart failure type, but not as monotherapy because they do not change mortality rates.[34,35] Diuretics alter efficacy and toxicity of other heart failure medications, especially in the elderly.[2] Dosing is best guided by daily body weight measurement. Complications include electrolyte depletion (e.g., Na^+, K^+, Mg^{2+}), to which the elderly are more susceptible,[2, 33] as well as hypotension and azotemia. Excessive diuresis should be avoided in the elderly because of a high frequency of diastolic dysfunction.

Diuretic dosing in ED patients with acute dyspnea and pulmonary congestion should be double the daily oral dose of furosemide administered intravenously (maximum 180 mg), so long as the patient is not hypotensive. If there has been no prior loop diuretic use, 40 mg is an adequate initial dose. Alternatively, 1 mg bumetanide equals 40 mg furosemide.[36] After 2 to 3 hours, if urine output is poor, the dose should be doubled and repeated. Output goal is 500 mL within 2 hours; if the creatinine level is greater than 2.5 mg/dL, then the output goal is halved. Diuretic response predicts outcome. In acute pul-

monary edema, poor diuresis is associated with higher mortality,[37] and net urine output of less than 1 L is more common in those failing observation unit therapy.[38]

Nesiritide

As the first natriuretic peptide for heart failure treatment, nesiritide is indicated for the intravenous treatment of acutely decompensated heart failure in patients with dyspnea at rest or with minimal activity. Physiologically, it is a balanced vasodilator, with effects on the arteries, veins, and coronary arteries. This causes decreases in preload and afterload and improvements in both dyspnea and global clinical status. It is predominately metabolized by a protein receptor and neutral endopeptidases. Because renal elimination is a relatively minor metabolic pathway, it may be used in patients with renal insufficiency. Significantly, it is a neurohormonal antagonist and decreases levels of norepinephrine, aldosterone, and endothelin in heart failure patients. Finally, it is a weak diuretic, resulting in natriuresis, and is synergistic with loop diuretics.

In the choice of either inotropic agents or vasodilators for heart failure treatment, the latter are clearly superior for mortality reduction. Compared with dobutamine, a commonly used inotrope for heart failure, nesiritide has better effects on dyspnea, produces fewer ventricular arrhythmias, and results in a significantly lower 6-month mortality.[39] This may be due in part to the fact that nesiritide has no inotropic, chronotropic, or proarrhythmic effects. These are important considerations because heart failure is the greatest risk factor for sudden death.

In the largest studies, nesiritide is used in combination with standard treatment. This includes loop diuretics, ACE inhibitor, beta blockers, digoxin, and spironolactone. Consequently, barring contraindications, these medications are recommended to be continued when nesiritide is instituted, provided that the patient is not hypotensive.

In decompensated heart failure, nesiritide produced greater dyspnea reduction than standard care by 3 hours and was superior to standard care and nitroglycerin by 24 hours.[30] Nesiritide use results in a small decrease in systolic blood pressure, usually within the first hour, after which there are minimal changes in vital signs. Consequently, invasive monitoring is unnecessary, and patients may be able to be admitted on a telemetry unit rather than an intensive care unit.

The most common significant complication of nesiritide is hypotension. Symptomatic hypotension after 3 hours of therapy occurred in 0.5 percent of nesiritide patients compared with 1 percent of those treated with nitroglycerin. By 24 hours, the hypotension rates were similar (4 percent for nesiritide, 5 percent for nitroglycerin). In the majority of patients, hypotension was asymptomatic and only required dose reduction. If hypotension is symptomatic and does not respond to stopping the infusion, a fluid bolus may be indicated. If further treatment for hypotension is required, dopamine is recommended; however, this is usually unnecessary. Persistent hypotension suggests that other causes (e.g., coronary ischemia) should be considered.

Nesiritide is contraindicated in hypotension, cardiogenic shock, and when vasodilation would be inappropriate (e.g., HOCM). In patients with acute pulmonary edema and extreme hypertension, for whom intubation is an early consideration, initial treatment may be nitroglycerin or nitroprusside. This is due to the necessity for rapid titration to reduce blood pressure. While nesiritide can be titrated, it is only recommended to be done at 3-hour intervals. Once the hypertension is controlled, nitroglycerin may be changed to nesiritide.

ACE Inhibitors

ACE inhibitors are the cornerstone of heart failure therapy. Powerful vasodilators have failed to benefit patients with heart failure, whereas less potent vasodilators, such as ACE inhibitors, have changed the course of this disease. The effects of ACE inhibitors on heart failure are not due solely to their vasodilating effects. ACE inhibitors work mainly by suppressing levels of angiotensin II and augmenting levels of endothelium-protective bradykinins. ACE inhibitors also prevent ventricular remodeling, a benefit that continues despite failure to chronically suppress angiotensin II levels.

In the absence of contraindications, all elderly patients with heart failure should be treated with an ACE inhibitor. Patients with asymptomatic left ventricular dysfunction also may derive benefit from ACE inhibitors.[40] ACE inhibitors have been shown to decrease the overall mortality and combined endpoint of death or hospitalization due to heart failure.[41]

Despite data supporting the quality-of-life and mortality benefit of ACE inhibitors in both younger and older patient populations, they may be underused in the elderly.[24,42] The reasons are unclear; however, concerns regarding hypotension or worsening of renal function may play a role. Although the benefit of ACE inhibitors in both diabetic and nondiabetic renal insufficiency is well established,[43] there is some concern that ACE inhibitors may

have less clinical benefit in elderly patients with heart failure and moderate to severe renal insufficiency.[44] Since most ACE inhibitors are cleared renally, dosage should be adjusted for the degree of renal insufficiency.

Symptomatic hypotension is not a common event in elderly patients treated with ACE inhibitors.[45] Since diuresis may sensitize patients to the hypotensive effect of ACE inhibitors, initiation of therapy should be delayed during aggressive diuresis. In the absence of postural symptoms, hypotension is relatively well tolerated. If a patient experiences symptomatic hypotension with ACE inhibitor, diuretic doses can be decreased or dosing can be separated from other blood pressure–lowering agents.

Angiotensin-Receptor Blockers

Angiotensin-receptor blockers (ARBs) produce blockade of the angiotensin-receptor subtype AT1.[46] Stimulation of the AT1 receptor by angiotensin II promotes aldosterone release, left ventricular remodeling, arterial vasoconstriction, and renal damage.[47] Enzymatic systems other than the ACE system can produce angiotensin II (i.e., chymase system), and angiotensin II production may escape ACE inhibition secondary to local tissue ACE activity and upregulation of AT1 receptors. By blocking the AT1 receptor independent of angiotensin II production, these agents may have a theoretical advantage in the treatment of angiotensin II–induced diseases.[47]

ARBs are effective in the management of hypertension, are very well tolerated, and may be more effective than beta blockers at reducing left ventricular hypertrophy.[48,49] Because the incidence of cough and angioedema are very rare with ARBs, the therapeutic indication in heart failure is for patients intolerant to ACE inhibitors secondary to cough or angioedema.

Hydralazine–Isosorbide Dinitrate

The combination of hydralazine–isosorbide dinitrate decreases both preload and afterload,[50] and one study demonstrated a significant mortality reduction over placebo.[51] The use of hydralazine–isosorbide dinitrate is considered only in those intolerant to ACE inhibitors.

Digoxin

Once a primary agent for heart failure, digoxin is now used primarily in heart failure with atrial fibrillation.

Digoxin may be useful for symptomatic therapy while beta blockers and ACE inhibitors are being up titrated. Digoxin therapy does not produce a mortality benefit; however, it improves symptoms and decreases hospitalizations.[52] Levels should be monitored closely if there is concomitant renal insufficiency; in addition, there are important drug interactions (amiodarone, spironolactone, verapamil, and macrolides).

Beta Blockers

Once contraindicated in heart failure, beta blockers provide mortality reduction similar to and even better than some ACE inhibitors. In the MERIT heart failure trial, metoprolol provided a 34 percent reduction in 1-year overall mortality for NYHA class II and III heart failure. Additionally, there was a 41 percent decrease in sudden death compared with placebo.[53] Beta- blocker therapy provides impressive clinical benefit for patients with NYHA class II, III, and even IV heart failure.[54] Although carvedilol (a combined alpha and beta blocker) has mortality benefits in class IV patients, the use of beta blockers in end-stage heart failure patients is best left to a heart failure specialist.

Spironolactone

This is an aldosterone antagonist and weak diuretic. The RALES trial of NYHA class III and IV heart failure was stopped early secondary to a 30 percent decrease in all-cause mortality.[55] Current recommendations for spironolactone are limited to NYHA class IV patients. A serum creatinine level of more than 2.5 mg/dL and a potassium leve of more than 5 mmol/L are important contraindications to the use of spironolactone.

In the elderly, multiple simultaneous disease processes are common. This complicates management and contributes to the high rehospitalization rate. Heart failure 90-day readmission rates are 33 to 47 percent[34,53]; in Medicare patients older than age 65, nearly 50 percent are readmitted within 3 to 6 months. Table 12-5 lists predictors of increased 90-day readmission.[56]

No strict admission criteria exist, but suggested intensive care unit admission criteria are listed in Table 12-6. Severe electrolyte abnormalities also may require a monitored bed. A low admission threshold should be used in the very elderly, in the presence of severe comorbidity, or if the home environment precludes successful outpatient management.

Table 12-5. Factors Increasing 90-Day Readmission Rates

Age
Male
Heart failure admission within 6 months
Initial admission length of stay > 1 week
Failed social support system
Inadequate follow-up
Dietary noncompliance
Medication noncompliance

Observation Unit

Stable patients with heart failure who meet the criteria in Table 12-7 may be considered for treatment in the observation unit. Since heart failure management is complicated, it is recommended that an observation unit protocol be used to assist in management. In the observation unit, a heart failure management protocol increased discharge rates by 50 percent[57] and decreased both 90-day ED heart failure revisits by more than 50 percent and heart failure readmission by two-thirds.[58,59] If the patient is congested and unable to attain urinary output goals, or if dyspnea is unrelieved after therapy, admission is warranted.

Patients with a good diuretic response, resolution of their dyspnea, and edema improvement are expected to do well. Ambulation prior to discharge is an effective method to evaluate functional reserve. Suggested discharge criteria from the observation unit are listed in Table 12-8.

Table 12-6. Intensive Care Unit Admission Indications

Sustained ventricular tachycardia
Symptomatic arrhythmia
Cardiogenic shock
Unstable vital signs unresponsive to treatment
ECG or serum marker evidence of myocardial ischemia
  or infarction
Ischemic chest pain
Multiple severe comorbidities
Unstable airway

Table 12-7. Observation Unit Heart Failure Entry Criteria (Must Have at Least One from Each Category)

1. **History**
   Orthopnea
   Dyspnea on exertion
   Paroxysmal nocturnal dyspnea
   Shortness of breath
   Swelling of legs or abdomen
   Weight gain
2. **Physical examination**
   JVD or elevation in pulsation
   Positive abdominal jugular reflux
   S_3/S_4
   Inspiratory rales
   Peripheral edema
3. **Chest radiograph**
   Cardiomegaly
   Pulmonary vascular congestion
   Kerley B lines
   Pulmonary edema
   Pleural effusion

Observation unit exclusion criteria

1. Unstable vital signs (blood pressure > 220/120 mmHg, respiratory rate > 25, heart rate > 130 bpm)
2. ECG or serum markers of myocardial ischemia
3. Unstable airway, or needing > 4 L/min supplemental O_2 by nasal cannula to keep Sao_2 > 90%
4. Complex decompensation: concomitant end-organ hypoperfusion, volume overload, and systemic vasoconstriction
5. Requiring continuous vasoactive medication (e.g., nitroglycerin, nitroprusside, dobutamine, or milrinone) to stabilize hemodynamics
6. Nonsustained VT not due to electrolyte imbalance
7. Acute mental status abnormality
8. Severe electrolyte imbalances

ADDITIONAL ASPECTS

The following are pitfalls in the management of heart failure:

- *Failure to recognize that patients with diastolic dysfunction are preload-dependent.* As a result, excessive diuresis or venodilation may result in hypotension.

- *Assuming that oxygen and diuretic therapy alone are sufficient for the heart failure patient who pres-*

Table 12-8. Observation Unit Heart Failure Discharge Guidelines

The use of these parameters is to suggest guidelines for the discharge of heart failure patients from the observation unit; they should not supersede good clinical judgment. Patients failing to meet all the following should be considered for inpatient treatment.

1. Patient reports subjective improvement
2. Ambulatory, without long suffering orthostasis
3. Resting heart rate < 100 beats per minute
4. Systolic blood pressure > 80 mmHg
5. Total urine output > 1000 mL and no new decrease in urine output below 30 mL/h (or <0.5 mL/kg/h)
6. Room air O_2 saturation > 90% (unless on home O_2)
7. Normal CK-MB and troponin T or I
8. No ischemic type chest pain
9. No new clinically significant arrhythmia
10. Stable electrolyte profile

ents in extremis. The expedient initiation of serial sublingual nitroglycerin therapy frequently precludes the need to intubate the patient in respiratory distress.

REFERENCES

1. Massie BM, Shah NB: Evolving trends in the epidemiologic factors of heart failure: Rationale for preventive strategies and comprehensive disease management. *Am Heart J* 133:703, 1997.
2. Friesinger GC: Cardiovascular disease in the elderly, in Friesinger GC (ed): *Cardiology Clinics.* Philadelphia, Saunders, 1999, p 648.
3. Rich MW: Epidemiology, pathophysiology, and etiology of congestive heart failure in older adults. *J Am Geriatr Soc* 45:968, 1997.
4. Krumholz HM, Parent EM, Tu N, et al: Readmission after hospitalization for congestive heart failure among medicare beneficiaries. *Arch Intern Med* 157:99, 1997.
5. Pulignano G, Del Sindaco D, Tavazzi L, et al: Clinical features and outcomes of elderly outpatients with heart failure followed up in hospital cardiology units: Data from a large nationwide cardiology database (Heart Failure Registry). *Am Heart J* 143:45, 2002.
6. Tresh DD: The clinical diagnosis of heart failure in older patients. *J Am Geriatr Sos* 45:1128, 1997.
7. Kitzman DW: Heart failure with normal systolic function. *Clin Geriatr Med* 16:489, 2000.

8. Lakatta EG: Cardiovascular aging in health. *Clin Geriatr Med* 16:419, 2000.

9. Gerstenblith G, Fredricksen J, Yin FCP, et al: Echocardiographic assessment of a normal adult aging population. *Circulation* 56:273, 1977.

10. Olivetti G, Melissari M, Capasso JM, et al: Cardiomyopathy of the aging human heart: Myocyte loss and reactive cellular hypertrophy. *Circ Res* 68:1560, 1991.

11. Nagai J, Metter EJ, Earley CJ, et al: Increased carotid artery intimal-medial thickness in asymptomatic older subjects with exercise-induced myocardial ischemia. *Circulation* 98:1504, 1998.

12. Ghali JK, Kadakia S, Cooper RS, Liao Y: Beside diagnosis of preserved versus impaired left ventricular systolic function in heart failure. *Am J Cardiol* 67:1002, 1991.

13. Hollenberg SM, Kavinsky CJ, Parrillo JE: Cardiogenic shock. *Ann Intern Med* 131:47, 1999.

14. Califf RM, Bengtson JR: Cardiogenic shock. *New Engl J Med* 330:172, 1994.

15. Jiang W, Alexander J, Christopher E, et al: Relationship of depression to increased risk of mortality and rehospitalization in patients with congestive heart failure. *Arch Intern Med* 161:1849, 2001.

16. Doughty R, Andersen V, Sharpe N: Optimal treatment of heart failure in the elderly. *Drugs Aging* 10(6):435, 1997.

17. Chakko S, Woska D, Marinex H, et al: Clinical, radiographic, and hemodynamic correlations in chronic congestive hart failure: Conflicting results may lead to inappropriate care. *Am J Med* 90:353, 1991.

18. Kono T, Suwa M, Hanada H, et al: Clinical significance of normal cardiac silhouette in dilated cardiomyopathy: Evaluation based upon echocardiography and magnetic resonance imaging. *Jpn Circ J* 56(4):359, 1992.

19. Peacock WF, Emerman CL, Doleh M, et al: The incidence of elevated cardiac enzymes in decompensated heart failure. *Acad Emerg Med* 5:552, 2001.

20. Freda BJ, Peacock WF, Lindsell CJ, et al: Outcomes in heart failure patients with elevated cardiac markers of ischemia. *J Heart Fail* (in press).

21. Peacock WF: The B-type natriuretic peptide assay: A rapid test for heart failure. *Cleve Clin J Med* 69(3):243, 2002.

22. Vinson JM, Rich MW, Sperry JC, et al: Early readmission of elderly patients with congestive heart failure. *J Am Geriatr Soc* 38:1290, 1990.

23. Sweitzer NK, Frishman WH, Stevenson LW: Drug therapy of heart failure caused by systolic dysfunction in the elderly. *Clin Geriatr Med* 16:513, 2000.

24. Havranek EP, Masoudi FA, Westfall KA, et al: Spectrum of heart failure in older patients: Results from the National Heart Failure Project. *Am Heart J* 143:412, 2002.

25. Richard C, Ricome JL, Rimallho A, et al: Combined hemodynamic effects of dopamine and dobutamine in cardiogenic shock. *Circulation* 67:620, 1983.

26. Hochman JS, Sleeper LA, Webb JG, et al: Early revascularization in acute myocardial infarction complicated by cardiogenic shock. *New Engl J Med* 341:625, 1999.

27. Hochman JS, Sleeper LA, White HD, et al: One-year survival following early revascularization for cardiogenic shock. *JAMA* 285:190, 2001.

28. Sanborn TA, Sleeper LA, Bates ER, et al: Impact of thrombolysis, intra-aortic balloon pump counterpulsation, and their combination in cardiogenic shock complicating acute myocardial infarction: A report from the SHOCK trial registry. *J Am Coll Cardiol* 36:1123, 2000.

29. Hasdai D, Holmes DR, Topol EJ, et al: Frequency and clinical outcomes of cardiogenic shock during acute myocardial infarction among patients receiving reteplase or alteplase: Results from GUSTO-III. *Eur Heart J* 20:128, 1999.

30. Publication Committee for the VMAC Investigators: Intravenous nesiritide versus nitroglycerin for treatment of decompensated congestive heart failure: The VMAC trial. *JAMA* 287(12);1531, 2002.

31. Howard PA, Dunn MI: Aggressive diuresis for severe heart failure in the elderly. *Chest* 119:807, 2001.

32. Mills RM, Young JB: Heart failure therapy: Not as complicated as it looks. *Clin Cardiol* 22:339, 1999.

33. Rich MW: Epidemiology, pathophysiology, and etiology of congestive heart failure in older adults. *J Am Geriatr Soc* 45(8):968, 1997.

34. Packer M, Cohn JN: Consensus recommendations for the management of chronic heart failure. *Am J Cardiol* 83:2A, 1999.

35. Clinical Practice Guideline Number 11: *Heart Failure: Evaluation and Care of Patients with Left-Ventricular Systolic Dysfunction.* AHCPR Publication No. 94–0612. Washington, US Department of Health and Human Services. June 1994.

36. Bumetadine, in *1998 Physician's Desk Reference,* 2441–43. Montvale, NJ, Medical Economics Company, 1999.

37. Le Conte P, Coutant V, N'Guyen JM, et al: Prognostic factors in acute cardiogenic pulmonary edema. *Am J Emerg Med* 17:329, 1999.

38. Peacock W, Aponte J, Craig M, et al: Predictors of unsuccessful treatment for congestive heart failure in the emergency department observation unit. *Acad Emerg Med* 4:494, 1997.

39. Burger AJ, Horton D, LeJemtel T, et al: Differential effects of nesiritide and dobutamine on ventricular arrhythmias: The Precedent study. *Am Heart J* 144:1102, 2002.

40. The SOLVD Investigators: Effect of enalapril on mortality and the development of heart failure in asymptomatic patients with reduced left ventricular ejection fraction. *New Engl J Med* 327:685, 1992.

41. The CONSENSUS Study Group: Effects of enalapril on mortality in severe heart failure. *New Engl J Med* 316:1429, 1981.

42. Johansson S, Wallander M, Ruigomez A, et al: Treatment patterns among newly diagnosed heart failure patients in general practice. *Eur J Clin Pharmacol* 57:813, 2002.

43. Remuzzi G, Ruggenenti P, Perico N: Chronic renal diseases: Renoprotective benefits of renin-angiotensin system inhibition. *Ann Intern Med* 136:604, 2002.

44. Philbin EF, Santella RN, Rocco TA: Angiotensin-converting enzyme inhibitor use in older patients with heart failure and renal dysfunction. *J Am Geriatr Soc* 47:302, 1999.

45. Portuguese Community Hospital Study Group on Heart Failure: A comparative study of the first dose hypotensive effects of captopril and perindopril in patients with heart failure. *Cardiovasc Drugs Ther* 15(6):501, 2001.

46. Packer M, Poole-Wilson PA, Armstrong PW, et al: Comparative effects of low and high doses of the angiotensin converting enzyme inhibitor, lisinopril, on mortality in chronic heart failure. *Circulation* 100:2312, 1999.

47. Ramahi TM: Expanded role for ARBs in cardiovascular disease and renal disease? Recent observations have far-reaching clinical implications. *Postgrad Med* 109:115, 2001.

48. Thurmann PA, Kenedi P, Schmidt A, et al: Influence of the angiotensin II antagonist valsartan on left ventricular hypertrophy in patients with hypertension. *Circulation* 98:2037, 1998.

49. Rochon PA, Tu JV, Anderson GM, et al: Rate of heart failure and 1-year survival for older people receiving beta-blocker therapy after myocardial infarction. *Lancet* 356:639, 2000.

50. Cohn JN, Archibald DG, Ziesche S, et al: Effect of vasodilator therapy on mortality in chronic congestive heart failure. *New Engl J Med* 314:1547, 1986.

51. Cohn JN, Johnson G, Ziesche S, et al: A comparison of enalapril with hydrolazine–tsosonbide dinitrate in the treatment of chronic congestive heart failure. *New Engl J Med* 325:303, 1991.

52. The Digitalis Investigation Group: The effect of digoxin on mortality and morbidity in patients with heart failure. *New Engl J Med* 28(336):525, 1997.

53. The MERIT Heart Failure Study Group: Effect of metoprolol CR/XL in chronic heart failure: Metoprolol CR/XL randomized intervention trial in congestive heart failure. *Lancet* 353:2001, 1999.

54. Packer M, Coats AJ, Fowler MB, et al: Effect of carvedilol survival in severe chronic heart failure. *New Engl J Med* 344:1651, 2001.

55. Pitt B, Zawnad F, Remme WJ, et al: The effect of spironolactone on morbidity and mortality in patients with severe heart failure. *New Engl J Med* 341:709, 1999.

56. Rich MW, Vinson JM, Sperry JC, et al: Prevention of readmission in elderly patients with congestive heart failure. *J Gen Intern Med* 8:585, 1993.

57. Krumholz HM, Parent EM, Tu N, et al: Readmission after hospitalization for congestive heart failure among Medicare beneficiaries. *Arch Intern Med* 157:99, 1997.

58. Albert NM, Peacock WF: Patient outcome and costs after implementation of an acute heart failure management program in an emergency department observation unit. *J Int Soc Heart Lung Transplant* 18(1): 92, 1999.

59. Peacock WF IV, Remer EE, Aponte J, et al: Effective observation unit treatment of decompensated heart failure. *Congest Heart Fail* 8(2):68, 2002.

13

Dysrhythmias

Thomas Lemke

HIGH-YIELD FACTS

- An elderly patient who suffers a rapid decline in consciousness or hemodynamic status has a high likelihood of experiencing a dysrhythmia.
- Most wide-complex tachycardias ultimately are diagnosed as ventricular tachycardia.
- With the exception of bypass tract disease and intranodal tachycardias, the incidence of both dysrhythmias and blocks rises in direct proportion to age.

The most common cause of death in the industrialized world is sudden cardiac death.[1,2] Recent developments in both the chemical and mechanical management of dysrhythmias have improved outcome dramatically. Before initiating treatment, however, the emergency physician must first recognize the dysrhythmia.

Among geriatric patients, certain dysrhythmias should be considered in more depth than others. Congenital defects, accessory pathway disease, and intranodal tachycardias present early in life and usually are diagnosed and managed long before the patient is advanced in years. Conversely, ventricular tachycardias, blocks (both sinoatrial and bundle branch), wide-complex tachycardias, and sick-sinus syndrome appear predominantly in the elderly.

EPIDEMIOLOGY

Many dysrhythmias are age-dependent to some degree. The paradigm is atrial fibrillation, where the single greatest factor influencing its development is age. The incidence varies from all but negligible in a healthy, young population to 16 percent in those over 90 years of age.[3–7] Similarly, atrial flutter, while occurring only one-tenth as frequently as atrial fibrillation,[8] also in-

creases with age.[9] Ventricular dysrhythmias increase with age but more as secondary to the development of coronary artery disease. The mean age for the development of ventricular tachycardia is in the mid-50s, coinciding with the age at which coronary artery diseases begins to manifest itself.[10,11] Unlike the ventricular dysrhythmias, the incidence of bundle branch-blocks peaks at later ages.[12] Bundle-branch blocks are caused by myocardial fibrosis due to aging as well as fibrosis caused by coronary artery disease. Atrioventricular (AV) blocks do not exhibit the strong relation to age seen by these other dysrhythmias.

PATHOPHYSIOLOGY

Causes of cardiac dysrhythmias in the geriatric population are numerous, including both endogenous (e.g., coronary artery disease, congenital diseases, and myocardial fibrosis) and exogenous (e.g., endocrine effects, medications, and infections). Viewed from a cellular level, destruction, suppression of function, and irritability all may be the end result. Irritability usually results in depolarization at a more rapid rate than normal, leading to a tachydysrhythmia. Destruction of myocardium may cause block at any level or loss of pacemaker activity. Suppression of function is the common cause of many bradydysrhythmias. Successful treatment depends on recognizing which one of these mechanisms is operative and attempting to reverse the pathology on a cellular level or to bypass the malfunctioning area entirely.

CLINICAL FEATURES

Although the term *dysrhythmia* covers a wide span of rhythms, the history provided by the patient may have a great deal of common ground. Whether too fast or too slow, the end result is usually malperfusion of organ systems, with the central nervous system (CNS) being affected most. The most common effect of decreased perfusion of the CNS is syncope. Because cardiac rhythm can change so rapidly, symptoms characteristically are of rapid onset. While syncope in an elderly patient may be the result of a myriad of causes, an abrupt change from normal to unconscious should suggest a cardiac etiology as opposed to a neurologic or metabolic cause.

After the CNS, the heart itself is the next most common victim of such malperfusion. The tachydysrhythmias

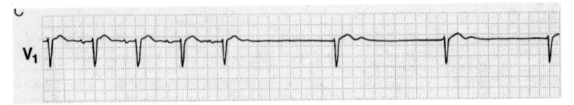

Fig. 13-1   Sinus pause with junctional takeover.

particularly are capable of stressing the heart to levels it is unable to bear, causing patients to present with chest pain as their primary complaint. Conversely, the pulmonary system suffers from hydrostatic pressures that rise rapidly, with transudation of fluid into the alveolar space. The resulting shortness of breath due to congestive heart failure may be what prompts the patient to seek attention.

The physical examination is often sufficient to make the correct diagnosis of the dysrhythmia well in advance of the electrocardiogram (ECG). The vital signs invariably will be abnormal. Rapid or slow heart rates, often accompanied by hypotension, usually point to a dysrhythmia. The patient may present with unconsciousness, diaphoresis, or pallor. Neck vein distension and pulmonary rales suggest that the heart is unable to pump efficiently. The irregularly irregular rhythm noted on both cardiac examination and palpation of the pulse should strongly point to the diagnosis of atrial fibrillation. A tell-tale intermittent pulse wave visualized in the neck veins is caused by an atrium contracting against a valve closed by concomitant ventricular contraction, thereby making the diagnosis of AV dissociation at the bedside.

DIAGNOSIS AND DIFFERENTIAL

Supraventricular Dysrhythmias

The sinoatrial (SA) node may be the source of a variety of dysrhythmias. Although a number of SA blocks and dysrhythmias exist, the main concern for elderly patients is sick-sinus syndrome. The patient develops periods of sinus arrest that may result in syncope or death. If sinus node dysfunction were the only problem, the syndrome would not exist. For a patient to develop the full syndrome, lack of prompt AV nodal takeover also must be present. The diagnosis is made electrocardiographically by noting periodic absence of sinus activity. The lack of nodal takeover yields the appearance of prolonged periods with no electrical activity whatsoever (Fig. 13-1). Occasionally, this syndrome may take the form of a "tachy-brady" pattern, with periods of tachycardia interposed with periods of no electrical activity (Fig. 13-2).

Diagnosis usually is attained through outpatient Holter monitoring. The diagnostic yield through electrophysiologic testing remains unimpressive primarily because the stress of undergoing the procedure raises the level of patient anxiety, which, in turn, increases both sympathetic tone and circulating catecholamines. This combined ef-

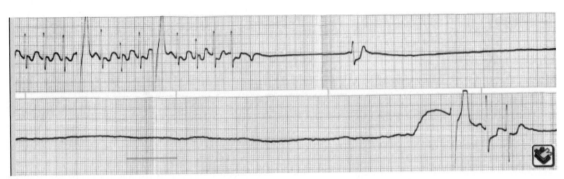

Fig. 13-2   "Tachy-brady" pattern of sick-sinus syndrome. *(Courtesy of Michael Rosengarten, M.D., F.R.C.P.(C), McGill University.)*

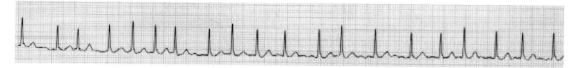

Fig. 13-3   Atrial fibrillation.

fect is usually enough to stimulate the sinus node to function normally.[13]

Moving down the conduction pathway, the next area encountered is the atrium. Atrial fibrillation is a common problem in the elderly and usually poses few diagnostic dilemmas on ECG (Fig. 13-3). Other causes of an irregularly irregular rhythm exist, but atrial fibrillation is the diagnosis in more than 99 percent of the cases.

Atrial flutter, however, may pose some difficulty on diagnosis. The rhythm is regular and tachycardic. P waves usually are not visualized; therefore, differentiating it from paroxysmal atrial tachycardia may be difficult. The following three features may help in differentiating atrial flutter (Fig. 13-4): First, since the atrium tends to flutter at or around 300 beats per minute, the ventricular rate (due to the protective AV block) is usually around 150. Tachycardias with a rate of around 150 beats per minute should be suspected of atrial flutter. Second, the baseline in the inferior leads is virtually never isoelectric; the baseline is either moving up or down, not level. Third, it is often possible to trace the flutter waves right through the QRS complexes. The flutter wave hits the QRS complex higher than normal and can be seen coming out low after the complex.

Two types of atrial tachycardias may present in the elderly. One is paroxysmal supraventricular tachycardia

(PSVT), which usually has been diagnosed during the patient's youth. The second type of atrial tachycardia, nonparoxysmal atrial tachycardia (PAT), is much more common in the elderly population and frequently is due to unintentional digitalis toxicity. The term *PAT with block* has been considered pathognomonic of this condition. The terminology, however, is incorrect in that this dysrhythmia is not paroxysmal but rather comes on gradually and then slows gradually as the digitalis level falls.[14] The diagnosis is straightforward when nonconducted P waves are seen clearly between normal complexes. If, however, the nonconducted P waves are buried in the T waves of the preceding complexes, the diagnosis becomes more difficult. In these cases, examination of previous ECGs allows the clinician to discern the malformed T wave and make the correct diagnosis (Fig. 13-5).

The final level of supraventricular dysrhythmias is the AV junction. When pacemaker function in both the SA node and the atrium fail, a junctional escape rhythm prevents the patient's rapid demise. The complexes appear normal except for the total absence of P waves (Fig. 13-6). The rate is usually between 40 and 60 beats per minute, which is the rate associated with the junction's intrinsic pacemaker function. Diagnostic efforts should ignore junctional activity and focus rather on

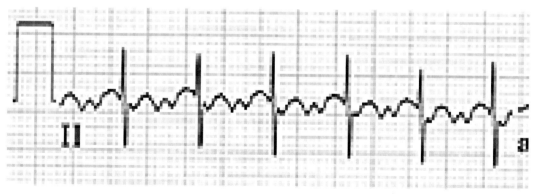

Fig. 13-4   Atrial flutter. *(Courtesy of Frank Yanowitz, M.D., The Alan Lindsay ECG Learning Center, http://medstat.med.utah.edu /kw/ecg.)*

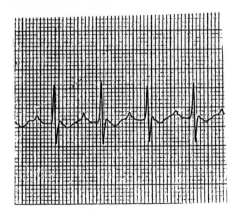

Fig. 13-5 "PAT with block." *(Courtesy of Alfred Buxton, M.D., Brown University.)*

what is wrong with the areas of the conduction system above it.

Conversely, if the junction is irritated, its intrinsic pacemaker activity increases, often to the point where it becomes the driving pacemaker for the heart (Fig. 13-7). This is not a healthy rhythm, and its cause must be sought. Most commonly, junctional tachycardia is a manifestation of digitalis toxicity.[15] Digitalis-toxic junctional tachycardia is seen most commonly during the management of atrial fibrillation. Because of digitalis's narrow therapeutic window, overdose is not uncommon. The treating physician should suspect a toxic rhythm when the rate switches from irregularly irregular to regular. If not diagnosed, the rhythm (now a junctional tachycardia) will increase in rate. This may make the treating physician believe that more digitalis is required for rate control. Unless recognized, this pattern will spiral down to progressively more dangerous ventricular rhythms and death.

Ventricular Dysrhythmias

The most common ventricular dysrhythmia is premature ventricular contractions (PVC). Recognition is usually straightforward if the complex is premature, has a major deflection opposite that of the complexes surrounding it, and exhibits the classic compensatory pause (Fig. 13-8).

However, in that the timing of a premature ventricular discharge is governed only by the irritability of the ventricle and the recovery period of the surrounding tissue, it is possible for a PVC to occur between two normally conducted beats and not disrupt the normal rate. These are known as *interpolated PVCs* (Fig. 13-9). While the timing of this type of premature complex may pose a modicum of difficulty in diagnosis, a longer rhythm strip usually can resolve the issue. Considerable odds must be overcome for a PVC to fall in the precise spot such as to not disrupt the underlying rhythm.

The next most common dysrhythmia that a clinician must manage is ventricular tachycardia (Fig. 13-10). In making the diagnosis, the most common mistake made is the assumption that ventricular tachycardia is a short-lived dysrhythmia that quickly degenerates into ventricular fibrillation. While this may be true in some cases, patients often remain in this rhythm for prolonged periods of time.[16] In one study, the average duration of sustained ventricular tachycardia was approximately 14 minutes.[17]

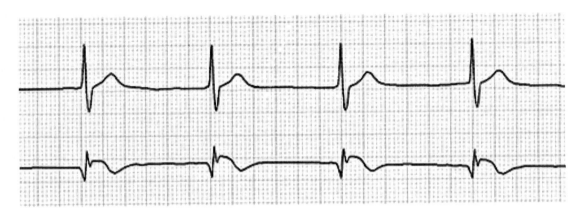

Fig. 13-6 Junctional Escape Rhythm. *(Courtesy of Frank Yanowitz, M.D., The Alan Lindsay ECG Learning Center, http://med-stat.med.utah.edu/kw/ecg and GE Medical Systems, Information Technologies.)*

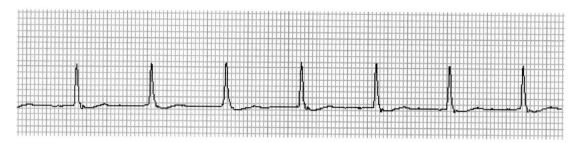

Fig. 13-7 Junctional tachycardia. *(Courtesy of Frank Yanowitz, M.D., The Alan Lindsay ECG Learning Center, http://medstat.med.utah.edu/kw/ecg, and GE Medical Systems, Information Technologies.)*

A common problem is the diagnosis and management of a wide-complex tachycardia. Clearly, this rhythm could be either a supraventricular tachycardia with conduction abnormalities or ventricular tachycardia. If the patient is having symptoms secondary to the dysrhythmia (e.g., angina, increasing congestive heart failure, decreased level of consciousness, etc.), it matters little whether the origin of the dysrhythmia is supraventricular or ventricular; the patient needs to undergo cardioversion. If the patient is not in extremis, clinicians should be aware that the vast majority of wide-complex tachycardias ultimately are diagnosed as ventricular tachycardia.[17] Also, the patient's history may provide clues. One study assessed patients with ventricular tachycardia and asked two questions: (1) "Have you ever had a heart attack?" and (2) "Did you ever have this rapid rhythm before your heart attack?" Patients answering yes to the first question and no to the second were correctly diagnosed as having ventricular tachycardia in 28 of 29 cases.[18]

The ECG also offers several clues as to the origin of the tachycardia. One approach is to consider ABCDEF of the rhythm.[19] A is for axis, B is for "bunny ears," C is for concordance, D is for dissociation, E is for elongation, and F is for fusion beats. An axis in "no man's land" (−90 to −180 degrees) strongly supports the diagnosis of ventricular tachycardia. "Bunny ears" represents the two peaks often present in the anterior lead complexes. The wide complexes often have one peak taller than the other. If the left peak is higher than the right, this favors the diagnosis of ventricular tachycardia (Figs. 13-11 and 13–12). Concordance means that the major deflection of all the anterior leads is in the same direction. When present, concordance provides strong evidence of ventricular tachycardia (Fig. 13-13). Anytime P waves and QRS complexes bear no relationship to one another (dissociated), the likelihood for ventricular tachycardia is high. Elongation features, specifically the period from the onset of the R wave to the deepest part of the S wave, are specific for ventricular tachycardia.[20] Finally, fusion beats, when present, offer near-conclusive evidence of a ventricular origin of the tachycardia. Fusion beats (Fig. 13-14) are a fusion of an

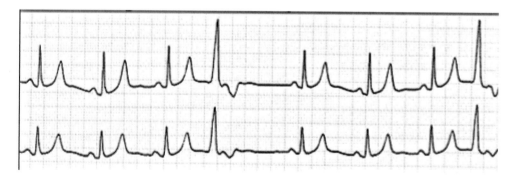

Fig. 13-8 PVCs. *(Courtesy of Frank Yanowitz, M.D., The Alan Lindsay ECG Learning Center, http://medstat.med.utah.edu/kw/ecg, and GE Medical Systems, Information Technologies.)*

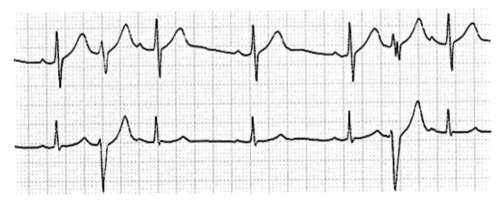

Fig. 13-9 Interpolated PVCs. *(Courtesy of Frank Yanowitz, M.D., The Alan Lindsay ECG Learning Center, http://medstat.med.utah.edu/kw/ecg, and GE Medical Systems, Information Technologies.)*

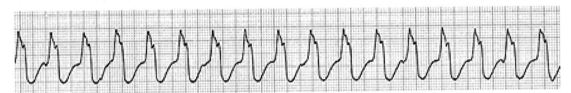

Fig. 13-10 Ventricular tachycardia. *(Courtesy of Frank Yanowitz, M.D., The Alan Lindsay ECG Learning Center, http://medstat.med.utah.edu/kw/ecg.)*

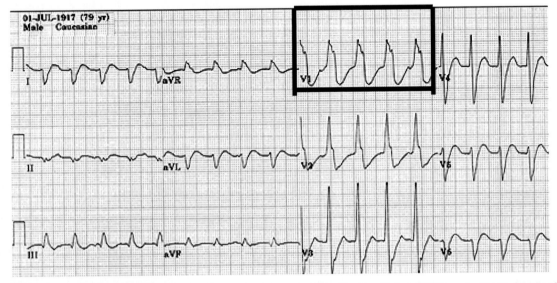

Fig. 13-11 Left ventricular tachycardia. *(Courtesy of Frank Yanowitz, M.D., The Alan Lindsay ECG Learning Center, http://medstat.med.utah.edu/kw/ecg.)*

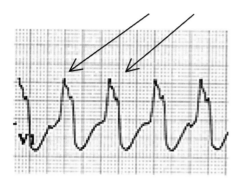

Fig. 13-12 "Bunny ears."

ectopic beat and a normal beat, producing a complex that shares features of both.

Pacemakers

Pacemakers offer a challenge in that they involve both the atrium and the ventricle. The most straightforward ap-

proach to pacemaker problems in the emergency department (ED) is a simplistic one. Acutely, two questions must be answered: (1) "Is it capturing?" and (2) "Is it sensing?" Every pacer spike must be followed by a QRS complex (full capture), and no pacer spike should occur immediately after or during another complex (adequate sensing). If either of these conditions is not met, the patient must be further assessed, usually by electronic pacer interrogation (Figs. 13-15 and 13-16).

Blocks

Blocks can be classified by the area in which they occur: SA, AV, intraventricular, or bundle branch. SA blocks and AV blocks in the elderly are diagnosed and managed in a similar fashion as those in a younger population. The aging process, however, produces problems primarily in the intraventricular system and creates complexity in the differential diagnoses of these entities. Intraventricular blocks can be divided into two areas: major (complete left and right bundle-branch blocks) and minor (anterior and

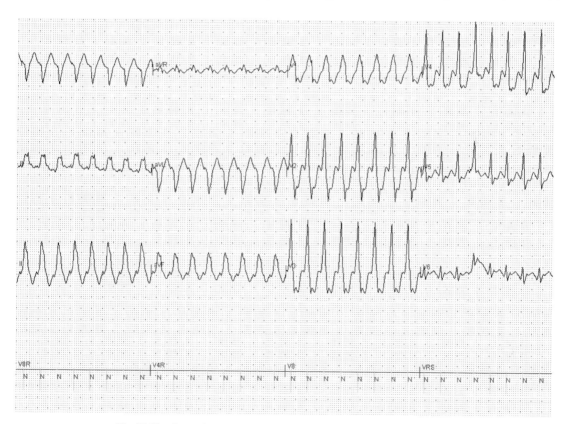

Fig. 13-13 Concordance *(Courtesy of Alfred Buxton, M.D., Brown University.)*

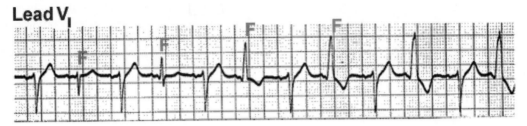

Fig. 13-14   Fusion beat. *(Courtesy of Frank Yanowitz, M.D., The Alan Lindsay ECG Learning Center, http://medstat.med.utah. edu/kw/ecg.)*

posterior fascicular blocks). All these blocks occur with increased frequency in the elderly population.

Looking first at the major blocks, their diagnoses are facilitated by dividing the QRS complex in half. The first half of the complex tends to represent left bundle activity and the latter half right bundle activity. Using this model, a left bundle-branch block (LBBB) should alter the QRS complex immediately, whereas a right bundle-branch block (RBBB) should affect only the latter portion of the complex, marked by a wide, slurred S wave. These differences are best appreciated in leads I and V_6 (Fig. 13-17).

Axis is the key to the diagnosis of the minor blocks (left anterior fascicular block (LAFB) and left posterior fascicular block (LPFB)). Unexplained marked left-axis deviation (greater than −45 degrees) is LAFB and unexplained marked right-axis deviation (greater than 110 degrees) is LPFB unless proven otherwise. Other causes of axis shift exist as well. Emphysema, right ventricular hypertrophy, RBBB, dextrocardia, ventricular ectopic rhythms, and Wolff-Parkinson-White syndrome also can produce marked right-axis deviation. Congenital cardiac abnormalities, LBBB, Wolff-Parkinson-White syndrome, hyperkalemia, and ventricular ectopic rhythms are capable of producing marked left-axis deviation.[21] The history, physical examination, laboratory analysis, and ECG can aid in excluding virtually all these alternative diagnoses. Once they are eliminated, marked left-axis deviation is LAFB and marked right-axis deviation is LPFB (Figs. 13-18, Fig. 13-19).

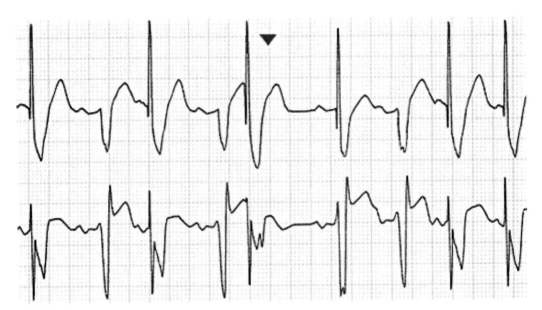

Fig. 13-15   Failure to sense. *(Courtesy of Frank Yanowitz, M.D., The Alan Lindsay ECG Learning Center, http:// medstat.med.utah.edu/kw/ecg, and GE Medical Systems, Information Technologies.)*

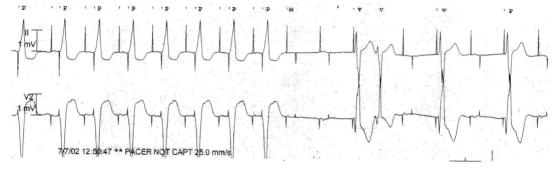

Fig. 13-16 Pacemaker-failure to capture.*(Courtesy of Alfred Buxton, M.D., Brown University.)*

Lead I   **Lead V6**

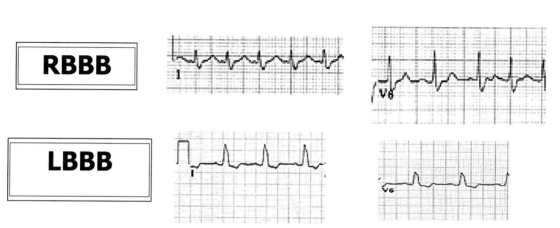

Fig. 13-17 Bundle-branch block.

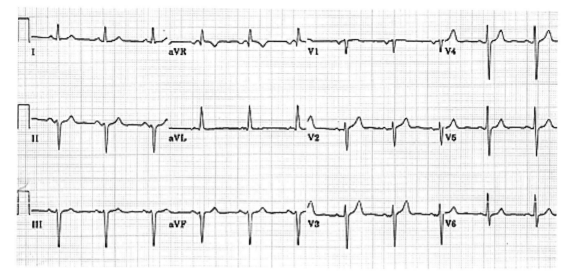

Fig. 13-18 Left anterior fascicular block. *(Courtesy of Frank Yanowitz, M.D., The Alan Lindsay ECG Learning Center, http://med-stat.med.utah.edu/kw/ecg.)*

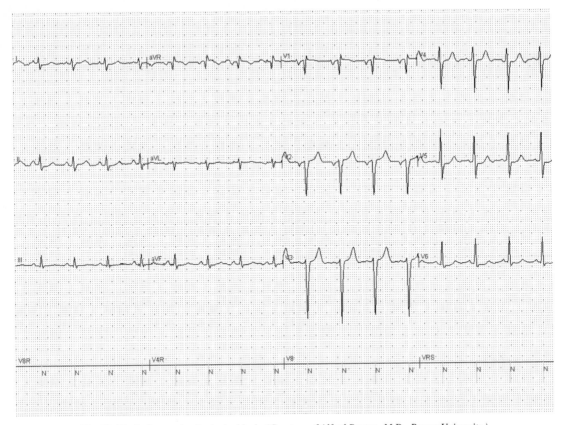

Fig. 13-19 Left posterior fascicular block. *(Courtesy of Alfred Buxton, M.D., Brown University.)*

EMERGENCY DEPARTMENT CARE AND DISPOSITION

If the patient is doing well (asymptomatic, normal vital signs, etc), then the clinician has time to probe the dysrhythmia carefully. Conversely, the unstable or decompensating patient demands immediate therapy.

In general, four forms of therapy are available to the emergency physician: electricity, antidysrhythmic agents, electrical pacing, and medications that modify conduction at the AV junction. Direct cardiac stimulants used to treat certain forms of bradydysrhythmias have fallen out of favor, but drugs such as atropine that act by reducing parasympathetic influence on the heart remain useful.

Electricity, in the form of cardioversion or defibrillation, should be used for all tachydysrhythmias in unstable or decompensating patients. This is true regardless of whether the tachydysrhythmia originates in the ventricle, the junction, or the atrium. For sinus tachycardia, of course, defibrillation/cardioversion has little to offer. This dysrhythmia is merely the body's response to pathology elsewhere that must be identified and treated. Hypovolemia is commonly the reason, but fever, thyrotoxicosis, drug ingestion, and the like also must be considered.

For bradydysrhythmias, pacemakers are the bedrock of management. While passage of a transvenous pacer wire remains the "gold standard" for this form of therapy, it can be both difficult and time-consuming. External pacer pads, on the other hand, can be applied in a few seconds. In most cases, these will be able to drive the heart at a rate necessary to stabilize the patient long enough for a transvenous wire to be placed under more controlled circumstances. If external pacing fails to achieve capture, then a transvenous pacer must be placed as an emergency procedure. Most EDs are equipped with balloon-tipped pacer catheters. The balloon allows the catheter to pass the tricuspid valve with more ease than a catheter not so equipped, allowing the procedure to be performed without fluoroscopy. The position of the catheter can be determined by observing the cardiac monitor while the wire is being passed. After the catheter reaches the central circulation, the pacer is turned on and the balloon inflated. As the catheter is advanced, the ECG is observed first for atrial activity and then for ventricular pacing. Once in the ventricle, the ECG should look like any other ECG performed on a patient with a ventricular pacemaker. The balloon can then be deflated and the catheter advanced slightly with the intent of firmly lodging it in the trabeculae of the right ventricle.

With antidysrhythmic medications, the emergency physician must first determine if the rhythm in question needs suppression. In the case of escape rhythms, suppression is the last thing that the patient needs. This decision is made easier because most escape rhythms beat at a slow rate, which usually discourages suppressive therapy. Ectopic tachydysrhythmias, however, often need chemical suppression, and the choice of medications may be crucial.

In the ventricle, ectopic beats are best managed acutely with drugs such as lidocaine and amiodarone. For the long term, however, attempts to use medications to suppress ventricular dysrhythmias have not proven to be successful. Proarrhythmic drug effects often increased, rather than decreased, patient mortality. Mechanical management, usually in the form of automatic internal cardiac defibrillators (AICDs), now dominates the long-term treatment for these dysrhythmias.

The need for short-term management of atrial dysrhythmias is virtually nonexistent; control of ventricular response should be the main priority. In an elderly patient, the ventricle often is incapable of handling the same response rate as that of a younger person's ventricle. In these cases, a medication designed to increase the conduction time of the junction (and thereby slow the ventricular response) is needed. Digoxin, in the past, was the primary agent used for this purpose. While it remains a viable choice, an increase in sympathetic tone or circulating catecholamines can overcome its effects. Calcium channel blockers have supplanted digoxin as the primary agent administered in these patients. Early cardioversion of new-onset atrial fibrillation is rarely an option in the elderly. Concomitant diseases, clot formation, and remodeling of the atrial architecture preclude this approach in most elderly patients.

For atrial fibrillation in the presence of accessory tract disease, the chaotic atrial impulses are not conducted through the AV junction but via a bypass bundle. Administering AV blocking agents in this case will ensure that all impulses are transmitted via the bypass tract, often increasing the already rapid rate. In this case, procainamide is the drug of choice.

REFERENCES

1. Thomas AC, Knapman PA, Krikler DM, Davies MJ: Community study of the causes of "natural" sudden death. *Br Med J* 297:1453, 1988.
2. Leach IH, Blundell JW, Rowley JM, Turner DR: Acute ischaemic lesions in death due to ischaemic heart disease. An autopsy study of 333 cases of out-of-hospital death. *Eur Heart J* 16:1181,1995.
3. Busby DE, Davis AW: Paroxysmal and chronic atrial fibrillation in airman certification. *Aviat Space Environ Med* 47:185, 1976.
4. Lake FR, Cullen KJ, de Klerk NH, et al: Atrial fibrillation and mortality in an elderly population. *Aust NZ J Med* 19:321, 1989.
5. Fisch C, Genovese PD, Dyke RW, et al: The electrocardiogram in persons over 70. *Geriatrics* 12:616, 1957.
6. Camm AJ, Evans KE, Ward DE, Martin A: The rhythm of the heart in active elderly subjects. *Am Heart J* 99:598, 1980.
7. Golden GS, Golden LH: The "nona" electrocardiogram: Findings in 100 patients of the 90 plus age group. *J Am Geriatr Soc* 22:329, 1974.
8. Katz LN, Pick A: The arrhythmias, part I, in Lea R(ed): *Clinical Electrocardiography*. Philadelphia, Lippincott, 1956, p 43.
9. Makinson DH, Wade G: Aetiology and treatment of auricular flutter. *Lancet* 1:105, 1950.
10. Armburst CA, Levine SA: Paroxysmal ventricular tachycardia: A study of one hundred and seven cases. *Circulation* 1:28, 1950.
11. Morady F, Shen EN, Bhandari A, et al: Clinical symptoms in patients with sustained ventricular tachycardia. *West J Med* 142:341, 1985.
12. De Bacquer D, De Backer G, Kornitzer M: Prevalences of ECG findings in large population based samples of men and women. *Heart* 84(6):625, 2000.
13. Friedman PA, Cardiology, part III, in Prakash UBS (ed): *Mayo Internal Medicine Board Review 2000–2001.* Philadelphia, Lippincott, Williams & Williams, 2000, p 72.
14. Lown B, Wyatt NF, Levine HD: Paroxysmal atrial tachycardia with block. *Circulation* 21:129, 1960.
15. Ma G: Electrocardiographic manifestations: Digitalis toxicity. *J Emerg Med* 20(2):145, 2001.
16. Kilpatrick TR, Moore CB, Maza E: Drug-resistant ventricular tachycardia of 62 days duration. *JAMA* 197:762, 1966.
17. Anderson KP, Walker R, Dustman T, et al: Spontaneous sustained ventricular tachycardia in the Electrophysiologic Study Versus Electrocardiographic Monitoring (ESVEM) Trial. *J Am Coll Cardiol* 26:489, 1995.

18. Tchou P, Young P, Mahmud R, et al: Useful clinical criteria for the diagnosis of ventricular tachycardia. *Am J Med* 84:53, 1988.

19. Coley, Andrew: Personal communication, 2002.

20. Brugada P, Brugada J, Mont L, et al: A new approach to the differential diagnosis of a regular tachycardia with a wide QRS complex. *Circulation* 83:1649, 1991.

21. Marriott HJL Electrical Axis: in *Practical Electrocardiography* 8th ed.. Baltimore, Williams & Wilkins, 1987, p 39.

14

Valvular Heart Disease

Stefanie R. Ellison

HIGH-YIELD FACTS

- Aortic stenosis is the most common valvular disorder in the geriatric population and the third most common cardiovascular cause of death.
- Patients with aortic stenosis, mitral stenosis, or mitral valve prolapse have an increased risk of sudden cardiac death.
- In hemodynamically compromised aortic regurgitation, aortic balloon counterpulsation is relatively contraindicated.
- The cardiac examination for aortic stenosis and mitral stenosis in the geriatric patient differs from that of the younger patient. The decreased compliance of the geriatric heart may make the classic auscultatory findings more subtle.

The geriatric patient population is living longer with comorbidities that contribute to cardiac disease. There is a greater prevalence of hypertension, pulmonary disease, and diabetes, which all contribute to valvular heart disease. The heart's tremendous ability to adapt allows patients to remain asymptomatic from valvular disorders for years.

The normal function of the cardiac valves is to direct forward flow and prevent backflow in the heart. The valves open and close based on varied phases of systole and diastole. The mitral valve is a bicuspid valve; in contrast, the aortic, pulmonary, and tricuspid valves are all tricuspid structures. Valves that are physiologically intact allow no leakage when they are closed. The valves each open in sequence to a specific surface area, opening to provide flow into or out of the cardiac chambers. Valvular disorders arise when the valves do not close adequately or open to their normal surface capacity. Papillary muscles and chordae tendineae attach to the tricuspid and mitral valves to close the valves in sequence with the beating heart. Any abnormality to the valves or structure of the heart can result in hemodynamic compromise.

AORTIC STENOSIS

Aortic stenosis is the most common valvular disease in the geriatric population. It ranks behind only atherosclerosis and hypertension as a cardiovascular cause of death.[1] One of the reasons it is a significant source of morbidity is that patients are often asymptomatic for a long period of time. The gradual narrowing of the aortic valve and accompanying increased obstruction lead to eventual cardiac hypertrophy. Severe congestive heart failure in the elderly should prompt clinicians to investigate for occult aortic stenosis.

Epidemiology

Aortic stenosis in general is more common in men, older persons, and patients with hypercholesterolemia. In a random sample of men with an average age of 80 years, it was shown to be present in 14 percent by echocardiography.[2] However, 50 to 60 percent of elderly patients with calcific aortic stenosis are female, compared with 20 percent in younger individuals.[3]

Pathophysiology

In the elderly, aortic stenosis most often occurs from calcification of the aortic valve with subsequent stenosis. This is different from the etiology of aortic stenosis in younger individuals, where the most common cause is a congenital bicuspid valve.

The aortic valve is normally a tricuspid valve with three leaflets. The normal functional area is 3 to 4 cm^2. When this area is reduced by sclerosis to one-quarter of its normal valve area, severe obstruction to cardiac outflow results in a progressive pressure overload on the left ventricle.

The pressure gradient across the aortic valve can be determined by the pressure difference between the left ventricle and the central aorta. This can be measured by echocardiography or cardiac catheterization. Symptoms usually are present when the mean aortic valve gradient exceeds 50 mmHg or if the aortic valve area is no larger than 1 cm.[2,3]

The heart responds to the increased ventricular pressure with myocardial hypertrophy to maintain cardiac output. The ventricular pressure eventually exceeds the ability of the thickened myocardium to compensate, and an increase in afterload results. This is the cause of the systolic dysfunction seen in aortic stenosis.[4] The hypertrophy is additionally maladaptive because this portion of the myocardium has decreased coronary blood flow and is at risk for ischemia. Eventual systolic and diastolic dysfunction of the hypertrophic myocardium further predisposes the patient to congestive heart failure.

Three general etiologies are responsible for aortic stenosis in the elderly: (1) degenerative calcification of a previously normal valve, (2) atherosclerotic aortic valvular stenosis, and (3) calcification of a bicuspid aortic valve. The first is responsible for aortic stenosis in more than 90 percent of patients over age 65.[1] The commissural fusion seen in younger patients with aortic stenosis is usually absent in older patients. The pathophysiology of aortic stenosis shows that the calcification in the congenitally abnormal valve will lead to significant stenosis in the younger patient a decade before degenerative calcification in the older patient.[5]

Clinical Features

Most patients present with symptoms in the sixth and seventh decades of life. The cardinal symptoms of obstruction in severe aortic stenosis are angina pectoris, syncope, presyncope, and congestive heart failure. Gastrointestinal bleeding, atrioventricular conduction defects leading to complete heart block, calcific cerebral emboli, and bacterial endocarditis are also serious manifestations. Syncope related to aortic stenosis can be attributable to a number of causes (Table 14-1).

The presence of a narrow pulse pressure is common in the patient with hemodynamically significant aortic stenosis. The progressive increase in peripheral vascular resistance in the aging process may lead to a higher systolic pressure component and less of narrowed pulse pressure, as seen in the younger patient. In severe aortic stenosis, the carotid upstroke may be slowed, and there is usually a palpable shudder in the carotid vessel. Systemic hypertension and sclerotic vessels of the geriatric patient can mask this sign.

On cardiac examination, there is not a significant displacement of the left ventricular impulse until late in the course. Concentric left ventricular hypertrophy will make the hypertrophy less appreciable. It is important to palpate for an atrial filling wave. The fourth heart sound heard in the younger age group is less reliable in the elderly. The elderly patient has a less mobile calcific valve, making the ejection sound difficult to hear. A fourth heart sound occurs in 70 to 80 percent of patients over age 70.[3] This sound may be present physiologically from decreased compliance of the left ventricular wall that occurs with aging.

The harsh systolic ejection murmur is loudest at the upper-right sternal border. There also may be a palpable thrill in that area. The murmur also may be transmitted to the carotid vessels. A higher-pitched apical murmur may be heard as well. Clues that the disease is at least moderate in severity include peaking of the murmur late in systole, delayed carotid upstroke, and a soft single heart sound.[5] The second heart sound is soft or absent due to the decreased mobility of the aortic leaflets. There can be a paradoxical splitting of the second heart sound from prolonged left ventricular ejection (Fig. 14-1 and Table 14-2).

Following the onset of symptoms, the patient's life expectancy is approximately 4 years. The presenting symptoms can be prognostic as well. Angina pectoris has an average of 5 years before death, whereas congestive heart failure patients may survive for 2 years following the onset of symptoms.[2,3] Patients who present with syncope have a 1- to 18-year survival rate.[6]

Up to 15 percent of patients with significant aortic stenosis suffer sudden cardiac death. Up to 5 percent of patients die without preceding symptoms, whereas the others have heralding symptoms that necessitate evaluation.[2,6]

Table 14-1. Causes of Syncope in Aortic Stenosis

1. Paroxysmal supraventricular or ventricular tachyarrhythmias with subsequent poor cardiac output
2. Reduced peripheral vascular resistance and the inability to increase cardiac output sufficiently to maintain perfusion pressure
3. Development of atrioventricular conduction abnormalities
4. Increased vagal sensitivity that may lead to bradyarrhythmias, heart block, and hypotension
5. Medications, such as nitroglycerin, that can further reduce peripheral vascular resistance

Diagnosis and Differential

The electrocardiogram (ECG) may be normal even in the presence of hemodynamically significant disease. Prolonged PR interval, left ventricular hypertrophy, and ST- and T-wave changes are most common. Calcification also may result in degeneration of the conduction system, resulting in first-, second-, and third-degree heart block, left bundle-branch block, and left anterior hemiblock.

Aortic Stenosis

Loud crescendo-decrescendo systolic murmur
Diminished intensity of S_2
May have paradoxical splitting of S_2
Murmur transmits to carotid vessels

Aortic Regurgitation

High-pitched "blowing murmur"
An S_3 may be present

Mitral Stenosis

Mid-diastolic rumbling murmur
Loud S_1
Opening snap

Mitral Regurgitation

Usually an S_3 and S_4 will be heard
Harsh apical systolic murmur from S_1 to S_2

Mitral Valve Prolapse

Mid-systolic click
Click may be followed by systolic murmur
S_2 may be diminished by murmur

Fig. 14-1   Auscultation of heart murmurs.

Special attention should be directed toward identifying the presence of a calcified aortic valve on the chest radiograph. There also may be an annular calcification of the mitral valve. Poststenotic dilatation of the ascending aorta may be seen.

Echocardiography remains the most useful noninvasive study for evaluation of aortic stenosis. The valve can be assessed directly for thickened immobile aortic cusps. Left ventricular performance also can be quantitated.

Cardiac catheterization can evaluate the severity of aortic stenosis and any associated coronary atherosclerosis. All operative candidates for valve replacement should undergo cardiac catheterization to evaluate the severity of the valvular disorder as well as their cardiac risk for surgery. Comparing pressure differences between the left ventricle and the central aorta by flow can help determine which patients to consider for operative intervention. A pressure gradient over 40 mmHg or a calculated valve area of 0.75 cm^2 or less would indicate need for operative intervention. In addition, 25 to 50 percent of patients with severe aortic stenosis and angina pectoris have associated coronary atherosclerosis.[2]

Emergency Department Care and Disposition

Coronary ischemia should be treated with nitroglycerin, with the patient's hemodynamic status monitored carefully. In the elderly patient, lowering the peripheral vascular resistance may decrease perfusion pressure. Congestive heart failure should be managed with diuresis and decreasing afterload for more effective cardiac output.

Syncope may require admission for continuous cardiac monitoring and to investigate the comorbidities as a cause of syncope. The workup should evaluate for conduction abnormalities and the development of hemodynamically significant tachyarrhythmias.

In patients presenting in cardiogenic shock, there is a role for an aortic counterpulsation balloon. While it may be difficult to place this device beyond a stenotic valve, these valves respond well to the balloon pump.[7]

Patients with symptoms of hemodynamically significant aortic stenosis should undergo aortic valve replacement. With improved intraoperative technique and postoperative care, patients over age 65 have a favorable outcome with a low operative mortality. Optimal results are achieved when the procedure is elective and in patients without severe compromise of left ventricular func-

Table 14-2. Clinical Signs of Aortic Stenosis and Its Variation in Geriatric Patients

Clinical Signs of Aortic Stenosis	Variation of Clinical Features in the Elderly
Slow carotid upstroke	Normal to brisk carotid upstroke
Narrowed pulse pressure	Normal pulse pressure
Apical impulse thrust	Apical murmur more prominent
Basal systolic ejection murmur	Atrial gallop "normal" S_4
Left ventricular hypertrophy on ECG	Nonspecific ECG
Calcified aortic valve on chest x-ray	Symptoms due to other organ disease

tion (New York Heart Association functional class III or IV).[8] Even patients with severe left ventricular dysfunction can benefit from valve replacement with an acceptable mortality and morbidity. For patients 80 years of age and older, the operative mortality is 0.2 percent for aortic valve replacement and 20.9 percent when combined with coronary artery bypass surgery.[9,10]

AORTIC REGURGITATION

Pathophysiology

Infective endocarditis accounts for the majority of acute aortic regurgitation cases. Aortic dissection from the aortic root accounts for the rest. The immediate backflow of blood from the aorta to the left ventricle can cause acute heart failure. The geriatric population with hypertension is at greatest risk for this valvular disorder and its complications. Aortic regurgitation has been discovered on echocardiography in 32 percent of men with an average age of 80.[1]

Causes of chronic aortic regurgitation include rheumatic heart disease and congenital abnormalities. Other inflammatory causes include syphilis, Reiter syndrome, and ankylosing spondylitis. There is an association with fenfluramine, phentermine, or dexfenfluramine.

Chronic aortic regurgitation is seen in a male-to-female ratio of 3:2. In chronic disease, the ventricle dilates to handle the regurgitant volume. This results in eventual ventricular hypertrophy and a fall in the diastolic blood pressure. Peripheral vasodilation also occurs. When the heart rate is increased, the time in diastole is decreased, and thus the regurgitation volume is decreased and cardiac output is nearly normalized. Geriatric patients are more likely to have symptoms in times of stress or febrile illness when greater cardiac output is needed or dehydration exacerbates symptoms.

Clinical Features

Acute Aortic Regurgitation

Aortic regurgitation from endocarditis may present with fever, rigor, dyspnea, or pulmonary edema. Aortic dissection presents with chest pain that is severe and radiating to the midscapular region. Diaphoresis, tachycardia, tachypnea, rales, and signs of stroke may be present .

On cardiac examination, there is a high-pitched "blow-ing" murmur heard immediately after S_2. It is best heard in the right second intercostal area near the sternum. An S_3 also may be present along with a systolic flow murmur (see Fig. 14-1).

Electrocardiographic changes may include acute myocardial infarction if the coronary arteries are involved in aortic dissection. Acute pulmonary edema without cardiac enlargement can be seen on the chest radiograph. Signs of aortic dissection would show a widened mediastinum, blurred aortic contour, apical cap, or left pleural effusion.

Chronic Aortic Regurgitation

Patients may complain of palpitations from premature ventricular contractions or the large stroke volume from the regurgitation. Other symptoms include chest pain, fatigue, and dyspnea. Up to 70 percent of patients may be asymptomatic despite significant regurgitation. Sudden death is common in patients with acute and chronic aortic regurgitation

Signs include a wide pulse pressure. Patients may have a head bob due to a strong ventricular impulse. The classic "water-hammer pulse" is a peripheral pulse sign that has a strong, quick upstroke followed by collapse. The Duroziez sign is a palpable to-and-fro murmur best heard at the femoral artery. Quincke pulse is capillary pulsations that are visible in the proximal nailbed when pressure is placed distally on the nail. The ECG may demonstrate left ventricular hypertrophy or congestive heart failure. Chest radiography may reveal left ventricular hypertrophy, evidence of heart failure, and aortic dilatation.

Emergency Department Care and Disposition

Initial treatment should focus on stabilization of the airway, breathing, and circulation. Standard congestive heart failure therapy should be started. The patient should be treated with intravenous afterload reducers, and the emergency physician should consult cardiology for emergent echocardiography. Intraaortic balloon counterpulsation is contraindicated in severe aortic regurgitation. If the regurgitant lesion is critical, emergency surgery may be required.

Patients with fever and acute aortic regurgitation should be suspected of having infective endocarditis. Blood cultures should be obtained, and broad-spectrum antibiotics should be administered.

MITRAL STENOSIS

Epidemiology

Mitral stenosis is a narrowing of the outflow path of the left ventricle. The stenosis can stem from thickened mitral valves, fused commissures, or thickened and shortened chordae tendineae. The cause of mitral stenosis is most commonly rheumatic fever. Prevalence of mitral stenosis in the United States has decreased with the decline of rheumatic fever cases. Other less frequent causes are congenital mitral stenosis, rheumatoid arthritis, bacterial endocarditis, and systemic lupus erythematosus. Geriatric patients who have lived with these chronic conditions are particularly at risk for developing mitral stenosis. This disease is seen less commonly in the geriatric population; one study found that 4 percent of men with an average age of 80 years had rheumatic mitral stenosis.[1]

Pathophysiology

Scarring from rheumatic endocarditis causes fusion of the commissures and matting of the chordae tendineae. This scarring interferes with valve closure. Further calcification over time makes the valve less mobile. This combination leads to stenosis. The normal valve area measures 4 to 6 cm^2; with stenosis, the area is reduced to 2 cm^2. This leads to increased left atrial pressure to maintain flow into the left ventricle. Once the stenosis has reached a critical level, the natural progression is increased pressures across the left atrium into the pulmonary vessels, resulting in pulmonary hypertension. This increased pressure can carry across the heart to cause pulmonary and tricuspid insufficiency, and eventual right-sided heart failure results.

The increased pressure on the left atrium increases the risk of developing a mural thrombus and possible embolization, especially in the elderly population. Atrial fibrillation subsequently develops in up to 40 percent of patients with mitral stenosis. This further increases the risk of mural thrombus formation.[9] Patients with atrial fibrillation also have decreased cardiac output. The propensity of atrial fibrillation to have a rapid ventricular response also decreases cardiac filling, resulting in a further decrease in cardiac output. These events, paired with the decreased wall motion of the geriatric heart, further compromise cardiac output. The older population has a greater risk of complications if mitral stenosis is present in the later years of life.

Clinical Features

Generally, mitral stenosis is a chronic condition. Symptoms may arise when there are increased demands on cardiac output. Exertion, tachycardia, anemia, infection, and atrial fibrillation can induce symptoms. Exertional dyspnea is the most common presenting symptom. Paroxysmal nocturnal dyspnea can occur with more severe disease. Hemoptysis is the second most common presenting symptom from pulmonary hypertension and bronchial vein rupture. Other symptoms include orthopnea and palpitations from premature atrial contractions and atrial fibrillation. Systemic emboli may occur from an atrial thrombus with resulting myocardial, kidney, or central nervous system infarction. With progression of disease, right-sided heart failure symptoms also may develop.

On cardiac examination, the signs of mitral stenosis include a mid-diastolic rumbling murmur with crescendo toward the S_2. With atrial fibrillation the presystolic accentuation of the murmur may disappear. Typically, the S_1 is loud, and the murmur is preceded by a loud opening "snap." This sound is best heard over the apex (see Fig. 14-1). A prominent *a* wave may be seen in the neck. An early systolic parasternal lift may be felt due to the right-sided heart pressure overload. The apical impulse is small and tapping, secondary to an underfilled left ventricle. Systemic blood pressure may be normal or low. Rales may be heard as the disease progresses. With pulmonary hypertension, signs include a thin body habitus, peripheral cyanosis, and cool extremities from the low cardiac output. When pulmonary hypertension is present, the auscultatory findings are less evident.

The ECG may demonstrate a notched or diphasic P wave with right-axis deviation. The chest radiograph may reveal straightening of the left heart border from left atrial enlargement. Eventually, pulmonary congestion is evident with cephalization of the pulmonary vessels, Kerley B lines, and an increase in vascular markings.

The suspected diagnosis should be confirmed with an echocardiogram and consultation with a cardiologist. A transesophageal echocardiogram (TEE) yields a more complete analysis of dysfunction, especially for the mitral valve. The urgency for formal diagnosis is based on the severity of symptoms and the suspected diagnosis.

Emergency Department Care and Disposition

The most common presentation requiring treatment is atrial fibrillation with rapid ventricular response. With silent valvular disease this may precipitate the symptoms of mitral stenosis. Heart rate control should be accomplished with intravenous diltiazem or digoxin; intravenous propranolol or verapamil may be considered, but their negative inotropic action may cause problems of inadequate cardiac output. Cardioversion may be needed in severely compromised patients. The most common cause of the dysrhythmia is the dilated atrium. This remains unchanged after cardioversion, so recurrence of the dysrhythmia is common. The danger of embolization is greater with long-standing atrial fibrillation.

Hemoptysis can accompany pulmonary edema. If pulmonary hypertension is present, gross hemoptysis may require emergent management of the airway, blood transfusion, pulmonary vessel embolization, and emergency surgery.

Embolic stroke is also a risk from concurrent atrial fibrillation. Independent predictors of cerebrovascular events are age, atrial fibrillation, and severe aortic stenosis.[11,12] In the event of ischemic stroke, anticoagulation should be initiated with intravenous heparin. Other embolic events, such as bowel ischemia, renal infarct, myocardial infarction, and peripheral ischemia, should be considered, especially in the geriatric patient.

Definitive treatment of mitral stenosis is replacement or repair of the valve. There is an increase in the average age of patients undergoing surgical procedures because of comorbid conditions and mixed cardiac indications for surgery in older patients. Replacement of the valve may be accomplished by either a mechanical valve or a biologic prosthetic valve. In treating mitral valve stenosis, percutaneous balloon mitral commissurotomy also has had successful results. A study of Medicare-aged patients demonstrated that this procedure had similar survival and complication rates at 4 years compared with younger patients undergoing the same procedure.[13]

MITRAL REGURGITATION

Epidemiology

Mitral regurgitation, which is retrograde flow of blood from the left ventricle into the left atrium, is a relatively common valve disorder in the geriatric population. Doppler echocardiography demonstrated the prevalence of mitral regurgitation to be 32 percent in a population of men with a mean age of 80 years.[1] This valvular abnormality should be considered in any patient with evidence of heart failure.

Pathophysiology

The mitral valve itself is made up of anterior and posterior leaflets, an annulus, chordae tendineae, papillary muscles, and a portion of the wall of the left ventricle. The mitral valve apparatus is important to the contraction of the left ventricle and is responsible for about 10 percent of the ejection fraction. Disruption of this apparatus results in significant changes in cardiac output.

The etiologies of mitral regurgitation are most commonly infective endocarditis or myocardial infarction. Myocardial infarction causes acute rupture of the chordae tendineae and papillary muscles or perforation of the valve leaflets. Inferior myocardial infarction is the most common cause of ischemic mitral valve incompetence. The ischemic etiology of mitral regurgitation is the most common acute presentation in the geriatric population. Trauma is an occasional cause of acute mitral valve regurgitation. Patients with acute mitral regurgitation deteriorate rapidly.

Rheumatic heart disease is the most common cause of chronic mitral incompetence in the geriatric population. The use of appetite suppressant drugs, such as fenfluramine, phentermine, or dexfenfluramine, has been found to be associated with mitral and aortic cardiac valve incompetence. The pathophysiology has been determined to be plaque deposition on valves.[14]

Acute mitral regurgitation with a noncompliant left atrium quickly elevates pressures and causes pulmonary edema. With chronic mitral regurgitation, the left atrium dilates so that left atrial pressure rises in a controlled rate. The heart adapts by increasing left ventricular stroke volume. Effective forward flow into the aorta is maintained despite the regurgitation across the incompetent mitral valve.

Clinical Features

Acute Mitral Regurgitation

In acute mitral regurgitation, patients present with dyspnea, tachycardia, and pulmonary edema. Patients may deteriorate quickly to cardiogenic shock or cardiac arrest. They may present with acute respiratory distress and pulmonary edema, with asymptomatic periods in between. The pronounced dyspnea of these attacks may mask the angina and ischemia causing the intermittent regurgitation (see Table 14-3).

On cardiac examination, an S_3 and S_4 sound usually will be auscultated along with a harsh apical systolic murmur, starting with S_1 and ending before S_2. Patients may have an active apical impulse, systolic thrust, and thrill

Table 14-3. Signs and Symptoms of Acute versus Chronic Mitral Regurgitation

Acute Mitral Regurgitation	Chronic Mitral Regurgitation
Presents with pulmonary edema	Presents with dyspnea, atrial fibrillation
Results from acute myocardial infarction	Results from rheumatic fever, endocarditis
Harsh systolic murmur	High-pitched holosystolic murmur
Apical impulse, thrill	Radiates to the axilla
ECG: myocardial ischemia/infarction	ECG: left atrial/ventricular hypertrophy
Chest radiograph: pulmonary edema	Chest radiograph: left ventricular hypertrophy

at the apex. Jugular venous distension may be seen, with a prominent *a* wave and a left parasternal lift (see Fig. 14-1).

The ECG may show evidence of acute inferior wall myocardial infarction (more common than anterior infarction in this setting). Acute mitral regurgitation from papillary muscle rupture may demonstrate an enlarged left atrium and pulmonary edema on chest radiograph. The cardiac silhouette would be less impressive than expected from chronic heart failure.

Chronic Mitral Regurgitation

Chronic mitral regurgitation can be tolerated for years. Usually the first symptoms are exertional dyspnea and those associated with atrial fibrillation. Systemic emboli can occur in 20 percent of patients with atrial fibrillation. Endocarditis is a possible complication (See Table 14-3).

On cardiac examination, a high-pitched holosystolic murmur is best auscultated in the fifth intercostal space and mid-left thorax, and it radiates to the axilla. The first heart sound can be decreased due to the murmur. The intensity of the murmur is increased by squatting and leg elevation. An S_3 can be heard if left ventricular failure is present.

The ECG may reveal left atrial and left ventricular hypertrophy. The chest radiograph may demonstrate left ventricular and atrial enlargement proportional to the severity of the regurgitation. Two-dimensional echocardiography and Doppler flow studies enhance assessment of the severity of mitral regurgitation and its mechanism. Valvular incompetence can be determined by using Doppler studies to measure the regurgitant fraction; the study also may reveal ischemic contribution to the valve dysfunction.

Right-sided heart catheterization assists in evaluating mitral regurgitation and managing patients with decompensated heart failure resulting from myocardial infarction. Hemodynamic evidence of left ventricular failure, manifested by low cardiac output, elevated pulmonary artery wedge pressure, and pulmonary hypertension, in mitral regurgitation can help direct therapy.[15]

Emergency Department Care and Disposition

Treatment of acute mitral regurgitation from myocardial infarction should begin by addressing the underlying problem. If the patient meets inclusion criteria, infusion of fibrinolytic agents will improve blood flow to the papillary muscle and facilitate valvular competence. Coronary angioplasty is another reperfusion technique that can serve to improve mitral regurgitation.

Another goal is to decrease the valvular incompetence volume. This may be accomplished by reducing afterload. Since acute pulmonary edema is usually present, the initial treatment should include afterload reduction. Patients with mitral regurgitation can benefit from intravenous nitroprusside or nitroglycerin therapy. The reduction in afterload can help relieve both the regurgitation and the pulmonary edema. Swan-Ganz catheter insertion should be considered to optimize management. If medical management fails, intraaortic balloon counterpulsation should be considered.

Aspirin therapy and other treatments for the acute coronary syndrome should be implemented as well. In mitral regurgitation from cardiac ischemia, beta blockers should be avoided. By slowing the cardiac cycle, the volume of regurgitation will increase and worsen symptoms.

If infective endocarditis is in the differential diagnosis, standard workup and treatment for this disorder should be initiated in the emergency department.

Emergency surgery should be considered in patients with decompensation of acute or chronic mitral regurgitation. Since patients are usually acutely ill, the emergency physician needs to expeditiously initiate treatment while arranging for emergent cardiology and cardiothoracic surgery consultation.

MITRAL VALVE PROLAPSE

Epidemiology

Mitral valve prolapse is the most common valvular heart disease in the United States, affecting nearly 3 percent of the population. The etiology is currently unknown but is suspected to be congenital. Women and men have a nearly equal occurrence of mitral valve prolapse.[16]

Pathophysiology

There is disruption of collagen bundles in the leaflets and chordae tendineae of the mitral valves. Mitral valve prolapse is seen in 57 percent of patients with Marfan's syndrome. It also occurs in Ehlers-Danlos and osteogenesis imperfecta. Hypertrophic cardiomyopathy and pulmonary hypertension are the most common secondary causes of mitral valve prolapse in the elderly population.

Clinical Features

Patients are usually asymptomatic. Presenting symptoms may include chest pain, panic attacks, palpitations, fatigue, and dyspnea unrelated to exertion. There is an increased incidence of sudden death and dysrhythmia in patients with mitral valve prolapse. If over the age of 45, patients are at increased risk of transient ischemic attack. In mitral valve prolapse without mitral regurgitation, it occasionally can be induced by exercise. Leaner body mass index and lower waist-to-hip ratio are seen typically in patients with mitral valve prolapse.[16]

The classic cardiac finding in mitral valve prolapse is a midsystolic click. The second heart sound may be diminished by the late portion of the systolic murmur. The ECG and chest radiograph are usually normal. Echocardiography is diagnostic and can determine if there is coexisting mitral regurgitation. Screening with this diagnostic tool is recommended when symptoms are suspected from concomitant regurgitation.

Emergency Department Care and Disposition

Emergency physicians need to reassure patients with mitral valve prolapse of the benign nature of the disease. Geriatric patients need to follow up with a cardiologist to confirm the diagnosis. It is important to warn patients of the remote possibility of sudden cardiac death and dysrhythmias. Geriatric patients are more likely to have enlarged atria or ventricles from coexisting disease, which predispose them to complications of mitral valve prolapse. Patients with comorbidities should have other life-threatening causes excluded before attributing them to mitral valve prolapse.

RIGHT-SIDED VALVULAR HEART DISEASE

Right-sided heart disease is relatively uncommon. For geriatric patients, the most common causes would be rheumatic heart disease leading to mitral valve disease and left-sided heart failure resulting in right-sided heart failure, and tricuspid regurgitation. Tricuspid disease also can be associated with mitral valve disease. This is due to a functional relationship between the tricuspid annulus and transmission of mechanical insufficiency from the mitral valve across the fibrous septum. Pulmonary regurgitation is most often a result of pulmonary hypertension. There is also a correlation of tricuspid and pulmonary valve stenosis from carcinoid disease.[17]

The symptoms of right-sided valvular heart disease are most commonly dyspnea and orthopnea. Cardiac examination of tricuspid regurgitation reveals a soft blowing holosystolic murmur. In tricuspid stenosis, the murmur is a crescendo-decrescendo diastolic murmur. Both are best auscultated at the left sternal border. Treatment should focus on stabilization of heart failure and reduction of hypertension.

PROPHYLAXIS FOR VALVULAR DISEASE

Patients with existing cardiac valvular disease or prosthetic valves require antibiotic prophylaxis for the prevention of infective endocarditis. Minor procedures in the emergency department that require pretreatment with antibiotics are incision and drainage of an abscess, urethral catheterization in the presence of infection, and dental procedures known to cause bleeding. Intubation alone does not require prophylactic antibiotics.

The choice of antibiotics is based on the microorganism most likely to be present. *Streptococcus, Enterococcus, Staphylococcus, Haemophilus, Actinobacillus, Cardiobacterium, Eikenella, Kingella, Coxiella, Brucella, Legionella, Bartonella,* and fungi are all species pathologic to the endocardium. For dental procedures, amoxicillin 2.0 g orally or ampicillin 2.0 g intravenously or intramuscularly 30 minutes before the procedure is a standard regimen. For the penicillin-allergic patient, clindamycin 600 mg, cephalexin 2.0 g, cefadroxil 2.0 g, or azithromycin 500 mg orally is appropriate. Medications administered orally should be given 1 hour prior to the procedure.

For urethral catheterization in the presence of infection, ampicillin 2.0 g intravenously or intramuscularly plus gentamicin 1.5 mg/kg intravenously or intramuscularly should be administered 30 minutes prior to the procedure. This should be followed by ampicillin 1.0 g intravenously or intramuscularly after the procedure. Vancomycin 1.0 g intravenously over 1 hour in combination with gentamicin is an alternative.

For incision and drainage of infected tissue, cefazolin 1.0 g intravenously or intramuscularly, cephalexin 2.0 g orally, or cefadroxil 2.0 g orally is appropriate. Vancomycin 1.0 g intravenously over 1 hour plus gentamicin 1.5 mg/kg intravenously or intramuscularly 30 minutes prior to the procedure is an alternate regimen.[7,18]

MANAGING PROSTHETIC VALVE COMPLICATIONS

Use of prosthetic cardiac valves to treat hemodynamically significant valvular disease is becoming a more common procedure in the United States, especially in the geriatric patient. Elderly patients benefit from valve replacement and are at no greater risk if they lack comorbidities.[8,9] Complications of prosthetic valves include endocarditis, thromboembolism, anticoagulant-related hemorrhage, and mechanical hemolytic anemia. Failure of the prosthetic valve is also a life-threatening complication that needs to be recognized and treated immediately in the emergency department.

Mechanical valves are either mechanical or fashioned from biologic tissue. The three mechanical valves encountered most commonly are (1) the caged-ball valve, (2) the single-leaflet valve, and (3) the bileaflet valve. The most common bileaflet valve is the St. Jude. Biologic tissue valves are made from porcine valves or bovine pericardium. Biologic valves are less thrombogenic than mechanical valves and are a better choice in elderly patients who are intolerant of anticoagulation.[19] Tissue prosthetic valves may degenerate, calcify, or develop thrombus formation.

Primary failure of mechanical valves can occur from thrombus formation or breakage of valve components. The valve components can embolize and cause further complications. There also may be breakdown of the suture line to the valve causing acute regurgitation.

Acute failure of an aortic valve is similar to the presentation of acute aortic regurgitation. It presents with ventricular volume overload. The increased pressure in the left ventricle results in pulmonary congestion and edema, which leads to poor cardiac output. Myocardial ischemia can occur even in patients without coronary artery disease due to the acute regurgitation.

When the mitral valve fails acutely, the left atrium receives a volume overload, and pulmonary congestion and edema ensue. Cardiac output is decreased due to the acute regurgitation into the left atrium. Increased sympathetic tone from the stress also can increase peripheral vascular resistance and heart rate. This leads to further decompensation from decreased filling time in diastole and increased work for left ventricular outflow, respectively. This results in worse regurgitation.

Prosthetic valve endocarditis may develop into a ring abscess and cause dehiscence or a valve leak. Conduction disorders, valve stenosis, and pericarditis can result from direct extension of the abscess, which is more common in the mechanical valves. Valve tears or leakage commonly result from endocarditis. Glomerulonephritis, mycotic aneurysms, and sepsis also may develop.

Treatment of acute prosthetic valvular insufficiency should focus on stabilizing the patient for surgical replacement of the malfunctioning valve. Afterload reduction and inotropic support are the main goals of treatment. If the patient's mean arterial pressure is greater than 70 mmHg, sodium nitroprusside can reduce the impedence to forward flow. If the patient's pressure is less than 70 mmHg, then dobutamine or amrinone is a helpful adjunct. Intraaortic balloon counterpulsation may be useful in cases of acute mitral regurgitation as a stabilizing measure before surgical intervention.

Vancomycin and gentamicin should be administered to patients suspected of prosthetic valve endocarditis after blood cultures have been ordered. Anticoagulation should be considered due to the high risk of embolization in endocarditis. Echocardiography should be performed to check for an unstable valve and in all patients in heart failure.

Fibrinolytic therapy should be considered for patients with a thrombosed prosthetic valve. Since valve location and valve type play a role in the indication for fibrinolytic therapy, cardiology consultation should be obtained prior to its administration.

REFERENCES

1. Otto CM, Lind BK, Kitzman DW, et al: Association of aortic valve stenosis with cardiovascular mortality and morbidity in the elderly. *New Engl J Med* 341:142, 1999.

2. Aronow WS: The older man's heart and heart disease. *Med Clin North Am* 83:1291, 1999.

3. Thompson ME, Shaver JA: Aortic stenosis in the elderly. *Geriatrics* 38:50, 1983.

4. Gunther S, Grossman W: Determinants of ventricular function in pressure-overload hypertrophy in man. *Circulation* 59:676, 1979.

5. Carabello BA: Aortic stenosis. *New Engl J Med* 346(9):677, 2002.

6. Morrow AG, Roberts WC, Ross J Jr, et al: Obstruction to left ventricular outflow: Current concepts of management and operative treatment. *Ann Intern Med* 69:1255, 1968.

7. Cline DM: Valvular emergencies and endocarditis, in Tintinalli JE (ed): *Emergency Medicine: A Comprehensive Study Guide,* 5th ed. New York, McGraw-Hill, 2000, pp 376–387.

8. Connolly HM, Oh JK, Orszulak TA, et al Aortic valve replacement for aortic stenosis with severe left ventricular dysfunction: Prognostic indicators. *Circulation* 95:2395, 1997.

9. Sprigings DC, Forfar JC: How should we manage symptomatic aortic stenosis in the patient who 80 or older? *Br Heart J* 74:481, 1995.

10. Rahimtoola SH: Severe aortic stenosis with low systolic gradient: The good and bad news. *Circulation* 101:1892, 2000.

11. Braunwald E: Valvular heart disease, in Isselbacher KJ (ed): *Harrision's Principles of Internal Medicine.* New York, McGraw-Hill, 1991, pp 938–942.

12. Petty GW, Khandheria BK, Whisnant JP, et al: Predictors of cerebrovascular events and death among patients with valvular heart disease: A population-based study. *Stroke* 31:2628, 2000.

13. Krasuski RA, Warner JJ, Peterson G, et al: Comparison of results of percutaneous balloon mitral commissurotomy in patients aged over 65 years with those in patients aged less than 65 years. *Am J Cardiol* 88:994, 2001.

14. Gardin JM, Weissman NJ, Leung C, et al: Clinical and echocardiographic follow-up of patients previously treated with dexfenfluramine or phentermine/fenfluramine. *JAMA* 286:2011, 2001.

15. Scott RL: Native Mitral valve regurgitation: A proactive management can improve outlook. *Postgrad Med* 110:57, 2001.

16. Freed LA, Levy D, Levine RA, et al: Prevalence and clinical outcome of mitral valve prolapse. *New Engl J Med* 341:1, 1999.

17. Lundin L: Carcinoid heart disease. *Acta Oncol* 30:499, 1991.

18. Delahaye F, Hoen B, McFadden E, et al: Treatment and prevention of infective endocarditis. *Expert Opin Pharmacother* 3:131, 2002.

19. Demirag M, Kirali K, Omeroglu SN, et al: Mechanical versus biological valve prosthesis in the mitral position: A 10-year follow-up of St Jude Medical and Biocor valves. *J Heart Valve* 10:78, 2001.

15

Hypertensive Emergencies

Timothy D. Babbitt
Matthew C. Gratton

HIGH-YIELD FACTS

- A hypertensive emergency is not defined by a specific blood pressure reading but by evidence of impending end-organ damage in the presence of hypertension.

- Elderly patients are at an increased risk for end-organ damage due to their aged organ systems.

- The cerebral autoregulatory curve is shifted to the right in patients with long-standing hypertension; therefore, the mean arterial pressure should be lowered no more than 25 percent during the initial treatment phase.

- Careful titration of blood pressure is of critical importance because sudden precipitous drops in blood pressure or excessive blood pressure reduction can lead to serious consequences.

Hypertension is one of the most common chronic medical conditions encountered in the United States.[1,2] True hypertensive emergencies tend to arise in patients with poorly controlled chronic hypertension rather than in previously normotensive patients. Although less than 1 percent of patients with hypertension will develop a hypertensive emergency, the morbidity and mortality are very high.[3–6] Furthermore, epidemiologic data have demonstrated that elevations in blood pressure are associated with an increased morbidity and mortality in people over 65 years of age due to the decreased end-organ reserve seen in the elderly.[1,7] Organ systems at increased risk for damage due to uncontrolled blood pressure include the cardiovascular, cerebral, renal, and optic systems. Although the rates of hypertensive crises have seen a downward trend since the 1940s because of effective treatment of hypertension,[8] the decreased organ system reserve seen

in the elderly and the expanding proportion of elderly patients in our country may lead to an increase in the complications of acute hypertension.

Traditionally, hypertensive crises have been divided into hypertensive emergencies and hypertensive urgencies.[8] A *hypertensive emergency* is defined as a condition in which there is evidence of end-organ damage due to an elevated blood pressure. Examples of hypertensive emergencies include hypertensive encephalopathy, aortic dissection, acute coronary syndromes, acute left ventricular failure, stroke syndromes, and acute renal failure. In order to limit damage to vital organ systems during a hypertensive emergency, current treatment guidelines suggest an expeditious, smooth reduction in blood pressure, generally in less than 1 hour.[1,3,9] It is important to note that the absolute level of the blood pressure is not the determining factor in the definition of hypertensive emergency or in the decision to treat; damage to end-organ system functioning is the crucial defining factor. Some patients may tolerate very high blood pressures with few or no symptoms and signs, yet others may manifest end-organ damage at lower pressures. The blood pressure reading along with the clinical status of the patient and laboratory and radiographic assessment of end-organ functioning determines the seriousness of the situation and how quickly treatment should be instituted.

Hypertensive urgency is more loosely defined but generally is considered to be a condition in which the diastolic blood pressure is greater than 120 mmHg without evidence of end-organ damage.[10] Despite the risk for morbid complications if not treated aggressively, most authorities recommend extending the time frame for blood pressure reduction in hypertensive urgencies to 24 hours.[1,3,5,11–13] In fact, precipitous reduction of blood pressure in a hypertensive urgency may be harmful and thus should be avoided.[5,14] Hypertensive urgencies are much more common than emergencies and frequently are discovered during routine evaluation of asymptomatic patients.

EPIDEMIOLOGY

The prevalence of hypertension in the general population is thought to be 20 to 30 percent, with an estimated 60 million persons in the United States affected.[3,6,9,15] Blood pressure tends to increase with age in most countries, and the actual prevalence of hypertension in the geriatric population is estimated to be as high as 64 percent in persons aged 65 to 74 years.[7,12] Hypertensive emergencies comprise only a small fraction of hypertensive complications, approximately 1 percent.[3,4,16] The prevalence of hypertension in the African-American population is 1.5 to 2 times that of Caucasians, and the incidence of hypertensive crises is higher among African Americans and the elderly.[3,12] Isolated systolic hypertension is particularly common in the elderly. Epidemiologic data confirm that both systolic and diastolic blood pressure elevations are associated with an increased morbidity and mortality in persons over 65 years of age.[7] Improved control of chronic hypertension should lead to the decreased incidence of hypertensive emergencies due to the fact that hypertensive complications arise more often in patients with uncontrolled or poorly treated hypertension. The Framingham Heart Study confirms that tight management of blood pressure lowers the incidence of hypertensive complications.[12] Failure to identify hypertensive patients and inadequate treatment of hypertensive patients who receive regular care increase the risk of complications.[17]

PATHOPHYSIOLOGY

The cerebral, cardiovascular, renal, and optic organ systems are the most susceptible to damage from acute elevations in blood pressure. An alteration in autoregulation to dependent tissue beds is the primary pathophysiologic abnormality seen in a hypertensive emergency. The process of autoregulation provides dependent tissue beds with a near-constant blood flow over a range of blood pressures by regulating vascular tone. Blood flow is thus regulated over a range of mean arterial pressures (MAPs). A MAP above or below this range overwhelms the system. For example, the cerebral circulation is maintained over mean arterial pressures [MAP = DBP + (SBP − DBP)/3, where SBP is systolic blood pressure and DBP is diastolic blood pressure] ranging from 60 mmHg to over 150 mmHg.[11,18,19] Cerebral blood flow (CBF) is directly related to the MAP through the relationship CBF = MAP − ICP, where ICP is the intracranial pressure.[20] As the blood pressure falls, cerebral vasodilation occurs in order to maintain an adequate cerebral blood flow. As blood pressure rises, cerebral vasoconstriction occurs to prevent extravasation and cerebral edema. This vasodilatation and constriction are likely mediated by stretch receptors in the smooth muscle of cerebral arterioles.[11,19] Signs and symptoms of cerebral ischemia will not be seen until autoregulation fails.

As the upper limits of autoregulation are surpassed, severe elevations in blood pressure will cause direct damage to the vascular endothelium. The endothelium attempts to respond to the elevated blood pressure by

releasing vasodilator molecules such as nitric oxide. The compensatory mechanisms are overwhelmed when faced with sustained or severe hypertension that leads to direct endothelial damage.[6,12] As platelets encounter damaged areas of endothelium, they adhere, aggregate, and initiate the clotting cascade. The platelets release vasoreactive substances, including thromboxane, that stimulate further aggregation of platelets and fibrin. Blood flow to the vascular beds is interrupted due to the platelet plugging and fibrin deposition. The increase in vascular reactivity also stimulates the migration and proliferation of myointimal cells in the damaged areas. This results in further narrowing and damage to the vascular system.[6,15] This cycle of damage, reactivity, and proliferation is called *fibrinoid necrosis*. The further release of vasoreactive substances and proinflammatory cytokines results in a cycle of homeostatic failure.[12] Prompt reduction of blood pressure in a hypertensive emergency can circumvent this cycle and prevent further end-organ damage.

A caveat in hypertensive emergencies is that chronically hypertensive patients tolerate a higher MAP, and a higher MAP is required to maintain blood flow to dependent vascular beds. This is due to a compensatory rightward shift in the chronically hypertensive patient's autoregulatory curve that allows the patient to tolerate a seemingly dangerously high blood pressure. In addition, the rightward shift of the autoregulatory curve precludes acute reductions of blood pressure to normotensive levels because tissue bed hypoperfusion may result. It has been shown that the lower limit of cerebral autoregulation is about 25 percent below the resting MAP.[11] The goal of treatment in a hypertensive emergency thus should be a reduction of MAP by no more than 25 percent in the first minutes to hours.[4,11,13,21] The timing of the blood pressure reduction depends on the type of hypertensive crisis. A reduction beyond 25 percent places the hypertensive patient at risk for hypoperfusion.

In the kidneys, impaired autoregulation secondary to elevated blood pressure results in decreased renal perfusion. Poor renal perfusion leads to the activation of the renin-angiotensin-aldosterone system. The juxtaglomerular cells of the afferent arterioles respond by releasing renin. Renin, a potent enzyme, stimulates the formation of angiotensin I, which is subsequently split into angiotensin II and amino acids by angiotensin-converting enzyme (ACE). Angiotensin II works through two mechanisms to increase blood pressure. First, angiotensin II is a potent vasoconstrictor of the arterioles and to a lesser degree of the venous system. The increase in peripheral resistance results in an increased arterial pressure. Second, angiotensin II stimulates aldosterone secretion and thus sodium retention, leading to an increased blood volume and increased blood pressure.[6]

Several unique features must be considered in the treatment of the geriatric hypertensive emergency. Atherosclerosis, common in the elderly, can greatly complicate the management of hypertensive patients. The loss of vascular reactivity due to atherosclerotic plaques may reduce the ability of the cerebral, cardiac, and renal vasculature to autoregulate blood flow. This may result in large fluctuations in blood flow and subsequent vascular events. Secondary hypertension caused by renal artery stenosis also may be seen due to significant atherosclerosis. Other considerations unique to the elderly include lower circulating blood volume, lower plasma renin activity, and increased peripheral vascular resistance.[1]

CLINICAL FEATURES

History

The initial approach to a patient with an elevated blood pressure is to focus on differentiating between a true hypertensive emergency, hypertensive urgency, or transient hypertension. A hypertensive emergency is an elevation in blood pressure that requires immediate reduction to prevent or limit end-organ damage. A hypertensive urgency is a condition in which the diastolic blood pressure is greater than 120 mmHg without evidence of end-organ damage. Transient hypertension is simply a fluctuation in blood pressure that can be seen in many conditions such as anxiety, dehydration, medication overdoses, and alcohol withdrawal.[5] Treatment of the underlying condition will correct transient hypertension. The differentiation between these entities is crucial because it determines the need for treatment, the speed of blood pressure reduction, the medication given, the route of administration of that medication, and eventual disposition of the patient. Moreover, the clinician must recognize that the rate of elevation of the blood pressure is more important than the absolute level of the pressure.[3] Acute elevations in blood pressure have the potential for more significant damage than a gradual rise that has stimulated compensatory mechanisms.

While obtaining the history of present illness, questions should be directed to elicit any symptoms that would suggest impending or ongoing end-organ pathology. The clinician should obtain an accurate, targeted past medical history; in particular, any history of hypertension, hypertensive emergencies, retinopathy, cardiovascular, cerebrovascular, or renal disease should be elicited. A thorough history of all medications prescribed and taken, including over-the-counter medications such as stimulants, nonsteroidal anti-inflammatory agents, and decongestants, should be obtained. Since the elderly are often on multiple medications, potential pharmacologic interactions should be assessed. Furthermore, compliance with the medication regimen may provide a clue to the etiology of the patient's blood pressure elevation. A drug history should be obtained because illicit use of cocaine, amphetamines, and PCP may be responsible for acute blood pressure elevations, even in the elderly.

A brief review of systems focusing on the cardiovascular, cerebrovascular, and renal systems may indicate compromise of end-organ functioning. Blurred vision, diplopia, hemiparesis, seizures, headache, or dizziness may indicate central nervous system compromise. Symptoms such as chest pain, dyspnea, nausea, back pain, orthopnea, or paroxysmal nocturnal dyspnea may indicate cardiopulmonary involvement. Hematuria and decreased urinary output, including anuria, may be elicited in patients with end-organ damage to the kidneys.

Physical Examination

As with any patient encounter in the emergency department (ED), an initial assessment of airway, breathing, and circulation should be performed. If any significant airway, ventilation, or circulatory problems are discovered, they should be addressed immediately. An accurate blood pressure reading should be obtained, which may require an appropriately sized blood pressure cuff to ascertain a true blood pressure reading. The cuff should be placed against the bare upper arm, and the cuff bladder should surround 80 percent of the upper arm. Any abnormal reading should be confirmed with repeat blood pressure measurements. Furthermore, the blood pressure should be taken in both upper and lower extremities to delineate any possible structural abnormalities such as coarctation of the aorta or aortic dissection. A rare, confounding condition may be seen in the elderly. The term *pseudohypertension* describes a condition of severe medial sclerosis in the brachial artery limiting the compressibility of the artery during blood pressure measurement. Pseudohypertension should be suspected when the blood pressure measurements are very high in the absence of any signs or symptoms of end-organ failure.[1,7]

A focused physical examination will help the emergency physician determine the status of end-organ function. Palpation of peripheral pulses may identify vascular disorders such as aortic dissection. Auscultation over the carotid arteries may reveal a bruit, raising the suspicion of cerebrovascular disease in the appropriate setting. A bruit over the aorta and flank or a palpable, pulsatile mass may be discovered during the abdominal examination. Cardiac auscultation may reveal murmurs, extra heart sounds, and rubs. An S_3 indicates left or right ventricular failure, whereas an S_4 indicates a noncompliant left ventricle, usually seen in the setting of left ventricular hypertrophy. Pulmonary auscultation may reveal rales associated with left ventricular failure. The neurologic examination may reveal focal neurologic deficits or mental status changes indicative of stroke or encephalopathy.

The funduscopic examination should not be overlooked because it may provide the only physical examination finding consistent with end-organ involvement. The fundus is the only area that allows for a direct visual assessment of the arterial system.[1] The optic disk should be assessed for the presence of papilledema. Acute elevations in blood pressure may lead to flame hemorrhages seen in the superficial nerve fiber layer of the retina. Cotton wool spots suggest microinfarcts of the nerve fiber layer. Evaluation of the fundus may be complicated in the elderly due to the presence of cataracts. Mydriatic agents should be used cautiously in elderly patients with previous cataract surgery because they may cause angle-closure glaucoma or lens dislocation.[1]

Hypertensive Encephalopathy

Currently, hypertensive encephalopathy is thought to result from a rapid rise in blood pressure exceeding the upper limits of cerebral autoregulation. As blood pressure surpasses the upper limits of the autoregulatory curve, a "forced dilatation" of the cerebral vasculature occurs with loss of the integrity of the blood-brain barrier at the arteriole. Extravasation of fluid results in cerebral edema, hemorrhage, and microinfarction.[4,5,11,12] Previously normotensive patients may surpass their autoregulatory curve at lower MAPs, whereas chronically hypertensive patients may not exceed autoregulation until the MAP reaches 160 to 180 mmHg.[4] This shifting of the autoregulatory curve offers a protective mechanism for the hypertensive patient to help tolerate much higher MAPs.

Hypertensive encephalopathy usually presents with an insidious onset of headache, nausea, vomiting, altered mental status, visual change, and occasionally, focal neurologic deficits. Seizures, both focal or generalized, may be present. The diagnosis should be suspected in a hypertensive patient with gradually developing signs and symptoms over 1 to 2 days. This differentiates hypertensive encephalopathy from an acute intracranial hemorrhage or infarction, which usually presents with an abrupt onset and evolution of symptoms. Magnetic resonance imaging (MRI) characteristically shows posterior leukoencephalopathy affecting the white matter of the parieto-occipital regions, and computed tomography (CT) may show posterior cerebral changes.[12] Acute intracranial hemorrhage often is demonstrated as hyperdensities on CT. Appropriate reduction in the MAP commonly will lead to the resolution of symptoms during hypertensive encephalopathy, whereas other intracranial processes will not resolve and may worsen with blood pressure reduction. Reduction of MAP by 25 percent should be accomplished in 1 to 3 hours, and neurologic status should improve during the first 12 to 24 hours if permanent damage has not occurred.[4,5,11,22] If not treated as a true medical emergency, hypertensive encephalopathy may progress to death.

The medication most commonly used for treating hypertensive encephalopathy is nitroprusside at a dose titrated from 0.5 to 10 µg/kg/min. With a constant titratable infusion, the blood pressure should be cautiously lowered, but not by more than a 25 percent reduction in MAP.[11] If the patient's clinical status deteriorates with a MAP reduction, then the blood pressure should be elevated to the lowest pressure where clinical improvement was seen. Labetalol has been used as an alternate therapy to nitroprusside in the treatment of hypertensive encephalopathy.

Acute Coronary Syndromes

Uncontrolled hypertension in a patient with an acute coronary syndrome constitutes another hypertensive emergency. The increase in peripheral vascular resistance represents an increase in afterload; an increase in afterload leads to an increased left ventricular end-diastolic pressure and myocardial oxygen demand.[4] The elevation of left ventricular end-diastolic pressure may lead directly to the development of anginal complaints due to the reduction of subendocardial blood flow. This is extremely dangerous in an infarcting patient because subendocardial blood flow is already compromised. Moreover, patients with fixed coronary artery lesions may not be able to compensate for the increase in myocardial oxygen demand by coronary artery dilatation. Consequently, blood pressure reduction becomes imperative in order to optimize blood flow to ischemic myocardium. Close hemodynamic monitoring is required to reduce blood pressure to an acceptable level without further compromise of coronary artery perfusion.

Intravenous, sublingual, or transdermal nitroglycerin remains the agent of choice in acute coronary syndromes because it augments coronary perfusion through vasodilation of the coronary arteries and reduces blood pressure by dilation of the venous capacitance vessels. Beta blockers should be considered as well because they reduce myocardial oxygen demand through their negative inotropic and chronotropic effects. Other standard measures include oxygen, morphine sulfate, anticoagulation, and reperfusion strategies, as indicated. Relative contraindications to the use of fibrinolytic agents include uncontrolled hypertension (180/110 mmHg) and age greater than 75 years.[23] Sodium nitroprusside should be avoided unless the blood pressure cannot be controlled with other pharmacologic measures because of the potential for coronary steal. Coronary steal is thought to be the result of generalized relaxation of unaffected resistance vessels in the coronary system. Areas of coronary vasculature with fixed atherosclerotic lesions are unable to dilate appropriately in the face of ischemia. This leads to decreased coronary perfusion to ischemic areas of myocardium.[11] Since atherosclerosis progresses with age, the likelihood of coronary steal increases due to the prevalence of fixed atherosclerotic stenoses.

Aortic Dissection

Acute aortic dissection is the result of a tear in the aortic intimal layer that allows blood to propagate into the media. Occasionally, the pressure may rupture the adventitial layer, but most commonly, there is a second intimal layer tear, creating a double-barreled aorta. The dissection may propagate proximally and result in coronary ischemia, acute aortic valvular insufficiency, or cardiac tamponade. Distal propagation of the dissection may involve the renal or spinal arteries. A strong correlation between aortic dissection and hypertension exists; the treatment is aimed at reducing the shearing force on the dissecting aortic wall. Acute aortic dissection is associated with a history of hypertension in more than 90 percent of patients regardless of what their blood pressure is on presentation to the ED.[5] The aged vasculature and high prevalence of hypertension predispose the geriatric population to this problem.

Although the location of the pain varies depending on the site of dissection, the classic presentation of aortic dissection is the acute onset of tearing chest pain radiating to the midscapular region. Dissection of the descending aorta may present as abdominal or back pain. Blood pressure and pulse differences between the arms or between the up-

per and lower extremities due to vascular obstruction may be discovered. Aortic dissections have been classically described in the Stanford classification: Type A dissections involve the ascending aorta, and type B dissections involve the descending aorta. Uncomplicated dissection of the descending aorta (type B dissections) is usually treated with medical management, whereas more proximal dissections (type A dissections) usually require definitive surgical repair.[4,11] Intravenous antihypertensive therapy should be initiated in all hypertensive patients with suspected acute aortic dissection.[3] Aggressive management is imperative to limit propagation of the dissection and potential deterioration in the patient. Blood pressure should be controlled rapidly within 15 to 60 minutes to a target systolic blood pressure of 100 to 120 mmHg.[6,11,22] Caution must be exercised because this goal may be below the lower limits of autoregulation in a chronically hypertensive patient.

The therapeutic goal is limitation of the shearing forces on the compromised aorta, thus preventing the propagation of the dissection. Pharmacologic agents that reduce vascular resistance and the left ventricular ejection forces have been used to accomplish this goal. The combination of sodium nitroprusside to reduce vascular resistance with labetalol to block the reflex tachycardia and to decrease cardiac contractility has been used extensively in the treatment of dissections. Other options include labetalol alone or the substitution of labetalol with beta blockers such as esmolol. Trimethaphan also has been used successfully for the treatment of aortic dissection. A surgical consultation should be obtained in all cases of dissection.

Acute Left Ventricular Failure

Regardless of the etiology, an increase in total peripheral vascular resistance (i.e., afterload) due to increased circulating vasoconstrictors plays a vital role in acute left ventricular failure.[5] The failing left ventricle will be unable to provide sufficient forward blood flow, which may result in pulmonary edema. The release of vasoactive substances in response to the pulmonary edema further increases afterload by causing vasoconstriction and increasing peripheral vascular resistance. The increase in afterload causes increased myocardial oxygen demand and may decrease coronary blood flow by increasing left ventricular end-diastolic pressure.[5] In rare cases, an acute rise in blood pressure leads to acute left ventricular failure and resulting pulmonary edema. Controlled reduction of the blood pressure must be achieved in order to circumvent this process. Any evidence of left ventricular failure in a hypertensive patient requires prompt blood pressure reduction.[13]

Pharmacologic agents that reduce both preload and afterload are needed to reduce myocardial oxygen demand and improve cardiac output.[5,6] Standard therapies for the treatment of pulmonary edema and myocardial ischemia should be initiated as first-line treatments because these measures typically reduce preload and afterload. Nitroglycerin will provide a vasodilatory effect with subsequent increases in coronary perfusion. Diuresis can be achieved with intravenous furosemide, whereas intravenous morphine may block the sympathetic release of catecholamines. Supplemental oxygen should be administered as well. If standard treatments fail, then nitroprusside may be used to control the refractory hypertension.[4,6] Nitroprusside is an excellent choice in the setting of acute left ventricular failure because it produces dilatation of both arterioles and venous capacitance vessels. Favorable hemodynamic effects of nitroprusside on the failing left ventricle have been demonstrated even when hypertension is minimal or absent.[11] ACE inhibitors also are effective due to their afterload-reducing properties.

Renal Failure

Blood pressure is influenced directly by the function of the renal system. Uncontrolled hypertension can contribute to kidney dysfunction, and chronic renal disease results in hypertension. Renal perfusion determines the status of the renin-angiotensin-aldosterone system, which influences blood pressure by causing vasoconstriction and altering volume status. Low renal perfusion activates the system, whereas increased perfusion shuts down the system through negative feedback. Chronic renal failure leads to volume overload through excessive sodium retention and subsequent hypertension. With the advent of dialysis and transplantation, hypertension has become a larger problem in the chronic renal failure patient due to prolonged life expectancies. Dialysis may be required to reduce blood pressure in the chronic renal failure patient with a hypertensive emergency.

Any deterioration in renal function, seen as elevations in the blood urea nitrogen (BUN) and creatinine levels, proteinuria, and/or red cells and red cell casts in the urine, in the face of an elevated blood pressure should be considered a hypertensive emergency requiring immediate reduction of blood pressure.[5,6,20] Nitroprusside remains the drug of choice in acute renal failure secondary to a hypertensive crisis because of its rapid onset of action as well

as its predictable and easily controlled dose-response relationship.[20] Nitroprusside metabolism releases cyanide, which is converted to the less toxic metabolite thiocyanate. Thiocyanate is excreted through the kidneys; thus the clinician must be aware of the increased risk of thiocyanate toxicity with the prolonged use of nitroprusside in the setting of renal failure.[3]

Fenoldopam may change the treatment strategy in severely hypertensive patients with impaired renal function. Fenoldopam has been shown to improve creatinine clearance, urine flow rates, and sodium excretion in severely hypertensive patients with both normal and impaired renal function.[3,20] While nitroprusside provides excellent blood pressure reduction, the favorable renal effects are not seen, and thiocyanate toxicity, although rare, is more likely in patients with renal dysfunction. The risk for thiocyanate toxicity is elevated with prolonged administration of the drug (24 to 48 hours) and infusion rates greater than 10 μg/kg/min.[9,10] Labetalol also has been used with success in the treatment of hypertensive emergencies with renal failure.

Stroke Syndromes

Hypertension and the stroke syndromes are intimately related. Although chronic hypertension is an independent risk factor for stroke, the hypertensive episode during the acute cerebrovascular event is often the physiologic response to hypoperfusion of an ischemic area. The initial event results in increased edema and pressure in the corresponding tissue. Blood flow in the damaged area becomes pressure-dependent as cerebral autoregulation is lost. In order to maintain cerebral perfusion pressure to the salvageable cerebral tissue in the face of increased intracranial pressure, the physiologic response is a corresponding increase in blood pressure. Blood pressures after acute stroke usually are mildly elevated, with a gradual decrease to prestroke levels over time without intervention.[6] There is no evidence that mild hypertension has a negative effect during the acute phase of ischemic stroke.[3] Thus aggressive blood pressure reduction is detrimental and could extend the area of damage by causing hypoperfusion.

Occasionally, the emergency physician will be presented with a stroke patient with a severely elevated blood pressure (diastolic pressure > 130 mmHg).[3,5] The blood pressure should be monitored closely during an acute intracranial event. The American Heart Association suggests that hypertension in the setting of ischemic stroke should be treated "rarely and cautiously."[8] In the rare case of a diastolic blood pressure greater than 130 mmHg, cautious MAP reduction of 20 to 25 percent is suggested with close monitoring of neurologic status.[3,5,6] Any deterioration in neurologic status with blood pressure reduction should result in immediate limitation or cessation of treatment. Short-acting, titratable agents such as sodium nitroprusside and labetalol have been advocated for blood pressure control with the caveat that nitroprusside may increase intracranial pressure.[3,11]

Hypertension seen with hemorrhagic stroke usually is a transitory phenomenon but may result in a significant rise in blood pressure. Increased intracranial pressure and activation of the autonomic nervous system lead to the rise in blood pressure seen with hemorrhagic strokes. Although the benefits of antihypertensive therapy in preventing rebleeding or edema are lacking, cautious, gradual lowering of systolic blood pressure greater than 200 mmHg and diastolic blood pressure greater than 120 mmHg is suggested.[3] Once again, if the neurologic status of the patient deteriorates during therapy, the treatment should be stopped. Treatment strategies for intracranial hemorrhage are controversial but generally have included nimodipine for vasospasm associated with subarachnoid hemorrhage. Nitroprusside has been used to address severe elevations in blood pressure unresponsive to nimodipine.[11]

DIAGNOSIS AND DIFFERENTIAL

Objective evidence of end-organ damage should be sought in all potential cases of hypertensive emergencies. Laboratory confirmation of a suspected hypertensive crisis should never delay the initiation of treatment. If available, previous baseline studies provide a benchmark of previous organ system functioning. Appropriate laboratory evaluation, including a complete blood count (CBC); determinations of BUN, creatinine, electrolytes, and blood glucose; and urinalysis, should be obtained to determine potential end-organ involvement. The CBC may reveal a microangiopathic hemolytic anemia suggesting vascular damage. Damage to the renal system may be seen as elevations in the BUN and creatinine levels, hematuria, and proteinuria. A normal creatinine level may be seen in the elderly patient with the renal dysfunction due to the age-related decrease in glomerular filtration and lean muscle mass; thus suspicion for renal injury must remain high.[1]

Electrolyte abnormalities may explain changes in mental status or place the patient at risk for arrhythmias. A blood glucose level should be checked in the setting of mental status changes because hypoglycemia mimics

many central nervous system processes. Evidence of ischemia, infarction, left ventricular hypertrophy, or electrolyte changes may be detected on the 12-lead electrocardiogram (ECG). Signs of congestive heart failure or aortic dissection may be seen on the chest radiograph. CT of the head should be done immediately on patients with neurologic changes to detect intracranial processes. CT and MRI may show cerebral edema and a posterior leukoencephalopathy in hypertensive encephalopathy. Areas of hemorrhage and edema may be seen with acute intracranial hemorrhage. Ischemic infarcts may be detected as well. The differential diagnosis depends on the organ system involved and the diagnostic findings present.

EMERGENCY DEPARTMENT CARE AND DISPOSITION

After a primary survey has been completed, a thorough history, physical examination, and laboratory evaluation of the elderly patient will help the emergency physician delineate whether a hypertensive episode is an emergency, urgency, or transient elevation. Institution of therapy and ultimate disposition rest on this distinction. Because of the risk of impending end-organ damage, hypertensive emergencies must be treated with parenteral agents, with the goal of blood pressure reduction being minutes to hours depending on the status of end-organ functioning. If the clinical status of the patient deteriorates with the reduction in blood pressure, then the blood pressure should be allowed to rise to higher levels in order to maintain perfusion.

Treatment of hypertensive emergencies in the elderly is challenging. Comorbid conditions, seen frequently in the geriatric population, may predispose the elderly patient to a hypertensive emergency and complicate management. The elderly tend to be sensitive to rapid reductions in blood pressure, predisposing them to cardiac ischemia, transient ischemic attack, and stroke. Moreover, the blunted baroreceptor reflex places the geriatric patient at higher risk for orthostasis and subsequent falls after antihypertensive therapy initiation.[1] All patients with hypertensive emergencies should be admitted to the intensive care unit with close monitoring of their blood pressure, preferably with an arterial line. Parenteral antihypertensives can be titrated closely to achieve the desired rate and endpoint of decline in blood pressure. Treatment should be initiated carefully at low doses and titrated upward to avoid unwanted side effects.

Pharmacologic Therapy

Sodium Nitroprusside

Sodium nitroprusside is a potent short-acting arterial and venous vasodilator that requires a constant infusion (0.3 to 10 μg/kg/min) to titrate blood pressures to the desired level. Nitroprusside is the "gold standard" titratable antihypertensive agent against which all other agents are measured.[8,20] The mechanism of action of nitroprusside is thought to be a reaction with cysteine to form nitrocysteine. Nitrocysteine activates guanylate cyclase, leading to the formation of cyclic guanosine monophosphate. The latter relaxes smooth muscle, particularly in the systemic circulation.[3] Despite the vasodilatory effects of the drug, cardiac output is maintained due to a reflex tachycardia. The onset of action is within seconds to minutes, and the half-life is about 2 minutes.[10,20] Rapid onset and short duration of action make this drug well suited for intravenous titration of blood pressure to a desired clinical range.

The most common side effect seen with the use of nitroprusside is hypotension due to the rapid onset of action and potency of the drug. Hypotension can be reversed quickly by slowing or stopping the infusion. Tissue and erythrocyte sulfhydryl groups release free cyanide radicals from nitroprusside, creating the potential for cyanide toxicity. Normally, the cyanide radicals are rapidly converted to thiocyanate, 100 times less toxic than cyanide, by the liver. Thiocyanate is largely excreted by the kidneys but may cause toxicity if excretion is impaired or levels increase.[3,9,10,11] Prolonged administration (24 to 48 hours) or infusion rates greater than 10 μg/kg/min in association with renal and hepatic failure place a patient at a higher risk for cyanide toxicity.[9,10] The cerebral vasodilatory effects of sodium nitroprusside place patients at risk for elevated intracranial pressure.

Labetalol

Labetalol is a combined blocker of the α_1, β_1, and β_2 adrenergic receptors. Blockade of the α_1 receptors results in a decrease in peripheral vascular resistance. The beta-blocking effects prevent a reflex tachycardia expected with a decrease in peripheral vascular resistance. The beta-blocking effects are much more pronounced than the alpha blockade.[3,9,20] Peripheral blood flow, including cerebral, renal, and coronary, is maintained despite the reduction in peripheral vascular resistance.[3] Intravenous administration of labetalol provides a controlled reduction in blood pressure. Boluses of labetalol 20 mg intra-

venously are administered every 10 minutes (maximum cumulative dose is 300 mg) until the desired blood pressure is achieved; an infusion of 1 to 2 mg/min is then started. The onset of action of labetalol is 5 to 10 minutes when it is given intravenously, and its duration of action varies dramatically from 4 to 24 hours.[9,20] The peak hypotensive effect is seen within 5 to 15 minutes.[3] Labetalol is metabolized primarily by the liver.

The use of labetalol in patients with asthma or emphysema should be undertaken cautiously due to the nonselective beta blockade potentially resulting in bronchospasm. Other contraindications to the use of labetalol are heart block greater than first degree, decompensated congestive heart failure, and bradycardia. Large bolus injections should be avoided to avoid large, precipitous drops in blood pressure. Labetalol occasionally has caused orthostatic hypotension due the α-adrenergic antagonist effects.

Esmolol

This drug is an ultrashort-acting β_1-selective adrenergic blocker that has rapid distribution and elimination half-lives of 2 and 9 minutes, respectively.[10,20] The rapid metabolism of this drug is through hydrolysis by red blood cells rather than hepatic or renal clearance. The virtually immediate onset of action, short duration of action, and cardioselectivity make esmolol an excellent choice in the management of critically ill patients.[3] The use of esmolol in hypertensive crises is relatively new. A loading dose of 500 μg/kg over 1 minute is followed by an infusion at 25 to 50 μg/kg/min titrated every 10 to 20 minutes, with a maximum of 300 μg/kg/min. Esmolol does not cause excessive reductions in diastolic blood pressure and reflex tachycardia that are commonly seen with sodium nitroprusside.[10] Esmolol has been used in combination with other antihypertensive agents in the treatment of hypertensive crises. This drug should not be used in the treatment of cocaine-induced hypertension due to the possibility of unopposed α-receptor stimulation.

Nitroglycerin

The mode of action of intravenous nitroglycerin is primarily dilation of the venous capacitance vessels. At high doses, nitroglycerin also will cause a dilatation of arterial smooth muscle to a lesser degree than venodilatation.[16,24] The dilation of the coronary vasculature is particularly advantageous for myocardial ischemia in the setting of hypertension. The dilation of the coronary arteries, as opposed to nitroprusside, promotes a favorable distribution of coronary blood to ischemic myocardium.[20] This effect is mainly through the reduction of preload, which decreases left ventricular end-diastolic pressure and thus myocardial wall tension. Nitroglycerin offers many of the advantages of sodium nitroprusside but does not carry the risk of cyanide toxicity. The onset of action is almost immediate, and the half-life is 1 to 4 minutes.[1] Titration of the nitroglycerin drip from 5 to 100 μg/min allows for careful control over the absolute blood pressure.

Side effects associated with the use of nitroglycerin include headache, nausea, and vomiting. Careful attention must be paid to the use of nitroglycerin in the hypovolemic patient because it may cause hypotension and a reflex tachycardia. Discontinuation of the infusion and fluid replacement will correct the hypotension. Prolonged infusions of high doses may lead to methemoglobinemia.[20] The exact effects on cerebral and renal perfusion are unknown, but a reduction in cardiac output is usually seen and may compromise cerebral and renal perfusion.[3]

Fenoldopam

Fenoldopam selectively activates postsynaptic dopaminergic receptors (DA_1), resulting in potent vasodilative and natriuretic properties.[10,22] Fenoldopam can be titrated until sufficient vasodilatory effect is seen without the side effects of α- and β-adrenergic activation due to its specificity for the DA_1 receptors. Activation of the DA_1 receptors on the proximal and distal kidney tubules results in inhibition of sodium resorption, leading to diuresis and natriuresis.[3] In clinical trials, fenoldopam has been shown to have equal efficacy with nitroprusside in the treatment of hypertensive emergencies.[3] Additionally, fenoldopam improves creatinine clearance, diuresis, and natriuresis, possibly making it the drug of choice in a patient with a hypertensive emergency and renal impairment. Effects of the drug are seen within 5 minutes, and maximal response is seen within 15 minutes. Fenoldopam's short half-life is due to rapid conjugation in the liver to inactive substances.

The initial recommended dosage of fenoldopam is 0.1 μg/kg/min. The dosage may be titrated in increments of 0.05 to 0.1 μg/kg/min to a maximum of 1.6 μg/kg/min. As compared with sodium nitroprusside, the side-effect profile is minimal, with 25 percent of patients receiving the drug experiencing headache and flushing.[10] Other side effects seen with the use of fenoldopam include dizziness, reflex tachycardia, hypotension, and volume depletion.

As fenoldopam becomes used more extensively, it may become a competitor with nitroprusside for the treatment of most hypertensive emergencies.

ADDITIONAL ASPECTS

The following are pitfalls in the management of hypertensive emergencies in the elderly:

- Excessive reduction or precipitous drops in MAP during a hypertensive emergency may result in ischemic complications.

- Overtreating of isolated systolic hypertension (without evidence of end-organ dysfunction) as a hypertensive emergency is common.

- The pharmacokinetics of some drugs may be altered due to the age-related decrease in blood volume and total body water.

REFERENCES

1. Thacker HL, Jahnigen DW: Managing hypertensive emergencies and urgencies in the geriatric patient. *Geriatrics* 46:26, 1991.
2. Joint National Committee (JNC) on Prevention, Detection, Evaluation, and Treatment of High Blood Pressure: The sixth report of the Joint National Committee on Prevention, Detection, Evaluation, and Treatment of High Blood Pressure. *Arch Intern Med* 157: 2413, 1997.
3. Varon J, Marik P: The diagnosis and management of hypertensive crises. *Chest* 118:214, 2000.
4. McRae RP Jr, Liebson PR: Hypertensive crisis. *Med Clinics North Am* 70:749, 1986.
5. Jackson RE: Hypertension in the emergency department. *Emerg Med Clin North Am* 6:173, 1988.
6. Rubenstein E, Escalante C: Hypertensive crisis. *Crit Care Clin* 5:477, 1989.
7. The Working Group on Hypertension in the Elderly: Statement on hypertension in the elderly. *JAMA* 256:70, 1986.
8. Prisant LM, Carr AA, Hawkins DW: Treating hypertensive emergencies, controlled reduction of blood pressure and protection of target organs. *Postgrad Med* 93:92, 1993.
9. Garcia JY, Vidt DG: Current management of hypertensive emergencies. *Drugs* 34:263, 1987.
10. Abdelwahab W, Frishman W, Landau A: Management of hypertensive urgencies and emergencies. *J Clin Pharm* 35:747, 1995.
11. Gifford RW: Management of hypertensive crises. *JAMA* 266:829, 1991.

12. Vaughn C, Delanty N: Hypertensive emergencies. *Lancet* 356:411, 2000.

13. Hirschl MM: Guidelines for the drug treatment of hypertensive crises. *Drugs* 50:991, 1995.

14. Grossman E, Messerli F, Grodzicki T, Kowey P: Should a moratorium be placed on sublingual nifedipine capsules given for hypertensive emergencies and pseudoemergencies? *JAMA* 276:1328, 1996.

15. Houston M: Hypertensive emergencies and urgencies: Pathophysiology and clinical aspects. *Am Heart J* 111:205, 1986.

16. Smith MB, Flower LW, Reinhardt CE: Control of hypertensive emergencies. *Postgrad Med* 89:111, 1991.

17. Zampaglione B, Pascale C, Marchisio M, Cavalio-Perin P: Hypertensive urgencies and emergencies, prevalence and clinical presentation. *Hypertension* 27:144, 1996.

18. Strandgaard S, Olesen J, Skinhoj E, Lassen N: Autoregulation of brain circulation in severe arterial hypertension. *Br Med J* 1:507, 1973.

19. Gifford RW: Effect of reducing elevated blood pressure on cerebral circulation. *Hypertension* 5(suppl III):III-17, 1983.

20. Murphy C: Hypertensive emergencies. *Emerg Med Clin North Am* 13:973, 1995.

21. Kaplan N: Management of hypertensive emergencies. *Lancet* 344:1335, 1994.

22. Elliot W: Hypertensive emergencies. *Crit Care Clin* 17:435, 2001.

23. Part 7: The era of reperfusion. Section 1: Acute coronary syndromes (acute myocardial infarction). *Circulation* 102:I-183, 2000.

24. Vidt D, Gifford R: A compendium for the treatment of hypertensive emergencies. *Cleve Clin Q* 51:421, 1984.

16

Sudden Cardiac Death and Resuscitation

Stefanie R. Ellison

HIGH-YIELD FACTS

- Sudden cardiac death has a more favorable survival rate for the geriatric patient if the patient is not home-bound at the time of cardiac arrest and the event is witnessed, has prompt initiation of cardiopulmonary resuscitation (CPR) and early defibrillation, results from a ventricular arrhythmia, and occurs with concurrent cardiac ischemia.

- The implantable cardioverter-defibrillator is successful in preventing sudden cardiac death in patients at risk regardless of age.

Sudden cardiac death (SCD) is the state of cessation of effective cardiac activity and cardiac output. Each year in the United States, 400,000 to 600,000 persons die of unexpected SCD.[1] It is estimated that up to 85 percent of these patients are in the geriatric age group (age > 65 years). Multiple changes in resuscitation and emergency medical services (EMS) guidelines have occurred but with little change in survival rates for SCD. The survival rate is 3 to 30 percent for all cardiac arrest patients.[2] The variation in survival is based on age, comorbidity, rhythm at the time of arrest, time to cardiopulmonary resuscitation (CPR), time to defibrillation, and location of arrest.

EPIDEMIOLOGY

SCD is more common among men 50 to 75 years of age. The majority of SCDs occur outside the hospital. One study found that 80 percent of cardiac arrests occurred at home, were witnessed 60 percent of the time, and resulted in a survival rate of 8 percent, compared with 18 percent for cardiac arrests that occurred outside the home.[2] Nearly 45 percent of the patients who were resuscitated successfully in the out-of-hospital setting and over 55

percent of in-hospital resuscitation patients were over 70 years of age.[3]

It is estimated that up to 80 percent of SCD patients have underlying structural cardiac disease. This can include, but is not limited to, coronary atherosclerosis, valvular heart disease, cardiomyopathy, cardiomegaly, and primary conduction abnormalities. Of the patients with SCD, 50 to 85 percent have coronary atherosclerosis; within this subgroup, 50 percent suffer SCD from a ventricular tachyarrhthmia.[4] Fewer than half of all patients who experienced SCD had a concurrent acute myocardial infarction. Patients with a history of myocardial infarction are at greater risk to suffer an SCD event.[2] While the effects of plaque rupture or thrombus formation in promoting SCD are not clearly understood, patients with this pathology are certainly at greater risk for ischemic cardiac events and subsequent SCD.

SCD has an occurrence that changes with circadian rhythms. There is an increased incidence of SCD and myocardial infarction in the first few hours after awakening, which is due to increased sympathetic stimulation. One study found that there is a common circadian variation of out-of-hospital cardiac arrest, regardless of underlying etiology, when the presenting rhythm is any dysrhythmia other than ventricular fibrillation (VF). This is different from the circadian variation of cases of cardiac etiology presenting with VF. The circadian variation of VF, and consequently survival, may be affected by the availability of bystander CPR and the speed of ambulance response.[5]

There is also a seasonal variation to the incidence of SCD. Both SCD and myocardial infarction are more likely to occur during winter. One study indicated that cardiac-related mortality was 15 to 18 percent higher during winter months for those over age 75.[6] This may be accounted for by the increase in respiratory disease during the winter months.

PATHOPHYSIOLOGY

During SCD, the ensuing circulatory arrest results in tissue hypoxia of the vital organs. The most susceptible organ is the brain, followed by the heart and kidneys. A poor return of neurologic function can be expected following cardiac arrest that remains untreated for longer than 10 minutes.

During cardiac arrest, tissue hypoxia triggers anaerobic metabolism for energy production. This inefficient energy-producing method results in cellular energy depletion. In the myocardium, the cardiac rhythm during the arrest state determines how quickly this energy depletion occurs. The fibrillating heart depletes energy stores faster than in asystole or pulseless electrical activity (PEA) states. The eventual energy depletion of cells results in the generation of free radicals, intracellular calcium overload, activation of catabolic enzymes, and inflammation. These injury pathways become more significant during the postresuscitation period.

Experimental findings suggest that the decreased autonomic tone of geriatric patients may decrease their ability to develop and sustain a serious cardiac arrhythmia. In addition, the myocardial cells of geriatric patients may suffer from chronic or intermittent ischemia, rendering them more resistant to ischemic insult and cardiac arrhythmias. However, underlying disease may render geriatric patients even more susceptible due to their lack of physiologic reserve.

Ventricular Tachyarrhythmias

Arrhythmic events can be triggered by structural abnormalities of the heart or electrophysiologic disturbances. Approximately 85 percent of SCD cases are due to a ventricular tachyarrhythmia.[7,8] The two most common initial rhythms of SCD are pulseless ventricular tachycardia (VT) and VF.[7]

Both VT and VF can be triggered by ventricular irritability seen in myocardial ischemia, left ventricular dysfunction, and cardiomegaly, which are all more prevalent in the geriatric population. Geriatric patients also have a higher prevalence of preexisting comorbid conditions, the most common of which are cardiovascular disease, pulmonary disease, and diabetes. Geriatric patients have progressive stiffening of the myocardium and decreased overall pumping efficiency. An 80-year-old has 50 percent of the cardiac output of a 20-year-old. The myocardium of geriatric patients is also more sensitive to endogenous and exogenous catecholamines. Factors in myocardial ischemia that change the depolarization and repolarization of the myocardial tissue are "islands" of irritable ventricular cells. The irritable focus can trigger a circuitous movement of electrical reentry into the conductive cells. This reentry can initiate and sustain ventricular tachyarrhythmias.

Prolonged QT-interval syndrome is also associated with SCD. This rhythm can be congenital or acquired from electrolyte disturbances (hypokalemia, hypomagnesemia, and hypocalcemia), cardiac ischemia, central nervous system pathology, and medications (terfenadine-ketoconazole combinations, antipsychotics, or antiarrhythmic drugs such as amiodarone). Taking multiple medications places the geriatric population at a higher risk of SCD.

One medication used widely by elderly men is sildenafil citrate (Viagra). Cases of SCD associated with sildenafil citrate have been reported in men with coronary artery disease and mild chronic heart failure. Sildenafil citrate has a direct effect on cardiac repolarization and sinus autonomic and vascular control. The medication reduces vagal modulation and increases sympathetic modulation through a reflex vasodilatory action. At doses above what is usually taken for erectile dysfunction, the autonomic system could be altered to affect QT-interval dynamics. Both these effects can result in lethal ventricular arrhythmias.[9]

Bradydysrhythmia, Pulseless Electrical Activity, and Asystole

While the most common causes of SCD are tachyarrhythmias, there is a small proportion caused by bradydysrhythmias, PEA, or asystole.[10] *Bradycardia* is defined as a rhythm that is slower than 60 beats per minute. The distinction between PEA and asystole is the presence of a rhythm; both are pulseless. The distinction of PEA from a bradycardic rhythm is the absence of a pulse for each QRS complex. Asystole is the eventual rhythm of all nonresuscitated cardiac arrests.

SURVIVAL

Old age is not the sole determinant of prognosis or outcome after SCD.[2,3,7,8,11–14] This has been demonstrated for elderly patients who had timely out-of-hospital CPR and defibrillation for tachyarrhythmias. Early defibrillation is the most useful link in the chain of survival because 50 to 85 percent of SCD is due to ventricular tachyarrhythmias.[8,13] If defibrillation is achieved within 8 minutes of collapse due to VF in a patient with few comorbid conditions, then the prognosis is promising regardless of age.[13] There is also evidence that recovery of cerebral function is not adversely affected by old age after a SCD event.[15–17] Other indicators of improved survival in the elderly who experience SCD include a high level of self-care and if the tachyarrhythmia was caused by angina or myocardial infarction.[18] It has been shown that ambulatory elderly patients have a greater than 10 percent chance of surviving to discharge after out-of-hospital CPR in cities with well-established EMS systems.[19] One study found that 14 percent of out-of-hospital patients over 70 years of age who presented initially with VF or VT survived to discharge. Of those patients younger than age 70 who had VF or VT, 20 percent survived to discharge.[20]

Another study also found that patients older than age 70 had as great a likelihood of surviving out-of-hospital VF or VT as those under age 70.[19]

Independent indicators of poor survival after SCD were stroke or renal failure associated with the SCD event and if the initial rhythm was asystole, PEA, or a bradydysrhythmia. Previous comorbid diseases, such as diabetes mellitus, also contribute negatively to patient outcome following resuscitation The reported survival from tachyarrhythmias has been reported to be as high as 30 percent in the geriatric population; for nontachyarrhythmic causes, survival is less than 5 percent.[16,18]

Evidence exists that out-of-hospital arrest survival is different in octogenarians and nonagenarians. In patients who had out-of-hospital arrest due to a cardiac cause, patients younger than 70 years of age had higher hospital discharge rates than octogenarians, who also had higher hospital discharge rates than nonagenarians (19.4 versus 9.4 versus 4.4 percent, respectively). Survival to hospital discharge also was higher for all comparatively when their initial rhythm was VF or VT (36 versus 24 versus 17 percent, respectively). Even with the lower survival of octogenarians and nonagenarians, age was a weaker predictor of survival than other factors such as initial cardiac rhythm.[21] Therefore, decisions regarding resuscitation should not be based solely on age.

PREVENTION

Determining which patients are at risk for SCD is challenging. In one study, 71 percent of patients who survived SCD had no prodromal symptoms.[22] In another study, only half the patients who experienced SCD prior to EMS arrival reported having symptoms.[23] Disruption in cardiac conduction is more likely to have no associated symptoms prior to cardiac arrest. The medications of the geriatric population also may blunt some of these symptoms.

Use of electrophysiology, Holter monitoring, and other diagnostic tests to predict patients at risk for SCD has only identified 15 to 30 percent of at-risk patients.[24,25] Patients with a history of cardiac ischemia and heart failure are clearly at risk. SCD appears to strike less compromised heart failure patients (New York Heart Association functional class I) more often.

The most promising intervention for SCD is to ensure timely out-of-hospital response to witnessed cardiac arrest. The use of a two-tiered EMS response system can improve time to initial CPR as well as availability of defibrillation. Since there are more first responders than advanced cardiac life support (ACLS)–trained EMS personnel, their availability can improve initial response to the patient.[11,26,27] These systems use automated external defibrillators (AEDs) to defibrillate patients with VF or pulseless VT. Increased availability of AEDs in nursing homes, airport terminals, and other public facilities can improve time to defibrillation for ventricular tachyarrhythmias.

The implantable cardioverter-defibrillator (ICD), introduced into clinical practice in 1980, has improved survival in patients presenting with sustained VT or VF. Multiple studies conclusively demonstrated a benefit of the ICD in preventing SCD in patients with ischemic heart disease, left ventricular dysfunction, and inducible sustained ventricular tachycardia.[28,29] It has proven to be superior to pharmacologic therapy alone in preventing SCD.[30–32]

Up to 70 percent of patients with ICDs require concomitant antiarrhythmic medication to minimize the frequency of device discharges.[33] Antiarrhythmic agents can positively influence the defibrillation threshold of the ICD, making shocks more effective at terminating the dysrhythmia. This has been seen consistently with class III agents, with the exception of amiodarone. Class I agents, such as lidocaine, flecainide, and encainide, have demonstrated a rise in the defibrillation threshold and a subsequent decrease in the effectiveness of the ICD. Class III agents and to some extent the class II agents can be used as front-line agents in patients with ICDs.[33]

"DO NOT RESUSCITATE"

Each year approximately one-third of the 2 million patients who ultimately die after a SCD event are resuscitated initially before being pronounced dead.[34] Addressing advance directives with patients has taken on a greater importance. Advanced age alone was a reason for wanting CPR to be withheld in 25 percent of elderly patients surveyed.[35] Elderly patients under the care of primary care physicians were less likely to have a do-not-resuscitation (DNR) order than those managed by geriatricians.[36] One study showed that elderly patients on hospital admission wanted to be consulted about advance directives.[35] A full discussion of this issue is contained in Chap. 7.

RECOVERY

The ability of geriatric patients to withstand the stress of an SCD event and the associated mechanical trauma of

CPR has raised many questions. Complications of CPR include rib fractures, pulmonary contusion, pneumothorax, vertebral compression fracture, and liver or splenic injury. Geriatric patients are predisposed to these complications due to underlying osteoporosis, arthritis, and lung disease. They have less physiologic reserve to handle both tissue hypoxia and the stress of CPR than younger patients.

In patients who are resuscitated after an SCD event, anoxic neurologic injury is the primary cause of morbidity and mortality. Permanent neurologic sequelae after SCD are seen in up to 30 percent of survivors of out-of-hospital cardiac arrest.[37,38] However, patients over 70 years of age who experience an SCD event are no more likely to suffer an adverse neurologic outcome than younger survivors of SCD with similar premorbidity.[17,18]

REFERENCES

1. Zheng ZJ, Croft JB, Giles WH, et al. Sudden cardiac death in the United States, 1989–1998. Circulation 104:2158, 2001.
2. de Breede-Swagemakers JJ, Gorgels AP, Dubois-Arbouw WI, et al: Out-of-hospital cardiac arrest in the 1990s: A population-based study in the Maastricht area on incidence, characteristics and survival. *J Am Coll Cardiol* 30:1500, 1997.
3. Juchems R, Wahlig G, Frese W: Influence of age on the survival rate of out-of-hospital and in-hospital resuscitation. *Resuscitation* 26:23, 1993.
4. Niemann JT, Stratton SJ, Cruz B, Lewis R: Outcome of out-of-hospital post-countershock asystole and pulseless electrical activity versus asystole and pulseless electrical activity. *Crit Care Med* 29:2366, 2001.
5. Soo LH, Gray D, Young T, Hampton JR: Circadian variation in witnessed out of hospital cardiac arrest. *Heart* 84:370, 2000.
6. Stewart S, McIntyre K, Capewell S, McMurray JJ: Heart failure in a cold climate: Seasonal variation in heart failure-related morbidity and mortality. *J Am Coll Cardiol* 39:760, 2002.
7. Holmberg M, Holmberg S, Herlitz J: Incidence duration and survival of ventricular fibrillation in out-of-hospital cardiac arrest patients in Sweden. *Resuscitation* 44:7, 2000.
8. Bayes de Luna A, Coumel P, Leclercq JF: Ambulatory sudden cardiac death: Mechanisms of production of fatal arrhythmia on the basis of data from 157 cases. *Am Heart J* 117:151, 1989.
9. Piccirillo G, Nocco M, Lionetti M, et al: Effects of sildenafil citrate (Viagra) on cardiac repolarization and on autonomic control in subjects with chronic heart failure. *Am Heart J* 143:703, 2002.
10. Hays LJ, Lerman BB, DiMarco JP: Nonventricular arrhythmias as precursors of ventricular fibrillation in patients with out-of-hospital cardiac arrest. *Am Heart J* 118:53, 1989.
11. Pepe PE, Levine RL, Fromm RE Jr, et al: Cardiac arrest presenting with rhythms other than ventricular fibrillation: Contribution of resuscitative efforts toward total survivorship. *Crit Care Med* 21:1813, 1993.
12. Defibrillation: Guidelines 2000 for cardiopulmonary resuscitation and emergency cardiovascular care. International consensus on science. *Circulation* 102:90, 2000.
13. Ardagh MW: Resuscitation from out-of-hospital cardiac arrest: Past, present and future. *Aust NZ Med J* 109:153, 1996.
14. Gazmuri RJ: Outcome after cardiopulmonary resuscitation: Is age a factor? *Crit Care Med* 27:2295, 1999.
15. Lee KH, Angus DC, Abramson NS: Cardiopulmonary resuscitation: What cost to cheat death? *Crit Care Med* 24:2046, 1996.
16. Dautzenberg PL, Broekman TC, Hooyer C, et al: Review: Patient-related predictors of cardiopulmonary resuscitation of hospitalized patients. *Age Ageing* 22:464, 1993.
17. Rogove HJ, Safar P, Sutton-Tyrrell K, et al: Old age does not negate good cerebral outcome after cardiopulmonary resuscitation: Analysis from the brain resuscitation clinical trials: The brain resuscitation clinical trials I and II study groups. *Crit Care Med* 23:18, 1995.
18. de Vos R, Koster RW, de Haan RJ, et al: In-hospital cardiopulmonary resuscitation: Prearrest morbidity and outcome. *Arch Intern Med* 159:845, 1999.
19. Longstreth WT, Tresch DD, Thakur RK, et al: Comparison of outcome of paramedic-witnessed cardiac arrest in patients younger and older the 70 years. *Am J Cardiol* 65:453, 1990.
20. Eisenberg MS, Harwood BT, Cummins RO, et al: Cardiac arrest and resuscitation: A tale of 29 cities. *Ann Emerg Med* 19:170, 1990.
21. Kim C, Becker L, Eisenberg MS: Out-of-hospital cardiac arrest in octogenarians and nonagenarians. *Arch Intern Med* 60:3439, 2000.
22. Goldstein S, Mendendorp SV, Landis JR, et al: Analysis of cardiac symptoms preceding cardiac arrest. *Am J Cardiol* 58:1195, 1998.
23. Eisenberg MS, Cummins RO, Litwin PE, Hallstrom AP: Out-of-hospital cardiac arrest: Significance of symptoms in patients collapsing before and after arrival of paramedics. *Am J Emerg Med* 4:116, 1986.
24. Molnar J, Weiss JS, Rosenthal JE: Does heart rate identify sudden death survivors? Assessment of heart rate, QT interval, and heart rate variability. *Am J Ther* 9:99, 2002.
25. Edston E, Grontoft L, Johnsson J: TUNEL: A useful screening method in sudden cardiac death. *Int J Legal Med* 116:22, 2002.
26. Eisenberg MS, Harwood BT, Cummins RO, et al: Cardiac arrest and resuscitation: A tale of 29 cities. *Ann Emerg Med* 19:170, 1990.
27. Herlitz J, Estrom L, Wennerblom B, et al: Survival Among patients with out-of-hospital cardiac arrest found in electromechanical dissociation. *Resuscitation* 29:97, 1995.

28. Moss AJ, Hall WJ, Cannom DS, et al: Improved survival with an implanted defibrillator in patients with coronary disease at high risk for ventricular arrhythmia. Multicenter Automatic Defibrillator Implantation Trial Investigators. *New Engl J Med* 335:1933, 1996.

29. Buxton AE, Lee KL, Fisher JD, et al: A randomized study of the prevention of sudden death in patients with coronary artery disease. Multicenter Unsustained Tachycardia Trial Investigators *New Engl J Med* 342:24, 2000.

30. Connolly SJ, Gent M, Roberts RS, et al: Canadian Implantable Defibrillator Study (CIDS): A randomized trial of the implantable cardioverter-defibrillator against amiodarone. *Circulation* 101:1297, 2000.

31. Kuck KH, Cappato R, Siebels J, Russpel R: Randomized comparison of antiarrhythmic drug therapy with implantable defibrillators in patients resuscitated from cardiac arrest: The Cardiac Arrest Study Hamburg (CASH). *Circulation* 102:748, 2000.

32. Kadish A: Primary prevention of sudden death using ICD therapy: Incremental steps. *J Am Coll Cardiol* 39:788, 2002.

33. Qi X, Dorian P: Antiarrhythmic drugs and ventricular defibrillation energy requirements. *Chin Med J* 112:1147, 1999.

34. Council on Ethical and Judicial Affairs, American Medical Association: Guidelines for the appropriate use of do-not-resuscitation orders. *JAMA* 265:1868, 1991.

35. Watson DR, Wilkinson, TJ, Sainsbury, R, Kidd JE: The effect of hospital admission on the opinions and knowledge of elderly patients regarding cardiopulmonary resuscitation. *Age Aging* 26:429, 1997.

36. Smith EM, Hastie IR: Resuscitation status of the elderly. *J R Coll Phys Lond* 26:377, 1992.

37. Safar PJ: Therapeutic hypothermia after cardiac arrest. *New Engl J Med* 346:612, 2002.

38. Safar PJ: Resuscitation of the ischemic brain, in Albin MS (ed): *Textbook of Neuroanesthesia: With Neurosurgical and Neuroscience Perspectives.* New York, McGraw-Hill, 1997, pp 557–593.

17

Acute Dyspnea

T. Paul Tran

HIGH-YIELD FACTS

- Dyspnea in geriatric patients may be a late presentation of cardiorespiratory diseases due to blunted sensitivity to hypoxic and hypercarbic stimuli, attenuated inflammatory response, and decreased perception of dyspnea.
- Dyspnea may be the sole symptom of myocardial infarction.
- Most geriatric patients with significant dyspnea will need further care as inpatients.
- Be prepared for end-of-life care in the emergency department (ED).

The human respiratory system is an integrative organ system composed of airways (upper and lower), lung vasculature and lymphatics (blood circulation and fluid balance), lung parenchyma (main lung function), respiratory muscles, and breathing control centers.[1] While its primary function is to effect gas exchange, the respiratory system also works as an endocrine and a phagocytic organ. Lung function and gas exchange, however, decline with age.[2,3] There are various anatomic, structural, and chemical changes in senescent lungs, chest wall, and respiratory muscles. These changes are thought to be due to normal aging and acquired lung damage from cumulative environmental exposure over time.

Dyspnea, a cardinal symptom of cardiorespiratory diseases, is perhaps the most common cardiorespiratory complaint by geriatric patients presenting to the ED.[4] It is an important symptom that requires prompt medical attention because it can be the harbinger of serious cardiorespiratory diseases. *Dyspnea,* derived from "disor-

dered" (*dys-*) "respiration" (*-pnea*), refers to a sense of breathlessness or air hunger experienced by patients. It occurs when the respiratory drive in the brain stem and cortex is activated and increased disproportionately to the work of breathing or metabolic demand.

Dyspnea is difficult to quantitate. Numerous descriptors (e.g., "suffocating," "chest tightness," "not getting enough air," "out of breath") are used by patients to describe the feeling of dyspnea. Moreover, patients of different ethnic/cultural backgrounds living in different parts of the United States use different descriptors to describe dyspnea.[5] To help standardize the degree of dyspnea, various dyspnea-quantifying scales have been proposed. These scales use various questionnaires to rate patients' experience of breathlessness after a life event. For example, the Borg scale[6] gives a dyspnea score after exercise; the Baseline Dyspnea Index[7] gives a dyspnea score for daily living activities; the Quality of Life in Asthma scale[8] gives a quality-of-life score for asthmatics; and the Cincinnati Dyspnea Questionnaire[9] gives a composite dyspnea score for asthmatic patients during physical and verbal activities. While these scales may be helpful in certain clinical settings, none is consistently satisfactory in all settings, especially in the ED.

Since medical history is most important in establishing a diagnosis in clinical medicine, lacking a common language of dyspnea poses a significant diagnostic impediment. Even though most geriatric patients can provide a reliable medical history, a significant minority may not be able to give a complete history due to altered mental status, cognitive and hearing impairment, or other comorbid conditions. The emergency physician often has to take the medical history from a proxy informant (e.g., family, friend, or caregiver) who may not be entirely reliable. This lack of a precise language and reliable history, coupled with a broad differential diagnosis from the trivial to the most serious cardiorespiratory conditions, renders the evaluation of a dyspneic geriatric patient in the ED setting difficult. In the initial stage, however, the emergency physician can limit the management of dyspnea to ruling out and stabilizing the most potentially life-threatening conditions and defer the diagnostic workups until after the patient is admitted to the hospital.

GERIATRIC RESPIRATORY PHYSIOLOGY

The human respiratory system continually undergoes functional and structural changes from infancy to adulthood to the senescent years.[1,3] The senescent changes reflect the combined effects of the normal physiology of aging and environmental insults accumulated over time. With advanced age, the chest wall is stiffened due to calcification of the costal cartilages. Lung elastic recoil is reduced due to changes in the elastin and collagen fibers along with changes in the surface-tension forces. Respiratory muscle strength is weakened, and kyphoscoliotic changes are exaggerated. Consequently, the functional residual capacity (FRC) and residual volume (RV) are both increased. On the other hand, vital capacity (VC) and forced expiratory volume at 1 second (FEV_1) are decreased—about 30 percent lower in a 70-year-old compared with a 20- year-old cohort. The resulting age-related airflow limitation, premature closure of terminal bronchioles during tidal breathing, and ventilation-perfusion mismatch are believed to contribute to the age-related reductions in cardiovascular adaptability and arterial oxygen tension in the elderly. Interestingly, since age-related changes in alveolar oxygen tension are minimal,[10] the alveolar-arterial (A-a) gradient is widened in the elderly. The A-a gradient can be approximated by the equation $A\text{-}a = 0.36 \times age - 4.3$ mmHg.[11]

Ventilatory responsiveness to hypoxia and hypercapnia are both reduced by approximately 50 percent in older individuals (65–79 years) compared with the younger cohorts.[12] This is probably due to decreased chemosensitivity, reduced neural output to respiratory muscles, and lower mechanical efficiency and deconditioning.[3] There are also proportional reductions in mouth occlusion pressure in response to chemical stimuli.[12] Additionally, sensitivity to resistive [e.g., chronic obstructive pulmonary disease (COPD)] and elastic [e.g., congestive heart failure (CHF)] loads is attenuated in the elderly (>60 years).[13,14] This reduced sensitivity to mechanical loads is thought to be due to differences in the integration and processing of respiratory stimuli in the breathing centers rather than alterations in the muscle force. Separately, the immune system is altered. Both mucociliary clearance in the upper and lower airways is diminished and inflammatory reaction to infections is blunted. Results of these studies together suggest that geriatric patients may suffer greater impairment of the respiratory system before they experience respiratory discomfort[15] and may explain the relative lack of symptoms in geriatric presentation. Signs and symptoms of infection (e.g., dyspnea, cough, fever, chest pain, etc) and other cardiopulmonary diseases (e.g.,

hypoxia and hypercapnia) may be absent until the disease process is well advanced.[15]

EPIDEMIOLOGY

Studies have shown that respiratory symptoms are among the most common reasons for geriatric patients to seek medical care. In the United States, the number of persons older than 65 years of age approached 35 million in 2000, making up 12.5 percent of the total population.[16] Over time, these elderly patients are at an increased risk of developing cardiorespiratory diseases. In fact, more than half of adults older than age 60 have at least one respiratory symptom annually.[17] All of this accounts for many geriatric visits to the ED for respiratory-related ailments. Dyspnea and wheeze, however, epidemiologically are symptoms not only of common obstructive lung disorders (e.g., asthma or COPD) but also of cardiac, metabolic, infectious, and central nervous system (CNS) pathology. Seventy percent of patients with CHF report dyspnea as the main symptom that prompts them to go to the ED. Of these, 88 percent require admission to the hospital.[4] On the other hand, only half of COPD exacerbations actually are brought to the attention of a health care professional.[18] The majority of COPD patients who seek care, however, need hospitalization. Annually, more than 700,000 patients older than age 65 are hospitalized for CHF, and another half-million patients require hospitalization for COPD. The rates of readmission to the hospital within 6 months for both CHF and COPD approach 50 percent.[19]

PATHOPHYSIOLOGY

Breathing is controlled by the autonomic centers in the cortex and brain stem, which automatically adjust the level of ventilation to match that of metabolic demands. Normal persons are usually not aware of the act of breathing when they are at rest or even when they are subjected to mild or moderate loads of physical activity. However, individuals generally feel dyspneic when their respiratory drive in the brain stem and cortex is activated and increased disproportionately to the work of breathing or metabolic demand.

This activation seems to be the result of complex interactions between various stimuli and breathing centers in the brain stem and cortex[20] (Fig. 17–1). In this model of dyspnea, the breathing control centers, located in the medulla oblongata and cortex, receive information via an afferent limb and send out effector signals via an efferent

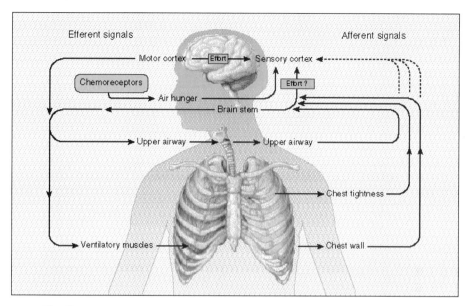

Fig. 17-1   Proposed neural circuit of dyspnea. (Modified with permission from Manning.[20])

limb that not only gives signals to the respiratory muscles but also provides feedback to the breathing control centers themselves. The afferent limb is composed of two groups[21,22]: (1) respiratory sensors and (2) sensory and mechanoreceptors. The respiratory sensors include the central chemoreceptors of hypercapnia ($Paco_2$)—a measure of acidosis, located at the medulla—and peripheral chemoreceptors of anoxia (Pao_2)—located at the carotid and aortic bodies. The sensory and mechanoreceptor sensors include the various receptors in the joints, tendons, and muscles in the chest wall and respiratory muscles, nonspecific receptors in the upper airways, irritant receptors in the airway epithelium, pulmonary stretch receptors in the smaller airways, C-fiber receptors in the lungs, and vascular receptors in the right atrium, ventricle, and pulmonary artery. Sensory signals in the afferent limb are transmitted to the brain stem and sensory cortex via various neural pathways, including the vagus nerve. Effector signals from the motor cortex reach the respiratory muscles via the efferent limb to complete the respiratory control circuit.

It is believed that different clinical conditions (e.g., pulmonary embolus, COPD, CHF, and anxiety neurosis) invoke different afferent stimuli, which are then processed by more than one mechanism in the breathing centers to produce the unique experience and intensity of dyspnea for a patient. Mechanistically, the sense of respiratory effort is believed to arise from the outputs from the motor cortex and brain stem going to the sensory cortex. The sense of air hunger, on the other hand, seems to arise, in part, from increased activation in the brain stem. Breathlessness also seems to result from a mismatch between incoming afferent sensory signals and outgoing efferent motor signals to the effector respiratory muscles.[20]

CLINICAL FEATURES

Geriatric patients who present to the ED with dyspnea may already have clinical evidence of cardiorespiratory disease. Although the etiology of dyspnea may be clear in some patients after an abbreviated history and physical examination, differentiating the two major causes of dyspnea—pulmonary and cardiac dyspnea—can be particularly challenging even after an exhaustive evaluation.

It is important to note the time of onset of dyspnea and its time course. Acute onset would suggest trauma or an acute medical disorder such as pneumothorax, myocardial ischemia, or pulmonary embolism (PE), for example. An abrupt onset with a history of exposure to an allergen raises the possibility of an anaphylactoid reaction or even anaphylaxis. Subacute onset, on the other hand, suggests a more indolent disease process such as pneumonia or an exacerbation of some chronic disorders such as CHF or COPD. A history of dietary indiscretion or medication noncompliance in the setting of CHF or tobacco use in a setting of COPD would be useful. For chronic diseases, it is also important to note the pattern and time course of the current exacerbation, how it affects daily activity, as well as aggravating and relieving factors. Any associated symptoms such as syncope, chest pain, location and characterization, palpitations, and nausea and vomiting would be particularly helpful in the dichotomy of cardiorespiratory disease. It is noteworthy that up to one-third of geriatric patients with myocardial infarction may present without chest pain,[23] and dyspnea can be the proxy presentation for acute coronary syndrome.[24] Other symptoms that should be elicited include fever, wheezing, cough, hemoptysis, leg pain or swelling, night sweats, and weight changes.

Although the language of dyspnea is imprecise, how patients describe their breathlessness can be helpful in establishing a diagnosis. Table 17-1 lists the descriptors that patients use to describe the different cardiopulmonary disorders.

The physical examination should be focused first on the general appearance, level of respiratory distress and mentation, use of accessory muscles, and presence of diaphoresis and cyanosis. Note the vital signs for tachypnea, fever, and any desaturation in pulse oximetry. The basic pulmonary examination should include inspection for asymmetry of chest movement; palpation for subcutaneous emphysema, tactile fremitus, or tenderness; percussion; and auscultation for stridor, rales, wheezes, or adventitious breath sounds. Basic cardiac examination should include checking for evidence of jugular venous distension or peripheral pulses and the presence of any extracardiac heart sounds, pathologic murmurs, pulsatile abdominal masses, leg edema, and any calf warmth, cord, or tenderness.

DIAGNOSIS AND DIFFERENTIAL

The range of pathologic conditions that lead to dyspnea is quite diverse, ranging from nonurgent to life-threatening and sometimes exotic diagnoses.[25] Table 17-2 lists the more important diagnoses to consider in the ED. High on the differential diagnostic list are cardiorespiratory disorders that should be the focus of ED evaluation and workup. True respiratory emergencies may originate from disorders in the airways and pulmonary parenchyma. Cardiovascular emergencies include angina equivalent, acute coronary syndrome, arrhythmias, disorders of thoracic vessels, pericardial effusion,[26] and myocardial infarction. Geriatric patients with the complaint of dyspnea should be triaged to the main ED for immediate medical attention. While the patient is undergoing the initial assessment, stabilization steps, including bedside pulse oximetry, oxygen therapy by nasal cannula or mask, cardiac monitor, and intravenous access, should occur simultaneously. The initial assessment should focus on airway patency, adequacy of ventilation, level of respiratory distress, and level of mentation. This is followed by a more thorough examination looking for signs and symptoms of trauma to the head or chest; any abnormal chest movement or chest trauma; hemo/pneumothorax; and signs and symptoms of pulmonary edema, COPD, pneumonia, angina equivalent, ischemic heart disease, or PE. As in other medical emergencies, emergent treatment and stabilization maneuvers should be started and should precede diagnosis for patients in acute dyspnea (e.g., imminent acute respiratory failure).

A 12-lead electrocardiogram (ECG) and a chest radiograph are essential tools in the evaluation of a geriatric patient with dyspnea. A complete blood count (CBC),

Table 17-1. Descriptors Most Commonly Used by Patients in Selected Cardiorespiratory Disorders

Descriptor	CHF	COPD	ASTHMA	PE	ILD
I feel "out of breath"	x	x			x
My breath does not go in (or out) all the way	x				
My breathing is "shallow"/I cannot take a deep breath				x	
My breathing requires "work" or "effort"	x	x			x
I cannot get enough air/I feel a hunger for air			x	x	
My chest feels "tight" or "constricted"			x		
My breathing is "rapid"					x

Note: CHF = congestive heart failure; COPD = chronic obstructive pulmonary diseases; PE = pulmonary embolism; ILD = interstitial lung diseases.
Source: Modified with permission from Mahler et al.[33]

Table 17-2. Differential Diagnoses for Acute Dyspnea

Organ System	Examples	Comments
Upper airway	Upper airway obstruction (aspiration syndrome, angioedema, tumor, anaphylaxis, epiglottitis, fibrotic stenosis)	Stridor, retraction of supraclavicular fossae with inspiration
Lower airway	Asthma, chronic bronchitis, emphysema, bronchiectasis	Patients usually have a known history of the disease
Lung parenchyma	Solitary nodular lung disease (infectious, neoplasms, Wegener's granulomatosis, rheumatoid nodule, vascular malformation, bronchogenic cyst) Diffuse nodular lung disease (metastatic neoplasm, infectious, pneumoconiosis, eosinophilic granuloma) Infiltrate (infectious pneumonias, neoplasm, radiation pneumonitis, BOOP, bronchocentric granulomatosis, pulmonary infarction) Interstitial (infectious, pulmonary fibrosis, sarcoid, pneumoconiosis, hypersensitivity syndrome, eosinophilic granuloma) Alveolar (infectious, pulmonary edema, ARDS, sarcoidosis, pulmonary hemorrhage syndromes)	Differential diagnosis is grouped by findings on chest radiography for ease of categorization. The list can be extensive. Most common pulmonary causes of geriatric dyspnea include COPD, asthma, infectious pneumonias, bronchiectasis, pulmonary embolism, pleural effusion, neoplasms, carcinomatosis, and pneumothorax
Pulmonary vessel	Pulmonary embolism	Lower extremity DVT usually source of emboli
Brain, chest wall, and respiratory muscles	Impaired respiratory drive (stroke, brain stem infarction, hemorrhage, trauma; drugs, etc.) Impaired neuromuscular system (cervical cord injury, Guillain-Barré, myasthenia gravis, organophosphate poisoning) Impaired ventilatory apparatus (flail chest, hemopneumothorax, kyphoscoliosis)	
Heart	Pulmonary edema, angina equivalent, acute coronary syndrome, myocardial infarction, cardiomyopathies, arrhythmias, valvular heart disease, pericardial effusion and tamponade, pericarditis, cardiomyopathy, acute cor pulmonale	JVD, rales, extracardiac (or muffled) heart sounds, murmur on auscultation
Blood	Anemia, carbon monoxide poisoning	
Endocrine	Electrolyte abnormalities, metabolic acidosis, DKA, thyroid disease	
Abdomen	Hypotension (ruptured abdominal aortic aneurysm, perforated viscus, urosepsis or sepsis from other organs, etc.)	

Source: Modified with permission from Drazen and Weinberger.[34]

chemistry, and urinalysis (UA) are appropriate initial screening studies. Arterial blood gas (ABG) determination should be considered in cases of significant dyspnea. Determinations of cardiac enzymes, b-type natriuretic peptide, calcium, magnesium, and phosphorus and sputum examination and studies (Gram stain and culture) can be ordered selectively as clinical condition warrants. If PE is suspected, a second-generation D-dimer test can be used as a screening test, and a ventilation-perfusion ($\dot{V}/\dot{Q}$) scan or spiral computed tomographic (sCT) scan and pulmonary vascular imaging modality such as pulmonary angiography can be used as confirmatory tests.[27] Echocardiography also can be used to assess regional wall-motion abnormalities, pericardial effusion, pulmonary vascular pressure, and any valvular disorders. Soft tissue examination of neck with or without laryngoscopy, in collaboration with appropriate surgical consultant, is indicated for suspected epiglottitis or airway blockage with any foreign body.

EMERGENCY DEPARTMENT CARE AND DISPOSITION

Since disease-specific emergency care and dispositions are discussed in other chapters, only a general approach to dyspnea will be discussed here. Patients with imminent acute respiratory failure should be treated with oxygen therapy, ventilatory support with noninvasive positive-pressure ventilation (NPPV), endotracheal intubation, needle cricothyrotomy, surgical airway, or tube and needle thoracostomy as appropriate. Pharmacologic interventions may include, in addition to supplemental oxygen, aerosolized β_2-agonists (e.g., albuterol, racemic epinephrine), anticholinergic bronchodilators (e.g., ipratropium bromide), diuretics or hydration, and inotropic or antiarrhythmic agents as indicated clinically. In consultation with the patient's primary care physician or geriatrician, the few patients who have reversible airway disease, who no longer feel dyspneic, whose examination is at baseline, who can resume daily activities, and who have good support systems can be discharged to home from the ED. The rest of the patients should be admitted to the hospital for further care.

END-OF-LIFE CARE IN THE ED

Occasionally the emergency physician is confronted with a situation in which a patient is brought to the ED for dyspnea, but the situation rapidly evolves into a terminal end-of-life care issue in the ED. The role of emergency physi-

cian in this phase of care has been discussed extensively elsewhere[28] (see Chap. 7). Even though it may be very difficult to make decisions to withhold, terminate, or even withdraw care for patients while in the ED, the emergency physician should make every attempt to support those dying patients and their loved ones. The U.S. Supreme Court has ruled that there is no constitutional right to physician-assisted suicide. Nevertheless, patients who clearly demonstrate the expressed wish of "do not resuscitate" or who clearly derive no benefit from further futile medical care can be given supportive care in the appropriate setting (ED, hospital, hospice, home). The principles of medical ethics—respect for autonomy, beneficence (principle of doing good), nonmaleficence (principle of first do no harm), and justice (principle of distributive justice or equal care for equal condition)—should govern these end-of-life care decisions.[29] Even though medical care is crucial and should remain the primary focus of the emergency physician while a patient is in the ED, dying patients and their families tend to view end-of-life care as a process shaped by broader psychosocial and life-long personal experiences.[30]

Communication skills and empathy are crucial in this phase of care. Von Gunten and colleagues[31] outlined a seven-step plan for improving communication with dying patients and their families. All EDs should have an appropriate environment (family or consultation room) for this occasion. The emergency physician in charge should assemble as many facts as possible in consultation with the patient's geriatrician. This physician should attempt to establish a congenial alliance with the family and then discuss the facts with the appropriate family members. In general, information should be delivered in a sensitive, clear, and straightforward manner. During this briefing, the physician should listen attentively to questions from the family members and be prepared to respond to the emotional reactions from the family. Attention to this step conveys respect and support and strengthens the patient-physician relationship.[31]

Dyspnea is distressing to terminal patients and should be treated aggressively and properly. The underlying cause of dyspnea should be determined and reversed if possible. If a reversible cause of dyspnea cannot be determined, low doses of narcotics such as morphine, titrated up to effects, can be used safely to treat dyspnea by reducing the air hunger.[32] Since dyspnea is exacerbated by anxiety, anxiolytics such as benzodiazepines also can be used as adjunct agents. Airway secretion can be managed with suctioning. Mucolytic agents (hyoscyamine 0.125 mg orally or sublingually) or drying agents (atropine 1–2 mg intramuscularly/intravenously or scopolamine (0.3–0.6 mg intramuscularly or subcutaneously) also can be used.[32]

REFERENCES

1. Johnson BD: Age-associated changes in pulmonary reserve, in Evans JG, Wiliams TF, Beattie BL, et al. (eds): *Oxford Textbook of Geriatric Medicine,* 2d ed. Oxford, England, Oxford University Press, 2000, p 483

2. Pack AI, Millman RP: The lungs in later life, in Fishman AP (ed): *Pulmonary Diseases and Disorders,* New York, McGraw-Hill 1998; p 79

3. Chan ED, Welsh CH: Geriatric respiratory medicine. *Chest* 114:1704, 1998.

4. Parshall MB: Adult emergency visits for chronic cardiorespiratory disease: Does dyspnea matter? *Nurs Res* 48:62, 1999.

5. Hardie GE, Janson S, Gold WM, et al.: Ethnic differences: Word descriptors used by African-American and white asthma patients during induced bronchoconstriction. *Chest* 117:935, 2000.

6. Borg GA: Psychophysical bases of perceived exertion. *Med Sci Sports Exerc* 14:377, 1982.

7. Mahler DA, Weinberg DH, Wells CK, et al: The measurement of dyspnea: Contents, interobserver agreement, and physiologic correlates of two new clinical indexes. *Chest* 85:751, 1984.

8. Juniper EF, Guyatt GH, Ferrie PJ, et al: Measuring quality of life in asthma. *Am Rev Respir Dis* 147:832, 1993.

9. Lee L, Friesen M, Lambert IR, et al: Evaluation of dyspnea during physical and speech activities in patients with pulmonary diseases. *Chest* 113:625, 1998.

10. Sorbini CA, Grassi V, Solinas E, et al: Arterial oxygen tension in relation to age in healthy subjects. *Respiration* 25:3, 1968.

11. Raine JM, Bishop JM: A-a Difference in O_2 tension and physiological dead space in normal man. *J Appl Physiol* 18:284, 1963.

12. Peterson DD, Pack AI, Silage DA, et al: Effects of aging on ventilatory and occlusion pressure responses to hypoxia and hypercapnia. *Am Rev Respir Dis* 124:387, 1981.

13. Tack M, Altose MD, Cherniack NS: Effect of aging on respiratory sensations produced by elastic loads. *J Appl Physiol* 50:844, 1981.

14. Tack M, Altose MD, Cherniack NS: Effect of aging on the perception of resistive ventilatory loads. *Am Rev Respir Dis* 126:463, 1982.

15. Silvestri GA, Mahler DA: Evaluation of dyspnea in the elderly patient. *Clin Chest Med* 14:393, 1993.

16. Day JC: Population projections of the United States, by age, sex, race, and Hispanic origin: 1995–2050. Current Population Reports Series P25, No. 1130. Washington, DC, U.S. Government Printing Office, 1996.

17. Lebowitz MD, Knudson RJ, Burrows B: Tucson epidemiologic study of obstructive lung diseases: I. Methodology and prevalence of disease. *Am J Epidemiol* 102:137, 1975.

18. Seemungal TA, Donaldson GC, Bhowmik A, et al: Time course and recovery of exacerbations in patients with chronic obstructive pulmonary disease. *Am J Respir Crit Care Med* 161:1608, 2000.

19. Feldman DE, Thivierge C, Guerard L, et al: Changing trends in mortality and admissions to hospital for elderly patients with congestive heart failure in Montreal. *CMAJ* 165:1033, 2001.

20. Manning HL, Schwartzstein RM: Pathophysiology of dyspnea. *New Engl J Med* 333:1547, 1995.

21. Tobin MJ: Dyspnea: Pathophysiologic basis, clinical presentation, and management. *Arch Intern Med* 150:1604, 1990.

22. Wasserman K, Casaburi R: Dyspnea: Physiological and pathophysiological mechanisms. *Annu Rev Med* 39:503, 1988.

23. Canto JG, Shlipak MG, Rogers WJ, et al: Prevalence, clinical characteristics, and mortality among patients with myocardial infarction presenting without chest pain. *JAMA* 283:3223, 2000.

24. Gregoratos G: Clinical manifestations of acute myocardial infarction in older patients. *Am J Geriatr Cardiol* 10:345, 2001.

25. Thomson CC, Tager AM, Weller PF: Clinical problem-solving: More than your average wheeze. *New Engl J Med* 346:438, 2002.

26. Blaivas M: Incidence of pericardial effusion in patients presenting to the emergency department with unexplained dyspnea. *Acad Emerg Med* 8:1143, 2001.

27. Kline JA, Johns KL, Colucciello SA, et al: New diagnostic tests for pulmonary embolism. *Ann Emerg Med* 35:168, 2000.

28. Schears RM: Emergency physicians' role in end-of-life care. *Emerg Med Clin North Am* 17:539, 1999.

29. Escalante CP, Martin CG, Elting LS, et al: Medical futility and appropriate medical care in patients whose death is thought to be imminent. *Support Care Cancer* 5:274, 1997.

30. Steinhauser KE, Christakis NA, Clipp EC, et al: Factors considered important at the end of life by patients, family, physicians, and other care providers. *JAMA* 284:2476, 2000.

31. von Gunten CF, Ferris FD, Emanuel LL: The patient-physician relationship: Ensuring competency in end-of-life care. Communication and relational skills. *JAMA* 284:3051, 2000.

32. Keay TJ, Lynn J: Care of the dying patient, in Hazzard WR, Blass JP, Ettinger WH Jr, et al (eds): *Principles of Geriatric Medicine and Gerontology,* 4th ed. New York, McGraw-Hill, 1999, p 537

33. Mahler DA, Harver A, Lentine T, et al: Descriptors of breathlessness in cardiorespiratory diseases. *Am J Respir Crit Care Med* 154:1357, 1996.

34. Drazen JM, Weinberger SE: Approach to the patient with disease of the respiratory system, in Braunwald E, Fauci AS, Kasper DL, et al (eds): *Harrison's Principles of Internal Medicine,* 15th ed. New York, McGraw-Hill, 2001, p 1443

18

Geriatric Pneumonia

Scott T. Wilber

HIGH-YIELD FACTS

- Older patients are more likely to have pneumonia from typical bacteria (*Streptococcus pneumoniae* most common) and aerobic gram-negative bacilli.

- The sensitivity of fever is only 30 percent and leukocytosis is only 60 percent, so the absence of these findings should not be used to rule out pneumonia.

- Antibiotic choices must be made empirically and should cover all likely pathogens.

- Extended-spectrum fluoroquinolones are recommended for older outpatients and for monotherapy of inpatients (general medical ward) with pneumonia.

- Patients admitted to the intensive care unit require coverage with a β-lactam/β-lactamase inhibitor or a cephalosporin *plus* a fluoroquinolone or a macrolide.

- Disposition decisions should take into account risk stratification (Pneumonia Severity Index), as well as other medical and psychosocial factors.

Despite advances in antimicrobial treatment and supportive care, pneumonia continues to have a significant impact on older persons. Pneumonia is the fourth leading cause of hospitalization and the fifth leading cause of death in patients over age 65.[1] As the population ages, emergency physicians will be called on increasingly to diagnose and manage older patients with pneumonia.

As a result of recent studies and published guidelines,[2,3] there will be increasing pressure to manage patients with pneumonia as outpatients. Understanding which elderly patients with pneumonia are appropriate for outpatient management will allow the emergency physician to respond to these pressures in a proactive, patient-centered manner. Additionally, the prompt administration of an-

tibiotics will be expected. This requires the emergency physician to have knowledge of the usual microbial etiologies of pneumonia in older patients, their resistance patterns, and the spectrum of coverage of antibiotics.

This chapter emphasizes the differences between older and younger patients in microbial etiology and clinical features of pneumonia. Most important, diagnosis, risk stratification, and treatment will be emphasized so that emergency physicians can provide high-quality care to the geriatric patient with pneumonia.

EPIDEMIOLOGY

The incidence of pneumonia requiring hospitalization in persons older than age 65 is over 2 percent and is six times higher than any other age group.[4] The incidence is higher in males and increases with age.[1] One-third of physician visits for pneumonia in patients over age 65 result in hospital admission (>750,000 admissions in 2000),[4] and 42 percent of patients older than age 65 who have pneumonia are seen in an emergency department (ED).[5]

Following a long period of declining mortality from pneumonia in the antibiotic era, mortality rates for pneumonia have increased in the past two decades.[6] One explanation for this is the aging of our population. The risk of death from pneumonia increases with age.[1,7,8] Pneumonia is the seventh leading cause of death in those aged 65 to 74 years, the sixth in those aged 75 to 84 years, and the fourth in those age 85 and older.[7] Elderly patients who survive pneumonia initially are twice as likely to die in the next 10 years than those without pneumonia.[9]

PATHOPHYSIOLOGY

Pneumonia develops when microorganisms gain access to the epithelium of the lower respiratory tract, overcome host defenses, and establish infection. This may occur via hematogenous or direct spread or by direct inoculation. Direct inoculation is most common method and may occur through bacterial colonization of the upper respiratory tract mucosa with subsequent aspiration or direct inhalation of aerosolized microorganisms into the lower respiratory tract.

"Typical" bacterial pathogens usually gain access to the lower respiratory tract by colonization and aspiration. Older patients are more likely to have risk factors for oropharyngeal colonization and aspiration.[10–12] Infection may be occur following the aspiration of as little as 0.01

mL of oropharyngeal secretions, and 50 percent of normal persons aspirate small amounts of oropharyngeal secretions during sleep.[13]

Microorganisms also may gain access to the lower respiratory tract via direct inhalation. This is the common method by which viruses, atypical bacteria, mycobacteria, and fungi initiate pneumonia. The inhalation of as few as 5 to 50 mycobacteria may cause disease.[13]

Host defenses that prevent the development of pneumonia include removal of microorganisms from the upper airways through salivary flow, epithelial cell loss, coughing and sneezing, mucociliary transport to remove secretions and microorganisms from the conducting airways, and local humoral defenses (IgA and IgG) and alveolar macrophages to fight pathogens that gain access to the lower respiratory tract.[13]

Microbial Etiology

The microbial etiology of pneumonia in older patients differs from that in younger patients. *Streptococcus pneumoniae* is responsible for a greater proportion (up to 50 percent) of cases and is the most common pathogen.[10,14,15] Infection by the other "typical" bacterial pathogens *Hemophilus influenza*, *Staphylococcus aureus*, and *Moraxella catarrhalis* is also more common.[10,15]

Older patients have an increased risk of pneumonia due to aerobic gram-negative bacilli, including *Enterobacter*, *Acinetobacter*, *Escherichia coli*, *Klebsiella*, *Serratia*, *Proteus*, and *Pseudomonas* species.[10,15] Risk factors for oropharyngeal colonization and pneumonia from aerobic gram-negative bacilli include underlying cardiopulmonary or neoplastic disease, broad-spectrum antibiotics, and declining functional status.[10–12]

"Atypical" bacterial pathogens (*Legionella*, *Mycoplasma*, and *Chlamydia*) are responsible for a smaller proportion of pneumonias in the elderly.[10,15] *Legionella* pneumonia occurs more commonly in patients with pneumonia severe enough to require hospitalization.[15] A recent study did show an increased prevalence of *Mycoplasma pneumoniae* infections in patients over age 65.[14] *C. pneumoniae* occurred less commonly in this group.[14]

Polymicrobial and anaerobic pneumonias occur infrequently but are more common in patients requiring hospitalization for their pneumonia.[15]

No microbial etiology is found in 40 to 60 percent of patients in studies to determine the etiology of pneumonia, despite extensive testing. Multiple organisms are found in 2 to 5 percent of patients.[3,10,14,15]

CLINICAL FEATURES

Historical features of typical bacterial pneumonias include the sudden onset of fever and chills, dyspnea, pleuritic chest pain, and cough with purulent sputum. Fatigue, anorexia, headache, and myalgias may also be present. Older patients usually have a longer duration of symptoms, and the prevalence of all these symptoms is lower than in younger patients.[10,16] The elderly present more commonly with vague, nonspecific complaints, including weakness, falls, confusion, delirium, anorexia, abdominal pain, or functional decline.[10,11]

Vital signs in patients with pneumonia include fever, tachycardia, and tachypnea. Tachypnea is common in the older pneumonia patient, with 65 percent having a respiratory rate of 30 or higher.[10,16] The sensitivity of fever (>38°C) is only 30 percent for the diagnosis of pneumonia, so a normal temperature should not be used to "rule out" pneumonia.[16]

Physical examination of the chest may provide clues to the diagnosis of pneumonia. Inspection of the chest may show asymmetrical chest expansion. Tactile fremitus, elicited by palpating the chest wall while the patient speaks, will be increased in patients with pneumonia but decreased in patients with pleural effusions or pneumothorax. Dullness to percussion may be present in pneumonia or pleural effusion. Auscultation of the lungs may reveal bronchial breath sounds in the area of pneumonia. Crackles, or rales, are nonmusical lung sounds that may occur in patients with pneumonia. Consolidation of the lung may produce increased transmission of whispered or normal speech, known as *whispered pectoriloquy* or *bronchophony*, respectively. Similarly, a change in the sound of vowels from *e* to *a*, known as *egophony*, may occur.[17]

The value of the chest examination is diminished by its subjectivity. Interobserver reliability, or the agreement between physicians accounting for chance, is poor for tactile fremitus and whispered pectoriloquy and fair for dullness to percussion, wheezes, and rales.[17,18] Lack of cooperation in elders with confusion, altered mental status, or weakness further diminishes the value of the physical examination. For these reasons, the ability to diagnose pneumonia based solely on history and physical examination is limited.

It has been taught traditionally that "typical" pneumonias can be differentiated from "atypical" pneumonias by history and physical examination. However, clinical features are neither sensitive nor specific for determining the etiology of pneumonia.[15,19] Certain elements of the history and physical examination are important for the risk stratification of patients with pneumonia and are discussed below under "Risk Stratification."

It is important to remember that although appropriately treated younger patients' fevers usually resolve within 2 to 5 days, older patients may take longer to resolve, and 35 to 85 percent of patients will still have some symptoms of pneumonia after 1 month.[3,20]

DIAGNOSIS AND DIFFERENTIAL

Pneumonia is a clinical and radiographic diagnosis, and no other laboratory studies are required. Patients diagnosed with pneumonia should have some of the preceding symptoms of acute infection accompanied by the presence of an acute infiltrate on chest radiograph.[3]

Chest Radiography

The chest x-ray is the primary diagnostic test for pneumonia. Treatment of patients without a confirmatory radiograph is discouraged in published clinical guidelines, based on the limitations of physical examination in diagnosing pneumonia noted earlier.[3,15] Ideally, a posteroanterior (PA) and lateral chest x-ray should be performed. Portable anteroposterior (AP) chest x-rays may be easier to perform in older patients but decrease the quality of the film.[11]

The radiographic appearance of pneumonia is divided into lobar, bronchopneumonia, and interstitial patterns.[21] However, these patterns are of limited usefulness in determining the etiology of pneumonia.[10,22] Studies show that the different patterns are approximately equal in distribution in pneumococcal pneumonia rather than the traditionally taught lobar infiltrate.[21,22] Radiologists cannot reliably distinguish viral from bacterial pneumonia.[21,23]

Many patients who present with lower respiratory tract symptoms do not have pneumonia. The chest x-ray can suggest other common causes of lower respiratory tract symptoms in older patients, such as congestive heart failure, malignancy, atelectasis, pleural effusion, pulmonary embolism, or infarct.

Complications of pneumonia identified on chest x-ray include parapneumonic effusions, abscess formation, and mass lesions causing postobstructive pneumonia. Parapneumonic effusions may be sterile or may represent empyema, an infection of the pleural space.

A widely held axiom is that chest x-rays may be negative in patients with dehydration,[10] a common finding in geriatric patients with pneumonia. There is little clinical

evidence to support this theory, and animal studies have yielded conflicting results.[21] Similarly, it has been suggested that elderly patients with pneumonia less commonly have infiltrates on initial chest x-rays as compared with younger patients.[10,11,24]

Laboratory Testing

While laboratory testing is not required to diagnose pneumonia, routine studies are helpful to determine the severity of disease. The complete blood count (CBC) may show leukocytosis, although the sensitivity of this finding is only 60 percent.[19] Both high and low white blood cell (WBC) counts have been associated with more severe disease, although neither was shown to be a predictor of mortality in a recent large study.[8] A low hematocrit has been associated with more severe disease.[8]

Chemistry panels (electrolytes, blood urea nitrogen, creatinine, and glucose) may be helpful in assessing patients with pneumonia. Findings associated with higher mortality include elevated blood glucose, elevated blood urea nitrogen (BUN), and decreased sodium.[8]

Microbial Testing

Microbial testing is performed to determine the etiology of pneumonia so that therapy may be directed at the specific pathogen. Pathogen-specific therapy can limit the consequences of antibiotic overuse, including cost, antibiotic resistance, and adverse drug reactions.[3] Additionally, microbial studies constitute less than 1 percent of admitted patient's hospital bill.[3] However, as noted earlier, pathogens are only identified in about half of the cases, and therefore, the value of this testing in patients with pneumonia remains controversial.[2,3,15] Some studies of the benefit of diagnostic testing have reported no benefit in adults with community-acquired pneumonia (CAP),[26] yet others have found that obtaining blood cultures within the first 24 hours in elderly patients with pneumonia was associated with lower 30-day mortality.[27]

Sputum Gram Stain and Culture

The yield of sputum Gram stain is approximately 30 to 40 percent, primarily limited by the fact that most patients are unable to produce acceptable sputum samples.[3] Sensitivity for *S. pneumoniae* is 50 to 60 percent, and specificity is greater than 80 percent.[3] A sputum sample for microbiologic tests should be a grossly purulent, deep-cough specimen obtained in the presence of the physician or nurse. The specimen should be examined within 1 to 2 hours by an experienced observer. Specimens with less than 10 squamous epithelial cells and more than 25 polymorphonuclear leukocytes (PMNs) per low-powered field are considered acceptable. The sputum should be obtained before antibiotic therapy, if possible, because prior antibiotic therapy may decrease the sensitivity and specificity of the test. However, the treatment of acutely ill patients should not be delayed due to difficulty in obtaining sputum specimens.[3,28] If an adequate sputum specimen is obtained and a predominant organism is identified on Gram stain, directed antimicrobial therapy may be appropriate.[3,28]

Sputum cultures generally are ordered in conjunction with the Gram stain, although contamination and overgrowth limit the sensitivity and specificity of standard culture techniques determining the etiology of pneumonia.[3,28]

Blood Cultures

Blood cultures have a low yield for etiologic agents in pneumonia (4–18 percent).[28] However, they are recommended by most authorities in patients admitted to the hospital with pneumonia.[2,3,15] They cite the low cost, ease of obtaining blood cultures, the specificity in identifying the causative organism, and the ability to test for antimicrobial sensitivity. Antimicrobial therapy may be altered in up to 50 percent of patients with positive blood cultures.[29] Obtaining blood cultures within 24 hours of admission in patients with CAP also has been associated with lower mortality.[27] Consequently, this has been used as an indicator of quality of care for patients with CAP.[2,3] Since the yield of blood cultures is lowered by prior antibiotic therapy, they should be obtained before antibiotic therapy is instituted.

Differential Diagnosis

The differential diagnosis of pneumonia depends on presenting symptoms. Patients who present with respiratory symptoms (cough, dyspnea) may have an upper respiratory tract infection, acute or chronic bronchitis, congestive heart failure, pulmonary embolism, malignancy, or a pleural effusion as the cause of their symptoms.

Patients who present primarily with nonrespiratory symptoms (such as confusion, fever, falls, or functional decline) must be evaluated for other infections (urinary tract infection, meningitis, cellulitis, bacteremia, etc.) and noninfectious causes (electrolyte abnormalities, cerebrovascular accident, subdural hematoma, encephalopathy).

EMERGENCY DEPARTMENT CARE AND DISPOSITION

Nonpharmacologic Management

Supportive care of the older patient with pneumonia must be provided in a timely fashion, frequently in conjunction with history, examination, and diagnostic testing. The assessment and treatment of respiration (oxygenation and ventilation) and perfusion are the emergency physician's primary concern.

Oxygenation should be assessed rapidly using pulse oximetry. Patients with arterial oxygen saturations of less than 90 percent should receive oxygen. Arterial blood gas determinations may be helpful if hypercarbia is suspected (i.e., patients with chronic obstructive pulmonary disease, decreased mental status, and fatigue). Patients whose hypoxia does not respond to supplemental oxygen and those with significant respiratory acidosis may require mechanical ventilation. Recent studies have shown noninvasive bilevel positive-pressure ventilation (BiPAP) to be successful in treating patients with respiratory failure due to pneumonia.[30] This may avert the need for endotracheal intubation and its potential complications when available. Patients with evidence of bronchospasm on examination or a history of obstructive airways disease (asthma or chronic obstructive pulmonary disease) may benefit from inhaled bronchodilator therapy.

Inadequate perfusion may range from dehydration with mild tachycardia to life-threatening hypotension due to septic shock. Patients with septic shock have signs of decreased tissue perfusion (confusion and oliguria) but a hyperdynamic circulation. Initial therapy of inadequate perfusion consists of intravenous crystalloids (normal saline or lactated Ringer's solution) administered through a large-bore intravenous line. In older patients, fluid overload is a potential complication, and it is wise to administer intravenous fluids in judicious boluses and frequently assess the patient's response. Patients who do not respond to crystalloid infusion may require treatment with vasopressors.

Antibiotic Therapy

There are over 30 antibiotics approved by the Food and Drug Administration (FDA) for the treatment of pneumonia.[2] Ideally, one should use narrow-spectrum, etiology-specific antibiotics. However, given the inability of history, physical examination, and radiographic features to determine the etiology of pneumonia, the initial antibiotic treatment is usually empirical. Empirical antibiotic regimens must cover likely pathogens, and therefore, such factors as the setting, age of the patient, severity of illness, comorbidities, and the likelihood of drug resistance must be taken into account when selecting empirical antibiotics for pneumonia in older patients. Table 18-1 suggests appropriate antibiotic choices for the treatment of pneumonia in older adults based on recent guidelines.[3]

Antibiotics should be administered as soon as possible in the ED. Studies have shown that delayed antibiotic administration (>8 hours) results in increased mortality in patients with pneumonia.[2,3,27] Development of clinical pathways for the treatment of pneumonia in the ED may reduce delays in antibiotic treatment.[31]

Recommended duration of antibiotic therapy varies by pathogen. For *S. pneumoniae*, treatment should be continued for 7 to 14 days or until the patient is afebrile for 72 hours. Atypical pathogens should be treated for 10 to 21 days.[3] Empirical treatment of older outpatients therefore should continue for a minimum of 10 to 14 days.

Specific Antibiotics

Fluoroquinolones

Available quinolones for the treatment of pneumonia include ciprofloxacin, ofloxacin, levofloxacin, sparfloxacin, moxifloxacin, gatifloxacin, and trovafloxacin. Levofloxacin, sparfloxacin, moxifloxacin, gatifloxacin, and trovafloxacin provide increased coverage of *S. pneumoniae* compared with ciprofloxacin and ofloxacin.[3] Penicillin-resistant *S. pneumoniae* (PRSP) are also susceptible to these "enhanced spectrum" fluoroquinolones.

Table 18-1. Antibiotic Treatment of Older Patients with Pneumonia

Setting	Antibiotic
Outpatients	Fluoroquinolone* (preferred)
	or
	Doxycycline or macrolide† (alternative)
Inpatients	
General medical ward	β-Lactam/β-lactamase inhibitor‡ + macrolide†
	or
	Extended-spectrum cephalosporin§ + macrolide†
	or
	Fluoroquinolone* (alone)
Intensive care unit	β-Lactam/β-lactamase inhibitor‡
	or
	Extended-spectrum cephalosporin§
	plus
	Fluoroquinolone* *or* macrolide†
Modifying factors	
Structural lung disease	Pipericillin, pipericillin-tazobactam, carbapenem, or cefepime
	plus
	Fluoroquinolone* (including high-dose ciprofloxacin)
β-Lactam allergy	Fluoroquinolone* ± clindamycin
Suspected aspiration	Fluoroquinolone* (trovafloxacin, moxifloxacin, and gatifloxacin have in vitro activity against anaerobes and may not require combination therapy)
	with or without
	Clindamycin, metronidazole or β-lactam/β-lactamase inhibitor‡

*Levofloxacin, moxifloxacin, gatifloxacin, or other fluoroquinolone with enhanced activity against *S. pneumoniae*.
†Azithromycin or clarithromycin.
‡Ampicillin-sulbactam or piperacillin-tazobactam.
§Cefotaxime or ceftriaxone.
Source: Used with permission from Bartlett et al.[3]

Coverage also includes gram-negative bacilli, *H. influenzae*, *M. catarrhalis*, *Legionella*, *M. pneumoniae*, and *C. pneumoniae*, making them excellent choices for single-drug treatment of pneumonia.[3]

Trovafloxacin use has been significantly restricted by the FDA due to severe and sometimes fatal hepatotoxicity. Sparfloxacin is not available for intravenous use, causes more photosensitivity, and can prolong the QT interval.[3,32]

Macrolides

Macrolides provide excellent coverage of atypical bacterial infections, including *M. pneumoniae*, *C. pneumoniae*, and *Legionella*. *S. pneumoniae* is increasingly resistant to macrolides (10–20 percent). The rate of resistance is much higher in PRSP.[3]

Erythromycin use has multiple disadvantages for the treatment of pneumonia in elders, including more frequent dosing and increased gastrointestinal side effects. Erythromycin is also relatively ineffective against *H. influenzae*, a more common pathogen in the elderly.[3]

Better choices for pneumonia treatment in this group are azithromycin and clarithromycin. Azithromycin is more active against *H. influenzae*, *Legionella*, and *M. pneumoniae*, whereas clarithromycin provides better coverage of *S. pneumoniae* and *C. pneumoniae*.[3,32] Advantages to azithromycin include a simplified dosing schedule of once daily for 5 days and the availability of an intravenous preparation.

β-Lactams

Although penicillin remains the drug of choice for the treatment of susceptible strains of *S. pneumoniae* [3], β-lactam/β-lactamase inhibitors are the members of this class recommended for empirical treatment of pneumonia. Intravenous preparations include ticarcillin-clavulanate, ampicillin-sulbactam, and piperacillin-tazobactam. These drugs provide activity against *H. influenzae*, anaerobes, *M. catarrhalis*, *S. pneumoniae*, and *S. aureus*.[13] Atypical organisms are not covered. Ticarcillin is less active against *S. pneumoniae* than other penicillins and therefore is not recommended by the Infections Disease Society of America (IDSA) for empirical treatment of pneumonia.[3] Piperacillin offer the best coverage of *Pseudomonas*.[3]

Risk factors for infection with PRSP include the use of β-lactams in the past 3 months, immunosuppression, hospitalization within 6 months, and nosocomial pneumonia.[32]

Cephalosporins

Many cephalosporins have been studied for the treatment of pneumonia. Cefotaxime and ceftriaxone have the best activity against *S. pneumoniae;* cefuroxime is less active.[3] Cefepime is recommended for those with underlying structural lung disease due to its enhanced activity against *Pseudomonas*.[3]

Other Antimicrobials

Doxycycline is one of the recommended antibiotics in the IDSA guidelines for the outpatient treatment of CAP. Twice-daily dosing, good bioavailability, and low cost are advantages. Coverage is excellent for the atypical organisms; however, there are concerns over increasing resistance to *S. pneumoniae* (~15 percent).[3]

Trimethoprim-sulfamethoxazole was previously included in guidelines for the outpatient treatment of pneumonia.[15] However, currently it is not recommended due to increasing resistance to *S. pneumoniae* (20–25 percent, ≥70 percent of PRSP) and lack of coverage of atypical organisms.[3]

Risk Stratification and Disposition

Determining whether to admit or discharge patients with pneumonia is the most costly decision emergency physicians make.[5] For this reason, there have been increasing efforts to treat patients with CAP as outpatients.[33–36] The disposition decision should take into account the severity of the pneumonia, as well as other medical and psychosocial factors.[8] Geriatric patients considered for management as outpatients must be able to take oral fluids and antibiotics, comply with outpatient care, and be able to carry out activities of daily living (ADLs) or have adequate home support to assist in ADLs.[8]

Although there have been many efforts at assessing severity and risk of death in patients with pneumonia, the most commonly recommended is the Pneumonia Severity Index (also referred to as the PORT criteria).[8] This prediction rule was derived and validated with data on over 52,000 inpatients and then validated with a second cohort of 2287 inpatients and outpatients as part of the Pneumonia PORT study.[8] Subsequent validation has been performed with geriatric patients and nursing home residents.[37,38] Patients are assigned to one of five risk classes (1 is lowest risk, 5 is highest risk) based on a point system that considers age, coexisting disease, abnormal physical findings, and abnormal laboratory findings. Elderly patients cannot be assigned to class 1 because a requirement is age less than 50 years. Table 18-2 shows the point scoring system for assignment to classes 2 to 5, associated mortality rates and recommended disposition.[8]

In older patients, age contributes the most points to the overall score. In the study by Fine and colleagues,[8] patients assigned to classes 1 and 2 typically were younger patients (median ages 35–59 years), and patients in classes 3 to 5 were older (median ages 72–75 years).

Originally, outpatient management was suggested for classes 1 and 2, brief inpatient observation for class 3, and traditional hospitalization for classes 4 and 5.[8] Other

authors, including guidelines from the American College of Emergency Physicians and the Infectious Disease Society of America, have suggested outpatient management for class 3 patients.[2,3]

Other risk factors for morbidity or mortality from pneumonia were not significant predictors in the Pneumonia Severity Index. These include other comorbid illnesses (diabetes mellitus, chronic obstructive pulmonary disease, postsplenectomy state), aspiration, chronic alcohol abuse or malnutrition, and evidence of extrapulmonary disease, as well as laboratory studies such as

Table 18-2. Pneumonia Severity Score for Elderly Patients

Characteristic	Points
Historical findings	
Age	
Men	Age (years)
Women	Age (years) − 10
Nursing home resident	10
Coexisting disease	
Neoplastic disease	30
Liver disease	20
Congestive heart failure	10
Cerebrovascular disease	10
Renal disease	10
Physical examination findings	
Altered mental status (acute)	20
Respiratory rate ≥ 30	20
Systolic BP < 90 mmHg	20
Temperature < 35°C or ≤ 40°C	15
Pulse ≥ 125/min	10
Diagnostic testing findings	
Arterial pH < 7.35	30
BUN ≥ 30 mg/dL	20
Sodium < 130 mmol/L	20
Glucose ≥ 250 mg/dL	10
Hematocrit < 30%	10
Pao_2 < 60 mmHg (or Sao_2 < 90%)	10
Pleural effusion	10

Risk Class	Point Score	Mortality (%)	Disposition
2	≤70	0.6	Outpatient
3	71–90	2.8	Outpatient or Brief inpatient
4	91–130	8.2	Inpatient
5	>130	29.2	Inpatient

Source: Used with permission from Fine et al.[8]

WBC count less than 4,000/mm^3 or greater than 30,000/mm^3, absolute neutrophil count 1,000/mm^3 less than 1, elevated prothrombin time or partial thromboplastin time, decreased platelet count, or radiographic evidence of multilobar involvement, cavitation, and rapid spreading.[15]

Severe pneumonia may require intensive care unit (ICU) admission. American Thoracic Society guidelines define severe pneumonia as the presence of at least one of the following: respiratory rate greater than 30, severe respiratory failure (Pao$_2$/Fio$_2$ < 250), mechanical ventilation, bilateral or multilobar infiltrates, shock, vasopressor requirement, or oliguria (urine output < 20 mL/h).[15] The presence of at least one of these is highly sensitive (98 percent) but only 32 percent specific for the need for ICU management.[39] In the study by Fine and colleagues,[8] 6 percent of patients in class 3, 11 percent of patients in class 4, and 17 percent of patients class 5 required ICU admission.

The preceding guidelines for admission should not supersede individual clinical judgment of the need to hospitalize patients.

ADDITIONAL ASPECTS

Prevention

Prevention of pneumonia in older patients is highly desirable given its morbidity, mortality, and economic cost. Immunizations against influenza and *S. pneumoniae* are effective at reducing hospitalization and death from pneumonia by as much as 63 and 81 percent, respectively,[40] and are recommended for all persons 65 years of age and older. However, only 65 percent of patients over age 65 are immunized against influenza and 45 percent against *S. pneumoniae*.[41] Studies in one urban ED showed that only 28 percent of high-risk patients reported immunization against influenza, and only 3 percent reported immunization against *S. pneumoniae*.[42]

Prior ED studies have shown that ED-based immunization programs are feasible and beneficial. Length of stays were not affected because the median time needed for all immunization-related activities was only 4 minutes.[42,43] Other studies have estimated significant cost savings for such programs.[44] The American College of Emergency Physicians has recently published a policy that "supports the immunization of high-risk patients against influenza and pneumococcal disease in the emergency department." [45]

Nursing Home-Acquired Pneumonia

The most common microbial etiology of nursing home-acquired pneumonia is gram-negative bacilli, causing 30 to 40 percent of pneumonias. *S. pneumoniae* remains the most common individual bacterial cause (20–30 percent of cases). *H. influenzae* causes 10 to 20 percent of nursing home-acquired pneumonias, and *S. aureus* pneumonia occurs with greater frequency (5–12 percent) in this population. Atypical organisms and viruses are less common but may cause outbreaks of pneumonia in nursing homes.[10,11,46] Antibiotic treatment should take these differences into account.

Risk factors for the development of pneumonia in nursing home patients include increasing age, male sex, swallowing difficulty, and inability to take oral medications. Influenza vaccination is protective.[47]

Nursing home patients were included in the derivation of the Pneumonia Severity Index,[8] and it has been evaluated independently in this population.[38]

Although nearly all older patients with nursing home-acquired pneumonia would meet criteria for admission based on the recommendations of the Pneumonia Severity Index, other studies have shown that the mortality rate may not be affected by hospitalization.[48] The abilities of nursing homes to provide hydration, intravenous antibiotics, oxygen, and other skilled nursing care varies, and the decision to admit these patients should be made in conjunction with the patient's physician and nursing home staff.

Tuberculosis

Persons over age 65 have a higher prevalence of tuberculosis (TB) than any other age group (12.8 cases per 100,000 population in 1998).[49] The risk is higher in nursing home patients than in community-dwelling elders.[50]

Typical symptoms of active TB include fatigue, weight loss, low-grade fever, night sweats, and cough, which may last for months. Again, older patients frequently present atypically. Weight loss is more common, but fever, night sweats, and hemoptysis occur less often. [50] Older patients more frequently have middle or lower lobe infiltrates or miliary disease on chest x-ray rather than the classic apical infiltrate.[50]

TB skin tests, sputum smears for acid-fast bacilli, symptoms, and chest x-ray can provide presumptive evidence of infection. The diagnosis of TB requires culture, but 4 to 6 weeks are required for growth. [50]

Drug therapy consists of a combination of isoniazid,

rifampin, pyrazinamide, ethambutol, or streptomycin. The duration of therapy is 6 to 9 months. [50]

REFERENCES

1. Desai MM, Zhang P, Hagan-Hennessy C: Surveillance for morbidity and mortality among older adults—United States, 1995–1996. *MMWR* 48(SS-8):7, 1999.
2. American College of Emergency Physicians: Clinical policy for the management and risk stratification of community-acquired pneumonia in adults in the emergency department. *Ann Emerg Med* 38:107, 2001.
3. Bartlett JG, Breiman RF, Mandell LA, et al: Practice guidelines for the management of community-acquired pneumonia in adults. *Clin Infect Dis* 31:347, 2000.
4. Hall MJ, Owings MF: *2000 National Hospital Discharge Survey: Advance Data from Vital and Health Statistics,* no 329. Hyattsville, MD, National Center for Health Statistics, 2002.
5. Niederman MS, McCombs JS, Unger AN, et al: The cost of treating community-acquired pneumonia. *Clin Ther* 20(4):820, 1998.
6. Armstrong GI, Conn LA, Pinner RW: Trends in infectious disease mortality in the United States during the 20th century. *JAMA* 281(1):61, 1999.
7. Minino AM, Arias E, Kochanek KD, et al: *Deaths: Final Data for 2000: National Vital Statistics Reports,* vol 50, no 15. Hyattsville, MD, National Center for Health Statistics, 2002.
8. Fine MJ, Auble TE, Yealy DM, et al: A prediction rule to identify low-risk patients with community-acquired pneumonia. *New Engl J Med* 336:243, 1997.
9. Koivula I, Sten M, Makela PH: Prognosis after community-acquired pneumonia in the elderly. *Arch Intern Med* 159:1550, 1999.
10. Feldman C: Pneumonia in the elderly. *Clin Chest Med* 20(3):563, 1999.
11. Sims RV: Bacterial pneumonia in the elderly. *Emerg Med Clin North Am* 8(2):207, 1990.
12. Stein D: Managing pneumonia acquired in nursing homes: Special concerns. *Geriatrics* 45(3):39, 1990.
13. Mason CM, Nelson S: Pulmonary host defenses: Implications for therapy. *Clin Chest Med* 20(3):475, 1999.
14. Marston BJ, Plouffe JF, File TM, et al: Incidence of community-acquired pneumonia requiring hospitalization: Results of a population-based active surveillance study in Ohio. *Arch Intern Med* 157:1709, 1997.
15. American Thoracic Society: Guidelines for the initial management of adults with community-acquired pneumonia: Diagnosis, assessment of severity, and initial antimicrobial therapy. *Am Rev Respir Dis* 148:1418, 1993.
16. Metlay JP, Schulz R, Li YH, et al: Influence of age of symptoms at presentation in patients with community-acquired pneumonia. *Arch Intern Med* 157:1453, 1997.
17. Metlay JP, Kapoor WN, Fine JM: Does this patient have community-acquired pneumonia? Diagnosing pneumonia by history and physical examination. *JAMA* 278(17):1440, 1997.
18. Wipf JE, Lipsky BA, Hirchmann JV, et al: Diagnosing pneumonia by physical examination: Relevant or relic? *Arch Intern Med* 159:1082, 1999.
19. Ruiz M, Ewig S, Marcos MA, et al†: Etiology of community-acquired pneumonia: Impact of age, comorbidity, and severity. *Am J Respir Crit Care Med* 160:397, 1999.
20. Metlay JP, Atlas SJ, Borowsky LH, et al: Time course of symptom resolution in patients with community-acquired pneumonia. *Respir Med* 92:1137, 1998.
21. Katz DS, Leung AN: Radiology of pneumonia. *Clin Chest Med* 20(3):549, 1999.
22. Kantor HG: The many radiologic facies of pneumococcal pneumonia. *AJR* 137(6):1213, 1981.
23. Tew J, Calenoff L, Berlin BS: Bacterial or nonbacterial pneumonia: Accuracy of radiographic diagnosis. *Radiology* 124(3):607, 1977.
24. Esposito AL: Community-acquired bacteremic pneumococcal pneumonia: Effect of age on outcome. *Arch Intern Med* 144:945, 1984.
25. Fine MJ, Stone RA, Singer DE, et al: Processes and outcomes of care for patients with community-acquired pneumonia. *Arch Intern Med* 159:970, 1999.
26. Sanyal S, Smith PR, Saha AC, et al: Initial microbiologic studies did not affect outcome in adults hospitalized with community-acquired pneumonia. *Am J Respir Crit Care Med* 160:346, 1999.
27. Meehan TP, Fine MJ, Krumholz HM, et al: Quality of care, process, and outcomes in elderly patients with pneumonia. *JAMA* 278(23):2080, 1997.
28. Skerrett SJ: Diagnostic testing for community-acquired pneumonia. *Clin Chest Med* 20(3):531, 1999.
29. Wilber ST, Domers TA, Garrity DA, et al: The yield of blood cultures in patients with community-acquired pneumonia (abstract). *Acad Emerg Med* 5(5):426, 1998.
30. Confalonieri M, Potena A, Carbone G, et al: Acute respiratory failure in patients with severe community-acquired pneumonia: A prospective randomized evaluation of noninvasive ventilation. *Am J Respir Crit Care Med* 160:1585, 1999.
31. Benenson R, Magalski A, Cavanaugh S, et al: Effects of a pneumonia clinical pathway on time to antibiotic treatment, length of stay, and mortality. *Acad Emerg Med* 6(12):1243, 1999.
32. Mandell LA: Antibiotic therapy for community-acquired pneumonia. *Clin Chest Med* 20(3):589, 1999.
33. Hoe LK, Keang LT: Hospitalized low-risk community-acquired pneumonia: Outcome and potential for cost savings. *Respirology* 4:307, 1999.
34. Marrie TJ, Lau CY, Wheeler SL, et al: A controlled trial of a critical pathway for treatment of community-acquired pneumonia. *JAMA* 283(6):749, 2000.

35. Dean NC, Suchyta MR, Bateman KA: Implementation of admission decision support for community-acquired pneumonia: A pilot study. *Chest* 117:1368, 2000.

36. Flanders WD, Tucker G, Krishnadasan A, et al: Validation of the Pneumonia Severity Index: Importance of study-specific recalibration. *J Gen Intern Med* 14:333, 1999.

37. Ewig S, Kleinfeld T, Bauer T, et al: Comparative validation of prognostic rules for community-acquired pneumonia in an elderly population. *Eur Respir J* 14:370, 1999.

38. Mylotte JM, Naughton B, Saludades C, et al: Validation and application of the Pneumonia Prognosis Index to nursing home residents with pneumonia. *J Am Geriatr Soc* 46:1538, 1998.

39. Ewig S, Ruiz M, Mensa J, et al: Severe community-acquired pneumonia: Assessment of severity criteria. *Am J Respir Crit Care Med* 158:1102, 1998.

40. Nichol KL: The additive benefits of influenza and pneumococcal vaccinations during influenza seasons among elderly persons with chronic lung disease. *Vaccine* 17:S91, 1999.

41. Influenza and pneumococcal vaccination levels among adults aged > 65 years—United States, 1997. *MMWR* 47(38):797, 1998.

42. Slobodkin D, Zielske PG, Kitlas JL, et al: Demonstration of the feasibility of emergency department immunization against influenza and pneumococcus. *Ann Emerg Med* 32(5):537, 1998.

43. Slobodkin D, Kitlas JL, Zielske PG: A test of the feasibility of pneumococcal vaccination in the emergency department. *Acad Emerg Med* 6:724, 1999.

44. Stack SJ, Martin DR, Plouffe JF: An emergency department-based pneumococcal vaccination program could save money and lives. *Ann Emerg Med* 33:299, 1999.

45. American College of Emergency Physicians: Immunizations in the emergency department. *Ann Emerg Med* 34:576, 1999.

46. Stein D: Managing pneumonia acquired in nursing homes: Special concerns *Geriatrics* 45(3):39, 1990.

47. Loeb M, McGeer A, McArthur M, et al: Risk factors for pneumonia and other lower respiratory tract infections in elderly residents of long-term care facilities. *Arch Intern Med* 159:2058, 1999.

48. Thompson RS, Hall NK, Szpiech M, et al: Hospitalization and mortality rates for nursing home-acquired pneumonia. *J Fam Pract* 48(4):291, 1999.

49. Progress toward the elimination of tuberculosis—United States, 1998. *MMWR* 48(33):732, 1999.

50. Hocking TL, Choi C: Tuberculosis: A strategy to detect and treat new and reactivated infections. *Geriatrics* 52(3):52, 1997.

19

Chronic Obstructive Pulmonary Disease (COPD)

T. Paul Tran

HIGH-YIELD FACTS

- Chronic obstructive pulmonary disease (COPD) exacerbations are commonly precipitated by tracheobronchitis.

- Ischemic heart disease, myocardial infarction, congestive heart failure, acute cor pulmonale, pulmonary embolus, and pneumothorax are important causes of acute dyspnea to consider in the emergency department (ED).

- A short course of steroids and antibiotics, anticholinergic and sympathomimetic bronchodilators, oxygen, and ventilatory support form the mainstays of treatment of acute COPD exacerbations.

- Noninvasive positive-pressure ventilation (NPPV) is the first mode of ventilatory support for COPD patients at risks for acute respiratory failure (ARF)

- COPD patients on oxygen therapy should be monitored to keep pulse oxymetry $\geq 90\%$ (Pao_2 60 to 65 mm Hg) and pH ≥ 7.26 to avoid hypercapnic respiratory failure.

- Age, presence of comorbid conditions, refractoriness to the ED therapy, altered level of consciousness, gas-exchange disturbance, arterial blood gas deviation from baseline, poor home support system, lower pretreatment or posttreatment FEV_1, and previous history of outpatient failure portend risks of outpatient failure and should influence the decision to hospitalize.

Chronic obstructive pulmonary disease (COPD) represents an "umbrella term used to encompass several more specific respiratory conditions," including chronic (obstructive) bronchitis and emphysema.[1] It is a syndrome characterized by minimally reversible, progressive expiratory airflow obstruction punctuated by periodic exacerbations. In the Western world, COPD is principally caused by smoking, although genetics (e.g., α_1-antitrypsin deficiency), environmental and occupational exposures, and possibly airway hyperresponsiveness may be causative in a minority of cases.

COPD patients typically have a blend of chronic bronchitis and emphysema, although tradition holds that approximately 85 percent of these patients have chronic bronchitis and the remaining 15 percent have emphysema. While both chronic bronchitis and emphysema share expiratory airflow obstruction, chronic bronchitis is defined clinically by the presence of chronic cough with productive sputum for at least 3 months during 2 consecutive years. Patients may look overweight, edematous, and cyanotic ("blue bloater"). In contrast, emphysema is defined anatomically as permanent destructive changes of airways terminal to bronchioles. Patients may be thin and barrel-chested but usually noncyanotic ("pink puffer"). A cigarette smoke-induced inflammatory process underlies the pathogenesis of the majority of pathologic lesions associated with COPD.

COPD exacerbations are characterized by worsening dyspnea, increased cough, sputum production, and wheezing. Precipitating factors for a COPD exacerbation are not well understood but most commonly include tracheobronchitis, continued smoking, medication noncompliance or medication error, decompensated congestive heart failure (CHF), and air pollution. In the emergency department (ED), the less common but potentially catastrophic causes of dyspnea such as ischemic heart disease, myocardial infarction, pulmonary embolus, atelectasis, and pneumothorax are important considerations for the emergency physician.

COPD exacerbations should raise serious clinical consideration for the emergency physician. In contrast to popular beliefs, only half of COPD exacerbations are actually reported by patients and evaluated by medical professionals.[2] Those who seek care, however, frequently need to be hospitalized. The hospitalization course is often prolonged, with inpatient mortality up to 4 percent for low-risk patients and up to 24 percent for patients admitted to the intensive care unit (ICU).[3] The 6-month rate of rehospitalization after a COPD exacerbation approaches 50 percent.[4]

EPIDEMIOLOGY, NATURAL HISTORY, AND PROGNOSIS[5]

Studies have illustrated the disease burden of COPD on patients and health care resources. In the United States, there are currently more than 16 million patients with COPD, accounting for more than half a million annual hospitalizations and $18 billion in annual direct health care costs.[6] Smoking is responsible in up to 90 percent of all cases of COPD. COPD is currently the fourth leading cause of death (after heart disease, cancer, and stroke), accounting for 107,000 deaths in 1998.[7]

Human lung function, measured by force expiratory volume at 1 second (FEV_1), declines by about 35 mL per year after reaching a summit at 20 years of age. Smoking, however, accelerates this decline by two- to fivefold in susceptible individuals. Because of large lung function reserve, symptomatic COPD is largely limited to patients entering the fifth decade and older. Figure 19-1 is reproduced from the classic study by Fletcher[8] showing the natural progression of lung function and the effects of smoking in susceptible patients. From the graph, one can see that smoking cessation is beneficial at any age, although the earlier the better. Dyspnea on exertion becomes evident when FEV_1 falls to about 60 percent of predicted—approximately 1.5 L—and death occurs within a few years when FEV_1 falls to below 20 percent of predicted (approximately 500 mL). The American Thoracic Society (ATS) defines stable COPD as mild (stage I) if $FEV_1 \geq 50$ percent of predicted, moderate (stage II) if ≥ 35 percent $FEV_1 \leq 49$ percent, and severe (stage III) if $FEV_1 < 35$ percent.[9]

PATHOPHYSIOLOGY

Permanent, minimally reversible, slowly progressive obstruction of expiratory airflow and destructive changes of terminal airway units of the lung parenchyma are hallmarks of COPD, setting it apart from other pulmonary obstructive conditions such as asthma. Airway obstruction, more prominent in chronic bronchitis, is caused by airway inflammation, epithelial metaplasia, mucus gland hypertrophy and mucus hypersecretion, and structural changes in the bronchi. Narrowing of the airways caused by the inflammatory process leads to exponential increases in airway resistance and corresponding decreases in airflow. Destruction of lung parenchyma, a prominent feature in emphysema, leads to increased collapsibility of small airways, augmented dynamic compression, decreased lung elastic recoil, and consequently, reduced expiratory driving pressure. As expiratory airflow drops off, airtrapping occurs, resulting in hyperinflation of chest and lung. By the time a patient begins to experience dyspnea from COPD, some degree of airway obstruction can always be demonstrable on bronchoscopic examination.

Cigarette smoking is overwhelmingly the etiologic agent in causing COPD in the industrialized world, whereas environmental pollution appears to play a more

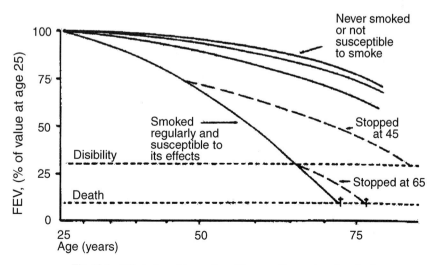

Fig. 19-1 Effect of smoking, and smoking cessation, on lung function.[8]

important role in the developing countries. Occupational exposure (cadmium), passive smoking, airway hyperresponsiveness, and bacterial and viral (rhinovirus) chronic lung infections are other risk factors. Genetics plays a yet to be defined role in the development of COPD, but the fraction of COPD attributable to genetic variants is relatively small (about 1 percent).[10] Deficiency of α_1-antitrypsin, a serine proteinase inhibitor, is the only known genetic disorder firmly liked to the development of emphysema. Additionally, only 15 percent of white and .5 percent of Asian smokers are susceptible to developing COPD. How do environmental agents (such as cigarette smoke) lead to the development of COPD in genetically susceptible individuals? There are currently two interrelated concepts to explain this question: (1) the presence of an imbalance of protease-antiprotease in the lung and (2) the presence of a chronic oxidative stress induced by environmental agents such as cigarette smoke. Both these concepts stem from a predominantly neutrophilic inflammatory process as the common underlying pathogenetic mechanism.[11]

In genetically susceptible individuals, cigarette smoke initially activates epithelial cells and alveolar macrophages in peripheral airways (bronchioles) and lung parenchyma.[11] Neutrophil chemotactic factors, including interleukin 9 (IL-9) and leukotriene B$_4$, are released, and cytotoxic CD8+ T cells and neutrophils are recruited. This leads to a buildup of proteinases such as neutrophil elastase, cathepsins, proteinase 3, matrix metalloproteinases (MMPs), and others. Concurrently, antiproteases such as α_1-antitrypsin, secretory leukoprotease inhibitor, elafin, and tissue inhibitors of MMP (TIMP-1, TIMP-2, TIMP-3) are not produced in sufficient amounts to counteract the proteinases, resulting imbalance of protease-antiprotease. This imbalance is believed to lead to the two main pathologic lesions observed: mucus hypersecretion (bronchitis) and alveolar wall destruction (emphysema). Interdependently, the same inflammatory cells and cigarette smoke stimulate the production of reactive oxygen species such as superoxide anion (O_2^-), hydrogen peroxide (H_2O_2), hydroxyl radial (OH^-), and peroxynitrite ($ONOO^-$). This increased oxidative stress is believed to produce many of the features of COPD, including lowering levels of antiproteases, increasing mucus secretion, leaking plasma to the surrounding tissue, direct bronchoconstriction, stimulating production of isoprostanes (which, in turn, causes more plasma leak and bronchoconstriction), and activation of nuclear factor κB, which leads to the release of IL-8 and tumor necrosis factor α (TNF-α). TNF-α, in turn, may play an important role in amplifying the effects of cytokines and neutrophil recruitment, perpetuating the inflammatory process.

Patients during the early stages of COPD have mild airway inflammation, mild airflow obstruction, and mild hypoxemia. As the disease progresses, however, two clinical patterns emerge. At one end of the spectrum is a group of patients with a predominantly bronchitis pattern. These patients tend to respond to airway inflammation and higher resistive load by limiting their minute ventilation. This hypoalveolar ventilation leads to hypercapnia, hypoxia, and hypoxemia, with the latter exacerbated by ventilation-perfusion ($\dot{V}/\dot{Q}$) mismatch. The ventilatory drive in response to hypoxemia and hypercapnia is also blunted. As a result, these patients develop pulmonary vasoconstriction and pulmonary arterial hypertension (from chronic hypoxia), acidosis (from hypercapnia), secondary polycythemia (from chronic hypoxemia), right ventricular hypertrophy, cor pulmonale and its associated stigmata (leg edema, hepatic congestion, elevated jugular venous distension). Clinically, these patients present with dyspnea and productive cough as primary symptoms. This group of patients looks overweight, cyanotic, and edematous and bears the clinical rubric of "blue bloater."[12]

At the other end of the spectrum is a group of patients who have emphysema as the primary lung disorder. These patients have relatively little airway disease, and the airflow limitation is related primarily to destructive changes in lung parenchyma. Both expiratory driving pressure and cross-sectional area available for flow are decreased due to reduced lung recoil, augmented dynamic compression, and increased airway collapsibility. Since destruction of alveolar walls also leads to destruction of alveolar pulmonary capillaries bed, ventilation-perfusion is relatively preserved. Shunt hypoxemia is unusual. In contrast to the patients with bronchitis, these patients tend to have enhanced ventilatory drive in response to hypoxemia and hypercapnia. As a result, emphysematous patients tend to have only mild to moderate hypoxemia ($Po_2 > 65$ mmHg) and usually normocapnea. Reactive erythrocytosis consequently does not develop, pulmonary arterial vasoconstriction is minimal, pulmonary hypertension is mild, and cor pulmonale develops only infrequently. Apart from these cardiovascular changes, diffusing capacity for carbon dioxide is reduced (due to the lung destruction). Clinically, these patients present with dyspnea as the primary symptom. This group of patients looks thin, even cachectic, barreled-chested from loss of lung recoil, and noncyanotic and bears the clinical rubric of "pink puffer."[12]

CLINICAL FEATURES

Most COPD patients have the disease diagnosis established by the time they present to the ED for COPD exacerbations. Patients commonly have a prolonged history of cigarette smoking, usually exceeding one pack per day for more than 20 years. Dyspnea, cough, and sputum production are the usual chief complaints, although perception of dyspnea may be blunted in geriatric patients. Sputum volume is usually less than 2 oz/day and can be mucoid to purulent in appearance. Sputum volume more than 2 oz/day suggests other pulmonary disorders such as bronchiectasis. The majority of patients experience exertional dyspnea when their FEV_1 falls below 40 percent of predicted. Symptoms of dyspnea at rest, hypercapnia, and cor pulmonale become more prevalent when FEV_1 falls below 40 percent of predicted.

Physical examination may show the findings of predominantly bronchitis at one end to those of predominantly emphysema at the other end of the COPD spectrum. Most commonly, however, mixed findings of both pathophysiologic disorders are present as part of the COPD syndrome. The emphysematous patient may be thin, anxious, dyspneic, tachypneic, sitting forward, sometimes on elbows and knees, struggling for breaths ("tripod") with pursed-lip breathing and use of accessory muscles. The chest and lungs are hyperinflated on percussion. Breath sounds are diminished with faint wheezes or end-expiratory rhonchi. Cardiac examination may reveal a hypodynamic heart. The patient may have near-normal arterial blood gases (ABGs) and a pink color despite the respiratory distress.

The predominantly bronchitic patient may be overweight, edematous, cyanotic, and even irritable. Stigmata of (chronic) cor pulmonale include distended jugular veins, prominent a waves and v waves, Kussmaul's sign (distended neck vein with inspiration), parasternal or subxiphoid heave, accentuated pulmonic component of the second heart sound, an S_3 or S_4 of the right ventricle, murmur of tricuspid regurgitation or pulmonic ejection click, or even a Graham Steell murmur of pulmonic regurgitation. If acute cor pulmonale is suspected, an echocardiogram is needed to confirm the diagnosis. Echocardiographic findings consistent with acute cor pulmonale may include right ventricular dilatation, tricuspid regurgitation, septal flattening with paradoxical septal motion, and left ventricular diastolic dysfunction.[12]

Factors leading to COPD exacerbations are still poorly understood, but most are thought to be the result of infection of the tracheobronchial tree.[13] Continued smoking, medication noncompliance or medication interaction and/or error (e.g., newly prescribed β_2-blocker eye drop for glaucoma), and air pollution are other common causes. Exacerbations also can be caused by, and must be distinguished from, other potentially catastrophic causes. These include ischemic heart disease and myocardial infarction, left ventricular failure, pulmonary thromboembolism, atelectasis, traumatic chest injury, and pneumothorax.

Most of the infections are bacterial in origin or superimposed bacterial infections on viral infections. Isolates from sputum studies during COPD exacerbations showed *Haemophilus influenzae* (22 percent), *Pseudomonas aeruginosa* (15 percent), *Streptococcus pneumoniae* (10 percent), *Moraxella catarrhalis* (9 percent), and other gram-negative bacteria (7 percent) in one series.[14] Also in this study, non-potentially pathogenic microorganisms such as *H. parainfluenzae* account for 36 percent of the sputum isolates. *Chlamydia pneumoniae, Mycoplasma pneumoniae,* and viral infections are also implicated in other studies.[13,15,16]

DIAGNOSIS AND DIFFERENTIAL

Routine laboratory evaluations include a complete blood count (CBC) and chemistry with cardiac enzymes and theophyline level as clinically indicated.[17] ABGs are not needed routinely for mild COPD exacerbations but should be performed for patients in stage II or stage III COPD. Since the majority of COPD patients are carbon dioxide retainers, a Po_2 of less than 60 mmHg and a normal or alkalemic pH from respiratory alkalosis ($Pco_2 <$ 35 mmHg) actually suggest ventilatory insufficiency. Hypoxemia and subsequent respiratory acidosis strongly suggest impending acute respiratory failure from respiratory muscle fatigue. Ventilatory support may be urgently needed in these patients. The decision to initiate invasive airway support is based on the overall clinical assessment of the patient and not the ABGs. Traditionally, however, acute hypoxemic respiratory failure (type I ARF) is defined as an arterial oxygen tension (Po_2) of less than 60 mmHg and acute hypercapnic respiratory failure (type II ARF) if the arterial carbon dioxide tension (Pco_2) is greater than 50 mmHg.

A chest radiograph and electrocardiogram (ECG) should be routine as part of the evaluation of COPD exacerbation.[17] Changes of COPD on chest films include hyperlucency and hyperinflation of the lungs, paucity of vascular and parenchymal markings in the upper lobes, flattened diaphragm, increased retrosternal and retrocardiac airspace, and a small, elongated cardiac silhouette. Radiolucencies (>1 cm) surrounded by radiopaque lines suggest bullae and blebs, diagnostic features of emphysema. Prominent or "plump" pulmonary arteries in the hila with rapid tapering to narrow segmental arteries suggest pulmonary hypertension. Most important, chest films may reveal catastrophic causes of exacerbation such as infiltrate, pneumothorax, effusion, pulmonary edema, atelectasis, or nodular diseases. If pneumonia is confirmed on chest x-ray, sputum studies are indicated.[17]

ECG may reveal acute changes or chronic abnormalities of COPD.[18] Acute changes include signs of cardiac ischemia, acute cor pulmonale (lead III with prominent Q wave, slight ST-segment elevation, inversion of T wave), multifocal atrial tachycardia (MAT), or signs of digitalis toxicity ("pill drop" ST-segment depression, flattened T wave, decreased QT_c interval). Changes of COPD include the effects of increased pulmonary blood flow resistance, right atrial enlargement, and right ventricular hypertrophy (P pulmonale in leads II, III, and aVF; slight ST-segment depression in leads II, III, and and aVF due to early atrial repolarization; poor R-wave progression in the precordial leads; rightward shift of the QRS axis in the frontal plane; negative Q'RS in lead I; right-axis deviation; and low QRS voltage in left precordial leads).

Differential considerations in a geriatric patient presenting with symptoms of COPD exacerbation (dyspnea, productive cough) are centered on cardiopulmonary and infectious disorders. Table 19-1 tabulates the common differential diagnoses by organ system. While geriatric patients with COPD usually have the diagnosis established by the time they come to the ED, these patients often have comorbid conditions that can make a definitive diagnosis challenging. A good history from the patient or proxy informant (in consultation with the patient's geriatrician or primary care physician supplemented by physical examination, knowledge of geriatric respiratory pathophysiology, and laboratory and radiologic studies) focusing on the most emergent causes of dyspnea, remains the best diagnostic tool available to the emergency physician.

EMERGENCY DEPARTMENT CARE AND DISPOSITION

Geriatric patients presenting with dyspnea should be triaged to the main ED for immediate medical attention. While the patient is undergoing the primary survey, stabilization steps, including bedside pulse oximetry, oxygen therapy by nasal cannula or mask, cardiac monitor, and intravenous access, should be obtained simultaneously. The primary survey should include an inspection of patient's airway for patency and assessment of the patient's level of mentation and state of ventilation. Airway support and pharmacologic intervention can be administered as clinically indicated after the primary survey.

The secondary survey covers a detailed history and physical examination, investigation of the severity of the patient's COPD, evaluation of comorbid conditions, identification of the cause of the exacerbation, and an assessment of patient's response to therapy in the ED. The ED evaluation is punctuated by an assessment of the patient's overall clinical condition for disposition. Consultation with the patient's primary care physician or geriatrician and with patient's family is crucial to ensure a seamless continuity of care, accountability, patient's and family's participation in health care, and an up-to-date assessment of risk and prognosis.

Most geriatric patients with acute COPD exacerbations need hospitalization. The few patients with mild COPD exacerbations who return to baseline, are clinically stable, and have good home support can be discharged home. These patients should be given an outpatient regimen that includes bronchodilators, antibiotics, and steroids. Bronchodilators should include an anticholinergic as the first-line medication in combination with a sympathomimetic. While anticholinergics should be taken every 4 to 6 hours, sympathomimetics can be taken as often as every 20 minutes. The preferred delivery method is a metered-dose inhaler (MDI) with a spacer. A 10-day course of steroids, usually 20 to 40 mg/day of prednisone without taper, is currently recommended by COPD authorities.[19] Antibiotics usually include a 7- to 10-day course of a first-generation macrolide, the extended-spectrum penicillins, the tetracyclines, or trimethoprim-sulfamethoxazole.[12]

Geriatric patients who are at risk for failed outpatient management should be hospitalized. Risk stratification studies have been conducted and collectively suggest the following risk factors for outpatient failures: lower pretreatment or posttreatment FEV_1, patient refractoriness to the ED therapy (manifested by increased bronchodilator and corticosteroid requirements), and previous history of outpatient failure.[6] Other risk factors include advanced age, presence of comorbid conditions, change in level of consciousness, gas-exchange disturbance, arterial blood gas deviation from baseline, and poor home support system. Patients with these features should be admitted to the hospital for further care.

Table 19-1 Common Considerations for Symptoms of COPD Exacerbations

Organ System	Examples	Comments

Airway/Lung	Asthma
	Aspiration syndrome
	Acute respiratory distress syndrome (ARDS)
	Bronchiectasis
	Infectious
	    Bacterial
	    Viral
	    Atypical
	    TB/fangal
	Neoplasm and carcinomatosis
	Pumionary embolism
		Past medical history of asthma, bronchiectasis, or COPD helpful
		Fever, productive cough, pleuritic chest pain suggest infectious

Chest wall and respiratory muscles (impaired ventilatory apparatus)	Clinical rib fracture Pneumothorax Pleural effusion Chronic pneumothorax/bullae disease Kyphoscoliosis	A history of subclinical trauma may be elicited; thoracostomy is contraindicated in chronic pneumothorax
Heart	Pulmonary edema Acute cor pulmonale Angina equivalent; acute coronary syndrome, myocardial infarction Arrhythmias Cardiac tamponade Valvular heart disease Cardiomyopathy	JVD, rales, extracardiac (or muffled) heart sounds, murmur on auscultation
Brain/nervous System	Impaired respiratory drive (stroke, brainstem infarction, hemorrhage, trauma, medication) Impaired neuromuscular system (cervical cord injury, Guillain-Barré, myasthenia gravis, organophosphate poisoning)	
Blood	Anemia Carbon monoxide poisoning	
Endocrine/others	Electrolyte abnormalities Diabetic ketoacidosis Thyroid disease Sepsis syndrome	

Pharmacologic Intervention

In the ED, pharmacologic interventions in the management of an acute COPD exacerbation are aimed at reversing the patient's respiratory symptoms, stabilizing other derangements related to hypoxemia, and obviating the need for ventilatory support. Five classes of therapeutic agents are commonly used: oxygen, bronchodilators (β_2 agonists and anticholinergics), corticosteroids, methylxanthines, and antibiotics.

Oxygen

Patients with acute COPD exacerbations who are hypoxemic should be given oxygen therapy immediately. Oxygen therapy helps restore cardiac output and improve oxygen delivery to the heart, brain, and other critical organs. Specifically, oxygen improves pulmonary vasoconstriction and right ventricular strain, cerebral hypoxemia, and any myocardial ischemia caused by hypoxemia. Since injudicious use of oxygen can lead to hypercapnia and acute respiratory failure, these patients should be monitored closely. On the other hand, oxygen therapy should never be withheld if the patient is hypoxic. Various mechanisms proposed to explain this hypercapnic respiratory failure include blunting of the hypoxia drive, increased dead space due to reduced tidal volume, deranged $\dot{V}/\dot{Q}$ mismatch, and the Haldane effect (oxygenated erythrocytes carrying less CO_2). COPD patients who present to the ED hypoxemic and acidemic are at greatest risk of developing carbon dioxide retention and acute respiratory failure on supplemental oxygen.[20] Oxygen therapy can be given via nasal canula or face mask, although preference is given to the method with titratable fractional inspiratory oxygen concentration (FIO_2). FIO_2 is titrated to keep pulse oxymetry at 90 percent or greater (PaO_2 between 60 and 65 mmHg) and pH at 7.26 or higher.[21–23] Venturi mask can be used on patients at risk for CO_2 retention.

Bronchodilators

Even though COPD is mostly an obstructive airways disease with minimal reversibility, most COPD patients will improve with a 12 to 15 percent increase in maximal expiratory flow when treated properly with bronchodilators.[24] Besides oxygen, bronchodilators are the cornerstone of drug therapy in the treatment of COPD exacerbations. Two classes of bronchodilators are available: anticholinergics and β_2 agonists (Table 19-2). Of the two, the anticholinergics are more effective than the sympathomimetics in COPD and should be the first-line drugs.[9,12] In addition to improving the FEV_1, bronchodilators also improve exercise tolerance and dyspnea by reducing hyperinflation. Nebulized anticholinergic and sympathomimetic bronchodilators can be given together every 4 to 6 hours. In addition, sympathomimetic bronchodilators can be given as often as every 20 minutes. Side effects include hypokalemia, tremor, palpitation, tachycardia, headache, nausea, and vomiting. Side effects of anticholinergics are milder and include dry mouth, urinary retention, and tremors. Pre- and post-bronchodilator peak expiratory flow should be determined.[21,25] Anticholinergics exert their bronchodilatory

Table 19-2 Bronchodilators in common use in North America

Bronchodilator	MDI Dose/puff (ug)	Nebulized Dose	Time to Onsets* (min)	Time to Peak Effect† (mn)	Duration (hr)
β_2 Agonists					
Albuterol	90	2.5 mg	5-15	10–60	1–3
Levalbuterol	–	0.63 or 1.25 mg	5–15	10–60	1–3
Metaproterenol	650	0.3 ml (5%)	5–15	60–12	3–6
Terbutaline	200	2 mg	5–30	60–12	3–6
Bitolterol	370	0.5–1 ml (0.2%)	5–10	60–90	5–8
Pirbuterol	200	–	5–10	30–60	3–5
Salmeterol†	21	–	30–60	60–180	10–14
Formotero1†	12	–	36–60	60–120	10–14
Anticholinergics					
Ipratropium	18	0.5 mg	5–30	60–120	4–8
Combination					
Albuterol-ipratropium	90/18	3 mg/0.5 mg	5–15	60–120	6–8

*Data for MDI only
†Not for acute bronchospasm.
Source: Modified with permission from Ferguson[26]

effects by blocking periganglionic muscarinic receptors (M_1) in the parasympathetic ganglion and muscarinic receptors (M_3) on airway smooth muscle. β_2 Agonists, on the other hand, effect their bronchodilation by stimulating the membrane-associated β_2 receptors on airway smooth muscle.[26]

The long-acting β_2 agonists salmeterol and formoterol have been shown to improve lung function and FEV_1 in COPD[27,28] and may help reduce infective exacerbations by reducing bacterial adhesion such as *P. aeruginosa* and *H. influenzae* to airway epithelial cells.[11,29]

In the ED, the nebulized method of delivering bronchodilators is preferred to MDI, although the two methods of delivering bronchodilators, if used properly, appear to be equally efficacious.[30]

Corticosteroids

The predominantly neutrophilic inflammatory response in COPD differs markedly from that of asthma, with differences in inflammatory cells, mediators, and response to corticosteroids. Theoretically, corticosteroids are expected to provide little benefit in the case of pure emphysema given the underlying pathophysiology of parenchymal lung destruction. They should, however, reduce airway inflammation, mucus hypersecretion, and bronchial reactivity in chronic and asthmatic bronchitis. Studies have shown that systemic (intravenous and oral) administration of corticosteroids reduces length of hospitalization (by 1 to 2 days) and improves clinical outcome (e.g., improves FEV_1 by 100 mL, reduces treatment rate by 10 percent) in acute COPD exacerbations.[31,32] For acute COPD exacerbations that may require hospitalization, an initial dose of 125 mg intravenously of methylprednisolone is adequate. A 10-day course of 20 to 40 mg prednisone is appropriate for outpatient management.

Inhaled corticosteroids are recommended for those with moderate to severe COPD and for patients with frequent exacerbations.[33] They are widely prescribed for chronic COPD in North America.[11] In a recent study, inhaled triamcinolone improved respiratory symptoms, decreased the number of exacerbations, and decreased the use of health care resources in patients with COPD.[34] It did not, however, slow the rate of decline in pulmonary function, as measured by FEV_1. Other smaller studies produce more contradictory results. In one study, COPD patients on inhaled fluticasone (500 μg twice daily) had a small increase in FEV_1, fewer exacerbations, and a slower decline in health status.[35] In another study, inhaled budesonide (800 mg twice daily for 2 weeks) and oral prednisolone (30 mg daily for 2 weeks) provided no clinical benefit in either lung function or symptom scores and no significant change in the inflammatory indices.[36]

Methylxanthines

Methylxanthines deserve special attention mostly because of their historical role. In fact, theophylline (and caffeine) has been used to treat respiratory illness and COPD for decades. In its peak, theophylline was used in 63.4 percent of COPD patients in 1987 but has fallen out of favor in the recent years, down to 29 percent in 1995.[37] The main reason for this decline is the persistent controversy about its risk-benefit ratio.[38] Theophylline is a phosphodiesterase (PDE) inhibitor and was thought to possess bronchodilatory effects via cAMP-induced smooth muscle relaxation. This mechanism was later deemed untenuous at the usual pharmacologic dosages. Recent proposed mechanisms suggest that theophylline exerts its bronchodilatory effects via selective inhibition of specific PDE receptors (type III and IV) present on specific cells in the airway. Blockade of these receptors is believed to lead ultimately to bronchodilation.[26] In addition to its bronchodilatory effects, theophylline is also thought to improve peripheral ventilation, diaphragm function, exercise tolerance, pulmonary vasoconstriction, gas trapping, and dyspnea.[26] Latest guidelines from the ATS and leading authors on COPD still recommend that theophylline be used as a second-line medication if response to anticholinergics and B_2 agonists is inadequate.[17,26] In fact, more than one-third of patients report symptomatic improvement when theophylline is added to high-dose combination of inhaled salbutamol and ipratropium bromide.[39] Downsides of theophylline include narrow therapeutic range, arrhythmias, tremor, gastrointestinal disorders, interactions with other medications (Dilantin, erythromycin, etc.), and seizures, which can occur in the elderly at blood levels as low as 14 mg/L.[40]

Antibiotics

Since approximately half of COPD exacerbations are precipitated by bacterial infection of the tracheobronchial tree, a 7- to 10-day course of antibiotics benefits patients with acute COPD exacerbations.[6,13] Antibiotics seem to reduce the severity of lung deterioration and the duration of the exacerbation. Patients in stage I COPD ($FEV_1 \geq 50$ percent of predicted) can be treated empirically with a first-generation macrolide, amoxicillin, ampicillin, tetracycline, or trimethoprim-sulfamethoxazole.[12] Patients in stage II and III COPD ($FEV_1 < 50$ percent of predicted), who are older, or who have comorbid conditions harbor resistant pathogens. Broad-spectrum antibiotics such as a second-generation macrolide, second-generation cephalosporin, quinolones, or β-lactam with β-lactamase inhibitor are indicated for these high-risk patients.

Ventilatory Support

Not uncommonly, COPD patients who show signs and symptoms of acute respiratory failure (ARF, type I or type II) or who deteriorate clinically despite maximal pharmacologic support are candidates for positive ventilatory support. Positive-pressure ventilation can be provided noninvasively via facial or nasal mask or invasively via either nasal or oral intubation of the trachea.[41] Regardless of the means, the goals of mechanical ventilation are (1) to restore potentially life-threatening blood gas abnormalities and (2) to provide support for the tiring respiratory muscles, allowing them to rest and recover from fatigue. Absolute indications for tracheal intubation include cardiorespiratory arrest, inability to protect the airway, and failure of noninvasive positive-pressure ventilation. Relative indications for tracheal intubation include impaired mental status or patient at risk of aspiration from a variety of sources, including excessive secretions.

Noninvasive positive-pressure ventilation (NPPV) is the method of choice for ventilatory support because it reduces the need for endotracheal intubation (26 versus 74 percent in one series), length of the hospital stay, and in-hospital mortality rate.[42] Patients who have excessive secretions, altered mental status, or hemodynamic compromise are not good candidates for NPPV. A fractional inspired oxygen (FIO_2) of 24 to 40 percent should be adequate to keep pulse oxymetry at 90 percent or greater. Pressure support can be set at 10 to 20 cmH_2O and adjusted to achieve the desired clinical parameters (patient tolerance and comfort, pH $\geq$ 7.26). For example, an expired tidal volume of 5 to 7 mL/kg is well tolerated and safe and yet provides good patient comfort. Positive end-expiratory pressure (PEEP) can be set at 5 to 10 cmH_2O.

Endotracheal intubation (ET) may become necessary when conservative measures fail. Oral ET is preferred to nasal ET due to risks of sinusitis,[43] increased airway resistance, and reduced drug delivery associated with the latter.[23] Ventilator settings should aim to minimize dynamic hyperinflation (stacking) due to expiratory airflow obstruction and maximize respiratory muscle rest. Typical settings include tidal volumes of 8 to 10 mL/kg and respiration rates to keep pH at 7.26 or higher, avoiding the "normal" PCO_2. Again, an FIO_2 of 24 to 40 percent should be adequate to keep the pulse oxymetry at 90 per-

cent or greater and PO_2 at 60 to 65 mmHg. A detailed discussion of mechanical ventilation in COPD is beyond the scope of this chapter, and readers are referred elsewhere for more detail on the subject.[23]

Special Management Principles

Mucus hypersecretion and production is pathophysiologically important in the clinical manifestation of COPD. Routine medications that increase viscosity and impede mucus clearance—antihistamines, cough suppressants, and decongestants—therefore should be used with caution in COPD patients.[26] Expectorants, mucolytics, and mucokinetic agents (e.g., guaifenesin, oral iodide, domiodol, bromhexine, ambroxol, oral hydration, inhaled hypertonic saline, S-carboxymethylcysteine, N-acetylcysteine) as mucus-clearance strategies might improve symptoms of acute COPD exacerbations but have not been found to shorten the course of treatment.[6] Similarly, chest percussion as part of physical and respiratory therapies generally is ineffective and may even be harmful.[6]

Combining anticholinergic and β₂-agonist bronchodilators at standard doses has been shown to be superior to either agent alone[44] and to have fewer side effects associated with higher doses of either agent. Adding theophylline to a combination of anticholinergic and β₂-agonist bronchodilators can be beneficial.[45]

Dyspnea, anxiety, depression, and insomnia can be disabling but often are overlooked and unrecognized in the overall treatment of patients with COPD.[26] Opiates have been used successfully with careful monitoring to treat dyspnea in COPD. Serotonin selective reuptake inhibitors (SSRIs) are preferred to tricyclic antidepressants (TCAs) for the treatment of depression and anxiety. Hypnotic agents should be prescribed only after careful investigation of the cause of the insomnia.

Of interest, antioxidant vitamins may have a marginal role in improving symptomatology of patients with chronic bronchitis. Respiratory stimulants and respiratory muscle relaxants are of no proven benefits.[26]

Prevention

A cigarette smoke-induced inflammatory process underlies the pathogenesis and clinical progression of COPD. The disease burden of COPD on patients and health care resources can only be reduced with smoking cessation. It is a sobering fact that the inflammation and tissue destruction in COPD are irreversible and relentlessly progressive. Except for long-term administration of supplemental oxygen, no treatments are proven to favorably alter the course of COPD progression. As shown by Fletcher (Fig. 19-1) and others,[8,46] smoking cessation, even in the geriatric population, slows the progression of the disease to those of their nonsmoker cohorts and can be the most important intervention administered by the emergency physician.

COPD exacerbations also can be reduced by annual vaccinations against influenza, pneumococcus, and *H. influenzae.* Patients should be educated about medication compliance and should be referred for pulmonary rehabilitation and follow-up with a pulmonologist or geriatrician.

ADDITIONAL ASPECTS

The following are common pitfalls in the management of COPD:

- Failure to recognize that COPD, different from asthma, is minimally reversible
- Failure to recognize that a "normal" blood gas may signal ventilatory insufficiency
- Failure to adequately correct hypoxemia in the older patient with comorbid cardiovascular conditions
- Failure to recognize the risks of hypercapnic respiratory failure via injudicious administration of oxygen
- Failure to rule out potentially catastrophic causes of acute dyspnea
- Failure to incorporate input from patient's geriatrist and patient's family in the final disposition

REFERENCES

1. Petty TL, Weinmann GG: Building a national strategy for the prevention and management of and research in chronic obstructive pulmonary disease. National Heart, Lung, and Blood Institute Workshop Summary. Bethesda, Maryland, August 29–31, 1995. *JAMA* 277:246, 1997.
2. Seemungal TA, Donaldson GC, Bhowmik A, et al: Time course and recovery of exacerbations in patients with chronic obstructive pulmonary disease. *Am J Respir Crit Care Med* 161:1608, 2000.
3. Seneff MG, Wagner DP, Wagner RP, et al: Hospital and 1-year survival of patients admitted to intensive care units with acute exacerbation of chronic obstructive pulmonary disease. *JAMA* 274:1852, 1995.
4. Connors AF Jr, Dawson NV, Thomas C, et al: Outcomes following acute exacerbation of severe chronic obstructive lung disease. The SUPPORT investigators (Study to Un-

derstand Prognoses and Preferences for Outcomes and Risks of Treatments). *Am J Respir Crit Care Med* 154:959, 1996.
5. Adair N: Chronic airflow obstruction and respiratory failure in Hazzard WR, Blass JP, Ettinger WH Jr, et al (eds): *Principles of Geriatric Medicine and Gerontology.* New York, McGraw-Hill, 1999, p 745.
6. McCrory DC, Brown C, Gelfand SE, et al: Management of acute exacerbations of COPD: A summary and appraisal of published evidence. *Chest* 119:1190, 2001.
7. Monthly Report: *Monthly Vital Statistics Report, 1979–1998.* Hyattsville, MD, National Center for Health Statistics, 1998.
8. Fletcher C, Peto R: The natural history of chronic airflow obstruction. *Br Med J* 1:1645, 1977.
9. American Thoracic Society: Standards for the diagnosis and care of patients with chronic obstructive pulmonary disease. *Am J Respir Crit Care Med* 152:S77, 1995.
10. Anto JM, Vermeire P, Vestbo J, et al: Epidemiology of chronic obstructive pulmonary disease. *Eur Respir J* 17:982, 2001.
11. Barnes PJ: Chronic obstructive pulmonary disease. *New Engl J Med* 343:269, 2000.
12. Staton GW, Ingram RH: Chronic obstructive diseases of the lung, in Dale DC, Federman DG (eds): *Web MD: Scientific American Medicine.* 2001.
13. Sethi S, Murphy TF: Bacterial infection in chronic obstructive pulmonary disease in 2000: A state-of-the-art review. *Clin Microbiol Rev* 14:336, 2001.
14. Miravitles M, Espinosa C, Fernandez-Laso E, et al: Relationship between bacterial flora in sputum and functional impairment in patients with acute exacerbations of COPD. Study Group of Bacterial Infection in COPD. *Chest* 116:40, 1999.
15. Beaty CD, Grayston JT, Wang SP, et al: *Chlamydia pneumoniae,* strain TWAR, infection in patients with chronic obstructive pulmonary disease. *Am Rev Respir Dis* 144:1408, 1991.
16. Seemungal T, Harper-Owen R, Bhowmik A, et al: Respiratory viruses, symptoms, and inflammatory markers in acute exacerbations and stable chronic obstructive pulmonary disease. *Am J Respir Crit Care Med* 164:1618, 2001.
17. Ferguson GT: Recommendations for the management of COPD. *Chest* 117:23S, 2000.
18. Wagner GS: Miscellaneous conditions, in Wagner GS (ed): *Marriott's Practical Electrocardiography,* 9th Ed. ed. Baltimore, Williams & Wilkins, 1994; p 174.
19. Honig EG, Ingram RH: Chronic bronchitis, emphysema, and airways obstruction, in Braunwald E, Fauci AS, Kasper DL, et al (eds): *Harrison's Principles of Internal Medicine,* 15th ed. New York, McGraw-Hill, 2001, p 1491.
20. Bone RC, Pierce AK, Johnson RL Jr: Controlled oxygen administration in acute respiratory failure in chronic obstructive pulmonary disease: A reappraisal. *Am J Med* 65:896, 1978.
21. The COPD Guidelines Group of the Standards of Care Com-

mittee of the BTS: BTS guidelines for the management of chronic obstructive pulmonary disease. *Thorax* 52(suppl 5):S1, 1997.

22. Stoller JK, Lange PA: Inpatient management of chronic obstructive pulmonary disease. *Respir Care Clin North Am* 4:425, 1998.

23. Hill NS: Noninvasive ventilation in chronic obstructive pulmonary disease. *Clin Chest Med* 21:783, 2000.

24. Dorinsky PM, Reisner C, Ferguson GT, et al: The combination of ipratropium and albuterol optimizes pulmonary function reversibility testing in patients with COPD. *Chest* 115:966, 1999.

25. Siafakas NM, Vermeire P, Pride NB, et al: Optimal assessment and management of chronic obstructive pulmonary disease (COPD). The European Respiratory Society Task Force. *Eur Respir J* 8:1398, 1995.

26. Ferguson GT: Update on pharmacologic therapy for chronic obstructive pulmonary disease. *Clin Chest Med* 21:723, 2000.

27. Mahler DA, Donohue JF, Barbee RA, et al: Efficacy of salmeterol xinafoate in the treatment of COPD. *Chest* 115:957, 1999.

28. Maesen BL, Westermann CJ, Duurkens VA, et al: Effects of formoterol in apparently poorly reversible chronic obstructive pulmonary disease. *Eur Respir J* 13:1103, 1999.

29. Dowling RB, Johnson M, Cole PJ, et al: Effect of salmeterol on *Haemophilus influenzae* infection of respiratory mucosa in vitro. *Eur Respir J* 11:86, 1998.

30. Turner MO, Patel A, Ginsburg S, et al: Bronchodilator delivery in acute airflow obstruction: A meta-analysis. *Arch Intern Med* 157:1736, 1997.

31. Niewoehner DE, Erbland ML, Deupree RH, et al: Effect of systemic glucocorticoids on exacerbations of chronic obstructive pulmonary disease. Department of Veterans Affairs Cooperative Study Group. *New Engl J Med* 340:1941, 1999.

32. Davies L, Angus RM, Calverley PM: Oral corticosteroids in patients admitted to hospital with exacerbations of chronic obstructive pulmonary disease: A prospective randomised controlled trial. *Lancet* 354:456, 1999.

33. Mapp CE: Inhaled glucocorticoids in chronic obstructive pulmonary disease. *New Engl J Med* 343:1960, 2000.

34. The Lung Health Study Research Group: Effect of inhaled triamcinolone on the decline in pulmonary function in chronic obstructive pulmonary disease. *New Engl J Med* 343:1902, 2000.

35. Burge PS, Calverley PM, Jones PW, et al: Randomised, double-blind, placebo-controlled study of fluticasone propionate in patients with moderate to severe chronic obstructive pulmonary disease: The ISOLDE trial. *Br Med J* 320:1297, 2000.

36. Keatings VM, Jatakanon A, Worsdell YM, et al: Effects of inhaled and oral glucocorticoids on inflammatory indices in asthma and COPD. *Am J Respir Crit Care Med* 155:542, 1997.

37. Van Andel AE, Reisner C, Menjoge SS, et al: Analysis of inhaled corticosteroid and oral theophylline use among patients with stable COPD from 1987 to 1995. *Chest* 115:703, 1999.

38. Barr RG, Rowe BH, Camargo CA Jr: Methyl-xanthines for exacerbations of chronic obstructive pulmonary disease. *Cochrane Database Syst Rev* 1:CD002168, 2001.

39. Nishimura K, Koyama H, Ikeda A, et al: The additive effect of theophylline on a high-dose combination of inhaled salbutamol and ipratropium bromide in stable COPD. *Chest* 107:718, 1995.

40. Shannon M: Life-threatening events after theophylline overdose: A 10-year prospective analysis. *Arch Intern Med* 159:989, 1999.

41. Sethi JM, Siegel MD: Mechanical ventilation in chronic obstructive lung disease. *Clin Chest Med* 21:799, 2000.

42. Brochard L, Mancebo J, Wysocki M, et al: Noninvasive ventilation for acute exacerbations of chronic obstructive pulmonary disease. *New Engl J Med* 333:817, 1995.

43. Michelson A, Schuster B, Kamp HD: Paranasal sinusitis associated with nasotracheal and orotracheal long-term intubation. *Arch Otolaryngol Head Neck Surg* 118:937, 1992.

44. The COMBIVENT Inhalation Solution Study Group: Routine nebulized ipratropium and albuterol together are better than either alone in COPD. *Chest* 112:1514, 1997.

45. Karpel JP, Kotch A, Zinny M, et al: A comparison of inhaled ipratropium, oral theophylline plus inhaled beta-agonist, and the combination of all three in patients with COPD. *Chest* 105:1089, 1994.

46. Anthonisen NR, Connett JE, Kiley JP, et al: Effects of smoking intervention and the use of an inhaled anticholinergic bronchodilator on the rate of decline of FEV_1. The Lung Health Study. *JAMA* 272:1497, 1994.

20

Pulmonary Embolism

Janet Poponick

HIGH-YIELD FACTS

- The incidence of venous thromboembolism, including pulmonary embolism (PE), is significantly increased in persons over 65 years of age and increases again (twofold higher) in those over 85 years of age.
- Major risk factors for PE include increased age, major joint replacement surgery, trauma, malignancy, and recent travel history.
- Ventilation-perfusion scans are a primary screening tool for PE; however, diagnostic yield decreases with age (from approximately 70 percent in younger patients to approximately 40 percent in the oldest patients).
- Anticoagulation therapy, unless contraindicated, should be initiated in the emergency department (ED) using weight-based dosing protocols for unfractionated or low-molecular-weight heparin in patients with moderate to high clinical suspicion for PE.

Venous thromboembolism (VTE) is a common disease affecting over 2 million people each year.[1] With an incidence in the United States of 1 in 1000,[2] VTE may present as deep venous thrombosis (DVT), which is the more common presentation, or pulmonary embolism (PE). There are approximately 600,000 patients each year who develop PE and 60,000 deaths due to this disease.[1] Unfortunately, these statistics have not changed in three decades despite aggressive diagnostic evaluations, evidence-based treatment protocols, and improved prophylaxis.

The incidence of VTE increases with age, and PE represents an increasing proportion of total cases of VTE. Among those aged 65 to 69 years, the annual incidence of PE is approximately 1.3 per 1000 and that of DVT is approximately 1.8 per 1000.[3] These rates are twice as great in persons aged 85 to 89 years. Age alone is an important risk factor for VTE, but comorbid conditions also

increase the risk. Immobilization due to chronic illness or due to an acute medical condition requiring hospitalization will greatly increase the risk of VTE in this population.

Therefore, it is important to recognize patients who are at risk of VTE in their emergency department (ED) presentation and initiate an appropriate evaluation and treatment plan. In the elderly patient, differentiating PE from exacerbations of underlying disease is essential. Also, instituting prophylaxis against VTE becomes important to improving overall survival of the elderly patient.

EPIDEMIOLOGY

While this chapter primarily will discuss PE, it is important to recognize that PE and DVT are manifestations of the same disease process, venous thromboembolism (VTE). Of patients diagnosed with DVT, approximately 30 percent develop symptomatic PE. Asymptomatic PE occurs in 40 to 60 percent of patients with diagnosed DVT. Conversely, 80 percent of those with documented PE also will have DVT. Therefore, DVT and PE often will be seen together, and patients should be evaluated with this in mind.[4]

In one long-term (10 years) study of hospitalized elderly patients, survival rates declined with advancing age. In this study, the diagnosis of PE was divided into those with PE as the primary diagnosis and those with PE as a secondary diagnosis with other comorbid conditions listed. The overall median survival time for a primary diagnosis of PE was approximately 5 years (rates for 1, 5 and 10 years were 70, 50, and 36 percent, respectively). For those with a secondary diagnosis of PE, the median survival time was l year (1-, 5-, and 10-year survival rates were 50, 34, and 25 percent, respectively).[5] Therefore, a PE in the elderly patient with a serious underlying condition results in a higher mortality risk. The major comorbid conditions included congestive heart failure, chronic obstructive pulmonary disease (COPD), cancer, stroke, and myocardial infarction. As the number of comorbidities increases, this risk of mortality increases for all elderly patients with PE.

PATHOPHYSIOLOGY

PE occurs when thrombus embolizes to the pulmonary circulation. This embolus travels from a distant site, usually from the veins of the legs, but also may arise in the pelvic veins, inferior vena cava, or the veins of the arms.[1]

A thrombus originates as a local fibrin-platelet-red blood cell aggregate that breaks off and travels to the pulmonary circulation causing obstruction of a portion of the pulmonary vasculature. This aggregate, or thrombus, causes endothelial damage and changes in the clotting system that may increase the size of the clot.

Major risk factors for VTE include increased age, venous stasis from any cause, and any type of trauma, including childbirth and hypercoagulable states[1] (Table 20-1). Inherited deficiencies of antithrombin, protein C, and protein S have been recognized for years. Factor V(Leiden) is a point mutation on factor V in which an Arg is substituted for Gln, causing coagulation factor resistance to degradation by protein C. This is the most common cause of thrombophilia, having been identified in 50 percent of those with recurrent VTE. Those who have this mutation have a twofold increased risk of VTE,[6] and the risk of recurrence is 40 percent over 8 years. Prothrombin mutation has been recognized recently as another inherited cause of thrombophilia. This mutation causes higher plasma prothrombin levels and is associated with an increased risk to form thrombi through amplification of the coagulation system. The mutation occurs in 2 to 4 percent of the general population.[6] Those with the mutation have a two- to fourfold increased risk of VTE.

Table 20-1. Risks for VTE

Inherited
Antithrombin deficiency
Proteins C and S deficiency
Factor V Leiden
Prothrombin mutation

Acquired
Age
Surgery and major trauma
Pregnancy
Oral contraceptives/hormone-replacement therapy
Prolong immobilization
    Bed rest
    Paralysis
    Travel

Medical illnesses
History VTE
Obesity
Stroke
Chronic lung disease
Congestive heart failure
Malignancy
Serious infections

Transient risks of VTE include pregnancy, hormone-replacement therapy, and prolonged immobilization.[6] Surgery is a very common and well-recognized transient risk factor, especially orthopedic and neurosurgical procedures. Without prophylaxis, 45 to 70 percent of patients develop DVT after total knee or hip replacement surgery. Major trauma, especially involving the head, the spinal cord, or the pelvis, is often complicated by VTE. PE is the third most common cause of death in trauma patients who survive 24 hours. Almost 60 percent of major trauma patients will develop a DVT.[6]

Travel by any means for greater than 4 hours duration is associated with an increased risk for VTE, even in patients without significant risk factors. Unfortunately, most studies related to travel are small in numbers or are poorly documented cases. Recently, a study from France examined patients arriving at the airport and requiring transport to the hospital.[7] Of the 170 people transported, 56 (33 percent) were found to have PE. Only 4 of the 56 confirmed cases were considered to be at high risk for PE due to other medical problems or recent surgery. The risk is higher for those who traveled more than 6 hours or greater than 5000 km. With air travel being the most common means of travel, the *economy-class syndrome* has become a popular term for travel-related VTE. Immobility from prolonged sitting in areas of limited space are assumed to be the risk.

Malignancy is a well-recognized risk factor for VTE. All forms of cancer predispose a patient to thromboembolic disease; however, adenocarcinoma of the visceral organs is the most commonly recognized malignancy. Idiopathic VTE may be the first sign of an underlying malignance; such individuals have a 10 to 20 percent chance of developing cancer over a 2-year period.[6,8]

Various medical conditions add to the risk of VTE, especially in the hospitalized patient. Immobilization prior to admission or during hospitalization for another medical problem places patients at risk. Congestive heart failure, COPD, and stroke are among the top comorbid conditions associated with the risk of VTE.[5]

CLINICAL FEATURES

PE symptoms are often indistinguishable from other life-threatening disorders of the cardiorespiratory system (Table 20-2). The presentation of PE is nonspecific, and symptoms may include dyspnea, anxiety, pleuritic chest pain, and hemoptysis. Sudden onset of symptoms should raise suspicion, especially in those with known risk factors. Tachypnea remains the most common sign of PE,

Table 20-2. Differential Diagnosis of PE

Acute myocardial infarction
Aortic dissection
Musculoskeletal disorders
    Chest contusion
    Costochondritis
    Rib fracture
Obstructive pulmonary disease (including asthma)
Pericardial disease
Pneumonia
Pneumothorax

occurring in 70 percent of patients, whereas tachycardia occurs in only one-third of patients.[9] Syncope, sudden hypotension, or sudden death are signs of massive PE but also may be attributed to cardiac tamponade, aortic dissection, or acute myocardial infarction.[9]

DIAGNOSIS AND DIFFERENTIAL

The history, physical examination, and risk assessment are the most important steps in the evaluation of a patient with suspected PE. In the PIOPED study,[10] clinical assessment for the likelihood of disease was important in the process of evaluating the patient. Recently, a clinical model of probability of disease has been proposed that stresses assessment of the patient for other causes of the signs and symptoms.[11] Simple tests such as chest x-ray, electrocardiogram, and arterial blood gas determination are the next step in the evaluation process to exclude other diagnoses (see Table 20-2).

The chest x-ray is helpful in excluding the diagnoses of pneumonia and pneumothorax. The patient with PE may demonstrate atelectasis, an elevated hemidiaphragm, or pleural effusion on chest x-ray. These findings are nonspecific and do not make a diagnosis of PE. The classic findings of Hampton's hump or Westermark sign (decreased vascularity) are seen infrequently. The chest x-ray may even be normal. Such a finding in a patient without underlying cardiopulmonary findings presenting with chest pain, dyspnea, and hypoxemia makes PE more likely.

The electrocardiogram (ECG) is nonspecific and cannot make the diagnosis of PE. However, the ECG remains useful in diagnosing or excluding acute myocardial infarction or acute pericarditis. Sinus tachycardia is the most frequent ECG finding in PE. Other findings may include nonspecific ST-T wave changes, left- or right-axis

deviation, and rarely, signs of acute cor pulmonale with a $S_1Q_3T_3$ pattern, right bundle-branch block, P-wave pulmonale, or right-axis deviation.[9]

The arterial blood gas (ABG) determination is another nonspecific test. The findings of hypoxemia, hypocarbia, and an elevated alveolar-arteriolar gradient raise the suspicion of PE but also can be seen in pneumonia. In young, healthy patients, the ABGs may be entirely normal; in fact, 20 percent of those with proven PE had normal ABGs. A pitfall in using ABG determination is relying too heavily on finding abnormalities. The other pitfall is the patient with COPD who is hypoxic with a normal carbon dioxide tension. This blood gas could be the patient's baseline ABG, or the "normal" P_{CO_2} actually may represent new hyperventilation suggestive of PE. Comparing the ABG with baseline status is mandatory in the evaluation of COPD patients. Furthermore, the arterial blood oxygen tension (Pa_{O_2}) decreases predictably with physiologic age-associated changes alone. The average decline can be estimated with the following equation: $Pa_{O_2} = 109 - 0.43 \times age$ (years).

The next step in making the diagnosis of PE is arriving at a pretest clinical probability of disease (Table 20-3). In most patients, clinical evaluation along with the simple tests noted above will exclude other possibilities, and the emergency physician can arrive at a reasonable clinical likelihood of PE. Unfortunately, arriving at the final diagnosis is still a challenge because no one test is available to exclude PE with complete certainty.

The "gold standard" for the diagnosis of PE remains pulmonary angiogram. However, the test is invasive and costly and has been associated with contrast reactions, re-

Table 20-3. Predicting Pretest Probability for PE

Clinical Features	Score*
Clinical signs and symptoms of DVT	3.0
Heart rate > 100 beats/min	1.5
Immobilization (for ≥3 consecutive days)	1.5
Surgery in the previous 4 weeks	1.5
Previous diagnosis of DVT or PE	1.5
Hemoptysis	1.0
Cancer (treatment ongoing or within 6 months, or palliative)	1.0
PE as likely or more likely than another diagnosis	3.0

*Analysis: High-probability score >6.0; moderate, 2–6.0; low, <2.0.

Source: Used with permission from Wells et al.[13]

nal failure, and death in 0.2 to 0.5 percent of patients.[10] Unfortunately, the elderly patient already may have some degree of renal insufficiency, and a contrast study is not the best option at this time in the evaluation.

Several noninvasive studies are available to aid the physician. Again, no single noninvasive study reliably excludes PE; therefore, combinations of noninvasive testing and clinical suspicion are used to evaluate the patient with suspected VTE.

Ventilation-Perfusion ($\dot{V}/\dot{Q}$) Scan

A nuclear medicine study or $\dot{V}/\dot{Q}$ scan is the primary screening tool for patients with suspected PE.[3,9,10] An advantage is that it is simple for the patient to perform. The test has been used for decades, and many radiologists have considerable experience with interpretation. The most important study documenting the utility of $\dot{V}/\dot{Q}$ scanning is the PIOPED study.[10] In that study, 98 percent of those with PE had an abnormality on the $\dot{V}/\dot{Q}$ study. However, specificity is poor, with 72 percent of the study population having nondiagnostic studies. Among patients with angiographic documentation of PE, only 41 percent had a high-probability scan, and 16 percent had a low-probability scan.[10]

The final interpretation of the $\dot{V}/\dot{Q}$ scan may be normal or near-normal, high-probability, or nondiagnostic. Normal studies or high-probability studies, along with clinical assessment, help the clinician decide on management. It is agreed that a normal or near-normal scan excludes PE, and a high-probability scan is sufficient for diagnosis and treatment of PE. The large group with nondiagnostic studies (50 percent of all $\dot{V}/\dot{Q}$ scans) is more challenging and will require further testing. If angiography were performed on all patients with nondiagnostic scans, only 25 percent would be diagnosed with PE.[10,11]

In the elderly population, more $\dot{V}/\dot{Q}$ scans are read as nondiagnostic or high probability. Those with normal or near-normal studies generally were younger patients (61 percent in those younger than 40 years, 11 percent in those 80 years of age or younger). The diagnostic yield of $\dot{V}/\dot{Q}$ scans decreases with age (68 percent in the youngest to 42 percent in the oldest age groups).[3]

Venous Ultrasonography

For those with a nondiagnostic $\dot{V}/\dot{Q}$ scan, bilateral ultrasound of the legs is performed.[3] Compression ultrasonography of the common femoral vein and popliteal vein is highly sensitive (95 percent) and specific (96 per-

cent) for proximal venous thrombosis in the popliteal vein or more proximally. A noncompressible segment of vein will accurately diagnose DVT.[12] If the ultrasound is normal, pretest clinical probability is used to decide on further testing. The high clinical pretext probability group would require angiography. With low clinical probability and normal ultrasound of the legs, PE generally can be excluded from the diagnosis. The moderate-probability group should be further elevated with serial ultrasound or angiography or even helical computed tomography (CT).[11,13]

D-Dimer

This is a noninvasive blood test measuring fibrin degradation products. The test is useful as an adjunct to the diagnosis of VTE; however, it may be a better test for the diagnosis of PE due to the higher load of fibrin products. The test is performed by different methods at different institutions: latex agglutination (least sensitive), enzyme-linked immunosorbent assay (ELISA) techniques, and new rapid methods.[13,14] Unfortunately, different techniques have been used in the literature, which makes it difficult to compare study results.

When using ELISA methods, the test is highly sensitive (99 percent) for VTE when the cutoff value is 500 μg/L. A lower value essentially excludes VTE and has been used recently to avoid further testing in patients with low clinical suspicion.[13,14] However, ELISA testing is labor-intensive and takes time to obtain results. Furthermore, an elevated D-dimer is not very specific for PE. Conditions that may cause an elevated D-dimer include cancer, inflammation, infection and older age due to multiple comorbid conditions.[3,14,15] While overall sensitivity (99.6 percent; 95 percent confidence interval: 98–100 percent) was good in all age groups, specificity was age-dependent, decreasing from 67 percent (95 percent confidence interval: 60–74 percent) to as low as 10 percent (95 percent confidence interval: 5–18 percent) in patients older than age 80.[3]

Helical CT

In most institutions, $\dot{V}/\dot{Q}$ scan remains the initial test for evaluation of PE. In outlying facilities, CT scan may be the only choice available, and therefore, it may be used as the initial study. In a cooperative patient who is able to do a single-breathhold maneuver, the procedure can be performed quickly. A contrast bolus must be used; therefore, CT scan is contraindicated in patients with allergies to contrast material or those who have renal insufficiency. Filling defects within contrast-filled vessels identify acute thrombi.

The main advantage of CT over other methods is that it is very accurate at diagnosing other pulmonary disorders that may account for the patient's symptoms, including emphysema, cancer, pulmonary edema, aspiration pneumonia, and bronchiolitis. Most agree that a positive study is adequate to diagnose PE; however, a negative CT scan should be interpreted with clinical suspicion.[9,16] Helical CT scans may diagnose another cause for the patient's symptoms and, in the context of clinical suspicion, can exclude the diagnosis of PE.[16]

Echocardiography

When patients with known PE undergo echocardiography, 40 percent will have abnormalities of the right ventricle. However, this is a nonspecific finding. Finding thrombus in the main pulmonary artery is helpful but an unusual finding. At this time, echocardiographic evaluation is not indicated for all patients but may be a valuable bedside test for critically ill patients with hypotension to help exclude other diagnoses, such as myocardial infarction, valvular disorders, aortic dissection, or cardiac tamponade.[9] In the evaluation of a major PE, angiography is undertaken to quickly evaluate the anatomy and start definitive treatment. Helical CT also would be accurate in the diagnosis of major PE. Its utility in such cases remains to be validated.

EMERGENCY DEPARTMENT CARE AND DISPOSITION

Immediate Priorities

All patients presenting to the ED with signs and symptoms of PE should be evaluated promptly to exclude life-threatening conditions and initiate proper treatment. As with all life-threatening conditions, attention should be given to airway, breathing, and circulation. Supplemental oxygen and intravenous access should be instituted. All elderly patients should have an ECG and chest x-ray, as well as routine laboratory tests such as a complete blood count with platelets, coagulation studies, renal panel, and possibly cardiac enzymes. In the process of obtaining these tests, the physician should begin the process of developing a pretest probability of disease based on history, physical examination, and the results of initial studies (see Tables 20-2 and 20-3).

Initial ED Management

Heparin

For patients with a moderate to high clinical likelihood of PE, anticoagulation should be initiated while waiting to obtain further tests. Anticoagulation is usually started in the ED with heparin unless contraindications exist. Active bleeding and potential to bleed, such as active peptic ulcer disease, recent surgery, trauma, or intracranial hemorrhage, are relative contraindications to starting heparin.

The goals of anticoagulant therapy include prevention of PE, recurrence of DVT, and propagation of thrombus. Heparin prevents further clotting by binding to antithrombin. This antithrombin-heparin complex inactivates other coagulation factors (IIa, Xa, IXa, and XIIa). Heparin also binds to platelets, inhibiting aggregation, which contributes to its bleeding effects.[17,18]

Weight-adjusted protocols are the current recommendation for using heparin. In most patients, the weight-adjusted dosage regimen is effective at achieving a partial thromboplastin time (aPTT) of 60 to 80 seconds, or 1.5 to 2.5 times control. The usual dose is an initial bolus of 80 μ/kg, followed by a continuous infusion at 18 μ/kg/hr. Further adjustments are based on the aPTT after 6 hours of therapy.[17,18] Heparin is continued for 5 to 7 days and is as effective as the old 10-day regimen. Oral anticoagulation with warfarin generally is begun on the first or second day. When dose adjustment of warfarin achieves an appropriate level of anticoagulation, the heparin may be stopped. This approach is effective and reduces hospitalization by 3 to 5 days, and the recurrence rate of VTE is low. Inadequate anticoagulation correlates with the rate of recurrence; in fact, the rate of recurrence may be 15 times higher in those who do not achieve adequate anticoagulation in the first 24 hours. Therefore, adequate anticoagulation within the first day is important, and weight-adjusted nomograms achieve this goal.

There are many limitations to heparin therapy. First, it requires careful laboratory monitoring of the aPTT to achieve adequate anticoagulation. Therapy is unpredictable in some patients due to binding to plasma proteins. The anticoagulant effect may vary among different patients depending on age, sex, weight, smoking history, and renal function. Finally, heparin affects the platelets by inhibiting anticoagulation, causing bleeding problems. Heparin-induced thrombocytopenia is an antibody-mediated adverse reaction that occurs in a small percentage of patients. It may be associated with arterial thrombosis and extension of thrombus.[24,25]

Low-Molecular-Weight Heparin (LMWH)

LMWH is safe, effective, and cost-effective in appropriately chosen patients. LMWHs are prepared by chemical or enzymatic depolymerization of heparin. It exerts its anticoagulant effect by inactivation of factor Xa. LMWH has a small effect on thrombin and a negligible effect on the aPTT; therefore, monitoring is not necessary.[18] The smaller size of the molecules (molecular weight 4000–5000 Da) prevents binding to plasma proteins, acute-phase reactants, and endothelium. The result is a more predictable anticoagulant effect and a longer half-life. Also, LMWH has minimal effects on platelets, therefore decreasing the incidence of thrombocytopenia.

Several LMWHs are available, with the most common being enoxaparin (Lovenox). Administration is by the subcutaneous route at a fixed dose based on weight and given usually twice daily, but some of the newer LMWHs can be used once per day. LMWHs are excreted by the kidneys and therefore are more difficult to use in patients with renal problems. Monitoring generally is not performed but may be required in those with renal failure or obesity. LMWHs generally are not used in patients with serum creatinine levels in excess of 3 mg/dL. Active bleeding and the potential for bleeding are also relative contraindications to therapy.[18]

Multiple studies from the early 1990s document safety with regard to bleeding complications and equal efficacy with regard to recurrence rate when comparing LMWH with traditional heparin therapy.[18,19] The largest study available randomized over 1000 patients to receive LMWH or heparin followed by a coumarin derivative for 12 weeks.[20] Approximately one-third of patients had PE. The results of the two groups were very similar with respect to outcome variables, including recurrent events, bleeding, or death. The investigators concluded that LMWH and heparin are equally safe and effective for the treatment of VTE.

While LMWH itself is quite expensive, the overall cost generally is lower than costs with heparin due to the need for laboratory monitoring and hospitalization with heparin therapy. It is estimated that 5 to 6 days of hospital charges can be saved with outpatient therapy.[18,19] Patients managed as outpatients require close monitoring and appropriate support from family and home health providers. At this time, treatment of massive PE has not been studied.

Disposition

Patients with a diagnosis of PE generally are admitted to the hospital for continued therapy. Those with signs of hemodynamic instability or severe hypoxia will require admission to the intensive care unit. Selected patients may be candidates for LMWH as an outpatient. The logistics of arranging home health care and giving appropriate instruction to family/caregivers may be difficult in the ED setting. Such patients should be admitted overnight to observation status while completing all the arrangements necessary.

Subsequent Care

Generally, warfarin is continued for at least 3 months after PE. For those with significant risk factors, such as the hereditary thrombophilias, anticoagulation should continue for life. Oral anticoagulation generally is safe and effective at preventing thrombus formation. Warfarin is the most commonly used coumarin preparation. It is absorbed well from the gut and transported to the liver. Warfarin inhibits the synthesis of vitamin K-dependent factors II, VII, IX, and X and protein C and S. Warfarin requires several days to be effective until coagulation factors are cleared from the blood.[17]

Warfarin usually is started on day 1 or 2 with heparin. The initial dose is 5 mg/day, and adequacy of anticoagulation is monitored using the international normalized ratio (INR), with the goal therapeutic range of an INR of 2.0 to 3.0. Beginning oral therapy early in the course decreases the length of heparin or LMWH to 7 days. The heparin may be discontinued once the warfarin achieves an appropriate INR. Warfarin is never used alone in the treatment of VTE because it may cause a paradoxical increase in hypercoagulability and increase the risk of recurrent VTE.

Multiple drugs and foods interact with coumarin therapy and change the state of anticoagulation. Instruction on maintaining a stable diet with a consistent amount of vitamin K is important, as well as avoiding alcohol. Warfarin generally is well tolerated. However, in those with partial protein-C deficiency, microvascular thrombosis leading to skin necrosis may occur and requires discontinuation of therapy. Vitamin K is the antidote for overanticoagulation with a coumarin preparation. For serious bleeding, fresh-frozen plasma or cryprecipitate should be given and will reverse the effects of warfarin.

ADDITIONAL ASPECTS

Pitfalls

Failure to consider pretest clinical suspicion or changing the pretest suspicion without sufficient evidence is a major pitfall. Another broad category of pitfalls is overreliance on any one physical examination finding or diagnostic test to safely exclude or make the diagnosis. For instance, bronchospasm will lead to $\dot{V}/\dot{Q}$ mismatching, making the test less reliable in a patient with COPD or asthma. Large central or saddle embolus may cause a false-negative $\dot{V}/\dot{Q}$ scan. All diagnostic tests discussed in this chapter are most useful as complementary tests taken together with clinical probability of VTE. When history, physical examination, and risk factors are used to arrive at the pretest clinical probability of disease, the ED physician can choose appropriate diagnostic tests and arrive at the correct diagnosis.

Prophylaxis

Prevention of VTE is a well-known practice in the surgical fields, especially in patients undergoing orthopedic procedures. The elderly patient with a hip fracture undergoing total hip replacement surgery will be bedridden for a period of time and is most susceptible to fatal PE.[1,9,21] Therefore, it is important to risk stratify patients who are hospitalized for prevention strategies. VTE is nonspecific in presentation and may be masked by other disease processes. VTE may be unrecognized and lead to considerable morbidity and mortality.

It is important to establish which patients are at risk for VTE and may require prophylaxis when hospitalized. Those receiving lifelong anticoagulation for thrombophilia should continue while in the hospital. Those with cancer who are undergoing treatment should receive prophylaxis. Patients admitted to the hospital for surgery also should receive prophylaxis. The high-risk patient is one who is having major surgery, age greater than 40 years, who has had VTE in the past, cancer, or a hypercoagulable state.[21] Patients admitted for knee or hip arthroplasty, hip fracture surgery, major trauma, or spinal cord injury all benefit from VTE prophylaxis.[9,21] Non-major surgery in patients over age 60 also carry an increased risk of VTE, and prophylaxis should be considered.[21]

While prophylaxis for VTE in surgical patients is accepted and considered safe and effective, the prophylaxis of medical patients only recently has been shown to be effective and appropriate. It has been the teaching on the medical services to use VTE prophylaxis with 5000 units of heparin subcutaneously twice daily for those who will be bedridden for a prolonged period of time. However, risk assessment based on underlying disease was not considered.

In one study, 384 patients developed VTE while hospitalized or within 30 days of discharge.[22] This was a retrospective chart review to determine whether prophylaxis was given. Most patients were on the general medical service, with 52 percent receiving prophylaxis. Unfractionated heparin alone or in combination with mechanical measures was used in approximately 65 percent of patients (LMWH in only 1.5 percent). Most patients received prophylaxis of some kind, and deaths from PE were due to failed prophylactic measures. The authors recommended close follow-up of high-risk patients, especially medical patients.

The largest study to date is the MEDENOX trial, which evaluated enoxaparin at 40 or 20 mg or placebo for 6 to 14 days.[23] This was a double-blinded, randomized study of three treatment regimens used to prevent VTE in medical patients. All patients with risk factors and chronic medical illness (see Table 20-1) were included in the study. Outcomes were development of VTE between days 1 and 14. Follow-up was for 3 months. By day 14, the placebo group had a 14.9 percent incidence of VTE, placing these medically ill patients at moderate risk. The enoxaparin 40 mg/day group had a 5.5 percent incidence of VTE, representing a 63 percent relative risk reduction (97 percent confidence interval: 37–78 percent; $P = 0.0002$) without increasing the risk of hemorrhage. A subgroup analysis of the enoxaparin group demonstrated a VTE risk reduction of 72 percent in patients with acute heart failure (95 percent confidence interval, 19–92 percent; $P = 0.01$), 74 percent in those with chronic heart failure (95 percent confidence interval, 9–93 percent; $P = 0.022$), and 78 percent in all patients older than age 75 (95 percent confidence interval, 49–91 percent; $P = 0.0001$).[24] This trial supports the use of VTE prophylaxis with enoxaparin in medical patients hospitalized with cardiopulmonary disease, infectious diseases, or rheumatic disorders.

A meta-analysis of prophylactic strategy in general medical patients compared heparin and LMWH.[25] On review of all the literature, heparins were effective in preventing VTE in medical patients. There seems to be no difference between heparin and LMWH, except that LMWH may be associated with less risk of hemorrhage. Currently, a large trial is underway evaluating heparin and LMWH for prevention of VTE in immobilized patients with respiratory or cardiac diseases. Therefore, elderly patients with chronic medical illnesses should be considered for VTE prophylaxis with heparin or LMWH while hospitalized.

REFERENCES

1. Hirsh J, Hoak J: Management of deep vein thrombosis and pulmonary embolism. *Circulation* 93:2212, 1996.
2. Silverstein MD, Heit JA, Mohr DN, et al: Trends in the incidence of deep vein thrombosis and pulmonary embolism. *Arch Intern Med* 158:585, 1998.
3. Righini M, Goehring C, Bounameaux H, et al: Effects of age on the performance of common diagnostic tests for pulmonary embolism. *Am J Med* 109:357, 2000.
4. Moser KM, Fedullo PF, LitteJohn JK, et al: Frequent asymptomatic pulmonary embolism in patients with deep venous thrombosis. *JAMA* 271:223, 1993.
5. Siddique RM, Amini SB, Connors AF, et al: Race and sex differences in long-term survival rates for elderly patients with pulmonary embolism. *Am J Public Health* 88:1476, 1998.
6. Martinelli I: Risk factors in venous thromboembolism. *Thromb Haemost* 86:395, 2001.
7. Lapostolle F, Surget V, Borron SW, et al: Severe pulmonary embolism associated with air travel. *New Eng J Med* 345:779, 2001.
8. Sorensen HT, Mellemkjar L, Steffensen FH, et al: The risk of a diagnosis of cancer after primary deep venous thrombosis or pulmonary embolism. *New Engl J Med* 338:1169, 1998.
9. Goldhaber SZ: Pulmonary embolism. *New Engl J Med* 339:93, 1998.
10. The PIOPED Investigators: Value of the ventilation/perfusion scan in acute pulmonary embolism. *JAMA* 263:2753, 1990.
11. Wells PS, Ginsberg JS, Anderson DR, et al: Use of a clinical model for safe management of patients with suspected pulmonary embolism. *Ann Intern Med* 129:997, 1998.
12. Kearon C, Ginsberg JS, Hirsh J: The role of venous ultrasonography in the diagnosis of suspected deep venous thrombosis and pulmonary embolism. *Ann Intern Med* 129:1044, 1998.
13. Wells PS, Anderson DR, Rodger M, et al: Excluding pulmonary embolism at the bedside without diagnostic imaging: Management of patients with suspected pulmonary embolism presenting to the emergency department by using a simple clinical model and D-dimer. *Ann Intern Med* 135:98, 2001.
14. Bounameaux H, DeMoerloose P, Perrier A, et al: D-Dimer testing in suspected venous thromboembolism: An updated. *Q J Med* 90:437, 1997.
15. Tardy B, Tardy-Poncet B, Viallon A, et al: Evaluation of D-dimer ELISA test in elderly patients with suspected pulmonary embolism. *Thromb Haemost* 79:38, 1998.
16. Mayo JR, Remy-Jardin M, Muller NL, et al: Pulmonary embolism: Prospective comparison of spiral CT with ventilation-perfusion scintigraphy. *Radiology* 205:447, 1997.
17. Hirsh J, Anand SS, Halperin JL, et al: Guide to anticoagulant therapy: Heparin. *Circulation* 103:2994, 2001.
18. Hirsh J, Warkentin TE, Shaughnessy SG, et al: Heparin and low-molecular-weight heparin. *Chest* 119:64S, 2001.
19. Ageno W, Huisman MV: Low-molecular-weight heparins in the treatment of venous thromboembolism. *Curr Control Trials Cardiovasc Med* 1:102, 2000.
20. The Columbus Investigators: Low-molecular-weight heparin in the treatment of patients with venous thromboembolism. *New Engl J Med* 337:657, 1997.
21. Geerts WH, Heit JA, Clagett GP, et al: Prevention of venous thromboembolism. *Chest* 119:132S, 2001.
22. Goldhaber SZ, Dunn K, MacDougall RC: New onset of venous thromboembolism among hospitalized patients at Brigham and Women's Hospital is caused more often by prophylaxis failure than by withholding treatment. *Chest* 118:1680, 2000.
23. Samama MM, Cohen AT, Darmon JY, et al: A comparison of enoxaparin with placebo for the prevention of venous thromboembolism in acutely ill medical patients. *New Eng J Med* 341:793, 1999.
24. Alikhan R, Cohen A, Conabe S, et al: Benefits of enoxaparin in medical patients: A subgroup analysis. Abstract no 1118, available at *www.abstracts-on-line.com,* March 2002.
25. Mismetti P, Laporte-Simitsidis S, Tardy B, et al: Prevention of venous thromboembolism in internal medicine with unfractionated or low-molecular-weight heparins: A meta-analysis of randomized clinical trials. *Thromb Haemost* 83:14, 2000.

21

Abdominal Pain

Jeffrey N. Glaspy
O. John Ma
Robert A. Schwab
Stephen W. Meldon

HIGH-YIELD FACTS

- Approximately 60 percent of elderly patients presenting to the emergency department (ED) with abdominal pain require admission, and 40 percent require surgical intervention.

- Although leukocytosis is associated with significant intraabdominal infections, it should be noted that the white blood cell count has limited ability to differentiate serious from nonserious illnesses.

- Ultrasonography has a sensitivity of nearly 100 percent for detecting abdominal aortic aneurysm.

- Abdominal surgery in the elderly results in morbidity and mortality rates two to three times greater than those seen in younger patients.

Evaluation of elderly patients with acute abdominal pain can be challenging even to the experienced emergency physician. The number of disease entities that can cause abdominal pain in the elderly is extensive, and the spectrum of diseases differs from that of younger age groups. In addition, the high prevalence of underlying chronic abdominal diseases further confounds the clinical assessment. Elderly patients at baseline may have cholelithiasis, diverticular disease, gastritis, or a stable abdominal aortic aneurysm (AAA). The presence of these comorbidities, along with any decline in the immune system, has led to a significantly worse clinical outcome for geriatric patients presenting with abdominal pain.

EPIDEMIOLOGY

Elderly adults comprise 12 to 21 percent of all ED visits.[1] As the proportion of the population shifts toward a higher elderly component, this figure is likely to grow. Abdominal pain is the chief complaint in 5 to 10 percent of ED visits.[2] Given these figures, encounters with elderly patients complaining of abdominal pain will become increasingly common.

The morbidity, mortality, and diagnostic accuracy associated with geriatric abdominal pain are particularly concerning. It has been reported that 63 percent of elderly patients (age > 65 years) presenting to the ED with abdominal pain required admission, and 42 percent required surgical intervention.[3] The mortality rate of elderly adults with abdominal pain has been demonstrated to be between 5 and 11 percent.[4,5] Furthermore, one study found that diagnostic accuracy declined in the geriatric age group. The diagnostic accuracy was reported to be 59 percent in patients younger than age 12; in contrast, the diagnostic accuracy for patients older than age 80 was 29 percent.[6]

PATHOPHYSIOLOGY

Although the pathophysiology of abdominal pain does not differ between elderly and younger persons, both the perception and underlying cause of pain do vary markedly with age. There are three types of abdominal pain perceptions. The first type is *visceral pain,* which is caused by the stretching of hollow organs or distension of the capsules of solid organs. Visceral pain is transmitted by autonomic nerves. This type of pain generally is difficult to describe and localize. The second type is *somatic pain,* which is caused by irritation of the parietal peritoneum. Somatic pain is transmitted by peripheral nerves. This type of pain is better localized and generally is described as constant, sharp, or intense. The third type is *referred pain,* which is defined as pain perceived at a site distant from its origin. Referred pain can be caused by either visceral or somatic causes.

Pain perception decreases with aging.[7] Elderly adults often present with vague, diffuse abdominal pain that is more consistent with visceral origin. However, because of the alterations in pain perception, vagueness does not necessarily indicate one origin over another.

Complicating matters further, elderly adults often have chronic comorbid conditions that alter their presentation. Cholelithiasis, peptic ulcer disease, diverticulosis, urogenital disease, and AAA all occur more frequently in the elderly.[2] These chronic underlying conditions may make the timely determination of the etiology of abdominal pain more difficult in the elderly. The presence of gallstones, for example, may or may not explain the etiology of a patient's diffuse abdominal pain. It may be necessary to exclude other causes, such as AAA, before attributing the pain to a baseline condition, making the workup more time-consuming and costly.

Because of their comorbid conditions, elderly adults also may take medications that can cloud their clinical presentations. Nonsteroidal anti-inflammatory medications and steroids inhibit inflammation and may further decrease an already hindered pain response. Cardiovascular medications may inhibit the normal tachycardic response to life-threatening conditions. Diuretics may exacerbate dehydration. Chronic narcotic therapy also may inhibit pain response. Therefore, it is necessary to obtain a complete listing of all medications, including over-the-counter preparations.

CLINICAL FEATURES

History

A precise history may be difficult to obtain because of underlying cognitive impairments or communication difficulties. Important sources for the history besides the patient include family, other caregivers, and nursing home personnel. In general, the main elements of the history are no different in elderly patients. The key features of onset, severity, description, duration, quality, location, progression, radiation, prior episodes, and precipitating and relieving factors should be sought.

Other aspects of the history are equally important. In addition to obtaining a complete list of medications, taking a thorough social history and review of systems are essential. Any history of drug or alcohol abuse needs to be elicited. Alcohol and cocaine are substances that have been reported to be abused in the elderly population. A complete review of systems may provide clues that the abdominal pain is due to pathology in an organ system outside the gastrointestinal system.

Physical Examination

The approach to the abdominal examination does not differ from that of younger patients. Particular attention should be paid to the general appearance and vital signs. An ill-appearing elderly patient demands immediate evaluation and resuscitation. Abnormal vital signs also should raise concern for serious life-threatening disease. It is important, however, to remember that a well-appearing elderly patient with normal vital signs may still have a catastrophic illness.

The abdominal examination should begin with inspection. The presence of scars may yield clues to past surgical procedures. Distension of the abdomen should raise suspicion for bowel obstruction or liver disease. The presence of erythema may indicate an abdominal wall cellulitis. The presence of a skin lesion consistent with herpes zoster may elucidate the etiology of the pain.

Auscultation of the abdomen may reveal high-pitched "rushes and tinkles" in patients with bowel obstruction. Lack of abdominal sounds may be present in patients with ileus or peritonitis. Presence of a bruit may indicate a dissection or aneurysm of the abdominal aorta, renal artery, or splenic artery.

The location and severity of tenderness should be elicited with palpation. The location of tenderness generally is predictive of underlying disease origin in elderly patients. Although the pain perception is altered with aging, elderly patients generally retain the ability to localize tenderness to palpation. Elderly patients with appendicitis have been found to exhibit right lower quadrant tenderness in 94 percent of patients.[5] The associated signs of peritonitis, however, are often absent, even in the presence of severe intraabdominal pathology. Only 21 percent of elderly patients with perforated gastroduodenal ulcer were found to present with epigastric rigidity.[5] The routine abdominal examination of elderly patients also should include palpation for a pulsatile mass. The presence of a large pulsatile mass should raise immediate concern for the presence of a leaking AAA.

A detailed cardiovascular, pulmonary, and urogenital examination is essential; abdominal pain in this population often stems from disease in other organ systems. A rectal examination should be included in the evaluation of all elderly adults with abdominal pain. The presence of gross or occult blood, prostate tenderness, or localization of pain with rectal examination may help in making an accurate diagnosis. A pelvic examination is necessary in the evaluation of elderly women presenting with abdominal pain. Vaginal, cervical, uterine, and ovarian malignancy or infections all may present with a chief complaint of abdominal pain.

DIAGNOSIS AND DIFFERENTIAL

Evaluation of abdominal pain in the elderly begins with a careful history and physical examination. The differential diagnosis of abdominal pain (Table 21-1) is more expansive in the older population, as is the prevalence of concurrent medical conditions, which may obscure, accentuate, or contribute to various aspects of the disease process. Because of these factors and the fact that the history and physical examination may be more unreliable in pinpointing the disease process, the scope of imaging and laboratory investigation should be expanded.

Tools for evaluating acute abdominal pain in this patient population include laboratory studies, plain radiographs, ultrasonography, and computed tomographic (CT) scanning. Also, a 12-lead electrocardiogram (ECG) should be obtained if acute coronary syndrome is considered.

Laboratory Evaluation

A complete blood count (CBC) should be obtained in patients with suspected serious intraabdominal disease. Although leukocytosis and an elevated band count (>1000 cells/mm^3 or >6 percent) are associated with significant infections and bacteremia, it should be noted that the white blood cell (WBC) count has limited ability to differentiate serious from nonserious illnesses. A significant number of patients with acute cholecystitis or acute appendicitis have normal WBC counts.

Another important and commonly obtained test is a urinalysis. When interpreting this test, it should be noted that asymptomatic pyuria is common in the elderly female population and may not signify disease.

Serum amylase and lipase determinations often are useful in the diagnosis of pancreatitis. Hyperamylasemia, however, can occur in a wide variety of disorders in the elderly, including pneumonia, renal insufficiency, and peptic ulcer disease.[2] While liver function tests may be useful in the evaluation of biliary tract disease, they are neither sensitive nor specific in diagnosing acute cholecystitis. Alkaline phosphatase levels can be elevated 2.5 times normal in otherwise healthy patients. Other liver enzymes and the total bilirubin, however, change minimally with increased age. Although findings of elevated serum phosphatase and serum lactic acid levels can be seen in acute mesenteric ischemia, their absence cannot be used to exclude this process.

Plain Radiographs

Plain radiographs of the abdomen are obtained often in the evaluation of acute abdominal pain; however, they

Table 21-1. Differential Diagnosis of Abdominal Pain in the Elderly

Inflammatory
Appendicitis
Cholecystitis
Cystitis
Diverticulitis
Esophagitis
Hepatitis
Inflammatory bowel disease
Pancreatitis
Prostatitis
Pyelonephritis

Obstructive
Bowel obstruction
Choledocholithiasis
Ureterolithiasis
Volvulus

Vascular
Abdominal aortic aneurysm
Mesenteric ischemia

Other Intraabdominal disorders
Constipation
Gastroenteritis
Hernia
Irritable bowel syndromes
Genitourinary tract disorders
Gynecological disorders
Peptic ulcer disease
Perforated viscus

Extraabdominal disorders
Acute myocardial infarction
Herpes zoster
Hypercalcemia
Lower lobar pneumonia
Pleural effusions
Pulmonary embolism

generally have limited usefulness. Positive findings are seen in fewer than 25 percent of all patients with abdominal pain.[8] Predictors of positive findings on plain films include a history of prior abdominal surgery, abnormal bowel sounds, abdominal distension, peritoneal signs, and suspicion for a foreign body. Plain radiographs are most useful when bowel obstruction or hollow viscus perforation is suspected. Even in these settings, plain films may be misleading. In one series, plain radiographs failed to demonstrate the presence of pneumoperitoneum in 39 percent of elderly patients with documented perforated peptic ulcer disease.[5] In an acute abdominal series, the chest radiograph may demonstrate a lower lobe infiltrate or pleural effusion, both of which may be the source of the abdominal pain.

Ultrasonography

Abdominal sonography is a valuable diagnostic adjunct for detecting intraabdominal pathology in the elderly. Ultrasonography is highly accurate in evaluating the biliary tract. This modality has a high sensitivity (86 percent) and specificity (98 percent) for detecting acute cholecystitis and is nearly 100 percent sensitive for detecting cholelithiasis.[9] In addition, abnormalities also will be present in most patients with acute cholangitis, emphysematous cholecystitis, and gallbladder perforation. Ultrasonography also has been shown to be sensitive and specific for acute appendicitis, although body habitus and failure to visualize the appendix may limit this modality in older patients. Ultrasonography is also an important diagnostic tool for detecting AAA, with a sensitivity approaching 100 percent. Ultrasonography, however, has a limited ability to detect a leaking AAA; for stable patients, CT scan is the procedure of choice.[8] Ultrasonography also may be useful for evaluation of mesenteric ischemia, especially when Doppler flow measurements of the celiac and superior mesenteric arteries are employed.

Computed Tomography

CT scan has become the diagnostic modality of choice in most patients with abdominal pain. It is capable of identifying free intraperitoneal fluid, pneumoperitoneum, air within the bowel wall or retroperitoneum, inflammatory changes, and vascular abnormalities. Both oral and intravenous contrast agents are often needed for accurate studies. CT scan appears to be the optimal diagnostic tool for detecting acute appendicitis, aneurysmal rupture in stable patients, diverticulitis, intraabdominal abscess formation, and perforated hollow viscus. In addition, non-contrast-enhanced spiral CT scanning has become the "gold standard" procedure for detecting nephrolithiasis and hydronephrosis.[8]

A general approach to acute abdominal pain in older patients has been recommended.[10] After performing a careful history and physical examination, it is suggested that laboratory tests, including CBC, electrolytes, renal studies, liver function tests, lipase, and urinalysis, be obtained. If clinically indicated, plain radiographs of the abdomen (flat plate and upright abdomen and chest radiographs) should be ordered. For patients with upper abdominal pain, nausea, vomiting, or possible atypical myocardial ischemia, an ECG should be obtained. Blood cultures should be ordered for patients with suspected serious intraabdominal infection. For patients with right upper quadrant abdominal pain, an ultrasound examination of the biliary tract is recommended. Patients with diffuse abdominal pain or right or left lower quadrant pain should undergo a CT scan of the abdomen. Although diagnostic imaging tests have improved localization, treatment, and outcomes of several abdominal disease entities (such as appendicitis and diverticulitis), diagnostic imaging should not delay surgical intervention for patients with generalized peritonitis or those who are deteriorating rapidly.

EMERGENCY DEPARTMENT CARE AND DISPOSITION

The first priority for elderly patients with abdominal pain is to ensure the integrity of the airway, breathing, and circulation. Patients with ischemic bowel, ruptured AAA, significant gastrointestinal bleeding, viscus perforation, or sepsis may present with a diminished level of consciousness and require intubation to protect their airway. They also may present with unstable vital signs and require rapid resuscitation via intravenous crystalloid infusion. Blood and component therapy may be required in patients with significant blood loss. Blood cultures should be obtained from patients thought to have perforation or sepsis. Empirical antibiotic coverage effective against gram-negative and anaerobic bacteria should be administered pending the results of diagnostic studies.

Most elderly patients with abdominal pain will be hemodynamically stable In these patients, initial ED management will include intravenous hydration, analgesics, and antibiotics. Since many elderly patients with abdominal pain will require urgent or emergent surgical interventions, nothing should be given by mouth in the ED.

Fluid status should be assessed by paying close attention to the history of oral intake and by evaluating the moisture content of mucous membranes and skin. In the absence of underlying renal dysfunction, determination of blood urea nitrogen and creatinine blood levels may be useful. Urine specific gravity can be assessed relatively rapidly and provides a rough estimate of hydration status. Bladder catheterization, although invasive, provides an immediate urine specimen and allows for ongoing urine output monitoring to assess the effectiveness of rehydration.

Initial rehydration usually can be accomplished by administering serial small intravenous boluses (250 mL) of crystalloid solution. Patients, especially those known to have underlying cardiac disease, should be monitored and reassessed carefully to prevent significant fluid overload. Patients with high fever and those who are found to have bowel obstruction may have larger fluid deficits and thus should be rehydrated more vigorously. Bladder catheterization is indicated in these patients so that fluid status can be monitored continuously.

Nasogastric suction should be initiated in all patients with confirmed bowel obstruction, as well as in patients thought to have upper gastrointestinal tract bleeding. Nasogastric suction is also indicated for patients with significant vomiting; unlike antiemetics, nasogastric suction does not affect mental status and thus will not interfere with ongoing evaluation of the patient's clinical status.

Analgesia should be given early and in adequate amounts to control discomfort. The ideal agent would have a rapid onset of action, few side effects, and a brief duration of action so that reassessment of patient status could be performed frequently. Fentanyl probably approaches this ideal more than any other analgesic agent. Given in small doses (0.5–1.0 μg/kg), it provides rapid improvement in patient comfort without significant hemodynamic effects. Respiratory depression can occur; oxygen saturation should be monitored during administration of fentanyl. Nausea also can occur and may require coadministration of an antiemetic. The duration of effect is typically 30 to 60 minutes, which provides time for diagnostic studies and allows for accurate reassessment of physical findings by the ED physician and consultant at frequent intervals. Meperidine and morphine are more likely to cause undesirable side effects, including hypotension and respiratory depression, and therefore should be considered second-line analgesics in elderly patients with abdominal pain.

Empirical antibiotic coverage should be directed against typical colonic flora, including gram-negative and anaerobic species, particularly *Bacteroides fragilis* and *Escherichia coli*. Intravenous regimens should include clindamycin or metronidazole in combination with an aminoglycoside or a third-generation cephalosporin.

Most elderly patients with abdominal pain will require hospitalization, regardless of whether a specific diagnosis is made in the ED or not. Hospitalization is always indicated for unstable patients, patients with active gastrointestinal bleeding, and patients with fever or peritoneal signs on physical examination. Patients who cannot tolerate oral intake, whose pain cannot be managed with oral analgesics, or who do not have a supportive home environment also should be admitted. Immunocompromised patients and patients with other significant comorbidities should be treated in an inpatient setting. Laboratory data that should contribute to the decision to admit include leukocytosis and a falling hematocrit in the presence of Hemoccult-positive stool. Consultation with a surgeon should be considered in all cases, although admission to an internist or gastroenterologist is often appropriate depending on the admitting diagnosis.

Outpatient therapy, although fairly common in younger patients, should be the exception in the geriatric population. If symptoms are mild, physical examination findings are limited to mild localized tenderness without peritoneal signs, and extensive diagnostic evaluation demonstrates no complications, patients can be considered for outpatient management, provided that oral intake is adequate, pain can be controlled, and the home environment is supportive. Patients treated at home should be instructed to rest and take a clear liquid diet initially. In addition, patients should have adequate transportation and the ability to follow up with a primary care physician within 24 hours. The case should be discussed with the primary care physician by telephone whenever possible. The patient should be instructed to return immediately for fever, increased pain, or inability to tolerate oral medications or liquids.

ADDITIONAL ASPECTS

The following are pitfalls in the management of patients with abdominal pain:

- *Failure to appreciate the severity of undifferentiated abdominal pain in the elderly.* Unlike younger patients with undifferentiated abdominal pain, elderly patients most often have significant disease and always require a thorough diagnostic evaluation, including laboratory testing and diagnostic imaging. Sound clinical judgment and an understanding of the natural history of undifferentiated abdominal pain in the elderly will prevent overreliance on negative diagnostic tests.

- *Failure to secure timely outpatient follow-up for elderly patients with abdominal pain.* The decision to discharge an elderly patient with abdominal pain should be made only after a negative exhaustive evaluation of a highly reliable patient with good home support and certain continuity of care.

REFERENCES

1. Aminzadeh F, Dalziel WB: Older adults in the emergency department: A systematic review of patterns of use, adverse outcomes and effectiveness of interventions. *Ann Emerg Med* 39:238, 2002.
2. Sanson TG, O'Keefe KP: Evaluation of abdominal pain in the elderly. *Emeg Med Clin North Amer* 14:615, 1996.
3. Bugliosi TF, Meloy TD, Vukov LF: Acute abdominal pain in the elderly. *Ann Emerg Med* 19:1383, 1990.
4. Marco CA, Schoenfeld CN, Keyl PM, et al: Abdominal pain in geriatric emergency patients: Variables associated with adverse outcomes. *Acad Emerg Med* 5:1163, 1998.
5. Fenyo G: Acute abdominal disease in the elderly: Experience from two series in Stockholm. *Am J Surg* 143:751, 1982.
6. Adams ID, Chan M, Clifford PC, et al: Computer-aided diagnosis of abdominal pain: A multicenter study. *Br Med J* 293:800, 1986.
7. Li SF, Greenwald PW, Gennis P, et al: Effect of age of acute pain perception of a standardized stimulus in the emergency department. *Ann Emerg Med* 38:644, 2001.
8. Mayo-Smith WW: Imaging the patient with acute abdominal pain: Current concepts. *Med Health* 82:202, 1999.
9. Parker LJ, Vukov LF, Wollan PC: Emergency department evaluation of geriatric patients with acute cholecystitis. *Acad Emerg Med* 4:51, 1997.
10. Abi-Hanna P, Gleckman R: Acute abdominal pain: A medical emergency in older patients. *Geriatrics* 52:72, 1997.

22

Peptic Ulcer Disease and Gastrointestinal Bleeding

Mark E. Hoffmann

HIGH-YIELD FACTS

- Geriatric patients have higher morbidity and mortality due to complications of peptic ulcer disease and its delayed diagnosis.
- The elderly have less ability to compensate for acute hemorrhage, and the majority of deaths from gastrointestinal bleeding occur in elderly patients.
- Physical examination findings associated with peritonitis, including fever and leukocytosis, may be diminished or completely absent in the elderly.

Peptic ulcers are mucosal ulcerations that penetrate to the submucosa in either the stomach or duodenum and result in pain, bleeding, or perforation. These ulcerations are a direct result of destruction of the defensive barrier and tissue damage caused by gastric acid and pepsin. Ten percent of adults have peptic ulcer disease in the United States[1]; the associated morbidity and mortality rates are higher in the elderly population. The use of nonsteroidal anti-inflammatory drugs (NSAIDs), *Helicobacter pylori* infections, and Zollinger-Ellison syndrome are important etiologic factors. Clinical presentation in the elderly may be atypical, and up to half of elderly patients may not experience pain. Complications include bleeding, gastric outlet obstruction, penetration into adjacent organs, and perforation. Endoscopy is the most sensitive and specific test for assessing the presence and degree of peptic ulcer disease.

Gastrointestinal (GI) bleeding in the elderly has significant morbidity and mortality. Bleeding proximal to the ligament of Treitz defines upper GI bleeding, which usually presents as hematemesis or melena. Bleeding distal to the ligament of Treitz, most commonly colonic or rectal in nature, defines lower GI bleeding; patients present with hematochezia. The elderly have differences in their clinical presentation compared with younger populations. The differential diagnosis is broad, and the location of the bleeding may be obscure. Complications include aspiration, hypovolemic shock, and end-organ damage associated with underperfusion.

EPIDEMIOLOGY

The elderly have greater risk factors for gastric and duodenal ulcers and experience increased complications and mortality.[2] Mortality from GI bleeding as a complication of peptic ulcer disease is 4 to 10 times greater in the elderly than in younger patients.[3] The prevalence of *H. pylori* infection at 60 years of age is 50 percent.[4] Approximately 40 percent of people over age 65 are prescribed NSAIDs, and up to 8 percent are hospitalized with a GI complication within the first year of therapy.[5] One-third of patients with Zollinger-Ellison syndrome, a condition marked by hypergastrinemia and gastric hypersecretion due to a tumor, are elderly. Persons older than 60 years account for up to 45 percent of cases of acute upper GI bleeding.[6] The incidence of lower GI bleeding increases with age, with a greater than 200-fold increase from the twenties to the eighties.[7]

PATHOPHYSIOLOGY

Peptic Ulcer Disease

The mucosa of the stomach is protected from gastric acid and pepsin by a bicarbonate layer that acts as a buffering zone. Mucus neck cells secrete mucus and bicarbonate to maintain this buffering-zone. Parietal cells in the gastric mucosa secrete hydrochloric acid and are stimulated by histamine, gastrin, and acetylcholine (parasympathetic vagal nerve stimulation). It was believed previously that with aging gastric acid secretion and the protective buffer decrease. However, this was prior to the understanding of how *H. pylori* affects the gastric environment. Gastric acid secretion is maintained in more than 80 percent of elderly,[8] and one study suggested that gastric acid secretion in some men may increase with age.[9]

H. pylori is a urease-positive, gram-negative rod that attaches to the mucus-secreting cells of the gastric mucosa. Ammonia production from urea, coupled with an inflammatory response, not only diminishes the protective bicarbonate layer but also leads to mucosal ulceration. *H. pylori* has been identified in approximately 90 percent of patients with gastric ulcers and 95 percent of patients with duodenal ulcers.

NSAIDs cause gastric inflammation and may lead to GI bleeding and perforation. This process is a result of diminished gastric blood flow, increased cell permeability to acids, and reduced prostaglandin levels (vital for maintaining bicarbonate layers and diminishing gastrin). Fifteen percent of patients taking NSAIDs chronically will develop gastric or duodenal ulcers.[10] Bleeding occurs in 15 percent of these patients and most commonly in elderly patients.

The prevalence of Zollinger-Ellison syndrome increases with age and is associated with elevated levels of gastrin and hydrochloric acid. Gastrin-secreting tumors represent up to 1 percent of peptic ulcer disease. Ulcers and symptoms usually are persistent despite medical interventions.

Upper GI Bleeding

Two-thirds of GI bleeding is proximal to the ligament of Treitz (upper GI bleeding) and results in melena. Melena is digested hemoglobin that appears as tarry and dark-colored stool. Melena results from peptic ulcer bleeding, esophageal varices, Mallory-Weiss tear, esophagitis, duodenitis, drug ingestion, and aortoenteric fistula. Most deaths occur in the elderly, who have less ability to compensate for acute hemorrhage and hypovolemia.[11]

Peptic ulcers are the most common cause of upper GI bleeding; gastric or duodenal ulcers are the cause of upper GI bleeding in an estimated 45 percent of cases.[12] Bleeding is five times more common after age 50. Not all patients experience pain after eating, and acute hemorrhage is often painless. Blood acts as a cathartic, and bright red rectal blood may be seen during brisk bleeding. Erosion of an ulcer into an adjacent vessel initiates the process. Ten percent of ulcer perforations are associated with upper GI bleeding.[13] Gastritis-related bleeding ranges from slight to massive, has an 8 percent mortality,[14] and accounts for 2 percent of bleeding-related deaths.[15]

Esophageal varices are dilatations in veins that become engorged due to collateral blood flow in portal hypertension. When bleeding does occur, it is usually massive. Alcoholism and cirrhosis are the most common etiologies. Esophageal varices occur less frequently in the elderly than in younger patients. Variceal bleeding accounts for one-third of deaths in upper GI bleeding.[15]

Mallory-Weiss tears account for less than 10 percent of patients with massive upper GI bleeding.[16] Alcoholics and younger patients suffer from Mallory-Weiss tears more frequently than the older population. Forceful vomiting and retching increase the intraabdominal pressure,

and longitudinal tears in the mucosa (1–5 cm) occur at the level of the gastroesophageal junction and distal esophagus. Bleeding is usually mild and stops spontaneously.[17]

Esophagitis and duodenitis are common diseases, but they account for only a small percentage of upper GI bleeding in the elderly. Rebleeding occurs in up to 10 percent of patients, and hemorrhage is usually self-limited.

Drug ingestion (NSAIDs and aspirin) can increase the risk of GI bleeding. Elderly patients are more likely to be prescribed these medications for arthritic pain and cardiovascular disease. Aspirin may cause gastric ulceration, but it more commonly leads to gastritis and mucosal erosion.[18] Acetaminophen has not been associated with either peptic ulcer disease or GI bleeding.[19]

Elderly patients, usually men, who have undergone grafting of the aorta or repair of an abdominal aortic aneurysm have an increased risk for massive upper GI bleeding from an aortoenteric fistula. The "herald bleed" is usually a small amount of hematemesis and is followed by massive exsanguinating hemorrhage.[20]

Lower GI Bleeding

Lower intestinal bleeding in the elderly is one-third as common as upper GI bleeding and, in general, less severe. Lower intestinal bleeding stops spontaneously in 80 percent of cases. Up to 15 percent of apparent lower GI bleeding is from an upper GI source. The most common sources of lower GI bleeding in the elderly include colonic diverticulosis, angiodysplasia, NSAID-induced bleeding, colonic ischemia, colitis, proctitis, constipation, hemorrhoids, tumors, and polyps.

Colonic diverticula account for roughly 45 percent of cases of lower intestinal hemorrhage in the elderly. The prevalence of colonic diverticula increases with age, and half the people over the age of 80 have disease[21]; less than 5 percent will experience bleeding.[22] Most serious bleeding occurs in the proximal colon. Most diverticula do not rebleed, and patients usually are treated conservatively without surgery.

Angiodysplasia is a result of dilated submucosal veins due to increased intraluminal pressure.[23] Two-thirds occur in people older than age 70 with equal frequency in men and women. They are usually less than 5 mm and tend to bleed from the proximal ascending colon.[24] Only 15 percent of patients present with massive lower GI bleeding, and 90 percent stop bleeding spontaneously.[25]

NSAIDs have been implicated as a cause in colitis and diverticular bleeding. Patients with diverticular bleeding were more likely to be taking a combination of NSAIDs and aspirin.[26]

Colonic ischemia causes between 3 and 9 percent of cases of acute lower GI bleeding.[27] Angiography rarely demonstrates significant abnormalities and plays a small role in the evaluation of suspected ischemic colitis. Patients present with sudden onset of lower crampy abdominal pain followed by bloody diarrhea within 24 hours. Massive hemorrhage suggests another etiology. Patients do not appear toxic, as they do in acute mesenteric ischemia. Perforation and stricture formation may occur.

Inflammatory bowel disease may present in the elderly as bloody diarrhea. The onset of ulcerative colitis and Crohn's disease has a second peak occurring around age 70. Infectious colitis is common in the elderly. *Salmonella* and *Escherichia coli* may lead to bloody diarrhea.[28] Older people are more susceptible to pseudomembranous colitis due to age and increased exposure to antibiotics. Lower GI bleeding is rare and generally not severe. Patients undergoing radiation therapy for prostate cancer may present with proctitis and mild lower intestinal bleeding. The onset of bleeding can be delayed up to 15 months after radiotherapy.

Hemorrhoids are present in 75 percent of lower GI bleeding evaluations but only account for less than 10 percent of the cases. Bleeding is due to excoriation of the hemorrhoidal tissue. Blood is present in small amounts outside the stool, appearing in the toilet water or on the toilet paper; on occasion, bleeding can be severe.

Constipation in the elderly may cause intestinal bleeding from stercoral ulcers, which cause adherence of stool to the colonic mucosa. Bleeding can be massive following manual disimpaction of hard stool.

Approximately 10 percent of significant lower GI bleeding is due to a neoplasm. Polyps and postpolypectomy bleeding account for 5 percent of lower GI bleeding. Bleeding may occur up to 2 weeks after the procedure.

CLINICAL FEATURES

Peptic ulcer disease in the elderly may present with dyspepsia or pyrosis 1 to 2 hours after meals. However, up to 50 percent of patients taking NSAIDs may present without pain. The pain classically is described as an epigastric, nonradiating, burning discomfort occurring 1 to 2 hours after meals. Patients may awake at night with pain and find relief by eating food or antacids. These symptoms are much less frequent in the elderly population. With perforation, physical examination findings, such as peritonitis, fever, and leukocytosis, may be absent in the elderly.[2] In the setting of altered mental status or dementia, the history may be completely unreliable. These factors can lead to a delayed diagnosis and increased morbidity and mortality if perforation or bleeding occurs.

Perforation occasionally may erode into adjacent organs, such as the pancreas, leading to pancreatitis with peritonitis. Less commonly, a gastric ulcer may be located in the pyloric channel and lead to gastric outlet obstruction. Severe colicky epigastric pain with persistent vomiting after meals is seen generally.

Upper GI bleeding may present with hematemesis, melena, or hematochezia. These symptoms often present with associated anemia and hypovolemia. Patients may be orthostatic or have experienced syncope. The signs of shock may be present with tachypnea, tachycardia, hypotension, and depressed mentation. Elderly patients may not have a corresponding tachycardia if they are taking beta blockers. If hematemesis is present in combination with depressed mentation or compromised protective airway reflexes, aspiration may occur. Melena may result from as little as 60 mL of blood[29] and usually requires at least 8 hours in the digestive tract to turn the stool black.[30]

Lower GI bleeding may present with bloody diarrhea or hematochezia. Blood from the proximal colon may take on a darker, more maroon color. If bleeding is massive enough, symptoms of hypovolemia and shock may be present. Orthostatic changes in vital signs may be the only initial clue to large volume loss.

DIAGNOSIS AND DIFFERENTIAL

Peptic Ulcer Disease

The differential diagnosis of dyspepsia, pyrosis, and epigastric pain seen in peptic ulcer disease includes esophageal disease, acute myocardial infarction or ischemia, pericarditis, pulmonary disease, renal disease, pancreatitis, hepatitis, cholecystitis, cholelithiasis, splenic rupture, surgical causes of peritonitis, acute mesenteric ischemia, diverticulitis, constipation, obstipation, small bowel obstruction, and dissecting or ruptured aortic aneurysm.

The diagnosis of peptic ulcer disease requires endoscopy or an upper GI series, which usually can be ordered on an outpatient basis via the patient's primary physician. Endoscopy has the highest sensitivity and specificity. Advantages include its ability to biopsy suspicious-looking ulcers for malignancy; detect *H. pylori*; diagnose esophagitis, gastritis, or duodenitis; electrocautery bleeding; and measure gastric pH. An upper GI series with barium may identify up to 80 percent of peptic ulcers and is less invasive and less expensive.

Laboratory studies, such as a complete blood count (CBC) and chemistry panel, may identify anemia or co-morbid states. In the setting of perforation, leukocytosis may be present. A 12-lead electrocardiogram (ECG) should be performed on all elderly patients with epigastric pain.

Plain abdominal radiographs may detect viscus perforation or small bowel obstruction but have no diagnostic role in peptic ulcer disease. If the initial upright chest radiograph is normal and perforation is still strongly suspected, a nasogastric tube may be inserted and 300 mL of air insufflated; a repeat upright chest radiograph or a left lateral decubitus radiograph should be taken in 10 minutes. Pneumoperitoneum may be identified in up to 80 percent of cases of perforated viscus on plain radiograph. A computed tomographic (CT) scan with water-soluble contrast material may identify perforation missed by plain radiographs. Perforations into areas such as the lesser sac or retroperitoneum (the first three segments of the duodenum are retroperitoneal) are more easily identified on CT scan.

Upper and Lower GI Bleeding

A nasogastric tube with gastric lavage may demonstrate bleeding or the presence of "coffee grounds" associated with upper GI bleeding. A nonbloody nasogastric aspirate may be seen in 16 percent of patients with upper GI bleeding, usually from a duodenal source.[31] Hemoccult-positive stools suggest the presence of GI blood loss. The "gold standard" for diagnosis and treatment of upper GI bleeding is upper endoscopy.

A history of hematochezia suggests the presence of lower GI bleeding. The rectal examination, including the use of a rigid proctoscope or anoscope, may show rectal or hemorrhoidal bleeding. In the majority of cases, the presence of blood in the rectal vault above the plastic anoscope is all that is visualized. Forty percent of rectal carcinomas diagnosed by rigid proctoscopy are palpable on digital rectal examination.[32] Definitive diagnosis requires the use of colonoscopy. Barium enema examinations in the elderly often are suboptimal.[33]

Laboratory evaluation should include a CBC, chemistry panel, liver panel, coagulation studies, and blood type and crossmatch. An elevated blood urea nitrogen to creatinine ratio (>30:1) with the absence of significant clinical dehydration suggests upper GI bleeding due to protein digestion. A CBC will identify anemia if sufficient time has elapsed from initiation of the GI bleeding. The liver panel and coagulation studies can identify underlying causes.

Angiography and radionuclide scanning with technetium-99m can be helpful when other diagnostic modalities have failed to reveal a source of bleeding. Angiography also allows for therapeutic interventions such as the use of local vasopressor agents and embolization. Radionuclide scanning detects some bleeding that angiography has missed and allows for repeat imaging up to 24 hours later for intermittent lower GI bleeding.

EMERGENCY DEPARTMENT CARE AND DISPOSITION

Peptic Ulcer Disease

Abdominal pain of gastroduodenal origin can range from mild to severe. A through history and physical examination should be performed, and potential life-threatening entities in the differential diagnosis need to be considered. In the elderly, attention to volume status and assessment of orthostatic vital signs are important. The patient should be placed on a cardiac monitor and a 12-lead ECG obtained. A rectal examination with evaluation of stool for blood is mandatory. A nasogastric tube is indicated in the setting of hematemesis, suspected perforation, or volvulus. If perforation is suspected, then intravenous access should be established, intravenous H_2 receptor antagonist and antibiotics administered, and expedient surgical consultation obtained. Gastric lavage is contraindicated in the setting of perforation.

Most patients with peptic ulcer disease have normal vital signs and are stable. A GI cocktail of viscous lidocaine and Maalox may be given for symptomatic relief. This maneuver does not exclude an acute coronary syndrome even if it provides relief of the epigastric pain. An H_2 receptor antagonist may help relieve symptoms and generally is safe and effective. Proton pump inhibitors are even safer in the elderly population and improve ulcer and mucosal healing times, but they are more expensive. Sucralfate coats the mucosa and helps prevent pain. Referral to a gastroenterologist is recommended if conservative therapy has failed. In order to facilitate continuity of care, the antibiotic treatment of *H. pylori* ought to be initiated in consultation with the patient's primary physician. Elderly patients with intractable abdominal pain and signs of dehydration or who are in general debilitated and malnourished should be admitted into the hospital.

GI Bleeding

Elderly patients who present to the ED with a history suggestive of an acute upper or lower GI bleed should be placed on a cardiac monitor and pulse oximetry. Two large-bore intravenous lines should be established, with blood drawn for a type and screen (if stable) or type and crossmatch (if unstable). Patients should receive supplemental oxygen while they are being assessed. The patient's airway, breathing, and circulation status should be assessed carefully.

The assessment of circulation is of particular importance. Overall skin color (paleness) or diaphoresis may represent hypovolemic shock. The central and peripheral capillary refill may provide a clinical clue that peripheral vasoconstriction (elevated peripheral vascular resistance) is attempting to shunt available volume centrally for organ perfusion. The jugular venous pressure can reflect volume depletion and diminished central venous pressure (CVP). A central line not only can provide ample venous access (if peripheral lines are inadequate or unobtainable), but it also can allow measurement of CVP and direct volume resuscitation. A Foley catheter should be placed to monitor end-organ perfusion and effective resuscitation.

If signs of hypovolemic shock are present and the patient's mental status is altered, an initial intravenous crystalloid bolus (20 mL/kg) should be administered and 2 units of O-negative packed red blood cells transfused while crossmatched blood is being prepared. If patients demonstrate continued hemodynamic instability, then they should be intubated to protect their airway, especially if upper endoscopy is planned.

In addition to the administration of packed red blood cells, platelet transfusion and reversal of coagulopathy may be required. Platelets should be administered when active bleeding persists and the platelet count is below 50,000/mm³. Patients on coumadin who are overanticoagulated should receive fresh-frozen plasma and vitamin K (5–10 mg subcutaneously or intramuscularly). Patients on heparin should have the heparin held and should be administered protamine sulfate (1 mg per 100 units of heparin; maximum dose 50 mg at a rate of 5 mg/minute intravenously).

An H_2 antagonist should be administered intravenously; this therapy reduces morbidity and mortality associated with GI bleeding.[34] In the elderly, H_2 antagonists can cause bradycardia and confusion.[35] However, an initial dose in the ED will not likely produce this effect.

Vasopressin (0.2–0.4 units/minute intravenously) has been used to treat esophageal variceal bleeding when a delay in endoscopy is anticipated; however, overall mortality may not be much improved.[36,37] Intravenous nitroglycerin has been used to counteract the side effects of vasopressin.[38] Somatostatin has been shown to be superior to vasopressin in treating bleeding varices, but it does not decrease the need for surgery and it does not reduce the rebleeding rate.[39] Octreotide has been demonstrated to be as effective as emergent sclerotherapy for the initial control of bleeding varices.[40] If a patient is exsanguinating and endoscopy is delayed or fails, placement of a Sengstaken-Blakemore tube may be indicated; this procedure usually controls hemorrhage in 75 percent of cases.[41]

Patients with massive lower GI bleeding should undergo angiography with embolization of arterial bleeding if lower endoscopy is unsuccessful. This treatment can control bleeding in up to 80 percent of cases. If this procedure is unsuccessful, a subtotal colectomy may be indicated. Consultation with a surgeon should be obtained if a patient with upper or lower GI bleeding fails to respond to volume expansion, blood products, medical therapy, and endoscopy.

ADDITIONAL ASPECTS

The following are pitfalls in the management of peptic ulcer disease and GI bleeding:

- Failure to consider myocardial ischemia in patients who present with epigastric pain

- Assuming a negative nasogastric tube lavage completely excludes an upper GI bleed and failing to refer patients to their primary physician or gastroenterologist for further outpatient follow-up

- Assuming that normal hemoglobin and hematocrit levels indicate insignificant blood loss

REFERENCES

1. NIH Consensus Development Panel on *Helicobacter pylori* in peptic ulcer disease. *JAMA* 272:65, 1994.
2. McCarthy D: Acid peptic disease in the elderly. *Clin Geriatr Med* 7:231, 1991.
3. Gilinsk NH: Peptic ulcer disease in the elderly. *Scand J Gastrenterol* 23:191, 1988.
4. Graham DY, Malaty HM, Evans DG, et al: Epidemiology of *Helicobacter pylori* in an asymptomatic population in the United States: Effect of age, race, and socioeconomic status. *Gastroenterology* 100:1495, 1991.
5. Griffin MR: Epidemiology of nonsteroidal anti-inflammatory drugs-associated gastrointestinal injury. *Am J Med* 104:23, 1998.
6. Cooper BT, Weston CF, Neumann CS: Acute upper gastrointestinal hemorrhage in patients aged 80 years or more. *Q J Med* 68:765, 1988.

7. Longstreth GF: Epidemiology and outcome of patients hospitalized with acute lower gastrointestinal hemorrhage: A population-based study. *Am J Gastroenterol* 92:419, 1997.

8. Hurwitz A, Brady DA, Schaal SE, et al: Gastric acidity in older adults. *JAMA* 278:269, 1997.

9. Goldschmidt M, Barrnett CC, Schwarz BE, et al: Effect of age on gastric acid concentration in healthy men and women. *Gastroenterology* 101:997, 1991.

10. Raskin JB, Chong J: NSAID-induced ulcerations, in Bayless TM (ed): *Current Therapy in Gastroenterology and Liver Disease.* St Louis, Mosby, 1994, p 675.

11. Bordley DR, Mushlin AI, Dolan JG, et al: Early clinical signs identify low risk patients with acute upper gastrointestinal hemorrhage. *JAMA* 253:382, 1985.

12. Gilbert DA, Silverstein FE, Tedesco FJ: The national ASGE survey on upper gastrointestinal bleeding, *Gastrointest Endosc* 27:73, 1981.

13. DeBakey M: Acute perforated gastroduodenal ulcer. *Surgery* 8:852, 1940.

14. Gogel HK, Tandenberg D: Emergency management of upper gastrointestinal bleeding. *Am J Emerg Med* 4:150, 1986.

15. Chalmers TC: Fatal gastrointestinal hemorrhage: Clinicopathologic correlation in 101 patients. *Am J Clin Pathol* 22:634, 1952.

16. Sugawa C, Benishek D, Watt AJ: Mallory-Weiss syndrome: A study of 224 patients. *Am J Surg* 145:30, 1983.

17. Graham DY, Schwartz SJ: The spectrum of the Mallory-Weiss tear. *Medicine* 57:307, 1978.

18. Levy M: Aspirin use in patients with major gastrointestinal bleeding and peptic ulcer disease: A report from the Boston University Medical Center. *New Engl J Med* 290:1185, 1974.

19. Levy M: Major upper gastrointestinal bleeding: Relation to the use of aspirin and other nonnarcotic analgesics. *Arch Intern Med* 148:281, 1988.

20. Low RN, Wall SD, Jeffery RB Jr, et al: Aortoenteric fistula and perigraft infection: Evaluation with CT. *Radiology* 175:157, 1990.

21. Morson BC: Pathology of diverticular disease of the colon. *Clin Gastroenterol* 4:37, 1975.

22. McGuire HH, Haynes BW: Massive hemorrhage from diverticulosis of the colon. *Ann Surg* 175:847, 1972.

23. Boley SJ, Sammartano R, Adams A, et al: On the nature and etiology of vascular ectasias in the colon: Degenerative lesions of aging. *Gastroenterology* 72:650, 1977.

24. Richter JM, Christensen MR, Colditz GA, et al: Angiodysplasia: Natural history and efficacy of therapeutic intervention. *Dig Sci* 34:1542, 1989.

25. Boley SJ, DiBase A, Brandt LJ, et al: Lower intestinal bleeding in the elderly. *Am J Surg* 137:57, 1979.

26. Foutch PG: Diverticular bleeding: Are nonsteroidal anti-inflammatory drugs risk factors for hemorrhage and can colonoscopy predict outcome for patients. *Am J Gastroenterol* 90:1779, 1995.

27. Longstreth GF: Epidemiology and outcome of patients hospitalized with acute lower gastrointestinal hemorrhage: A population-based study. *Am J Gastroenterol* 92:419, 1997.

28. Carter AO, Borczyk AA, Carlson JAK, et al: A severe outbreak of *Escherichia coli* O157:H7-associated hemorrhagic colitis in a nursing home. *New Engl J Med* 317:1496, 1984.

29. Daniel A Jr, Egan S: Quantity of blood required to produce tarry stool. *JAMA* 113:2232, 1939.

30. Bogoch A: Bleeding, in Berk JE (ed): *Gastroenterology.* Philadelphia, Saunders, 1985, p 439.

31. Cueller RE, Gavaler JS, Alexander JA, et al: Gastrointestinal tract hemorrhage. *Arch Intern Med* 150:1381, 1990.

32. Steer ML, Silen W: Diagnostic procedures in gastrointestinal hemorrhage. *New Engl J Med* 309:646, 1983.

33. Gurwitz JH, Noonan JP, Sanchez M, et al: Barium enemas in the frail elderly. *Am J Med* 92:41, 1992.

34. Collins R, Langman M: Treatment with histamine H_2 antagonists in acute upper gastrointestinal hemorrhage: Implications of randomized trials. *New Engl J Med* 313:660, 1985.

35. Freston JW: Cimetidine II: Adverse reactions and patterns of use. *Ann Intern Med* 97:573, 1982.

36. Forgel MR, Knauer CM, Andres LL: Continuous intravenous vasopressin in active gastrointestinal bleeding. *Ann Intern Med* 96:565, 1982.

37. Mutchnik MG: Vasopressin in the management of variceal hemorrhage, in Fiddian-Green RG, Turcotte JG (eds): *Gastrointestinal Hemorrhage.* New York, Grune and Stratton, 1980, p 634.

38. Terlanche J, Burroughs AK, Hobbs KEF: Controversies in the management of bleeding esophageal varices. *New Engl J Med* 320:1393, 1989.

39. Jenkins SA, Baxter JN, Corbett W: A prospective randomized controlled clinical trail comparing somatostatin and vasopressin in controlling acute variceal hemorrhage. *Br Med J* 290:275, 1985.

40. Sung JYJ: Octreotide infusion or emergency sclerotherapy for variceal hemorrhage. *Lancet* 342:637, 1993.

41. Chojkler M, Conn HO: Esophageal tamponade in the treatment of bleeding varices: A decade progress report. *Dig Dis Sci* 25:267, 1980.

23

Esophageal Emergencies

Mark E. Hoffmann

HIGH-YIELD FACTS

- Dysphagia has a prevalence of 50 percent in elderly persons living in nursing homes.
- Gastroesophageal reflux disease is more debilitating in the elderly.
- With the exception of esophageal perforation, most causes of esophageal chest pain are not life-threatening and usually do not require hospitalization.
- Barium or Gastrografin contrast studies and endoscopy are key diagnostic procedures in the evaluation of esophageal disease.

Swallowing is a highly coordinated process that involves facial, oral, cervical, laryngeal, and esophageal muscle contractions to transport ingested material to the stomach. Aging affects these various phases to some degree. Impairment of swallowing occurs in several anatomic, muscular, and neurologic disorders that commonly affect the elderly. Dysphagia, the sensation of impaired passage of food from the oropharynx to the stomach, can occur at any age. It is the most common esophageal complaint in the elderly and is estimated to occur in up to 50 percent of patients in long-term care facilities.[1]

Oropharyngeal dysphagia is difficulty in initiating swallowing or transferring food from the oropharynx to the upper esophagus. Disease may arise from stroke, central nervous system tumors, multiple sclerosis, botulism, Zenker's diverticulum, foreign-body obstruction, or the rare cervical osteophytic compression.

Esophageal dysphagia is difficulty in swallowing when ingested material cannot be transported from the hypopharynx through the esophagus into the stomach. Neuromuscular causes of esophageal dysphagia include achalasia, esophageal spasm, and progressive systemic sclerosis. Obstructive causes of dysphagia include foreign bodies, strictures, esophageal rings and webs, aortic compression, and tumors. Disorders of the esophagus that may not necessarily present with dysphagia but rather with pain or bleeding include esophagitis, esophageal varices, gastroesophageal reflux disease (GERD), and esophageal perforation.

EPIDEMIOLOGY

Poor appetite, reduced appreciation for food, and diminished physical activity encompass anorexia-related to aging.[5] Disorders of the esophagus lead to malnutrition and increase the risk of aspiration. Studies have shown dysphagia to have a prevalence of 50 to 60 percent among persons in nursing homes[1] and 10 to 30 percent among those on general medical wards.[6,7] Several studies have demonstrated that the prevalence of heartburn and endoscopic esophagitis increases after age 50.[8,9]

PATHOPHYSIOLOGY

Swallowing is a complex event requiring voluntary and involuntary muscle activity. The process is governed by afferent and efferent cranial nerves. Swallowing can be divided into oral, pharyngeal, and esophageal phases. In the oral phase, salivation with mastication prepares and lubricates a food bolus. The tongue and the buccal muscles direct the bolus to the posterior of the oropharynx. The oral phase exhibits a wide range of pressure variation in the supralingual and intralingual aspects. The effect of aging on deglutitive lingual peristaltic pressure is not well established. Transit time, however, has been reported to be longer in elderly people than in younger people.[10] Stroke (drooling and seventh cranial nerve dysfunction), diseases of the tongue (angioedema, amyloidosis, trauma), difficulty with salivation (drugs, Sjögren's), and dentures can limit this phase. An age- and dentition-related increase in effort during swallowing has been reported.[11]

The pharyngeal phase is marked by voluntary contraction of the tongue against the hard and soft palates with elevation of the larynx and hyoid bone, sealing off the nasopharynx and supralaryngeal/tracheal entrance. The upper esophageal sphincter relaxes, and involuntary peristaltic waves sweep the bolus into the proximal esophagus. The upper esophageal sphincter opening in the elderly tends to be smaller than in younger persons.[12] Dysphagia from upper esophageal lesions is usually perceived within 2 to 4 seconds. Disorders of the pharyngeal phase can lead to regurgitation, aspiration, or obstruction.

During the esophageal phase, the food bolus is propelled by peristalsis through the esophagus and past the relaxed lower esophageal sphincter into the stomach. In the elderly, there is a high rate of lower esophageal sphincter incompetence associated with hiatal hernia and GERD, which becomes more prevalent with advancing age. Several disease states may exist along this conduit. Narrowing of the esophagus by strictures, webs, malignancy, or achalasia may result in progressive dysphagia and lead to complete obstruction by solid foods. Obstruction of esophageal transit also may occur from extrinsic compression by tumors, the aortic arch, or the left main bronchus. Dysphagia from lower esophageal lesions occurs between 4 and 10 seconds after swallowing.

Odynophagia, or pain with swallowing, is mediated by sympathetic afferent fibers. These sensations are detected initially by chemoreceptors, thermoreceptors, mechanoreceptors, and nociceptors. Pain is produced by distension of the esophageal lumen, spasm of muscular layers, or stimulation of the mucosa.

CLINICAL FEATURES

Dysphagia, odynophagia, and pyrosis (heartburn) are the principal symptoms of esophageal disease. The elderly also may complain of respiratory difficulties, chest pain, regurgitation, vomiting, or weight loss. Each disease has certain historical and clinical clues; however, many disorders present vaguely and may have overlapping symptoms.

A Zenker's diverticulum is a posterior herniation of the hypopharynx through the triangular area just above the upper esophageal sphincter. It is encountered once per every 1000 routine upper gastrointestinal (GI) studies. It is more common in men, and approximately 85 percent of the cases occur in people over age 50.[13] Up to 50 percent of these patients have associated esophageal motor disorders.[14] Lateral pharyngeal diverticula and esophageal diverticula also may be encountered. Increased intraluminal pressures and traction from peristalsis are thought to be important etiologic factors. Symptoms usually develop insidiously. An irritation in the back of the throat may be the first complaint. Later, a patient may experience regurgitation and dysphagia. A persistent halitosis also may be present.

Diffuse esophageal spasm is characterized by dysphagia and chest pain.[15,16] Esophageal manometry demonstrates normal peristalsis interrupted by simultaneous disorganized esophageal contractions. Focal distal esophageal contractions ("nutcracker esophagus") also may be seen. Clinically, patients can have chest pain that may be indistinguishable from cardiac pain. Approximately 30 percent of patients

who undergo cardiac catheterization are found to have normal coronary arteries; of these patients, roughly 50 percent have esophageal abnormalities.[2,3] Nonprogressive and intermittent dysphagia is the usual complaint.

Achalasia is a disease of the esophagus resulting from the absence of ganglion cells in the smooth muscle myenteric plexus (Auerbach's plexus). This motor disorder results in a narrowed distal esophagus ("bird beak") at the level of the lower esophageal sphincter. Achalasia becomes more prevalent with advancing age.[17] Symptoms include dysphagia for solids and liquids, pyrosis, regurgitation, and respiratory complaints. In later stages, weight loss and malnutrition become apparent.

Cervical hypertrophic osteoarthropathy occurs in 20 to 30 percent of the general population, most frequently in the elderly. Dysphagia from osteophyte compression on the esophagus occurs rarely. In addition to obstruction from compression, the esophagus may become inflamed and result in a periesophagitis. Patients experience dysphagia and odynophagia predominately.

Foreign bodies may result in complete obstruction of the esophagus; these are most commonly related to a food bolus that becomes impacted. Foreign bodies tend to lodge in areas of narrowing: the cricopharyngeus muscle, the site of the aortic arch, the level of the left primary bronchus, and the diaphragm. In the nonpediatric population, pieces of meat, cartilage, bone, or dentures are usually involved.[18] In the elderly, the higher risk of obstruction is related to underlying anatomic abnormalities. Complete obstructions present with the inability to swallow liquids or even oral secretions. Drooling and spitting is common. Patients experience chest pain with the associated esophageal spasms in the location of the foreign body.

An esophageal ring is a 2- to 4-mm mucosal structure causing a ringlike narrowing of the distal esophagus. The most common is a Schatzki's ring at the gastroesophageal junction. An esophageal web occurs in the middle or upper esophagus as a result of membrane formation from squamous epithelium. Intermittent dysphagia occurs when the diameter of the esophagus approaches 13 mm or less.[19] Commonly, the first clinical presentation involves the proverbial "steakhouse syndrome" after ingestion a large piece of meat. Symptoms are that of complete esophageal obstruction. The incidence of esophageal webs increases with age, and many are incidental findings at endoscopy.

Strictures are a localized narrowing of the esophagus. Strictures of the distal esophagus result from long-standing GERD and repeated irritation of the esophagus by gastric acid. In addition to acid reflux as a source of injury, pill-induced esophagitis can lead to irritation and scarring. Injury-induced strictures also may result from alkali or acidic chemical ingestion. Alkali ingestion, which involves liquefaction necrosis, has a higher risk of esophageal perforation. Dysphagia with solids results over time. Intermittent pyrosis is also encountered.

GERD tends to be more aggressive in the elderly, and studies suggest that elderly patients (age > 60) have milder heartburn in the setting of more severe disease. Mechanisms involve anatomic abnormalities (hiatal hernia), functional abnormalities (lower esophageal sphincter dysfunction), reduced salivary bicarbonate production, and prolonged exposure of the esophagus to refluxed acid. Most esophageal pain requiring evaluation in the emergency department (ED) is caused by GERD.[20] Pyrosis with positional changes is important. Bending forward, lying in the supine position, and straining with defecation tend to exacerbate the pain. Radiation of the pain is an inconsistent finding in GERD. Patients also may experience nausea, shortness of breath, and diaphoresis.

Esophageal malignancy may cause progressive dysphagia and weight loss. Benign tumors of the esophagus are rare. Squamous carcinoma is four times higher in African-Americans. The two major environmental factors that predispose to squamous carcinoma are smoking and alcohol. Adenocarcinoma is less common but generally arises from dysplastic cells associated with Barrett's epithelium. Barrett's esophagitis results from chronic repeated distal esophageal injury from GERD.

Mallory-Weiss syndrome involves longitudinal tears in the mucosa (1–5 cm) at the level the gastroesophageal junction and distal esophagus. Alcohol overuse and repeated retching are significant risk factors. This is one of the most common causes of upper GI bleeding. Bleeding is usually mild and stops spontaneously.[21]

Esophageal varices are related to venous dilatation associated with collateral venous flow resulting from portal hypertension. Variceal bleeding accounts for approximately one-third of deaths associated with massive upper GI bleeding.

Esophagitis results from infection of the esophageal mucosa. HIV disease, malignancy, immunosuppressants, diabetes, alcoholism, or advanced age may weaken host defenses against these infections.[22] Chest pain and dysphagia predominate. Infectious agents include *Candida albicans,* herpes simplex virus, cytomegalovirus, varicella-zoster virus, and mycobacteria.

Esophageal perforation is the most immediately life-threatening esophageal disease. Approximately 50 percent of all esophageal perforations are iatrogenic (endoscopy, nasogastric tube placement, endotracheal intubation, or surgery). Other causes include caustic injury, severe esophagitis, foreign bodies, penetrating trauma, or Boerhaave's syndrome. Boerhaave's syndrome is spontaneous perforation that results from repeated forceful vomiting usually associated with alcohol ingestion.[23] Saliva, ingested material, and bacteria gain access to the mediastinum, and life-threatening sepsis may ensue. Symptoms include substernal chest pain described as a burning sensation, dyspnea, tachycardia, and fever. Patients often experience neck, chest, and abdominal pain. Mediastinal emphysema may be appreciated when auscultating the chest (Hamman's sign). Subcutaneous air also may be noticed when palpating the neck.

DIAGNOSIS AND DIFFERENTIAL

The diagnosis of esophageal disorders can be challenging. Depending on the presentation and the stage at which a patient becomes symptomatic, historical and physical examination findings may be subtle. The majority of disorders will be detected by either radiographic swallow studies or directed visualization under endoscopy.

Dysphagia may be caused by a number of disorders, including stroke, myasthenia gravis, scleroderma, multiple sclerosis, polio, diphtheria, botulism, tetanus, rabies, amyotrophic lateral sclerosis, central nervous system tumor, diabetic neuropathy, lead poisoning, and Parkinson's disease.

Pyrosis, chest pain, or shortness of breath may be due to myocardial ischemia, myocardial infarction, pericarditis, pericardial effusion, pneumothorax, pulmonary emboli, pneumonia, pneumonitis, gastritis, peptic ulcer disease, biliary disease, hepatitis, pancreatitis, or a perforated viscus.

Less specific symptoms such as nausea, vomiting, and anorexia involve a much larger differential diagnosis in the elderly population and warrant a systematic approach to those complaints.

Depending on the history and physical examination, laboratory studies are more useful in the evaluation of diseases suspected in the differential and in determining the degree of complication related to esophageal disease rather than the actual diagnosis. For example, a white blood cell count may suggest an infectious or more serious cause of symptoms. A complete blood cell count with a cell differential may indicate degree and type of associated anemia. Determination of electrolytes and the blood urea nitrogen to creatinine ratio may help assess hydration status and evaluate comorbid states such as renal disease. If hepatic, pancreatic, or biliary causes are suspected, then liver function tests and lipase level determination would be appropriate. When an acute cardiac syndrome is even remotely suspected, an electrocardiogram and cardiac enzymes should be obtained.

Radiographic studies such as a soft tissue neck and chest radiograph can help identify radiopaque foreign bodies, including their shape, size, and location. Radiographs also may reveal subcutaneous air, large anatomic abnormalities (tumor with mass effect, hiatal hernia, osteophytic impingement), or potential cardiopulmonary diseases. Esophageal perforation can be associated with left-sided pleural effusion, subcutaneous air, pneumomediastinum, pneumopericardium, or pneumothorax. Computed tomographic (CT) scans also may aid in the detection of perforation. These studies can be helpful under certain clinical conditions but are unreliable and insufficient in excluding esophageal disease.

Barium- or Gastrografin-contrasted swallow studies are helpful in the evaluation of esophageal disease. These are usually performed under the care of a gastroenterologist. Contrasted swallow studies can show both intrinsic and extrinsic (compressive) anatomic deformities. Caution should be used when there is a risk for aspiration or esophageal perforation If a patient is able to swallow liquids or his or her secretions, these studies usually can be performed on an outpatient basis.

Endoscopy has become the diagnostic and therapeutic procedure of choice in most settings. It allows for direct visualization of the anatomy and the mucosa. Biopsy can be obtained for histologic study in the setting of tumor or esophagitis. Direct treatment of esophageal bleeding is possible, as well as the removal of a foreign body. Again, with the exception of foreign-body removal, most studies can be performed on an outpatient basis under the care of a gastroenterologist.

EMERGENCY DEPARTMENT CARE AND DISPOSITION

Patients with inflammatory or neuromuscular causes of dysphagia who can tolerate fluids or their own secretions can be discharged with close follow-up. If they have evidence of malnutrition, dehydration, or aspiration, then further therapy and workup are appropriate.

Patients with a foreign body that is oropharyngeal in nature should undergo removal of the foreign body in the ED. Using radiographs, a dental mirror, or a fiberoptic nasopharyngeal scope, the location of the foreign body may be identified. With topical sprays and sufficient oropharyngeal mucosal anesthesia, foreign-body removal with a

Kelly clamp or bayonet forceps may be possible. Failure to remove the foreign body requires endoscopic removal under the care of a specialist.

Foreign bodies that are impacted in the esophagus (usually food) may be passed through to the stomach with facilitation by glucagon and effervescent liquids (soft drinks). Glucagon 0.5 mg intravenously (up to 2.0 mg total) may relax the smooth esophageal muscles to allow passage in 50 percent of patients.[24] The combined use of soft drinks and glucagon can result in the passage of the obstructive food bolus in up to 80 percent of patients undergoing treatment.[25] Glucagon should be avoided in patients with risk for airway aspiration. Side effects of glucagon include hyperglycemia, nausea, vomiting, hypotension, and flushing. Contraindications to glucagon use include patients with a known insulinoma or pheochromocytoma. Patients relieved of their obstruction need outpatient endoscopy to assess for underlying disease.

Patients with a sharp-edged foreign-body obstruction in the esophagus or who have failed to pass an obstructive esophageal food bolus should undergo endoscopic removal in the ED. Studies have suggested that use of the "push technique" (food bolus is pushed through the esophagus to the stomach) is safe, effective, and efficient.[26,27] Objects in the esophagus longer than 5 cm or wider than 2 cm rarely pass spontaneously.

If esophagitis is suspected, treatment should be targeted toward symptomatic relief. Referral should be made for identification of causative pathogen and for initiation of appropriate antimicrobial therapy. Patients who are debilitated, excessively dehydrated, at risk for aspiration, or experiencing intractable pain or who have no follow-up care may require hospitalization. Antacids, H_2 blockers, topical anesthetics, or sucralfate may provide temporary relief.

Treatment of patients with diagnosed esophageal motility disorders such as esophageal spasm may respond to various medications. Nitroglycerin may help relax smooth muscle spasm. Anticholinergic drugs such as Bentyl or Levsin and calcium channel blockers may decrease the intensity of esophageal spasm. However, these medications also reduce the lower esophageal sphincter tone and may delay gastric emptying, resulting in the reflux of gastric contents and worsening symptoms.

Patients with suspected GERD should be provided symptomatic relief in the ED after the more life-threatening causes of their symptoms have been carefully addressed. H_2 blockers or a cocktail of Maalox and viscous lidocaine may help relieve symptoms. Patients should be instructed on lifestyle and behavioral issues.

Sleeping with the head of the bed elevated, avoiding exercise after meals, avoiding eating before sleep, eliminating smoking and alcohol use, limiting caffeine intake, and eating low-fat meals assist in controlling GERD symptoms.

Patients with GERD who are taking medications that decrease lower esophageal sphincter tone (anticholinergics or calcium channel blockers) may need to be switched to a different medication. Proton pump inhibitors should be considered for disease refractory to H_2 blockers. Sucralfate is a mucosal barrier therapy taken before meals and at bedtime. It absorbs and inactivates bile salts that may be refluxing as well. Prokinetic agents (metoclopramide, cisapride) increase lower esophageal sphincter tone and promote gastric emptying, thus decreasing the reflux of gastric contents.

Patients with suspected GERD need referral to a specialist for further evaluation and treatment. A gastroenterologist may perform an upper GI series or endoscopy. Peptic ulcer disease, the presence of *Heliobacter pylori*, lesions suspicious for malignancy, and Barrett's esophagitis will require further treatment. Patients who have GERD that is refractory to medical management umay ltimately undergo surgical treatment (Nissen fundoplication or other surgical intervention).

Esophageal perforation requires aggressive evaluation and treatment. Expedient airway management may be required to protect the airway. If the patient appears septic, intravenous fluid or pressor may need to be administered to support the patient's hemodynamic status. An intravenous dose of antibiotics should be administered during the evaluation if a high suspicion for perforation exists. The use of a second-generation cephalosporin in combination with an aminoglycoside provides sufficient antimicrobial coverage.[28] Emergent surgical consultation is required. Mortality rates of 45 and 20 percent were found in esophageal perforation patients undergoing conservative and operative management, respectively.[29]

ADDITIONAL ASPECTS

The following are common pitfalls in the management of esophageal disease:

- Failure to consider cardiac ischemia in the evaluation of nonspecific chest symptoms
- Failure to refer elderly patients with GERD or mild dysphagia for an appropriate workup with a gastroenterologist

REFERENCES

1. Trupe EH, Siebens H, Siebens A: Prevalence of feeding and swallowing disorders in a nursing home. Paper presented at the American Congress of Rehabilitation Medicine, Boston, 1984.
2. Castell DO: Chest pain of undetermined origin: Overview of pathophysiology. *Am J Med* 92:2, 1992.
3. Davies HA: Anginal pain of esophageal origin: Clinical presentation, prevalence, and prognosis. *Am J Med* 92:5, 1992.
4. Morley JE: Anorexia of aging: Physiologic and pathologic. *Am J Clin Nutr* 66:760, 1997.
5. Groher ME: The prevalence of swallowing disorders in two teaching hospitals. *Dysphagia* 1:3, 1986.
6. Layne KA, Lsinski DS, Zenner PM, et al: Using the Fleming Index of dysphagia to establish prevalence. *Dysphagia* 4:39, 1989.
7. Thompson WG, Keaton KW: Heartburn and globus in apparently healthy people. *Can Med Assoc J* 126:46, 1982.
8. Brunner PL, Karmody AM, Needham CD, et al: Severe peptic esophagitis. *Gut* 10:831, 1969.
9. Cook IJ, Weltman MD, Wallace K, et al: Influence of aging on oral-pharyngeal bolus transit and clearance during swallowing: Scintigraphic study. *Am J Physiol* 266:G972, 1994.
10. Feldman RS, Kapur KK, Alman JE, et al: Aging and mastication: Changes in performance and in the swallowing threshold with natural dentition. *J Am Geriatr Soc* 28:97, 1980.
11. Kern MS, Bardan E, Arndorfer R, et al: Comparison of upper esophageal sphincter opening in healthy asymptomatic young and elderly volunteers. *Ann Otol Rhinol Laryngol* 108:982, 1999.
12. Holinger PH, Schild JA: The Zenker's (hypopharyngeal) diverticulum. *Ann Otol* 78:679, 1969.
13. Kaye MD: Esophageal motor dysfunction in patients with diverticula of the mid-thoracic esophagus. *Thorax* 29:666, 1974.
14. Castell DO: Achalasia and diffuse esophageal spasm. *Arch Intern Med* 136:571, 1976.
15. Richter JE, Castell DO: Diffuse esophageal spasm: A reappraisal. *Ann Intern Med* 100:789, 1981.
16. Sonnenberg A, Massey BT, McCarty DJ, et al: Epidemiology of hospitalization for achalasia in the United States. *Dig Dis Sci* 38:233, 1993.
17. Webb WA: Management of foreign bodies of the upper gastrointestinal tract. *Gastroenterology* 94:204, 1988.
18. Schatzki R: The lower esophageal ring: Long-term follow-up of symptomatic and asymptomatic rings. *AJRl* 90:805, 1963.
19. Castell DO: The lower esophageal sphincter: physiologic and clinical aspects. *Ann Intern Med* 83:390, 1975.
20. Graham DY, Schwartz SJ: The spectrum of the Mallory-Weiss tear. *Medicine* 57:307, 1978.

21. Baehr PH, McDonald GB: Esophageal infections: Risk factors, presentation, diagnosis, and treatment. *Gastroenterology* 106:509, 1994.

22. Henderson JA, Peloquin AJ: Boerhaave revisited: Spontaneous esophageal perforation as a diagnostic masquerader. *Am J Med* 86:559, 1989.

23. Glauser J, Lilja GP, Greenfeld B, et al: Intravenous glucagon in the management of esophageal food obstruction. *J Am Coll Emerg Phys* 8:228, 1979.

24. Robbins MI, Shortsleeve MJ: Treatment of acute esophageal food impaction with glucagon, an effervescent agent, and water. *AJR* 162:325, 1994.

25. Vicari JJ, Johanson JF, Frakes JT: Outcomes of acute esophageal food impaction: Success of the push technique. *Gastrointest Endosc* 53:178, 2001.

26. Weinstock LB, Shatz BA, Thyssen SE: Esophageal food bolus obstruction: Evaluation of extraction and modified push techniques in 75 cases. *Endosopy* 31:421, 1999.

27. Oringer MB: Tumors, injuries, and miscellaneous conditions of the esophagus, in Greenfield LJ (ed): *Surgery: Scientific Principles and Practice*. Philadelphia, Lippincott, 1993, p 564.

28. Okten I, Cangir AK, Ozdemir N, et al: Management of esophageal perforation. *Surg Today* 31:36, 2001.

24

Diverticular Disease

Robert A. Schwab
Kary Kaltenbronn

HIGH-YIELD FACTS

- Diverticulitis is associated with advanced age and a low-fiber diet.
- Only 15 to 20 percent of patients with diverticular disease become symptomatic.
- Diverticular hemorrhage is the most common cause of major lower gastrointestinal bleeding in the elderly.
- Computed tomographic (CT) scanning is the most useful diagnostic study.
- Follow-up colonoscopy is mandatory to exclude carcinoma.

Acute abdominal pain in the elderly patient presents the clinician with a diagnostic challenge. The differential diagnosis is broad and includes many potentially life-threatening disorders. Diverticular disease always should be included in the differential diagnosis in this patient population because the prevalence of this disorder is greater than 50 percent, particularly in Western societies.[1]

The presentation of diverticular disease in the elderly patient may range from mild discomfort to massive lower gastrointestinal hemorrhage. For the most part, the history and physical examination are nonspecific, and diagnostic testing is required to establish a definitive diagnosis. Fortunately, available diagnostic studies are quite accurate.

Treatment of mild, uncomplicated episodes of diverticulitis and painful diverticulosis is straightforward, but most cases in the elderly will require admission and treatment by a specialist. The emergency physician's knowledge of the epidemiology and pathophysiology of diverticular disease will ensure accurate diagnosis, management, and disposition and assist in preventing recurrent episodes of this common disorder.

EPIDEMIOLOGY

Diverticulosis is a disease primarily affecting elderly members of modern industrialized societies. Rarely reported before the beginning of the twentieth century, diverticular disease is now recognized as a common acquired disorder that is found in more than half of all adults over age 60.[1] The prevalence seems to be roughly equal in men and women, although some studies report a higher prevalence in women.[2]

The association between diet and the development of diverticular disease is well established. The highest rates of diverticulosis are seen in the United States, Europe, and Australia, all modern societies with a Western diet that is high in fat and refined carbohydrates.[1,3] Conversely, in poorly developed African countries where the diet contains more dietary fiber, much lower rates of diverticular disease are observed.[1,3] Studies in countries that have recently undergone westernization have shown sharply increasing rates of diverticulosis paralleling the availability of more processed foods.[3]

Ethnicity appears to play a role in the development of this disease as well. Within a given geographic location, Europeans demonstrate a much higher prevalence of diverticulosis than do adults of African, Indian, or East Asian descent.[3] There is also a difference in the anatomic distribution of the disease: Asian populations have a much higher prevalence of ascending colonic involvement,[2,4] whereas members of Western societies manifest disease in the sigmoid colon almost exclusively.[5] These changes have persisted despite changes in diet, suggesting that there are genetic determinants of diverticular disease as well.[3]

Patients with collagen-vascular disorders appear to have an increased incidence of diverticular disease, and collagen disorders are frequently found in association with young adults and even children diagnosed with diverticulosis.[2] Immunocompromised patients do not have an increased risk of developing diverticular disease, but the complications of the disease are harder to detect and often more severe.[1] As advances in medicine allow immunocompromised patients to live longer, the clinical characteristics of diverticular disease may change in important ways.

PATHOPHYSIOLOGY

The pathophysiology of diverticular disease is related to alterations in bowel wall anatomy and intraluminal pressure.[1,5] Colonic diverticula are herniations of mucosa and submucosa through weaknesses in the circular muscle layer of the colonic wall. Since these herniations do not contain all layers of the bowel wall, *pseudodiverticula* is the more precise descriptive histologic term.

Diverticula typically occur in rows between the mesenteric and lateral tenia, or longitudinal muscle layers external to the circular layer.[1,2,5] Herniation is usually observed at the site of penetration of vessels supplying the submucosa because this is the area of greatest muscular weakness.[1,5] Gross examination of pathologic specimens from patients with diverticular disease reveals marked thickening of both muscle layers.[6] Microscopic examination shows the thickening to be due to increased elastin deposition between the muscle cells rather than due to hypertrophy of the muscle cells themselves.[7] Elastin causes contraction of the tenia and bunching of the circular muscle layers; the net effect is narrowing of the colonic lumen and production of multiple isolated bowel segments, a deformity called *myochosis*.[8]

Other anatomic changes related to aging contribute to the pathophysiology of diverticulosis. Atherosclerosis may cause deterioration of the elastin fibers in the circular muscle layer, and age-related increases in collagen cross-linking further decrease the tensile strength of the bowel wall.[2,5] The net effect of these anatomic abnormalities is an increase in intraluminal colonic pressure.

The forces acting on the colonic wall are explained by the law of Laplace, which states that intraluminal pressure varies inversely with the radius of a cylinder and directly with the cylinder wall thickness.[2] The narrowest portion of the colon is the sigmoid; myochosis produces segmental complete occlusion of its lumen with marked increases in intraluminal pressures within each isolated "little bladder."[8] Herniation of mucosa can then occur in areas of relative muscle weakness. Other age-related factors contributing to increased intraluminal pressure include lower stool weights (often related to low-fiber diet as well as age); increased gastrointestinal transit time, which increases water absorption; and constipation, which is aggravated by a sedentary lifestyle and polypharmacy.[2,5]

Diverticulitis is thought to occur as a result of diverticular neck obstruction by inspissated stool. Inflammation ensues due to irritation of the mucosa by the fecalith, with resulting vascular obstruction and colonic bacterial proliferation. The thin-walled diverticulum is highly susceptible to vascular compromise, ischemia, and ultimately, microperforation, which is characteristic of diverticulitis. Microperforations usually are contained by the mesentery or pericolic fat, resulting in peridiverticulitis, or uncomplicated diverticulitis. Complicated diverticulitis occurs when the infection and inflammation produce intestinal obstruction, free perforation into the peritoneal cavity, or fistula or abscess formation.

CLINICAL FEATURES

Although diverticulosis is quite common in the geriatric population, most patients will remain asymptomatic; overall, 15 to 20 percent of patients with diverticular disease will present clinically.[2] Most of the symptomatic patients will present with painful diverticulosis, whereas the remaining small percentage will present with diverticulitis, complicated diverticulitis, or diverticular hemorrhage.

Painful diverticulosis produces lower abdominal pain often accompanied by bloating and a change in bowel habits. Constipation is more common than diarrhea.[2] The pain is frequently located on the left side, may be colicky or steady, and often is exacerbated by eating and relieved by defecation. Physical examination reveals no fever or peritoneal signs, although there is often left lower quadrant tenderness with or without a palpable distended sigmoid colon.

Diverticulitis often begins with abdominal pain in the hypogastrium that later localizes to the left lower quadrant, although right-sided disease can occur. The pain may be constant or intermittent and associated with a change in bowel habits. Anorexia, nausea, vomiting, or hematochezia may be present. If the affected bowel segment lies near the urinary bladder, dysuria, frequency, and urgency can occur. Signs associated with diverticulitis include fever, which is seen in the majority of cases,[5] and localized tenderness, usually in the left lower quadrant, often accompanied by guarding and rebound tenderness confined to the area.[1,2,5] A mass may be palpable in the area. Rectal examination may reveal tenderness in the left pelvis with or without a palpable mass, and the stool may test positive for the presence of blood; gross bleeding is uncommon in acute diverticulitis, however.[5]

Patients with complicated diverticulitis may present with many of the same symptoms as patients with uncomplicated disease or may present with a much more dramatic clinical picture in the presence of uncontained perforation into the peritoneal cavity. Free perforation or rupture of a peridiverticular abscess should be suspected when patients present with unstable vital signs including hypotension, tachycardia, tachypnea, and fever. The presence of diffuse signs of peritoneal irritation suggest free perforation as well.

Less dramatic presentations also may be seen in patients whose diverticulitis produces other complications. Patients with colovesicular fistulas will present with pneumaturia, fecaluria, or recurrent urinary tract infections.[2] Patients with obstruction related to diverticular disease usually will present with abdominal pain, distension, and constipation or obstipation. Nausea and vomiting may be present, and physical examination will reveal distension with tympany, altered bowel sounds, and localized tenderness.

Diverticular hemorrhage is associated primarily with diverticulosis and is not often seen in the presence of diverticulitis.[5] Although less than half of all patients with diverticular disease will experience occult or gross bleeding at some point, the incidence of bleeding increases with advanced age; diverticular hemorrhage is the most common cause of major lower gastrointestinal tract bleeding in the elderly.[9]

The bleeding is usually painless or associated with only mild, crampy pain.[2] Patients often complain of melena or bright red blood in the stool. Depending on the amount of blood loss, vital signs may be normal or consistent with significant hypovolemia. Less than 5 percent of patients require transfusion, so clinical shock is uncommon.[5]

As with other abdominal disorders, the presentation of diverticular disease and its complications may be muted in the elderly patient population. Physiologic changes associated with aging combined with the effects of comorbidities and polypharmacy may mask many of the classic signs and symptoms of diverticulitis and its complications. The classic (and unhelpful) admonition to "maintain a high index of suspicion" should be abandoned in favor of a recommendation to lower one's threshold for ordering imaging studies in elderly patients with abdominal complaints and in demented or obtunded older patients with a decline in their level of functioning.

DIAGNOSIS AND DIFFERENTIAL

The differential diagnosis of patients with signs and symptoms related to diverticular disease is broad (Table 24-1). The most important emergent conditions to exclude in the elderly are abdominal aortic aneurysm, ischemic colitis, volvulus, and acute appendicitis. Symptomatic diverticulosis can mimic any cause of vague abdominal pain, including bacterial and viral enteritis, inflammatory bowel disease, irritable bowel syndrome, and ovarian pathology in women.[2,5] Definitive differentiation of these entities often requires imaging procedures and further evaluation by consultants. When fever and more localized pain and tenderness typical of diverticulitis are present, the differential diagnosis should include acute appendicitis, inflammatory bowel disease, other types of

Table 24-1. Differential Diagnosis of Diverticular Disease and Its Complications

Abdominal aortic aneurysm
Acute appendicitis
Arteriovenous malformation hemorrhage
Carcinoma of the colon
Colitis: ischemic, pseudomembranous, amebic, ulcerative
Crohn's disease
Ovarian pathology: hemorrhagic cyst, painful cyst, torsion, tumor
Pelvic inflammatory disease
Perforated viscus
Polyposis with hemorrhage
Pyelonephritis
Volvulus

colitis (ischemic, pseudomembranous, and amebic), pyelonephritis, pelvic inflammatory disease, or other intraabdominal infections.

In complicated diverticulitis, the differential diagnosis depends on the specific complication. Free perforation may mimic perforated peptic ulcer, whereas obstruction may suggest the presence of a tumor or volvulus. Fistula formation can be seen with inflammatory bowel diseases. Gastrointestinal bleeding should lead the clinician to consider arteriovenous malformations, colonic polyps, and carcinoma of the colon as possible etiologies.

In mild cases of symptomatic diverticulosis, a presumptive diagnosis and empirical treatment with close follow-up may be appropriate. However, patients with more severe symptoms and elderly patients most often will require diagnostic testing during the emergency department (ED) visit to help guide appropriate treatment and disposition.

Diagnosis

Complete Blood Count

Leukocytosis is a common finding in diverticulitis. Various studies report sensitivities between 70 and 85 percent.[10] The specificity of this test is extremely low, however, and its predictive value (positive or negative) in the elderly is not high enough to make it a strong discriminator. An elevated white blood cell (WBC) count should prompt further investigation and will provide support for involving consultants in the management of the patient. Ultimately, the patient's clinical presentation is far more important than a blood test; a normal WBC count never excludes serious pathology, especially in the elderly.

Urinalysis

Pyuria, bacteriuria, and fecaluria may be seen if colovesical fistulas are present, and pyuria also may exist when inflammation adjacent to the ureter or bladder is present. Given the high prevalence of asymptomatic pyuria, bacteriuria, and urinary tract infection in the geriatric population, these abnormal urinary findings are potentially more dangerous than helpful because they may distract the clinician from more aggressive pursuit of the proper diagnosis.

Abdominal Radiographs

Plain abdominal films may be helpful in the diagnosis of complicated diverticular disease. Frank pneumoperitoneum is seen in only 10 percent of patients with acute diverticulitis,[2,5] and the overall sensitivity for any abnormality is less than 50 percent,[2,5] but findings of bowel dilatation, ileus, bowel wall thickening, and obstruction may be seen. These findings may guide consultation and disposition but more often are indications for further diagnostic evaluation.

Computed Tomography

The most useful diagnostic modality for ED diagnosis of diverticular disease is computed tomographic (CT) scanning.[1] CT scanning provides noninvasive visualization of transluminal and extraluminal disease and also can be useful therapeutically to guide percutaneous drainage of abscesses. Risks are confined to those associated with the use of intravenous contrast material, which should be used unless contraindicated.

Uncomplicated diverticula appear as outpouchings from the colonic wall; these outpouchings contain air, enteroliths, or contrast material. Muscular wall thickening highlighted by contrast-filled diverticula give the colon a characteristic "sawtooth" pattern.[11] Diverticulitis produces focal colonic wall thickening, pericolonic fat stranding, free fluid, and in cases of abscess formation, phlegmon, air bubbles, and free fluid.[2] The abscess itself appears as a thick-walled fluid collection often containing air. Fistulas are identifiable as contrast-filled tracts extending from the affected segment of the colon to adjacent structures. The "arrowhead sign" is an arrowhead-shaped collection of contrast material adjacent to focally inflamed colonic wall. This sign, reported in 17 percent of patients

with diverticulitis, is seen only if rectal contrast material is administered.[12]

CT scanning also can assist is distinguishing diverticular disease from other entities such as carcinoma, in which fluid collections are seen less often and which often is accompanied by pericolic lymph node enlargement. A completely normal-appearing CT scan of the sigmoid colon should prompt a search for an alternate diagnosis because the overall high sensitivity of CT scanning (69–98 percent) has been demonstrated in multiple trials.[13,14] Although specificity is also high (75–100 percent),[13,14] follow-up endoscopic examination should be performed after resolution of symptoms to exclude colonic neoplasia.

Ultrasonography

Ultrasonography is a noninvasive, low-cost alternative to CT scanning for diagnostic imaging in patients with suspected diverticular disease. Diverticula can be seen along with associated inflammatory changes, including hypoechoic bowel wall thickening and hyperechogenicity surrounding the bowel wall.[15] Use of a graded compression technique, which identifies focal tenderness and displaces bowel gas, increases the accuracy of the examination.[16] Sensitivity and specificity have been reported to be 80 to 98 percent in several studies[16–18]; this rate compares favorably with the performance of CT scanning as a diagnostic modality for diverticular disease. Ultrasonography remains a second-line diagnostic modality, however, because its diagnostic accuracy is highly operator-dependent and because performance of the examination is more painful than performance of CT scanning.[1] In direct comparative studies, CT scanning appears to perform as well or better.[19,20]

Other Diagnostic Studies

Contrast enemas were the diagnostic study of choice for many years but have been largely replaced by CT scanning. Although diverticula are readily visualized with the use of water-soluble contrast material, extraluminal disease is not well delineated, and differentiation of diverticular disease and carcinoma is difficult. In addition, performance of the examination is associated with an increased risk of perforation. Similarly, endoscopy carries a higher risk of perforation when performed in the acute phase of diverticular disease.[5] Colonoscopy should be deferred until the acute symptoms have resolved (6–8 weeks after the initial presentation) but is mandatory in all patients to exclude neoplastic disease.

Recent studies suggest that magnetic resonance imaging (MRI) may provide excellent diagnostic accuracy in the evaluation of suspected diverticular disease.[21] It is more expensive and less available than CT scanning but may assume a more prominent diagnostic role in the future.

EMERGENCY DEPARTMENT CARE AND DISPOSITION

As for all ED patients, the first priority for patients with diverticular disease is to ensure the integrity of the airway, breathing, and circulation. Patients with significant gastrointestinal bleeding, free intraperitoneal perforation, or sepsis may present with diminished level of consciousness and require intubation or may present with unstable vital signs and require rapid resuscitation via large-bore intravenous lines. Blood and component therapy may be required in patients with hemodynamically significant gastrointestinal bleeding.

Blood cultures should be obtained from patients thought to have perforation or sepsis. Empirical antibiotic coverage effective against gram-negative and anaerobic bacteria should be administered pending the results of diagnostic studies.

More commonly, diverticular disease will manifest as a hemodynamically stable patient with abdominal pain. Initial ED management will include intravenous hydration, analgesics, and antibiotics. All patients with suspected diverticular disease should be given nothing by mouth pending the results of diagnostic studies.

Fluid status should be assessed by paying close attention to the history of oral intake and by evaluating the moisture content of mucous membranes and skin. In the absence of underlying renal dysfunction, blood urea nitrogen and creatinine blood level determinations may be useful. Urine specific gravity can be assessed relatively rapidly and provides a rough estimate of hydration status. Bladder catheterization, although invasive, provides an immediate urine specimen and allows for ongoing urine output monitoring to assess the effectiveness of rehydration.

Initial rehydration usually can be accomplished with 0.45% normal saline at a rate of 250 to 500 mL/h. This rate, which should be adjusted to achieve adequate urine output, provides adequate maintenance fluids and replaces 1 to 2 L during a typical ED visit. Although significant fluid overload is unlikely with this regimen, the clinician should factor in any history of cardiovascular disease. Patients with high fever and those who are found

to have bowel obstruction may have larger fluid deficits and thus should be rehydrated more vigorously. Catheterization is indicated in these patients so that fluid status can be monitored continuously.

Analgesia should be given early and in adequate amounts to control discomfort. The ideal agent would have a rapid onset of action, few side effects, and a brief duration of action so that reassessment of patient status could be done frequently. Fentanyl probably approaches this ideal more than any other agent. Given in small doses (0.5–1.0 μg/kg), it provides rapid improvement in patient comfort without significant hemodynamic effects. Respiratory depression can occur; oxygen saturation should be monitored during administration of fentanyl. Nausea also can occur and may require coadministration of an antiemetic. The duration of effect is typically about 1 hour, which provides time for diagnostic studies and which allows for accurate reassessment of physical findings by the emergency physician and consultant at frequent intervals. Meperidine has been recommended due to its effects on intraluminal pressure, and morphine generally is not recommended because it can produce colonic spasm.[1] Both these agents can cause hypotension and significant respiratory depression in addition to nausea and vomiting.

Antibiotic coverage should be directed against typical colonic flora, including gram-negative and anaerobic species, particularly *Bacteroides fragilis* and *Escherichia coli*.[22] Intravenous regimens should include clindamycin or metronidazole in combination with an aminoglycoside or a third-generation cephalosporin. Oral therapy with metronidazole or clindamycin combined with a fluoroquinolone for 7 to 10 days should provide adequate coverage.

Hospitalization is indicated in unstable patients, patients with active gastrointestinal bleeding, and patients with diverticular disease who cannot tolerate oral intake, whose pain cannot be managed with oral analgesics, who have fever or peritoneal signs on physical examination, or who do not have a supportive home environment. Immunocompromised patients and patients with other significant comorbidities should be treated in an inpatient setting. In addition, patients whose diagnostic studies indicate complicated diverticulitis (obstruction, abscess, fistula) should be hospitalized. Laboratory data that should contribute to the decision to admit include leukocytosis and a falling hematocrit in the presence of guaiac-positive stool. Consultation with a surgeon should be considered in all cases, although admission to an internist or gastroenterologist is usually appropriate.

Outpatient therapy, although fairly common in younger

patients, should be the exception in the geriatric population. If symptoms are mild, physical findings are limited to localized tenderness without peritoneal signs, and diagnostic evaluation demonstrates no complications, patients can be considered for outpatient management, provided that oral intake is adequate, pain can be controlled, and the home environment is supportive. Patients treated at home should be instructed to rest, take a clear liquid diet for 48 hours, and expect improvement in 48 to 72 hours. In addition, patients should have adequate transportation and the ability to follow up with a primary care physician in 1 to 2 days. The patient should be instructed to return immediately to the ED for fever, increased pain, or inability to tolerate oral medications or liquids.

Painful diverticulosis can be treated with a high-fiber diet, which should be recommended to all patients with diverticular disease after the acute phase of their illness. Daily ingestion of 20 to 30 g of coarse bran has been shown to increase stool weight, speed transit time, and reduce intraluminal pressure in the colon.[2] If patients find it difficult to ingest that amount of daily fiber, bulk-forming agents such as psyllium can be substituted. Fiber can improve symptoms and help to prevent worsening of disease.

Definitive treatment of diverticular abscesses depends on the extent of the disease. A useful grading system has been described by Hinchey and colleagues[23] (Table 24-2). Patients with stage I disease are treated medically. Stage II disease requires drainage, which often can be performed percutaneously with CT guidance. Use of percutaneous drainage may avoid the need for a two-stage surgical procedure with colostomy. Stage III and stage IV disease involve free peritoneal contamination and thus require staged surgical intervention and creation of a colostomy for fecal diversion. The morbidity and mortality associated with this more extensive disease and more complicated management are high.

Table 24-2. Hinchey Diverticular Abscess Classification System

Stage I: Confined pericolic abscess
Stage II: Retroperitoneal or pelvic abscess
Stage III: Free peritoneal rupture without fecal contamination (noncommunicating)
Stage IV: Fecal peritonitis due to free perforation of a communicating diverticulum

Source: Adapted with permission from Hinchey EJ, Schaal PH, Richards MB: Treatment of perforated diverticular disease of the colon. *Adv Surg* 12:85, 1978.

ADDITIONAL ASPECTS

Most patients respond well to medical management of diverticular disease; for these patients, follow-up colonoscopy should be performed 8 weeks after the acute illness to exclude neoplastic disease. A high-fiber diet should be initiated to help prevent recurrence.

Recurrent attacks of diverticulitis occur in approximately 33 to 50 percent of patients.[24] Morbidity and mortality rates are higher with recurrent disease[2]; since surgical resection is often curative, the role and timing of surgical intervention are controversial. Most authorities do not recommend surgery for the initial attack of diverticulitis, but preliminary results from laparoscopic techniques may alter this recommendation in the future.[25,26] After a second episode of diverticulitis, surgery should be considered in all patients, and referral to a surgeon is mandatory.

Diverticular hemorrhage recurs in about 25 percent of patients.[2] Management generally is conservative, although urgent colonoscopic intervention has been advocated.[27] Surgery usually is reserved for patients who have failed medical, angiographic, or endoscopic therapies.

REFERENCES

1. Ferzoco LB, Raptopoulos V, Silen W: Current concepts: acute diverticulitis. *New Engl J Med* 338:1521, 1998.
2. Farrell RJ, Farrell JJ, Morrin MM: Gastrointestinal disorders in the elderly. *Gastroenterol Clin North Am* 30:475, 2001.
3. Chia JG, Wilde CC, Ngoi SS, et al: Trends of diverticular disease of the large bowel in a newly developed country. *Dis Colon Rectum* 34:498, 1991.
4. Katz DS, Lane MJ, Ross BA, et al: Diverticulitis of the right colon revisited. *AJR* 171:151, 1998.
5. Stollman NH, Raskin JB: Diverticular disease of the colon. *J Clin Gastroenterol* 29:241, 1999.
6. Whiteway J, Morson BC: Pathology of the aging: Diverticular disease. *Clin Gastroenterol* 14:829, 1985.
7. Whiteway J, Morson BC: Elastosis in diverticular disease of the sigmoid colon. *Gut* 26:158, 1985.
8. Painter NS: The etiology of diverticulosis of the colon with special reference to the action of certain drugs on behavior of the colon. *Ann R Coll Surg* 34:98, 1964.
9. Peura DA, Lanza FL, Gostout CJ, et al: The American College of Gastroenterology Bleeding Registry: Preliminary findings. *Am J Gastroenterol* 92:924, 1997.
10. Ambrosetti P, Robert JH, Witzig J, et al: Acute left colonic diverticulitis: A prospective analysis of 226 consecutive cases. *Surgery* 115:546, 1994.
11. O'Malley M, Wilson SR: Ultrasonography and computed tomography of appendicitis and diverticulitis. *Semin Roentgenol* 36:138, 2001.

12. Rao PM, Rhea JT: Colonic diverticulitis: Evaluation of the arrowhead sign and the inflamed diverticulum for CT diagnosis. *Radiology* 209:775, 1998.

13. Morris J, Stellato TA, Hagga JR, et al: The utility of computed tomography in colonic diverticulitis. *Ann Surg* 204:128, 1986.

14. Rao, PM, Rhea JT, Novelline RA, et al: Helical CT with only colonic contrast material for diagnosing diverticulitis: Prospective evaluation of 150 patients. *AJR* 170:1445, 1998

15. Wilson SR, Toi A: The value of sonography in the diagnosis of acute diverticulitis of the colon. *AJR* 154:1199, 1990.

16. Schwerk WB, Schwarz S, Rothmund M: Sonography in acute colonic diverticulitis: A prospective study. *Dis Colon Rectum* 35:1077, 1992.

17. Verbanck J, Lambrecht S, Rutgeerts L, et al: Can sonography diagnose acute colonic diverticulitis in patients with acute intestinal inflammation? A prospective study. *J Clin Ultrasound* 17:661, 1989.

18. Zielke A, Hasse C, Nies C, et al: Prospective evaluation of ultrasonography in acute colonic diverticulitis. *Br J Surg* 84:385, 1997.

19. Pradel JA, Adell J-F, Taourel P, et al: Acute colonic divrticulitis: Prospective comparative evaluation with US and CT. *Radiology* 205:503, 1997.

20. Eggesbo HB, Jacobsen T, Kolmannskog F, et al: Diagnosis of acute left-sided colonic diverticulitis by three radiological modalities. *Acta Radiol* 39:315, 1998.

21. Heverhagen JT, Ishaque N, Zielke A, et al: Feasibility of MRI in the diagnosis of acute diverticulitis: Initial results. *Magma* 12:4, 2001.

22. Brook I, Frazier EH: Aerobic and anaerobic microbiology in intraabdominal infections associated with diverticulitis. *J Med Microbiol* 49:827, 2000.

23. Hinchey EJ, Schaal PH, Richards MB: Treatment of perforated diverticular disease of the colon. *Adv Surg* 12:85, 1978.

24. Roberts PL, Veidenheimer MC: Current management of diverticulitis. *Adv Surg* 27:189, 1994.

25. Franklin ME, Dorman JP, Jacobs M, et al: Is laparoscopic surgery applicable to complicated colonic diverticular disease? *Surg Endosc* 11:1021, 1997.

26. Stevenson ARL, Stitz RW, Lumley JW, et al: Laparoscopically assisted anterior resection for diverticular disease: Follow-up of 100 consecutive patients. *Ann Surg* 227:335, 1998.

27. Jensen DM, Machicado GA, Jutabha R, et al: Urgent colonoscopy for the diagnosis and treatment of severe diverticular hemorrhage. *New Engl J Med* 342:78, 2000.

25

Bowel Obstruction

Walter N. Simmons
Gavin J. Putzer

HIGH-YIELD FACTS

- Elderly patients with bowel obstruction often present with symptoms that are atypical compared with younger adults, thus making an accurate initial diagnosis difficult.

- Large bowel obstructions are caused primarily by malignancy, volvulus, and diverticular disease.

- Patients with large bowel obstruction complain of diffuse abdominal pain and progressive abdominal distension; nausea and vomiting are not as common in comparison with patients with small bowel obstruction.

- The competence of the ileocecal valve is critical in determining the appearance of colonic obstruction radiographically.

Bowel obstruction is primarily a disease of the aged and is associated with a high mortality rate. The geriatric population suffers from a higher prevalence of both large and small bowel obstruction because they are more often affected by the causes of intestinal obstruction. Adhesions and hernias are well known as the usual causes of small bowel obstruction, whereas the three most common etiologies of large bowel obstruction include malignancy, diverticular disease, and volvulus. Large bowel obstruction is less common compared with that of the small bowel because of the small intestine's narrow lumen; in addition, adhesions and hernias are encountered more frequently in the small bowel compared with the large bowel.[1] In one series, both small bowel and large bowel obstructions secondary to malignancy were observed in 8 percent of patients.[2]

Bowel obstruction is associated most often with abdominal pain. The intestinal wall contains pain receptors that respond to distension and increased wall tension.[3] The pain typically described in bowel obstruction occurs in paroxysms, with the severity a function of the speed of onset as well as the degree of distension. Slowly developing obstruction (occurring over weeks) may be relatively subtle in presentation in comparison with acute obstruction, which produces a more dramatic picture.[4]

EPIDEMIOLOGY

Approximately 20 percent of surgical admissions for acute abdominal pain are for bowel obstruction. Adhesive bands are the most frequent cause of bowel obstruction for all age groups combined. Strangulated groin hernia is usually the second most common cause in younger age groups, whereas neoplasm is common in the geriatric population. Malignant disease accounts for a large portion of all cases of obstruction; adenocarcinoma is the predominant malignancy. Primary neoplasms are discovered more often in the colon than any other organ system.[5] Approximately 25 percent of patients who require laparotomy to treat their obstruction are found to have benign disease, and 4 percent have a new primary malignancy.[6] Diverticulitis is another prominent cause of obstruction in the older age groups, causing approximately twice as many large bowel obstructions as volvulus (20 versus 10 percent, respectively).[7] About 20 percent of patients with colorectal cancer present with obstructive symptoms, and half these patients will require emergency operative decompression.[8]

Other causes of bowel obstruction include fecal impaction; foreign bodies; inflammatory processes (e.g., radiation colitis, ischemic colitis, and Crohn's disease); paralytic ileus secondary to injury, medication, or illness; electrolyte abnormalities; and pseudo-obstruction. Pseudo-obstruction (also referred to as *Ogilvie's syndrome*) is an acute transient process in which the colon appears obstructed without a definable obstructive lesion. This is often seen in geriatric patients and may be a result of chronic illnesses, congestive heart failure, or hypothyroidism. Overall, approximately 25 percent of all patients presenting to an emergency setting with abdominal pain are found to have a serious condition that requires hospital admission.[9] In addition, Medicare data show that the frequency of hospitalization for major bowel procedures nearly doubles from age 65 to 74 to age 75 to 84.[10]

PATHOPHYSIOLOGY

The competence of the ileocecal valve is of utmost importance in colonic obstruction. As intraluminal pressures rise, a competent ileocecal valve results in a closed-loop obstruction. This occurs as intestinal secretions of fluid and gas, which normally are absorbed in the large intestine, are prevented from being decompressed through the ileocecal valve and cecum and into the small intestine. The colonic pressure can rise to the point that arterial flow is compromised, leading to colon wall ischemia and perforation. In an obstructed colon that becomes ischemic, bacteria can invade local nodes, leading to sepsis. The greatest dilatation will occur at the cecum. Cecal diameter allows for an estimation of potential rupture and ischemia. Cecal dilation of 12 to 14 cm is thought to be associated with a high risk for perforation. Expeditious decompression of the cecum when it reaches 10 cm is prudent because of the high potential for ischemia at that size.[11,12]

In addition to cecal dilatation and ischemia, large fluid losses into the obstructed large intestine can cause substantial dehydration.[13] Dehydration, often difficult to ascertain in the elderly patient, may be exacerbated by nausea, vomiting, and decreased or absent intake of any liquids. In addition, the thirst response to dehydration is diminished even among healthy elderly individuals.[14]

CLINICAL FEATURES

Success in the management of bowel obstruction depends on an accurate diagnosis in a timely manner. Emergency physicians should keep in mind that patients at extremes of age often present with symptoms that are atypical compared with younger adults. Large bowel obstruction often presents with symptoms that are more insidious than small bowel obstruction. This difference in presentation exists because of the increased reservoir capacity of the large bowel and the slower peristaltic transit time compared with the small bowel.[15] Because of the volume capacity of the large bowel and the competency of the ileocecal valve, vomiting may be late or absent as a symptom of obstruction.[1] Of note, patients who complain of nausea, vomiting, and fever may provide greater sensitivity and specificity for obstruction than complaints of abdominal pain.[16] Failure to pass flatus and feces (i.e., obstipation) is often indicative of bowel obstruction, whereas only a little over 50 percent of those older than 60 years of age complain of abdominal pain.[16] When abdominal pain is present, it is often described as diffuse and gradual in its development, often occurring over days.[17] The patient also may report a recent change in bowel habits, often with alternating diarrhea followed by constipation or generalized constipation. Finally, if the

obstruction is secondary to a neoplasm, the patient may report intermittent bloody stools.[18]

The past medical history should include previous intestinal neoplasm or obstruction, previous abdominal surgeries, and a history of diverticular or inflammatory bowel disease.

On physical examination, vital signs often are found to be within normal limits; however, a low-grade temperature (to 38.5°C) is seen commonly in obstructed patients. Hypothermia may indicate sepsis and portend a worse outcome. Alterations in the pulse and blood pressure may be indicative of significant pain, sepsis, or dehydration. Hypotension, persistent tachycardia, and high fever may suggest bowel perforation.[19]

Physical examination in obstruction is most remarkable for abdominal distension. Bowel sounds may be either hyperdynamic or absent, and the abdomen often is found to be diffusely tender; severe pain out of proportion to physical examination is worrisome for mesenteric ischemia.[20] Digital examination can be used to assess the presence of a fecal impaction. Many patients with bowel obstructions will present with Hemoccult-positive stool.[21]

DIAGNOSIS AND DIFFERENTIAL

Obstruction is usually secondary to an underlying condition. Patients presenting with symptoms consistent with bowel obstruction should be evaluated carefully and expeditiously. Perforation is always a risk, and early diagnosis helps prevent this complication. Diverticulitis, ischemic bowel, leaking aortic abdominal aneurysm, volvulus, fecal impaction, cholecystitis, and appendicitis are diagnoses that should be considered in the elderly with these symptoms.

Laboratory studies are often not helpful in the acutely obstructed patient but may become of greater value in the later stages of obstruction. A complete blood count (CBC) and electrolyte panel should be ordered; a urinalysis, lipase, liver enzymes, and lactate level should be considered as well. Although the white blood cell count is often normal, an elevation can broaden the differential diagnosis, assist in determining a cause for the obstruction, or alert the clinician to the possibility of the serious complication of ischemic bowel.

Obstruction is one of the few diagnoses of the elderly that can be confirmed by a flat and upright abdominal radiograph. Air-fluid levels are the most important criterion in the radiographic diagnosis of bowel obstruction. The competency of the ileocecal valve also aids in determining the radiograph's appearance. If the valve is competent, then the site of the colon obstruction to the cecum will be distended. If the valve is incompetent, then bowel gas will travel into the small bowel, which allows for partial decompression of the colon. In the case of an incompetent ileocecal valve, the colon should remain mildly enlarged in relation to that of the small bowel.[22] If the large bowel increases beyond 10 cm, then the risk of ischemia and perforation increases greatly. Free air from bowel perforation should be appreciated on the plain abdominal radiograph.

Computed tomographic (CT) scanning of the abdomen with a water-soluble contrast material also will detect bowel obstruction with a high degree of sensitivity and can accurately define the location and cause of the obstruction and detect signs of bowel ischemia. CT scans are also indicated if small bowel obstruction is suspected and plain films are equivocal.

EMERGENCY DEPARTMENT CARE AND DISPOSITION

Emergency department (ED) treatment of the patient with bowel obstruction should be directed at pain control, rehydration, and correcting electrolyte disturbances. Once the diagnosis of obstruction has been made, potent, short-acting analgesics (e.g., fentanyl) should be administered. Antiemetic medications may also provide symptomatic relief. Fluid resuscitation is often required because patients usually are depleted intravascularly from the persistent fluid loss into the large bowel. Small serial intravenous boluses of lactated Ringer's solution may begin to correct the volume status of these patients.[23] A nasogastric tube should be inserted to assist with decompression and symptomatic relief.

Critically ill patients mandate a more aggressive treatment regimen. First, the airway, breathing, and circulation status of the patient should be addressed. More aggressive fluid resuscitation may be required; an initial intravenous bolus of lactated Ringer's 10 mL/kg should be administered. It is often helpful to monitor the rate of urine output with a Foley catheter. Central venous or pulmonary wedge capillary pressure monitoring may be needed in some patients.

Preoperative prophylactic antibiotics should be administered. Antibiotics that are effective against a broad range of gastrointestinal tract organisms, including anaerobes, provide the optimal coverage. Cefotetan 2 g intravenously provides adequate preoperative coverage in a patient who is not toxic in appearance. In a septic patient, a combination of agents (e.g., gentamicin 1.5 mg/kg, ampicillin 2 g, and metronidazole 500 mg) is appropriate.

Expeditious surgical consultation is strongly advised because many patients require colon decompression.[24] The type of surgical procedure is based on the site of the obstruction and the underlying etiology and may range from hemicolectomy to colonoscopy. Patients with advanced cancer may have bowel obstruction that is found to be inoperable. This is often the case in colonic obstruction caused by extensive tumor and multiple partial obstructions.[25] In inoperable patients, expandable metal stents have been applied; colorectal, esophageal, gastroduodenal, and biliary stents have had varying degrees of success. These stents are placed under endoscopy and fluoroscopy.[26]

Prognosis depends on the age and general condition of the patient, extent of vascular impairment of the bowel, presence or absence of ischemia and perforation, cause of obstruction, and promptness of surgical management. The overall mortality rate of obstruction is estimated to be 20 percent.[27,28] Cecal perforation alone carries a 40 percent mortality rate.[27] In patients with significant obstruction (i.e., a radiograph demonstrating bowel wall dilated greater than 10 cm), extended delay in surgery often is associate with a steep increase in mortality.[27]

ADDITIONAL ASPECTS

The following are pitfalls in the management of bowel obstruction:

- Failure to recognize that comorbid disease processes may cause patients to have a limited physiologic reserve. Correction of electrolyte imbalances and volume status is essential.

- Assuming that the geriatric patient without frank peritoneal signs does not have an acute surgical abdomen. Patients with an acute bowel obstruction require expeditious surgical consultation.

REFERENCES

1. Richards WO, Williams LF: Obstruction of the large and small intestine. *Surg Clin North Am* 68:355, 1988.
2. Tang E, David J, Silberman H: Bowel obstruction in cancer patients. *Arch Surg* 130:832, 1995.
3. Higashi H: Pharmacological aspects of visceral sensory receptors, in Cervero F, Morrison JF (eds): *Visceral Sensation.* Amsterdam, Elsevier, 1986, p 21.
4. Manning AP: Towards positive diagnosis of the irritable bowel. *Br Med J* 2:653, 1978.
5. Cotran RS, Kumar V, Collins T: *Robbins Pathologic Basis of Disease,* 6th ed. Philadelphia, Saunders, 1999, p 825.

6. Osteen RT, Guyton S, Steele G Jr, et al: Malignant intestinal obstruction. *Surgery* 87:611, 1980.

7. Greenlee HB, Aranha GV, DeOrio A J: Neoplastic obstruction of the small and large intestine. *Curr Probl Cancer* 4:1, 1979.

8. Lo AM, Evans WE, Carey LC: Review of SBO at Milwaukee County General Hospital. *Am J Surg* 111:884, 1966.

9. Graff LG, Radford MJ, Werne C: Probability of appendicitis before and after observation. *Ann Emerg Med* 20:503, 1991.

10. Levinsky NG, Ash AS, Wei Y, et al: Patterns of use of common major procedures in medical care of older adults. *J Am Geriatr Soc* 47:131, 1999.

11. Turnage RH, Bergen PC: Intestinal obstruction and ileus, in Feldman M, Scharschmidt BF, Sleisenger MH, et al (eds): *Feldman: Sleisenger & Fordtran's Gastrointestinal and Liver Disease,* 6th ed. Philidelphia, Saunders, 1998, p 1799.

12. Baines M, Oliver DJ, Carter RI: Medical management of intestinal obstruction in patients with advanced malignant disease: A clinical and pathological study. *Lancet* 2:990, 1985.

13. Buechter KJ, Boustany C, Caillouette R, et al: Surgical management of the acutely obstructed colon: A review of 127 cases. *Am J Surg* 156:163, 1988.

14. Ahronheim JC: Special problems in the geriatric patient, in Goldman L, Bennett JC (eds): *Goldman: Cecil Textbook of Medicine,* 21st ed. St. Louis, Saunders, 2000, p 24.

15. Silen W: *Cope's Early Diagnosis of the Acute Abdomen,* 20th ed. New York, Oxford University Press, 1991, p 150.

16. Gibson SJ, Helme RD: Age-related differences in pain perception and report *Clin Geriatr Med* 17(3):433, 2001.

17. Sial SH, Catalano MF: Gastrointestinal tract cancer in the elderly. *Gastroenterol Clin North Am* 30(2):565, 2001.

18. Hardcastle JD, Chir M, Pye G: Screening for colorectal cancer: A critical view. *World J Surg* 13:38, 1989.

19. Lambright ES, Williams NN: Acute abdomen and common surgical abdominal problems, in Noble J, Greene HL, Levinson W, et al (eds): *Noble: Textbook of Primary Care Medicine,* 3d ed. St. Louis, Mosby, 2001, p 976.

20. Byrne TK: Complications of surgery for obesity. *Surg Clin North Am* 81(5):1181, 2001.

21. Richter JM: Evaluation of abdominal pain, in Goroll AH, Mulley AG (eds): *Goroll: Primary Care Medicine,* 4th ed. Baltimore, Lippincott Williams & Wilkins, 2000, p 375.

22. Davis M: The Colon, in Juhl JH, Crummy AB, Kuhlman JE (eds): *Juhl: Paul and Juhl's Essentials of Radiologic Imaging,* 7th ed. Baltimore, Lippincott Williams & Wilkins, 1998, p 491.

23. May HL, Aghababian R, Fleisher G: *Emergency Medicine,* 2d ed., Vol. 2. Boston, Little, Brown, 1992, p 1515.

24. Lamah M, Mathur P, Mckeown B, et al: The use of rectosigmoid stents in the management of acute large bowel obstruction. *R Coll Surg Edinb* 43:318, 1998.

25. Jung GS, Song HY, Kang SG, et al: Malignant gastroduodenal obstructions: Treatment by means of a covered expandable metallic stent-initial experience. *Radiology* 216(3):758, 2000.

26. Coco C, Cogliandolo S, Riccioni E, et al: Use of a self-expanding stent in the palliation of rectal cancer recurrences: A report of three cases. *Surg Endoscop* 14(8):708, 2000.

27. Throck TR: Small intestine, in Way LW (ed): *Current Surgical Diagnosis and Treatment,* 10th ed. East Norwalk CT,, Appleton & Lange, 1994, p 627.

28. Mercandante S: Assessment and management of mechanical bowel obstruction, in Portenoy RK, Bruera E (eds): *Topics in Palliative Care,* Vol. 1. New York, Oxford University Press, 1997, p 113.

26

Volvulus

Walter N. Simmons
Anika Parab

HIGH-YIELD FACTS

- A history of chronic constipation, inactivity, and institutionalization in an elderly patient should raise suspicion for colonic volvulus.
- Because the clinical features of intestinal obstruction in the elderly are often subtle, volvulus should be suspected in patients with even mild symptoms of distension, abdominal pain, vomiting, and constipation.
- In most cases, the diagnosis of sigmoid volvulus can be made based on history, physical examination, and plain abdominal radiographs alone.
- In the presence of viable bowel, the initial treatment for sigmoid volvulus is nonoperative endoscopic decompression. The management of cecal volvulus is surgical.
- Guarding and rebound tenderness are late findings that, in combination with fever and shock, indicate gangrenous bowel. Gangrene is the major determinant of mortality in colonic volvulus.

The growing geriatric population consists of a significant proportion of patients who present to the emergency department (ED) with acute abdominal emergencies.[1,2] The elderly patient with abdominal symptoms often presents with diffuse and nonspecific complaints. The evaluation of these complaints in the older patient typically demands more time and resources than in younger patients.[3] When compared with younger patients, older patients who visit the ED are more likely to present with urgent or life-threatening conditions.[2] In addition, the elderly patient often presents with subtle signs and symptoms that may understate a serious condition.[1-4] For example, the cardinal clinical features of intestinal obstruction, including abdominal pain, vomiting, distension, and obstipation,

are often masked in the elderly.[5] In evaluating the elderly patient with acute abdominal symptoms, it is important to consider colonic volvulus, which accounts for 3 to 5 percent of all intestinal obstructions in the geriatric population.[5] In the setting of an abdominal emergency such as volvulus, improved survival for the geriatric patient depends on early diagnosis, appropriate resuscitation, close monitoring, and expedient surgical intervention.[6]

EPIDEMIOLOGY

In the United States, volvulus is the third leading cause of large bowel obstruction after neoplasm and diverticular disease.[7] In the geriatric population, sigmoid volvulus is the most common type of colonic volvulus, accounting for 65 to 80 percent of cases.[5,8,9] Cecal volvulus is the second most common type of volvulus, accounting for 15 to 20 percent of cases.[8] Volvulus of the transverse colon and splenic flexure are rare and comprise only 2 to 5 percent of cases.[7,8,10] While cecal and sigmoid volvulus have similar incidence in patients younger than age 60, the incidence of sigmoid volvulus increases in patients older than age 60.[11] Studies have reported that the mean age of onset for sigmoid volvulus is 66 years, with a slight male predominance (64 percent), whereas cecal volvulus tends to have a younger age distribution (53 years is the mean age of onset) with no clear gender predisposition.[8,12,13] The presence of gangrene is the major determinant of mortality in colonic volvulus.[7] Sigmoid volvulus has a reported mortality rate of 35 percent and up to 53 percent mortality in the presence of gangrenous colon.[11,12,14] In one series, the overall mortality rate for cecal volvulus was 23 percent, ranging from 15 percent mortality with viable bowel to 41 percent mortality in the setting of gangrenous bowel.[9]

PATHOPHYSIOLOGY

Volvulus is an axial twist of a portion of the gastrointestinal (GI) tract around its mesentery. For volvulus to occur, the colon segment must be large and mobile in order to twist around its base.[5,9] This twisting causes a partial or complete obstruction of the bowel and a variable degree of arterial and venous occlusion. The colon is the most common site for volvulus, although the stomach and small bowel also may be affected.[7,11]

Sigmoid volvulus occurs in people with a floppy, redundant colon with narrow mesosigmoid parietal attachments.[8] A redundant sigmoid colon with a narrow mesocolon base may represent a congenital variation in anatomy that predisposes a patient to volvulus, although any condition associated with a redundant colon, such as chronic constipation, high-residue diet, Chagas' disease, or Hirschsprung's disease, can increase the likelihood of volvulus.[7,8,11]

Sigmoid volvulus should be suspected in inactive elderly patients with concurrent debilitating disease. In one series, 85 percent of elderly patients with sigmoid volvulus had some concomitant disease. The majority (63 percent) of patients had psychiatric or neurologic conditions, including previous cerebrovascular accident, Parkinson's disease, or seizure disorder. Forty-five percent of patients had cardiovascular disease, and 20 percent had diabetes mellitus.[14] Conditions that alter bowel motility, such as Parkinson's disease, multiple sclerosis, neurosyphilis, and pseudobulbar palsy are associated with volvulus.[8] Systemic diseases such as diabetic visceral neuropathy may produce autonomic dysfunction that affects bowel motility and therefore predisposes to volvulus.[8]

Approximately one-third of the cases of volvulus occur in institutionalized patients. Chronic constipation secondary to inactivity and use of neuropsychiatric drugs that alter bowel motility increase the likelihood of volvulus in these patients.[10,11] Common medications used in the elderly population that predispose to volvulus include excessive laxative use, tranquilizers, anticholinergic medications, ganglionic blocking agents, and antiparkinsonian drugs.[3,9] Adhesions from previous abdominal surgery also predispose the geriatric patient to volvulus.[11,12] The adhesion acts as a pivot around which the redundant colon can twist.[8]

Cecal volvulus is due to the failure of the right colon mesentery to fuse with the posterior abdominal wall, creating a freely mobile cecum. This excess mobility allows rotation to occur.[7] The suspicion of cecal volvulus is raised when distal small bowel obstruction is associated with an abdominal mass in debilitated, mentally retarded patients or in patients with previous abdominal surgery.[15] Predisposing factors for cecal volvulus include recent abdominal surgery, adhesions, congenital bands, and prolonged constipation.[3] Cecal or right colon volvulus also occurs in patients in whom distal obstruction from neoplasm or inflammation is present.[7]

The cecal bascule is a variant of cecal volvulus and represents 10 percent of cases of right colonic volvulus.[11] Because the cecum is mobile and the ascending colon is fixed, the cecum can fold transversely and superiorly over the ascending colon to form the cecal bascule. Contents from the small bowel are able to enter the cecum, but cecal contents are unable to exit distally. As a result,

massive cecal distension with subsequent gangrene can occur.[12]

Volvulus of the transverse colon and splenic flexure are rare. Congenital absence of the gastrocolic, phrenocolic, and splenocolic ligaments has been implicated in cases of volvulus of the transverse colon.[11]

CLINICAL FEATURES

Elderly patients who present to the ED with colonic volvulus are likely to present later in their illness. The geriatric patient with large bowel obstruction may have an insidious onset of abdominal complaints and may not seek medical attention until more obvious symptoms, such as abdominal distension or vomiting, develop several days later.[6] In one series, 57 percent of patients with sigmoid volvulus were in a nursing home when their volvulus occurred.[14] When compared with elderly patients admitted from home, institutionalized patients have a longer duration of symptoms before diagnosis.[14] Institutionalized patients often are unable to provide an accurate history and generally are difficult to interview and examine. Consequently, they tend to present to the ED later in the course of their illness.[10] In contrast to their nursing home counterparts who experienced symptoms for an average of 5.6 days before diagnosis, patients admitted from home had an average duration of symptoms of 3 days before diagnosis.[14] Factors contributing to the delay in presentation include the elderly patient's fear of hospitalization, possible institutionalization, and further loss of independence.[5]

Presenting Symptoms

The presentation of sigmoid volvulus is variable, but typically the onset of symptoms is gradual. Early symptoms of sigmoid volvulus include crampy abdominal pain (63 percent), followed by obstipation (51 percent), vomiting (35 percent), constipation (29 percent), and small-volume liquid stools.[12,14] Abdominal distension usually occurs later in the course. Other symptoms include nausea, anorexia, and weight loss.[14] A history of recurrent minor episodes of similar symptoms is found in 40 to 60 percent of patients.[11] A history of chronic constipation, nausea, vomiting, episodes of obstructive bowel symptoms, chronic drug use, and central nervous system, cardiac, or renal disease is common.[9,12] Occasionally, the patient with volvulus appears acutely ill.[9] In one series, 7 percent of patients with sigmoid volvulus presented in shock.[10]

While the initial symptoms of sigmoid volvulus may

be gradual in onset, cecal volvulus often has a more dramatic presentation with a shorter clinical history.[12] Cecal volvulus typically presents with signs of small bowel obstruction and abdominal pain (90 percent), distension (80 percent), constipation, and obstipation (60 percent), followed by nausea and vomiting (28 percent).[3,13] Symptoms of cecal volvulus may be intermittent, and a past history of several similar episodes is common.[7] Cecal volvulus constitutes an emergency because of the danger of cecal perforation.[9] If cecal volvulus is not recognized early, the lesion can progress to colonic ischemia, perforation, sepsis, and death.[15] The incidence of gangrenous bowel at the time of diagnosis of cecal volvulus is 25 percent.[12]

Atypical Presentation Unique to the Geriatric Patient

The evaluation of acute abdominal disorders in the geriatric patient is especially challenging for several reasons. Eliciting an accurate history from an elderly patient may be complicated by communication difficulties resulting from mental confusion, aphasia from previous stroke, hearing and speech difficulties, or neuropsychiatric disease.[5,6] In the geriatric patient, the signs of acute abdominal conditions are less obvious, and physical examination findings are less reliable. Because the elderly often have thin abdominal musculature with some amount of atrophy, the geriatric patient may demonstrate less splinting or muscle guarding on examination.[5] The emergency physician should suspect volvulus in elderly patients when even mild symptoms of distension, abdominal pain, vomiting, and constipation are present.[9]

Physical examination findings in colonic volvulus include abdominal tenderness, upper abdominal distension, and obstructive bowel sounds on auscultation.[14] In sigmoid volvulus, distension is often massive and more marked on one side of the abdomen than the other.[11,14] On occasion, the distended pelvic colon may be visible or palpable.[11] Patients with sigmoid volvulus also may present with dehydration, tympanum, visible peristalsis, empty rectum, and fecal odor to the breath.[5,12] In cecal volvulus, the cecum may be felt as a soft, rubbery mass palpable in the right lower quadrant or extending into the left side of the abdomen.[9] If fever and peritoneal signs are present, then the emergency physician should suspect infarcted bowel, perforation, and peritonitis. Peritoneal signs, fever, and shock indicate gangrenous bowel.[7] Once gangrene and perforation have occurred, severe constant abdominal pain, diffuse peritonitis, and lack of peristaltic sounds are common.[15]

DIAGNOSIS AND DIFFERENTIAL

Laboratory Findings

Routine laboratory data are important in evaluating a patient with acute abdominal pain.

Laboratory studies should include a complete blood count, electrolyte determinations, prothrombin time with international normalized ratio (PT/INR), and type and crossmatch.[6,9] Because the white blood cell (WBC) count is often lower for a given degree of inflammation in the elderly patient, the absence of leukocytosis does not rule out the possibility of a surgical abdomen.[6]

Imaging Studies

While the diagnosis of sigmoid volvulus can be based on history, physical examination, and plain abdominal radiographs alone, the definitive diagnosis of cecal volvulus often requires additional contrast studies. In one study, the diagnosis of sigmoid volvulus was made by plain abdominal radiographs alone in 85 percent of patients and in over 50 percent of patients with cecal volvulus.[7,10] In sigmoid volvulus, the dilated colon may have the appearance of an inverted-U shape or "bent inner tube" with its point directed to the right upper quadrant[7] (Fig. 26-1). A double air-fluid loop on abdominal plain film is diagnostic for sigmoid volvulus.[5,9] Additional diagnostic workup after abdominal plain films are unnecessary for sigmoid volvulus and may delay treatment.[10] Delay in treatment increases the risk of bowel necrosis, which, in turn, increases mortality.[10] If the diagnosis of sigmoid volvulus remains unclear after abdominal plain films, contrast enema or a computed tomographic (CT) scan with contrast material may help establish the diagnosis. Contrast enema should be used only when the diagnosis of volvulus is unclear because the enema increases the risk of perforation in the setting of compromised bowel.[10] An upright chest radiograph may demonstrate free air if perforation has occurred.

In cecal volvulus, the abdominal plain film may reveal a kidney-shaped distended loop located in the midabdomen. The point of this "coffee bean" colon is directed toward the left upper quadrant. The plain-film diagnosis of cecal volvulus is based on findings of a dilated cecum (98 percent) containing a single air-fluid level (72 percent), little or no gas in the distal colon (82 percent), an abnormally positioned cecum (56 percent), and dilatation of small bowel with air-fluid levels (55 percent)[15] (Fig. 26-2). While plain abdominal radiograph alone establishes the diagnosis of sigmoid volvulus in over 80 percent of cases, one study showed that the definitive diag-

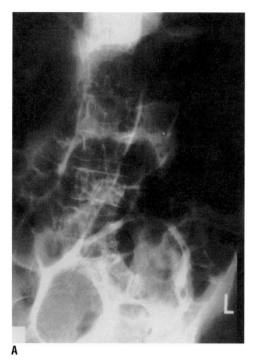

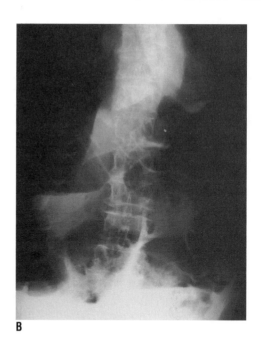

Fig. 26-1 *A.* Sigmoid volvulus on plain abdominal radiograph. *B.* Sigmoid volvulus. *(Courtesy of David Effron, M.D.,* *MetroHealth Medical Center; Cleveland, Ohio.)*

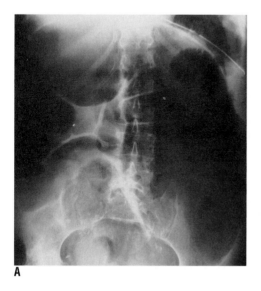

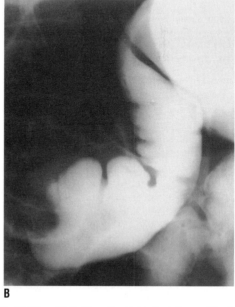

Fig. 26-2 *A.* Cecal volvulus on plain abdominal radiograph. *B.* Barium enema showing "bird's beak" appearance. *(Courtesy* *of David Effron, M.D., MetroHealth Medical Center; Cleveland, Ohio.)*

nosis of cecal volvulus based on plain abdominal radiograph alone was made in only 17 percent of patients.[7,15] The most reliable diagnostic procedure for cecal volvulus is the barium enema (88 percent accuracy).[15] Typical findings for cecal volvulus on barium enema include the "bird's beak" deformity with obstruction at the site of the colonic twist and no filling of the cecum. Contrast studies also may rule out concomitant distal colonic obstruction, which may have precipitated the colonic volvulus.[15] Barium enemas are more dangerous in cecal volvulus than in sigmoid volvulus and are rarely therapeutic.[12] Diagnosis of transverse colon or splenic flexure volvulus usually is made at laparotomy.[7]

Large bowel obstruction in the aged is most likely the result of carcinoma, diverticulitis, or volvulus and should be suspected in geriatric patients presenting with abdominal symptoms. The most common etiologies of acute abdomen in the elderly patient include biliary disease, intestinal obstruction, perforated peptic ulcer, diverticulitis, intussusception, and appendicitis.[6,12] Less common disorders include abdominal aortic aneurysm and acute intestinal ischemia.[6] Carcinoma of the distal colon, diverticulitis, ischemic colitis, primary mesenteric thrombosis, acute pancreatitis, strangulated internal hernia, toxic megacolon, bacterial infections, electrolyte imbalance, and spinal cord injuries can produce obstructive symptoms in elderly patients with the radiographic appearance of a grossly distended colon.[9]

EMERGENCY DEPARTMENT CARE AND DISPOSITION

ED management of colonic volvulus in the geriatric patient includes correction of fluid and electrolyte imbalances, nasogastric tube decompression, and administration of broad-spectrum preoperative antibiotics.[6,9] It is important to obtain early surgical consultation because delays in treatment increase mortality by increasing the risk of bowel necrosis, perforation, gangrene, and shock.

Provided that the bowel is viable and that there are no signs of peritonitis or gangrene, the primary therapy for sigmoid volvulus should be nonoperative. Initial treatment for sigmoid volvulus is sigmoidoscopy with volvulus reduction. Administration of a regular or barium enema and colonoscopy are also used in the treatment of sigmoid volvulus with a 70 to 90 percent success rate.[9–11] The majority of patients with sigmoid volvulus are decompressed initially by passing a proctoscope through the volvulus and inserting a rectal tube. A forceful release of gas and stool with proctoscopy or tube decompression confirms the diagnosis of sigmoid volvulus.[7,9] Because recurrence rates of sigmoid volvulus are as high as 90 percent after nonoperative reduction, elective resection is recommended several days after admission when the patient can be appropriately prepared for surgery.[14] Nonoperative treatment is contraindicated in patients with compromised bowel viability, obvious perforation with free air and peritonitis, or internal hernia with strangulation.[9] Surgery is required emergently if nonoperative decompression is unsuccessful or if gangrene is noted at proctoscopic or sigmoidoscopic examiantion.[7,11] Patients who present with sigmoid volvulus and peritoneal signs, blood per rectum, shock, or evidence of intraabdominal free air should undergo immediate exploratory celiotomy.[10]

The primary treatment for cecal volvulus is operative. Surgical interventions include some combination of detorsion, cecopexy, cecostomy, or resection. Resection has the lowest recurrence rate but the highest complication rate. The treatment of choice for splenic flexure or transverse colon volvulus is resection and anastamosis.[11]

ADDITIONAL ASPECTS

The following are pitfalls in the management of volvulus:

- Failure to recognize that elderly patients who present with constipation may have an early volvulus.

- Assuming that patients who lack significant abdominal tenderness or acute peritoneal signs do not have significant intraabdominal pathology, including volvulus.

REFERENCES

1. de Dombal FT: Acute abdominal pain in the elderly. *J Clin Gastroenterol* 19(4):331, 1994.
2. Lowenstein SR, Crescenzi CA, Kern DC, et al: Care of the elderly in the emergency department. *Ann Emerg Med* 15:528, 1986.
3. Sanson TG, O'Keefe KP: Evaluation of abdominal pain in the elderly. *Emerg Med Clin North Am* 14(3):615, 1996.
4. American College of Emergency Physicians: Clinical policy for the initial approach to patients presenting with a chief complaint of nontraumatic acute abdominal pain. *Ann Emerg Med* 23:906, 1994.
5. Phillips SL, Burns GP: Acute abdominal disease in the aged. *Med Clin North Am* 72(5):1213, 1988.
6. Vogt DP: The acute abdomen in the geriatric patient. *Clev Clin J Med* 57:125, 1990.

7. Jones IT, Fazio VW: Colonic volvulus: Etiology and management. *Dig Dis* 7(4):203, 1989.

8. Ballantyne GH: Review of sigmoid volvulus: Clinical patterns and pathogenesis. *Dis Colon Rectum* 25(8):823, 1982.

9. Avots-Avotins KV, Waugh DE: Colon volvulus and the geriatric patient. *Surg Clin North Am* 62:249, 1982.

10. Grossman EM, Longo WE, Stratton MD, et al: Sigmoid volvulus in Department of Veterans Affairs medical centers. *Dis Colon Rectum* 43(3):414, 2000.

11. Frizelle FA, Wolff BG: Colonic volvulus. *Adv Surg* 29:131, 1996.

12. Kauvar DR: The geriatric acute abdomen. *Clin Geriatr Med* 9:547, 1993.

13. Madiba TE, Thomson SR, Church JM: The management of cecal volvulus. *Dis Colon Rectum* 45:264, 2002.

14. Bak MP, Boley SJ: Sigmoid volvulus in elderly patients. *Am J Surg* 151(1):71, 1986.

15. Rabinovici R, Simansky DA, Kaplan O, et al: Cecal volvulus. *Dis Colon Rectum* 33(9):765, 1990.

27

Constipation

Walter N. Simmons
Gavin J. Putzer

HIGH-YIELD FACTS

- The causes of constipation are numerous, but in the emergency setting, patients often present with acute constipation due to medications or from painful perianal lesions.

- More than 25 percent of patients with colorectal carcinomas present with constipation. If colon cancer is suspected, referring the patient for colonoscopy is required.

- Significant complications from constipation or related treatment may occur and include hemorrhoids, anal fissure, rectal prolapse, stercoral ulcer, colonic perforation, colonic volvulus, ischemic colitis, fecal incontinence, urinary retention, melanosis coli, cathartic colon, cardiac and cerebrovascular dysfunction, and fecal impaction.

Constipation may be defined by a combination of changes in the frequency, size, consistency, and ease of stool passage, which leads to an overall decrease in volume of bowel movements. The American Academy of Gastroenterologists defines constipation as any two of the following: (1) staining to pass stool 25 percent of the time, (2) lumpy or hard stools 25 percent of the time, (3) incomplete sensation of evacuation 25 percent of the time, and (4) two or fewer stools per week.

Constipation can be difficult to define precisely because of the wide range of normal bowel habits. Constipation is endemic in nursing home residents.[1] The increase in constipation among the institutionalized elderly may be attributable to many factors such as immobility, decreased fluid and fiber ingestion, or the myriad of constipating medications taken. It is also a prevalent complaint in independently living elderly persons.[2] Among this subgroup, nearly one in two women and one in three men have symptoms of constipation or take laxatives or enemas.[2]

Most individuals who describe themselves as constipated complain of excessive straining or discomfort at defecation or the passage of hard stools, although frequency of defecation is within the normal range.[3] Studies demonstrated that self-reported constipation poorly corresponds with symptoms compatible with constipation.[2,4] Thus constipation is a common complaint that is quite subjective, and each individual has his or her own threshold level. Consequently, constipation is often improperly and erroneously self-diagnosed. Thus it is important to know what the patient means by constipation. The elderly present with one of several patterns of symptoms when they see a physician for the complaint of constipation. The first involves a diminished or lessened frequency of defecation than "normal." Normal stool frequency ranges from three to five bowel movements per week to two bowel movements per day.[5] The situation may be complicated when laxatives are used in such circumstances to induce defecation. Infrequency of spontaneous defecation best defines colonic inertia at a clinical level. Stool frequency alone, however, is insufficient to use because many constipated patients describe a normal frequency but have subjective complaints of excessive straining, hard stools, lower abdominal fullness, and a sense of incomplete evacuation.[6]

Another symptom in patients presenting with constipation is difficulty with evacuation, or dyschezia. Patients may have one or more bowel movements daily but experience difficulty initiating or completing a bowel movement. These symptoms may suggest the presence of an outlet problem, such as intrarectal intussusception or anismus. Patients often complain of the passage of harder stools than normal, but they often mean stools that are hard to pass or stools with pebble-like form.[7]

The importance of defining infrequency and dyschezia is that they have different implications for the possible mechanisms involved in constipation: colonic inertia, difficulty expelling feces from the rectum, and painful evacuation of feces. Since constipation is a symptom rather than a disease, it is necessary to identify the cause to effectively deliver the proper treatment and disposition. Constipation can be an acute problem complicating some other illness or a chronic problem.

EPIDEMIOLOGY

Most individuals with constipation are elderly, and the costs associated with constipation are considerable. In the United States, more than $800 million is spent for laxatives, and there are 2.5 million physician visits for constipation each year.[3]

The prevalence of constipation is higher at extremes of life (i.e., among infants/children and the elderly). Epidemiologic studies from the United States and elsewhere indicate that the point prevalence of constipation is higher in the elderly as compared with younger adults.[8] The epidemiology of chronic constipation in the elderly remains poorly defined.[2] Inadequate fluid intake may play a role because the elderly often have a decreased thirst mechanism even in the presence of dehydration. The high prevalence in the geriatric population is multifactorial and related to polypharmacy, a diet low or deficient in fiber, sedentary habits, and various disease processes that impair neurologic and motor control.[3]

PATHOPHYSIOLOGY

Normal Physiology

The gastrointestinal tract is presented with approximately 9 to 10 L of secretions and ingested fluids per day. The small intestine usually absorbs this entirely, except 500 to 600 mL. Each day the colon receives 1 to 1.5 L of fluid containing substantial amounts of salt, fiber, and other residues from the absorptive process in the small intestine.[9] Approximately 90 percent of the salt and water delivered to the colon is absorbed by the colonic mucosa. Approximately 100 g of stool is produced daily, containing 70 mL of water and 30 g of solids. Sodium is actively absorbed even against large concentration gradients. Water is passively absorbed following the osmotic gradient produced by the absorption of sodium. Because salt and water absorption and bacterial metabolism are time-dependent, slowing colon transit increases the time available for absorption and metabolism and reduces stool frequency and the amount of material entering the rectum each day. In most constipated patients, stools have about the same size and composition as stools produced by nonconstipated individuals, suggesting that a critical mass of feces must accumulate before the need to defecate is recognized.[6]

Physiologically, the process of normal defecation consists of a complex, coordinated series of events involving the (1) distension of the rectum, (2) relaxation of the internal sphincter, (3) contraction of the external sphincter, (4) relaxation of the puborectalis muscle with Valsalva, (5) mild ascent of the pelvic floor causing straightening of the anorectal angle and opening of the anal canal, and (6) increased intraluminal pressure produced by straining.[10]

Etiology

The causes of constipation are numerous but may be classified according to an acute or chronic state (Table 27-1). In the emergency setting, patients will present most often with acute constipation due to medications or painful perianal lesions (e.g., abscesses, fissures, hemorrhoids, herpes). Medications most often causing acute constipation include anticholinergics (e.g., antihistamines, tricyclic antidepressants, antiparkinsonian agents, antispasmodics), antacids (e.g., aluminum hydroxide, calcium carbonate), antihypertensives (e.g., calcium channel antagonists, clonidine, diuretics), narcotics, nonsteroidal anti-inflammatory agents, sympathomimetics (e.g., ephedrine, phenylephedrine, phenylpropanolamine, terbutaline), Dilantin, and sucralfate.

One of the most important external factors governing

Table 27-1. Etiologies of Acute and Chronic Constipation

Acute Constipation	Chronic Constipation
Anatomic	Amyotrophic lateral sclerosis
Barium	Bedridden, debilitated, or institutionalized
Bismuth	Dementia
Carcinoma	Diabetic autonomic neuropathy
Depression	Diverticulosis
Diet	Irritable bowel syndrome
Diverticulitis	Neurogenic
Drugs	Parkinson's disease
Deficient fiber intake	Psychogenic disorders
Deficient fluid intake	Spinal cord lesions
Immobility	Stroke
Iron	
Lack of exercise	
Laxative abuse	
Metabolic disorders (such as hypercalcemia, hypoadrenalism, hypokalemia, hypothyroidism)	
Painful perianal lesions (such as abscesses, fissures, hemorrhoids, herpes)	
Psychosis	
Stress	
Travel	

colonic function is diet and an adequate intake of fluid; fiber is also essential in preventing constipation. Constipation of any cause may be exacerbated by chronic illnesses, such as those commonly afflicting the elderly, which lead to physical or mental impairment and result in inactivity or physical immobility. However, in a large majority of patients with severe constipation, no obvious cause can be identified. Thus many cases of constipation remain undiagnosed after initial assessment yet respond to empirical therapy.

Many potential disorders of anorectal function are thought to contribute to disordered defecation. These disorders include megarectum, congenital aganglionosis (Hirschsprung's disease), pelvic floor dyssynergia (in which there is an unconscious contraction of striated muscles of the pelvic floor during defecation),[11,12] and some rectoceles (in which there is a misdirection of stool into pouches associated with weakness of the rectovaginal septum). It is important to distinguish such causes from voluntary inhibition of defecation, which may be psychologic or a response to painful disorders.

Slow colonic transit and pelvic floor dysfunction often play roles in certain cases, especially in middle-aged and elderly women with chronic intractable constipation. Inactivity is considered to predispose to constipation in the elderly.[13,14] Many constipated persons are also depressed[3,15]; aspirin intake, smoking, and alcohol abuse also may be implicated.[16–18] Rectosigmoid outlet difficulty or delay (obstructed defecation) due to structural or pelvic floor muscle abnormalities may produce difficulty with defecation requiring manual disimpaction of stool or a feeling of anal blockage with prolonged defecation.[19,20] The elderly also may ignore calls to stool, which results in fecal retention; because rectal sensation is then suppressed, the desire to defecate may be perceived only with large rectal masses that are very difficult to evacuate.[10,21]

CLINICAL FEATURES

A thorough, detailed history usually can elucidate the most likely cause of a patient's constipation. Patients usually present with abdominal cramping or distension. Pertinent historical information involves assessing the character of the stools (loose or hard), the timing and frequency of the stools, associated symptoms (e.g., occupation, sleep habits, appetite, daily activities, and mood), concurrent diseases, and exogenous factors (e.g., diet, exercise, and medications).

A precise description of symptoms and their duration should be obtained. Acute constipation is associated more often with organic disease than is chronic constipation. Constipation with a later onset in life suggests an acquired disease. A recent change in an adult's bowel habits with nausea and vomiting may result from an obstructing neoplasm. Also, diarrhea alternating with constipation and weight loss suggests an obstructing neoplasm or irritable bowel syndrome. Significant temperature elevation may be due to prolonged fecal impaction, inflammatory disease, or invasive infection. Generalized malaise or weakness may be associated with dehydration or an electrolyte imbalance. Flatulence and bloating concomitant with constipation may be a result of a malabsorption syndrome.

Evaluation begins with a definition of the size, character, nature, and frequency of bowel movements, followed by a determination of the chronicity of the problem. A history of prior laxative use should be obtained. The patient must be asked about symptoms that suggest an underlying gastrointestinal problem, such as abdominal pain (may be dull, crampy, or visceral), nausea, cramping, vomiting, weight loss, melena, rectal bleeding, rectal pain, and fever. Anorexia, bloating, belching, fatigue, flatus, mucus in the stool, headache, weakness, depression, and anxiety also should be recorded; these symptoms may be associated with constipation of any etiology but often accompany functional disorders. The most concerning symptoms associated with constipation are rectal bleeding and changes in the caliber of the stool, which suggest possible colorectal cancer.

It is helpful during the initial visit to elicit a history of working, eating, and bowel habits. Inquiry into dietary fiber intake and physical activity is essential. Use of medications, including nonprescription agents (especially laxatives and antacids), needs to be detailed. A careful psychosocial history should be obtained, with attention to emotional distress, evidence of anxiety, or affective disorders. Depression is relatively common in the elderly population and may compound the problem of constipation.[10,23]

The physical examination should be directed both toward the detection of nongastrointestinal diseases and physical findings of primary diseases, such as endocrinopathies and neurologic disorders, that may contribute to constipation. Skin should be checked for pallor and signs of hypothyroidism. The abdomen should be examined for masses, distension, tenderness, and high-pitched or absent bowel sounds. The abdominal examination is usually normal but may reveal tenderness, a mass, or distension and evidence of obstruction.

The rectal examination for anorectal conditions and an evaluation of the stool are two of the most important parts of the physical assessment. Rectal examination includes careful inspection and palpation for masses, fissures, inflammation, and the presence of hard stool. The lattermost finding excludes significant obstruction, and poor colonic motility suggests that the problem is inadequate rectal emptying. A digital rectal examination can assist in confirming the presence of anorectal outlet problems by considering the reaction of the pelvic floor muscles, sphincter muscles, and rectum when defecation is simulated. The digital rectal examination also can be used to assess the presence of a fecal impaction and the consistency of stool within the rectum. The stool should be noted for color and consistency and tested for occult blood. The patient should be asked to strain to demonstrate evidence of a rectocele or rectal prolapse. Disordered innervation of the anus is indicated if the anal canal opens wide when the puborectalis muscle is pulled posteriorly. Anoscopy is needed to identify internal hemorrhoids, fissures, tumors, and other local pathology.

If constipation is acute, the evaluation often can be stopped at this point because adjustments in medications, correction of metabolic derangements, or treatment of reversible medical problems may allow constipation to resolve. Laxatives of almost any kind can be used to manage acute constipation.

When constipation is chronic, diagnostic testing should be targeted to answer specific questions in the elderly. In contrast to younger patients, in whom the risk of colon cancer presenting with constipation is low, colon cancer is a common disease in the elderly and should be excluded. Patients suspected of having anorectal outlet problems should be referred for defecography, which can show lesions such as intrarectal intussusception, abnormal pelvic floor muscle relaxation, and rectal prolapse.[24]

DIAGNOSIS AND DIFFERENTIAL

Radiologic investigation is of limited use unless evidence from the history and physical examination points to bowel obstruction or other serious pathology as the cause of constipation. There are few cases of morbidity and even fewer cases of mortality for patients with the primary presentation of constipation; most adverse outcomes are due to a missed diagnosis of bowel obstruction or perforation.[3] Plain radiographs of the abdomen may help to discern the extent and nature of the problem. Constipation can be diagnosed easily with flat and upright abdominal radiographs. These films aid in evaluating for bowel obstruction, megacolon, volvulus, or mass lesions. Masses of stools typically have a bubbly or speckled appearance.

The acute onset of constipation requires excluding obstruction and ileus, especially when accompanied by abdominal discomfort. Plain supine and upright films of the abdomen, along with measurements of serum potassium and calcium levels, are indicated. Patients with acute constipation for which the cause is not readily apparent should be treated symptomatically and referred for outpatient diagnostic evaluation. This outpatient workup usually includes a sigmoidoscopy and a barium enema, preferably air contrast in nature, to evaluate for an underlying intrinsic bowel lesion. Possible endocrinologic or metabolic causes should also be investigated on an outpatient basis.

Chronic laxative abuse can present as acute constipation, and patients often do not divulge their laxative use. If laxative abuse is suspected, a sodium hydroxide test of the stool may be revealing. If 3% sodium hydroxide turns the stool red, and if the reaction is abrogated by the addition of hydrochloric acid, it is indicative of the presence of phenolphthalein, the most commonly abused laxative.

More chronic or recurrent forms of constipation should be assessed with a check of the serum glucose level for diabetes and of the serum thyroid-stimulating hormone (TSH) level for hypothyroidism. Greater than 25 percent of patients with colorectal carcinomas present with constipation. If colon cancer is suspected, referring the patient for colonoscopy is required.[3]

The differential diagnosis of chronic constipation is extensive because constipation secondary to other illnesses and therapies is common, and the elderly tend to have more of these other illness. Important considerations in the differential diagnosis include bowel obstruction, chronic intestinal pseudo-obstruction, hypothyroidism, diabetes, and side effects of drug therapy. Constipation-predominant irritable bowel syndrome can be present in the elderly, but characteristically there should be a history of abdominal pain and constipation going back many years. Other considerations in the differential diagnosis include functional outlet obstruction conditions such as anismus, hypertonic internal anal sphincter, solitary rectal ulcer syndrome, mucosal intussusception, and rectal prolapse. Neurologic diseases in the differential diagnosis include spinal cord injury, cauda equina tumor, multiple sclerosis, Parkinson's disease, autonomic neuropathy, and Hirschsprung's disease. The rectoanal diseases that should be considered include anal fissures, hemorrhoids, anal strictures; inflammatory bowel disease; proctitis; and myotonic dystrophy. The patient's medication list should be reviewed for drugs that may have a constipating side effect.

EMERGENCY DEPARTMENT CARE AND DISPOSITION

Symptomatic management is quite empirical and is appropriate for the patient with a suspected functional etiology but only after bowel obstruction and other forms of serious organic pathology have been excluded. The initial step is to educate patients about increasing dietary fiber, normal defecation patterns, exercise, the use of laxatives, and appropriate fluid intake. Routine use of laxatives over extended periods of time should be discouraged because of the risk of side effects such as damage to the myenteric plexus resulting in "cathartic colon" due to stimulant laxatives.

If the patient insists on medication, clinicians may recommend fiber supplements, such as a nondigestible fiber residue, or bulk-forming laxatives, such as ground psyllium seed (Metamucil), methylcellulose (Citrucel), or polycarbophil. These act to increase bulk by means of their hydrophilic properties, but they must be taken with plenty of fluids to prevent formation of an obstructing bolus.[25]

A few classes of laxatives are relatively safe and worth considering when simpler measures have failed. Sorbitol and lactulose are classified as nonabsorbable saccharide or bulk laxatives. These agents have been shown to be safe and effective when used on a long-term basis in the elderly.[26] They induce a potent osmotic effect, causing the retention of fluid in the bowel lumen and consequently softening the stool. The cost of sorbitol (30–60 mL daily at bedtime) is approximately one-tenth that of lactulose, and sorbitol has been shown in studies to be equal in effect and slightly better tolerated.[9,26] Side effects of these agents include bloating, cramping, and excessive flatulence.

Milk of magnesia and magnesium citrate are magnesium-containing laxatives that are also osmotically active, but they should be used more prudently because they may induce magnesium and sodium overload in the elderly with renal dysfunction. Magnesium-containing laxatives are less expensive than sorbitol. Surfactant laxatives, such as docusate, soften the stool by promoting the mixing of water and fat and may be efficacious in patients reporting hard stools.

Conversely, many laxatives should not be used on a regular basis because of the potential for adverse effects. The stimulant/irritant laxatives include the derivatives of diphenylmethane (bisacodyl), anthraquinone (senna), and cascara. These irritants trigger colonic contraction acutely. Extended or long-term use is associated with an increased risk for bowel refractoriness and exacerbation of existing constipation (i.e., laxative abuse syndrome). Cisapride, a prokinetic agent producing dopaminergic stimulation, is associated with an increased risk for ventricular dysrhythmias. Soapsuds enemas should be avoided because colitis has been reported with their use.

ADDITIONAL ASPECTS

The following are pitfalls in the management of constipation:

- A number of complications of constipation or its treatment may be the reason the patient seeks medical attention. These complications include hemorrhoids, anal fissure, rectal prolapse, stercoral ulcer, colonic perforation, colonic volvulus, ischemic colitis, fecal incontinence, urinary retention, melanosis coli, cathartic colon, cardiac and cerebrovascular dysfunction (i.e., angina, arrhythmias, syncope), and fecal impaction.

- Signs and symptoms of fecal impaction include an altered mental status, agitation, fever, paradoxical diarrhea that is caused by leakage around the area of impaction, and urinary retention and overflow incontinence. Any patient who presents to the ED with fecal impaction should be disimpacted prior to discharge. Treatment for fecal impaction includes enemas or, commonly, manual disimpaction. Patients with unrelieved fecal impaction often require admission for further therapy. Extreme cases (e.g., mechanical bowel obstruction) may mandate surgical intervention.[27]

REFERENCES

1. Robson KM, Kiely DK, Lembo T: Development of constipation in nursing home residents. *Dis Colon Rectum* 43:940, 2000.
2. Talley NJ, Fleming KC, Evans JM, et al: Constipation in an elderly community: A study of prevalence and potential risk factors. *Am J Gastroenterol* 91(1):19, 1996.
3. Wald A: Constipation. *Adv Gastroenterol* 84(5):1231, 2000.
4. Whitehead WE, Drinkwater D, Cheskin LJ, et al: Constipation in the elderly living at home: Definition, prevalence, and relationship to life style and health status. *J Am Geriatr Soc* 37:423, 1989.
5. Drossman DA, Sandler RS, McKee DC, et al: Bowel patterns among subjects not seeking health care: Use of a questionnaire to identify a population with bowel dysfunction. *Gastroenterology* 83:529, 1982.

6. Koch A, Voderholzer WA, Klauser AG, et al: Symptoms in chronic constipation. *Dis Colon Rectum* 40:902, 1997.

7. Aichbichler BW, Wenzl HH, Santa Ana CA, et al: A comparison of stool characteristics from normal and constipated people. *Dig Dis Sci* 43:2353, 1998.

8. Schiller LR: Constipation and fecal incontinence in the elderly. *Gastroenterol Clin North Am* 30(2):497, 2001.

9. Fine KD: Diarrhea, in Feldman M, Scharschmidt BF, Sleisenger MH (eds): *Sleisenger and Fordtran's Gastrointestinal and Hepatic Disease: Pathophysiology, Diagnosis, Management*, 6th ed. Philadelphia, Saunders, 1998, p 128.

10. Cullen N: Constipation, in Marx JA, Hockberger RS, Walls RM (eds): *Rosen's Emergency Medicine: Concepts and Clinical Practice*, 5th ed. St Louis, Mosby, 2002, p 209.

11. Velio P, Bassotti G: Chronic idiopathic constipation: Pathophysiology and treatment. *J Clin Gastroenterol* 22:190, 1996.

12. Rao SSC, Enck P, Loening-Baucke V: Biofeedback therapy for defecation disorders. *Dig Dis* 15(suppl 1):78, 1997.

13. Talley NJ, O'Keefe EA, Zinsmeister AR, et al: Prevalence of gastrointestinal symptoms in the elderly: A population based study. *Gastroenterology* 102:895, 1992.

14. Donald IP, Smith RG, Cruikshank JG, et al: A study of constipation in the elderly living at home. *Gerontology* 31:112, 1985.

15. Talley NJ, Weaver AL, Zinsmeister AR, et al: Functional constipation and outlet delay: A population-based study. *Gastroenterology* 105:781, 1993.

16. Scott AM, Kellow JE, Eckersley GM, et al: Cigarette smoking and nicotine delay postprandial mouth-cecum transit time. *Dig Dis Sci* 37:1544, 1992.

17. Wegener M, Schaffstein J, Dilger U, et al: Gastrointestinal transit of solid-liquid meal in chronic alcoholics. *Dig Dis Sci* 36:917, 1991.

18. Whitehead WE, Devroede G, Habib FI, et al: Functional disorders of the anorectum. *Gastroenterol Int* 5:92, 1992.

19. Grotz RL, Pemberton JH, Talley NJ, et al: Discriminant value of psychological distress, symptom profiles and segmental colonic dysfunction in outpatients with severe idiopathic constipation. *Gut* 35:798, 1994.

20. Brocklehurst JC, Khan MY: A study of fecal stasis in old age and the use of Dorbanex in its prevention. *Gerontol Clin* 11:293, 1969.

21. Whitehead WE, Chaussade S, Corazziari E, et al: Report of an international workshop on management of constipation. *Gastroenterol Int* 4:99, 1991.

22. Glia A, Lindberg G, Nilsson LH, et al: Clinical value of symptom assessment in patients with constipation. *Dis Colon Rectum* 42:1401, 1999.

23. Jones HJ, Swift RI, Blake H: A prospective audit of the usefulness of evacuating proctography. *Ann R Coll Surg Engl* 80:40, 1998.

24. Prokesch RW, Breitenseher MJ, Kettenbach J, et al: Assessment of chronic constipation: Colon transit time versus defecography. *Eur J Radiol* 32:197, 1999.

25. Bharucha AE: Functional abdominal pain in the elderly. *Gastroenterol Clin North Am* 30(2):517, 2001.

26. Richter JM: Approach to the patient with constipation, in Goroll AH, Mulley AG (eds): *Primary Care Medicine*, 4th ed. Philadelphia, Lippincott Williams & Wilkins, 2000, p 423.

27. Christiansen J, Rasmussen O: Colectomy for severe slow transit constipation in strictly selected patients. *Scand J Gastroenterol* 31:770, 1996.

28

Biliary Emergencies

Matthew A. Bridges
O. John Ma

HIGH-YIELD FACTS

- Disorders of the biliary tract are the most common cause of abdominal pain in the geriatric population.
- Gallstones are found in the gallbladder or bile ducts in 33 percent of the U.S. population by age 70.
- Gallbladder disease is the most common condition requiring intraabdominal surgery in the elderly.
- Ultrasonography is the most reliable diagnostic modality for diagnosing biliary tract disease. Computed tomography rarely adds to the diagnosis.
- Most patients with cholecystitis are afebrile at presentation, and approximately 30 to 40 percent of these patients fail to develop leukocytosis.

Biliary tract disease is frequently the etiology of abdominal pain in adults of all ages; however, in the elderly it is the most common cause of abdominal pain. The evaluation and treatment of biliary disease, as is the case with other abdominal processes, may be much more difficult in the elderly patient. Declines in visual acuity and hearing, as well as concurrent medical problems such as previous stroke or underlying neurologic disease, may make communication of the history more difficult. Certain medications may mask the symptoms, physical examination findings, and laboratory results associated with the disease process.

Furthermore, the elderly patient is likely to present at a more advanced stage of disease than the younger patient. This propensity for a later presentation is multifactorial. Fears of loss of independence and the surgical procedure, attitudes of the patient and family toward hospitals, and physician bias may all prolong the time to definitive treatment. This is exemplified by the finding

that 70 percent of elderly patients undergoing biliary tract surgery do so on an emergent or urgent basis.[1] The mortality of biliary tract surgery is increased from 4 to 10 percent in elective cases to 20 percent in emergent surgeries in the elderly.[2]

EPIDEMIOLOGY

Diseases of the gallbladder and biliary system are extremely common and important causes of abdominal pain in the elderly. In fact, cholelithiasis or choledocholithiasis is found in 33 to 50 percent of the U.S. population by 70 years of age.[1,2] Often this represents asymptomatic disease, and many of these cases are identified incidentally at autopsy. As people age, it stands to reason that they would have an increased likelihood of developing signs and symptoms, as well as some of the later complications, associated with cholelithiasis. This likely contributes to the finding that more than 25 percent of all elderly patients who undergo abdominal surgery for benign biliary disease are found to have acute cholecystitis.[1] The incidence of acute cholecystitis in the elderly patient with abdominal pain ranges in various studies from 12 to 41 percent, with the true number probably lying near 25 percent.[3,4] The gender distribution for biliary disease is different in elderly patients when compared with the general population. In a series of elderly patients diagnosed with acute cholecystitis, 52 to 58 percent of patients were female, whereas in the general population up to 70 percent of all patients with acute cholecystitis were female.[5–9]

PATHOPHYSIOLOGY

Bile is produced in hepatocytes and is stored in the gallbladder. It is then transported from the gallbladder through the cystic duct and common bile duct into the duodenum. There are three types of biliary stones. The most common is the cholesterol stone, which accounts for 70 percent of all biliary stones. The second most common type is the pigment stone, which accounts for 20 percent. The remainder of all biliary stones is of mixed composition.

Gallstones form in the gallbladder and enlarge. They eventually are expelled into the cystic duct and common bile duct, where they may become lodged and obstruct flow. Contractions of the gallbladder and biliary tree cause the initial biliary pain, which is usually colicky in nature. These contractions may dislodge the stone into the duodenum.

If the obstruction is not relieved, inflammation develops and leads to acute cholecystitis. Three factors lead to the clinical picture of cholecystitis: mechanical, chemical, and infectious. In the initial stages, mechanical factors, such as distension leading to ischemia of the gallbladder wall, predominate. This ischemia leads to the release of inflammatory mediators, a chemical factor. As stasis and inflammation continue, infectious factors become more important with the proliferation of various bacteria. *Escherichia coli* and *Klebsiella* are the most common pathogens involved in acute cholecystitis, whereas group D *Streptococcus*, *Staphylococcus*, *Clostridium*, and *Enterococcus* are less commonly involved pathogens. As in the general population, *E. coli* is the most commonly isolated pathogen from the biliary tract of elderly patients with acute cholecystitis.[1,10]

Left unchecked, this process eventually will lead to gangrene and perforation of the gallbladder wall. As biliary obstruction and bacterial proliferation persist, bacteria may move retrograde through the liver and into the systemic circulation, a condition known as *ascending cholangitis*. Gallstone pancreatitis is also related to persistent obstruction. Gallstones are a common cause of pancreatitis, but the pathophysiology is multifactorial and not well understood.

Emphysematous cholecystitis is different from acute cholecystitis in that the bacteria involved are gasforming. *Clostridium* is the most common pathogen isolated from patients with this disease (46 percent of isolates compared with 12 percent in acute cholecystitis). These bacteria penetrate the gallbladder wall, moving in fascial planes, and produce the characteristic appearance of air in the gallbladder, gallbladder wall, and adjacent tissues. Emphysematous cholecystitis is much less likely to be associated with gallstones than acute cholecystitis. Ischemia has been found to have a strong association with the disease, with blood vessel narrowing or blockage being discovered on pathologic examination in a much higher percentage than in acute cholecystitis.[9,11]

CLINICAL FEATURES

The classic description of the pain associated with biliary disease is colicky right upper quadrant abdominal pain, particularly after the ingestion of greasy foods. This pain may be associated with nausea and vomiting. As is the case in many conditions, the actual presentation for biliary disease is highly variable, with most patients exhibiting various combinations of signs and symptoms. For biliary tract disease, comparison of various case series in the literature reveal very little difference in the presenting complaints and physical examination findings between the geriatric population and the population in general.[7,8,12]

Up to 70 percent of all patients with biliary disease complain of right upper quadrant abdominal pain, with more than 10 percent reporting lower abdominal pain.[7,8] In contrast to the classic description of colicky pain, patients with gallstones are more likely than patients with nonbiliary pathology to report persistent pain. In one study, 83 percent of the patients reported episodes lasting longer than 30 minutes, with 64 percent reporting steady pain. Only 62 percent of the patients had pain associated with eating, whereas 59 percent reported pain after ingesting greasy foods, and 32 percent had pain without relation to food. Nausea was a complaint in 70 percent of patients.[8]

Multiple series have failed to demonstrate significant differences in presenting complaint and physical examination findings between geriatric and younger populations presenting with biliary disease. There is, however, a trend for symptoms and signs to be less severe or even absent in the elderly patient when compared with younger patients with similar severity of disease. In one series, the mean age of asymptomatic patients with cholelithiasis was 73.6 years, whereas the mean age of symptomatic patients was 63.6 years.[13] There are also data to suggest that the presence of multiple medical problems increases the likelihood of asymptomatic biliary disease. Conditions such as coronary artery disease, diabetes mellitus, and various malignancies also seem to decrease the likelihood of reporting symptoms associated with biliary disease.

The classic presentation of acute cholecystitis is the typical biliary pain described earlier associated with fever, a positive Murphy's sign, leukocytosis, and abnormal liver enzymes. Approximately 36 to 68 percent of patients with confirmed acute cholecystitis, however, will be afebrile.[5–7,12] Both fever and leukocytosis are absent in about a third of patients.[5,6] Age has not been shown definitively to have a statistically significant effect on fever; there is, however, a trend for higher white blood cell counts in patients over age 60.[6,12] On the physical examination, a Murphy's sign is highly sensitive (97 percent) but low in specificity (48 percent). Rebound tenderness and guarding are findings with a good positive predictive value but poor sensitivity.[5]

The patient with emphysematous cholecystitis presents in a similar fashion to the patient with acute cholecystitis. Approximately two-thirds of patients are febrile. The percentage of patients with leukocytosis does appear to be slightly higher in this group. Despite the high mortality associated with this disease, the patient may not necessarily present ill or septic-appearing.[9]

The classic findings of cholecystitis are commonly absent in patients with ascending cholangitis. The triad of right upper quadrant pain, fever, and jaundice is found in about 25 percent of all patients with ascending cholangitis. In general, patients present toxic in appearance and display signs and symptoms of sepsis.

Elderly patients occasionally may present with vague complaints, such as confusion, malaise, frequent falls, weakness, or declining mental functioning, and be found to have biliary disease, even in the complete absence of abdominal complaints or physical examination findings. Typically, these patients are diagnosed after discovery of abnormal screening laboratory tests, such as elevated liver enzymes and alkaline phosphatase. The exact mechanism of this process is unclear, but it has been postulated that a combination of decreased hepatic function and occult sepsis contributes to this pathophysiologic process.[14]

DIAGNOSIS AND DIFFERENTIAL

As with the general population, the diagnosis of biliary tract disease in the elderly can be quite challenging. The differential diagnosis is more expansive in the older population, as is the prevalence of concurrent medical conditions that may obscure, accentuate, or contribute to various aspects of the disease process. Because of these factors and the fact that the history and physical examination may be more unreliable in pinpointing the disease process, the scope of imaging and laboratory investigation must be expanded.

The differential diagnosis should consider common and uncommon causes of upper abdominal or back pain, which include pancreatitis, bowel obstruction, hepatitis, gastritis, gastric or duodenal ulcer, renal colic, pyelonephritis, perforated viscus, abdominal aortic aneurysm, traumatic injury, and various malignancies. If the pain is located in the lower abdomen, as is the case in more than 10 percent of patients with biliary disease, the differential is expanded to include appendicitis, diverticulitis, urinary tract infection, hernia, and genitourinary or gynecologic conditions. The possibility of myocardial or mesenteric ischemia also must be considered during the evaluation of elderly patients with abdominal pain.

When evaluating the elderly patient for biliary disease, laboratory studies that may prove helpful include a complete blood count, electrolytes, urinalysis, hepatic function tests, amylase, lipase, and coagulation studies. Obtaining an electrocardiogram and cardiac enzymes also should be strongly considered in this population. In general, laboratory testing has not been shown to be predictive of the presence or severity of biliary tract disease in the elderly patient; however, most situations will require broad diagnostic testing to exclude pathology outside the biliary system.[7,12]

In uncomplicated cholelithiasis, laboratory tests typically are normal but should be ordered to exclude other disease processes, as well as to evaluate for the complications of gallstones. In acute cholecystitis, there is a higher likelihood of leukocytosis in the elderly patient. Hepatic function tests also are more likely to be abnormal in the geriatric population but are only abnormal in about half of all elderly patients.[7,12]

As gallstone obstruction persists, laboratory values are more likely to be abnormal. If gallstone pancreatitis develops, the amylase and lipase levels should be elevated. The patient with gallstone pancreatitis also may demonstrate leukocytosis, anemia, or hypocalcemia in severe cases. If the obstruction is at the level of the common bile duct, liver enzymes are likely to be abnormal.

Patients with ascending cholangitis are more likely to develop leukocytosis than patients with acute cholecystitis. Hepatic enzymes are also more likely to be abnormal, and blood cultures are commonly positive. Similarly, with emphysematous cholecystitis, most elderly patients will develop leukocytosis. Hepatic enzymes are likely to be normal because the disease is often acalculous in nature. Blood cultures are positive approximately 50 percent of the time.[9,11]

The keystone for the diagnosis of biliary tract disease is ultrasonography. This applies to all age groups. Sonography has the ability to detect gallstones that are 2 mm in size or larger. It is noninvasive and does not require injection of contrast material or isotopes. Sonography is useful for identifying gallstones (Fig. 28-1), gallbladder distension, gallbladder wall thickening, distension of the common bile duct or hepatic ducts, gallbladder sludge, and free fluid. The sensitivity of ultrasound for acute cholecystitis (Fig. 28-2) approaches 90 percent.[7]

Use of computed tomographic (CT) scanning for the diagnosis of biliary diseases is increasingly common, especially in the elderly population, in which the source of the patient's pathology often is difficult to pinpoint clinically. For diseases of the biliary tract, CT scanning has not been demonstrated to be superior to ultrasound. In fact, several series have shown the ultrasound examination to be a superior tool for identifying both gallstones and the changes associated with acute cholecystitis.[7,15] CT scanning, however, is superior to ultrasound in evaluating for other causes of the patient's symptomatology,

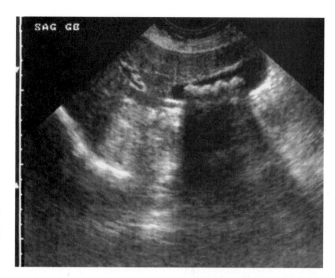

Fig. 28-1 Longitudinal view of the gallbladder demonstrating multiple moderate-sized stones resembling "peas in a pod" with prominent posterior acoustic shadowing. *(Courtesy of Lori Sens and Lori Green, Gulfcoast Ultrasound.)*

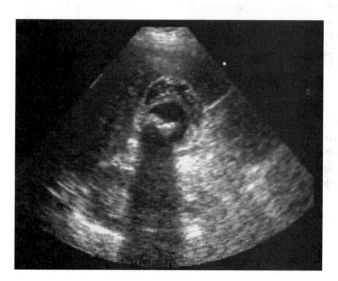

Fig. 28-2 Transverse view of the gallbladder shows marked thickening of the anterior wall and associated edema separating the layers of the wall. Cholelithiasis with shadowing is obvious. This patient was diagnosed with acute cholecystitis.

including pathology of the abdominal aorta and appendix, air in the biliary tree, pneumoperitoneum, and intraabdominal malignancies.

Plain radiographs of the abdomen typically do not add to the diagnosis of biliary pathology. They may identify gallstones, but ultrasonography remains a superior modality. Plain radiographs are useful for identifying air in the gallbladder, the gallbladder wall, or the tissues surrounding the gallbladder in the patient with emphysematous cholecystitis. They are also helpful in patients in whom bowel obstruction or perforation is a part of the differential diagnosis.

Hepatobiliary scintigraphy is an excellent confirmatory test for acute cholecystitis. It is more accurate than other imaging modalities in identifying cystic duct obstruction. For acute cholecystitis, the sensitivity is 90 to 100 percent with a specificity of 85 to 95 percent.

EMERGENCY DEPARTMENT CARE AND DISPOSITION

For the elderly patient with uncomplicated cholelithiasis, the mainstay of emergency department (ED) treatment is hydration, pain control, and antiemetics. Opiates are used commonly for pain control in this situation. While all narcotics have been demonstrated to increase the tone of the biliary sphincter, studies have shown that meperidine has a weaker spasmodic effect than other narcotic medications.[16–18] The clinical impact of this finding has not been well established; however, most would agree that it would be prudent to selectively use meperidine in the setting in which narcotic pain medications are necessary for the relief of biliary pain. Ketorolac also has been shown to be quite effective. Some patients may require nasogastric decompression of the stomach for relief. Patients may be discharged home if they appear nontoxic, have close follow-up care established, have their pain well controlled, appear well hydrated, and are able to take fluids by mouth. Establishing close follow-up care is crucial in this age group because the early stages of acute cholecystitis may be quite insidious.

There is disagreement as to the optimal disposition of the elderly patient with symptomatic cholelithiasis. Many surgeons and primary care physicians are reluctant to subject the elderly patient to elective surgery because there is a chance that the patient's symptoms will resolve without intervention and there will be no further episodes. However, more than half of all elderly patients with biliary pain that resolves initially will experience further episodes of biliary colic.[2] In addition, the elderly patient is much less able to tolerate emergent or urgent surgery than the younger population. For elderly patients, mortality increases from 4 to 10 percent in elective cases to 20 percent in emergent or urgent surgeries.[1] This is magnified by the finding that 70 percent of all elderly patients undergo surgery on an urgent or emergent basis.[2] Nearly 90 percent of all elderly patients undergoing biliary surgery have either had previous biliary surgery, established cholelithiasis, a history of biliary colic, or pancreatitis.[1,19]

Because of this debate, the patient with cholelithiasis who is discharged home should be referred to their primary care physician immediately. The decision on whether to refer to a surgeon may be made at a later date after discussion between the patient and his or her primary physician. This also allows the primary physician to optimize treatment of the patient's other medical problems prior to referral.

The patient with acute cholecystitis requires more urgent treatment. Extracellular volume repletion is important. Pain control often requires narcotic pain medications. Antibiotics should be administered after blood cultures are drawn (Table 28-1). The definitive treatment is typically surgical. In the toxic-appearing elderly patient with acute cholecystitis who has multiple comorbidities, endoscopic

Table 28-1. Antibiotic Regimens for Cholecystitis, Ascending Cholangitis, Emphysematous Cholecystitis, Biliary Sepsis, and Common Duct Obstruction

---

Piperacillin-tazobactam 3.375 g q6h or 4.5 g q8h IV
Ampicillin-sulbactam 3.0 g q6h IV
Ticarcillin-clavulanate 3.1 g q6h IV
Imipenem 0.5 g q6h IV
Meropenem 1.0 g q8h IV
Third-generation cephalosporin plus metronidazole
   1.0 g q12h IV or clindamycin 450–900 mg q8h IV
Aztreonam 2.0 g q8h IV plus clindamycin 450–900 mg
   q8h IV
Ampicillin 2.0 g q6h IV plus gentamicin 2 mg/kg load,
   then 1.7 mg/kg q8h IV

---

retrograde cholangiopancreatography (ERCP) has been shown to have lower complication and mortality rates when compared with emergent surgery.[2,20] The various treatment options should be discussed with the surgical consultant.

The patient with ascending cholangitis is more likely to be acutely ill and septic, so more aggressive resuscitation is often required. Intravenous fluids are important in the early stages of the resuscitation to restore intravascular volume. Vasopressors occasionally may be required to maintain cardiac output in the setting of sepsis and shock. Appropriate antibiotics should be administered in a timely fashion after cultures are drawn (see Table 28-1). A surgeon should be consulted early because definitive treatment typically is operative.

The ED treatment for emphysematous cholecystitis is similar to that for acute cholecystitis. These patients are much more likely to require an emergent surgical procedure than the patient with acute cholecystitis.

The treatment for gallstone pancreatitis is largely supportive, with extracellular volume repletion and pain control being most important. The patient should be given nothing by mouth. Nasogastric decompression of the stomach may be necessary for relief of discomfort. The patient should be admitted with surgical consultation.

ADDITIONAL ASPECTS

The following are pitfalls in the management of patients with biliary disease:

- The elderly patient may present with milder symptomatology at similar or more advanced stages of gallbladder disease. A higher index of suspicion should be maintained for those conditions, such as emphysematous cholecystitis, that are seen infrequently in younger patients. Emergency physicians should entertain the possibility of serious intraabdominal pathology even in elderly patients who appear well and nontoxic.

- The diagnoses of abdominal aortic aneurysm, myocardial ischemia, and mesenteric ischemia always must be considered, especially in the elderly patient with a presentation indicative of biliary disease and a negative biliary disease workup.

- Emergency physicians should not rely on a normal CT scan of the abdomen as an indication that biliary tract disease is absent.

REFERENCES

1. Harness JK, Strodel WE, Talsam SE: Symptomatic biliary tract disease in the elderly patient. *Am Surg* 52:442, 1986.
2. Siegel JH, Kasmin FE: Biliary tract diseases in the elderly: Management and outcomes. *Gut* 41:433, 1997.
3. Fenyo G: Acute abdominal disease in the elderly. *Am J Surg* 143:751, 1982.
4. Bugliosi TF, Meloy TD, Vukov LF: Acute abdominal pain in the elderly. *Ann Emerg Med* 19:1383, 1990.
5. Singer AJ, McCracken G, Henry MC, et al: Correlation among clinical, laboratory, and hepatobiliary scanning findings in patients with suspected acute cholecystitis. *Ann Emerg Med* 28:267, 1996.
6. Gruber PJ, Silverman RA, Gottesfeld S, Flaster E: Presence of fever and leukocytosis in acute cholecystitis. *Ann Emerg Med* 28:273, 1996.
7. Parker LJ, Vukov LF, Wollan PC: Emergency department evaluation of geriatric patients with acute cholecystitis. *Acad Emerg Med* 4:51, 1997.
8. Diehl AK, Sugarek NJ, Todd KH: Clinical evaluation for gallstone disease: Usefulness of symptoms and signs in diagnosis. *Am J Med* 89:29, 1990.
9. Mentzer RM, Golden GT, Chandler JG, Horsley JS: A comparative appraisal of emphysematous cholecystitis. *Am J Surg* 129:10, 1975.
10. Fukunaga FH: Gallbladder bacteriology, histology, and gallstones. *Arch Surg* 106:169, 1973.
11. Laor T, Deluca SA: Emphysematous cholecystitis. *Am Fam Phys* 38(4):157, 1988.
12. Burbige EJ, Moskowitz SA, Belber JP: Influence of age on the clinical presentation of acute biliary tract disease. *J Clin Gastroenterol* 5:29, 1983.
13. McSherry CK, Ferstenberg H, Calhoun WF, et al: The natural history of diagnosed gallstone disease in symptomatic and asymptomatic patients. *Ann Surg* 202(1):59, 1985.
14. Cobden I, Venables CW, Lendrum R, James OFW: Gallstones presenting as mental and physical debility in the elderly. *Lancet* 1:1062, 1984.
15. Fidler J, Paulson EK, Layfield L: CT evaluation of acute cholecystitis: Findings and usefulness in diagnosis. *AJR* 166:1085, 1996.
16. Greenstein AJ, Kaynan A, Singer A, Dreiling DA: A comparative study of pentazocine and meperidine on the biliary passage pressure. *Am J Gastroenterol* 58(4):417, 1972.
17. Pedersen SA, Oster-Jorgenson E, Kragland K: The effects of morphine on biliary dynamics. *Scand J Gastroenterol* 22(8):982, 1987.
18. Sherman S, Gottlieb K, Uzer MF, et al: Effects of meperidine on the pancreatic and biliary sphincter. *Gastrointest Endosc* 44(3):239, 1996.
19. Pigott JP, Williams GB: Cholecystectomy in the elderly. *Am J Surg* 155:408, 1988.
20. Ramirez FC, McIntosh AS, Dennert B, Harlan JR: Emergency endoscopic retrograde cholangiopancreatography in critically ill patients. *Gastrointest Endosc* 47(5):71, 1998.

29

Acute Appendicitis

Robert D. Sidman
Colleen N. Roche
Stephen W. Meldon

HIGH-YIELD FACTS

- Less than one-third of older patients will exhibit the classic presentation of periumbilical pain localizing to the right lower quadrant of the abdomen.
- Most patients present to the emergency department (ED) more than 24 hours after symptom onset.
- Twenty percent of patients do not have a leukocytosis, and 25 percent do not have a fever.
- Peritoneal signs may be subtle or absent in this age group.
- Computed tomographic (CT) scanning is the most useful imaging test for appendicitis and is recommended if the etiology of abdominal pain is uncertain.

Acute abdominal pain is one of the most common chief complaints in older patients presenting to the ED. Evaluation of these patients is often a daunting and complex task. The number of conditions that can cause acute abdominal pain in this group is extensive, and the etiologies differ when compared with those seen in a younger cohort. Although acute appendicitis is less common than other intraabdominal surgical emergencies, such as cholecystitis, it remains an important cause of abdominal pain in the elderly. Complication rates of acute appendicitis in the older population (age > 65 years) approach 50 percent.[1] This is due to several factors but is most commonly secondary to the delayed diagnosis of appendicitis, which has been shown to increase mortality from 8 to 19 percent.[2]

Diagnosing appendicitis in the elderly patient is particularly challenging. Although right lower quadrant abdominal pain in older patients with appendicitis is elicited in more than three-quarters of patients at some point during their examination, it may not be apparent on initial evaluation in the ED. The classic history of periumbilical pain that localizes to the right lower quadrant is seen in less than one-third of older patients.[1] Approximately one-quarter of older patients with proven appendicitis who are evaluated initially in the ED are misdiagnosed and discharged home.[3]

In addition to misdiagnosis, definitive care for older patients may be delayed because of patient delays in seeking medical care. This may be due in part to decreased pain perception but also may occur because of problems in communication, transportation, economic factors, dislike of hospitals, or the belief that pain and decline in function are an inevitable part of aging. Most patients older than age 65 present to the ED more than 24 hours after symptom onset.[4,5]

Factors that contribute to the delay in the diagnosis of appendicitis in this age group include limitations in history, the physiologic changes of aging, and physician bias. Obtaining a medical history from an elderly patient can be difficult because of cognitive impairment and communication difficulties. Although family members or nursing homes may not always provide accurate histories, these sources should be interviewed because the information they provide is often valuable. When available, additional history should be garnered by early acquisition of the patient's medical records and discussion with the patient's primary care physician.

Various physiologic changes seen in the elderly make the diagnosis of appendicitis both confusing and challenging. With age, the abdominal musculature decreases, and peritoneal irritation is less likely to manifest itself as guarding or rebound. Thus the elderly are more likely to present with vague complaints and a paucity of alarming signs and symptoms despite the presence of serious intraabdominal processes. It also has been speculated that the appendiceal wall in the elderly is weaker and more prone to perforation.

Another difficulty is physician bias with regard to certain diseases. For example, many physicians think of appendicitis as a disease of the young. In addition, few older patients with appendicitis will present classically. Horattas and colleagues[4] noted that only 20 percent of their older patients exhibited all the following features: anorexia, right lower quadrant pain, nausea or vomiting, fever, and elevated white blood cell (WBC) count with a left shift. Nausea and vomiting also occurred less commonly in the elderly than in younger patients presenting with appendicitis.

Since elderly patients with abdominal pain require

twice the rate of surgical intervention than younger patients, prompt diagnosis and treatment are paramount. One study showed that only half of older patients were diagnosed correctly with appendicitis at the time of admission and that only 70 percent had the diagnosis considered at the time of surgery.[4] Conversely, one-third of ED patients older than age 65 who were taken to the operating room with a preoperative diagnosis other than appendicitis were found to have appendicitis. Misdiagnosis and delays in diagnosis contribute to the increased morbidity and mortality of appendicitis in the elderly.

EPIDEMIOLOGY

Between 50 and 60 percent of elderly patients who present with abdominal pain are admitted. Approximately one-third of these patients will undergo a surgical procedure during their initial hospitalization.[6,7] Appendicitis comprises 14 percent of all abdominal emergencies in elderly patients compared with 80 percent in patients younger than age 50.[8] As the population ages, an increase in the number of older patients presenting with appendicitis is likely. In persons older than age 50, approximately 1 in 35 women and 1 in 50 men will develop appendicitis during the remainder of their lifetimes.[9]

PATHOPHYSIOLOGY

The chain of events responsible for acute appendicitis is initiated by luminal obstruction of the appendix. The most common etiology for obstruction is hyperplasia of lymphoid follicles (60 percent), followed by the presence of an appendicolith (35 percent). Numerous other factors can cause obstruction, including parasites, foreign bodies, tumors, inflammatory bowel disease, barium, appendiceal lymphadenopathy, and carcinomas. Although lymphoid hyperplasia is thought to have a major causative role in appendiceal obstruction in children, the appendix in the elderly is markedly atrophic with decreased lymphadenopathy. The elderly appendix is predisposed to obstruction and inflammation because of other factors, including a narrow or obliterated lumen, mucosal thinning and fibrosis, and fatty infiltrates. These characteristics, along with atherosclerosis, also lead to more rapid progression of the disease.

After obstruction has occurred, the appendix continues to secrete mucus until intraluminal pressure reaches 85 cmH$_2$O. This fluid accumulation increases intraluminal pressure, resulting in edema and stretching of the muscular layer. Venous stasis allows for increased bacterial growth, most commonly *Bacteroides* spp. or *Escherichia coli*, and the subsequent production of endotoxins and exotoxins. These toxins lead to mucosal ulceration, allowing bacteria to translocate into the muscular layers of the appendix. Polymorphonuclear cells invade the appendiceal wall as well. The increasing inflammation leads to a further increase in appendiceal pressure, which impedes arterial, venous, and lymphatic flow. Tissue infarction results.

Visceral autonomic nerves entering the spinal cord at the levels of T8 and T10 are stimulated by stretch fibers located in the muscular layer of the appendix. Patients then perceive pain as poorly localized to the periumbilical region, as referred by these dermatomes.

The disease process then spreads to adjacent intraabdominal structures and organs. Once the inflammation contacts the parietal peritoneum, somatic pain develops, and patients experience more localized pain, classically in the right lower quadrant. If the disease process is allowed to continue, perforation ensues with a release of pressure, and patients often experience a brief respite of symptoms. Perforation generally takes 24 to 36 hours to occur. Most commonly, perforation results in localized peritonitis and abscess formation. Pneumoperitoneum or bowel obstruction has been found in some cases.

CLINICAL FEATURES

In most cases of acute appendicitis, patients seek care 12 to 48 hours into the course of the illness, and the clinician needs only to conduct a thorough history and physical examination to make the diagnosis. Elderly patients often present later, with less reliable signs and symptoms, making appendicitis more difficult to distinguish from other disease processes.

In several series, more than 90 percent of elderly patients with appendicitis presented with a chief complaint of abdominal pain.[5,10] The increased number of underlying medical problems and medications common in older persons may complicate the presentation. Symptoms such as nausea, vomiting, anorexia, abdominal pain, diarrhea, and constipation are all encountered less commonly in the aged than what is expected for the general population. However, in one case-control study of 300 elderly patients with appendicitis, no significant differences were found when compared with the younger control cohort.[9]

The classic sequence of events of acute appendicitis begins with abdominal pain, then anorexia, nausea, and vomiting, followed by right lower quadrant pain and fever. Many patients will not exhibit every symptom. Most elderly patients will complain of anorexia, nausea, or vomiting. Constipation or diarrhea may be present. Constipation motivates many to use laxatives or enemas without relief. Abdominal pain usually precedes vomiting by several hours. Protracted vomiting is unlikely, and its presence should make the clinician question the diagnosis of appendicitis. Patients report the initial pain as dull, midepigastric, and periumbilical in nature, often awakening them from sleep. Although abdominal pain is usually the chief complaint, some patients will only report mild gastrointestinal upset. Men may report testicular pain. This initial pain is visceral and often somewhat subsides, only to reappear in the right lower quadrant as a severe ache that often increases with peritoneal irritation. The movement of pain is important to note. Unfortunately, the classic presentation of acute appendicitis occurs in less than one-third of cases in the elderly,[2,4] and approximately one-fifth of elderly patients never exhibit right lower quadrant pain.[4,5]

Physical examination findings usually coincide with the course of disease, depending on the degree of inflammation. On physical examination, most patients (75 percent) will have a temperature greater than 37.7°C (99.9°F), and a temperature greater than 38°C (100.4°F) usually occurs after transmural inflammation is present.[10] The temperature, however, may be normal or decreased in the elderly. Slight elevation in heart rate and blood pressure may occur in the apprehensive patient, but vital signs are often normal in uncomplicated cases or if the patient is taking medications, such as beta antagonists, that blunt the sympathetic response. Right lower quadrant abdominal tenderness is a frequent finding and is present in 80 to 90 percent of patients.[1,5] However, as has been noted previously, peritoneal signs may be absent or subtle.

The variable location of the appendix is also responsible for atypical presentations of acute appendicitis. The appendix can be located at any point 360 degrees around the cecum, and the variety of these positions may account for atypical presentations. With a pelvic appendicitis, the pain may begin in the epigastrium but quickly settle into the lower abdomen. Some patients present with only minimal abdominal pain but have localized tenderness found on rectal or pelvic examination. With a high retrocecal or retroiliac appendicitis, the inflamed structure is shielded from the anterior abdominal wall by the overlying cecum or ileum. The pain is often perceived as less intense, with less discomfort when ambulating. These patients may present with urinary frequency and right flank pain due

Table 29-1. Comparison of Clinical Features

	Young	Elderly
Time to presentation	Usually <24 h	Often >24 h
Abdominal pain	+++	++
Associated symptoms (N/V, anorexia)	+++	++
Fever and leukocytosis	+	+/−
Classic presentation	++	+ (<1/3)
Perforation on presentation	+	+++
Morbidity and mortality	+	+++

Source: Adapted with permission from Sidman RD, Roche CN, Duggal S: Acute appendicitis in the elderly. *Geriatr Emerg Med Rep* 1:91, 2000.

to proximity of the appendix to the ureter. In these cases, abdominal wall rigidity is usually absent and abdominal discomfort minimal. Rovsing's sign (right lower quadrant pain elicited by palpation in the left lower quadrant) is often present. A positive psoas sign is somewhat specific but insensitive. It is elicited by extension of the right hip or by flexion against resistance. A similar maneuver, the obturator sign, is performed by passive rotation of the hip with the knee flexed. Pain in response to the maneuver is considered positive. Either sign, when positive, represents irritation in the involved areas.

Duration of symptoms correlates directly with incidence of perforation and mortality in elderly patients. One study found that at the time of operation, fewer than 10 percent had simple, uncomplicated appendicitis, and most (85 percent) presented after 24 hours of pain.[11] Another study concluded that the elderly have a more rapidly progressive course with earlier abscess formation and rupture.[5] These findings account, in part, for the observed increase in mortality in older persons. A summary of clinical findings, with comparison between younger and older patients, is provided in the Table 29-1.

DIAGNOSIS AND DIFFERENTIAL

Although appendicitis classically has been considered to be a clinical diagnosis, this process becomes more difficult in the elderly. It is important to entertain this diagnosis in any older patient presenting with abdominal complaints because delays in diagnosis increase the risk for perforation and concomitant morbidity and mortality. There are multiple diagnostic studies to aid the emergency physician in the workup of suspected appendicitis, especially when the diagnosis is unclear.

Laboratory Investigations

A complete blood count (CBC) and urinalysis (UA) are appropriate initial studies. An evaluation of renal function may be indicated if the patient is to receive intravenous contrast material. If the clinical picture warrants (i.e., upper abdominal tenderness on examination), lipase and liver function tests may add useful information. Serum lactate levels are often obtained in this clinical situation, and although nonspecific, they are a sensitive indicator of poor tissue perfusion. Elderly patients often present with a history of abdominal pain that is not confirmed on physical examination. In such cases, a chest radiograph and electrocardiogram should be obtained to evaluate for the possibility of referred cardiopulmonary pathology.

The white blood cell (WBC) count, although limited by a lack of sensitivity and specificity, has some value when evaluating an elderly patient with undifferentiated abdominal pain. The WBC count may be normal in many elderly patients with infection, although in most such patients neutrophilia is present. An elevated WBC count is not specific for appendicitis. Serial WBC counts may increase sensitivity because WBC counts usually increase during the first 4 to 8 hours in patients with appendicitis.[12] The WBC count is elevated in 70 to 90 percent of patients with appendicitis at some point during the disease process. The mean WBC count in two studies involving older persons[4,6] was 14,000 to 15,000/mm^3. However, 12 percent presented only with immature forms (>10 percent bands), and another 8 percent had a normal WBC count and differential.[4] Therefore, it is important not to exclude the possibility of appendicitis in an elderly patient based solely on an initially normal WBC count. Conversely, leukocytosis in the setting of abdominal pain, while not diagnostic, should increase the index of suspicion for surgical pathology.

A UA should be obtained in all elderly patients with abdominal pain. The UA may be abnormal in 19 to 40 percent of patients with appendicitis.[1] Findings usually include mild pyuria (<20 WBCs per high-powered field), bacteriuria, or hematuria and are thought to occur due to direct contact between the inflamed appendix and the ureter. Importantly, false-positive findings can be noted in those with indwelling catheters and in elderly women, who often have asymptomatic bacteriuria and pyuria. If the emergency physician is not considering appendicitis, it may be easy to attribute these laboratory abnormalities to a urinary tract infection or nephrolithiasis.

C-reactive protein (CRP), an acute-phase reactant, has been studied in patients suspected of having appendicitis. The CRP level is often very high with bacterial infections and only minimally elevated in viral infections. An elevated CRP level alone has a sensitivity of 47 to 75 percent and a specificity of 56 to 82 percent for making the diagnosis of appendicitis.[12,13] It is also more likely to be elevated in acute appendicitis when symptoms have persisted more than 12 hours. Use of both the CRP and WBC count can improve diagnostic accuracy. The presence of leukocytosis or neutrophilia greater than 75 percent or an elevated CRP increased diagnostic sensitivity for appendicitis to 97 to 100 percent, with a specificity around 50 percent.[14] One group specifically looked at the CRP level and WBC count in elderly patients and found that if neither the CRP nor the WBC count were elevated, the diagnosis of appendicitis could be effectively excluded.[15]

Radiographic Investigations

Plain radiographs are obtained often in elderly patients with abdominal pain and can be useful when considering other diseases, such as lower lobe infiltrates, hollow viscus perforation, or intestinal obstruction. Plain radiographs, however, are not currently recommended in the workup of suspected appendicitis because of the lack of sensitivity and the presence of better diagnostic tests.

Computed tomographic (CT) scanning of the abdomen and pelvis is a much more useful imaging modality for older patients with abdominal pain. CT scanning of the abdomen and pelvis can reveal similar alternative diagnoses (e.g., bowel perforation and obstruction) as visualized on plain films while offering more complete information (e.g., intraabdominal masses or abscesses, vascular pathology) and improved sensitivity and specificity. CT scanning of patients suspected of having appendicitis is also cost-effective. Rao and colleagues[16] found that the cost per specific correct diagnosis of an abnormality was five times greater with plain radiographs than with appendiceal CT scan alone.

CT scans of the abdomen and pelvis on patients with suspected appendicitis have been found to be 96 to 98 percent sensitive and 83 to 89 percent specific.[17,18] Findings specific for appendicitis include a visualized abnormal appendix (dilated or thickened wall) or an appendicolith with pericecal inflammation or abscess. Findings suggestive of appendicitis include periappendiceal fat stranding, fluid collection in the right lower quadrant, abscess, adenopathy, and cecal apical changes. Use of CT scanning decreased the overall rate of nontherapeutic appendectomies from 20 to 7 percent and further decreased the rate of nontherapeutic appendectomies to 3 percent in patients who had a positive CT scan.[19] In patients in whom appendicitis was not diagnosed, an alternative diagnosis was discovered in 50 to 80 percent.[18,20]

Risks of CT scanning with intravenous contrast material include precipitating renal insufficiency and allergic reactions. There also may be site extravasation of contrast material. Oral contrast material may present an aspiration risk in the preoperative patient who will undergo anesthesia. The emergency physician needs to be aware these possibilities, and a serum creatinine level should be checked prior to the use of intravenous contrast material.

Ultrasound is another imaging test used for suspected appendicitis. It is advantageous in that it allows for visualization of other pathologic processes in the abdomen/pelvis and avoids ionizing radiation and the need for contrast material. It is readily accessible in most EDs and is relatively inexpensive. The diagnosis of appendicitis is made by ultrasound if a noncompressible, aperistaltic appendix with a diameter greater than 6 to 7 mm is seen or if an appendicolith is visualized.[17] Additional findings suggestive of appendicitis include gas in the appendiceal lumen, the presence of loculated or focally organized fluid collection, and loss of the echogenic submucosal ring. False-positive results occur when there is a dilated fallopian tube, muscle fibers from the psoas muscle mimic appendicitis, periappendiceal inflammation secondary to inflammatory bowel disease is present, or intussipated stool is present.

The overall sensitivity of graded compression ultrasound is reported to be between 76 and 85 percent with a specificity of 84 to 92 percent.[17,21,22] Because findings suggestive of appendicitis are present more commonly with an intact appendix, the sensitivity of ultrasound has been found to decrease with perforation. Additionally, false-negative results may occur if the appendix is not visualized, when inflammation is confined to the appendiceal tip, with retrocecal appendicitis, or if the appendix is markedly enlarged and, therefore, misconstrued as small bowel. Factors limiting the adequacy of the study include obesity, tense ascites, or pain. If the ultrasound is reported as suboptimal, indeterminate, or normal, or if perforation is suspected, a CT scan is recommended. Ultrasound should be employed primarily in the elderly when pathology of the biliary tree also is considered in the differential diagnosis.

Differential Diagnosis

A number of disorders may be confused with appendicitis. In the older patient these include bowel obstructions (especially an ileal obstruction), diverticulitis, cholecystitis, cecal carcinomas, and mesenteric vascular occlusions. Gastroenteritis and constipation are common early misdiagnoses.

EMERGENCY DEPARTMENT CARE AND DISPOSITION

If the diagnosis of appendicitis is high in the emergency physician's differential diagnosis, the patient should have intravenous access obtained and be kept nothing by mouth (NPO), and a surgeon should be consulted. The patient should receive intravenous antibiotics with aerobic and anaerobic coverage, such as cefotetan (1–2 g intravenously every 12 hours) or cefoxitan (1–2 g intravenously every 6–8 hours). Antibiotics have been shown to reduce postoperative wound infections and to decrease the incidence of postoperative abscesses if perforation has occurred.[23,24] Once the diagnosis is suspected, judicious use of analgesics, including short-acting narcotics, should not be withheld in the ED. Taking patients promptly to the operating room can minimize the chance of perforation.

However, in many older patients the diagnosis of acute appendicitis will not be so clear-cut. If the diagnosis is still considered after the initial evaluation (careful history, complete physical examination, and laboratory tests), the patient should be evaluated with a CT scan of the abdomen and pelvis. Findings consistent with acute appendicitis warrant an urgent surgical consult.

If the ED workup of an elderly patient with abdominal pain is inconclusive, the patient should be admitted for observation, for serial abdominal examinations, and serial WBC counts. A high index of suspicion must be maintained because the longer the delay to an accurate diagnosis of appendicitis, the higher is the risk of perforation and subsequent morbidity and mortality. A management algorithm based on the clinical likelihood for the diagnosis of appendicitis is shown in the Fig. 29-1.

Patients suspected of having acute appendicitis should be admitted to the care of a surgeon. The patient's primary care provider and medical specialists (cardiologist, pulmonologist, nephrologist, etc.) should be notified so as to assist in preoperative and postoperative medical care. Emergency physicians should rapidly facilitate and coordinate the patient's emergency care.

ADDITIONAL ASPECTS

Most younger patients diagnosed with undifferentiated abdominal pain have a benign course, with quick resolu-

ALL PATIENTS

- History and physical examination

- NPO

HIGH SUSPICION

- Judicious intravenous fluid resuscitation

- CBC and urinalysis

- Antibiotics (cefotetan or cefoxitin)

- Pain control

- Surgical consultation

- Appendectomy

MODERATE SUSPICION

- Intravenous rehydration as needed

- CBC and urinalysis (lipase, lactate, renal, and liver function tests as indicated)

- Ultrasound if biliary pathology suspected

- Plain radiographs of the abdomen if perforation or obstruction is suspected

- CT scanning of the abdomen/pelvis

    - If positive, appendectomy or treat other pathology as indicated

    - If negative, admit for observation and serial examinations and WBC counts

- Surgical consultation

Fig. 29-1   Management algorithm for elderly patients with possible appendicitis. *(Adapted with permission from Sidman RD, Roche CN, Duggal S: Acute appendicitis in the elderly. Geriatr Emerg Med Rep 1:91, 2000.)*

tion of symptoms (1–2 weeks) and very low morbidity.[25] In contrast, older patient presenting with undifferentiated abdominal pain often should be observed in the hospital setting. When the emergency physician is unable to identify the etiology of a patient's abdominal complaints, caution should be exercised before sending that patient home. Discharged patients generally should have a reevaluation within 24 hours. Emergency physicians must be patient advocates when discussing cases with a patient's primary caregiver or surgeon. Consultation with a surgeon should not be delayed and narcotics not withheld. Failure to consider appendicitis as an etiology of abdominal pain in this population not only will result in a poorer patient outcome but also may prompt medicolegal consequences.

REFERENCES

1. Fenyo G: Diagnostic problems of acute abdominal diseases in the aged. *Acta Chir Scand* 140:396, 1974.
2. Fenyo G: Acute abdominal disease in the elderly: Experience from two series in Stockholm. *Am J Surg* 143:751, 1982.
3. Rogers J: *Abdominal Pain: Foresight.* Dallas, American College of Emergency Physicians, Issue 3, December 1986.
4. Horattas MC, Guyton DP, Wu D: A reappraisal of appendicitis in the elderly. *Am J Surg* 160:291, 1990.
5. Freund HR, Rubinstein E: Appendicitis in the aged: Is it really different? *Ann Surg* 50:573, 1984.
6. Bugliosi TF, Meloy TD, Vukof LF: Acute abdominal pain in the elderly. *Ann Emerg Med* 19:1382, 1990.
7. Brewer RJ, Golden GT, Hitch DC, et al: Abdominal pain: An analysis 0f 1000 consecutive cases in a university hospital emergency room. *Am J Surg* 131:219, 1976.
8. Reiss R, Deutsch A: Emergency abdominal procedures in patients above 70. *J Gerontol* 40:154, 1985.
9. Peltokallio P, Jauhianinen K: Acute appendicitis in the aged patient. *Arch Surg* 100:140, 1970.
10. Owens JO, Hamit HF: Appendicitis in the elderly. *Ann Surg* 187:392, 1978.
11. Williams JS, Hale HW: Acute appendicitis in the elderly: Review of 83 cases. *Ann Surg* 162:208, 1965.
12. Hals G: Acute appendicitis: Meeting the challenge of diagnosis in the emergency department. *Emerg Med Rep* 20:71, 1999.
13. Eriksson S, Ganstrom L, Bark S: Laboratory tests in patients with suspected acute appendicitis. *Acta Chir Scand* 115:117, 1989.
14. Marachand A, Van Lente F, Galen GS: The assessment of laboratory tests in the diagnosis of acute appendicitis. *Am J Clin Pathol* 80:369, 1983.
15. Gronroos JM: Is there a role for leukocyte and C-reactive protein measurements in the diagnosis of acute appendicitis in the elderly? *Maturitas* 31:255, 1999.
16. Rao PM, Rhea JT, Rao JA, et al: Plain abdominal radiography in clinically suspected appendicitis: Diagnostic yield, resource use, and comparison with CT. *Am J Emerg Med* 17:325, 1999.
17. Balthazar EJ, Birnbaum BA, Yee J, et al: Acute appendicitis: CT and ultrasound correlation in 100 patients. *Radiology* 190:31, 1994.
18. Balthazar EJ, Megibow AJ, Siegel SE, et al: Appendicitis: Prospective evaluation with high resolution CT. *Radiology* 180:21, 1991.
19. Rao PM, Rhea JT, Rattner DW, et al: Introduction of appendiceal CT: Impact on negative appendectomy and appendiceal perforation rates. *Ann Surg* 229:344, 1999.
20. Rao PM, Rhea JT, Novelline RA, et al: Helical CT technique for the diagnosis of appendicitis: Prospective evaluation of a focused appendix CT examination. *Radiology* 202:139, 1997.
21. Wade DS, Morrow SE, Balsara ZN, et al: Accuracy of ultrasound in the diagnosis of acute appendicitis compared with the surgeon's clinical impression. *Arch Surg* 128:1039, 1993.
22. Skaane P, Amland PF, Nordshus T, et al: Ultrasonography in patients with suspected acute appendicitis: A prospective study. *Br J Radiol* 3:787, 1990.
23. Meller JL, Reyes HM, Loeffs DS, et al: One-drug versus two-drug antibiotic therapy in pediatric perforated appendicitis: A prospective randomized study. *Surgery* 110:764, 1991.
24. Bauer T, Vennits B, Holm B, et al: Antibiotic prophylaxis in acute non-perforated appendicitis. *Ann Surg* 209:307, 1989.
25. Lukens TW, Emerman CL, Effron D: The natural history and clinical findings in undifferentiated abdominal pain. *Ann Emerg Med* 22:690, 1993.

30

Mesenteric Ischemia

Jeffrey A. Manko
Phillip D. Levy

HIGH-YIELD FACTS

- The classic triad for mesenteric ischemia is severe abdominal pain, gastric emptying (vomiting and/or diarrhea), and a history of cardiac disease.
- Timely diagnosis and initiation of treatment are the best predictor of outcome for patients diagnosed with mesenteric ischemia.
- Lactate is a sensitive nonspecific marker for ischemia that becomes elevated late in the course of the disease.
- Angiography should be considered and initiated before "hard" physical examination findings are present.
- Computed tomographic (CT) scanning is an acceptable modality to use in stable patients to diagnose mesenteric ischemia when there is moderate suspicion or angiography is unavailable; however, a normal CT scan does not exclude the diagnosis of mesenteric ischemia.

The geriatric population continues to increase in the United States, bringing a concomitant increase in diseases that predominantly affect them. Mesenteric ischemia is one such disease. Geriatric patients with mesenteric ischemia who present to the emergency department (ED) have an extremely high mortality rate and can be most challenging to diagnose. A high index of suspicion is required to make a timely diagnosis of mesenteric ischemia. The emergency physician should consider the diagnosis of mesenteric ischemia in every elderly patient who presents to the ED with an abdominal complaint. Early diagnosis and expedient treatment greatly improve survival rates. Failure to recognize the risk factors and early signs of the disease ultimately will result in high mortality rates.[1,2] The challenge is to accurately make the diagnosis before it becomes obvious. Classic findings such as peritonitis, hypotension, elevated lactate level, and occult fecal blood all signify extensive disease that portends a poor prognosis.

EPIDEMIOLOGY

The elderly are the fastest growing segment of the population. Between 1990 and 2010, it is estimated that the population over the age of 85 will balloon to three to four times its present number.[3,4] This will have a tremendous effect on the prevalence of diseases such as mesenteric ischemia that predominantly affect the geriatric population. Mesenteric ischemia is reported to be the cause of approximately 1.0 percent of all acute abdomen admissions and 0.1 percent of all hospital admissions.[5]

Risk factors for mesenteric ischemia are the diseases most commonly seen in the elderly, such as cardiovascular comorbidities and increased intensive care unit admissions. The eventual outcome of these patients generally is determined by the underlying etiology and the timeliness of diagnosis and treatment. The prognosis all too often is dismal due to the inability to recognize mesenteric ischemia in the early stages before irreversible damage has occurred.

PATHOPHYSIOLOGY

Anatomy

It is vital to understand the vascular anatomy of the abdomen in order to comprehend fully the pathophysiology of mesenteric ischemia. Three major branches off the abdominal aorta supply the entire intestine: the celiac artery, the superior mesenteric artery (SMA), and the inferior mesenteric artery (IMA).

The celiac artery exits perpendicular from the ventral abdominal aorta at the level of T12. Its diameter is large, and its length is short. The celiac artery is responsible for supplying blood to the foregut (distal esophagus to the second portion of the duodenum). The splenic, left gastric, and common hepatic arteries branch off the celiac artery. The gastroduodenal artery, which branches off the common hepatic artery, provides important collateral circulation between the celiac and superior mesenteric arteries via the pancreaticoduodenal arteries. The celiac artery's shape, short and wide, coupled with excellent collateral circulation, makes the foregut a rare level for ischemia to occur.

The SMA branches off the abdominal aorta at a 45-degree angle at the L1 level. The SMA supplies the midgut (latter duodenum through the large bowel up to the splenic flexure). The inferior pancreaticoduodenal, middle colic, right colic, ileocolic, jejunal, and ileal arteries all branch off the SMA. The SMA has important anastomoses with the IMA that include the marginal artery of Drummond and the arc of Riolan. If vascular insufficiency exists over a prolonged period of time, increased collateral circulation develops.

The IMA arises at the L3 level prior to the bifurcation of the aorta into the iliac arteries. The IMA supplies the hindgut, beginning with the transverse colon and extending to the rectum. Its branches include the left colic, sigmoidal, and hemorrhoidal arteries and ends as the superior rectal artery. The IMA anastomoses with the SMA, as above, and also with lumbar arteries that branch off the aorta and internal iliacs.

The venous system of the abdomen closely mirrors the arterial system. The inferior mesenteric vein drains into the splenic vein, which joins the superior mesenteric vein to form the portal vein. This is the venous drainage for the midgut and hindgut before entering the inferior vena cava.

Etiologies

Mesenteric ischemia is often categorized by chronicity and etiology: acute versus chronic and occlusive versus nonocclusive. Acute presentations of mesenteric ischemia occur more commonly than chronic ones. Acute arterial occlusion accounts for approximately 65 percent of cases of mesenteric ischemia; venous occlusion is responsible for another 15 percent of cases. Nonocclusive mesenteric ischemia (NOMI) represents about 20 percent of mesenteric ischemia cases. Acute SMA emboli account for the largest percentage of acute etiologies of mesenteric ischemia (~50 percent).[6]

Underlying cardiovascular disease often contributes to the formation of SMA emboli. The left atrium is most frequently the source of emboli due to dysrhythmias, most commonly atrial fibrillation, or ventricular/septal thrombi as a result of a myocardial infarction.[7,8] Valvular thrombi also can contribute to SMA emboli, but this etiology has been continuing to diminish as the incidence of rheumatic fever has continued to decline steadily. The emboli lodge most frequently in the SMA just distal to where the middle colic artery branches off. This is the portion of the SMA where the diameter begins to taper and explains why the proximal small intestine is often spared during an embolic event.

Another source of mesenteric ischemia is SMA thrombi. This etiology most often occurs in patients with atherosclerotic vascular disease. The acute event involves the breaking off of a plaque that then acts as the nidus for thrombus formation. The thrombus often begins at the origin of the SMA, which distinguishes this presentation from that of an embolus. The SMA thrombus usually evolves over time. This gradual onset often allows for collateral circulation to develop, thereby decreasing the extent of the ischemia.

Mesenteric venous thrombosis is the least frequent etiology of mesenteric ischemia and usually results from an underlying medical condition. Mesenteric venous thrombosis may result from hypercoagulable states such as protein deficiencies, malignancies, sepsis, or liver disease that results in portal hypertension or disturbances in the portal blood flow. Patients with mesenteric venous thrombosis have a much lower mortality rate (38 versus 82 percent) compared with patients who developed mesenteric ischemia from other etiologies.[9]

NOMI is believed to result from conditions that produce a low cardiac output state, such as congestive heart failure. NOMI is frequently associated with patients in intensive care units who suffer from conditions such as sepsis, dehydration, or other causes of hypotension. NOMI also has been linked to certain drugs, including digitalis, cocaine, ergotamines, and vasopressors.[10,11] Geriatric patients account for a large percentage of intensive care unit patients, and they are the most at risk for NOMI.

Risk Factors

Evaluating the risk factors for mesenteric ischemia is a crucial step to making a timely diagnosis (Table 30-1). Acute mesenteric ischemia has been closely linked to cardiovascular disease. Cardiac entities that predispose a patient to form emboli or thrombi, such as dysrhythmias, recent myocardial infarction, or valvular disease, account for the majority of cases of acute mesenteric ischemia.[12,13] Atrial fibrillation and recent myocardial infarction are the most common cardiac risk factors.[14]

NOMI has separate and distinct risk factors to contemplate. Contributing factors are those which predispose the patient to low cardiac output states. Congestive heart failure, sepsis, and dehydration are all entities that can lead to hypotension and contribute to the onset of NOMI. Vasoconstrictive drugs such as cocaine and medications such as digitalis, diuretics, and vasopressors can exacerbate NOMI.

Chronic mesenteric ischemia has the same set of risk factors as coronary artery disease, including hypertension, diabetes, and tobacco use. Patients with known cardiovascular and peripheral vascular disease certainly are more at risk for chronic mesenteric ischemia.

Table 30-1. Risk Factors for Acute Mesenteric Ischemia

Cardiovascular disease	*Pharmacotherapy*
Arrhythmias	Amitryptiline
Atherosclerosis	Cocaine
Congestive heart failure	Digitalis
Myocardial infarction	Diuretics
Valvular disease	Dextroamphetamine
Shock	Ergot alkaloids
	Estrogen/oral contraceptives
Thromboembolic potential	Methamphetamine
Atrial fibrillation	Pitressin
Deep vein thrombosis	Propranolol
Hypercoaguable states	Vasopressors
Anticardiolipin antibody	
Antithrombin III deficiency	*Abdominal disease*
Factor V Leiden mutation	Bowel obstruction
Protein S or C deficiency	Cholangitis
Prothrombin 20210A mutation	Crohn's disease
Neoplasms	Diverticulitis
Polycythemia vera	Intussusception
Pregnancy	Gastrointestinal bleeding
Sickle cell disease	Peritonitis
Thrombophlebitis	Portal hypertension
	Parasitic infection
Systemic disorders	Trauma
Collagen-vascular diseases	Volvulus
Vasculitides	
Sepsis	

Finally, mesenteric venous thrombosis needs to be suspected in patients who are at risk for hypercoagulable states. These risk factors include malignancy, protein deficiencies, sepsis, and liver disease. The risk factors alone do not make the diagnosis, but when present, they should alert the emergency physician to the possibility of mesenteric ischemia.

CLINICAL FEATURES

Obtaining a comprehensive history of present illness can be particularly challenging in the geriatric population, the subset most likely to have mesenteric ischemia, due to many potential confounding factors. Geriatric patients often have comorbidities, such as dementia, that limit their ability to provide a cogent history. Frequently, family members and caregivers may be the sole source of historical information. Geriatric patients may adopt a stoic manner and minimize their complaints in order to avoid admission to the hospital. Changes in mental status, acute or

chronic, and communicating difficulties, such as hearing and speech impairment, may hinder the physician's ability to obtain a thorough history. Despite these challenges, the history is essential for providing valuable information to help elucidate the diagnosis of mesenteric ischemia.

The classic historical triad for mesenteric ischemia is severe abdominal pain, gastric emptying (vomiting and/or diarrhea), and previous cardiac disease. The pain is often described as unbearable. When the ischemia results from an embolic event, the onset of pain is sudden and severe. Patients often can pinpoint the exact time it began. The pain is often followed by gastrointestinal symptoms: nausea and anorexia (80 percent), vomiting (60 percent), and diarrhea (50 percent).[15] Cardiac disease is routinely present, with 25 to 33 percent of patients having suffered from a prior embolic event.[16,17]

Various etiologies of mesenteric ischemia will present with different features. Patients with chronic mesenteric ischemia often will complain of postprandial abdominal pain, also referred to as *intestinal angina*. Eating is a stress test for the intestines, with large meals exacerbating the pain. These patients eat smaller meals more frequently (small-meal syndrome) and develop weight loss.[18–20] Over time, the pain becomes more predictable and reproducible. Risk factors are similar to those for cardiac ischemia, including tobacco use, diabetes, and hypertension.

Obtaining a medication history often can yield information about the patient's medical history that was not discovered previously. Prior embolic events or cardiac disease (ischemia, congestive heart failure, or dysrhythmias) can be critical pieces of information for pointing the clinician in the right direction. Patients who take diuretics, digoxin, or anticoagulants should be suspected of being at risk for mesenteric ischemia, either occlusive or nonocclusive.

The physical examination of the geriatric patient is often considered more complex and difficult to perform than comparable examinations on younger patients. Confounding factors such as dementia, stroke, or polypharmacy, as well as diminished pain perception, often result in delayed presentations to the ED. These delays result in higher morbidity and mortality rates. The physical examination must be comprehensive. The initial physical examination of a patient with early mesenteric ischemia may not yield any positive abdominal findings. The clues may come from an examination that reveals evidence of embolic disease, low-flow states, or cardiac abnormalities without pronounced abdominal tenderness.

The vital signs may be normal in the early stage of mesenteric ischemia, with the first signs being mild tachycardia or a low-grade fever. Elderly patients may not mount a febrile response, so being afebrile does not exclude mesenteric ischemia as a possible diagnosis. In fact, geriatric patients often will become hypothermic instead of hyperthermic as they become more critically ill.

Heart rate is considered to be the most sensitive vital sign. A patient's heart rate may increase from any combination of pain, fever, and dehydration. The physician should identify tachycardia as an early sign of illness and recognize that patients taking beta blockers may have a blunted response. Elderly patients with abdominal pain and tachycardia, a nonspecific finding, should alert the physician to the risk of a severe intraabdominal process such as mesenteric ischemia.

An increased respiratory rate is often the marker for a deteriorating condition. Tachypnea is the autonomic response to compensate for a metabolic acidosis that may be due to increasing lactate from ischemia. The longer the ischemia is left untreated, the lactate buildup and worsening acidosis lead to even more pronounced tachypnea.

Hypotension signifies critical illness with a rapidly increasing morbidity and mortality. These patients appear toxic, and the diagnosis often is apparent. Unfortunately,

at this stage the prognosis is dismal. The key is to recognize the impending deterioration and seek immediate surgical or interventional radiology consultation for emergent diagnosis and treatment.

The abdominal examination in the geriatric patient often can be misleading. The classic presentation of mesenteric ischemia is said to be "pain out of proportion to the examination." This can be particularly difficult when the patient is unable to communicate. Wincing or expressions of discomfort may be all that is elicited during abdominal palpation. The examination may yield a local area or diffuse tenderness. Bowel sounds are often normal or hyperactive, although if the ischemia is due to an obstruction, they may be absent. Initially, peritoneal signs are absent. This is a late finding and represents prolonged ischemia. Peritonitis may signify progression to infarction.

The rectal examination is helpful in determining if mucosal sloughing has begun. A patient will develop occult fecal blood as the ischemia progresses. A normal rectal examination without occult fecal blood does not exclude the diagnosis of mesenteric ischemia. This is a late finding and often represents a poorer prognosis when present.

The cardiac examination can be particularly helpful in making the diagnosis. The presence of murmurs or arrhythmias may suggest that the patient is at high risk for embolic events. Stigmata of previous embolic disease, such as a stroke, also may help direct the physician to the possibility of mesenteric ischemia.

Other forms of ischemia, such as NOMI, must be considered in patients demonstrating signs of congestive heart failure or hypovolemia. Rales, peripheral edema, or dehydration accompanying abdominal pain can provide early clues to the diagnosis of NOMI.

The mortality rate of mesenteric ischemia is reported to be about 70 percent. The survival rate in one study was close to 90 percent when patients with mesenteric ischemia received early angiography before the development of peritonitis.[21] The emergency physician should not wait until the diagnosis is apparent with "hard" physical findings. The longer the diagnosis is delayed, the worse is the potential outcome. The hard signs generally present later in the course of the disease and make survival less likely.

DIAGNOSIS AND DIFFERENTIAL

The differential diagnosis for abdominal pain in the elderly is both broad and diverse. Appropriate consideration of other disease entities is the leading factor that leads to a delay in the diagnosis and evaluation of mesenteric ischemia. Accurate and prompt diagnosis relies on a high index of clinical suspicion in the geriatric population. Irreversible bowel infarction may occur within 8 to 10 hours of the onset of ischemia, and intestinal viability has been shown to correlate with a time to intervention of less than 12 hours.[10,22] In addition, diagnosis and treatment within 12 to 24 hours of the onset of symptoms clearly reduces overall mortality.[22] In response to this, an early, aggressive method of management has been adopted by some, resulting in a reported improvement in survival of 50 percent.[23] This approach, coupled with advancements in diagnostic and interventional technology, has had limited impact on the overall prognosis.[22] Mortality rates remain as high as they were nearly 80 years ago, and debate persists regarding the most efficient means of diagnosis.

The initial approach to the geriatric patient with abdominal pain should include basic resuscitative measures in conjunction with the history and physical examination. An electrocardiogram should be obtained to search for evidence of cardiac ischemia or arrhythmias.

Basic laboratory studies, including a complete blood cell count (CBC), metabolic and hepatic panels, coagulation profiles, and urinalysis, should be obtained. These tests may be useful for diagnosing more common disorders but provide limited information for the detection of mesenteric ischemia. The CBC may provide information supporting but not confirming the diagnosis. A white blood cell (WBC) count greater than 15,000/mL is present in up to 75 percent of patients with evidence of mesenteric ischemia.[14,23] Unfortunately, leukocytosis is an extremely nonspecific finding and frequently accompanies a multitude of intraabdominal infections and disorders. More important, leukocytosis has a negligible negative predictive value, and its absence should not be used to exclude the diagnosis of intestinal ischemia. Elevation of various enzymes in the serum, such as amylase, creatinine phosphokinase (CPK), alkaline phosphatase (ALP), lactate dehydrogenase (LDH) and aspartate transferase (AST), are common but of limited value in diagnosing mesenteric ischemia; they should not be relied on for such purposes.[24,25]

Hyperphosphatemia may be found in approximately 25 percent of patients with mesenteric ischemia, especially those with extensive bowel necrosis.[24,26] The mechanism may be related to the release of inorganic phosphate as the bowel mucosa begins to slough under conditions of hypoperfusion. An elevation in the serum phosphate level should heighten clinical suspicion of mesenteric ischemia as well as predict a poor outcome. A normal serum phosphate concentration, however, should not be used to exclude the diagnosis.[24,26]

The role of serum lactate is controversial. While an elevated serum lactate concentration has a sensitivity ranging from 96 to 100 percent and is highly predictive of mesenteric ischemia, it carries a specificity of only 38 to 42 percent.[26,27] Normal lactate levels are seen frequently during the early stages of mesenteric ischemia and do not exclude the diagnosis. Elevated lactate levels, however, have been found to be accurate predictors of impending fatality in patients with mesenteric ischemia. It represents a late finding associated with progression to frank infarction and loss of intestinal viability.[10,26] As a result, the clinical implications of serum lactate levels are somewhat difficult to interpret. Absence of elevated lactate may represent a point in time that is "too early" in the ischemic process, whereas its presence may signal that it is "too late" to salvage. Clearly, the clinician's goal is to make the diagnosis without delay before irreversible damage occurs. Optimally, the diagnosis of mesenteric ischemia should be made before a substantial rise in serum lactate occurs.

Other serologically identifiable predictors of intestinal ischemia are emerging. The intestinal fatty acid binding protein, a product of mature enterocytes released early in the course of intestinal injury, has shown promise but requires highly specialized assays with limited availability.[28] Serum D(−)-lactate is a by-product of bacterial metabolism easily distinguished by serum assays from its mammalian counterpart and may be detectable during periods of bacterial overgrowth in ischemic segments of bowel.[29] D-Dimer assay elevations have been proposed recently as a potential indicator of thromboembolic causes of occlusive mesenteric ischemia.[30]

Plain radiographs generally are unhelpful in diagnosing mesenteric ischemia; 25 to 50 percent of abdominal radiographs obtained in patients with mesenteric ischemia lack abnormalities.[25] The primary utility of plain abdominal radiographs is to exclude other potential etiologies such as small bowel obstruction. Pathologic findings generally are nonspecific for ischemia and represent advanced disease with associated mortality rates near 78 percent.[22] The most common findings include adynamic ileus, air-fluid levels, and dilated loops of bowel.[25] The exceptions are "thumb printing," caused by mucosal edema and hemorrhage, and pneumatosis intestinalis, resulting from intramucosal perforation, which are considered to be pathognomonic findings.[25]

Computed tomographic (CT) scanning of the abdomen has become common in the ED evaluation of undifferentiated acute abdominal pain. CT scanning has been shown to be useful for the evaluation and diagnosis of numerous intraabdominal disorders and allows clear delineation of potentially confounding pathology. Early studies of the capabilities of CT scanning for the detection of mesenteric ischemia, however, yielded unsatisfactory results.[22,31] Subsequent analysis using later-generation CT scanners with advanced technology in conjunction with intravenous contrast agents resulted in only modest improvement, with a reported sensitivity of 64 percent, specificity of 92 percent, and overall accuracy of 75 percent.[31] The most common CT abnormalities, bowel wall thickening with or without a "target sign" and small bowel dilatation, are relatively nonspecific findings.[32] Other more specific CT abnormalities include the absence of intravenous contrast enhancement of the bowel wall, parietal pneumatosis, pneumobilia, blurring of the mesenteric adipose tissue, arterial or venous thrombosis, or embolic vessel occlusion.[31,32] Many of the CT findings consistent with mesenteric ischemia are noted in advanced disease. CT scanning should not be the diagnostic modality of choice in patients with early, high clinical suspicion for mesenteric ischemia.[22] One notable exception is the case of mesenteric venous thrombosis, where the vessel occlusion often precedes signs of ischemia; CT scanning has been shown to be 82 to 100 percent sensitive for this diagnosis and is considered the first-line test for its evaluation.[22,25]

No conclusive studies have been conducted using spiral CT scanners or CT angiography. Further evaluation may yield new insights into the actual diagnostic potential of these modalities. Additionally, further advancements in CT technology, such as the multi-detector row scanners, are currently available and will allow even better visualization of the mesenteric vasculature.[33] These scanners employ rapid three-dimensional reformatting capabilities and provide highly detailed examinations of the small bowel and mesentery. This may allow for early identification of the etiology of suspected mesenteric ischemia.[33]

Doppler ultrasonography may be a useful adjunct for the evaluation of mesenteric vascular flow. Measurements of the peak systolic flow and the end-diastolic velocity have been shown to be accurate criteria for detecting vessel narrowing.[34,35] In chronic mesenteric ischemia, ultrasonography has been shown to have a sensitivity of 100 percent for both celiac artery and SMA stenosis greater than 70 percent, with a specificity of 87 and 98 percent, respectively.[34] Careful interpretation of these results is important because splanchnic vessel occlusion can be found in a number of asymptomatic patients. To confirm the diagnosis of chronic mesenteric ischemia, two of the three main branches (celiac, superior mesenteric, inferior mesenteric) off the aorta must be involved.[22] Although some report the ability to accurately identify acute filling defects in the SMA, attempts to diagnose acute mesenteric ischemia have been less successful.[35] This is largely due to sonographic visualization of the SMA being limited to the proximal root, just short of where emboli tend to lodge. This area is also often easily obscured by bowel gas secondary to an accompanying ileus.[22,35] Identification of NOMI by ultrasonography is considered futile and is not recommended.[22]

Magnetic resonance imaging (MRI) allows superior resolution of bowel wall edema and the ability to differentiate individual bowel wall layers but offers limited assessment of intramural or portal venous gas.[25,36] Diagnosis by MRI relies on the ability to detect tissue water changes in the face of ischemia, findings that are suggestive of but nonspecific for mesenteric ischemia.[25] Magnetic resonance angiography (MRA) using gadolinium contrast material has vast practical applicability and can provide detailed information about mesenteric vasculature.[36,37] MRA has been reported to have a sensitivity of 100 percent and a specificity of 95 percent for the diagnosis of chronic mesenteric ischemia and is currently being used by some clinicians in a screening capacity.[37] Due to limited use, diagnostic criteria have yet to be developed for either MRI or MRA; although promising, their role in the diagnosis of mesenteric ischemia has not been precisely determined.

Angiography has been the "gold standard" for the detection and treatment of mesenteric ischemia for over two decades. It is the only modality (other than laparotomy) that reliably allows early diagnosis before bowel ischemia becomes irreversible.[22,25] Angiography has the added advantage of offering options for therapeutic intervention as well.[22,23,25] With sensitivities ranging from 74 to 100 percent and a specificity routinely close to 100 percent, angiography is highly accurate.[22]

The findings on angiography depend on the etiology of the ischemia. SMA embolic disease is best seen on the anteroposterior views and can be identified by a mercury meniscus sign 3 to 8 cm distal to the vessel origin.[25] Thrombosis appears as a vessel narrowing more proximal to the SMA root and is best seen on lateral views.[25] In addition, the chronic nature of thrombotic lesions results in prominent collateralization.[25] The identification of NOMI often can only be made by angiography.[22,23,25] Reliable signs include diffuse narrowing of multiple branches of the SMA, alternating segments of dilatation and narrowing along various intestinal branches (known as the "string of sausage sign"), vasospasm of the mesenteric arcade, and diminished intramural vessel filling.[23,25] In the presence of systemic shock or concurrent vasopressor therapy, interpretation of these findings is compromised. This limits the value of the angiogram until either has been resolved.[22,23,25] Angiographic diagnosis of chronic mesenteric ischemia requires the finding of stenosis of any combination of the celiac artery, SMA, and IMA or all three in a symptomatic patient.[22,23,25] Again, the presence of collaterals indicates chronicity. Mesenteric venous thrombosis is difficult to diagnose using angiography but may be noted by the presence of contrast material reflux into the aorta, absence of mesenteric venous drainage, or SMA spasm.[25] CT scanning is the test of choice for mesenteric venous thrombosis.

Angiography is limited to diagnosing vascular pathology and is not useful in detecting other types of intraabdominal pathology. If intestinal ischemia is not the leading diagnosis, another imaging modality should be chosen. Alternatively, angiography should be obtained expeditiously when there is a high suspicion for mesenteric ischemia, especially if NOMI is suspected. Acceptance of negative studies, in an effort to achieve higher survival rates and bowel viability, has formed the cornerstone of an early, aggressive approach.[22,23,25] The complication rates of angiography are generally low, with approximately 5 percent developing local hematomas, 2 percent experiencing transient hypotension or arrhythmias, and a mortality rate less than 0.03 percent.[8] Acute tubular necrosis from the intravenous dye load has been reported, as well as rare anaphylactic reactions.

Diagnostic laparoscopy may be considered in patients unable to undergo angiography.[23] Laparoscopy may be too insensitive to make the diagnosis because only the serosal surface of the bowel is visualized and can appear relatively normal in early cases.[23] Tonometry has received considerable attention, especially in the intensive care unit setting, for the detection of mesenteric hypoperfusion with subsequent development of NOMI.[24,39] Continuous automated measurement of intramucosal CO_2 and intramural pH is now possible and can provide real-time information.[39] Endoscopy may be of some use, particularly with IMA occlusions or isolated right colonic ischemia secondary to SMA branch embolism, but it has not been evaluated extensively.[24] Use of superconducting quantum interference devices (SQUIDs) to detect alterations in the underlying basic electric rhythm of the gastrointestinal tract may be a noninvasive alternative in the future.[40]

EMERGENCY DEPARTMENT CARE AND DISPOSITION

All patients with suspected acute mesenteric ischemia should be treated with an initial focus on general resuscitative management in conjunction with early surgical consultation. Although the etiologies of the disease differ, the management strategy in the ED should be the same (Fig. 30-1). Providing oxygen supplementation and addressing volume status are essential. Invasive monitoring may be required, and hypotension refractory to fluid administration may necessitate the use of vasopressor agents. Alpha-adrenergic agonists such as phenylephrine, norepinephrine, and dopamine may be used to maintain the patient's blood pressure but must be used with caution due to their effects on the splanchnic circulation. Cardiac arrhythmias may require rate control, but digoxin should be avoided. Nasogastric tube decompression should be considered, and patients must be kept NPO. Early initiation of broad-spectrum antibiotics directed at covering enteric flora is advised and may help to prevent bacterial overgrowth and translocation.[23] Once a diagnosis has been obtained, management is directed at treating the underlying cause and should be initiated immediately. The various etiologies of mesenteric ischemia will have different definitive management strategies.

SMA Embolism

Rapid intervention is critical when SMA embolus is diagnosed. Patients should be started immediately on intravenous heparin. Treatment depends on the presence or absence of peritonitis, the extent of embolic vessel occlusion, and the size and location of the embolus.[22] If peritoneal signs are present, laparotomy is indicated.[22] Preoperative angiography, if not already obtained, is recommended, and prompt institution of an intraarterial vasodilator, such as papaverine 30 to 60 mg/h, is used to treat associated vasoconstriction.[22,23,25] In general, revascularization by embolectomy precedes bowel resection, and adequate time is given to assess viability.[23] When peritonitis is absent, options include laparotomy with embolectomy or intraarterial infusion of fibrinolytic agents.[22,25] Experience with fibrinolytic therapy for this indication is limited but has been shown to be successful in cases of partial occlusion, embolism within the SMA distal to the ileocolic origin, or when a branch vessel of the SMA is involved.[22]

Nonocclusive Mesenteric Ischemia

Early diagnosis by angiogram allows for the prompt initiation of treatment in NOMI. Unlike other etiologies of intestinal ischemia, the principal management of NOMI is pharmacologic. Heparin therapy should be started immediately.[22] With the angiogram catheter in place, an in-

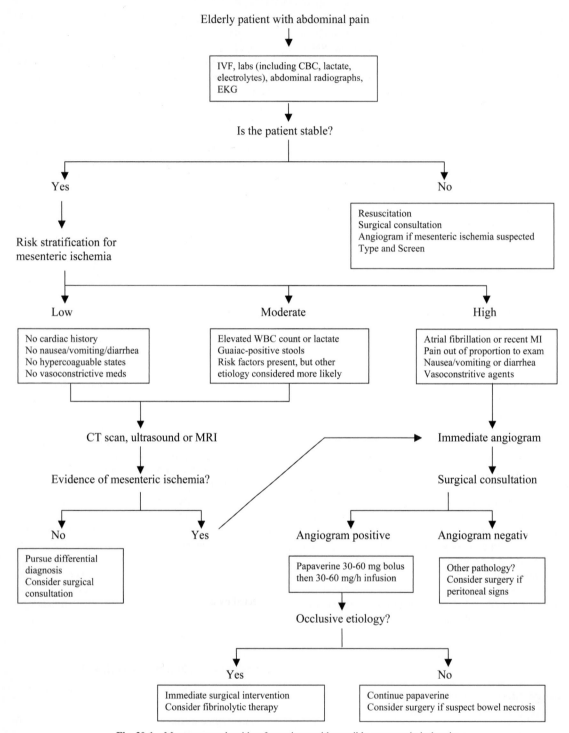

Fig. 30-1 Management algorithm for patients with possible mesenteric ischemia.

fusion of papaverine is begun at 30 to 60 mg/h and continued for 24 hours.[22,23,25] Subsequent infusion of normal saline takes place for 30 minutes and is followed by repeat angiography.[22,23,25] If persistent vasoconstriction is noted, or if the patient is still symptomatic, the papaverine infusion is restarted for another 24 hours.[22,23,25] If peritoneal signs are present, the infusion is continued while the patient undergoes exploratory laparotomy with necrotic bowel resection as required.[22,23,25] In situations where intraarterial papaverine cannot be administered, glucagon (2–4 mg/h) may be given peripherally.[25]

SMA Thrombosis

Although generally a more indolent disorder, acute occlusion of the SMA with thrombus may produce acute mesenteric ischemia. Differentiation from an embolism by angiography may be confusing and requires the evaluation of collateral vessels. Papaverine and heparin are initiated early, and the primary goal of treatment is SMA revascularization.[22,25,41] Bypass grafting and thrombectomy offer the best overall results and have replaced endarterectomy.[22,25] Successful treatment by percutaneous transluminal mesenteric angioplasty has been reported but is associated with repeat thrombosis and is not considered the standard approach for treatment.[22,23,41]

Mesenteric Venous Thrombosis

Anticoagulation with heparin has been shown to improve survival and limit thrombus propagation in patients with mesenteric venous thrombosis. This is often the only therapy required.[22,25] Some success has been reported with the use of transjugular or transhepatic vein infusion of fibrinolytic agents, but the necessity of this intervention is unclear.[22,42] In patients with peritoneal signs, operative intervention with wide-excision bowel resection and possible venous thrombectomy is recommended.[22,25] Long-term use of coumadin has been shown to reduce the postoperative recurrence rate from 40 to 5 percent.[25] The diagnosis of mesenteric venous thrombosis should prompt the search for underlying hypercoagulable causes.

Chronic Mesenteric Ischemia

Acute intervention is rarely required for chronic mesenteric ischemia. Patients may present with the sequelae of long-term malnourishment requiring parenteral nutrition.[25] In general, elective multivessel surgical revascularization is the treatment of choice for chronic mesenteric ischemia.[22,25] Not all patients with chronic

mesenteric ischemia warrant intervention, and several guidelines have emerged to help assess the risks and benefits.[25] Patients likely to benefit from surgery are those who have intestinal anginal symptoms, documented weight loss, and angiographic evidence of stenosis of two of three major splanchnic vessels.[25] This approach results in clinical success rates ranging from 59 to 100 percent and recurrence rates of 0 to 26 percent.[22] Percutaneous transluminal mesenteric angioplasty is an alternative method of establishing vessel patency and is particularly useful in patients who are operative risks or do not meet all criteria.[22,25] Percutaneous transluminal mesenteric angioplasty has been shown to be equivalent to surgery in relieving symptoms but has recurrence rates ranging from 10 to 67 percent.[22] Endovascular stent placement is associated with much lower rates of restenosis and may be a superior intervention to percutaneous transluminal mesenteric angioplasty.[22,43]

ADDITIONAL ASPECTS

The following are pitfalls in the management of mesenteric ischemia:

- Failure to consider the diagnosis of mesenteric ischemia because "hard evidence" was lacking clinically. In the case of mesenteric ischemia, time is of the essence, and rapid diagnosis and treatment are paramount to optimize a positive outcome.

- Ordering an abdominal CT scan because there is resistance in performing angiography. Time should not be spent preparing the patient for a CT scan of the abdomen when definitive treatment can be initiated in the operating room or angiography suite. In hemodynamically stable patients, CT scanning is certainly an acceptable option, with the caveat that a negative scan does not definitively exclude mesenteric ischemia. The CT scan also may provide evidence of alternative diagnoses that would not be detected by angiography.

REFERENCES

1. Fenyo G: Acute abdominal disease in the elderly: Experience from two series in Stockholm. *Am J Surg* 143:751, 1982.
2. Bender JS: Approach to the acute abdomen. *Med Clin North Am* 73:1413, 1989.
3. Sanders AB: Care of the elderly in the emergency department: Where do we stand? *Ann Emerg Med* 21:792, 1992.

4. US Bureau of the Census: *Statistical Abstract of the United States: 1990,* 110th ed. Washington, US Government Printing Office, 1990.

5. Klein HM, Lensing R, Klosterhalfen B: Diagnostic imaging of mesenteric infarction. *Radiology* 197:79, 1995.

6. Stoney RJ, Cunningham CG: Acute mesenteric ischemia. *Surgery* 114:489, 1993.

7. Ottinger LW, Austen WG: A study of 136 patients with mesenteric infarction. *Surg Gynecol Obstet* 124:251, 1967.

8. Sachs SM, Morton JH, Schwartz SI: Acute mesenteric ischemia. *Surgery* 92:646, 1982.

9. Clavien PA, Durig M, Harder F: Venous mesenteric infarction: A particular entity. *Br J Surg* 75:252, 1988.

10. Newman TS, Magnuson TH, Ahrendt SA, et al: The changing face of mesenteric ischemia. *Am Surg* 64:611, 1998.

11. Sai Sudhakar CB, Al-Hakeem M, MacArthur JD: Mesenteric ischemia secondary to cocaine abuse: Case reports and literature review. *Am J Gastroenterol* 92:1053, 1997.

12. McKinsey JF, Gewertz BL: Acute mesenteric ischemia. *Surg Clin North Am* 77:307, 1997.

13. Boley SJ: Early diagnosis of acute mesenteric ischemia. *Hosp Pract* 16:63, 1981.

14. Potts FE, Vukov LF: Utility of fever and leukocytosis in acute surgical abdomens in octagenerians and beyond. *J Gerontol* 54:M55, 1999.

15. Pierce GE, Brockenbrough EC: The spectrum of mesenteric infarction. *Am J Surg* 119:233, 1970.

16. Kazmers A: Operative management of acute mesenteric ischemia. *Ann Vasc Surg* 12:187, 1998.

17. Moore WM, Hollier LH: Mesenteric artery occlusive disease. *Cardiol Clin* 9:535, 1991.

18. Johnston KW, Lindsay TF, Wlaker PM: Mesenteric arterial bypass grafts: Early and late results and suggested surgical approach for chronic and acute mesenteric ischemia. *Surgery* 118:1, 1995.

19. Hollier LH, Bernatz PE, Pairolero PC: Surgical management of chronic intestinal ischemia: A reappraisal. *Surgery* 90:940, 1981.

20. McAfee MK, Cherry KJ, Naessens JM: Influence of complete revascularization on chronic mesenteric ischemia. *Arch Surg* 164:220, 1992.

21. Boley SJ, Sprayregan S, Siegelmann SS: Initial results from an aggressive approach roentgenological and surgical approach to mesenteric ischemia. *Surgery* 82:848, 1977.

22. Brandt LJ, Boley SJ: AGA technical review on intestinal ischemia. *Gastroenterology* 118:954, 2000.

23. Kaleya RN, Boley SJ: Acute mesenteric ischemia: An aggressive diagnostic and therapeutic approach. 1991 Roussel Lecture. *Can J Surg* 35:613, 1992.

24. Kurland B, Brandt LJ, Delany HM: Diagnostic tests for intestinal ischemia. *Surg Clin North Am* 72:85, 1992.

25. Ruotolo RA, Evans SRT: Mesenteric ischemia in the elderly. *Clin Geriatr Med* 15:527, 1999.

26. Lange H, Jackel R: Usefulness of plasma lactate concentra-tion in the diagnosis of acute abdominal disease. *Eur J Surg* 160:381, 1994.

27. Lange H, Toivola A: Warning signals in acute abdominal disorders: Lactate is the best marker of mesenteric ischemia. *Lakartidningen* 94:1893, 1997.

28. Lieberman JM, Sacchettini J, Marks C, Marks WH: Human intestinal fatty acid binding protein: Report of an assay with studies in normal volunteers and intestinal ischemia. *Surgery* 121:335, 1997.

29. Murray MJ, Barbose JJ, Cobb CF: Serum D(−)-lactate levels as a predictor of acute intestinal ischemia in a rat model. *J Surg Res* 54:507, 1993.

30. Acosta S, Nilsson TK, Bjorck M: Preliminary study of D-dimer as a possible marker of acute bowel ischemia. *Br J Surg* 88:385, 2001.

31. Taourel PG, Deneuville M, Pradel JA, et al: Acute mesenteric ischemia: Diagnosis with contrast-enhanced CT. *Radiology* 199:632, 1996.

32. Clark RA: Computed tomography of bowel infarction. *J Comput Asst Tomogr* 11:757, 1987.

33. Horton KM, Fishman EK: Multi-detector row CT of mesenteric ischemia: Can it be done? *Radiographics* 21:1463, 2001.

34. Lim HK, Lee WJ, Kim SH, et al: Splanchnic arterial stenosis or occlusion: Diagnosis at doppler US. *Radiology* 211:405, 1999.

35. Danse EM, Van Beers BE, Goffette P, et al: Acute intestinal ischemia due to occlusion of the superior mesenteric artery: Detection with Doppler sonography. *J Ultrasound Med* 15:323, 1996.

36. Baden JG, Racy DJ, Grist TM: Contrast-enhanced three-dimensional magnetic resonance angiography of the mesenteric vasculature. *J Magn Reson Imag* 10:369, 1999.

37. Meaney JFM, Prince MR, Nostrant TT, Stanley JC: Gadolinium-enhanced MR angiography of visceral arteries in patients with suspected chronic mesenteric ischemia. *J Magn Reson Imag* 7:171, 1997.

38. Hessel SJ, Adams DF, Abrams LH: Complications of angiography. *Radiology* 138:273, 1981.

39. Knichwitz G, Rotker J, Mollhoff T, et al: Continuous intramucosal Pco_2 measurement allows the early detection of intestinal malperfusion. *Crit Care Med* 26:1550, 1998.

40. Seidel SA, Bradshaw LA, Ladipo JK, et al: Noninvasive detection of ischemic bowel. *J Vasc Surg* 30:367, 1999.

41. Endean ED, Barnes SL, Kwolek CJ, et al: Surgical management of thrombotic acute intestinal ischemia. *Ann Surg* 233:801, 2001.

42. Divino CM, Park IS, Angel LP, et al: A retrospective study of diagnosis and management of mesenteric vein thrombosis. *Am J Surg* 181:20, 2001.

43. Matsumoto AH, Angle JF, Spinosa DJ, et al: Percutaneous transluminal angioplasty and stenting in the treatment of chronic mesenteric ischemia: Results and long-term follow up. *J Am Coll Surg* 194:S22, 2002.

31

Renal Emergencies

Jeffrey Cox

HIGH-YIELD FACTS

- Renal function declines with age. However, the concomitant loss of lean body mass leads to a relatively normal serum creatinine level.

- Occurrences of acute renal failure (ARF) are increasing and afflicting more older patients than any other group.

- Medicines play a large role in causing ARF in older patients; of particular concern are nonsteroidal anti-inflammatory drugs (NSAIDs), angiotensin-converting enzyme (ACE) inhibitors, and radiologic contrast material.

- Precontrast hydration can reduce the incidence of ARF. Patients with ARF can have life-threatening complications requiring emergency management, such as acute pulmonary edema and hyperkalemia, which require immediate recognition.

Age-related changes in the kidneys limit their functional reserve, rendering them more susceptible to renal insults. These changes alter the anatomic structure as well as the cellular function of the kidneys. Due to these changes, the elderly have an increasing incidence and differing patterns of renal diseases. Regardless of cause, the number one issue for emergency physicians is recognizing and managing acute renal failure (ARF), which is characterized by a rapid deterioration of kidney function over a short period of time. ARF recognized and treated promptly can be reversible.

The kidneys are responsible for maintaining homeostasis of the internal environment. They achieve this by eliminating the nitrogenous waste products of metabolism and adjusting excretion of water and electrolytes to match intake and production. The kidneys are able to regulate the excretion of water, sodium, potassium, and hydrogen through tubular reabsorption or secretion. Thus the kidneys are able to maintain water and electrolyte balance and control acid-base status. The kidneys secrete renin, angiotensin II, prostaglandins, and bradykinin to regulate renal and systemic hemodynamics; erythropoietin to stimulate red blood cell production; and 1,25-dihydroxyvitamin D to control calcium, phosphorus, and bone metabolism.

EPIDEMIOLOGY

Acute renal failure (ARF), is a significant problem for the elderly. The ARF case rate is 140 to 486 per million population per year. Survival is 54 to 56 percent to discharge from hospital and 47 to 54 percent at 3 months.[1,2] The rate of hospital-acquired ARF also is increasing from 4.9 percent of patients admitted in 1979 to 7.2 percent in 1996.[3] The mean age of patients diagnosed with ARF has increased from 41 years between 1956 and 1959 to 61 years between 1980 and 1988.[4] Age is an independent risk factor for developing ARF. Presentation is more likely after age 70. The increased prevalence of renal failure in the elderly is a consequence of growth of the elderly population and the decrease in renal function that occurs with aging.[5]

PATHOPHYSIOLOGY

The aging kidney loses up to one-quarter of its mass by age 80.[6] A significant portion of this loss occurs in the renal cortex, involving both the glomeruli and the tubules. Progressive sclerosis of glomeruli and afferent arterioles occurs with increasing age. Interstitial fibrosis occurs simultaneously with loss of tubules. The ongoing sclerosis and fibrosis result in a decline in glomerular filtration and tubular function.[7] Vascular changes also occur in the aging kidney. These changes result in both loss of functioning glumeruli in the cortex and asymmetrical blood flow between the cortex and juxtamedullary region. This dysfunction lessens the aging kidney's ability to reabsorb or secrete sodium.[8]

During normal conditions, renal blood flow (RBF) and glomerular filtration rate (GFR) remain constant over a range of blood pressures from 90/70 to 260/140 mmHg due to renal vascular autoregulation.[9] This constant RBF allows appropriate solute and water excretion during fluctuations in blood pressure. Autoregulation is a complex process that is modified by prostaglandins, the renin-angiotensin-aldosterone system, the nervous system, and serum atrial natriuretic factor (ANF). ANF is a renal protective hormone and diuretic that appears to play a key role in balancing renal vasoconstriction and vasodilatation and may be particularly important in renal function in the elderly.[10]

Due to the decrease in RBF and sclerosis and atrophy of glumeruli, GFR declines with age.[11] This results in a parallel decline in creatinine clearance, from 140 mL/min/1.73 m^2 at age 30 to 97 mL/min/1.73 m^2 at age 80.[12] However, there is a wide variation in renal function from individual to individual with age.[13] While some elders have a rapid decline in function, 30 percent show minimal decline in GFR at age 80. This decline in creatinine clearance is not accompanied by a rise in serum creatinine.[14] Daily creatinine production falls as muscle mass decreases with age. This fall in creatinine production occurs simultaneously with the decline in creatinine clearance. Therefore, serum creatinine levels remain rather constant throughout life. The decrease in GRF of 50 percent seen with aging would be expected to increase the serum creatinine level from 1.0 to 2.0 mg/mL.[15]

The serum creatinine level is used commonly to estimate renal function or GFR.[16] One hundred percent of creatinine is filtered across the glomerulus and neither reabsorbed nor metabolized by the kidney. However, approximately 10 to 15 percent of creatinine is cleared by tubular secretion, and as GFR falls, tubular secretion can increase to clear 35 percent of creatinine.[16–18] Certain drugs (ciprofloxacin, cimetidine, and trimethoprim) block tubular creatinine secretion, elevate the serum creatinine level, and give a false impression of decreased renal function and ARF.[19]

Creatinine clearance can be calculated after a 24-hour urine collection. Cockcroft and Gault[20] developed a formula to predict creatinine clearance based on the single serum creatinine level. Creatinine clearance = [(140–age) × weight (kg)]/[72 × serum creatinine (mg/dL)]. The value is multiplied by 0.85 in women to take into account their small muscle mass. This formula takes into account the decline in creatinine production with age and changes in body weight. It more accurately reflects renal function.[16]

With age, changes in the tubular system limit the ability of the kidneys to maintain sodium, potassium, and acid-base homeostasis under conditions of stress.[14] The proximal tubules reabsorb the majority of filtered solute required to maintain fluid and electrolyte homeostasis. The distal tubules are responsible for the elimination of potassium, free water, and hydrogen ions. Proximal sodium absorption is impaired in the elderly. During periods of restricted salt intake, the elderly require up to three times as long to bring sodium excretion back into balance. This is due in part to the decreased concentrating ability of the tubular system and to decreased levels of and responsiveness to renin and aldosterone. Because of this decrease in concentrating ability, water conservation is also impaired. The elderly have a higher thirst threshold, making them particularly prone to volume depletion and sodium wasting.[8]

The kidneys excrete potassium principally in the distal tubules. Potassium handling is complex and interrelated with water and sodium.[21] Potassium excretion depends on an adequate number of functioning distal tubules, the delivery of sodium and water to the distal tubules, and the function of aldosterone. Hyperkalemia is seen in up to 10 percent of elderly people due in part to changes in the kidneys that occur with aging.[15,22] The decrease in renal mass limits the number of functioning tubules. Renin levels are decreased, and angiotensin and aldosterone generation is lessened. Additionally, the distal tubules appear to have a blunted response to the effects of aldosterone. All these factors taken together place the elderly patient at risk for hyperkalemia. Hyperkalemia results most frequently from the use of potassium-altering medications in an already susceptible senescent renal system.[15]

Acute Renal Failure

ARF is defined as a sudden decrease in the ability of the kidneys to excrete the body's nitrogenous waste produces and to maintain water and electrolyte homeostasis. Common markers of ARF include an increase in serum creatinine of more than 50 percent from baseline, a rise in serum creatinine of greater than 5 mg/dL, or a more sensitive indicator among elders, a decrease in creatinine clearance of 50 percent.[23] ARF can be further classified by the amount of urinary output as anuric, oliguric, or nonoliguric. *Anuric failure* refers to a urine output of less than 50 mL/24 hours, whereas in *oliguric failure* the urine output is less than 400 mL/24 hours. Oliguric renal failure may be associated with an increased risk of the need for renal-replacement therapy and mortality.[24] The duration of ARF is longer in oliguric failure, averaging 14 days versus 7 days in nonoliguric failure.[25]

Renal failure is also classified as prerenal, intrinsic renal, postrenal, or obstructive failure. *Prerenal failure* is the result of diminished renal blood flow. Prerenal ARF may be due to either intravascular depletion, decreased effective circulating volume, or agents (drugs) that impair renal blood flow. Some forms of prerenal failure also have been referred to as *vasomotor disorders* because they impair GFR by reducing glomerular capillary pressure.[26] Prerenal ARF is considered a reversible process because there is no damage to renal tissue. Renal function returns to normal with rapid correction of the underlying process. When the cause of prerenal ARF is not corrected quickly, acute tubular necrosis (ATN) may result. Sustained prerenal insufficiency is a common factor leading to ischemia-induced ATN in the elderly.[8] ATN is the result of ARF in 23.4 percent of elderly patients as compared with 15.1 percent of younger patients.

Prerenal Failure

In the elderly, 60 percent of cases of community-acquired ARF are due to prerenal conditions.[27] In hospitalized patients, elders had a significantly greater incidence of prerenal failure than younger patients.[27] Because of the limited functional reserve of the aging kidney, excessive fluid loss due concurrent illness may lead to ARF. Sepsis, congestive heart failure (CHF), and cirrhosis are responsible for a decrease in effective renal perfusion leading to ARF in hospitalized patients.[23] Of concern in the elderly is the use of three medications: nonsteroidal anti-inflammatory drugs (NSAIDs), cyclooxygenase 2 (COX-2) inhibitors, and angiotensin-converting enzyme (ACE) inhibitors. These medications alter glomerular hemodynamics leading to prerenal failure.

Nonsteroidal Anti-inflammatory Drugs (NSAIDs)

NSAIDs are used widely for their anti-inflammatory properties. They are the second leading cause of drug-induced ARF. Between 10 and 15 percent of elderly use NSAIDs on a regular basis.[28] In normal individuals, renal prostagladins are vasodilatory but do not play an important role in regulating renal hemodynamics. Under certain conditions (CHF, cirrhosis, and diuretic use), vasodilatory prostanglandins maintain renal blood flow and GFR by counterbalancing vasoconstriction. During volume depletion, production of angiotensin II and vasopressin increase, and catecholamine release occurs. This results in vasoconstriction with a reduction of RBF and GFR, as well as increased water and sodium reabsorption and renin release. Under these conditions, renal prostaglandins are released to counterbalance these effects.

Since NSAIDs inhibit renal prostaglandin formation, patients whose RBF and GFR depend on prostaglandins are at risk for ARF when NSAIDs are used. Elders are at increased risk of nephrotoxicity from these drugs. In one study, hospitalization increased fourfold in patients using NSAIDs.[29] Another study showed that 60 percent of patients with ARF from NSAID use were age 70 or older.[30] The effects are usually seen within 3 to 5 days after beginning NSAID use or during periods of volume depletion in patients already taking these medications. Additionally, NSAIDs may cause intrinsic renal failure in the form of an acute interstitial nephritis that may lead to chronic interstitial fibrosis.

Cyclooxygenase 2 (COX-2) Inhibitors

NSAIDs block both COX-1 and COX-2 enzymes. COX-1 activity was thought to be homeostatic, whereas COX-2 enzyme activity was thought to be inflammatory.[31] Therefore, COX-2 inhibitors were introduced for their gastrointestinal safety while maintaining their anti-inflammatory efficacy. COX-2 inhibitor drugs have nephrotoxicity similar to NSAIDs.[32,33]

Angiotensin-Coverting Enzyme (ACE) Inhibitors

ACE inhibitors are one the most frequently used classes of antihypertensive agents.[9] They are also used to manage CHF and chronic renal disease and now are well recognized for their ability to cause ARF.[27] In one study, ACE inhibitors were second only to antibiotics as a cause of a drug-related ARF. Patients particularly at risk are similar to those at risk from NSAIDs.

During periods of decreased renal perfusion, angiotensin II is released. This causes vasoconstriction of the postglomerular efferent arterioles to a greater degree than the preglomerular afferent arterioles. What follows is an increase in GFR despite the decreased renal blood flow. Additionally, angiotensin II increases proximal tubular reabsorption of sodium and causes sodium to be reabsorbed in the collecting ducts by its effect on aldosterone release.

During ACE inhibitor use there is a fall in systemic vascular resistance and a reduction in mean arterial pressure

(MAP). Renal vascular resistance also falls, and RBF increases. GFR remains stable or falls slightly because of a greater dilatory effect on postglomerular efferent arterioles. In patients with CHF there is increase in urinary sodium secondary to reduced proximal tubule reabsorption of sodium and reduced aldosterone-dependent sodium reabsorption in the collecting ducts.

ARF can occur on initiation of ACE inhibitor therapy or months to years after treatment has begun.[9] The initiation of ACE inhibitor therapy may decrease MAP to a level that does not sustain RBF and thus results in ARF. If MAP falls below 55 mmHg, there is a high probability of renal failure occurring. In patients who are volume depleted from diuretic therapy, ACE inhibitors commonly lead to ARF. In a patient started on ACE inhibitors who is volume depleted, adequate GFR may be achieved by angiotension II, and ARF may ensue.[34] Patients taking NSAIDs are also at risk for developing ARF when ACE inhibitors are added to the treatment regime. Between 6 and 38 percent of patients with severe renovascular disease develop ARF when started on ACE inhibitors.[35] ARF occurs with bilateral renal artery stenosis or renal artery stenosis of a single or dominate kidney. By this mechanism, ACE inhibitors can cause ARF in renal transplant patients. Renal artery stenosis needs to be investigated in any patient who develops ARF after the initiation of ACE inhibitors.[27]

ARF in patients on chronic ACE inhibitor therapy usually occurs with a decrease in circulating volume or after a vasoconstricting agent (NSAID) is administered.[9] In these circumstances, GFR becomes dependent on angiotensin II, which is blocked, leading to ARF. Examples are patients with worsening CHF, overdiuresis, volume depletion from vomiting or diarrhea, or osmotic diuresis from hyperglycemia. Sepsis also can decrease effective circulating volume, leading to ARF in patients treated with ACE inhibitors.

Intrinsic Renal Failure

Intrinsic renal failure can result from glomerular, vascular, tubular, or interstitial problems. Some authors place tubular and interstitial processes together as tubulointerstial diseases. Intrinsic causes are the second most cited cause of renal failure in the elderly. Injury to the tubules represents the number one cause of intrinsic renal failure and the number two cause of ARF in the elderly.[8,36] Drug-induced interstitial nephritis is the next most common form of ARF, usually seen in hospitalized patients, frequently as the result of administration of antibiotics or NSAIDs. Supportive care usually is all that is required after stopping the offending agent. Glomerular and vascu-

lar disorders are an uncommon cause of ARF in the elderly.[5]

Tubular injury is usually the result of toxins or ischemia. Prolonged prerenal insufficiency leads to tubular ischemia. The proximal tubules are located in the outer medullary portion of the kidney and are susceptible to ischemia due to their high energy requirements. As ischemia occurs, there is disruption of cell structure and increased cell permeability, and cell death occurs with intratubular shedding, leading to tubular obstruction and a fall in GFR. Reversibility depends on the degree of cell death and injury. Ischemia- and toxin-induced tubular dysfunction is termed *acute tubular necrosis* (ATN).[37]

Contrast Material–Induced Renal Failure

Contrast material–induced renal failure is an important cause of renal failure in the elderly.[3] Contrast material–induced renal failure has been considered either prerenal or intrinsic. In one study of hospital-acquired renal failure, contrast material–induced renal failure was implicated as the cause in 11 percent of patients.[3] Contrast material given during cardiac catheterization was responsible in 49 percent of cases, and contract material given during computed tomographic (CT) scans was responsible in 33 percent of cases. Although age is not considered a risk factor, the elderly are subjected to a variety of procedures requiring the use of contrast material. They are prone to contrast material–induced ARF secondary to decreased renal function and their propensity for volume depletion. Both are risk factors for ATN. Other risk factors are preexisting renal insufficiency, diabetes, and the concurrent use of NSAIDs and ACE inhibitors or other nephrotoxic drugs.[38]

With contrast material–induced renal insufficiency there is renal vasoconstriction and direct injury to renal tubular cells.[27] After injection of contrast material, there is an initial rise in renal blood flow followed by a longer decrease. Alterations in renal vasoconstrictor agents and the high osmolality of contrast agents appear to play a role. Contrast agents also have a direct toxic effect on renal tubular cells.[39] In ARF after contrast material administration, serum creatinine levels rise in the first 24 to 48 hours and peak at around day 5. Most patients have a low excretion of sodium, less than 1 percent, indicating intact tubular function. The urine may be bland or reveal granular casts and mild proteinuria.

Multiple strategies have been attempted to prevent contrast material–induced ARF, including hydration, furosemide, mannitol, dopamine, atrial nariuretic peptide, calcium channel blockers, and theophylline.[40] Of these, the only currently recommended regimen is hydration prior to contrast administration.[41] Another recently described method for prevention of contrast material–induced renal failure is the use of *N*-acetylcysteine given the day prior to the procedure.[42] Both methods require a significant pretreatment time before contrast material may be given.

Multiple Myeloma

Myeloma is a less common cause of community-acquired renal failure in the elderly.[43] The annual incidence is 20 to 40 cases per million, with an average age of 70 years.[44] Up to 50 percent of patients will have renal failure during the course of the disease. ARF may be the initial presentation in up to 50 percent of the patients.[44] ARF is usually due to tubular dysfunction secondary to protein cast formation and direct tubule cell damage from intracellular crystals. Hypercalcemia occurs in 15 percent of patients and also may directly cause ARF.[45]

Embolic Renal Failure

Another form of intrinsic ARF seen typically in white males over the age of 60 is artheroembolic renal disease.[26] Cholestesterol from atheroscerotic aortic plaques embolizes to the small vessels of the kidneys. Although embolization may occur spontaneously, it typically occurs after angiographic procedures or vascular surgery. After arterial manipulation, ARF usual occurs within days or weeks. Embolization to other organs is a common finding, particularly to the lower extremities, causing livedo reticularis, purple or blue toes with normal pulses. Mircoembolism to the retina (Hollenhorst plaques) may be seen.[34] Constitutional symptoms may be present and consist of fever and malaise. Renal failure usually is slow to progress but can occur acutely.

Postrenal Failure

Obstructive renal failure is responsible for less than 10 percent of ARF occurring in the elderly patients.[36] Obstructive renal failure may occur anywhere along the urinary outflow tract. It may be intrarenal in cases of crystal and protein precipitation that obstructs the renal tubules or pelvis. Extrarenal failure can result from bilateral ureter obstruction, bladder outlet obstruction, or urethral obstruction. Bilateral ureter obstruction may occur in the setting of retroperitoneal fibrosis or tumor. Bladder outlet obstruction occurs in the setting of uterine or cervical carcinoma. Outlet obstruction also can occur after the administration of anticholinergic medications. In elderly males, postrenal failure is usually secondary to prostatic hypertrophy or carcinoma. Obstruction causes backpressure in the renal tubules decreasing GFR secondary to hydrostatic effects in the glomerlus and also alters renal hemodynamics negatively.[46]

CLINICAL FEATURES

History

Elderly patients presenting with ARF may be asymptomatic or complain of vague and nonspecific complains. Malaise, muscular pain, tiredness, or decreased appetite may be their only complaint. ARF is often discovered when patients present with another acute disease process.

The history can aid in determining the cause of ARF. Important clues to be gleaned from the history include the use of nephrotoxic drugs, in particular antibiotics, NSAIDs, and ACE inhibitors, and recent angiographic or diagnostic studies requiring contrast material. Nausea, vomiting, diarrhea, or a recent decrease in oral intake is associated with volume depletion and prerenal failure. A recent skin rash may be a clue to an allergic reaction and interstitial nephritis. A history of suprapubic pain, distensions, and difficulty voiding suggests obstruction. Bone pain in the elderly could suggest multiple myeloma. An elderly patient "found down" may have muscle breakdown and rhabdomyolysis with secondary pigment nephropathy.

Resting tachycardia and hypotension are the findings in volume-deleted patients or in patients with decreases in effective circulating volume such as sepsis and prerenal failure. Beta blockers are common medications in elderly patients and may inhibit a tachycardic response to volume depletion. Hypertension may be seen with glomerulonephritis or malignant hypertension. Fevers are not common in ARF.

Evaluation of the volume status is the key element of the physical examination. Tachycardia and hypotension are obvious clues. Findings of CHF or cirrhosis are important because of their association with decreased effective volume and prerenal failure. However, anuric or oliguric renal failure may result even with volume overload and signs of CHF. Costovertebral angle tenderness and a distended bladder may indicate an obstructive etiology for failure. Other finding suggestive of obstruction are prostatic enlargement or a rectal or pelvic mass. The skin should be examined for rashes associated with interstitial nephritis. Livedo reticularis is indicative of embolic renal failure. Retinal lesions are also seen with embolic disease. Bruises and ecchymosis of the trunk and extremities suggests rhabdomyolysis, whereas purpura suggests vasculitis.

EMERGENCY DEPARTMENT CARE AND DISPOSITION

ARF is usually recognized by an elevation in the serum creatinine or blood urea nitrogen (BUN) level; therefore, an electrolyte panel should be obtained in patients at risk for and suspected of ARF. The elderly are prone to hyperkalemia during ARF, which can be life-threatening. A BUN-to-creatinine ratio greater than 20 suggests prerenal failure but also can be seen in gastrointestinal bleeding.

Other blood tests that may be indicated include determinations of calcium, phosphorus, uric acid, and creatinine kinase and a liver panel. The history and physical examination should guild the ordering of these tests; e.g., hypercalcemia may be an important clue to myeloma as the cause of renal failure, particularly in patients complaining of bone pain.

A urinalysis and determination of urine electrolytes are useful in ascertaining the type of ARF. Normal or bland urine with no sediment is more indicative of nonintrinsic ARF.[5] Renal tubular cells form granular casts and are present in ATN. Red blood cells may originate anywhere along the entire renal system. Gross hematuria is typically nonglomerular in origin but may be the presenting complaint for renal cell carcinoma.[47] Red blood cells, red cell casts, and proteinuria usually are seen in glomerulonephritis. Dysmorphic red blood cells usually are seen in glomerular disorders.[48] Red cell casts with urinary eosinophils are indicative of vasculitis.[5] Urinary protein is associated with glomerular dysfunction, but trace amounts may be seen with interstitial nephritis. The urine dipstick only detects the protein albumin and not the immunoglobulin light chains found in myeloma.[48] Crystals in the urine may imply acute crystal nephropathy. White blood cells and casts with bacteria indicate pyelonephritis.

The kidney's response to decreased renal blood flow is water and sodium conservation. When the kidney can concentrate urine, urine osmolality typically is over 500 mOsmol in prerenal failure. This represents preserved tubular function and the effects of antidiuretic hormone. In cases of ATN, there is an early loss of concentrating ability, and urine osmolality usually is below 350 mOsmol.

Urine sodium tends to be low in prerenal states. Levels of less than 20 meq/L are seen in prerenal failure, and levels higher than 40 meq/L are seen in other conditions. There may be considerable overlap because water reabsorption will affect urine sodium concentrations. Urine sodium concentrations may be low with tubular dysfunction, because water may not be conserved. The fractional

excretion of sodium (FE_{Na}) is a better test to determine the integrity of the tubular system.[25]

FE_{Na} is calculated with this formula: [(urine sodium × serum creatinine)/(serum sodium × urine creatinine)] × 100. In prerenal failure, sodium is avidly reabsorbed. Calculating the FE_{Na} can help distinguish volume depletion as a cause of ARF. A fractional excretion of sodium of less than 1 percent indicates sodium retention and prerenal ARF (Table 31-1).

The initial goal of the emergency management of ARF in the elderly is to optimize fluid status. As treatment is started, the cause of failure should be sought. After assessment and treatment of any respiratory impairment, the circulatory status should be addressed. Concurrently, treatment should be initiated to identify and treat any life-threatening complications of acute ARF. The two most common complications in patients with ARF are volume overload and hyperkalemia.[23] Treatment of these conditions is no different from that in younger individuals.

Volume overload is particularly common in oliguric or anuric ARF patients. Patients who present with fluid overload or develop rales, edema, and increased venous pressure should be given a loop diuretic to improve urine output.[24] Vasodilators also should be used to reduce preload.[43] If urine output does not improve or if pulmonary edema persists with an increasing oxygen requirement, the patient should be transferred to an intensive care setting for dialysis.[34] In facilities in which dialysis is not readily available, venisection or phlebotomy may be attempted in life-threatening situations.[43]

Hyperkalemia is common in ARF secondary to reductions in GFR and tubular function.[15] Treatment depends on the serum level of potassium and electrocardiogram (ECG) changes. Patients with serum potassium levels greater than 6.5 meq/L or ECG changes (peaked T waves, QRS complex widening, flattened P waves, heart block, or ventricular fibrillation) should be treated aggressively. Temporary measures to treat hyperkalemia include the

Table 31-1. Prerenal and Renal Failure Laboratory Tests

	Prerenal ARF	**Intrinsic ARF**
BUN/creatinine	> 20:1	< 20:1
Urine osmolarity	> 500 mOsmol	< 400 mOsmol
Urine Na	< 10 meq/L	> 20 meq/L
Urine/plasma creatinine	> 20	< 20
FE_{NA}	< 1	> 1

following: intravenous calcium, insulin, and glucose; intravenous sodium bicarbonate; and a nebulized beta-adrenergic agonist. Increased excretion should be attempted with either oral or rectal sodium polystyrene sulfonate. Loop diuretics also may be used in an attempt to increase renal excretion of potassium. If these measures fail, dialysis should be started.

ARF may be secondary to a variety of insults to other systems. Low cardiac output from CHF, myocardial infarction, arrhythmias, hemorrhagic shock from an acute gastrointestinal bleed, or sepsis all may cause ARF. Identification of the type of renal failure should be a secondary priority. The focus is to identify prerenal and obstructive forms of ARF. Prerenal causes are the most common type of ARF in the elderly. Rapid infusion of saline is essential to restore circulating volume and often all that is needed to treat prerenal failure if no further insult occurs. Accurate determination of fluid status is critical because ARF can result in fluid overload. Fluid resuscitation should be monitored closely, particularly in the elderly with poor cardiac reserves. Central venous pressure (CVP) catheters may be needed to guide adequate fluid resuscitation.

Initially, as the patient's volume status is being evaluated, urinary obstruction must be ruled out as the cause of failure. A postvoid residual volume can be obtained by insertion of a Foley catheter. Outlet obstruction is suggested by a postvoid residual volume of greater than 100 mL.[8] If no urine is obtained with a functional catheter, renal ultrasonography should be performed. Renal ultrasonography is the imaging study of choice in the patient presenting with ARF.[24] Renal ultrasound is essential to rule out postobstructive ARF but has a sensitivity of only 80 to 85 percent.[4] A nondilated collecting system may be present if obstruction is associated with volume depletion. Obstructive findings also may be absent in patients in whom the ureters are encased in fibrosis. If obstruction is the cause of failure, postobstructive diuresis may occur, with urine output exceeding 500 to 1000 mL/hour.[2] Urine output needs to be monitored and replaced with intravenous fluids to prevent hypovolemia and further renal insult.

Renal ultrasonography also should be considered in all cases of ARF.[24] Doppler ultrasound has the ability to differentiate reversible prerenal failure from ATN.[49] Additionally, there are intrarenal echogenicity differences on ultrasound that help to determine the various types of intrinsic renal pathologies.[50]

There is no clinical evidence that diuretics improve outcome in ARF unless the patient is volume overloaded. Since elderly individuals present with ARF secondary to prerenal causes, the optimal management of ARF is correction of volume status. Numerous studies have shown the beneficial effects of fluid resuscitation in preventing prerenal azotemia from progressing to ATN.[10] Once ATN develops, the mainstay of treatment is conservative. Any potential renal toxin should be withheld. Patients who are hemodynamically stable with no sign of complications should be admitted for observation. Most patients with significant renal impairment and symptoms will require admission, often to intensive care.

CONCLUSION

Elder patients have a progressive loss of renal function that is not reflected by an increased serum creatinine level. They are vulnerable to develop ARF particularly when NSAIDs, ACE inhibitors, or radiologic contrast material is used. Occurrences of contrast material–induced ARF can be reduced by preprocedure hydration. Patients present with subtle signs of ARF, and often it is found with laboratory test results. The volume status of patients with ARF should be evaluated carefully because they can be hypovolumic or volume overloaded. Life-threatening consequences such as acute pulmonary edema and hyperkalema should be anticipated, identified early, and treated.

REFERENCES

1. Stevens PE, Tamimi NA, Al-Hasani MK, et al: Nonspecialist management of acute renal failure. *Q J Med* 94(10):533, 2001.
2. Round A, Hamad S: Incidence of severe ARF in adults: Results of a community-based study. *Br Med J* 306(6867):483, 1993.
3. Nash K, Hafeez A, Hou S: Hospital-acquired renal insufficiency. *Am J Kidney Dis* 39(5):930, 2002.
4. Turney JH, Marshall DH, Brownjohn AM, et al: The evolution of acute renal failure, 1956–1988. *Q J Med* 74(273):83, 1990.
5. Brown WW, Schmitz PG: Acute and chronic kidney disease. *Clin Geriatr Med* 14(2):211, 1998.
6. McLachlan M, Wasserman P: Changes in size and distensibity of the aging kidney. *Br J Radiol* 54(642):488, 1981.
7. Beck LH: The aging kidney: Defending a delicate balance of fluid and electrolytes. *Geriatrics* 55(4):26, 2000.
8. Macias-Nunez JF, Lopez-Novoa JM, Martinez-Maldonado M: Acute renal failure in the aged. *Semin Nephrol* 16(4):330, 1996.
9. Schoolwerth AC, Sica DA, Ballermann BJ, et al: Renal considerations in angiotensin converting enzyme inhibitor theraphy: A statement for health care professionals from the

Council on the Kidney in Cardiovascular Disease and the Council for High Blood Pressure Research of the American Hearth Association. *Circulation* 104(16):1985, 2001.

10. Sladen RN: Anesthesia and renal considerations. *Anesthesiol Clin North Am* 18:739, 2000.

11. Novis BK, Roizen MF, Aronson S, et al: Association of pre-operative risk factors with postoperative acute renal failure. *Anesth Analg* 78(1):143, 1994.

12. Rowe JW, Andres R, Tobin JD, et al: The effect of age on creatinine clearance in men: A cross-sectional and longitudinal study. *J Gerontol* 31(2):155, 1976.

13. Lindeman RD, Tobin J, Shock NW: Longitudinal studies on the rate of decline in renal function with age. *J Am Geriatr Soc* 33(4):278, 1985.

14. Beck LH: Changes in renal function with aging. *Clin Geriatr Med* 14:199, 1998.

15. Sica DA: Renal diseases, electrolyte abnormalities, and acid-base imbalance in the elderly. *Clin Geriatr Med* 10(1):197, 1994.

16. Ohashi M, Fulio N, Nawata H, et al: High plasma concentrations of human atrial natriuretic polypeptide in aged men. *J Clin Endorcrinol* 64(1):81, 1987.

17. Gault MH, Longerich LL, Harnett JD, et al: Predicting glomerular function from adjusted serum creatinine. *Nephron* 62(3):249, 1992.

18. Doolan PD, Alpen EL, Theil GB: A clinical appraisal of the plasma concentration and endogenous clearance of creatinine. *Am J Med* 32:65, 1962.

19. Edwards BF: Postoperative renal insufficiency. *Med Clin North Am* 85(5):1241, 2001.

20. Cockcroft DW, Gault MH: Prediction of creatinine clearance from serum creatinine. *Neprhron* 16(1):31, 1976.

21. Mulkerrin BK: Potassium homeostasis in the elderly. *Q J Med* 90:487, 1997.

22. Thadhani R, Pascual M, Bonventre JV: Medical progress: Acute renal failure. *New Engl J Med* 334(22):1448, 1996.

23. Mindell JA, Chertow GM: A practical approach to acute renal failure. *Med Clin North Am* 81(3):731, 1997.

24. Gilbert BR, Vaughan ED Jr: Pathophysiology of the aging kidney. *Clin Geriatr Med* 6(1):13, 1990.

25. Abuelo JG: Diagnosing vascular causes of renal failure. *Ann Intern Med* 123(8):601, 1995.

26. Albright RC Jr: Acute renal failure: A practical update. *Mayo Clin Proc* 76(1):67, 2001

27. Pascual J, Orofino L, Liano F, et al: Incidence and prognosis of acute renal failure in older patients. *J Am Geriatr Soc* 38(1):25, 1990.

28. Perez-Gutthann S, Garcia-Rodriguez LA, Railford DS, et al: Nonsteroidal anti-inflammatory drugs and the risk of hospitalization for acute renal failure. *Arch Intern Med* 156(21):2433, 1996.

29. Evans JM, McGregor E, McMahon AD: Nonsteroidal anti-inflammatory drugs and hospitalization for acute renal failure. *Q J Med* 88(8):551, 1995.

30. Harris RC: Cyclooxygenase-2 in the kidney. *J Am Soc Nephrol* 11:2387, 2000.

31. Nzerue CM: The coxibs, selective inhibitors of cyclooxygenase-2. *New Engl J Med* 345(23):1708, 2001.

32. Perazella MA, Tray K: Selective cyclooxygenase-2 inhibitors: A pattern of nephrotoxicity similar to traditional nonsteroidal anti-inflammatory drugs. *Am J Med* 111(1):64, 2001.

33. Agrawal M, Swartz R: Acute renal failure. *Am Fam Phys* 61(7):2077, 2000.

34. Molitoris BA, Sandoval R, Sutton TA: Endothelial injury and dysfunction in ischemic acute renal failure. *Critic Care Med* 30(5s):s235, 2002

35. Barrett BJ, Parfrey PS: Prevention of nephrotoxicity induced by radiocontrast agents. *New Engl J Med* 331(21):1449, 1994.

36. Field TS, Gurwitz JH, Gylnn RJ, et al: The renal effects of nonsteroidal anti-inflammatory drugs in older people: Findings from the Established Populations for Epidemiologic Studies of the Elderly. *J Am Geriatr Soc* 47(5):507, 1999.

37. Diaz-Sandoval LJ, Kosowsky BD, Losordo DW: Acetylcysteine to prevent angiography-related renal tissue injury (the APART Trail). *Am J Cardiol* 89(3):356, 2002.

38. Murphy SW, Barrett BJ, Parfrey PS: Contrast nephropathy. *J Am Soc Nephrol* 11(1):177, 2000.

39. Mueller C, Buerkle G, Buettner HJ: Prevention of contrast media–associated nephropathy: Randomized comparison of two hydration regimens in 1620 patients undergoing coronary angioplasty. *Arch Intern Med* 162(3):329, 2002.

40. Tepel M, van der Giet M, Schwarzfeld C: Prevention of radiographic-contrast-agent-induced reductions in renal function by acetylcysteine. *New Engl J Med* 343(3):180, 2000.

41. Irish AB, Winearls CG, Littlewood T: Presentation and survival of patients with severe renal failure and myeloma. *Q J Med* 90(12):773, 1997.

42. Kapoor K, Chan GZ: Malignancy and renal disease. *Crit Care Clin* 17(3):571, 2001.

43. Glynne PA, Lightstone L: Acute renal failure. *Clin Med* 1(4):266, 2001.

44. Martinez-Maldonado M, Kumjian DA: Acute renal failure due to urinart tract odstruction. *Med Clin North Am* 74(14):919, 1990.

45. Sokolosky MC: Hematuria. *Emerg Med Clin North Am* 19(3):621, 2001.

46. Chang BS: Red cell morphology as a diagnostic aid in hematuria. *JAMA* 252(13):1747, 1984.

47. Bazari H, Mauiyyedi S: Weekly clinicopathological exercises. Case 42002: A 75-year-old man with acute renal failure five months after cystoprostatectomy and urethrectomy for carcinoma. *New Engl J Med* 346(5):353, 2002.

48. O'neill WC: Sonographic evaluation of renal failure. *Am J Kidney Dis* 35(6):1021, 2000.

49. Abrass CK: Renal biopsy in the elderly. *Am J Kidney Dis* 35(3):544, 2000.

50. Haas M, Spargo BH, Wit EC, et al: Etiologies and outcome of acute renal insufficiency in older adults: A renal biopsy study of 259 cases. *Am J Kidney Dis* 35(3):433, 2000.

32

Urologic Emergencies

Charles F. Pattavina

HIGH-YIELD FACTS

- Renal colic symptoms may indicate a more severe underlying illness, such as abdominal aortic dissection. Computed tomographic (CT) scan may help rule out other pathology.

- Urinary retention is easily treated by catheterization in the emergency department (ED), but an underlying cause such as a medication effect should be considered.

- Obstruction secondary to penile pathology may require simple surgical procedures by the emergency physician.

- Infection of the scrotum can progress rapidly, particularly in diabetic patients, to become a necrotizing cellulitis.

- Unexplained hematuria even with anticoagulation should prompt outpatient evaluation for urinary tumors in older patients.

In the elderly, symptoms attributable to urologic emergencies are a frequent cause of emergency department (ED) visits. This chapter addresses those conditions which might be expected to lead an older person to seek emergency care or to need emergent intervention. The entities are arranged by disease or symptom.

RENAL CALCULUS DISEASE

Epidemiology

Although stones may form at any level, acute flank pain, described as colicky and usually severe, is caused most often by stones formed in the kidney. Pain usually occurs when a stone exits the kidney and enters the ureter, causing distension or obstruction as waves of peristalsis pass over the stone. Severity and referred location of pain vary as the calculus moves down the tract. Pain also results from distension of the renal capsule when high-grade obstruction is present. Once a patient is treated with analgesics, it can be difficult to tell whether improvement is spontaneous or due to the medications. A thorough medical history, laboratory studies, and prudent imaging are keys to making the diagnosis, thus avoiding missing other more life-threatening conditions that produce similar symptoms.

Conditions that precipitate calcium are invoked most often because 75 percent of renal calculi contain that element.[1] There are associations, such as excess excretion of oxalate—as in inflammatory bowel disease—or increased concentration of the urine and its calcium content. In particular, the incidence of symptomatic kidney stones in the United States is greatest during the summer months and is more prevalent in the warmest regions of the country.

Differential Diagnosis

Other conditions causing ureteral obstruction and therefore the same type of pain include sloughing of a renal papilla, as seen in diabetics; analgesic abuse or chronic infection; and a blood clot from a renal tumor. Of particular concern in the older patient with flank pain and hematuria is aortic or renal artery aneurysm or dissection. Intravenous contrast material may be needed to delineate dissection on computed tomographic (CT) scan. Renal artery embolism (as seen in atrial fibrillation, mural thrombosis, and septal defects), as well as renal vein thrombosis or even bleeding into a renal tumor, can produce a similar pain.[2] Pulmonary embolism, pulmonary infarct, and even pneumonia can mimic the flank pain of renal colic. Acute pyelonephritis is seen more commonly in women and tends to be more gradual and moderate than renal stone disease. Perinephric abscess can cause a similar presentation but usually produces fever. Muculoskeletal back pain and intraabdominal processes such as cholecystitis, diverticulitis, and appendicitis must be considered.

Clinical Features

Patients typically relate symptoms as the sudden onset of severe, unilateral flank pain that may wax and wane regardless of attempts to achieve comfort. Nausea, vomiting, and chills may result from severe pain, but in the absence of infection, actual fever is not typical. Hematuria also may be present. A distinction often pointed out is that patients with renal colic will be writhing in pain, moving all about attempting to feel better, in contrast to most patients with peritonitis, who tend to remain still in order to minimize their pain. Often there is a history of previous episodes of renal colic. There also may be a history of predisposing metabolic disease or medications such as protease inhibitors,[3] although currently these medications are not used commonly by the elderly. A history of abdominal aortic aneurysm or other vascular disease should be ascertained, as well as any predisposition to pulmonary embolism.

Other than monitoring the general appearance of a person in severe pain, the severity of which may vary during examination, the physical examination should be essentially normal. The emergency physician may observe pallor, diaphoresis, and vomiting, as well as a patient who is either standing or pacing. Findings that should encourage consideration of coexisting problems or other emergencies include fever, dyspnea, abdominal tenderness, significant flank tenderness, or a pulsatile abdominal mass.

Emergency Department Care

Urinalysis may show microscopic or gross hematuria. Pyuria suggests concurrent infection or a diagnosis of pyelonephritis, as does an elevated white blood cell count. In renal colic, the complete blood count (CBC) should be normal. Typically, a blood ureanitrogen and creatinine determination is done to check renal function, especially if the patient may need to receive intravenous contrast material or medications such as nonsteroidal anti-inflammatory drugs (NSAIDs). All urine should be strained for calculi, which will help with the acute diagnosis as well as long-term therapy directed at preventing recurrent stones.

Helical CT scanning has emerged as the imaging method of choice where and when it is available.[4] Noncontrast-enhanced CT scanning offers very high specificity and sensitivity for renal stone disease—as well as for demonstrating aneurysm. It can suggest other diagnoses such as pyelonephritis or a sloughed renal papilla. While there is radiation involved, non-contrast-enhanced CT scanning is otherwise completely safe. Ultrasound (US) imaging offers similar safety and demonstrates secondary signs of renal colic (hydronephrosis, hydroureter, etc.) as well.[5] The use of US by emergency physicians is expanding rapidly across the country. Emergency US is very helpful in facilities where 24-hour CT scanning is not available. The intravenous pyelogram has all but disappeared from ED use where these other tests are available. When done properly, it can be very helpful; however, it carries the increased risk associated with the administration of intravenous contrast material.

The goal of treatment is to relieve the patient's pain while making the diagnosis. Analgesics are the mainstay of treatment. However, the presence of nausea can be aggravated by typical analgesics unless an antiemetic is given first or concomitantly. Subcutaneous or intravenous morphine or Dilaudid are used commonly. In recent years, intravenous ketorolac has seen use in younger patients, but it should be used at lower doses in the elderly and only after ensuring that renal function is normal. Pain and nausea control can be achieved with injected medications. Then oral medications may be given to determine if they will control the patient's pain at home. Intravenous fluid—mainly normal saline—can help to ensure adequate hydration, but there is no benefit to excessive hydration. It may be detrimental, particularly in those with cardiac disease.

Although most patients with uncomplicated renal calculi can go home with analgesics and a urology follow-up, one must consider the effects of the stress of such severe pain on elderly patients, particularly those with other significant health problems. Reasons for admission include pain not controllable by outpatient medications, uncontrolled emesis, and obstruction of the patient's only functioning kidney. Reasons to consider admission include concurrent infection, particularly with high-grade obstruction, and the presence of a significant underlying disease.

URINARY RETENTION

Epidemiolgy

Occurring largely in a problem of older males, acute urinary retention can cause extreme distress for the patient. Symptoms include inability to void, extreme suprapubic discomfort, and dribbling and frequency. Most commonly it results from an anatomic cause at some level, although other factors, especially medications, may be found. Relief comes from establishing drainage of the bladder.[6]

An enlarged prostate is the most common cause and generally is due to benign hyperplasia. Carcinoma, bladder neck contracture, and prostatitis with severe swelling are other causes. Urethral causes—especially in women—include stricture, meatal stenosis, tumor, foreign body, clots, or calculus. Penile causes usually are fairly obvious to the examiner, including phimosis, paraphimosis, and external constriction. Medications, from over-the-counter cold preparations (which often contain antihistamines and α-adrenergic stimulators) to anticholinergics and cyclic antidepressants, are among the nonstructural causes of retention that can be persistent. Neurologic causes include neurogenic bladder (as seen most often in diabetics) and paralytic spinal problems.[2]

Clinical Features

It is common for men to experience a gradual, almost imperceptible decrease in urinary flow and stream power consistent with benign prostatic hypertrophy. This may be followed by frequency and dribbling from overflow incontinence and eventually acute obstruction and distension, leading to presentation at the ED. Sudden interruption of the stream suggests obstruction by a renal or bladder stone, whereas that symptom with frank hematuria suggests a blood clot. A history of any of the suspect medications or of recent anesthesia should lead one to consider a medication-related problem. A history of urologic surgery or procedure—including Foley catheterization—suggests the possibility of urethral stricture or bladder neck contracture.

The patient may be in acute distress from discomfort and anxiety, particularly on first presentation for this problem, and the vital signs may reflect that distress. Other than suprapubic tenderness and distension (which on occasion has been mistaken for a mass), the only findings may be at the meatus or penis. Phimosis, paraphimosis, and constriction by an external foreign body will be apparent on general inspection, whereas meatal stenosis requires a closer inspection. Rarely, a stone, mass, or foreign body may be palpable within the urethra and can be gently "milked" out, but this usually requires urologic consultation in the ED. Stones found during the examination may have formed anywhere in the tract from the bladder up to the renal pelvis, or occasionally, foreign bodies may be found. Urethral narrowing due to stricture, periurethral abscess (seen in patients with indwelling Foley catheters or following difficult instrumentation), or a foreign body may not be apparent and may prevent passage of a new catheter, necessitating urologic consultation.

Whereas plain radiographs may reveal radiopaque foreign bodies, ultrasound may show an abscess and estimate postvoid residual. The main intervention—gentle passage of a urethral catheter soon after the last attempt to void—is both therapeutic and diagnostic. The passage of urine relieves the patient's distress. With urinary obstruction postvoid urine of one liter or more is common, although as little as 250 mL may cause symptoms. Urinalysis is always indicated, although the results may reveal hematuria, crystals, or a normal study. The complete blood count should be normal. The blood ureanitrogen and creatinine are helpful in assessing renal function. Coagulation studies may be helpful for those with hematuria, especially when the patient is on anticoagulation therapy.

Emergency Department Care

Passage of a no. 16 French Foley catheter (no. 12 French if urethral stricture is suspected) should provide dramatic relief. A Coudé catheter, one with the distal 3 cm at an angle to the rest of the device, is designed to be aimed cephalad to pass over the median lobe of the prostate. Therefore, it can be useful when significant benign prostatic hyperplasia is suspected. If significant hematuria is part of the presentation, then a larger three-way catheter should be placed to allow copious irrigation and free drainage. The catheter always should be passed all the way into the bladder, with drainage of urine observed, before the balloon is inflated. If two or three gentle attempts to pass a catheter are unsuccessful, urologic consultation should be sought because repeated attempts may cause unnecessary discomfort. There is also danger of creating a false passage, which will not relieve the patient and may be a source of significant bleeding and a site for infection. Antibiotics should be reserved for those with evidence of infection. Whenever possible, treatment should be given for any underlying cause, including discontinuation of potentially causative medications.

A urology consultation or follow-up is important in order to continue the workup, including detection of prostate and other malignancy. Patients who have obtained relief with catheter placement usually can be sent home with a leg bag and instructions for its use and follow-up with a urologist within 5 days. Those who are unable to perform this self-care and for whom home care cannot be arranged may need placement in a rehabilitation facility—or even hospital admission if there is significant comorbidity, including acute infection or functional decline. Those with significant nonclearing hematuria, especially with clots, usually require admission to the urology service for continued irrigation and workup.[6]

PENILE CONDITIONS

Phimosis

Phimosis, a potential cause of urinary retention in the elderly, is an acquired condition, particularly in uncircumcised diabetics. The foreskin cannot be retracted because it is adherent to the glans, and obstruction may result. Often dilation of the meatus with a small hemostat suffices in the ED, and follow-up circumcision is definitive. In some cases, a dorsal slit procedure of the foreskin may need to be done after local anesthesia.[7]

Paraphimosis

While paraphimosis is the inability to reduce the foreskin over the glans, it, too, can cause obstruction due to compression by the edematous foreskin and glans. This edema of the retracted foreskin may occur after failure to reduce the foreskin following catheterization or after manipulation of the penis, including intercourse. Once the edema has developed, gentle pressure on the glans along with traction on the foreskin may not be adequate for reduction because of the presence of constricting bands. A 2-in Kling (rolled gauze) may be impregnated with xylocaine jelly and wrapped gently but firmly around the glans for about 15 minutes. After removal, the glans often will be small enough to allow reduction with the benefit of the lubrication and topical anesthesia. A similar-sized elastic wrap also may be tried. Other methods include anesthetizing the base of the penis and squeezing edema fluid out of the foreskin or making punctures in the glans with a small hypodermic needle and then squeezing edema fluid from the glans.[8]

Balanitis and Posthitis

These occur together as a result of poor hygiene. Balanitis and posthitis are, respectively, inflammations of the glans, penis, and foreskin. Cases range from mild inflammation—which responds to conservative measures such as cleansing and topical antibiotics—to severe cases that resemble cellulitis and track proximally. Severe cases can result in phimosis, which ultimately may require circumcision.

Penile Swelling

Generalized edema, anasarca, pelvic deep vein thrombosis, or tumor may produce edema of the penis and scrotum. Radiation to the pelvic nodes, as well as tumor obstruction, may block lymphatic flow and manifest as lymphedema. While problems can require intervention, these conditions improve when the underlying cause—nodal, penile, and scrotal—is treated.

SCROTAL PAIN

Fournier's Gangrene

Fournier's gangrene may develop from or even begin as an apparently benign localized infection such as cellulitis or abscess. However, it can progress rapidly to a severe and very painful necrotic process.[9] Although a hallmark of this condition is said to be "pain out of proportion to the physical findings," the gross appearance of true Fournier's gangrene would seem adequate to justify the most severe pain. In moderate stages, there is a marked swelling of the scrotum and penis with sharply demarcated black areas of gangrene. Surrounding tissues, including the higher urinary tract, can be affected very quickly, especially since those most susceptible are diabetics and the immunocompromised. One should have a high index of suspicion for this condition when diagnosing abscess or cellulitis at or near the scrotum in these patients, particularly when pain is a prominent feature.

Arising in the skin, rectum, or penis, the infection may contain a variety of organisms, including gram-positive and gram-negative rods and anaerobes. Appropriate antibiotics, fluid resuscitation, and prompt urologic consultation are required. Wide surgical debridement is needed to prevent significant tissue loss.

Epididymitis

Epidemiology

Epididymitis is a painful inflammation resulting from trauma and/or a variety of microbial agents. It is treated easily in the early stages when the diagnosis is made.

Urinary pathogens are the most common causative agents in the older age group, but the usual sexually transmitted pathogens should be considered when the history suggests them. Epididymitis may be the first sign of bladder outflow obstruction because stricture or prostatic hypertrophy causing urinary stasis with infection result in either epididymitis or urinary tract infection.

Differential Diagnosis

Other conditions should be considered when an elder presents with testicular pain. Testicular torsion can occur in older males but usually causes a more rapid onset of pain than epididymitis. Bleeding into a tumor is more sudden in onset. Hydroceles, while usually asymptomatic, can present with pain, particularly when they complicate epididymitis, trauma, or carcinoma.[10]

Clinical Features

Patients note a gradual onset of pain, usually in just one testicle. There may be a history of relatively minor trauma, such as recent lifting. There may be suprapubic or generalized lower abdominal discomfort. Fever and severe pain are usually late findings.

Early in the disease the only finding may be mild tenderness at the epididymis. Typically, later there will be more prominent tenderness and swelling, which can make accurate palpation more difficult. The overlying scrotal skin may show some erythema, but frank cellulitis or abscess should lead one to consider other diagnoses.[2]

Diagnostic Studies

Diagnosis is usually evident on examination. Urinalysis may show white blood cells, but it can be normal. If a sexually transmitted disease is a consideration, appropriate cultures and testing should be obtained. Should it be necessary to distinguish epididymitis from testicular torsion (which can occur at any age) or other painful masses, ultrasonography should be obtained.[10]

Emergency Department Care

NSAIDs in appropriate dose for the patient's age and rest with icepacks are mainstays of treatment. Antibiotics directed toward the likely pathogens are indicated. Stronger analgesics are needed often, and a scrotal support is helpful as the patient resumes ambulation. Follow-up with the primary physician within a few days is suggested and with a urologist as needed.

Patients with fever and chills or who appear toxic should be considered for hospital admission. Those for whom the diagnosis is not certain should have at least a telephone consultation with the urologist in order to guide further workup.

HEMATURIA

Epidemiolgy

Hematuria is blood in the urine, which may be either gross or microscopic. It is a *symptom* that can be confirmed by simple laboratory testing. When a patient is said to be complaining of hematuria, he or she usually has noted that the urine is discolored to somewhere between pink and looking just like whole blood. It is important to note that hematuria refers to actual red blood cells in the urine. *False hematuria* can be caused by pigments discoloring the urine with no red cells visible on microscopic examination.[11]

Hematuria can be produced at any level in the urinary tract and by many processes. Among nontraumatic causes, infection, usually cystitis, is common in this age group. Cancer of the bladder, prostate, and kidney are next, followed by benign prostatic hypertrophy and calculus.[6] Recent urologic surgery or instrumentation is another frequent cause in ED patients. Anticoagulant therapy is often a factor, whether it causes bleeding in a normal tract or unmasks bleeding from an existing occult lesion.

Clinical Features

The history to gather includes the extent and duration of bleeding, presence of any pain or fever, recent instrumentation or surgery, existing urologic or bleeding disorders, and recent anticoagulant therapy. A history of eating beets should be noted in those who turn out to have false hematuria because this food can discolor the urine red.

Most patients who present to the ED with this symptom have significant hematuria. Long, stringy clots suggest ureteral bleeding, whereas larger-sized casts suggest a source at or near the bladder. Of course, flank pain suggests renal calculus disease, whereas painless hematuria may be due to malignancy, occult cystitis, benign prostatic hypertrophy, or bleeding disorders, including excessive anticoagulation.

There may be few or no clues as to the origin of the problem on physical examination. Heart rate and blood pressure may be elevated from anxiety. Shock is unlikely unless bleeding has been severe and prolonged. There may be flank tenderness if infection or obstruction and distension are present, whereas suprapubic tenderness suggests cystitis. There is often gross blood visible in the area of the meatus. Vaginal or rectal bleeding *suggests* nonurologic causes. Ecchymoses and easy bruising may be noted when a coagulation disorder is present.

The urinalysis demonstrates red blood cells as the cause of the discoloration. White blood cells may suggest infection. A CBC is helpful in establishing the presence of any new or preexisting anemia or thrombocytopenia, as well as providing information about systemic infection. SMA-7 determination checks renal function and the degree of hydration. Coagulation studies are helpful in diagnosing a new coagulation disorder and are required when the patient has a known coagulopathy, including warfarin therapy. Blood type and crossmatch should be done when the bleeding is severe and prolonged. Ultrasound and plain CT scanning can be helpful in locating obstruction of the tract and some masses. Contrast material may be needed for others. Urologic evaluation will be needed for all but the most straightforward cases because cancer is a possible diagnosis, and cystoscopy is likely needed.

Emergency Department Care

Whether or not they already have a urethral catheter in place, these patients often obstruct from blood clots. If there is significant bleeding, especially with clots, and there is even the suggestion of impending obstruction, a larger-sized (approximately no. 22 French) three-way Foley catheter should be placed and continuous irrigation with normal saline begun. If a regular Foley catheter is already in place, irrigation should be attempted; however, replacement with a three-way will be needed unless the blood and clots clear promptly. Treatment of any underlying cause should commence—low platelets, excessive anticoagulation, infection, etc. Fluid and blood replacement should be considered but usually are not needed.

Patients whose bleeding does not clear promptly with irrigation will need admission for continuous irrigation and further urologic evaluation. Those with renal failure, significant anemia, or an important comorbidity—such as heart disease—should be considered for admission.[6] If there is any question about the patient being physically or otherwise unable to comply with the treatment plan at home or adequate home services cannot be arranged, admission may be warranted.

CONCLUSION

The variety of urinary emergency conditions is limited. The emergency physician should be aware of the common syndromes and be wary of missing other life-threatening conditions. The relief of pain associated with many of these conditions can be rewarding for the physician and patient.

REFERENCES

1. Coe FL, Parks JH, Asplin JR: The pathogenesis and treatment of kidney stones. *New Engl J Med* 327:1141, 1992.
2. Walsh PC, Retik AB, Vaughan, ED et al: *Campbell's Urology,* 7th ed. Philadelphia, Saunders, 1998.
3. Kopp JB, Miller KD, Mican JAM, et al: Crystalluuria and urinary tract abnormalities associated with Indinavir. *Ann Intern Med* 127:119, 1997.
4. Smith RC, Rosenfeld AT, Choe KA, ED et al: Comparison of non-contrast-enhanced CT and intravenous urography. *Radiology* 194:789, 1995.
5. Koelliker SL, Cronan JJ: Acute urinary tract obstruction: Imaging update. *Urol Clin North Am* 24:571, 1997.
6. O'Donnell PD: *Geriatric Urology.* Boston, Little Brown, 1994.
7. Hashmat AI, Das S: *The Penis.* Philadelphia, Lea & Febiger, 1993.
8. Williams JC, Morrison PM, Richardson JR: Paraphimosis in elderly men. *Am J Emerg Med* 13:351, 1995.
9. Clayton MD, Fowler JE, Sharifi R, et al: Causes, presentation and survival of fifty-seven patients with necrotizing fasciitis of the male genitalia. *Surg Gynecol Obstet* 70:49, 1990.
10. Pryor JL, Watson LR, Day DL, et al: Scrotal ultrasound for evaluation of testicular torsion. *J Urol* 151:693, 1994.
11. Howes DS, Bogner MP: Hematuria and Hematospermia, in Tintinalli JE, Kelen GD, Stapczynski JS (eds): *Emergency Medicine: A Comprehensive Study Guide,* 5th ed. New York, McGraw-Hill, 2000.

33

Gynecologic Emergencies

Marc R. Toglia

HIGH-YIELD FACTS

- Atrophic vaginitis is the most common cause for vaginal bleeding in the elderly woman.
- Heavy vaginal bleeding in the elderly woman is worrisome for cervical carcinoma.
- The chance that postmenopausal bleeding indicates uterine cancer increases with a woman's age.
- Pelvic organ prolapse is commonly associated with urinary retention.
- Incomplete voiding in the elderly female can predispose her to chronic cystitis and urosepsis.

Evaluation of the elderly woman who presents with gynecologic complaints offers significant challenges for emergency physicians. Many women stop going for routine gynecologic examinations following menopause. The older woman may be reluctant to discuss pelvic problems or may ignore symptoms of incontinence or bleeding.

Gynecologic problems in the elderly woman encompass a wide variety of disorders that range from irritative vulvar and vaginal complaints to pelvic malignancies. Pelvic organ prolapse and incontinence affect a significant number of older women. Bleeding and irritation are two common reasons that an older woman may present to the emergency department (ED).

The emergency physician can play a pivotal role in the evaluation of these complaints. While these symptoms rarely represent true medical or surgical emergencies, they should not be ignored. One of the emergency physicians' goals is to identify patients with malignancy and refer them to appropriate clinicians for diagnosis and management.

EPIDEMIOLOGY

The proportion of postmenopausal women will increase from 23 percent of the population in 1995 to 33 percent in 2050. Gynecologic malignancies, as a group, account for about 13 percent of all cancers in women. The incidence of most gynecologic malignancies increases as a woman ages. Women decrease their frequency of gynecologic screening examinations as they get older, thus missing opportunities for early detection.[1] Endometrial cancer is the fourth most common cancer in women and the most common gynecologic neoplasm, with an incidence of approximately 36,000 cases per year.[2] About 3 percent of women will develop endometrial cancer in their lifetimes. Ovarian cancer is the fifth most common cancer in women but the leading cause of death from gynecologic cancer. The lifetime risk of ovarian cancer is 1 in 70, or 1.4 percent. Cervical cancer has been decreasing in incidence because of widespread use of the Pap smear. The most common presenting symptom of cervical cancer is postmenopausal bleeding. Vulvar and vaginal cancers are uncommon in the United States, each accounting for less than 1 percent of cancers in women. However, the mean age of a women developing vulvar or vaginal cancer is 65 years, making it an important part of the differential diagnosis in the elderly woman who presents with bleeding.

Pelvic floor disorders affect a significant number of elderly women. One recent study suggests that the largest age group to seek care for these problems is between 60 and 79 years of age. The study projects that demand for services to care for these disorders will increase at twice the rate of growth for this population.[3] The prevalence of urinary incontinence in community-dwelling older women ranges from 8 to 41 percent. It has been estimated that fewer than half of those affected seek care.

PATHOPHYSIOLOGY

Aging is associated with a decrease in physiologic function and reserve. In general, aging is associated with a decrease in tissue elasticity and vascularization as well as a decrease in muscle tone and strength. Women enter a hypoestrogenic state after menopause, resulting in additional alterations in function within the genital tract. Estrogen deficiency results in atrophy of the urogenital tract, including the mucosal surfaces and smooth muscles of the vulva, vagina, urethra, bladder, and uterus. Postmenopausal women experience an increase in irritative symptoms, as well as a decreased resistance to infection. Also, decreased urethral vascularity and muscle function may predispose a woman to urinary incontinence. Childbirth can damage the pelvic floor directly by stretching and tearing the supportive structures of the urogenital hiatus and indirectly by initiating a denervational injury to the pelvic floor and secondary muscle atrophy. Other factors such as obesity, constipation, and hysterectomy are thought to contribute to the development of pelvic organ prolapse and urinary incontinence.

CLINICAL FEATURES

The most common emergency gynecologic complaints of elderly women are bleeding, vulvovaginal irritation, pelvic pain, pelvic organ prolapse, and vague abdominal symptoms. Because many elderly women no longer have a gynecologist, they sometimes seek care at the ED. These women may seek care at the onset of symptoms (vaginal bleeding) but more often seen care late in the course of the disorder.

History

Obtaining an accurate history can be especially challenging. Older women may be reluctant to discuss vaginal symptoms or questions related to sexuality and incontinence. Declining cognitive function and memory, problems with communication and comprehension, and denial of symptoms or problems can complicate history taking. The emergency physician therefore must inquire specifically about bleeding, pain, discharge, and incontinence. A significant number of older women may be unable to remember events accurately, such as the age of menopause or age and indications for prior gynecologic surgery. It is important to have a caregiver available to help answer questions. A significant goal of the history taking is to gain the patient's confidence in preparation for the examination.

Bleeding is often noticed only following urination, and it should be established whether the bleeding is thought to be vaginal, urinary, or rectal. Vaginal discharge may be due to atrophy, infection, malignancy, or trauma. Vulvar and vaginal irritation may or may not be associated with a discharge and may be either pruritic or burning in quality. Pelvic pain is often vague in this age group.

Attention should be given to the patient's bowel and bladder habits. Incontinence, urinary frequency, nocturia, difficulty emptying the bladder or bowel, and constipation often are associated with pelvic floor disorders, including pelvic organ prolapse. Alarm symptoms include anorexia, weight loss, dyspepsia, abdominal distension, and sudden changes in bowel habits, which often accompany ovarian and endometrial malignancies.

It is important to know whether the patient is currently using any estrogen preparations (prescription or otherwise) or any topical medication in and around the vagina. In a patient who has an intact uterus, it is critical to establish whether she is using hormone-replacement therapy (HRT) (estrogen plus a progestin) or unopposed estrogen. Combination HRT is associated with a significant rate of breakthrough bleeding. Some women have discovered that omitting the progestin alleviates this problem. Unfortunately, unopposed estrogen therapy is associated with a significant risk of developing endometrial carcinoma.

Important historical data can help guide evaluation and management. Women often associate certain medical events in relationship to the ages of their children at that particular time. The physician should establish the number and route deliveries the woman has had. It should also be established early on whether or not the woman has previously undergone a hysterectomy, and if so whether it was performed through an abdominal incision vs. vaginally, and for what indication. The history of other procedures, including abnormal Pap smear, biopsies, dilation and curettage, vaginal reconstruction, and anti-incontinence procedures, should be obtained. The age of menopause should be determined. Finally, it should be established whether the woman has been receiving routine gynecologic care and, if so, when the last encounter occurred.

Sexual history is often overlooked during the history taking of the geriatric woman. However, it is important to recognize that many women remain sexually active all their adult lives and that sexual intercourse may be a source for vaginal bleeding, pruritis, dysuria, and other complaints. It is often best to transition into a sexual history after establishing whether the woman is married, single, or widowed. One approach is to bring up the issue of sexuality by asking, "Because your symptoms involve the female organs, I need to know if you are sexually active and whether you experience any discomfort with intercourse?"

Gynecologic Examination

A gynecologic examination must be performed in a comfortable and private setting. Elderly women may be embarrassed or unwilling to undergo pelvic examination. The examination should therefore begin with the physician explaining that a thorough but gentle examination is necessary because of the nature of the complaint. Reluctant patients should be advised that serious gynecologic problems, including cancer, could occur at any age.

Gynecologic examination begins with inspection and palpation of the abdomen. Pelvic masses, including fibroids, often can be palpated abdominally above the pubic bone. A mass palpable near the umbilicus or upper abdomen may be formed by omentum that is infiltrated with carcinoma. Abdominal distension and ascites are common features of advanced ovarian and colonic malignancies.

The lymph nodes along the inguinal chain should be palpated, noting any enlargement or tenderness. Lymphadenopathy secondary to inflammation or infection is typically soft, mobile, and tender, whereas that caused by carcinoma is often firm, fixed, and nontender.

Pelvic examination begins with observation of the external genitalia and skin surrounding the vulva, perineum, and anus. Fecal or urinary soiling should be noted. Erythema, discoloration, and ulcerations should be noted. The clinician should keep in mind that malignancies can involve the vulva. Pelvic organ prolapse may be readily visible at rest. The vagina should be examined using a small, lubricated vaginal speculum. The vaginal sidewalls and cervix should be observed for bleeding or lesions. A foreign body may be the cause of bleeding, discharge, or pain. The absence of a cervix typically indicates a prior hysterectomy, although in some women atrophic changes may cause the cervix to retract and become flush with the vaginal vault. Cotton-tipped swabs should be used to collect vaginal discharge for microscopic examination. Following the speculum examination or when speculum examination is not possible because of patient discomfort, a digital examination should be performed. First, the vaginal surfaces should be palpated for foreign bodies and any mucosal lesions. A cervix that was not visualized on speculum examination may be palpable. A uterus should be palpable at the top of the vagina between the vaginal finger and a hand placed against the lower abdominal wall. An irregular, mobile solid mass may represent a fibroid uterus, although an ovarian mass cannot be excluded. The ovaries of an elderly woman typically are atrophic and not palpable. Any palpable abnormality warrants further evaluation.

Examination of the woman with pelvic organ prolapse can be confusing due to the loss of normal anatomic landmarks and the distortion and swelling of the tissues. To identify prolapse, the labia should be separated slightly with two fingers, and the patient should be asked to strain outward or to cough. The cervix is usually readily identifiable by the presence of the cervical os (Fig. 33.1). On occasion, the anterior or posterior lip of the cervix may be elongated. Prolapse of the vagina anterior to the cervix typically represents a cystocele. Prolapse of

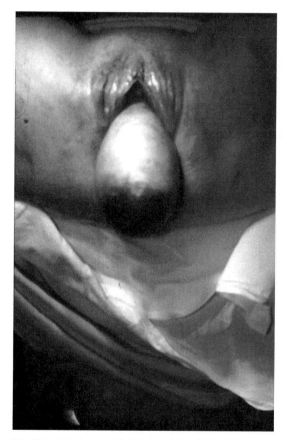

Fig. 33-1 Uterine procedentia. Complete eversion of the uterus and vagina through the vaginal introitus

the vagina posterior to the cervix may represent either a rectocele or an enterocele. Identification of the urethra may be difficult in a patient with a massive prolapse. Use of the posterior blade of a bivalve speculum can assist the examiner in identifying the anatomic defects associated with pelvic organ prolapse. The half speculum is lubricated and gently placed within the vagina. Depressing the speculum downward, toward the floor, allows the examiner to inspect the urethra, anterior vaginal wall, and cervix, if present. The patient should be asked to strain forcefully. The half speculum should then be removed, rotated 180 degrees and reinserted, and used to elevate the anterior vaginal wall. This allows the examiner to inspect the apex of the vagina and posterior vaginal wall for an enterocele and rectocele, respectively. Chronic exposure of a prolapsed vagina to external pressure may cause erosions or ulcerations that can be a source of bleeding.

Prolapse that extends beyond the vaginal opening can be reduced manually with a finger or a speculum. Reducing a large prolapse will allow the examiner to identify the urethra in most patients. After inspection, the physician should perform a bimanual examination. A large, cystic mass located anterior to the vagina and behind the pubic symphysis is often an overdistended bladder. This diagnosis can be confirmed rapidly by placing a Foley catheter to drain the bladder. On occasion, an old pessary or other foreign body may be found in the vagina. This can be the source of vaginal bleeding or discharge.

DIAGNOSIS AND DIFFERENTIAL

Vaginal Bleeding

Vaginal bleeding is the most common gynecologic reason that an elderly woman presents to the ED. Vaginal bleeding in this age group is rarely heavy or life-threatening. While most causes of vaginal bleeding in the postmenopausal woman are benign, the diagnosis of uterine, vaginal, cervical, and vulvar cancer must be entertained. It is most helpful to consider the differential diagnosis of bleeding with respect to the different anatomic structures within the pelvis (Table 33-1). A careful history taking often will provide valuable clues as to the site and cause of the bleeding—prior gynecologic surgery (including hysterectomy), use or past use of HRT, history of or treatment for abnormal Pap smears, timing of most recent gynecologic examination and Pap smear, and pattern of bleeding should all be elicited. Vaginal bleeding either will be observed on examination or not evident from the cervix, vagina, and vulva. If the source is not evident, a uterine source or nongynecologic source (e.g., urethra, bladder, or rectum) should be suspected. Hemorrhagic cystitis or rectal bleeding may be confused with vaginal bleeding. Heavy vaginal bleeding is uncommon in the geriatric patient but can arise from cervical or vaginal malignancy or acute trauma.

In one large series, atrophic vaginitis accounted for about half the women with a benign etiology vaginal bleeding.[4] It should be suspected in the elderly woman who does not have a recent history of HRT (either systemic or topical). Acute inflammatory processes, such as candidal infection and trichomoniasis, are other causes for bleeding originating from the vagina. Vaginal infections other than *Candida* are unusual in the elderly woman. Painless and sporadic bleeding episodes are the most common presenting symptom of squamous cell carcinoma. On examination, the woman usually is noted to

Table 33-1. Causes of Postmenopausal Bleeding

Vulvar
  Trauma
  Benign dermopathology (lichen sclerosus, vulvar
    dystrophy, condyloma)
  Vulvar carcinoma (squamous cell, melanoma)
Vaginal
  Atrophic vaginitis
  Infection (*Candida, Trichomonas*)
  Trauma (coitus, scratching)
  Squamous cell carcinoma
Cervical
  Endocervical polyps
  Cervical erosion
  Cervical carcinoma (squamous cell, adenocarcinoma)
Endometrial
  Atrophic endometrium
  Breakthrough bleeding on hormone-replacement
    therapy
  Endometrial polyps
  Endometrial carcinoma
  Submucus fibroids
  Endometritis
Systemic
Anticoagulation
Other
  Bladder source
  Bowel source

have an irregular and raised keratotic lesion that is easily friable. Trauma to the thin and fragile skin of the atrophic vagina also may result in bleeding. In general, a vaginal source can be confirmed by direct observation. It is important to rotate the speculum in both directions so that both the anterior and posterior vaginal walls can be visualized adequately.

Bleeding also may occur from an ulcerated area of vaginal prolapse. Any visible lesions should be referred for biopsy. The patient should be referred for Pap smear if it is not done in the ED. In a woman who previously underwent hysterectomy, a Pap smear of the vaginal cuff may be performed.

The endometrium also is a common source of postmenopausal bleeding. Atrophic endometrium can cause infrequent and sporadic bleeding because the lining is thin and fragile. The diagnosis is confirmed by endometrial biopsy. Breakthrough bleeding from HRT is common and is thought to be the result of progestin-induced atrophy of the endometrial lining. It occurs most commonly in the first 6 months after initiating therapy or if the scheduled pill taking becomes interrupted. Endometrial polyps are another common source of bleeding in this age group. They may be detected by endovaginal ultrasound.

Endometrial carcinoma typically is responsible for about 15 percent of cases of postmenopausal bleeding, with the likelihood of carcinoma increasing with advancing age. Women over age 80 who present with bleeding have a 60 percent chance of having endometrial cancer as compared with less than 1 percent of women with postmenopausal bleeding under age 50.[5] It is the most common malignancy of the female genital tract and occurs at a median age of 60 years. Risk factors include prolonged exposure to unopposed estrogen therapy or tamoxifen, obesity, and nulliparity. The vast majority of women with endometrial cancer will present with intermittent spotting or painless bleeding. Some women will complain of cramping associated with the bleeding. Endometrial hyperplasia may be a precursor to endometrial carcinoma and is also part of the differential diagnosis. The diagnosis of endometrial cancer typically is made by endometrial biopsy. Measurement of the endometrial thickness by vaginal ultrasonography may be a useful adjunct in the evaluation of postmenopausal bleeding. An endometrium with a total thickness of 5 mm or less has a 90 percent sensitivity and 95 percent specificity of excluding carcinoma. Endometrial thickness of 5 mm or greater requires endometrial sampling for histologic diagnosis, although carcinoma is extremely uncommon if the thickness is less than 8 mm. Vaginal ultrasonography is also useful in detecting both endometrial polyps and submucous fibroids.

The cervix is another common source of bleeding in elderly women. Endocervical polyps may bleed, especially following coitus. They appear as deep red polypoid tissue within the cervical canal. Cervical erosions may be caused by chronic inflammation, acute trichomoniasis, or uterine prolapse. Cervicitis also may be the result of chronic irritation from a pessary or poor hygiene. Cervical cancer unfortunately is a common cause of bleeding among postmenopausal women. Up to 90 percent of cervical cancers are squamous in histology, with the remainder being adenocarcinoma. Risk factors include prior abnormal Pap smears or an infection with human papillomavirus (HPV), early age of first coitus, and multiple sexual partners. Presenting symptoms include postmenopausal bleeding, intermenstrual bleeding, or bleeding following intercourse. A foul-smelling vaginal discharge from necrotic tissue may also occur. The physical examination will reveal a friable cervical mass that may extend along the upper vagina and pelvic sidewall.

Untreated cervical cancer may present with significant vaginal bleeding or even ureteral obstruction with uremia. Lymphatic blockage may result in edema of the lower extremities. Significant bleeding from cervical cancer may require packing the vagina and prompt consultation for hypogastric artery embolization or ligation or high-dose pelvic irradiation.

Vulvar sources of bleeding include both benign and malignant dermopathologies. Vulvar atrophy and lichen sclerosus are two common causes. Any irregular, raised, or discolored lesion should be referred for biopsy in order to rule out squamous cell carcinoma or malignant melanoma. Each of these entities will be discussed in detail in the following section.

Vulvovaginal Disorders

For the elderly woman, vulvovaginal disorders are a significant source of both discomfort and functionally disabling symptoms. The vulva and vagina should be thought of as separate and unique structures owing to their separate embryologic origins. The vulva (including the labiae minor and major) is derived from the ectoderm and develops into keratinized, stratified squamous epithelium. In contrast, the vaginal mucosa develops from endodermal-derived epithelium and consists of nonkeratinized mucous membrane. The clinical significance of this difference is that the vulvar and vaginal tissues respond differently to a variety of stimuli, notably sex steroids.

Atrophic vaginitis is perhaps the most commonly recognized clinical disorder affecting the vagina. In the absence of estrogen, the vaginal epithelium becomes thin, making it highly susceptible to trauma and infection. Common symptoms include dryness, burning, pruritis, painful intercourse, urinary frequency and urgency, and bleeding. On examination, the atrophic vagina appears pale, thin, and dry and loses the wrinkled appearance of the vagina rugae produced by the underlying fibromuscular layer.[6] The vaginal canal may be narrowed. In severe cases, there may be a thin white discharge referred to as *leukorrhea.*

Vaginal candidiasis occurs uncommonly in the elderly woman who is not on estrogen replacement. It is seen most often in women using systemic or topical estrogen therapy or in those who are wearing a pessary or estrogen-containing ring.

Vaginal carcinoma is uncommon, accounting for about 1 percent of all gynecologic cancers, but it occurs at a mean age of 60 to 70 years. Vaginal bleeding and discharge are the most common presentations. Vaginal carcinoma is locally invasive, and on examination, the physician will find a thickened area that bleeds easily. Advanced vaginal carcinoma may involve the bladder or rectum.

Vulvar disorders typically present with irritative symptoms, such as itching or burning, bleeding, or the appearance of a concerning lesion. The majority of vulvar disorders affecting the elderly are not malignant. Psoriasis, eczema, and seborrhea frequently involve the vulva. Lichen sclerosus, a thin, whitened, crinkling epithelium encircling the vulva and the anus, presents a "keyhole" or "hourglass" configuration. Squamous cell carcinoma can arise within the background of lichen sclerosus. Squamous cell hyperplasia from chronic skin irritation is characterized by pink-red vulvar skin with overlying gray-white keratin. Suspicious lesions should be biopsied. Benign lesions are treated with a topical steroid, such as betamethasone 0.1% or 0.1% triamcinolone cream, applied twice daily for 10 to 14 days.

Vulvar candidiasis in the elderly woman is typically the result of constant moisture and skin breakdown that accompanies urinary or fecal incontinence. The rash usually has a bright, beefy red appearance and may be associated with vertical fissuring of the skin. Diagnosis can be confirmed by microscopic examination of scrapings from vulvar lesions mixed with a drop of saline. Pseudohyphae or blastospores can be identified under low-power magnification. Treatment is with an azole-based cream for 7 days, such as terconazole or miconazole, or oral therapy with fluconazole 150 mg as a single dose. Severe cases may require prolonged or repetitive therapy.

The vulva is an uncommon site for malignancy, but it typically occurs in the geriatric age group. A long history of pruritis and sometimes bleeding without pain is typical. On examination, the lesion may appear as a wartlike growth, ulceration, or mass. The majority of vulvar carcinomas (90 percent) are squamous cell carcinomas. Suspicious lesions should be referred to a gynecologist for biopsy.

Pelvic Mass

Geriatric women may present to the ED with complaints of abdominal distension and discomfort, frequently accompanied by anorexia, nausea, and alteration of bowel habits. These symptoms are always suspicious for malignancy, including ovarian and colorectal carcinoma. Ovarian cancer occurs with greatest frequency in women 50 to 80 years of age. The most common presentation of ovarian cancer is abdominal distension associated with vague abdominal complaints, including dyspepsia, early

satiety, nausea, and abdominal pain. Physical examination reveals abdominal distension with either ascites or a palpable abdominopelvic mass. Other examination findings that are suspicious for a pelvic malignancy include enlargement of the adnexa. Ovarian cancer may cause ascites with no distinct pelvic mass. Sometimes a large omental cake filled with tumor will be palpable. Most patients with ascites also will be found to have pleural effusions. Others may present with symptoms suggestive of cholecystitis or small bowel obstruction. Initial diagnostic studies should include a complete blood count (CBC), blood ureanitrogen and creatinine determinations, liver function tests, and a chest x-ray. Computed tomographic (CT) scan of the abdomen and pelvis may be preferable to a pelvic ultrasound because it may more reliably detect lymphadenopathy and omental and liver involvement, as well as evaluate other structures, including the small and large bowel. Large ovarian masses (>10 cm) often represent benign tumors such as mucinous or serous cystadenomas. However, malignancy cannot be excluded without surgical exploration. In general, pelvic masses should not be decompressed or drained because this can spread malignant disease. However, careful aspiration of ascites by paracentesis can relieve symptoms, as well as allow a cytologic diagnosis to be made.

Occasionally, the ovary may be involved as a site for metastatic cancer. Both breast and colon cancers are recognized to occasionally involve the ovaries. Other gastrointestinal malignancies, including pancreatic and gastric carcinoma, also may metastasize to the pelvis.

Pelvic masses often are discovered as incidental findings during the evaluation of the postmenopausal woman for unrelated problems. These typically are discovered by pelvic ultrasound or CT scan or may be discovered on routine examination. Most pelvic masses are benign in etiology (Table 33-2). Simple serous ovarian cysts (typically < 5 cm) commonly occur in elderly women, as do asymptomatic fibroids. These findings should prompt referral to a gynecologist as an outpatient to determine the need for further testing.

Pelvic Organ Prolapse

Pelvic organ prolapse encompasses a range or combination of anatomic defects including uterine prolapse, cystocele (prolapse of the anterior vaginal compartment), rectocele (prolapse of the posterior vaginal compartment), and enterocele (prolapse of the vaginal apex with herniation of the peritoneum through the fibromuscular wall of the vagina). Prolapse of the vaginal vault following hysterectomy is commonly referred to as *vaginal*

Table 33-2. Causes of Pelvic Masses in the Elderly Woman

Gynecologic
  Uterine fibroids
  Benign ovarian serous cysts
  Benign ovarian neoplasms (serous and mucinous
    adenomas, fibromas)
  Malignant ovarian neoplasms
  Hydrosalpinx
Urinary
  Distended bladder
  Pelvic kidney
  Transplanted kidney
Gastrointestinal
  Stool within colon
  Diverticulitis
  Rectosigmoid cancer
Other
  Metastatic carcinoma (breast, colon, pancreas,
    uterus)

Table 33-3. Presenting Symptoms of Pelvic Organ Prolapse

Vaginal bulge or mass
Pelvic pain or pressure
Vaginal bleeding
Incomplete voiding (frequency, urgency, nocturia, poor
  stream)
Urinary retention (with or without urosepsis)
Fecal impaction
Incarceration of prolapsed tissue (rare)

EMERGENCY DEPARTMENT CARE AND DISPOSITION

The primary goals of the emergency physician when evaluating and managing an elder patient with gynecologic complaints should be to identify the cause for the patient's complaints, to screen for malignancy, and to ease the patient's suffering. Many nonemergent problems can be treated and referred to a gynecologist for further evaluation and management as an outpatient.

Typically, vaginal bleeding that is present on examination in the ED is easily treated. Bleeding that occurs from an epithelial surface such as the vulva, vagina, and cervix should be compressed initially. Silver nitrate can be applied to persistent bleeding using the commercially available applicator sticks. Absorbable Gelfoam®, Avitene®, and Surgicel® also can be applied to mucosal surfaces. Bleeding from ulceration of the vaginal mucosa may require placement of absorbable sutures. Bleeding that persists despite these maneuvers should prompt consultation. Heavy or persistent bleeding that appears to be uterine in etiology may require dilatation and curettage (D&C) and should be managed in consultation with a gynecologist.

A history of vaginal bleeding that cannot be confirmed by examination should be presumed to be uterine in etiology. A urine specimen should be obtained to rule out hemorrhagic cystitis. A rectal examination should be done to exclude rectal bleeding. A Pap smear can be performed, or the patient can be referred for Pap smear. If uterine bleeding is suspected, the patient should be referred to follow-up with a gynecologist. The woman should be asked to wear a tampon to verify or exclude a vaginal, cervical, or uterine source for the bleeding.

Vulvar skin conditions should be identified and treated. Candidiasis should respond to a 7-day course of terconazole or treatment with another azole-based product. Vulvar pruritis and burning may be treated with a topical ste-

vault prolapse. Pelvic organ prolapse can be associated with a variety of symptoms, including an obvious bulge, pelvic pressure, genital bleeding, and urinary incontinence or retention.

On occasion, women with pelvic organ prolapse may present to the ED for evaluation of a variety of symptoms, either prior to or following treatment (Table 33-3). Patients or family members may be alarmed by the appearance of a large mass protruding from the vagina, fearing that it represents cancer or the extrusion of the bladder or bowel. Most patients with pelvic organ prolapse report pelvic pressure and low back pain. Significant prolapse of the anterior vaginal compartment or uterus can cause acute urinary retention secondary to obstruction of the bladder neck or urethra. Incomplete bladder emptying may predispose the woman to chronic cystitis and urosepsis. It is therefore reasonable to catheterize all patients who present with vaginal prolapse extending beyond the vaginal introitus in order to check for infection and rule out urinary retention. Significant vaginal bleeding can occur from ulceration of the vaginal mucosa. Fecal impaction or severe constipation can result from prolapse of the posterior vaginal compartment or rectal prolapse.

Therapy for pelvic organ prolapse also can result in presentation to the ED. The use of pessaries may cause obstruction to both defecation and urination. Removal of the pessary will alleviate the problem.

roid applied twice daily for 10 to 14 days. Skin breakdown from excessive moisture can be treated with a barrier ointment containing zinc oxide. Atrophic vaginitis typically is treated with topical estrogens, which may be given as either a cream (Premarin® or Estrace®) or as vaginal tablets (Vagifem®). A reasonable course of therapy is to apply a fingertip full of cream just inside the vagina 2 or 3 nights a week. The elderly woman should be reminded that breast tenderness is common during the first few weeks of therapy until the vaginal mucosa has begun to thicken. Women in whom estrogen therapy is contraindicated may use an over-the-counter vaginal lubricant such as Replens® on an as-needed basis.

Large pelvic masses or masses suspicious for pelvic malignancy should prompt immediate gynecologic consultation. Large lower abdominal or pelvic masses should be evaluated by CT scan. Isolated ovarian masses are best evaluated by ultrasound. Ultrasound characteristics that are of concern for malignancy in an elderly woman include size greater than 3 cm, complex-appearing cyst (solid or solid and cystic components), the presence of septations or papillations, and the presence of ascites. Small, asymptomatic, simple-appearing ovarian cysts that are incidental to the presenting problem can be referred for outpatient evaluation and management.

Pelvic organ prolapse rarely requires emergency care. Frequently the prolapse can be reduced by gentle pressure. Sometimes a lubricant can be used to assist this maneuver. If the prolapse cannot be reduced easily, a Foley catheter should be placed, followed by another attempt at manual reduction. If this measure is unsuccessful, consultation with a gynecologist is appropriate. Nonsurgical long-term therapy typically consists of the use of a rubber pessary to hold the vagina in place. Surgical therapy for pelvic organ prolapse is very successful as long as all the anatomic defects are addressed.

It is reasonable to perform urinary catheterization in any patient with prolapse beyond the vaginal opening in order to rule out urinary retention. If the bladder volume exceeds 500 mL, consideration should be given to prolonged bladder drainage and referral to a urogynecologist, gynecologist, or urologist.

Bleeding from an ulcerated prolapse usually can be controlled with pressure or a hemostatic agent. More significant bleeding may require the placement of absorbable sutures or a vaginal pack.

REFERENCES

1. Kennedy AW, Flagg JS, Webster KD: Gynecologic cancer in the very elderly. *Gynecol Oncol* 32:49, 1989.
2. American Cancer Society: *Cancer Facts and Figures—2000.* Atlanta, ACS, 2000.
3. Luber KM, Boero S, Choe Y: The demographics of pelvic floor disorders: Current observations and future projections. *Am J Obstet Gynecol* 184:1496, 2001.
4. Dewhurst J: Postemopausal bleeding from benign causes. *Clin Obstet Gynecol* 26:769, 1983.
5. Marrow CP, Curtin JP, Townsend DE: *Synopsis of Gynecologic Oncology,* 4th ed. New York, Chirchill-Livingstone, 1993.
6. Capewell AE, McIntryre MA, Elton RA: Postmenopausal atrophy in elderly women: Is a vaginal smear necessary for diagnosis? *Age Ageing* 21:117, 1993.

34

Urinary Tract Infection

Michelle Blanda

HIGH-YIELD FACTS

- Urinary tract infections (UTIs) are the most common infections in elders and their most common cause of bacteremia

- Patients in nursing homes have a 16 percent incidence of UTI.

- Elders are more susceptible to UTI because of increased urinary stasis, obstruction, and use of indwelling bladder catheters.

- Fecal bacteria ascend the urethra from the perineum to cause most UTIs.

- Elders can present with a wide range of vague symptoms when serious UTI is present, such as change in mental or functional status, nausea, vomiting, abdominal pain, and respiratory symptoms.

- A urine dipstick or urinalysis and, when either is positive, a urine culture should be obtained in most cases when investigating an elder patient for UTI.

- Short courses of antibiotics are not recommended in older patients, and complicated infections should be treated with intravenous antibiotics based on local infection and susceptibility factors.

- Do not treat asymptomatic bacteriuria, which is common in older patients.

- Since indwelling catheters are associated with UTI, avoid placing them in elder patients.

Geriatric patients are a heterogeneous group ranging from fully functional community-dwelling elders to impaired, noncommunicative, immobile nursing home residents. Urinary tract infections (UTIs) are the most common infections seen in the elderly regardless of whether the patient is a community dweller or is institutionalized. UTIs are also the most common cause of bacteremia in the elderly, followed by respiratory infections.[1-4]

The diagnosis of UTI is a challenge in older patients because the disease may manifest in an obscure manner. Patients in this age group tend to have multiple medical problems and can present with several subtle somatic complaints. Because UTI is so common, it may be present when another disease brings the geriatric patient to the emergency department (ED). Thus the physician may diagnose UTI prematurely in a patient who actually has a different source of infection or another underlying problem.

DEFINITIONS

A number of definitions are used to describe infections involving the urinary tract (Table 34-1). *Bacteriuria* means that bacteria are in the urine with or without infection. *Urinary tract infection* (UTI) is defined as bacteriuria with infection that is manifested clinically by the presence of symptoms.[5] Symptoms of UTI include urgency, dysuria, and frequent urination, as well as lower abdominal pain, fever, and malaise. *Pyuria* is the presence of white blood cells (usually 10 per high-power field) in the urine and is found commonly with bacteriuria.

Pyelonephritis is an infection involving the kidneys,

Table 34-1. Definitions of Common Terms

Bacteriuria: Bacteria in the urine (usually > 10^5 cfu/mL)

Pyuria: Presence of white cells in the urine (usually > 5 WBC/hpf)

Complicated UTI: UTI associated with anatomic, functional, or pharmacologic factors predisposing to persistent or recurrent infection or to treatment failure

Uncomplicated UTI: Symptomatic bacteriuria in a patient without anatomic, functional or pharmacologic risk factors

Lower UTI: Infection of the bladder

Upper UTI: Infection of the kidneys or ureter, or perihephric infection

Pyelonephritis: Infection of the kidneys

Recurrent infection: Infection with different organisms subsequent to an initial infection

Relapse: Infection with the same organism after an initial infection characterized by the symptoms of UTI as well as flank pain and costovertebral angle tenderness. Pyelonephritis usually is an infection that has ascended from the bladder. Pyelonephritis can be a sequelae of a partially treated or untreated UTI. Recurrent UTI can be distinguished from relapse because the same organism causes a subsequent UTI relapse.

EPIDEMIOLOGY

Prevalence

In the general population, the incidence of UTIs in women is estimated to be about 10 times greater than that in men.[6] This disparity is less with age. The incidence of UTIs in elderly men closely matches that in elderly women. The prevalence of UTI is correlated with functional status, with the lowest prevalence among fully functional patients who live at home and the highest prevalence among patients who require care in long-term facilities.[7] For women who live in the community, the prevalence of bacteriuria at 70 years of age is 5 to 10 percent and increases to approximately 20 percent at 80 years of age.[6,8] In the same population of men aged 60 to 65 years, 1 to 3 percent have bacteriuria. Prevalence increases to over 10 percent for men older than 80 years of age.[9,10] In the institutionalized nonambulatory population, the incidence of bacteriuria exceeds 20 percent for both genders.[9] A 16 percent incidence of UTI was reported in a study of 13 nursing homes involving almost 2,000 patients.[11] The higher prevalence relates to the more debilitated patients.

Cost, Morbidity, and Mortality

UTIs remain a significant health care expense in all age groups.[12,13] It is estimated that the cost of treating U.S. women with UTIs in 1 year is approximately $1.6 billion.[13] UTIs are also the leading cause of gram-negative bacteremia.[14] However, compared with bacteremia from other sources, UTIs have the lowest mortality, 10 to 30 percent.[15–17] It is interesting to note that if other risks are controlled, advanced age does not significantly increase the risk of mortality from a UTI complicated by bacteremia. In one study, for patients aged 18 to 64 years, mortality was 15.2 percent; it was 14.8 percent in those aged 65 to 79 years and 20 percent in those aged 80 years and older.[18]

The frequency of concomitant chronic illness, decreased physiologic reserve, and impaired immune response in this age group may increase morbidity and mortality.[19] However, multiple studies have found that there is no increased incidence of death with asymptomatic bacteriuria or uncomplicated UTI among elders.[9,20–22] Characteristics associated with a higher mortality from bacteremic UTIs include male gender, concomitant illness, hospital acquisition of infection, gram-positive bacterial infection, and chronic presence of an indwelling bladder catheter.[9,18,23]

Risk Factors

Certain risk factors unique to the elderly population make them more susceptible to UTIs (Table 34-2). These contributing factors vary in importance among the diverse geriatric population. Stasis of urine flow contributes to attachment, colonization, and multiplication of pathogens in the genitourinary tract. Inflamation caused by immune response to pathogens can further compromise bladder and renal function. Therefore, obstruction to urine flow at any level of the urinary tract leads to stasis and contributes to UTI.

Increased residual volume both maintains and predisposes to bladder infection by providing a pool of stagnant urine that is suitable for bacterial growth. Structural genitourinary abnormalities, such as cystoceles, ureteroceles, and bladder diverticula, also lead to residual stagnant pools of urine and are risk factors for UTI among both elderly men and women, many of whom are fully functional. For community-dwelling men, prostatic hypertrophy with obstruction and bacterial prostatitis may contribute to development of UTI.[9,24]

The loss of estrogen is a more significant contributing factor for community-dwelling elderly women. When present, estrogen stimulates the proliferation of *Lactobacillus* in the vaginal epithelium. *Lactobacillus* reduces the pH of the genitourinary tract and interferes with col-

Table 34-2. Risk Factors for Urinary Tract Infections in the Elderly

Immobilization
Less frequent urination
Incomplete bladder emptying
Prostate disease (men)
Neuropathic diseases
Immune response deterioration
Renal, bladder, or prostatic calculi
Genitourinary procedures
Bladder catheterization

onization by preventing *Escherichia coli* attachment to the epithelium.[25] Some *Lactobacillus* strains produce hydrogen peroxide, which also contributes to lower bacteria counts.[26] Loss of estrogen results in the loss of normal protective lactobacilli, an elevated pH, and a uropathogen-dominant vaginal flora. The absence of estrogen also decreases the strength of the vaginal muscles. This results in laxity of the ligaments holding the uterus, pelvic floor, and bladder and impairs bladder emptying of a residual stagnant pool of urine.[27,28]

In the institutionalized elderly population, the risk factors for UTI include immobilization, functional impairment, prior antibiotic use, and bladder catheterization. Neurologic problems leading to decreased functional status, such as Alzheimer's disease, Parkinson's disease, and cerebrovascular accidents, are common among nursing home patients. Many of these patients have bacteriuria and a higher risk of UTI because their diseases can impair voiding, increase residual urine volumes, and cause vesicoureteral reflux.[9]

Other factors that affect the rate of UTI in all elderly patients are chronic illness and medications. Any chronic illness can contribute to bacteriuria. For example, diabetic women have three times the prevalence of bacteriuria as compared with women of the same age without diabetes.[9,29] This is so because glucose in the urine provides a better environment for bacterial growth. Alpha-adrenergic medications such as phenylpropanolamine and pseudoephedrine, common in over-the-counter medications, may cause an increase in urethral resistance and impair bladder emptying.[25] Antibiotics may change protective vaginal flora and select more exotic fecal pathogens that eventually cause UTI.

PATHOPHYSIOLOGY

Most UTIs follow an invasion of the urinary tract by fecal bacteria that colonize the perineum and then ascend the urethra. The virulence of the bacteria, the extent of colonization of the periurethral area, the inoculum size, and the inadequacy of host defenses determine if successful invasion of the urinary tract will occur.[29,30] UTI by the hematogenous route is uncommon in the elderly but is suggested by gram-positive organisms such as *Staphylococcus aureas* and *Streptococcus viridans*, as well as other pathogens, *Candida,* and tuberculosis.

In the older patient, a volume of fluid constantly present in a bladder with a compromised mucosa promotes bacterial growth. Diabetes may cause an autonomic neuropathy with urinary retention. The hyperglycemia also may produce an osmotic diuresis and ureterovesicular reflux and cause ascending UTIs. In addition, hyperglycemia causes a decrease in phagocytosis. Neurovascular disease with a decreased mental status can result in urinary retention and increased in perineal soiling. For women, the vaginal reservoir is also a additional source of uropathogens, but this is less important than fecal flora.

Urine naturally possesses characteristics that effectively diminish the survival of organisms in the urinary tract. Most organisms that normally colonize the urethra do not multiply in urine and are rarely responsible for UTI. For all ages except the neonate, *E. coli* is the most common cause of UTI.[31] In the oldest nursing home patients, however, *E. coli* causes only 40 to 60 percent of cases, as compared with 80 to 90 percent of cases for community-dwelling elderly wormen.[18] Rather, agents such as *Proteus, Klebsiella, Enterobacter, Serratia, Pseudomonas,* and *Enterococcus* become more common in older nursing home patients (Table 34-3). Both men and any patient with a chronic urinary catheter have higher proportions of UTI caused by non–*E. coli* gram-negative rods and gram-positive organisms.[18,24] *Enterococcus* is a particular concern for obstructed or instrumented men.[15,32] In addition, bacteriuria with multiple organisms is more common in the elderly than among younger patients.[33]

Prostate disease decreases bacterostatic and bactericidal secretions. For men it is felt that urinary tract pathogens may be prone to ascending the genitourinary tract because of decreased Tamm-Horsfall proteins, prostatic secretions that prevent bacteria from adhering to ureteral epithelial cells.

Traditionally, culture is considered "positive" with the growth of 100,000 colony-forming units (cfus) of one or more organisms from 1 mL of urine. However, lower counts may be significant in the presence of symptoms.[19] Recent studies suggest that counts as low as 100 cfu/mL

Table 34-3. Top Eight Organisms Causing Bacteremic UTI (in Order of Frequency)

E. coli
*S. aureus**
Klebsiella
Proteus
*Enterococcus**
Pseudomonas
Enterobacter
Citrobacter

*Gram-positive organisms.

may be significant if the organism is a uropathogen, the specimen is obtained by fresh catheterization, or the patient manifests pyuria and symptoms.[19] Hydration, urinary frequency, ureteral obstruction, or antibiotic therapy may influence the number of organisms that grow from a sample of urine.[3]

CLINICAL FEATURES

The elderly can present with symptoms of UTI that are very different from those of younger adults. Classically, lower tract symptoms include frequency, urgency, and dysuria; upper tract symptoms include fever, chills, flank pain, and tenderness. In the geriatric population, these classic symptoms may be altered or absent. Patients may lack fever and can be hypothermic.[11] Elderly patients with UTI can present with mental status deterioration, nausea, vomiting, abdominal pain, or respiratory distress.[2,19,27] Community-dwelling adults older than age 50 with bacteremia and UTI presented most commonly with confusion, cough, and dyspnea. New urinary symptoms were the chief complaint in only 20 percent of patients.[2] Acute pyelonephritis in the elderly typically presents as a septic syndrome with fever, tachycardia, and altered mental status.[27] In males, high fever, chills, perineal and back pain, dysuria, and urgency with frequency mark acute bacterial prostatitis. Chronic bacterial prostatitis is frequently asymptomatic and is the most common cause of relapsing UTI in men. Due to the wide range and often vague presenting symptoms, the misdiagnosis of UTI occurs in approximately 20 to 40 percent of patients, especially when patients present with nonurinary complaints.[19,34]

It may be clinically impossible to be certain that a fever is caused by an invasive UTI in the elderly patient who lacks urinary symptoms. Since UTIs are common, this source always should be considered when evaluating a febrile elderly patient. However, the majority of febrile episodes in the bacteriuric, noncatheterized elderly are unlikely to be caused by an invasive UTI.[9,14,35] Thus other sources must be sought as well.

Foul-smelling urine sometimes is considered a symptom in the elderly adult, especially in the institutionalized patient. Bacteria in the urine produce polyamines, which account for the odor. Management of incontinence and improved hygiene, especially in the institutionalized patient, usually solve this problem. Without other symptoms, foul-smelling urine from bacteria should not be treated as a UTI.[9]

EMERGENCY DEPARTMENT CARE AND DISPOSITION

It is always important to sample the urine for analysis in almost all older patients who are acutely ill because it may be the source of an infection causing the presentation. For both sexes, urine collection in a sterile container during normal voiding, after cleaning the periurethral region with water, is a reliable method for obtaining a sample.[36] Midstream clean-catch and catheterization methods of urine collection have a high concordance for findings of bacteria and positive tests for nitrites and leukocyte esterase, microscopic bacteriuria, and pyuria.[37] This approach will decrease the amount of unnecessary catheterizations undertaken in the elderly. Mixed flora found in midstream clean-catch urine samples suggest contamination. A repeat specimen by catheterization should be obtained if treatment is considered.[25]

Pyuria is the hallmark of inflammation and is easily and reliably detected by the leukocyte esterase dipstick test or by finding more than 10 white blood cells (WBCs) per high-power field (hpf) in the urinary sediment.[38] In asymptomatic men, pyuria (>10 WBCs/hpf) is 68 percent sensitive and 99 percent specific with a positive predictive value (PPV) of 88 percent, a negative predictive value (NPV) of 97 percent, and an efficiency of 94 percent for predicting bacteriuria.[41] In asymptomatic women, however, 61 percent of those with pyuria do not have bacteriuria. The PPV of pyuria in asymptomatic women is 39 percent, although the NPV remains at 95 percent.[42] In elderly women, pyuria and bacteriuria may represent a chronic situation with spontaneous resolution and frequent recurrences.[43] Although no studies have evaluated the predictive value of pyuria, leukocyte esterase, nitrites, or microscopic bacteriuria in febrile (i.e., symptomatic) elderly patients, the increased prevalence of bacteriuria in this population suggests a better PPV. Most patients with an infection will have more than 100 leukocytes per high-power field. If the clinical suspicion of UTI is high, a leukocyte esterase dipstick test may be helpful because it should have a high sensitivity. However, the sensitivity of the test is low when the clinical suspicion of UTI is low. These findings are also true of the dipstick test for nitrites.[39,40]

Microscopic and sometimes gross hematuria may be encountered in acute infection, but proteinuria is unusual. Gross hematuria is seldom directly attributable to hemorrhagic cystitis despite a high prevalence of bacteriuria in institutionalized patients with gross hematuria.[9,44] Alternate causes for gross hematuria, such as indwelling catheters, malignancy, ureterolithiasis, urinary retention, and bladder diverticula, should be considered.

A positive urine culture has a low specificity for the diagnosis of symptomatic UTI. Due to the high prevalence of bacteriuria in the elderly, a positive culture does not necessarily indicate an infection.[9] However, a negative culture is helpful to exclude an infection. Patients with symptoms of UTI (i.e., dysuria, urgency, increased frequency, incontinence, or gross hematuria) should have urine cultures sent if pyuria (>5–10 WBCs/hpf), leukocyte esterase, or nitrites are present or if organisms are noted on microscopic examination.[41] Pretreatment cultures are recommended in the elderly because the microbiology can vary, UTI may recur, and sepsis may develop. Culture results often aid subsequent treatment.

Other laboratory tests, such as a WBC count, may be elevated in elders with UTI. In one study, the rate of elevated WBC count was 70 percent[18] among community-dwelling elders with UTI. Older patients were as likely to have an elevated WBC count and temperature as younger patients on admission. However, a debilitated nursing home patient or a patient in an immunocompromised state may prevent elevation of the WBC count. Five factors (clinical and laboratory) have been associated with bacteremia. These include fever, elevated serum creatinine level, elevated WBC count, presence of diabetes mellitus, and low serum albumin level.[45]

Some clinicians believe that all elderly persons should undergo diagnostic testing for obstruction and anatomic problems. Most recommend that only patients at high risk be investigated, including those with recurrent or relapsing UTIs. Obstruction, if left untreated, can lead to renal parenchymal destruction, septic shock, and death. Obstruction should be suspected in a patient with persistent bacteremia, bacteriuria, and fever lasting more than 4 to 5 days.[3]

Symptomatic UTI should be treated regardless of age. However, strategies differ in the healthy community-dwelling elder as compared with the frail institutionalized patient. Susceptibility of the infecting organism, patient tolerance, severity of the illness, and cost will determine antimicrobial treatment. With institutionalized elderly patients, the emergency physician should know local patterns of infecting organisms and antimicrobial resistance, which should direct antimicrobial choices.[9]

While short-course antibiotic therapy is recommended in uncomplicated UTIs in young patients, it is less likely to be successful in the elderly patient and is not recommended for older men. Elderly women are less likely than younger women to be cured by any duration of therapy. Relapse and recurrence are most common in elderly institutionalized females.[9,46]

There are many options for treatment (Table 34-4). In the institutionalized patient, narrow-spectrum antibiotics

Table 34-4. Treatment Options

	Primary	**Days***	**Secondary**	**Days***
Acute	Trimethoprin-sulfamethoxazole	3	Doxycycline	3
uncomplicated	1 tab bid	3	Amoxicillin-clavulanate	3
UTI	FQ (ciproflox/norflox/oflox/levoflox)			
Acute pyelonephritis				
Outpatient	FQ (PO)	14	Amoxicillin-clavulanate	14
Inpatient	FQ (IV)	14	Ampicillin-sulbactam	14
	Ampicithin-gentamycin (IV)	14	Ticarcillin-clavulanate	14
	Cefotaxime (IV)	14		
Acute bacterial	FQ	14	Ampicillin-sulbactam (IV)	14
prostatitis	TMP-SMX	14†	P ceph 3 (IV)	14
			Ticarcillin-clavulanate (IV)	14
			Piperacillin-tazobactam (IV)	14
Chronic bacterial	FQ	28	TMP-SMX	30–90
Prostatitis				

*Days of therapy refers to *total* duration of therapy.
†May require 3 to 4 weeks of therapy.

should be avoided because many infections arise from organisms other than *E. coli*. For females, one option is a 3-day treatment and then retreatment if there is early recurrence (<4 weeks). However, a 7-day treatment is "also commonly suggested". Women who present with evidence of a more invasive infection such as pyelonephritis should be treated for at least 14 days. A 14-day treatment is appropriate for men as well, unless they present with recurrent symptomatic UTI. In this case, they need between 6 and 12 weeks of therapy.

ADDITIONAL CONSIDERATIONS

Asymptomatic Bacteriuria

Multiple studies have found asymptomatic bacteriuria to be benign and treatment to be unnecessary.[9,34,48,49] There are several reasons for this. First, symptomatic disease rarely develops in patients with asymptomatic bacteriuria.[48] The recurrence rate for asymptomatic bacteriuria after therapy is high in the elderly. There is no proof that keep-free intervals are maintained. Last, the adverse reaction rate to antimicrobial agents in this population is high. No morbidity is associated with asymptomatic bacteriuria.[48]

An exception to withholding treatment in asymptomatic bacteriuria, for both institutionalized and noninstitutionalized patients, is when patients are to undergo an invasive genitourinary procedure. In the presence of infected urine, procedures with mucosal trauma are likely to cause postprocedure bacteremia and, in some instances, death from septic shock.[9]

Urinary Incontinence

Urinary incontinence (involuntary loss of urine) in the presence of bacteriuria is used occasionally as an indication to treat with antibiotics.[50] The presumption is that the incontinence will improve with eradication of the bacteriuria. However, in the elderly, incontinence and bacteriuria can be unrelated. Incontinence should not be used as an indication to treat otherwise asymptomatic bacteriuria.[48] Chronic incontinence has not been shown to result from UTIs, even though many incontinent patients have bacteriuria.[27]

Indwelling Catheters

There are many reasons for urethral catheterization in elderly patients. These include surgery, urine output mea-

Table 34-5. Independent Risk Factors for Catheter-Associated Bacteriuria

Duration of catheterization
Absence of urimeter use
Colonization of drainage bag
Diabetes mellitus
Absence of antibiotic use
Female
Catheterization not for surgery
Abnormal serum creatinine
Errors in catheter care

surement, urinary retention, and urinary incontinence. Approximately 5 percent of the institutionalized elderly population has a chronic indwelling urinary catheter. The incidence of bacteriuria in this population is about 3 to 10 percent for each day of catheterization, the same magnitude as that found in hospitals.[51] Therefore, by the end of a 30-day catheterization, most patients will have bacteriuria.[51]

Bladder urine is not always reflected by urine obtained through the catheter.[52] Catheter urine has organisms that may not be present in the bladder, and this has been proven by comparing catheter specimens with suprapubic aspirate.[51] Urine specimens should be obtained from the catheter using a needle and syringe without opening the catheter–collection tube junction.

Table 34-5 outlines risk factors for catheter-associated bacteriuria.[11,27] Complications associated with short-term catheter use include symptomatic UTIs, trauma, urethritis, bacteriuria, pyelonephritis, and bacteremia. Patients may remain at risk for bacteriuria for at least 24 hours after catheter removal. Long-term catheterization is associated with catheter obstruction, nephrolithiasis, chronic renal inflammation, renal failure, and bladder cancer. Complications specific to men include urethritis, urethral fistulas, prostatitis, epididymitis, and scrotal abscess.

Many treatments have been suggested for bacteriuria associated with catheters, but discontinuing the catheter is the only effective method of eradicating the bacteriuria. Intermittent catheterization has shown a much lower infection rate than chronic indwelling catheterization.[53] Other catheterization options for prevention of bacteriuria are the use of condom catheters or suprapubic catheterization.

CONCLUSION

In our society, the proportion of elderly individuals is immense and will grow over the next few decades. UTIs will continue to be a major problem for the elderly, accounting for many emergency visits. The emergency physician needs to understand the signs and symptoms associated with UTIs in the elderly and how they differ from those in the younger population. Physicians also need to be able to interpret a urinalysis with respect to these symptoms. This is especially true when there is an indwelling catheter. Asymptomatic bacteriuria is common in the elderly, occurring more often in women and in the functionally impaired. To provide the best care for these patients, diagnostic and treatment options need to be tailored to the individual patient circumstance.

REFERENCES

1. Assantachai P, Gherunpong V, Suwanagool S: Urinary tract infection in the elderly: A clinical study. *J Med Assoc Thai* 80(12):753, 1997.
2. Barkham TMS, Martin FC, Eykyn SJ: Delay in the diagnosis of bacteraemic urinary tract infection in elderly patients. *Age Ageing* 25:130, 1996.
3. Gleckman RA: Urinary tract infection. *Clin Geriatr Med* 8:793, 1992.
4. Assantachai P, Ratanasuwan W, Suwunnagools S, et al: Septicemia in the elderly. *Siriraj Hosp Gaz* 46:10, 1994.
5. Howes DS: Urinary tract infections, in Tintinalli JE, Kelen GD, Stapczynski JS (eds): *Emergency Medicine: A Comprehensive Study Guide,* 5th ed. New York, McGraw-Hill, 1999.
6. Harwood-Nuss AL, Etheredge W, McKenna I: Urologic emergencies, in Rosen P, Barkin R (eds): *Emergency Medicine: Concepts and Clinical Practice,* 4th ed. St Louis, Mosby, 1998.
7. Matsumoto T, Kumazawa J: Urinary tract infection in geriatric patients. *Int J Antimicrob Agents* 11:269, 1999.
8. Boscia JA, Kobasa WD, Knight RA, et al: Therapy vs no therapy for bacteriuria in elderly ambulatory nonhospitalized women. *JAMA* 257(8):1067, 1987.
9. Nicolle LE: Urinary tract infection in the elderly. *J Antimicrob Chemother* 33(suppl A):99, 1994.
10. Nordenstam G, Sundh V, Lincoln K, et al: Bacteriuria in representative samples of persons aged 72–79 years. *Am J Epidemiol* 130:1176, 1989.
11. Barnett BJ, Stephens DS: Urinary tract infection: An overview. *Am J Med Sci* 314(4):245, 1997.
12. Orenstein R, Wong ES: Urinary tract infections in adults. *Am Fam Phys* 59(5):1225, 1999.
13. Foxman B, Barlow R, D'Arcy H, et al: Urinary tract infection: Self-reported incidence and associated costs. *Ann Epidemiol* 10:509, 2000.
14. Nicolle LE, McIntyre M, Zacharias H, et al: Twelve-month surveillance of infections in institutionalized elderly men. *J Am Geriatr Soc* 32:513, 1984.
15. Richardson JP: Bacteremia in the elderly. *J Gen Intern Med* 8:89, 1993.
16. Muder RR, Brennen CR, Wagener MM, et al: Bacteriuria in a long-term care facility: A five-year prospective study of 173 consecutive episodes. *Clin Infect Dis* 14:647, 1992.
17. Baldassarre JS, Kaye D: Special problems of urinary tract infection in the elderly. *Med Clin North Am* 75:375, 1991.
18. Ackermann RJ, Monroe PW: Bacteremic urinary tract infection in older people. *J Am Geriatr Soc* 44(8):927, 1996.
19. Nickel JC, Pidutti R: A rational approach to urinary tract infections in older patients. *Geriatrics* 47(10):49, 1992.
20. Nicolle LE, Henderson E, Bjornson J, et al: The association of bacteriuria with resident characteristics and survival in elderly institutionalized men. *Ann Intern Med* 106:682, 1987.
21. Heinamaki P, Haavisto M, Hakuline NT, et al: Mortality in relation to urinary characteristics in the very aged. *Gerontology* 32:165, 1986.
22. Nordenstam GR, Brandberg CA, Oden AS, et al: Bacteriuria and mortality in an elderly population. *New Engl J Med* 314:1152, 1986.
23. Ismail NH, Lieu PK, Lien CT, et al: Bacteraemia in the elderly. *Ann Acad Med Singapore* 26:593, 1997.
24. Wolfson SA, Kalmanson GM, Rubini ME, et al: Epidemiology of bacteriuria in a predominantly geriatric male population. *Am J Med Sci* 89:168, 1965.
25. Nygaard IE, Johnson JM: Urinary tract infections in elderly women. *Am Fam Phys* 53(1):175, 1996.
26. Klebanoff SJ, Hillier SL, Eschenbach DA, et al: Control of the microbial flora of the vagina by H_2O_2-generating lactobacilli. *J Infect Dis* 164:94, 1991.
27. Raz P: Urinary tract infection in elderly women. *Int J Antimicrob Agents* 10:177, 1998.
28. Cardozo L, Benness C, Abbott D: Low dose oestrogen prophylaxis for recurrent urinary tract infections in elderly women. *Br J Obstet Gynaecol* 105:403, 1998.
29. Sobel JD: Pathogenesis of urinary tract infection: Role of host defenses. *Infect Dis Clin North Am* 11(3):531, 1997.
30. Warren JW: Catheter-associated urinary tract infections. *Infect Dis Clin North Am* 11(3):609, 1997.
31. Aguirre-Avalos G, Zavala-Silva ML, Diaz-Nava A, et al: Asymptomatic bacteriuria and inflammatory response to urinary tract infection of elderly ambulatory women in nursing homes. *Arch Med Res* 30(1): 29-32 1999.
32. Warren JW: Guidelines for protecting the patient undergoing long-term urinary catheterization. *Nurs Home Med* 3:95, 1995.
33. Nicolle LE, Mayhew WJ, Bryan L: Prospective randomized comparison of therapy and no therapy for asymptomatic

bacteriuria in institutionalized elderly women. *Am J Med* 83:27, 1987.

34. Gleckman R, Blagg N, Hibert D, et al: Acute pyelonephritis in the elderly. *South Med J* 75:551, 1982.

35. Nicolle LE: Urinary tract infection in long-term care facility residents. *Clin Infect Dis* 31(3):757, 2000.

36. Michielsen WJS, Geurs FJC, Verschraegen GLC, et al: A simple and efficient urine sampling method for bacteriological examination in elderly women. *Age Ageing* 26:493, 1997.

37. Walter FG, Knopp RK: Urine sampling in ambulatory women: Midstream clean-catch versus catheterization. *Ann Emerg Med* 18:166, 1989.

38. Boscia JA, Abrutyn E, Levison ME, et al: Pyuria and asymptomatic bacteriuria in elderly ambulatory women. *Ann Intern Med* 110:404, 1989.

39. Kunin CM: Urinary tract infection in females. *Clin Infect Dis* 18:1, 1994.

40. Lachs MS, Nachamkin I, Edelstein PH, et al: Spectrum bias in the evaluation of diagnostic tests: Lessons from the rapid dipstick test for urinary tract infection. *Ann Intern Med* 117:135, 1992.

41. Norman DC, Yamamura R, Yoshikawa TT: Pyuria: Its predictive value of asymptomatic bacteriuria in ambulatory elderly men. *J Urol* 135:520, 1986.

42. Boscia JP, Abrutyn E, Levison ME, et al: Pyuria and asymptomatic bacteriuria in elderly ambulatory women. *Ann Intern Med* 110:404, 1986.

43. Monane M. Gurwitz JH, Lipsitz LA, et al: Epidemiologic and diagnostic aspects of bacteriuria: A longitudinal study in older women. *J Am Geriatr Soc* 43:618, 1995.

44. Nicolle LE, Orr P, Duckworth H, et al: Gross hematuria in residents of long term care facilities. *Am J Med* 94:611, 1993.

45. Leibovici L, Greenshtain S, Cohen O, et al: Toward improved empirical management of moderate to severe urinary tract infections. *Arch Intern Med* 152:2481, 1992.

46. Ikaheimo R, Siitonen A, Heiskanen T, et al: Recurrence of urinary tract infection in a primary care setting: Analysis of a 1-year follow-up of 179 women. *Clin Infect Dis* 22:91, 1996.

47. Stapleton A, Stamm WE: Prevention of urinary tract infection. *Infect Dis Clin North Am* 11(3):719, 1997.

48. Abrutyn E, Boscia JA, Kaye D: The treatment of asymptomatic bacteriuria in the elderly. *J Am Geriatr Soc* 36(5):473, 1988.

49. Boscia JA, Kobasa WD, Knight RA, et al: Epidemiology of bacteriuria in an elderly ambulatory population. *Am J Med* 80:208, 1986.

50. Bjornsdottir LT, Geirsson RT, Jonsson PV: Urinary incontinence and urinary tract infections in octogenarian women. *Acta Obstet Gynaecol Scand* 77:105, 1998.

51. Warren JW: The catheter and urinary tract infection. *Med Clin North Am* 75(2):481, 1991.

52. Nicolle LE, Muir P, Harding GKM, et al: Localization of urinary tract infection in elderly, institutionalized women with asymptomatic bacteriuria. *J Infect Dis* 157(1):65, 1988.

53. Lieu PK, Heng LC, Ding YY, et al: Carer-assisted intermittent urethral catheterisation in the management of persistent retention of urine in elderly women. *Ann Acad Med Singapore* 25:562, 1996.

35

Abdominal Aortic Aneurysm

Robert L. Rogers
Amal Mattu

HIGH-YIELD FACTS

- Patients with ruptured abdominal aortic aneurysm (AAA) may be hemodynamically stable initially and present with subtle findings such as back or flank pain.

- Although AAA is more common with advancing age and in white males, older women also are at risk for this disease.

- The classic triad of hypotension, abdominal or back pain, and pulsatile abdominal mass is seen in less than half of patients.

- Emergent bedside ultrasound and computed tomographic (CT) scanning are useful for confirming the diagnosis of AAA. Choice of radiographic imaging depends on the clinical presentation and stability of the patient.

One of the most feared clinical entities in emergency medicine practice is the ruptured abdominal aortic aneurysm (AAA). Patients with this vascular emergency may be hemodynamically stable initially and present with subtle findings, such as new-onset back pain, or with catastrophic intraperitoneal rupture and cardiovascular collapse. Emergency physicians should have a high index of suspicion for AAA in all patients older than age 50 who present with abdominal, back, or flank pain. The elderly patient population is at especially high risk for this catastrophic condition because as many as 4 to 8 percent of patients older than age 65 harbor an AAA.[1] As the population ages, emergency physicians can expect to encounter ruptured AAAs more frequently. Mortality rates for ruptured AAA may exceed 70 percent even when a diagnosis is made,[2,3] and the mortality increases further with delays in the diagnosis. This highlights the importance of expeditious diagnosis and treatment of ruptured AAA. Emergency physicians are in a unique position to make a rapid diagnosis in patients with both subtle and obvious presentations, perform resuscitative measures in the emergency department (ED), and rapidly involve surgeons in the care of the patient. An appreciation of the obvious and subtle presentations, as well as skill in rapid management, is critical to minimize mortality rates associated with this condition.

EPIDEMIOLOGY

AAAs tend to form in the sixth and seventh decades of life. They occur 4 to 7 times more commonly in males than in females, and they result in death 10 times more often in males. In addition, white males are affected substantially more often than black males. It is estimated that 4 to 8 percent of male patients over age 65 harbor an AAA. Women develop AAAs at an average of 10 years later than males. The average age overall at the time of diagnosis is 65 to 70 years.[8]

The risk of rupture is related to the size of the AAA; the larger aneurysms are at much higher risk of rupture. It should be emphasized, however, that smaller aneurysms can and do rupture. The yearly risk of rupture of AAAs that are less than 4 cm in diameter is 0.5 to 1.0 percent. This risk increases to 5 to 20 percent for aneurysm 4 to 5 cm in diameter. AAAs greater than 10 cm have a greater than 60 percent chance of rupture. Aneurysms typically expand at a rate of 3 to 5 mm per year, but individual variation exists. Factors that increase the risk of rupture include hypertension, tobacco use, and peripheral vascular disease.[10]

Ruptured AAA is associated with significant morbidity and mortality. Currently, rupture of an AAA is the thirteenth leading cause of death in the United States, causing 10,000 to 15,000 deaths annually. It is estimated that over 40 to 50 percent of patients with a ruptured AAA die before they reach the hospital. The average rate of mortality for a ruptured AAA is close to 80 to 90 percent. Morbidity rates are also high and relate to perioperative complications such as myocardial infarction and renal failure.[9,11]

PATHOPHYSIOLOGY

The descending thoracic aorta pierces the diaphragm at the twelfth thoracic vertebra and becomes the abdominal aorta. The abdominal aorta gives off many branches, including the celiac trunk, superior and inferior mesenteric arteries, renal arteries, and the greater radicular artery (artery of Adamkiewicz). The aorta is a retroperitoneal structure that bifurcates into the right and left common iliac arteries at the level of the umbilicus. Because the abdominal aorta lies in such close proximity to other structures, such as the ureters, spine, and nerves, patients may present with symptoms of urologic disease, back pain, and radiculopathy, respectively.

The aorta is composed of three layers: intima, media, and adventitia. Most authorities consider an aortic diameter greater than 3 cm or greater than 1.5 times the normal adjacent aorta to define an aneurysm.[4,7] Atherosclerosis formerly was thought to play a major role in aneurysm formation.[6] More recent evidence, however, suggests that aneurysm formation and rupture are controlled by a complex interaction of connective tissue constituents with degradative enzymes known as *metalloproteinases*. Metalloproteinase activity within the aortic media leads to weakening of the aorta and aneurysm formation.[5]

Several important risk factors have been found to be associated with AAA (Table 35-1). Among the most important risk factors are family history of AAA, male sex, advanced age, and presence of a connective tissue disease.[12,13] Other important associated factors include tobacco use, hypertension, and peripheral vascular disease.

Table 35-1. Risk Factors for AAA

First-degree relative with a AAA
Male sex
Age older than 60 years
Connective tissue disease
Tobacco smoking
Hypertension
Peripheral vascular disease

CLINICAL FEATURES

History

Unruptured Aneurysms

A large number of patients with an unruptured AAA present for medical evaluation because of symptoms that are attributable to the AAA. These are referred to as *symptomatic unruptured AAAs*. Patients also may have asymptomatic aneurysms detected during evaluation of an unrelated condition. When emergency physicians encounter these patients, they should use the opportunity to consult surgeons in order to prevent aneurysm rupture and its devastating consequences.

Symptomatic unruptured AAAs often present with symptoms that are similar to those of ruptured AAAs. These symptoms include abdominal "fullness," the sensation of abdominal pulsations, severe abdominal pain, and back or flank pain.[14] Ruptured or unruptured AAAs may produce symptoms that mimic those of renal colic. One proposed mechanism for this is that aneurysm rupture or expansion causes irritation of a ureter (usually the left ureter), producing pain down the length of the ureter from the flank to the lower abdomen or groin. Renal colic is the most frequent misdiagnosis of AAAs.

Ruptured Aneurysms

Approximately 40 percent of patients with AAAs present for the first time with rupture.[15] Classic teaching is that most patients will present with the triad of hypotension, abdominal or back pain, and a pulsatile abdominal mass. It is estimated that only 30 to 50 percent of patients will have this classic triad.[16] More often than not, patients will present with unexplained abdominal, back, or flank pain. Near-syncope or syncope also may be the sole manifestation of rupture. Physicians should consider the diagnosis of AAA in any patient over age 50 with abdominal pain, back pain, or syncope.

Free intraperitoneal rupture is rapidly fatal, and more than 50 percent of patients with this type of rupture die before they reach the hospital. Fortunately, retroperitoneal rupture is more common, occurring in 80 percent of cases, and often results in temporary tamponade of the bleeding within the confined retroperitoneal space. These patients frequently develop transient episodes of hypotension with light-headedness or syncope. However, patients often are able to compensate for this limited blood loss and temporarily may regain normal blood pressure before eventual hemodynamic collapse. More than two-thirds of patients will be normotensive initially at the time of presentation.[17] Unfortunately, the transient normal blood pressure may mislead the unwary physician into doubting the presence of this vascular catastrophe. Acute retroperitoneal AAA rupture should be suspected in any elderly patient who presents with acute onset of back or flank pain associated with light-headedness or syncope.

Physical Examination

The physical examination of patients with an AAA is fraught with difficulties. The classically reported examination findings include hypotension in the presence of a palpable abdominal mass. The examination may be misleading and lead to both false-positive and false-negative findings. Failure to detect an aneurysm during abdominal palpation does not exclude the diagnosis, especially in obese patients, in whom the examination is very difficult. On the other hand, thin patients with tortuous aortas may be mistakenly diagnosed with an AAA due to a prominent aortic pulse. It is important to realize that the physical examination may be completely normal, especially in patients with retroperitoneal rupture. Stable AAAs should be nontender; the presence of tenderness should suggest expansion or rupture.

The most clinically useful physical examination finding is the detection of an abnormally widened aortic pulse.[18] Another finding that might suggest AAA is detection of the aortic pulse to the right of the midline. The sensitivity of palpation increases as the diameter of the AAA increases. AAAs may be palpable in 29 percent of patients if they are 3 to 4 cm in diameter, 50 percent if they are 4.0 to 4.9 cm, and 76 percent if they are 5.0 cm or greater.[18–20] Aneurysms extending into or isolated to the iliac arteries may be palpated as a lower abdominal mass.

One last aspect of the physical examination warrants mentioning. Abdominal bruits are known to occur in patients with AAA in only 10 percent of cases. Palpation for unequal femoral pulses is also an insensitive test. Physicians should keep in mind the limitations of this part of the examination. Normal femoral and other lower extremity pulses do not rule out the presence of an AAA[18] (Table 35-2).

DIAGNOSIS

As the population ages, physicians can expect to encounter this disease more frequently. High morbidity and mortality rates are reported even when the diagnosis is

Table 35-2. Common History and Physical Examination Findings in Symptomatic AAA

Large, pulsatile abdominal aorta
Abdominal bruit
Unexplained hypotension
Microscopic hematuria
Peripheral embolization ("blue toe" syndrome)
Syncope
Diaphoresis
Left lower quadrant abdominal mass

made early. Emergency physicians should have a high index of suspicion for AAA in any patient over age 50 who presents to the ED with a complaint of abdominal, flank, or back pain. Rapid initiation of resuscitation measures, the initiation of appropriate radiographic studies, and consultation with a surgeon are crucial for the patient with a confirmed or suspected AAA. Knowledge of presenting features of ruptured AAAs and use of an appropriate diagnostic imaging strategy can help emergency physicians diagnose suspected AAA and maximize the chances of patient survival.

Radiographic Diagnosis

Plain Abdominal Radiography

Plain abdominal radiographs were used for years for the detection of AAA until more sophisticated imaging modalities arose. Aortic wall calcification is the most common abnormality seen in cases of AAA.

Advantages of plain radiographs include their low cost and the ability to perform them at the bedside as the patient undergoes resuscitation efforts. The main disadvantage of this modality is their poor sensitivity for detecting an AAA, ranging from 55 to 68 percent.[7] Plain radiographs also cannot identify aortic rupture, the extent of retroperitoneal hematoma, or branch vessel involvement. Performing plain radiographs to search for an AAA is a reasonable option if bedside ultrasound is not readily available.[23]

Ultrasound

Bedside ultrasound for the detection of symptomatic AAAs has become a popular imaging modality in recent years (Fig. 35-1). Ultrasound is rapid, sensitive (>90 percent for detecting AAAs), noninvasive, and inexpensive when used as a diagnostic tool in the ED. Many emer-

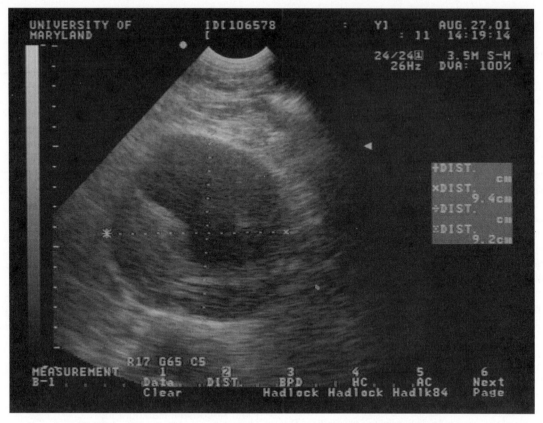

Fig. 35-1 Abdominal ultrasound showing a 9-cm AAA; note the echogenic mural thrombus.

gency medicine residency programs across the country have incorporated ultrasound training into their training curricula and have shown that emergency physicians are capable of detecting AAA with a high rate of accuracy.[24]

The main drawback of ultrasound as an imaging modality is its poor sensitivity for detecting the presence of aortic rupture. Other problems include the inability to obtain adequate views in obese patients or in patients with excessive bowel gas.[25]

Computed Tomography

Computed tomography has become the most reliable and readily available of the imaging modalities for the detection of AAAs and is considered the "gold standard" for diagnosis (Fig. 35-2). Abdominal computed tomographic (CT) scanning is highly sensitive for the detection of AAAs, is capable of defining branch vessel involvement, and reliably detects the presence or absence of rupture as well. Newer-generation CT scanners have improved the speed with which the test is done, and now scanning generally is completed within minutes.[26]

Potential problems with CT scanning are threefold. Patients must be transported out of the ED. This can be a problem especially if a patient is unstable. In addition, patients with a dye allergy or renal insufficiency should not undergo contrast-enhanced computed tomography.[27]

Magnetic Resonance Imaging

Magnetic resonance imaging (MRI) is highly sensitive for the evaluation of suspected AAA. It is a superior imaging modality for evaluating branch vessel involvement. It is also an option in patients with renal insufficiency or allergy to intravenous contrast material.

Several disadvantages of MRI exist. The test is fairly slow and, therefore, generally should not be used for patients who have a potential for becoming unstable. Patients must be transported out of the ED to have the study performed. Claustrophobic patients may have significant

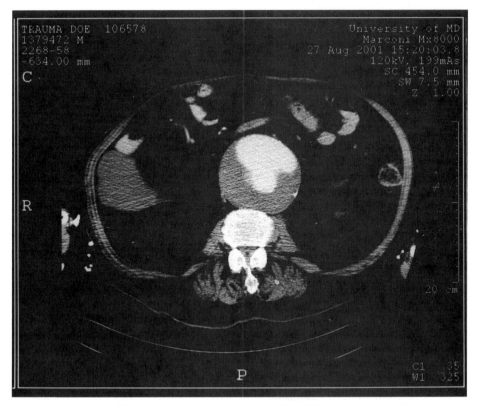

Fig. 35-2 Abdominal CT scan showing a 10-cm AAA.

difficulty in tolerating the procedure, often requiring sedation. MRI is also not available in all medical centers, especially during evenings, nights, and weekends. Lastly, because of the powerful magnet used, metal cannot be brought into the room, including monitoring equipment. This also excludes patients with metallic surgical clips and pacemakers from having the test.[28,29]

EMERGENCY DEPARTMENT CARE AND DISPOSTION

Unruptured Aneurysms

A significant number of unruptured AAAs are detected incidentally during the workup and evaluation of unrelated medical conditions, such as biliary colic. Alternatively, some patients present with symptoms, such as back pain or the new sensation of an abdominal pulsation. The most important aspect of management includes consultation with a surgeon so that follow-up plans can be arranged.

The size of an AAA that would mandate surgery is a matter of debate in the vascular surgery literature. Many surgeons will elect to operate when the aortic diameter reaches 4.5 to 5 cm or when the aortic diameter increases in size more than 0.5 cm within a 6-month period. Many patients are followed as outpatients with serial ultrasound examinations.

Ruptured Aneurysms

Treatment of a ruptured AAA often begins in the prehospital setting. Many patients already carry a diagnosis of AAA, and emergency medical personnel (EMP) are called because of diaphoresis, abdominal pain, and an expanding abdomen. Prompt notification of the receiving ED by EMP enables the ED to prepare for the patient's arrival and to have a surgeon and operating room available when the patient arrives.

Management of AAA rupture begins with attention to the ABCs of resuscitation. Unstable patients or patients going to the operating room should be intubated for airway protection. At least two large-bore intravenous lines should be established. A minimum of 10 to 12 units of packed red blood cells (PRBCs) should be typed and cross-matched in cases of AAA rupture. Intravenous crystalloid should be administered to try to maintain the patient's blood pressure. Hemodynamically unstable patients should be taken directly to the operating room without delay for exploratory laparotomy and AAA repair. Any delays in prompt surgical repair increase mortality significantly.[30]

Hemodynamically stable patients with suspected AAA rupture often are evaluated with radiologic testing in order to obtain a definitive diagnosis. In many centers, multislice CT scanning, which is even faster than spiral CT scanning, is the easiest and fastest test to obtain. A surgeon should be notified immediately that the diagnosis of AAA is being entertained because initially stable patients with an expanding or leaking AAA can become unstable very quickly. Patients with a suspected AAA should have the same early resuscitative measures instituted as those with a rupturing AAA. Airway management should take precedence if needed, and two large-bore intravenous lines should be placed.

Some patients with AAA expansion and rupture are not good candidates for open repair. Endovascular stent grafting, which involves placing a stent within the aortic lumen, has become an alternative to open repair in some medical centers. This approach is sometimes advocated in patients with multiple comorbidities who are considered to be poor surgical candidates.[31] More trials are needed to clarify the role of endovascular aortic stents.

ADDITIONAL ASPECTS

Failure to diagnose ruptured AAA is known to double the mortality.[17] Misdiagnosis is quite common and is estimated to occur in as many as 60 percent of cases.[11] Physicians should keep this diagnostic entity in mind when faced with an elderly patient with unexplained hypotension, syncope, or back, flank, or abdominal pain. This diagnosis also should be considered in elderly patients who present with suspected sepsis.

Several diagnostic entities can be confused with AAA (Table 35-3). The most common misdiagnosis is renal colic. Aneurysmal expansion and rupture simulating renal colic are well described in the medical and legal literature. Emergency physicians should consider all patients over age 50 who present with symptoms typical of renal colic to have a ruptured AAA until proven otherwise.

Table 35-3. Common Misdiagnoses for Ruptured AAA

Renal colic (most common)
Diverticulitis
Gastrointestinal bleed
Musculoskeletal back pain
Acute coronary syndrome
Sepsis
Other gastrointestinal disorders

Another common misdiagnosis is gastrointestinal bleeding, which may result if the aneurysm erodes into bowel lumen. Diverticulitis or appendicitis may be suspected initially in the patient who presents with severe lower abdominal pain. Pancreatitis also may be suspected initially due to the severity of the pain. Perforated viscus also may be suspected initially due to the abrupt onset of pain. Initial suspicion of any of these other gastrointestinal conditions can lead to significant delays in proper diagnosis and treatment, increasing morbidity and mortality.

Ruptured AAA also should be considered in the differential diagnosis in elderly patients who present with unexplained syncope, hypotension, or diaphoresis. When patients present without abdominal, back, or flank pain, the diagnosis often is not entertained. Instead, these patients frequently are evaluated for suspected acute coronary syndromes, leading to further delays in proper management. Initiation of anticoagulation therapy in these patients can have devastating consequences.

Other less common presentations should be considered as well. Rarely, patients may present with evidence of spinal cord dysfunction due to interruption of blood flow to the greater radicular artery (the artery of Adamkiewcz) or may have evidence of a femoral radiculopathy due to compression of the femoral nerve by an expanding AAA[22] (Table 35-4).

Table 35-4. Atypical Presentations of AAA

Flank pain mimicking renal colic
Left lower abdominal pain and/or mass mimicking diverticulitis
Testicular pain
Groin/thigh pain
Spinal cord ischemia
Aortic thrombosis with distal embolization
Lower extremity radiculopathy

Acute rupture is the most devastating complication of an AAA. However, there are other complications of AAA that should be remembered as well. One of the most common is the formation of an intramural thrombus and the development of "blue toe" syndrome. Most AAAs are complicated by intramural thrombus formation. Thrombi may embolize distally and occlude digital arteries, leading to ischemic digits. As many as 5 percent of patients with an AAA will present for evaluation with evidence of peripheral embolism.[7]

Occasionally, an AAA may erode into a segment of the duodenum and produce an aortoenteric fistula. Patients with aortoenteric fistula typically present with exsanguinating upper or lower gastrointestinal hemorrhage. Aortoenteric fistula formation is much more common in patients who have had prior surgical repair of an AAA. This diagnosis should be strongly considered in any patient who has undergone repair of an AAA who presents with gastrointesitinal bleeding.

Other complications are seen in patients who have undergone repair of an AAA as well. Recurrence of an AAA above or below the aortic graft should be considered in patients presenting after repair. Also, graft infection should be considered when patients present with unexplained fever after having had an AAA repair. This complication has a high mortality rate if it is not recognized early. Antibiotics should be started promptly when graft infection is suspected. The most common responsible organism is *Staphylococcus epidermidis*.

It was thought formerly that atherosclerosis was the primary underlying process behind AAA formation. Increasing evidence has shown that AAA rupture and expansion are caused by degradation of connective tissue components within the media of the aortic wall. Enzymes known as *metalloproteinases* reside within the media and continually break down normal components of the connective tissue matrix. Certain antibiotics, such as doxycycline, are known to inhibit this class of enzymes and are being used in some patients with AAA to prevent aneurysm expansion and rupture.[32] More studies are needed to clarify this prophylactic modality. Endovascular stent grafting, as mentioned earlier, is another area of research in AAA treatment. Risk-management "pearls" are shown in Table 35-5.

Table 35-5. Risk-Management Pearls (Salkin)

Flank, back, or abdominal pain in an elderly patient is a ruptured AAA until proven otherwise

Renal colic and diverticulitis are the two most common misdiagnoses

Urologic symptoms are present in up to 10 percent of patients

Ruptured AAAs may present with vague back or abdominal pain

Patients with ruptured AAAs may deteriorate rapidly

Physical examination is unreliable in excluding the presence of an AAA

REFERENCES

1. Beebe HG, Kritpracha B: Screening and preoperative imaging of candidates for conventional repair of abdominal aortic aneurysms. *Semin Vasc Surg* 12:300, 1999.
2. McNamara RM: Acute abdominal pain, in Sanders AB (ed): *Emergency Care of the Elder Person.* St Louis: Beverly Cracom Publications, 1996, p 219.
3. Sanson TG, O'Keefe KP: Evaluation of abdominal pain in the elderly. *Emerg Med Clin North Am* 14:615, 1996.
4. Grange JJ, Davis V, Baxter BT: Pathogenesis of abdominal aortic aneurysm: An update and look toward the future. *Cardiovasc Surg* 5:256, 1997.
5. Crowther M, Goodall S, Jones JL, et al: Localization of matrix metalloproteinase 2 within the aneurysmal and normal aortic wall. *Br J Surg* 87:1391, 2000.
6. Blanchard JF, Armenian HK, Friesen PP: Risk factors for abdominal aortic aneurysm: Results of a case-control study. *Am J Epidemiol* 151:575, 2000.
7. Rothrock SG, Green SM: Abdominal aortic aneurysm: Current clinical strategies for avoiding disasters. *Emerg Med Rep* 15:125, 1994.
8. Bessen HA: Abdominal aortic aneurysm, in Rosen P (ed): *Emergency Medicine: Concepts and Clinical Practice,* 4th ed. St Louis, Mosby–Year Book, 1998, p 1806.
9. Beebe HG, Kritpracha B: Screening and preoperative imaging of candidates for conventional repair of abdominal aortic aneurysms. *Semin Vasc Surg* 12:300, 1999.
10. van der Vliet JA, Boll AP: Abdominal aortic aneurysm. *Lancet* 349:863, 1997.
11. Johansen K, Kohler TR, Nicholls SC, et al: Ruptured abdominal aortic aneurysm: The Harborview experience. *J Vasc Surg* 13:240, 1991.
12. Verloes A, Sakalihasan N, Koulischer L, et al: Aneurysms of the abdominal aorta: Familial and genetic aspects in three hundred thirteen pedigrees. *J Vasc Surg* 21:646, 1995.
13. Walker JS, Dire D: Vascular abdominal emergencies. *Emerg Med Clin North Am* 14:571, 1996.
14. Fielding JWL, Black J, Ashton F, et al: Diagnosis and management of 528 abdominal aortic aneurysms. *B Med J* 283:355, 1981.
15. Martinez R, Garces D, Podeur L, et al: Ruptured abdominal aortic aneurysms: A ten year experience. *J Cardiovasc Surg* 38:1, 1997.

16. Banerjee A: Atypical manifestations of ruptured abdominal aortic aneurysms. *Postgrad Med* 69:6, 1993.

17. Rutherford RB, McCroskey BL: Ruptured abdominal aortic aneurysm: Special considerations. *Surg Clin North Am* 69:859, 1989.

18. Fink HA, Lederle FA, Roth CS, et al: The accuracy of physical examination to detect abdominal aortic aneurysm. *Arch Intern Med* 160:833, 2000.

19. Lederle FA, Walker JM, Reinke DB: Selective screening for abdominal aortic aneurysms with physical examination and ultrasound. *Arch Intern Med* 148:1753, 1988.

20. Beede SD, Ballard DJ, James EM, et al: Positive predictive value of clinical suspicion of abdominal aortic aneurysm. *Arch Intern Med* 150:549, 1990.

21. Karcz A, Holbrook J, Auerbach BS, et al: Preventability of malpractice claims in emergency medicine: A closed claims study. *Ann Emerg Med* 19:865, 1990.

22. Szilagyi DE, Hageman JH, Smith RF, et al: Spinal cord damage in surgery of the abdominal aorta. *Surgery* 83:38, 1978.

23. Laroy LL, Cornier RJ, Matalon TA, et al: Imaging of abdominal aortic aneurysms. *AJR* 152:785, 1989.

24. Kuhn M, Bonnin RL, Davey MJ, et al: Emergency department ultrasound scanning for abdominal aortic aneurysm: Accessible, accurate, and advantageous. *Ann Emerg Med* 36:213, 2000.

25. Frazee BW: The abdominal aorta, in Simon BC, Snoey ER (eds): *Ultrasound in Emergency and Ambulatory Medicine.* St Louis, Mosby–Year Book, 1997, p 190.

26. Bernstein EF: Computed tomography, ultrasound, and magnetic resonance imaging in the management of aortic aneurysm, in Hobson RW, Williams RA, Veith FJ, et al (eds): *Vascular Surgery: Principles and Practice,* 2d ed. New York, McGraw-Hill, 1994.

27. Greatorex RA, Dixon AK, Flower CD, et al: Limitations of computed tomography in leaking abdominal aortic aneurysm. *Br Med J* 297:284, 1988.

28. Tennant WG, Martnell G, Baird RN, et al: Radiologic investigation of aortic aneurysm disease: Comparison of three modalities in staging and the detection of inflammatory change. *J Vasc Surg* 17:703, 1993.

29. Durham JR, Hackworth CA, Tober JC, et al: Magnetic resonance angiography in the preoperative evaluation of abdominal aortic aneurysms. *Am J Surg* 166:173, 1993.

30. Donaldson MC, Rosenberg JM, Buckman CA: Factors affecting survival after ruptured abdominal aortic aneurysm. *J Vasc Surg* 2:564, 1985.

31. Guo W, Liang F, Zhang G, et al: Abdominal aortic aneurysm treated by endovascular stent-graft and conventional surgical repair: A comparison. *Zhonghua Wai Ke Za Zhi* 38(6):409, 2000.

32. Curci JA: Preoperative treatment with doxycycline reduces aortic wall expression and activation of matrix metalloproteinases in patients with abdominal aortic aneurysm. *J Vasc Surg* 31:325, 2000.

36

Aortic Dissection

Andrew K. Chang

HIGH-YIELD FACTS

- Aortic dissections are more common than ruptured abdominal aortic aneurysms (AAAs), and hypertension is the most common risk factor noted.

- Seventy-five percent of patients with dissection will die within 2 weeks if not treated.

- The classic presentation of "tearing" interscapular back pain is less common than sharp anterior chest pain.

- Although abnormalities such as a wide mediastinum are found commonly on the chest radiograph, a normal chest x-ray does not exclude the diagnosis.

- If suspicion for aortic dissection is high, reduction of blood pressure with a beta blocker and vasodilator should be promptly initiated.

Aortic dissection involves the longitudinal cleavage of the aortic media by a column of blood. Aortic dissection is sometimes mistakenly referred to as a *dissecting aortic aneurysm,* but this term has fallen out of favor because it is now known that the affected aorta is frequently not aneurysmal.[1] In addition, atherosclerosis is rarely involved at the site of dissetion.[2] Aortic dissection can be categorized as acute or chronic, with the 14-day period after onset being designated the *acute phase* because morbidity and mortality rates are highest and surviving patients typically stabilize during this time.[3]

Two commonly used classification systems include the Stanford and DeBakey systems. The Stanford classification is the simpler of the two and differentiates dissections based on whether they involve the ascending or descending aorta. Type A involves the ascending aorta, whereas type B is confined to the descending aorta beginning after the left subclavian artery. The DeBakey system uses three categories. Type I involves both the as-

cending and descending aorta, type II is confined to the ascending aorta, and type III is confined to the descending aorta distal to the left subclavian artery. These classification systems are used to help determine treatment options and prognosis.

EPIDEMIOLOGY AND ETIOLOGY

The incidence and prevalence of aortic dissection are likely underestimated due to underreporting of the condition.[4] In 1987, 7000 patients were discharged with a diagnosis of aortic dissection, which represents a prevalence of approximately 2.8 per 100,000 per year.[5] Aortic dissection is more common in men and increases with age.[3,6–8] Aortic dissections occur more often than ruptured abdominal aortic aneurysms (AAAs), making dissection the most common and most lethal aortic catastrophe. It is an uncommon disease before age 40 unless the patient has a preexisting condition, such as Marfan syndrome, Ehlers-Danlos syndrome, congenital heart disease, or giant cell arteritis.[9] The incidence also may increase in pregnancy,[10] although some authors dispute this association.[11] Hypertension is the most common risk factor and is seen in most patients.[3,6–8] Other risk factors include bicuspid aortic valve[2] and a history of cardiac surgery.[3] Although trauma can be a cause of aortic dissection,[12] blunt trauma from a high-speed deceleration injury usually causes traumatic aortic rupture as opposed to aortic dissection.[13] Iatrogenic aortic dissection, such as from cardiac surgical procedures and cardiac catheterization, cause up to 5 percent of cases.[14] Aortic dissection is not due to atherosclerotic disease. Overall, aortic dissection can be thought of as a multifactorial disease with hypertension as the principal risk factor.[15]

Mortality rates have been estimated to be 1 to 5 per 100,000 population per year.[16,17] Since aortic dissection can be a difficult diagnosis to make, many patients may have delayed diagnosis.[8,18] Untreated patients usually die from rupture of the aortic wall into the pericardial sac at the level of the right lateral wall of the aorta, where the adventitia is thinnest.[15] Death also may occur due to congestive heart failure or myocardial infarction. Approximately 75 percent of patients with untreated aortic dissection die within 2 weeks of the onset of symptoms.[19] The International Registry of Acute Aortic Dissection (IRAD) reveals that even today, the in-hospital mortality rate in type A dissection approaches 33 percent, even in centers that have extensive expertise and interest in the treatment of these high-risk patients.[20]

PATHOPHYSIOLOGY

The aortic wall consists of three layers: the intima, the media, and the adventitia. Dissection usually begins with an intimal tear that allows blood to penetrate down to the media, thus separating the intima from the adventitia. The site of the initial intimal tear is usually at the aortic root or between the origin of the left subclavian artery and the ligamentum arteriosum. This is so because these two areas are relatively fixed, and maximum stress is applied to these areas during systole as the heart swings from side to side. Dissection occurs through a degeneration of the media that is neither cystic nor necrotic; therefore, the term *cystic medial necrosis* is no longer used.[21,22]

Over time, the aortic intima weakens and medial degeneration worsens as blood is repeatedly ejected from the heart into the aorta. This process is augmented by the sustained hypertension that characterizes patients with aortic dissection. Since the hydrodynamic forces primarily affect the ascending aorta, type A dissections are more common (approximately 60 percent)[3,23] than type B dissections.

Once established, the dissection can propagate in either direction and may dissect the entire aorta in seconds. A false lumen can form from a reentry tear that occurs distal to the initial site, creating an alternate path for aortic blood flow. A rare spontaneous cure can occur if the dissection ruptures back into the true lumen. Otherwise, the dissection may propagate and rupture into the pericardial sac or pleural cavity. Because the outer wall of the aorta that contains the hematoma is thin, rupture is more likely to occur to the outside.[19] The dissection may dilate as blood flow through the false lumen increases or as the blood clots and a hematoma forms.[15]

CLINICAL FEATURES

It has been taught classically that the pain of aortic dissection is tearing or ripping in nature and located in the interscapular region. However, the results of a recent large international registry challenge these assumptions. In this registry it was found that the pain was described more often as sharp in character.[3] Also, since type A dissection is more common than type B, the location of the chest pain is usually in the anterior chest as opposed to the interscapular back region.

The location of the pain may help to localize the dissection. Anterior chest pain is associated with the ascending aorta, neck and jaw pain with the aortic arch, interscapular pain with the descending aorta, and abdominal or back pain with dissection below the diaphragm. Migratory pain is suggestive of propagation of the dissection, but this occurs in only 16 percent of patients.[3] Up to 20 percent of patients present without pain.[7] Most cases of painless aortic dissection are chronic in nature.[24]

Patients also may present with hoarseness (laryngeal nerve compression), dyspnea, stridor with wheezing (tracheal compression), or dysphagia (esophageal compression).[15] Gastrointestinal symptoms include midepigastric pain, hemorrhage, and melena secondary to splanchnic vessel infarctions.[15] Renal artery involvement may lead to hematuria, flank pain, and oliguria.

Syncope occurs in approximately 9 percent of patients and may be the sole presentation.[3] It can be an ominous presentation that indicates that the dissection has caused a pericardial tamponade, although it also can occur from interruption of blood flow to the brain. Other causes of syncope secondary to aortic dissection include hypovolemia, excessive vagal tone, and cardiac conduction abnormalities.

Neurologic symptoms such as focal weakness or mental status change occur in approximately 6 percent of patients.[3,24] Patients also may develop cranial nerve deficits secondary to carotid artery involvement, as well as motor deficits secondary to distal dissection of spinal arteries.[15] Vasovagal symptoms, such as diaphoresis, nausea, vomiting, light-headedness, and apprehension, often accompany the onset of dissection.

Most patients will have either a normal or elevated blood pressure. Hypotension, which occurs in approximately 25 percent of patients, may be an ominous sign that indicates pericardial tamponade or hypovolemia from rupture through the adventitia.[15] Some patients may have refractory hypertension if the dissection involves the renal arteries with subsequent renin release, although a recent retrospective review found that patients with refractory hypertension had infrequent involvement of the renal arteries.[25] Occasionally, pseudohypotension may occur. In this condition, the blood pressure in the arms is low or unobtainable, whereas the central arterial pressure is normal or high. This results from interruption of blood flow to the subclavian arteries.

Upper extremity blood pressure differentials occur in up to 24 percent[3,24] of patients due to involvement of one or both subclavian arteries. In one large study, pulse deficits in the brachialis, carotid, and femoral arteries were found in 30 percent of patients with type A aortic dissection.[26] Such patients are at increased risk of in-hospital events and mortality because pulse deficits imply that major arterial side branches are compromised by the flap itself or by compression of the true lumen by an expanding hematoma. This patient subgroup therefore is more likely to have organ hypoperfusion leading to more complications such as neurologic deficit, coma, altered mental status, hypotension, and renal failure.[26]

Aortic regurgitation occurs in approximately 30 percent of patients[3,24] and results from proximal dissection causing dilatation of the aortic valve ring and loss of commissural support of the aortic valve.[27] This can lead eventually to congestive heart failure.

DIAGNOSIS AND DIFFERENTIAL

The first radiologic study that should be performed is the chest radiograph. Abnormalities are found in approximately 65 to 85 percent of patients[24,27] and include a widened mediastinum, left-sided pleural effusion, or an indistinct aortic knob. The "calcium sign," in which the calcified aortic intima deviates from the outer wall by greater than 6 mm, is considered pathognomonic for dissection. In a recent retrospective review, 88 percent of patients had a pleural effusion that appeared on average 4.5 days after onset of the dissection.[28] Other suggestive signs include the double-density sign (a false lumen that is less radiopaque than the true lumen), tracheal deviation, and an irregular aortic contour. Since up to 12 percent of patients with aortic dissection have a normal chest radiograph,[3] it is important to keep in mind that a normal chest radiograph does not exclude the diagnosis of aortic dissection. Confirmation is usually required by computed tomography (CT), transesophageal echocardiogram (TEE), or aortography.

In some institutions, spiral CT is replacing aortography as the "gold standard" for the diagnosis of aortic dissection. Advantages of CT in general include superior visualization of fluid collections in the pericardium, pleura, and mediastinum; noninvasiveness; and demonstration of distal vessel patency.

Some advocate TEE as the imaging modality of choice because of its expediency, accuracy, and ability to perform the procedure at the patient's bedside while still in the emergency department (ED).[29–31] However, not all institutions have TEE readily available. TEE has reported sensitivities and specificities as high as 99 and 98 percent, respectively.[15] Radiation and contrast material are not required, and TEE is excellent at diagnosing pericardial effusion and aortic regurgitation.

Although the sensitivity and specificity are excellent, magnetic resonance imaging (MRI) is usually not performed because of the cost, length of time needed for the study, and relative unavailability.

Long considered the "gold standard" for diagnosing aortic dissection, nowadays aortography is used rarely as the initial diagnostic modality.[3] Indeed, some suggest that the sensitivity may be as low as 77 percent[32] because thrombosis of the false channel may prevent visualization of the intimal flap or double lumen.

The primary use of the electrocardiogram (ECG) is to exclude myocardial infarction. However, many patients with aortic dissection may have electrocardiographic abnormalities suggestive of cardiac ischemia,[3,33] especially if the dissection progresses proximally to involve the coronary arteries. Approximately 50 percent of patients with type A dissection and 20 percent of patients with type B dissection develop ST-T wave changes on their ECG.[33] Since most patients have long-standing hypertension, left ventricular hypertrophy is also found commonly on the ECG.

The differential diagnosis is extremely broad (Table 36-1). Because use of a thrombolytic agent would be disastrous in a patient with aortic dissection,[34] it is obviously important to exclude this diagnosis in patients presenting with myocardial infarction or stroke (for those presenting with neurologic symptoms).

Table 36-1. Differential Diagnosis of Aortic Dissection

Myocardial infarction
Stroke
Pulmonary embolism
Pneumothorax
Pneumonia
Pericarditis
Pancreatitis
Cholelithiasis
Cholecystitis
Perforated viscus
Peripheral vascular disease
Mediastinal cyst or tumor

EMERGENCY DEPARTMENT CARE AND DISPOSITION

If the index of suspicion is high, reduction of arterial blood pressure and the forceful contractility of the left ventricle should be started prior to confirmatory imaging studies. Two large-bore intravenous catheters should be placed. Since the medical therapy and surgical mortality rates for uncomplicated type B dissections are approximately the same (32–36 percent), medical therapy is used traditionally as first-line treatment in uncomplicated patients.[35] Therapy consists of using both beta blockers and afterload-reducing agents to decrease the risk of extension of the dissection. Intravenous narcotic analgesia also should be used to control pain and to decrease sympathetic tone.

The rate of dissection is directly proportional to the blood pressure and especially to the rate of rise of arterial blood pressure, which contributes to shearing forces. The blood pressure should be maintained at the lowest level compatible with adequate renal and cerebral perfusion, or at around 100 to 110 mmHg. Ideally, radial artery cannulation should be performed, and the mean arterial pressure should be maintained at approximately 60 to 70 mmHg.[36,37] The drug of choice is intravenous nitroprusside at an initial rate of 0.5 to 1.0 µg/kg/min. Patients who are treated initially with intravenous nitroglycerin for presumed cardiac ischemia–related hypertension should be switched over to nitroprusside once the diagnosis of aortic dissection is made. This is because nitroprusside is a more effective arterial dilator than intravenous nitroglycerin.

To prevent a rebound tachycardia that can occur with a drop in blood pressure, most authorities recommend first treating the patient with an intravenous beta blocker, which also reduces the force of cardiac contraction. The target heart rate is between 60 and 80 beats per minute. Typical agents include intravenous esmolol (0.5 mg/kg loading dose over 1 minute; infusion rate of 0.05 mg/kg/min) or intravenous propranolol (0.5- to 1.0-mg increments at 5-minute intervals).

Intravenous labetalol is a single agent that can be used as an alternative to the nitroprusside and beta-blocker combination. Incrementally increased boluses can be given every 5 to 10 minutes until a total of 300 mg has been given. Maintenance dosage is kept at 1 to 2 mg/h. Labetalol should not be used for patients with chronic obstructive pulmonary disease.

Type A dissections usually are treated surgically because complications include aortic rupture, cardiac tamponade, and aortic valve insufficiency. Type B dissections usually are managed medically, although some studies suggest that operative treatment may result in better outcomes in some patients.[38–42]

ADDITIONAL ASPECTS

The diagnosis of aortic dissection can be difficult to make. New research recently has dispelled long-standing beliefs, and we now realize that aortic dissection is not due to aneurysmal or atherosclerotic conditions at the site of the dissection. Recent findings of a large international registry have challenged beliefs regarding the classic clinical presentation of patients with aortic dissection and have shown that these patients present more typically with sharp anterior chest pain. Because it is the most frequent aortic catastrophe encountered, a high index of suspicion for this etiology should be maintained. Early therapy is critical and should be initiated while diagnostic tests are being performed.

REFERENCES

1. Dmowski AT, Carey MJ: Aortic dissection. *Am J Emerg Med* 17:372, 1999.
2. Larson EW, Edwards WD: Risk factors for aortic dissection: A necropsy study of 161 cases. *Am J Cardiol* 53:849, 1984.
3. Hagan PG, Nienaber CA, Isselbacher EM, et al: The International Registry of Acute Aortic Dissection (IRAD): New insights into an old disease. *JAMA* 283:897, 2000.
4. Kouchoukos NT, Dougenis D: Surgery of the thoracic aorta. *New Engl J Med* 336:1876, 1997.
5. Lytle B: Thoracic aortic dissections and aneurysms, in Sivak ED, Seiver A (eds): *The High-Risk Patient: Management of the Critically Ill.* Baltimore, Williams & Wilkins, 1995, p 700.
6. Sullivan PR, Wolfson AB, Leckey RD, Burke JL: Diagnosis of acute thoracic aortic dissection in the emergency department. *Am J Emerg Med* 18:46, 2000.
7. Torossov M, Singh A, Fein SA: Clinical presentation, diagnosis, and hospital outcome of patients with documented aortic dissection: The Albany Medical Center experience, 1986 to 1996. *Am Heart J* 137:154, 1999.
8. Meszaros I, Morocz J, Szlavi J, et al: Epidemiology and clinicopathology of aortic dissection. *Chest* 117:1271, 2000.
9. Evans JM, Bowles CA, Bjornsson J, et al: Thoracic aortic aneurysm and rupture in giant cell arteritis: A descriptive study of 41 cases. *Arthritis Rheum* 37:1539, 1994.
10. Roberts WC: Aortic dissection: Anatomy, consequences, and causes. *Am Heart J* 101:195, 1981.
11. Oskoui R, Lindsay J Jr: Aortic dissection in women < 40 years of age and the unimportance of pregnancy. *Am J Cardiol* 73:821, 1994.

12. Rogers FB, Osler TM, Shackford SR: Aortic dissection after trauma: Case report and review of the literature. *J Trauma* 41:906, 1996.

13. Newman RJ, Rastogi S: Rupture of the thoracic aorta and its relationship to road traffic accident characteristics. *Injury* 15:296, 1984.

14. Januzzi JL, Sabatine MS, Eagle KA, et al: Iatrogenic aortic dissection. *Am J Cardiol* 89:623, 2002.

15. Perry SJ: Aortic dissection and thoracic aortic aneurysms, in Harwood-Nuss A (ed): *The Clinical Practice of Emergency Medicine,* 3d ed. Philadelphia, Lippincott Williams & Wilkins, 2001, p 211.

16. Lilienfeld DE, Gunderson PD, Sprafka JM, Vargas C: Epidemiology of aortic aneurysms: I. Mortality trends in the United States, 1951 to 1981. *Arteriosclerosis* 7:637, 1987.

17. Johansson G, Markstrom U, Swedenborg J: Ruptured thoracic aortic aneurysms: A study of incidence and mortality rates. *J Vasc Surg* 21:985, 1995.

18. Klompas M: Does this patient have an acute thoracic aortic dissection? *JAMA* 287:2262, 2002.

19. Ankel F: Aortic dissection, in Marx J (ed): *Rosen's Emergency Medicine: Concepts and Clinical Practice,* Vol 2, 5th ed. St Louis, Mosby, 2002, p 1171.

20. Mehta RH, Suzuki T, Hagan PG, et al: Predicting death in patients with acute type A aortic dissection. *Circulation* 105:200, 2002.

21. Schlatmann TJ, Becker AE: Pathogenesis of dissecting aneurysm of aorta: Comparative histopathologic study of significance of medial changes. *Am J Cardiol* 39:21, 1977.

22. Schlatmann TJ, Becker AE: Histologic changes in the normal aging aorta: Implications for dissecting aortic aneurysm. *Am J Cardiol* 39:13, 1977.

23. Fuster V, Halperin JL: Aortic dissection: A medical perspective. *J Card Surg* 9:713, 1994.

24. Spittell PC, Spittell JA Jr, Joyce JW, et al: Clinical features and differential diagnosis of aortic dissection: Experience with 236 cases (1980 through 1990). *Mayo Clin Proc* 68:642, 1993.

25. Januzzi JL, Sabatine MS, Choi JC, et al: Refractory systemic hypertension following type B aortic dissection. *Am J Cardiol* 88:686, 2001.

26. Bossone E, Rampoldi V, Nienaber CA, et al: Usefulness of pulse deficit to predict in-hospital complications and mortality in patients with acute type A aortic dissection. *Am J Cardiol* 89:851, 2002.

27. Armstrong WF, Bach DS, Carey LM, et al: Clinical and echocardiographic findings in patients with suspected acute aortic dissection. *Am Heart J* 136:1051, 1998.

28. Hata N, Tanaka K, Imaizumi T, et al: Clinical significance of pleural effusion in acute aortic dissection. *Chest* 121:825, 2002.

29. Banning AP, Masani ND, Ikram S, et al: Transoesophageal echocardiography as the sole diagnostic investigation in patients with suspected thoracic aortic dissection. *Br Heart J* 72:461, 1994.

30. Wiet SP, Pearce WH, McCarthy WJ, et al: Utility of transesophageal echocardiography in the diagnosis of disease of the thoracic aorta. *J Vasc Surg* 20:613, 1994.

31. Sommer T, Fehske W, Holzknecht N, et al: Aortic dissection: A comparative study of diagnosis with spiral CT, multiplanar transesophageal echocardiography, and MR imaging. *Radiology* 199:347, 1996.

32. Bansal RC, Chandrasekaran K, Ayala K, Smith DC: Frequency and explanation of false negative diagnosis of aortic dissection by aortography and transesophageal echocardiography. *J Am Coll Cardiol* 25:1393, 1995.

33. Hirata K, Kyushima M, Asato H: Electrocardiographic abnormalities in patients with acute aortic dissection. *Am J Cardiol* 76:1207, 1995.

34. Marian AJ, Harris SL, Pickett JD, et al: Inadvertent administration of rtPA to a patient with type 1 aortic dissection and subsequent cardiac tamponade. *Am J Emerg Med* 11:613, 1993.

35. Miller DC: The continuing dilemma concerning medical versus surgical management of patients with acute type B dissections. *Semin Thorac Cardiovasc Surg* 5:33, 1993.

36. Ponraj P, Pepper J: Aortic dissection. *Br J Clin Pract* 46:127, 1992.

37. DeSanctis RW, Doroghazi RM, Austen WG, Buckley MJ: Aortic dissection. *New Engl J Med* 317:1060, 1987.

38. Gysi J, Schaffner T, Mohacsi P, et al: Early and late outcome of operated and nonoperated acute dissection of the descending aorta. *Eur J Cardiothorac Surg* 11:1163, 1997; discussion 1169.

39. Glower DD, Fann JI, Speier RH, et al: Comparison of medical and surgical therapy for uncomplicated descending aortic dissection. *Circulation* 82:IV39, 1990.

40. Kato M, Bai H, Sato K, et al: Determining surgical indications for acute type B dissection based on enlargement of aortic diameter during the chronic phase. *Circulation* 92:II107, 1995.

41. Perko MJ, Norgaard M, Herzog TM, et al: Unoperated aortic aneurysm: A survey of 170 patients. *Ann Thorac Surg* 59:1204, 1995.

42. Masuda Y, Yamada Z, Morooka N, et al: Prognosis of patients with medically treated aortic dissections. *Circulation* 84:III7, 1991.

37

Arterial Insufficiency

Chris J. Richter

HIGH-YIELD FACTS

- Claudication and peripheral arterial disease are associated with coronary artery disease, cerebrovascular disease, and diabetes.
- Many patients will not volunteer the symptoms because they are thought to be part of the normal aging process.
- The ankle-brachial index is an easy and effective screening tool that should be used on people with suggestive symptoms.

Arterial insufficiency, or peripheral vascular disease, is a very common disease among the older population. While arterial insufficiency frequently is not the presenting complaint, many common diseases seen in emergency department (ED) patients, such as coronary artery disease, cerebrovascular disease, and diabetes, are associated with or complicated by this disease. It is known that cardiovascular disease can be detected in up to 90 percent of patients with intermittent claudication,[1] that the prevalence of cerebrovascular disease is higher than 50 percent,[2] and that diabetes and diabetic foot ulcers often are associated with arterial insufficiency.

Ischemic pain in the lower extremities with exercise, or claudication, is relatively easy to elicit with a thorough history but often is not self-reported by older patients because they believe it is just part of the aging process. The diagnosis can be difficult to make in some elderly patients due to increasing dementia or aphasia from a cerebrovascular accident, but as the disease advances, the physical examination can be more helpful.

While this is a common disease, less than one-third of patients will require intervention of any kind, and only 5 percent will progress enough to have an amputation.[3] This may seem reassuring, but there is a 30 percent risk of death in 5 years and 50 percent within 10 years associated with claudication, mostly secondary to acute myocardial infarction or stroke.[3]

Claudication has a significant impact on quality of life and mobility, and patients often suffer from poorly healing leg ulcerations that are prone to serious infection. It is important to recognize the signs and symptoms of peripheral vascular disease in the ED for short- and long-term treatment, as well as for risk stratification.

EPIDEMIOLOGY

Like atherosclerosis in general, arterial insufficiency is a disease that predominantly affects the middle-aged to elderly patient. The prevalence of peripheral arterial disease is approximately 12 percent, with men and women being affected in equal numbers.[2] Prevalence increases steadily with age: 2.5 percent at ages 40 to 59, 8.3 percent at ages 60 to 69, and 18.8 percent at ages 70 to 79.[8] The annual incidence increases from approximately 0.12 to 0.19 percent in middle age to 0.94 percent after age 65.[4] Intermittent claudication is associated with a two- to fourfold increased risk of mortality,[5] with a cardiovascular cause likely to be responsible for up to 80 percent of those deaths.[1]

PATHOPHYSIOLOGY

The pathophysiology of arterial insufficiency effectively can be divided into two major types, which encompass the vast majority of patients.

Diabetic Microangiopathy

Patients with diabetes are more susceptible than the general population to atherosclerosis, but they also often suffer from poor microvascular circulation, especially in the distal lower extremities. While atherosclerosis is a structural lesion of the vessel, microvessel disease is mostly functional and is characterized by increased vascular permeability and impaired vascular tone. Basement membrane thickening and decreased capillary blood flow lead to an inability to vasodilate and a decreased hyperemic response to heat and injury.[13]

The normal endothelium of blood vessels is important in protecting the thrombogenic layers of the intima from exposure to blood products as well as producing prostacyclin, endothelin, prostaglandins, and nitric oxide, which play a large role in vasomotor tone.[6] In patients with diabetes, endothelial function is abnormal, which can lead to decreased vasodilatation and functional ischemia of the skin, making the lower extremity more susceptible to ulcer, injury, and infection and preventing effective and timely healing. Elderly patients with diabetes therefore are at risk for having both atherosclerosis and poor capillary circulation secondary to diabetes. Of note, patients with diabetes and atherosclerotic disease are more likely to have lesions of the infrageniculate arteries and sparing of the foot arteries, which makes them amenable to vascular bypass surgery.[7]

Atherosclerotic Disease

The pathophysiology of atherosclerosis is widely reported due to the prevalence of coronary artery and cerebrovascular disease. The most commonly accepted theory is based on the production of atherosclerotic plaque as a response to chronic endothelial and intimal injury. In this theory it is postulated that damage to the endothelial lining of arterial blood vessels secondary to high cholesterol, high blood pressure, turbulent blood flow, and even high blood levels of homocystiene is the sentinel event leading to intimal plaque formation. When endothelial cells are damaged, they no longer function effectively as a barrier, and potentially thrombogenic and inflammatory subendothelial tissues are exposed to the circulation. This exposure attracts circulating monocytes (which become tissue macrophages and absorb lipids) and platelets, which aggregate and form microthrombi. Macrophages and platelets then secrete cytokines and growth factors that stimulate smooth muscle cell growth and proliferation of connective tissue. Over time, continued injury and proliferation produce a fibrous plaque in the intimal layer of the vessel that eventually may reduce arterial lumen size enough to impede blood flow, initially during exercise and eventually at rest. These plaques can coalesce to form larger plaques or rupture and thrombose. Atheroembolic disease is due to micremboli consisting of cholesterol and platelet aggregation. The abdominal aorta is the most common site for plaque formation. Lower extremities sites are also very common, especially the femoral and popliteal arteries. In the peripheral vascular system, atheroembolism causes obstruction of very small vessels in the lower distal extremities, such as the digital arteries, resulting in the "blue toe" syndrome. Bilateral lower extremity involvement suggests an aortic site, whereas unilateral emboli usually result from a femoropopliteal or aortoiliac source.

CLINICAL FEATURES

As mentioned previously, patients do not always offer the symptoms of peripheral arterial disease because they equate them with normal aging. Furthermore, up to 50 percent of all patients with peripheral arterial disease over age 55 are asymptomatic.[9] Of the symptomatic patients, roughly 40 percent have intermittent claudication, and 10 percent have critical limb ischemia.[9] Chronic peripheral arterial disease may present with intermittent claudication or ischemic rest pain.

The most common symptom is intermittent claudication, which is usually described as calf or upper thigh and buttock pain on walking a certain, often well defined distance that is relieved by rest. When the patient walks, oxygen demand increases in the musculature, and when supply does not meet demand, pain ensues. Buttock, hip, and thigh pain occurs in patients with aortoiliac disease, and calf pain occurs in those with femoral or popliteal artery disease. Approximately 25 percent of these patients will have progressive claudication.[10] The 10 percent who go on to develop critical limb ischemia experience pain in their legs at rest that is often worse when supine and better with their legs hanging over the edge of a bed or chair. The latter characteristics are thought to be a product of gravity increasing flow in the dependent position. More than 50 percent of patients with peripheral arterial disease have enough leg pain to reduce ambulatory activity and quality of life.[11]

In contrast to chronic peripheral arterial disease, acute arterial occlusion often occurs in persons without significant atherosclerosis and may present with limb-threatening ischemia. A combination of pain, pallor, pulselessness, paresthesias, and paralysis (the five P's) is typically present.

Physical signs of chronic arterial insufficiency include decreased pulses distal to the constricting lesions, muscular atrophy, hair loss on lower extremities, smooth and shiny skin, and in more severe presentations, ischemic ulcers and gangrene. In acute embolic events, the involved limb is usually markedly pale, cool, and pulseless. Cyanosis may occur as ischemia progresses. Paresthesias and paralysis are ominous signs of limb-threatening ischemia. Atheroembolism from microembolic phenomena or "blue toe" syndrome presents with characteristic cool, painful, cyanotic toes.

The Fontaine classification is useful to describe clinical presentations of chronic peripheral arterial disease: stage I, asymptomatic; stage II, intermittent claudication; stage III, ischemic rest pain; and stage IV, ulceration or gangrene.

DIAGNOSIS

Although a thorough history and physical often can make the diagnosis of peripheral arterial disease, several confirmatory diagnostic tests are useful.

While the diagnostic "gold standard" remains arteriography, the ankle-brachial index is a simple, effective, and commonly used screening test. The *ankle-brachial index* (ABI) is a ratio of the systolic blood pressure in the upper limbs and in the lower limbs and is the most useful test for ED use. It has been shown in some epidemiologic studies that a low ABI is an independent predictor of all-cause and cardiovascular mortality.[14,15] Normally, the pressure in the lower extremity arterial system should be equal to or greater than that in the upper extremity, giving a ratio or 1.0 or greater. Patients with intermittent claudication will have an ABI in the range of 0.5 to 0.9, and those with critical limb ischemia will have a ratio below 0.5.[12] Medial arterial calcinosis can occur in diabetic patients, which results in poorly compressive arteries and artificially high arterial pressures and ABIs.[13] If the ABI is greater than 1.3, then other forms of testing should be considered.

Additional diagnostic tests include treadmill exercise testing, duplex ultrasound, angiography, and magnetic resonance angiography (MRA). Treadmill testing is an effective functional test that is often used to show improvement in symptoms in clinical therapeutic trials. Arteriography and MRA often are used as preoperative testing to map out lesions causing critical limb ischemia that may be amenable to bypass grafting or intraluminal stenting. However, with the exception of duplex ultrasound, these tests are not practical in the ED setting.

EMERGENCY DEPARTMENT CARE AND DISPOSITION

While this is a common disease in the elderly, there are, unfortunately, few therapies that can be offered by the emergency physician. However, patient education and disease prognosis are an important part of patient satisfaction, and the emergency physician should be well informed about the prognosis and definitive therapies that the patient may need in the future and should discuss them at the time of diagnosis and emergency care. If a patient has intermittent claudication, he or she should be referred to his or her primary physician, and the patient with critical limb ischemia should be referred to a vascular surgeon. Therapeutic measures can be divided into those which the emergency physician can do and those

for which the patient can be referred to a specialist. They can be subdivided further into lifestyle changes, pharmacotherapy, and invasive therapy.

Lifestyle Changes

Dietary changes may reduce the risk of death from coronary disease,[3] but it is not clear that they change the course of peripheral arterial disease. While diet may affect mortality by association, smoking cessation and exercise have been shown to have a direct effect on morbidity and mortality in patients with peripheral arterial disease. Patients who stop smoking have a twofold increase in their 5-year survival rate compared with those who continue to smoke.[15] Exercise has a definitive effect on morbidity. Most studies involve an exercise program that is 6 months or longer and show an improvement in pain-free walking and maximum walking distance.[16,17] A recent meta-analysis of six trials examining claudication and exercise programs noted a statistically significant difference in pain-free (increase of 139 m) and total walking distance (179.1 m).[18] It is clear that if a patient has claudication, the emergency physician should recommend smoking cessation if applicable and diet and exercise changes. It may even be beneficial to have, as part of the standard discharge instructions for claudication, a brief exercise program.

Pharmacotherapy

There are several antiplatelet drugs that are commonly considered for persons with peripheral arterial disease. However, only two, pentoxifylline and cilostazol are approved by the Food and Drug Administration (FDA) for peripheral arterial disease.

Aspirin is an important antiplatelet drug that is useful in the primary prevention of cardiovascular and cerebrovascular events that can be associated with peripheral arterial disease. In the Physicians' Health Study, aspirin reduced the need for peripheral arterial surgery.[20] Another study showed that aspirin significantly improved graft patency in patients treated with bypass grafting or intravascular stenting.[21] Despite this improvement in vascular flow, aspirin does not appear to have an effect on claudication.[19]

Pentoxifylline is a methylxanthine derivative and is one of the only two drugs that are FDA approved for the treatment of claudication symptoms. The drug functions to retard platelet aggregation, lower fibrinogen levels, and improve red cell deformability. In early trials it showed improvement in maximal walking distance.[22] A recent meta-analysis of nine trials showed a significant increase in pain-free walking distance and total walking distance.[18]

Clopidogrel inhibits platelet activation by blocking adenosine diphosphate receptors. This drug, like aspirin, has shown effectiveness in reducing the overall risk of morbidity and mortality from atherosclerosis-related illness. It showed an overall reduction of 8.7 percent when compared with aspirin.[23] There is a slight risk of thrombotic thrombocytopenic purpura with use of this drug.

Finally, cilostazol is a phosphodiesterase III inhibitor that has FDA approval for the treatment of claudication symptoms. This drug functions to improve vasodilatation, increase high-density lipoprotein (HDL) levels, and decrease plasma triglyceride levels and has antiplatelet activities.[16,25] In placebo-controlled trials, cilostazol showed a significant increase in treadmill walking distance and functional status, including community walking distance.[25–27] This drug appears to have the most clearly defined benefit in persons with claudication. The emergency physician should consider starting it, in consultation with the private physician, in those patients being discharged.

Invasive Therapy

Patients with worsening claudication and those who have developed critical limb ischemia, ulcerations, or gangrene require referral to a vascular surgeon. Prompt ED referral can be critical because endovascular stenting, bypass grafting, or amputation can help to restore mobility, reduce pain, and prolong the patient's life. Arteriographic lesions that are short in length and located in the iliac and superficial femoral arteries may be amenable to percutaneous transluminal angioplasty with stent placement. This approach has been shown to result in 1-year patency rates of 80 to 90 percent.[28] For longer or more distal lesions, bypass grafting with either Dacron, Gore-Tex, or autologous veins has shown 5-year patency rates of between 70 and 90 percent.[28] These procedures can have significant complications (such as reocclusion, infection, and thrombosis) that should be familiar to emergency physicians. If such complications are suspected, consultation with a vascular surgeon is suggested. If one is not available, transfer of the patient to a higher-level facility is recommended. Finally, for those patients with critical limb ischemia and gangrene or occlusions that are not amenable to bypass, below-knee amputation can be a lifesaving procedure. Patients with evidence of gangrene should be started on appropriate antibiotics and have an emergent vascular surgery consult.

ADDITIONAL ASPECTS

Remember that patients who have peripheral arterial disease are at risk for and are likely to have other significant comorbid illnesses such as coronary artery disease, cerebrovascular disease, and diabetes. It is good practice for the emergency physician to do an initial risk assessment on all patients in order to anticipate patterns of disease or complications that could necessitate urgent treatment or admission. Peripheral arterial disease should raise a red flag and suggest to the physician to consider these serious comorbid illnesses.

REFERENCES

1. TransAtlantic Inter-Society Consensus (TASC) Working Group: Management of peripheral arterial disease (PAD). *J Vasc Surg* 31(1):S5, 2000.
2. Criqui MH, Denenberg JO, Langer RD, Fronek A: The epidemiology of peripheral arterial disease: Importance of population at risk. *Vasc Med* 2:221, 1997.
3. Tierney S, Fennessy F, Hayes DB: Secondary prevention of peripheral vascular disease. *Br Med J* 320(7244):1262, 2000.
4. Kannel WB, Skinner JJ, Schwartz MJ, Shurtleff D: Intermittent claudication: Incidence in the Framingham Study. *Circulation* 41:875, 1970.
5. Kannel WB, McGee DL: Update on some epidemiologic features of intermittent claudication: The Framingham Study. *J Am Geriatr Soc* 33:13, 1985.
6. Vane JR, Anggard EE, Botting RM: Regulatory functions of the vascular endothelium. *New Engl J Med* 323:27, 1990.
7. Menzoian JO, LaMorte WW, Paniszyn CC, et al: Symptomatology and anatomic patterns of peripheral vascular disease: Differing impact of smoking and diabetes. *Ann Vasc Surg* 3:224, 1989.
8. Wietz JI, Byrne J, Clagett GP, et al: Diagnosis and treatment of chronic arterial insufficiency of the lower extremities: A critical review. *Circulation* 94:3026, 1996.
9. Imparato AM, Kim GE, Davidson T, Crowley JG: Intermittent claudication: Its natural course. *Surgery* 78:795, 1975.
10. McDermott MM, Mehta S, Liu K, et al: Leg symptoms, the ankle-brachial index, and walking ability in patients with peripheral arterial disease. *J Gen Intern Med* 14:173, 1999.
11. Orchard TJ, Strandness DE: Assessment of peripheral vascular disease in diabetes: Report and recommendations of an international workshop sponsored by the American Diabetes Association and the American Heart Association September 18–20, 1992, New Orleans, Louisiana. *Circulation* 88:819, 1993.
12. Akbari CM, LoGerfo FW: Diabetes and peripheral vascular disease. *J Vasc Surg* 30:373, 1999.
13. Sixth report of the Joint National Committee on detection,

evaluation, and treatment of high blood pressure (JNC-VI). *Arch Intern Med* 157:2413, 1997.

14. Newman AB, Sutton-Tyrrell K, Vogt MT, Kuller LH: Morbidity and mortality in hypertensive adults with a low ankle/arm blood pressure index. *JAMA* 270:487, 1993.

15. Regensteiner JG, Gardner A, Hiatt WR: Exercise testing and exercise rehabilitation for patients with peripheral arterial disease: Status in 1997. *Vasc Med* 2:147, 1997.

16. Gardner AW, Poehlman ET: Exercise rehabilitation programs for the treatment of claudication pain: A meta-analysis. *JAMA* 274:975, 1995.

17. Girolami B, Bernardi E, Prins MH, et al: Treatment of intermittent claudication with physical training, smoking cessation, pentoxifylline, or nafronyl: A meta-analysis. *Arch Intern Med* 159:337, 1999.

18. Antiplatelet Trialists' Collaboration: Collaborative overview of randomized trial of antiplatelet therapy: I. Prevention of death, myocardial infarction, and stroke by prolonged antiplatelet therapy in various categories of patients. *Br Med J* 308:81, 1994.

19. Goldhaber SZ, Manson JE, Stampfer MJ, et al: Low-dose aspirin and subsequent peripheral arterial surgery in the Physicians' Health Study. *Lancet* 340:143, 1992.

20. Collaborative overview of randomized trials of antiplatelet therapy: II. Maintenance of vascular graft or arterial patency by antiplatelet therapy. *Br Med J* 308:159, 1994.

21. Lingarde F, Jelnes R, Bjorkman H, et al: Conservative drug treatment in patients with moderately severe chronic occlusive peripheral arterial disease. Scandinavian Study Group. *Circulation* 80:1549, 1989.

22. CAPRIE Steering Committee: A randomized, blinded trial of colpidogrel versus aspirin in patients at risk of ischaemic events (CAPRIE). *Lancet* 348:1329, 1996.

23. Elam MB, Heckman J, Crouse JR, et al: Effect of the novel antiplatelet agent cilostazol on plasma lipoproteins in patient with intermittent claudication. *Arterioscler Thromb Vasc Biol* 18:1942, 1998.

24. Dawson DL, Cutler BS, Meissner MH, Strandness DE Jr: Cilostazol has beneficial effects in treatment of intermittent claudication: Results from a multicenter, randomized, prospective, double-blind trial. *Circulation* 98:678, 1998.

25. Money SR, Herd JA, Isaacsohn JL, et al: Effect of cilostazol on walking distances in patients with intermittent claudication caused by peripherial vascular disease. *J Vasc Surg* 27:267, 1998.

26. Beebe HG, Dawson DL, Cutler BS, et al: A new pharmacological treatment for intermittent claudication: Results of a randomized, multicenter trial. *Arch Intern Med* 159:2041, 1999.

27. Beard JD: Chronic lower limb ischaemia. *Br Med J* 320:854, 2000.

38

Venous Disorders

Natalie A. Kayani

HIGH-YIELD FACTS

- There is a higher incidence of venous disorders in the geriatric population.
- Geriatric patients have an increase in morbidity and mortality in the setting of thromboembolic diseases.
- One-fifth of patients with apparent superficial thrombophlebitis will have an occult associated deep venous thrombosis (DVT) at time of presentation.
- Prompt diagnosis and treatment are essential to prevent the long-term complication of postthrombotic syndrome
- Although D-dimer ELISA assays may be helpful in excluding DVT, they are often elevated because of age and comorbid illness in geriatric patients and thus of limited utility in this population.
- Outpatient low-molecular-weight heparin (LMWH) therapy for DVT is not a covered Medicare benefit, and home therapy with LMWH in the elderly has not been well studied.
- Most long-term care facilities are unable to absorb the cost of outpatient LMWH treatment for their residents.

The emergency department (ED) is a site for frequent visits from elderly patients with venous disorders because of the often subacute and frightening appearance of these disorders. The manifestations of venous disease most often seen in the ED include chronic venous insufficiency (CVI), superficial thrombophlebitis, and deep venous thrombosis (DVT).

It is especially important for the emergency physician to recognize and treat DVT quickly, particularly in the elderly, because the risk of embolism increases from 4 to 23 percent if the diagnosis is missed at the initial presen-

tation or a subtherapeutic dose of heparin is administered.[1] The geriatric patient is at significantly increased risk with a resulting increase in morbidity and mortality. This patient population is also more sensitive to the adverse effects of anticoagulant drugs because of age-related changes in pharmacokinetics and pharmacodynamics.

EPIDEMIOLOGY

In the United States there are approximately 7 million people with CVI and 2 million cases of venous thromboembolism per year.[2] Numerous studies have shown that the elderly have a significantly higher incidence of venous disorders,[3] with annual rates for DVT increasing from 0.5 percent for 50-year-olds to 3.8 percent for 80-year-olds.[4,5]

The incidence of complications of thromboembolism, such as recurrent DVT, postthrombotic syndrome, and death, also increases with age. The cumulative incidence of recurrent venous thromboembolic disease is 30 percent after 8 years of follow-up.[6] Patients with underlying malignancy or impaired coagulation systems have the highest risk of recurrence. Postthrombotic syndrome, characterized by venous ulceration, debilitating pain, or intractable edema, occurs in 20 to 60 percent of patients with DVT.[6,7] Mortality from all causes following a DVT increases with age, with a cumulative incidence of around 30 percent at 8 years.[3,6]

PATHOPHYSIOLOGY

Chronic Venous Insufficiency (CVI)

CVI can have no clear cause or be the result of an identifiable event, most commonly a previous DVT (which may have been undiagnosed or asymptomatic). Half the patients with CVI have had previous DVT, some form of serious leg injury in the past, or a family history of varicose veins or CVI. Weakened vein walls lead to dilatation and separation of valve cusps and eventually pooling of blood, venous hypertension, and capillary leakage.

Superficial Thrombophlebitis

Under normal circumstances, there is a continual balance between the formation and lysis of microthrombi throughout the vascular system. Pathology occurs when microthrombi escape the fibrinolytic system and are allowed to propagate and extend. Risk factors include venipuncture, trauma, and cancer. This kind of thrombosis can occur in any vein, but within the superficial venous system it occurs more commonly in varicose veins. The superficial system connects to the deep system through perforating veins, through which a thrombus can extend at any time. One-fifth of patients with apparent superficial thrombophlebitis will have an occult associated DVT at the time of presentation.[8]

Deep Venous Thrombosis (DVT)

The mechanism for DVT formation is similar to that for superficial thrombosis and differs mainly in location of the thrombus (superficial versus deep veins). The risk factors for DVT are related to Virchow's triad: venous stasis, hypercoagulability, and endothelial injury (Table 38-1). The most common risk factors noted are a history of DVT, recent surgery, immobilization, and cancer.[9,10] It is important to note that 25 to 33 percent of patients with femoral central lines develops DVT.[11] Although the risk factors for venous thromboembolic diseases are the same in younger adults as they are in older adults, elders generally have an increased number of these risk factors. However, it is important to note that thromboembolic disease occurs in many patients without known risk factors.

Resolution of thrombosis in the deep veins results in a valveless channel, leading to chronically elevated pressures and a clinical postphlebitic syndrome. Prompt diagnosis and treatment are essential to prevent the long-term complication of postthrombotic syndrome.[2]

CLINICAL FEATURES

Patients with chronic venous insufficiency usually present with complaints of long-standing swelling, cramping, throbbing, burning, aching, and leg fatigue, especially at the end of the day. Pain is usually relieved by walking and cold. Sudden increases in swelling in patients with CVI suggests DVT. Examination reveals hyperpigmentation, brawny edema, and sensitivity of the skin to minor trauma. Over time patients have replacement of the skin and subcutaneous tissue by fibrous scarring, which is called *lipodermatosclerosis.*

Superficial thrombophlebitis usually presents with pain and tenderness along the course of a vein, overlying warmth and erythema, and a palpable cord.

Patients with DVT present with complaints of gradual onset of pain and swelling. Examination often reveals swelling of greater than 1 cm in circumferential difference, tenderness on calf compression, warmth, and a palpable cord. However, the clinical examination has been shown to lack sensitivity and specificity for the diagnosis of DVT.[12] Even when these classic findings are present, only 50 percent of these patients have a DVT, and at least 50 percent of patients with DVT lack any of these findings.

Table 38-1. Risk Factors for Thromboembolic Disorders

Venous stasis
  Prolonged immobility
  Paralysis
  Obesity
  Varicose veins
Hypercoagulable states
  Cancer
  Protein deficiencies (C, S, antithrombin III)
  Factor V Leiden
  CHF/MI
  Sepsis
  Nephrotic syndrome
  Estrogen use
  Inflammatory or infectious conditions
Endothelial damage
  Surgery
  Trauma
  Use of indwelling devices (including pacemakers and
    central lines)
Smoking
Prior thromboembolism
Family history of DVT

DIAGNOSIS AND DIFFERENTIAL

Thrombosis in the superficial veins is generally benign and localized, but patients believed to have involvement of the greater saphenous vein should undergo diagnostic testing to rule out the presence of DVT. Physical examination is often unreliable for the diagnosis of DVT, and as such, clinical models for predicting pretest probability have been developed and validated[13,14] (Table 38-2). These models also can assist in interpreting results of radiographic tests. Further testing is needed if the pretest probability is discordant with test results. Clinical decision models can be useful in helping the emergency physician decide when to call in an ultrasound technician and radiologist during off hours, as well as when to order serial radiologic studies. When Wells and colleagues[14] tested this clinical model in patients with a high, moderate, or low pretest probability of DVT, they found a prevalence of disease of 85, 33, and 5 percent, respectively.

Radiologic Investigations

Duplex ultrasound (B-mode with compression) is the initial procedure of choice because it is rapid, inexpensive, and highly accurate in detecting proximal clot. B-mode ultrasound gives two-dimensional images of a vein, whereas Doppler flow combined with color images gives a visual and audible evaluation of blood flow. The combination of B-mode ultrasound and Doppler flow is referred to as a *duplex ultrasound*. This test has a sensitivity of 97 percent and a specificity of 94 percent for detecting proximal clots but is limited for detection of DVT in asymptomatic patients and patients with iliac thrombosis and isolated calf vein thrombosis because the calf veins are hard to compress.[15] Since 2 percent of patients with an initially normal ultrasound will have abnormalities on serial testing,[16] negative ultrasound in a high-risk patient may lead one to proceed to venogram.[17] In addition, only half of patients with proven pulmonary embolism will have a positive lower extremity duplex ultrasound. The use of ultrasound may be limited in patients who are obese or have edema or tenderness of their lower extremities.

Impedance plethysmography detects increased venous outflow resistance and therefore the rate of venous return in the deep veins of the proximal lower extremities. This test is performed by placing two sets of electrodes around the calf and a blood pressure cuff around the thigh. The electrodes sense a change in blood volume in the calf veins. An increase in blood volume decreases the electrical impedance and is recorded on a strip chart. However, this technique is insensitive to thrombi that do not decrease the rate of venous outflow, such as most calf and nonobstructing thrombi. In addition, it does not distinguish between thrombi and other causes of venous obstruction. False-positive results can occur from increased intrathoracic or intraabdominal pressure.

Contrast venography has been used historically as the "gold standard," with sensitivity and specificity of near 100 percent, and is the most sensitive test for calf DVT, but it is invasive, expensive, associated with dye reactions, and can precipitate phlebitis.

Magnetic resonance imaging (MRI) has excellent sensitivity and specificity for acute DVT, with sensitivity ranges of 90 to 100 percent and specificity ranges of 95

Table 38-2. Clinical Model for Predicting Pretest Probability for DVT

	Score
Active cancer (includes active treatment or within previous 6 months or palliative)	1
Paralysis, paresis, or recent plaster immobilization of the lower extremity	1
Recently bedridden for more than 3 days or major surgery within 4 weeks	1
Localized tenderness along the distribution of the deep venous system	1
Entire leg swollen	1
Calf swelling 3 cm bigger than asymptomatic side (measured 10 cm below tibial tuberosity)	1
Pitting edema confined to symptomatic leg	1
Collateral superficial veins (nonvaricose)	1
Alternative diagnosis as likely or greater than that of DVT	−2

Scoring: Low probability: 0; moderate probability: 1–2; high probability: > 3.
Source: Adapted with permission from Wells.[13]

to 100 percent. Because of its expense and the lack of large comparative trials with contrast venography, its use is still limited. Several small trials have shown its usefulness in acute pelvic vein thrombosis and upper extremity thrombosis.[17]

Laboratory Investigations

D-Dimers are breakdown products of cross-linked fibrin that are released into the bloodstream during acute thrombosis. Levels of D-dimer are increased with aging[18] and also can be elevated in other conditions, such as sepsis, recent myocardial infarction or stroke, recent surgery or trauma, disseminated intravascular coagulation, active collagen-vascular disease, metastatic cancer, and liver disease. In the elderly, assays for D-dimers with a cutoff value of 750 ng/mL for detecting DVT have a sensitivity around 98 percent but a specificity of only around 40 percent. Consequently, a normal D-dimer level (<750 ng/mL) is strong evidence against the presence of thromboembolism, with a negative predictive value of 95 percent.[19] Some studies suggest that the combination of results from a clinical decision model, an ultrasound, and a sensitive D-dimer assay may eliminate the need for invasive testing for some patients suspected of having DVT.[20,21] However, due to comorbidities often present in the geriatric population, only a few patients will present with D-dimer values of less than 750 ng/mL, making this test much less useful in this population.

Differential Diagnosis

The following can mimic DVT: cellulitis, torn muscles and ligaments, ruptured Baker's cyst, and lymphedema. If the history and physical examination are not sufficiently diagnostic, ancillary tests, such as duplex ultrasound, may be needed to help differentiate these conditions.

Two emergent venous thromboembolic disorders to recognize are phlegmasia alba dolens (painful white leg) and phlegmasia cerulea dolens (painful blue leg). Both are due to extensive obstruction of both superficial and deep venous systems that masquerade as arterial blockage. The former presents with a pale or white leg due to associated arterial spasm, and the latter presents with an extensively swollen, cyanotic leg from venous engorgement. These conditions can be limb-threatening if venous outflow is not reestablished.

EMERGENCY DEPARTMENT CARE AND DISPOSITION

The goals of ED care for chronic venous insufficiency are to counteract the pressure on the skin to prevent ulceration, which can be accomplished through leg compression, elevation, and protection. Arterial occlusive disease is a relative contraindication to leg compression. Most patients with venous insufficiency can be discharged home.

For superficial thrombophlebitis, it is important to rule out involvement of the deep venous system if there is clinical suspicion. Otherwise, thrombophlebitis can be managed with nonsteroidal anti-inflammatory drugs adjusted for renal clearance, warm compresses, elastic supports, and limb elevation.[22]

For patients with DVT, the goals of treatment are to prevent thrombus extension and embolization, as well as recurrence and postthrombotic syndrome. Anticoagulation via intravenous heparin or subcutaneous low-molecular-weight heparin (LMWH) needs to begin in the ED in order to reduce the risk of recurrent disease because it has been demonstrated that there is only a 4 to 6 percent recurrence rate if therapeutic levels are reached within the first 24 hours, compared with 23 percent if they are not.[1]

Inadequate Activated Partial Thromboplastin Time (APTT) levels in 45 percent of patients on fixed-dose he-

parin[23] prompted the development of a weight-based nomogram: 80 IU/kg bolus followed by continuous infusion of 18 IU/kg/h. Strong predictors of excessive prolongation of APTT are recent surgery, liver disease, severe thrombocytopenia, and concomitant antiplatelet therapy.[24]

Advantages of LMWH over unfractionated heparin include higher bioavailability, longer half-life, subcutaneous administration, absence of laboratory monitoring, less thrombocytopenia, less major bleeding, and improved mortality.[25–27] Previous studies have not shown an increased risk of bleeding in older patients. These drugs are excreted renally, and therefore the dose must be adjusted based on creatinine clearance.

A vena caval filter is indicated for patients with a contraindication to anticoagulation, such as active internal bleeding, uncontrolled hypertension, significant recent trauma or surgery, and central nervous system tumor or in whom there is recurrent DVT despite adequate anticoagulation. Although venal caval filters reduce the rate of pulmonary embolism, they increase the tendency for recurrent DVT.[28]

ADDITIONAL ASPECTS

Most trials that examined outpatient LMWH therapy to treat DVT excluded patients with significant comorbid illnesses. As such, these data cannot be extrapolated easily to most geriatric patients who present to the ED for treatment of DVT. Moreover, outpatient LMWH therapy for DVT is not a covered Medicare benefit. In addition, most long-term care facilities are unable to absorb the cost of outpatient LMWH treatment for their residents.

Although thrombolytic therapy produces more rapid symptom resolution and preserves venous valvular competency, which decreases the risk of postphlebitic syndrome, the elderly are at much higher risk for bleeding and therefore routinely should not be considered candidates for this mode of treatment. In addition, thrombectomy should be reserved for patients with limb-threatening disease, especially in light of the lack of clinical data to demonstrate its superiority over standard anticoagulation.

REFERENCES

1. Hull RD, Raskob GE, Brant RF, et al: Relation between the time to achieve the lower limit of the APTT therapeutic range and recurrent venous thromboembolism during he-

parin treatment for deep vein thrombosis. *Arch Intern Med* 157:2562, 1997.

2. Hirsh J, Hoak J: Management of deep vein thrombosis and pulmonary embolism: A statement for health care professionals for the Council on Thrombosis (in consultation with the Council on Cardiovascular Radiology), American Heart Association. *Circulation* 93:2212, 1996.

3. Nordstrom M, Lindblad B, Bergovist D, et al: A prospective study of the incidence of deep vein thrombosis within a defined urban population. *J Intern Med* 232:155, 1992.

4. Kniffin WD, Baron JA, Barrett J, et al: The epidemiology of diagnosed pulmonary embolism and deep venous thrombosis in the elderly. *Arch Intern Med* 154:861, 1994.

5. Hansson P, Welin L, Tibblin G, et al: Deep vein thrombosis and pulmonary embolism in the general population. *Arch Intern Med* 157:1665, 1997.

6. Prandoni P, Lensing AW, Cogo A, et al: The long-term clinical course of acute deep venous thrombosis. *Ann Intern Med* 125:1, 1996.

7. Ginsberg JS: Management of venous thromboembolism. *New Engl J Med* 335:1816, 1996.

8. Verlato F, Zuccheta P, Prandoni P, et al: An unexpectedly high rate of pulmonary embolism in patients with superficial thrombophlebitis of the thigh. *J Vasc Surg* 30:1113, 1999.

9. Heit JA, Silverstein MD, Mohr DN, et al: Risk factors for deep vein thrombosis and pulmonary embolism: A population-based case-control study. *Arch Intern Med* 160:809, 2000.

10. Anand SS, Wells PS, Hunt D, et al: An evidence-based approach to the diagnosis of deep vein thrombosis: Beyond the ultrasound report. *JAMA* 279:1094, 1998.

11. Dailey RH: Femoral vein cannulation: A review. *J Emerg Med* 2:367, 1985.

12. O'Donnell T, Abbott W, Athanasoulis C, et al: Diagnosis of deep vein thrombosis in the outpatient by venography. *Surg Gynecol Obstet* 150:69, 1980.

13. Wells PS, Hirsh J, Anderson DR, et al: Accuracy of clinical assessment of deep vein thrombosis. *Lancet* 345:1326, 1995.

14. Wells PS, Anderson DR, Bormanis J, et al: Value of assessment of pretest probability of deep-vein thrombosis in clinical management. *Lancet* 350:1795, 1997.

15. Tapson VF, Carroll BA, Davidson BL, et al: The diagnostic approach to acute venous thromboembolism. Clinical Practice Guideline. American Thoracic Society. *Am J Respir Crit Care Med* 160:1043, 1999.

16. Heijboer H, Buller HR, Lensing AWA, et al: A comparison of real-time compression ultrasonography with impedance plethysmography for the diagnosis of deep-vein thrombosis in symptomatic outpatients. *New Engl J Med* 320:1365, 1993.

17. Erdman WA, Jayson HT, Redman HC, et al: Deep venous thrombosis of extremities: Role of MRI in the diagnosis. *Radiology* 174:425, 1990.

18. Kario K, Matsuo T, Kobayashi H: Which factors affect D-dimer levels in the elderly? *Thromb Res* 62:501, 1992.

19. Le Blanche AF, Siguret V, Settegrana C, et al: Ruling out acute deep vein thrombosis by ELISA plasma D-dimer assay versus ultrasound in inpatients more than 70 years old. *Angiology* 50(11):873, 1999.

20. Lennox AF, Delis KT, Serunkuma S, et al: Combination of a clinical risk score and rapid whole blood D-dimer testing in the diagnosis of deep vein thrombosis in symptomatic patients. *J Vasc Surg* 30:794, 1999.

21. Bernardi E, Prandoni P, Lensing AW, et al: D-Dimer testing as an adjunct to ultrasonography in patients with clinically suspected deep vein thrombosis: Prospective cohort study. The Multicentre Italian D-Dimer Ultrasound Study Investigators Group. *Br Med J* 317:1037, 1998.

22. Messmore HL, Bishop M, Wehrmacher WH: Acute venous thrombosis: Therapeutic choices for superficial and deep veins. *Postgrad Med* 89(7):73, 1991.

23. Elliott CG, Hiltumen SJ, Suchyta M, et al: Physician-guided treatment compared with a heparin protocol for deep vein thrombosis. *Arch Intern Med* 154:999, 1994.

24. Levine MN, Raskob GE, Landefeld S, et al: Hemorrhagic complication of anticoagulant treatment. *Chest* 108(suppl):276s, 1995.

25. Gould MK, Dembitzer AD, Doyle RL, et al: Low-molecular-weight heparins compared with unfractionated heparin for treatment of acute deep venous thrombosis: A meta-analysis of randomized, controlled trials. *Ann Intern Med* 130:800, 1999.

26. Warkentin TE, Levine MN, Hirsh J, et al: Heparin-induced thrombocytopenia in patients treated with low-molecular-weight heparin or unfractionated heparin. *New Engl J Med* 332:1330, 1995.

27. Leizorovicz A: Comparison of the efficacy and safety of low molecular weight heparins and unfractionated heparin in initial treatment of deep venous thrombosis: An updated meta-analysis. *Drugs* 52:30, 1996.

28. Decousus H, Leizorovicz A, Parent F, et al: A clinical trial of vena caval filters in the prevention of pulmonary embolism in patients with proximal deep vein thrombosis. *New Engl J Med* 338:409, 1998.

39

Altered Mental Status

Fredric M. Hustey
Joseph LaMantia

HIGH-YIELD FACTS

- Mental status impairment is highly prevalent in elderly emergency department (ED) patients.
- Mental status impairment is often subtle in presentation and may be easily overlooked.
- ED patients with mental status impairment are at increased risk for morbidity and mortality.
- Toxic/metabolic abnormalities rather than structural brain lesions more often cause acute alteration in mental status in the elderly.
- Delirium is an acute emergency and is associated with high morbidity and mortality rates. Strong consideration should be given to hospitalizing such patients from the ED.

Every day in the United States approximately 6,000 people turn 65 years of age. In the next 10 years, that number is expected to reach 10,000.[32] Alteration in mental status is a very common presentation of elderly ED patients. Changes in behavior, affect, thought process and content, cognition, or level of consciousness may bring patients to the ED. The challenges in evaluation and management of these patients are many and include very diverse and often subtle presentations, a wide spectrum of etiologies, frequent coexistence of several underlying diseases, and interplay of predisposing and precipitating factors. Evaluation and treatment may be hindered by difficulties in obtaining an adequate history and physical examination.

Medications frequently play an important role and further complicate the presentation. There is significant risk for morbidity or mortality with alteration in mental status because this presentation may be a manifestation of a critical illness.

EPIDEMIOLOGY

Mental status impairment is highly prevalent in elderly patients seeking medical care. The most common form of mental status impairment encountered is dementia. Dementia affects approximately 10 to 17 percent of people aged 65 years and older,[1–4] and the prevalence increases dramatically with advancing age.[5] Nearly half of the population aged 85 and older in the United States is affected by dementia.[6] Dementia is even more common among elders who are seen in the ED. Estimated prevalence rates in this group of patients range from 16 to 22 percent.[7,8]

Delirium is also common among elderly patients seeking acute care. Approximately 10 percent of elders treated in the ED suffer from delirium.[7–10] Even higher prevalence rates occur in hospitalized elders. Approximately 10 to 24 percent of patients in general medical wards manifest delerium,[11] whereas nearly 35 to 65 percent of those hospitalized with acute hip fracture suffer from the syndrome.[12–14]

Mental status impairment in the elderly has a tremendous impact on both society and the health care system. Patients suffering from dementia have higher morbidity and mortality rates than the general population, corrected for age.[3,15] Dementia exceeds coronary artery disease and stroke as a leading contributor to loss of functional independence.[3] It is also one of the most common reasons for placement in extended care facilities. Family members caring for elders with dementia are also significantly affected, frequently suffering from depression and related social stress.[16] All these factors contribute to an increasing burden on society and the health care system.

Patients with delirium are at an increased risk for morbidity and mortality. Even after controlling for other comorbidities, hospitalized medical patients with delirium are more than 2½ times more likely to suffer death or require new nursing home placement after hospital discharge.[17] Delirium also has been shown to have an adverse impact on the recovery of elderly patients who are hospitalized with hip fracture. These patients have a slower progression to recovery and prolonged impairment of activities of daily living, and they are more likely to require new nursing home placement than counterparts without delirium.[12,18] They also have high rates of in-hospital complications.[19] While there are few studies regarding elders presenting to the ED with delirium, there is evidence that these patients are at risk for increased mortality after ED discharge as compared with counterparts without delirium.[9]

Psychiatric illness, including mood and anxiety disorders and psychosis, although seen less frequently than delirium or dementia, also must be considered in the elderly ED patient with altered mental status. The most common psychiatric condition in the elderly is depression.[20] Recent studies of elderly ED patients with depression have noted the same prevalence rate as in younger patients, i.e., 32 percent.[21–23] Depression in the elderly can have a significant impact; e.g., the rate of suicide is highest in men aged 65 to 74,[24] and all-cause mortality in depressed elderly is higher when compared with nondepressed elders in both institutional and outpatient settings.[25,26] In addition, late-life depression contributes significantly to health care costs and decreases functional ability and well-being.[27]

Late-life psychosis is also a common psychiatric condition in the older patient; it accounts for up to 10 percent of psychiatric admissions in patients over 60 years of age.[28,29] While elderly patients with this condition exhibit a lower mortality than those with depression, there is a significantly higher incidence of dementia in this group.

With the current rapid expansion of the geriatric population in the United States, the problems associated with mental status impairment are expected to increase exponentially over the next 20 to 40 years.[30,31]

PATHOPHYSIOLOGY

Etiologies of mental status impairment in elders vary widely. It is useful to subgroup these into various clinical syndromes to enhance understanding of this diverse topic. Identifiable syndromes causing mental status impairment most often fall into one or more of the following categories: delirium, dementia, and psychiatric illness.

Delirium is the result of an acute neurologic insult, usually in combination with other factors. Increasing age is one of the greatest risk factors for the development of delirium. As part of the normal aging process, elders suffer from decreased cerebral blood flow, neuron loss in the neocortex and hippocampus, and decreased neurotransmitter activity: norepinephrine, acetylcholine, dopamine, and gamma-aminobutyric acid (GABA).[33] Preexisting dementia is also highly associated with the development of delirium.[34] Other risk factors include sensory impairment, medication use, medical illness, male gender, and alcohol use.[34]

There are many causes of delirium, and delirium is usually multifactorial in origin. The most common contributors to the development of delirium are toxic and metabolic derangements. Infections (especially when associated with high fever or hypothermia), electrolyte abnormalities, endocrine dysfunction (such as disorders of thyroid function), and medication effects are all examples of these many derangements (Table 39-1). Acute neurologic injuries may also precipitate delirium, such as cerebrovascular infarct or hemorrhage, subdural hematoma, and primary or metastatic tumor with hemorrhage or edema.

The pathophysiology of delirium is not well understood. Prior theories have identified global cerebral impairment as the most common mechanism. More recently, delirium has been described as a final common symptom resulting from a variety of situation-specific neurotransmitter abnormalities.[33] Medications, substance withdrawal, medical illness, and stroke may alter neurotransmitter activity in the brain. Alterations of cholinergic, serotonergic, dopamine, GABA, glutamate, and cortisol activity all have been implicated in the development of delirium.[33]

In contrast to the acute nature of delirium, dementia is typified by a more chronic onset and slower progression. The greatest risk factor for the development of dementia is age. While dementia is extremely rare in the young, it affects approximately 10 to 17 percent of people age 65 and older.[1–4] The prevalence continues to increase dramatically with age,[5] affecting nearly half the population age 85 and older in the United States.[6] Degenerative brain disorders are responsible for most cases of dementia. Since these develop primarily with advancing age, they are responsible for the higher prevalence of dementia in this population.

While all patients suffering from dementia share similar signs and symptoms, etiologies that bring about the clinical syndrome vary widely. These etiologies may be broadly grouped into two categories: those in which the

Table 39-1. Examples of Potential Precipitants of Delirium

Etiologies	Examples
Metabolic	Electrolyte abnormalities, renal failure, hepatic encephalopathy, acid-base disturbance, hypoxemia, hypercapnea
Endocrine	Adrenal crisis, thyrotoxicosis, myxedema, hypoglycemia, diabetic ketoacidosis, hyperosmolar crisis
Medication intolerance or toxicity	Anticholinergics (amytryptylene), antihistamines (H_1 and H_2 blockers), beta blockers, benzodiazepine and other sedatives, antidepressants, neuroleptics, parkinsonian agents, and many others
Neurologic events	Cerebrovascular infarct or hemorrhage, subdural hematoma, cerebral edema
Infectious	Urosepsis, pneumonia, bacteremia, meningitis, cellulitis
Toxicologic	Substance abuse or withdrawal (especially alcohol or benzodiazepine withdrawal), overdosage

progression of dementia may be arrested or even reversed and those which are universally degenerative and progressive.[35] The most common single cause of dementia is Alzheimer's disease, accounting for 50 to 70 percent of all cases.[35,36] Vascular causes, including multi-infarct dementia, comprise the next largest group, accounting for 10 to 20 percent of dementia.[35] Less than 1 percent of all dementia is caused by potentially curable or reversible etiologies.[35,37]

Alzheimer's disease is the most widely recognized form of dementia. It is characterized by a progressive, irreversible decline in cognitive function. Short-term memory impairment is one of the earliest and most evident manifestations of Alzheimer's disease. Language impairment is also a hallmark of Alzheimer's dementia. Subtle findings may include difficulty with word finding in spontaneous speech. As the disease progresses, frank aphasia often develops. Impaired processing of visual and spatial information is also characteristic of Alzheimer's dementia. Patients often misperceive or are unable to recognize familiar objects or faces (such as mistaking shrubs or trees for people).[35] The inability to perform learned motor tasks (apraxia) is also a feature of Alzheimer's disease. Over time, patients become progressively more disoriented to time and place. This is a nearly universal finding in individuals with advanced disease.

Psychiatric symptoms can be part of Alzheimer's dementia as well. Patients may become withdrawn or increasingly hostile. Depression and suicidal ideation are common.[38] Psychotic features may be present. Hallucinations (predominantly visual) occur in up to 25 percent of patients,[35] whereas nearly half of all patients suffer from paranoid delusions.[39] Unlike other types of dementia, disorders of movement (tremor, rigidity) are uncommon in Alzheimer's disease.[35] The presence of these features early in the course of the dementia should lead to questioning of the diagnosis of Alzheimer's disease.

The pathophysiology of Alzheimer's disease involves many factors. Cognitive decline appears to be associated with a progressive deficit of cholinergic neurotransmitter activity in the brain.[40] Structural changes occur as well. Hyperphosphorylated tau proteins collect to form neurofibrillary tangles.[41] Pathologic formations of ß-amyloid plaque also have been implicated in the development of Alzheimer's disease.[42] These processes appear to be concentrated in specific regions of the brain. Nearly all patients with Alzheimer's disease have progressive atrophy of the hippocampal and parahippocampal regions of the temporal lobe. Metabolic and perfusion deficits in parietal and temporal lobes are also characteristic.[43,44]

Vascular dementia is second in frequency to Alzheimer's disease as a contributor to the development of dementia in the elderly. There are many causes of vascular dementia, including autoimmune and infectious vasculitis (as with systemic lupus erythematosus or neurosyphillis), subdural hematomas, and cerebrovascular infarcts. The most common of these is multi-infarct dementia. Unlike Alzheimer's dementia, disorders of movement are not uncommon in patients with multi-infarct dementia. Rigidity, masked facies, gait disturbance,[45] and other parkinsonian features may be evident. Dementia with focal neurologic deficits from prior cerebrovascular insults should arouse suspicion of multi-infarct dementia. The course typically fluctuates but is always progressive. There are currently no widely accepted criteria for the diagnosis of multi-infarct dementia.[35]

Another common cause of dementia is Parkinson's disease. Parkinson's dementia is characterized by movement disorders (cogwheel rigidity, bradykenesia, shuffling gait, postural instability) that precede the onset of dementia. When dementia is an early feature of parkinsonism, it often progresses much more rapidly than Alzheimer's dementia.[35] Diffuse Lewy body disease (DLBD) is another cause of parkinsonian-like dementia. It is characterized by the presence of Lewy bodies (intracytoplasmic eiosinophilic neuronal inclusion bodies) in the brain stem and cerebral cortex of affected individuals. However, in contrast to parkinsonism, symptoms of dementia precede evidence of movement disorder.

Occasionally, dementia may present with a predominance of psychiatric symptoms. This is the case with frontotemporal dementia (FTD). FTD occurs at an earlier age than most other degenerative dementias.[46] Subtle personality changes, disinhibition, psychotic features (hallucinations and delusions), and other psychiatric symptoms often precede frank dementia by several years.[46] This often leads to an initial psychiatric diagnosis early in the course of the disease.

Of all types of dementia, less than 1 percent are potentially reversible.[35,37] Among the reversible causes are normal-pressure hydrocephalus, vitamin B_{12} deficiency, hypothyroidism, and subdural hematoma.

Patients suffering from hypothyroidism may present with dementia.[35] History may reveal fatigue, cold intolerance, constipation, and weight gain. Evidence of a hypometabolic state, alopecia, or the classic delay in relaxation of deep tendon reflexes on physical examination may be found. With treatment, full recovery can occur, although reversal is usually partial.[47]

The classic triad of urinary incontinence, ataxia, and cognitive dysfunction is characteristic of normal-pressure hydrocephalus. However, the diagnosis should be entertained in all patients presenting with gait disturbance and dementia. A history of urinary incontinence may be lacking in up to 50 percent of patients.[48] Unlike Alzheimer's disease, apraxia and language impairment are extremely uncommon symptoms. Head computed tomographic (CT) scanning often will suggest the diagnosis, demonstrating enlarged ventricles without convolutional atrophy.

Profound vitamin B_{12} deficiency is another cause of dementia that can be arrested or reversed. A painful red tongue, peripheral neuropathy, or megaloblastic anemia also may be found with profound vitamin B_{12} deficiency. Abnormal cyanocobalamin levels confirm the diagnosis. As the deficiency progresses, there is less chance of reversal. Even with treatment, the prognosis is poor,[49] with recovery occuring rarely.[50]

The pathophysiologic basis for a number of psychiatric disorders in the elderly also has been studied extensively, and a number of mechanisms and anatomic correlates have been postulated. About one-half of patients with late-onset psychosis have identifiable underlying brain disease.[51] The frequent association of psychiatric symptoms with dementia was noted previously. Reported structural abnormalities in depressed elders include frontal cerebral atrophy, ventricular enlargement, and subcortical encephalomalacia, as well as alterations in frontal lobe vascular flow and metabolism.[52] Elderly patients with late-onset depression have significantly more white matter ischemic changes on magnetic resonance imaging (MRI) than age-matched controls.[53] Medical illness also may be a common precipitant for the development of major depression in the elderly.[54]

CLINICAL FEATURES

Clinical features of mental status impairment in the elderly vary widely with etiology. The most acute etiology of mental status impairment is delirium. Mental status changes usually occur over the course of hours to weeks but rarely are longer in duration. Symptoms typically fluctuate over the course of a day and often are more evident at night. During less severe periods, symptoms can be very subtle and easily may be overlooked. This may play a part in the poor recognition of this syndrome among acute care physicians.

Delirium is often far from obvious in acute care patients. ED chief complaints may be seemingly unrelated to mental status issues. However, clues obtained during the history and physical examination can reveal evidence of this acute emergency. Cardinal features of delirium include an attention deficit, illogical flow of ideas, and an altered level of consciousness. Careful attention to the level of consciousness during history taking may reveal a hyperalert or hypoactive patient. Elders who seem easily distracted or those having difficulty keeping track of questioning should be screened for delirium. Inappropriate or illogical responses to questioning may be evident. Family, caregivers, and nurses can provide valuable information, particularly about fluctuations in mental status. During their contacts with patients, these individuals may notice abnormal behaviors or subtle changes in cognition that are not evident during a brief examination by an emergency physician.

On physical examination, patients may be hyperactive and easily startled. In contrast, they may be hypoactive with a depressed level of consciousness. Hypoactive patients may be harder to appreciate, and this feature may be overlooked by the busy emergency physician. Hypoactive patients are also more likely to have a higher acuity of coexisting illness.[55] More commonly, a mixed hypoactive-hyperactive psychomotor pattern is present and manifests with a fluctuating course.

Other evidence of acute illness may be revealed during the physical examination as well. Abnormal vital signs including pulse oximetry in a confused patient are strong clues to the presence of delirium and a medical emergency. Poor hygiene or an unkempt appearance also may be found. However, the lack of any of these findings is not sufficient to exclude delirium from the diagnosis. The remainder of the physical examination, while not specific for delirium, may help to identify an etiology for the syndrome.

Dementia, in contrast to delirium, is characterized by a slower and more chronic deterioration in mental status. Mental status impairment usually develops over a period of months to several years. The hallmark of all elderly patients with dementia, regardless of etiology, is short-term memory impairment. While it is considered normal to have some degree of memory loss associated with aging,[56] memory loss in dementia differs in that it is severe enough to interfere with normal daily functioning. In order to confirm the diagnosis, patients also must exhibit at least one other deficit in cognitive function (Table 39-2). This may include a language disturbance (aphasia), agnosia (difficulty recognizing or identifying familiar objects despite intact sensory function), apraxia (difficulty executing learned motor tasks despite intact motor function), or impairment in executive functioning (planning, organizing, or abstracting).[57] The diagnosis of dementia cannot be made in a patient with delirium. Delirium must be excluded first as a potential etiology in all elderly patients with mental status impairment prior to making this diagnosis.

Patients with dementia rarely present with complaints directly related to mental status impairment. However, attention during history taking often reveals cognitive dysfunction. Patients may exhibit slow responses to questioning as they attempt to remember events. Inability to relay pertinent details related to the chief complaint and frequent contradiction of information by family members also may be subtle clues of impairment. Family members and caregivers can be extremely helpful in relaying evidence of dementia and can help to identify the acuity of onset of symptoms. Occasionally, family members may relay concerns of memory impairment when emergency staff are unconcerned about the patient's mental status. Caregivers usually are more aware of changes from a patient's baseline.

Depending on available home support, elders with moderate to severe dementia may have difficulty performing independent activities of daily living. Evidence of this may be seen in poor hygiene, inappropriate dress, or malnutrition. Abnormal clock drawing or figure copying during mental status testing can reveal impaired processing of visual and spatial information. Other findings may give clues to potential etiologies of dementia. Pathologic memory loss, urinary incontinence, and ataxia are suggestive of normal-pressure hydrocephalus. Painful red tongue, peripheral neuropathy, or megaloblastic anemia may signify vitamin B_{12} deficiency. Dementia in a patient with a hypometabolic state may be due to hypothyroidism.

The presentation of psychiatric illness may be atypical in the elderly patient. Whereas younger patients with depression commonly present with vegetative symptoms of diminished sleep, appetite, and energy and depressed mood and motivation, the older patient may manifest psychosis, agitation, irritability, or catatonia. Somatization, in which depression is manifested as chronic pain, fatigue, or hypochondriasis, also can be seen.[58] Patients with late-onset schizophrenia (age of onset between 40 and 60) and very late onset psychosis (onset after the age of 60) are less likely to present with a formal thought disorder without other psychiatric symptoms, such as a blunted affect.[59] Depression in the elderly also may result in significant cognitive impairment, dementia syndrome of depression (previously "pseudodementia").[60] Patients with this disorder can have rapidly progressive intellectual impairment, along with depressed motivation and affect and typical neurovegetative signs of depression. Persecutory delusions may also be present.[61]

The evaluation of psychosis in the elderly patient may pose several unique challenges. Because of the significant association of psychosis with delirium, dementia, and other medical illnesses, careful attention should be paid to evaluating the patient for an organic etiology to his or her symptoms. Medical conditions to consider include recreational drug or alcohol intoxication or withdrawal;

Table 39-2. Characteristics of Dementia

1. Chronic memory loss of such severity as to interfere with daily social or occupational activities.
2. The presence of at least one of the following additional deficits:
   a. Apraxa
   b. Aphasia
   c. Agnosia
   d. Impairment of executive functioning
3. Findings are not otherwise explained by acute illness or delirium.

medication side effects; central nervous system tumors, hemorrhage, or ischemia; disorders of calcium, thyroid, or glucose metabolism; seizure disorder; and vitamin deficiencies, among others.[62] Features that may make an organic etiology more likely include fluctuating symptoms, disordered attention, mood-congruent delusions, delusions that are poorly systematized, and visual, not auditory, hallucinations.[63,64]

DIAGNOSIS AND DIFFERENTIAL

The diagnosis of delirium is made clinically. However, delirium is an acute emergency and often a marker of severe underlying illness. An aggressive search for contributing factors is warranted. A thorough metabolic investigation, medication review, searches for underlying infection, assessment of oxygenation and ventilatory status, and neuroimaging are among some of the tests that should be considered. Findings from the history and physical examination may help to narrow the focus of the evaluation.

Dementia is primarily a clinical diagnosis as well. Further testing may be helpful in identifying reversible causes of dementia. The National Institutes of Mental Health and the National Institutes of Neurological Communicative Disorders recommend as part of the initial screening evaluation that all patients with dementia have a complete blood count, metabolic panel, set of electrolytes, thyroid function panel, vitamin B_{12} and folate determinations, serology for syphilis, urinalysis, chest radiograph, and electrocardiogram (ECG).[36] The routine use of neuroimaging studies for all patients with dementia is still controversial.[37,43,44,65,66] While these studies are costly and rarely diagnostic, they may help to identify potentially reversible causes of mental status impairment. Physical examination findings are not always reliable in excluding these etiologies from the differential diagnosis. Neuroimaging studies may also be helpful in identifying degenerative causes of dementia. Since treatment options vary with etiology, these studies may help to direct further therapy.

The diagnosis of psychiatric disease is also made primarily on clinical grounds. Features to help distinguish organic versus functional illness were noted earlier, although one must recognize that considerable overlap exists in these complexes of symptoms. In this regard, the importance of a careful history cannot be overemphasized. History should include past medical, psychiatric, medication, and substance abuse history and a thorough mental status and neurologic examination. Clues such as

ataxia could point to an organic cause for the patient's behavioral symptoms. A carefully directed diagnostic workup, considering toxic and metabolic causes, should be undertaken.

EMERGENCY DEPARTMENT CARE AND DISPOSITION

Of all identifiable syndromes of mental status impairment, delirium is associated with the highest short-term morbidity and mortality. Given this high acuity, a thorough and aggressive search for contributing factors is warranted in the ED. Metabolic profiles; pulse oximetry serum glucose sodium determinations; a complete blood count; urinalysis; an ECG; and medication levels should be considered in all patients. If there are any acute focal neurologic abnormalities, or if the initial evaluation fails to reveal a cause for delirium, neuroimaging should be considered. Further findings based on the history and physical examination may lead to additional testing, such as arterial blood gas determinations, to assess for hypercapnea or hypoxemia, blood and urine cultures, lumbar puncture, or cardiac enzyme determinations. While the most common contributors to the development of delirium are metabolic derangements and medication intolerance, a broad differential diagnosis should be considered.

Elders with delirium suffer a higher risk of morbidity and mortality than do their nondelirious counterparts.[9,11,12,17,67–72] Therefore, with few exceptions, patients with delirium should be hospitalized. Discharge to home should be considered only when the etiology of the delirium is known and easily reversible. There must be adequate home supervision and support for the patient to follow care plans.

Dementia is the least acute syndrome of mental status impairment and carries a lower risk of short-term morbidity and mortality. It is impractical to carry out a complete workup for dementia in the ED. The length of the evaluation should be guided by the chief complaint, history, and physical examination findings. These are often unrelated to the dementia. Many of the tests for causes of dementia are appropriately deferred to the physician to whom the patient is referred. However, a relatively recent onset of symptoms may carry a higher risk for morbidity and should result in a more aggressive search. The differential diagnosis should be reviewed for potentially reversible causes when formulating a care plan for each patient.

Dementia is often not the deciding factor in determining the patient's disposition from the ED. However, special circumstances should be considered when formulating a care plan for the patient with dementia. The effect of cognitive impairment on treatment compliance should be considered. Hospitalization should be strongly considered for patients with high-risk illnesses who lack adequate home support to assist with treatment. Patients who are incapable of performing necessary self-care functions and present with excessively poor hygiene (such as the presence of urine or feces in clothing), dehydration, or malnutrition may need to be hospitalized. Family or caregiver frustration may lead to abuse. Patients with dementia and suspected abuse should be hospitalized for further evaluation.

Patients with psychiatric illness and agitation may require immediate restraint, both physical and chemical, before further diagnostic evaluation. Initiating treatment with small doses of a short-acting benzodiazepines, such as lorazepam 0.5 to 1 mg parenterally, with or without a dose of neuroleptic such as haloperidol 1 to 5 mg parenterally,[73] may be necessary. While elderly patients with psychotic symptoms respond to neuroleptics and sedation, they frequently will need a thorough investigation for organic causes and generally require admission to a medical inpatient service for further medical and psychiatric evaluation.

EMERGENCY DEPARTMENT COGNITIVE ASSESSMENT TOOLS

There are a number of brief screening tools that can be useful to the emergency physician when assessing mental impairment. The Confusion Assessment Method (CAM) by Inouye and colleagues[74] can be used to screen for delirium; it has been validated against structured psychiatric interviews and shows a sensitivity of 94 to 100 percent and a specificity of 90 to 95 percent for the detection of delirium.[74] It also has been shown to have a high interobserver reliability.[74] The CAM evaluates for the presence of four criteria to differentiate delirium from dementia (Fig. 39-1): acute onset and fluctuating course, inattention, disorganized thinking, and an altered level of alertness. The Orientation Memory Concentration Test (OMC)[76] may be used to screen for potential dementia. The OMC consists of six items (Fig. 39-2), and it can be administered easily in the ED in less than 2 minutes.[77] It is reliable, valid,[76] and has sensitivity for milder levels of impairment than the short portable mental status questionnaire.[78] The modified Koenig scale is a screening tool for depression that has been studied in the ED. It consists of 11 brief questions requiring yes/no

responses.[21] All these tests are easy to conduct and can be completed quickly in the ED (Fig. 39-3).

ADDITIONAL ASPECTS

Failure to recognize mental status impairment is a common problem in the emergency department.[7-10,79] This is one of several potential pitfalls to avoid when evaluating the elderly ED patient. The pace of the ED often results in the urge to focus narrowly on the chief complaint. However, given the high prevalence of mental status abnormalities in geriatric ED often patients,[7-10] emergency physicians should expect to encounter these conditions when evaluating elders in the ED. Subtle evidence of mental status impairment should not be ignored. Individuals in close contact with the patient should be interviewed for additional information about cognitive baseline status and any recent changes. Patients are often unaware of cognitive difficulties and may deny problems when asked.

Failure to appreciate the increased morbidity and mortality associated with delirium may result in suboptimal ED workup and inappropriate discharge to home. Patients with delirium require a thorough and aggressive search for underlying illness in the ED. Strong consideration should be given to hospitalizing these patients.[7,79] Discharge to home is seldom appropriate.[7]

There are several pitfalls unique to dementia as well. Patients may be unreliable historians, and important components of the medical history may be missed unless caregivers are interviewed. Dementia patients may also have difficulty understanding and complying with medical treatment, even for simple medical problems such as urinary tract infection. Misperceiving dementia as a medically untreatable and terminal process may result in a lack of referral for further evaluation and treatment.[80] In cases of progressive and degenerative dementia, such as Alzheimer's disease, interventions can be initiated that slow cognitive deterioration and delay institutionalization. Cholinesterase inhibitors have been effective in the treatment of many Alzheimer's patients.[81-83] Early psychosocial intervention also has been shown to postpone institutionalization.[84] In patients with multi-infarct dementia, secondary prevention of cerebral infarcts also may be effective in slowing the course.[85] With potentially reversible dementia, early recognition and referral have an even greater importance. There is a much greater chance of curing a reversible dementia early in the course of the disease, and deficits may become more permanent as the dementia progresses.[80]

1.   Is there evidence of an acute change in mental status from the patient's baseline?

Yes ☐   No ☐

2a.   Did the patient have difficulty focusing attention, i.e., being easily distractable or having difficulty keeping track of what was being said?

Yes ☐   No ☐

2b.   (If present or abnormal)   did this behavior fluctuate during the interview, that is, tend to come and go or increase and decrease in severity?

Yes ☐   No ☐

3.   Was the patient's thinking disorganized or incoherent, such as, rambling or irrelevant conversation, unclear or illogical flow of ideas, or unpredictable switching from subject to subject?

Yes ☐   No ☐

4.   Overall, how would you rate this patient's level of consciousness?

☐ Alert (normal)

☐ Vigilant (hyperalert, easily startled)

☐ Lethargic (drowsy, easily aroused)

☐ Stupor (difficult to arouse)

☐ Coma (unarousable)

Delirium

☐ Presence of delirium (presence of features 1 and 2 with either 3 or 4)

☐ Absence of delirium (not meeting above criteria)

REFERENCE:

Inouye SK, van Dyck CH, Alessi CA, et al. Clarifying Confusion: The confusion assessment method.

Annals of Internal Medicine. 1990;113:941-948.

Fig. 39-1   The Confusion Assessment Method (CAM) algorithm for delirium. *(Used with permission from Inouye et al.[74])*

	Maximum Error	Score		Weight		Total Score
What year is it now?	1	☐	X	4		☐
What month is it now?	1	☐	X	3		☐

Repeat this phrase after me: John Brown, 42 Market Street, Chicago

About what time is it?	1	☐	X	3		☐
Count backwards from 20 to 1	2	☐	X	2		☐
Say the months in reverse order	2	☐	X	2		☐
Repeat the memory phase	5	☐	X	2		☐

TOTAL WEIGHTED SCORE ☐

0-10 = minimal to no impairment

11-20 = moderate impairment

21 or more = severe impairment

REFERENCE:

Katzman R, Brown T, Fuld P, Peck A, et al. Validation of a short orientation-memory-concentration test of cognitive impairment. *American Journal of Psychiatry*. 1983;140:734-739.

Fig. 39-2   The Orientation-Memory-Concentration Examination for cognitive impairment. *(Used with permission from Katzman et al.[76])*

Are you often bored?	**Yes** No
Are you often restless and fidgety?	**Yes** No
Are you in good spirits?	Yes **No**
Do you have more problems with memory than most?	**Yes** No
Can you concentrate easily when reading the newspaper?	Yes **No**
Do you prefer to avoid social gatherings?	**Yes** No
Are you often downhearted and blue?	**Yes** No
Are you happy most of the time?	Yes **No**
Do you often feel helpless?	**Yes** No
Do you feel worthless and ashamed of yourself?	**Yes** No
Do you often wish you were dead?	**Yes** No

❑ Responses indicative of depression are boldfaced.

❑ A cutoff score of 4 is indicative of depression.

REFERENCE:

Meldon, SW, Emerman CL, Schubert DSP: Recognition of Depression in Geriatric ED patients by Emergency Physicians Ann Emerg Med 1997 30:442-447.

Fig. 39-3 Depression scale. *(Used with permission from Meldon et al.[21])*

When dementia is readily apparent, the emergency physician should not assume that the primary care provider has already evaluated the dementia. Hustey and Meldon[7] found that nearly 70 percent of patients with mental status impairment in the ED had no prior history of dementia. While family members may recognize that there is a significant memory problem, they may not have arranged for further evaluation, believing that there is nothing medically that can be done. Finally, the perception of dementia as an illness of lower acuity may result in an incomplete or superficial evaluation.[86]

Practitioners also must remember the role that important medications may play in causing psychiatric symptoms and other forms of mental status impairment. Polypharmacy is a common occurrence in the elderly,[87] and many drugs can significantly affect cerebral function through a variety of indirect and direct mechanisms. Examples of the psychiatric effects of medications include hallucinations and psychosis with propranolol,[88] psychosis and delirium with antiparkinsonian agents,[89], and psychosis, depression, and cognitive impairment with nonsteroidal anti-inflammatory medications.[90] In one study, prednisone was found to be the most frequent drug-related cause of moderate or severe psychiatric side effects.[91] Finally, the effects of substance abuse, due either to intoxication or to withdrawal, should not be overlooked.

REFERENCES

1. Larson EB, Kukall WA, Katzman RL: Cognitive impairment: Dementia and Alzheimer's disease. *Ann Rev Pub Health* 13:431, 1992.
2. Erkinjuntti T, Ostbye T, Steenhuis R, Hachinski V: The effect of different diagnostic criteria on the prevalence of dementia. *New Engl J Med* 337:1667, 1997.
3. Aguero-Torres H, Fratiglioni L, Winblad B: Natural history of Alzheimer's disease and other dementias: Review of the literature in the light of the findings from the Kungsholmen Project. *Int J Geriatr Psychiatry* 13:755, 1998.
4. Fillenbaum GG, Landerman LR, Simonsick EM: Equivalence of two screens of cognitive functioning: The Short Portable Mental Status Questionnaire and the Orientation-Memory-Concentration test. *J Am Geriatr Soc* 46(12):1512, 1998.
5. Gao S, Henrie HC, Hall KS, Hui S: The relationship between age, sex, and the incidence of dementia and Alzheimer disease: A meta-analysis. *Arch Gen Psychiatry* 55(9):809, 1998.
6. Evans DA, Funkenstein HH, Albert MS, et al: Prevalence of Alzheimer's disease in a community population of older persons: Higher than previously reported. *JAMA* 226:2551, 1989.
7. Hustey FM, Meldon SW: The prevalence and documentation of impaired mental status in elderly emergency department patients. *Ann Emerg Med* 39:248, 2002.
8. Naughton BJ, Moran MB, Kadah H, et al: Delirium and other cognitive impairment in older adults in an emergency department. *Ann Emerg Med* 25:751, 1995.
9. Lewis LM, Miller DK, Morley JE, et al: Unrecognized delirium in ED geriatric patients. *Am J Emerg Med* 13:142, 1995.
10. Elie M, Rousseau F, Cole M, et al: Prevalence and detection of delirium in elderly emergency department patients. *Can Med Assoc J* 163:877, 2000.
11. Inouye SK: Delirium in hospitalized older patients (review). *Clin Geriatr Med* 14(4):745, 1998.
12. Marcantonio ER, Flacker JM, Michael M, Resnick NM: Delirium is independently associated with poor functional recovery after hip fracture. *J Am Geriatr Soc* 48:618, 2000.
13. Marcantonio ER, Flacker JM, Wright RJ, Resnick NM: Reducing delirium after hip fracture: A randomized trial. *J Am Geriatr Soc* 49:516, 2001.
14. Edlund A, Lundstrom M, Brannstrom B, et al: Delirium before and after operation for femoral neck fracture. *J Am Geriatr Soc* 49:1335, 2001.
15. Lanska DJ: Dementia mortality in the United States: Results of the 1986 National Mortality Followback Survey. *Neurology* 50(2):362, 1998.
16. Braekhus A, Oksengard AR, Engedal K, Laake K: Social and depressive stress suffered by spouses of patients with mild dementia. *Scand J Primary Health* 16(4):242, 1998.
17. Inouye SK, Rushing JT, Foreman MD, et al: Does delirium contribute to poor hospital outcomes? A three-site epidemiologic study. *J Geriatr Intern Med* 13(4):234, 1998.
18. Dolan MM, Hawkes WG, Zimmerman SI, et al: Delirium on hospital admission in aged hip fracture patients: Prediction of mortality and 2-year functional outcomes. *J Gerontol Med Sci* 55(9):M527, 2000.
19. Edlund A, Lundstrom M, Brannstrom B, et al: Delirium before and after operation for femoral neck fracture. *J Am Geriatr Soc* 49:1335, 2001.
20. Holt J, Alexopoulos G: Depression and the aged, in Robinson R, Rabins P (eds): *Depression and Coexisting Disease.* New York, Igaku-Shoin Medical, 1989, p 10.
21. Meldon SW, Emerman CL, Schubert DSP: Recognition of depression in geriatric ED patients by emergency physicians. *Ann Emerg Med* 30:442, 1997.
22. Meldon SW, Emerman CL, Schubert DSP, et al: Depression in geriatric ED patients: Prevalence and recognition. *Ann Emerg Med* 30:141, 1997.
23. Fabacher DA, Raccio-Robak N, McErlean MA, et al: Validation of a brief screening tool to detect depression in elderly ED patients. *Am J Emerg Med* 20:99, 2002.
24. Department of Health and Human Services: *Healthy People 2000.* Washington, US Government Printing Office, 1990.
25. Rovner BW, German P, Brant LJ, et al: Depression and mortality in nursing homes. *JAMA* 265:993, 1991.
26. Bruce ML, Leaf PJ: Psychiatric disorders and 15 month mortality in a community sample of older adults. *Am J Public Health* 79:727, 1989.
27. Callahan CM, Hui SL, Nienaber NA, et al: Longitudinal study of depression and health services use among elderly primary care patients. *J Am Geriatr Soc* 42:833, 1994.
28. Bridge TP, Wyatt RJ: Paraphrenia: Paranoid states of late life: I. European research. *J Am Geriatr Soc* 28:193, 1980.
29. Bridge TP, Wyatt RJ: Paraphrenia: Paranoid states of late life: II, American research. *J Am Geriatr Soc* 28:201, 1980.
30. Jorm AF: *The Epidemiology of Alzheimer's Disease and Related Disorders.* London: Chapman and Hall, 1990, p 54.
31. Jorm AF, Koren AE, Jacomb PA: Projected increases in the number of dementia cases for 29 developed countries: Application of a new method for making projections. *Acta Psychiatr Scand* 78:493, 1988.
32. *Ten Reasons Why America Is Not Ready for the Coming of Age Boom.* Alliance for Aging Research, Washington, DC February 2002.
33. Flacker JM, Lipsitz LA: Neural mechanisms of delirium: Current hypotheses and evolving concepts. *J Gerontol* 54A(6):B239, 1999.
34. Elie M, Cole MG, Primeau FJ, et al: Delirium risk factors in elderly hospitalized patients. *J Gen Intern Med* 13(3):204, 1998.
35. Geldmacher DS, Whitehouse PJ: Current concepts: Evaluation of dementia. *New Engl J Med* 335:330, 1996.
36. Johnson JC, Sims R, Gottlieb G: Differential diagnosis of dementia, delirium and depression. *Drugs Aging* 5:431, 1994.
37. Van Crevel H, van Gool WA, Walstra GJ: Early diagnosis of dementia: Which tests are indicated? What are their costs? *J Neurol* 246:73, 1999.

38. Draper B, MacCuspie-Moore C, Brodaty H: Suicidal ideation and the wish to die in dementia patients: The role of depression. *Age Ageing* 27(4):503, 1998.

39. Mendez MF, Martin R, Smyth KA, Whitehouse PJ: Psychiatric symptoms associated with Alzheimer's disease. *J Neuropsychistr Clin Neurosci* 2:28, 1990.

40. Schneider LS: New therapeutic approaches to cognitive impairment. *J Clin Psychiatry* 11:8, 1998.

41. Trojanowski JQ, Lee VM-Y: Phosphorylation of neuronal cytoskeletal proteins in Alzheimer's disease and Lewy body dementias. *Ann NY Acad Sci* 747:92, 1994.

42. Murphy GM, Tamminga CA: Amyloid plaques (Images in Neuroscience). *Am J Psychiatry* 152:1258, 1995.

43. Small GW, Leiter F: Neuroimaging for diagnosis of dementia. *J Clin Psychiatry* 11:4, 1998.

44. Scheltens P: Early diagnosis of dementia: neuroimaging. *J Neurol* 246(1):16, 1999.

45. Kotsoris H, Barclay LL, Kheyfets S, et al: Urinary and gait disturbances as markers for early multi-infarct dementia. *Stroke* 18:138, 1987.

46. Chow TW, Miller BL, Hayashi VN, Geschwind DH: Inheritance of frontotemporal dementia. *Arch Neurol* 56(7):817, 1999.

47. Haupt M, Kurz A: Reversibility of dementia in hypothyroidism. *J Neurol* 240:333, 1993.

48. Adams RD, Victor M: *Principles of Neurology*, 5th ed. New York, McGraw Hill, 1993.

49. Teunisse S, Bollen AE, Gool WA, van Walstra GJM: Dementia and subnormal levels of vitamin B$_{12}$: Effects of replacement therapy on severity of dementia. *J Neurol* 243:522, 1996.

50. Chatterjee A, Yapundich R, Palmer CA, et al: Leukencephalopathy associated with cobalamin deficiency. *Neurology* 46:832, 1996.

51. Miller BL, Lesser IM, Mena I, et al: Regional cerebral blood flow in late life onset psychosis. *Neuropsychiatr Neuropsychol Behav Neurol* 5:132, 1992.

52. Baxter LR, Phelps ME, Mazziotta J, et al: Reduction of prefrontal cortex glucose metabolism common to three types of depression. *Arch Gen Psychiatry* 46:243, 1989.

53. Coffey CE, Figiel GS, Djang WT, et al: Subcortical hyperintensity on magnetic resonance imaging: A comparison of normal and depressed elderly subjects. *Am J Psychiatry* 147:187, 1990.

54. Nelson JC: Treatment of major depression in the elderly, in Nelson JC (ed): *In Geriatric Pharmacology*. New York, Marcel Dekker, 1998 p 61.

55. O'Keefe ST, Lavan JN: Clinical significance of delirium subtypes in older people. *Age Ageing* 28(2):115, 1999.

56. Huppert F, Wilcock G: Ageing, cognition and dementia. *Age Ageing* 4:20, 1997.

57. *Diagnostic and Statistical Manual of Mental Disorders,* 4th ed. Washington DC, American Psychiatric Association, 1994.

58. Salzman C: Mood disorders, in Coffey CE, Cummings JL (eds): The American Psychiatric Press textbook of *Geriatric Neuropsychiatry,* 2d ed. Washington DC, American Psychology Press, 2002, p 313.

59. Robert H, Rabins PV, Seeman MV, et al: Late onset schizophrenia and very late onset schizophrenia—Like psychosis: An international consensus. *Am J Psychiatry* 157:172, 2000.

60. Folstein MF, McHugh PR: Dementia syndrome of depression, in Katzman R, Terry RD, Birch KL (eds): *Alzheimer's Disease: Senile Dementia and Related Disorders.* New York, Raven Press, 1978, p 87.

61. Reichman WE: Nondegenerative dementing disorders, in Coffee CE, Cummings L (eds): The American Psychiatric textbook of *Geriatric Neuro-psychiatry,* 2d ed. Washington, American Psychiatric Press, 2000, p 491.

62. Marsh CM: Psychiatric presentations of medical illness. *Psychiatr Clin North Am* 20(1):181, 1997.

63. Cutting J: The phenomenology of acute organic psychosis: Comparison with acute schizophrenia. *Br J Psychiatry* 151:324, 1987.

64. Forster PL, Buckley R, Phelps MA: Phenomenology and treatment of psychotic disorders in the psychiatric emergency service. *Psychiatr Clin North Am* 22:735, 1999.

65. George AE, de Leon MJ, Golomb J, et al: Imaging the brain in dementia: Expensive and futile? *Am J Neuroradiol* 18:1847, 1997.

66. Copeland JR: Assessment of dementia. *Lancet* 351(9105):769, 1998.

67. Inouye SK, Bogardus ST, Charpenter PA, et al: A multicomponent intervention to prevent delirium hospitalized older patients. *New Engl J Med* 340:669, 1999.

68. Pompei P, Foreman M, Rudberg MA, et al: Delirium in hospitalized older persons: Outcome and predictors. *J Am Geriatr Soc* 42:809, 1994.

69. Murray AM, Levkoff SE, Wetle TT, et al: Acute delirium and functional decline in the hospitalized elderly patient. *J Gerontol* 48:M181, 1993.

70. Marcantonio ER, Goldman L, Mangione CM, et al: A clinical prediction rule for delirium after elective noncardiac surgery. *JAMA* 271:134, 1994.

71. Francis J, Martin D, Kapoor WN: A prospective study of delirium in hospitalized elderly. *JAMA* 263:1097, 1990.

72. Levkoff SE, Evans DA, Liptzin B, et al: Delirium: The occurrence and persistence of symptoms among elderly hospitalized patients. *Arch Intern Med* 152:334, 1992.

73. Foster S, Kessel J, Berman ME, et al: Efficacy of lorazepam and haloperidol for rapid tranquilization in a psychiatric emergency room setting. *Int Clin Psychopharmacol* 12:175, 1997.

74. Inouye SK, van Dyck CH, Alessi CA, et al: Clarifying confusion: The confusion assessment method. *Ann Intern Med* 113:941, 1990.

75. Pfeiffer E: A short portable mental status questionnaire for the assessment of organic brain deficit in elderly patients. *J Am Geriatr Soc* 23:433, 1975.

76. Katzman R, Brown T, Fuld P, et al: Validation of a Short Orientation-Memory-Concentration Test of cognitive impairment. *Am J Psychiatry* 140:734, 1983.

77. Gerson LW, Counsell SR, Fontanarosa PB, Smucker WD: Case finding of cognitive impairment in elderly emergency department patients. *Ann Emerg Med* 23(4):813, 1994.

78. Fillenbaum GG, Landerman LR, Simonsick EM: Equivalence of two screens of cognitive functioning: The Short Portable Mental Status Questionnaire and the Orientation-Memory-Concentration test. *J Am Geriatr Soc* 46(12):1512, 1998.

79. Sanders AB: Missed delirium in older emergency department patients: A quality-of-care problem. *Ann Emerg Med* 39:338, 2002.

80. Hustey FM: Dementia in the elderly: Avoiding the pitfalls. *Geriatr Emerg Med Rep* 1:13, 2000.

81. Knopman D, Schneider L, Davis K, et al: Long-term tacrine (Cognex) treatment: Effects on nursing home placement and mortality, Tacrine Study Group. *Neurology* 47:166, 1996.

82. Minthon L, Gustafson L, Dalfelt G, et al: Oral tetrahydroaminoacridine treatment of Alzheimer's disease evaluated clinically and by regional cerebral blood flow and EEG. *Dementia* 4:32, 1993.

83. Nordberg A, Lilja A, Lundqvist H, et al: Tacrine restores cholinergic nicotinic receptors and glucose metabolism in Alzheimer patients as visualized by positron emission tomography. *Neurobiol Aging* 13:747, 1992.

84. Schneider LS: New therapeutic approaches to cognitive impairment. *J Clin Psychiatry* 11:8, 1998.

85. Amar K, Wilcock G: Vascular dementia. *Br Med J* 312:227, 1996.

86. Birrer R, Singh U, Kumar DN: Disability and dementia in the emergency department. *Emerg Med Clin North Am* 17(2):505, 1999.

87. Williams P, Rush DR: Geriatric polypharmacy. *Hosp Pract* 21:109, 1986.

88. Fleminger R: Visual hallucinations and illusions with propranolol. *Br Med J* 1:1182, 1978.

89. Young BK, Camicioli R, Ganzini L: Neuropsychiatric adverse effects of antiparkinsonian drugs: Characteristics, evaluation and treatment (review). *Drugs Aging* 10:367, 1997.

90. Hoppmann RA, Peden JG, Ober K: Central nervous system side effects of non-steroidal anti-inflammatory drugs: Aseptic meningitis, psychosis and cognitive dysfunction. *Arch Intern Med* 151:1309, 1991.

91. Boston Collaborative Drug Surveillance Program: Psychiatric side effects of non-psychiatric drugs. *Semin Psychiatry* 3:406, 1971.

40

Headache in the Elderly

Richard A. Walker
Michael C. Wadman

HIGH-YIELD FACTS

- A low threshold for neuroimaging is justified because the diagnostic yield will be higher and 15 percent of elders with headache in the emergency department (ED) will have serious underlying pathology.

- Subarachnoid hemorrhage incidence increases with age and is highest in women over age 70.

- Computed tomographic (CT) scanning and lumbar puncture (LP) are required to rule out subarachnoid hemorrhage.

- Subdural hematoma and giant cell arteritis should be considered in the differential diagnosis of older patients with headache.

- Tumors may be quite larger before they become symptomatic in the shrunken brain of elder patients.

- Fever and headache should prompt evaluation for encephalitis, brain abscess, and meningitis.

- Acute-angle-closure glaucoma may present as headache and must be considered in older patients.

- Chronic headaches such as migraine, cluster, tension, and trigeminal neuralgia occur in elders and on occasion can be treated symptomatically without further evaluation.

Headache is a common complaint in the elderly. Emergency physicians likely will see an increasing number of older patients presenting to the emergency department (ED) with headache. Initial onset of headache after age 65 accounts for only 5.4 percent of headaches and is more common in women.[1-3] Tension headache is a diagnosis of exclusion but remains the most common diagnosis in elderly patients with a headache.[4] However, headaches sec-

Table 40-1. Serious Headaches (To Be Ruled Out in Elders)

Subarachnoid hemorrhage
Subdural hematoma
Stroke
Temporal arteritis
Tumor
Metabolic or toxic headache
Glaucoma
Brain abscess
Encephalitis
Meningitis

ondary to serious illness account for 15 percent of headaches in elderly patients as compared with only 1.6 percent in patients under age 65.[2] The 1-year headache prevalence rate of the whole U.S. population is 51 percent, with 44.5 percent being tension headaches and 11.0 percent migraines. Headache prevalence rates decrease with advanced age: 56.7 percent for ages 65 to 74 years, 45.2 percent for ages 75 to 84 years, and 26.1 percent for ages 85 to 96 years.[5]

This chapter discusses headaches caused by emergency conditions first, such as subarachnoid hemorrhage, subdural hematoma, giant cell arteritis, stroke, tremor, encephalitis, abscess, meningitis, glaucoma, and tumor, and then more benign headaches, such as migraine, cluster, tension, cervicogenic, trigeminal neuralgia, and medicinal (Table 40-1).

SUBARACHNOID HEMORRHAGE

Epidemiology

Of all patients with headache presenting to the ED, 1 to 4 percent will have subarachnoid hemorrhage (SAH).[6] Seventeen percent of ED patients with the "worst headache" of their life and a normal neurologic examination have SAH.[8] This increases to 25 percent in patients with focal neurologic examinations.[7] The highest incidence of SAH is in women over age 70.[8]

The rate of initial misdiagnosis may be as high as 38 percent for patients presenting with headache as the only symptom, with the most common misdiagnoses being viral meningitis, migraine, and headache of uncertain etiology.[9] Risk factors include smoking, excessive alcohol consumption, and hypertension.[10] The use of hormone-replacement therapy (HRT) after menopause decreases the risk of SAH.[11] First-degree relatives of patients with SAH have a three- to sevenfold increased risk of suffering the same disease.[12] Most SAHs occur in the morning and evening hours.[10]

Clinical Features

Patients who are able to give a history may have the classic complaint of a "sudden onset" of a "thunderclap" headache or the "worst headache" of their life. The headache begins during exertion in a minority of patients (21 percent). Symptoms may include nausea and vomiting in approximately 75 percent of patients, transient loss of consciousness in 36 percent, neck pain in 24 percent, coma in 17 percent, confusion in 16 percent, lethargy in 12 percent, and seizures in 7 percent.[13] Sentinel headaches result from minor SAH leaks that precede definitive diagnosis of SAH by days or weeks and are found in up to 40 percent of patients.[7] These are the patients who present with headache as their only symptom and a completely normal physical examination.[10]

On physical examination, nuchal rigidity may be present (35 to 52 percent[16,17]) or may take hours to develop.[14] Hypertension may be seen in 32 percent and even fever (>37.5°C) in 5 percent.[15] Only 36 percent have a normal level of consciousness, and 28 percent are somnolent or confused. Focal motor weakness is detected in 10 percent[13] and cranial nerve palsies (third and sixth) in 9 percent.[7]

Half of all SAHs have minor bleeding and present with subtle features. The headache may occur in any location, may be mild, may resolve spontaneously, or may be relieved by analgesics.[16] Prominent vomiting may lead to a misdiagnosis of viral syndrome, gastroenteritis, influenza, or viral meningitis. The presence of blood irritating the cervical or lumbar theca may lead to a misdiagnosis of cervical strain or sciatica.[6]

Only half of patients with sentinel headaches are diagnosed correctly. Misdiagnosis of SAH is most likely in the setting of a normal neurologic examination, yet these patients with a small SAH have the best treatment outcomes.[9] Six hundred patients each year could be saved if all patients were diagnosed at the time of initial presentation.[17]

Emergency Department Care and Disposition

Evaluation of patients with the "worst headache" of their life requires computed tomographic (CT) scan and lumbar puncture (LP).[12] CT scan without contrast material is the diagnostic method of choice in suspected SAH. Thin cuts (3 mm thick) are recommended to avoid missing small amounts of blood.[6] LP should be performed in all patients suspected of SAH when the CT scan is negative or inadequate.[18,19] LP occasionally results in a traumatic tap, leading to a misdiagnosis of SAH. Traumatic taps may occur in up to 14 to 20 percent[20,21] of LPs depending on the experience of the operator. Differentiation between a traumatic tap and SAH may be difficult.

Once the diagnosis of SAH is made, prompt neurosurgical consultation for definitive therapy should occur.

CHRONIC SUBDURAL HEMATOMA

Chronic subdural hematoma (CSH) is defined as a hematoma that is more than 20 days old. CSH has a peak incidence in the sixth and seventh decades, with 70 to 80 percent ocurring in elderly men. It may occur after minor trauma, especially falls, and usually does not have associated underlying brain injury. Bilateral subdural hematomas are more frequent in the elderly. Fragility of the bridging veins in the subdural space, as well as brain atrophy, allows for increased movement of the brain within the skull. Anticoagulant therapy is a predisposing factor.

Headache is present in up to 90 percent of patients, but it is mild and generalized. Diagnosis is easy when findings include lethargy, papilledema, and focal neurologic symptoms. CSH should be considered in any elderly patient who has headache, especially with an acute change in mental or functional status, including a worsening of a preexisting dementia or a personality change.[22–25] Diagnosis is made by non-contrast-enhanced CT scan, but with an isodense hematoma, a delayed contrast-enhanced CT scan or magnetic resonance imaging (MRI) may be needed for diagnosis.

GIANT CELL ARTERITIS

Giant cell arteritis (GCA), commonly referred to as *temporal arteritis,* is the most common vasculitis in elderly patients. The incidence of GCA increases after 50 years of age, peaking at 70 to 80 years, and is most common in white females.[26]

Clinical Features

Classic presenting signs and symptoms for GCA include headache with fever, jaw or tongue claudication, and visual symptoms. Headache, the most common symptom, is described as intermittent or continuous throbbing at the temporal or occipital region.[27] Headache occurs in approximately two-thirds of patients, and about half report painful chewing secondary to jaw claudication. Permanent loss of vision, the most feared consequence of this disease, occurs in up to 20 percent of GCA patients, often early in the course of the disease.[28] Physical examination may reveal thickening, tenderness, nodularity, or erythema of the frontal or parietal branches of the temporal arteries.[29] Meeting four criteria—age greater than 50 years; new-onset headache; tenderness or decreased pulse of a temporal artery; and an erythrocyte sedimentation rate (ESR) of greater than 50 mm/h—has a sensitivity of 94 percent and a specificity of 91 percent for GCA.[30]

Emergency Department Care and Disposition

Prompt diagnosis and treatment may prevent loss of vision but usually will not reverse vision loss once it occurs. Corticosteroids are the first line of treatment of GCA. Treatment should be undertaken with a rhuematology consultant involved.

STROKE

Many elderly patients presenting with headache are concerned about the possibility of stroke. Although headache is an uncommon symptom of cerebrovascular disease, it occurs in approximately 17 percent of ischemic stroke patients. A "premonitory headache" preceding the onset of the readily recognized neurologic manifestation of stroke occurs in 10 percent of ischemic stroke patients, suggesting the potential for early detection of ischemic stroke in patients with new-onset headache.[31]

The headache in occlusive cerebrovascular disease may result from a variety of proposed mechanisms. Theories suggest that pain is produced by the dilatation of cerebral vessel by embolus, dilatation of pain-sensitive collateral vessels, or irritation of vessel walls by the release of vasoactive substances.[31,32] The headache usually is described as unilateral or focal, but it may be more diffuse and nonspecific. The quality of pain is described as dull or throbbing, with the severity of pain ranging from mild to severe.[31,32] The most common associated symptom is vomiting.

TUMOR

The incidence of primary and metastatic tumors increases with age, making tumor an important diagnosis to consider in an elderly patient with a headache. In the general population, the most common symptom of intracranial mass lesion is headache. In the elderly, however, intracranial masses lead to the complaint of headache less frequently than in younger patients. Symptoms are less likely to be seen secondary to the loss of brain substance that occurs with aging.[33] Intracranial masses cause headache by traction on pain-sensitive intracranial structures such as the meninges or blood vessels and elevation of the intracranial pressure (ICP). Headache is more likely to occur if the mass involves the leptomeninges or infratentorial compartment, leading to obstruction of cerebrospinal fluid (CSF) outflow.[32] In the elderly, most brain tumors are metastatic (61 percent).[33]

Clinical Features

The classic "brain tumor headache" (severe morning headache that worsens with positional changes and is associated with nausea and vomiting) is seen in a minority of patients with intracranial mass,[34] and tumor headache presentation changes with advancing age. Headache, when present, is most commonly described as bifrontal, closely resembling the quality and character of tension headache in most patients. In an elderly patient presenting with symptoms of tension-type headache (TTH), some features may help differentiate intracranial mass headache from TTH, such as worsening with bending over or positional changes and nausea and vomiting.[34] Patients with a new intracranial mass and a prior history of headaches may present with pain similar to that of the preexisting headache disorder, thus highlighting the need to thoroughly evaluate the elderly patient who reports to the ED with headache.[32] Any suspicious headache or abnormality on neurologic examination warrants neuroimaging.[35]

ENCEPHALITIS

Encephalitis is a diffuse infection of the brain most often caused by viruses, particularly enteroviruses. The brain damage caused by encephalitis is the result of intracellular viral replication and the host's inflammatory response.[36] Herpes simplex virus type 1 (HSV-1) causes 95 percent of all herpetic encephalitis and is the most common cause of sporadic encephalitis.[36] Approximately 25 percent of patients recovering from encephalitis have a permanent neurologic deficit and have an overall mortality of 10 percent.[36]

Clinical Features

Initial symptoms include headache, fever, and drowsiness with a progression to focal neurologic deficits, seizures, and death.[36] The symptoms are similar to those of meningitis and may include nuchal rigidity.[37] LP usually will show a lymphocytic pleocytosis, but herpes simplex encephalitis may be associated with hemorrhagic CSF.[37] MRI is the initial imaging study of choice for suspected encephalitis.[36] Acyclovir is indicated for herpes simplex encephalitis, but there is no specific antiviral therapy available for other causes of viral encephalitis. Specific antimicrobial therapy should be used for the nonviral causes of encephalitis. Supportive care with management of increased ICP is essential[37].

BRAIN ABSCESS

A *brain abscess* is a focal suppurative process within the brain parenchyma. It is a rare condition, with 1500 to 2500 cases diagnosed in the United States per year and an incidence of 1.3 per 100,000 person-years. The majority of cases occur within the third and fourth decades of life and have a male-to-female ratio of 2 to 3:1.[42] Half of brain abscesses result from the contiguous spread of infection from adjacent sites, with sinusitis and otitis being the most common. Hematogenous spread occurs in 25 percent, most commonly in association with endocarditis and pulmonary infections. Penetrating injury of the brain and neuosurgical procedures are additional risk factors.[40,42]

Clinical Features

Clinical findings depend on the location of the abscess. Headache, fever, and focal neurologic deficit constitute the classic triad for the clinical presentation of brain abscess, but the specific combination is seen in less than 50 percent of patients.[38] Since fever may occur in less than 50 percent of patients, absence of fever should not be used to exclude the diagnosis.[39] Other findings may include an altered level of consciousness (10–100 percent), seizures (12.4–47 percent), nausea and vomiting (31–77 percent), papilledema (6.3–50 percent), and nuchal rigidity (11

Table 40-2. Neuroimaging in Elder Headache Patients

Order CT for
  Onset after age 60
  Mental status or personality change
  Papilledema
  Focal neurologic defect
  Posttraumatic
  Seizure
Consider CT for
  First or worst headache
  Increasing frequency, severity, or change in chronic headache
  Unusual, prolonged, or persistent headache
Consider MRI for
  Nondiagnostic CT with posterior symptoms
  Suspected subdural, mass, arterial dissection or encephalitis

percent).[38] Headache is by far the most common presenting symptom and is often described as a poorly localized, dull aching.[39]

Emergency Department Care and Disposition

Diagnosis is made by head CT scan or MRI[38] (Table 40-2), but differentiation between brain abscess and necrotic neoplasm can be difficult.[36] Laboratory investigation is not helpful because patients frequently have normal leukocyte counts. Also, the ESR, although usually elevated, may be normal.[39]

A combined medical and surgical approach is appropriate for most patients. Antibiotics should be administered promptly. A combination of vancomycin, metronidazole, and ceftriaxone is recommended in patients without immune suppression. Empirical therapy in the immunosuppressed patient is dictated by the specific immune defect. Surrounding edema associated with the abscess may be extensive,[36] and consideration should be given to administration of steroids.[38] Prophylactic anticonvulsants should be given to reduce the risk of seizures, which may occur in 90 percent of untreated patients.[38]

MENINGITIS

Elders are at a greater risk of meningitis than are younger patients, with up to 56 percent of community-acquired meningitis occurring in patients age 50 and older.[40] Meningitis has an incidence of 3.0 per 100,000 person-life years over age 65.[41] An increasing proportion of adult meningitis is nosocomial rather than community-acquired, with risk factors including recent neurosurgery, indwelling shunts, and impaired immunity.[42] Mortality increases with advancing age. The overall mortality for meningitis in all age groups is 18 percent,[43] whereas mortality rates are as high as 50 to 70 percent in the elderly.[40] This may be due to the debility of elderly patients, difficulty of and delay in diagnosis, and an increased mortality related to specific pathogens.[44]

Pathogens associated with bacterial meningitis in patients over age 60 include *Streptococcus pneumoniae, Listeria monocytogenes, Neisseria meningitidis,* group B *Streptococcus,* and *Hemophilus influenzae.*[42] *L. monocytogenes* should be considered as a pathogen in adults over age 50.[40] Viruses are the most common cause of aseptic meningitis, with enteroviruses causing 55 to 70 percent of all cases.[42] Some drugs also can cause an aseptic meningitis that resolves with removal of the offending agent. These include nonsteroidal anti-inflammatory drugs (NSAIDs), intravenous immunoglobulin, monoclonal antibody infusions, antibiotics (e.g., ciprofloxacin, isoniazid, metronidazole, penicillin, phenazopyridine, sulfonamides, and trimethoprim), carbamazepine, azathioprine, and cytosine arabinoside.[42]

Clinical Features

The classic triad for clinical diagnosis of meningitis is headache, fever, and nuchal rigidity. The headache is severe and often frontal or retroorbital. Associated symptoms can include photophobia, nausea, vomiting, drowsiness, and general malaise.[42] A review of physical findings in patients of all ages with meningitis found that Kernig's sign and Brudzinski's sign do not accurately discriminate between patients with and without meningitis.[45] In addition, nuchal rigidity may be present in up to 35 percent of patients over age 62 without meningitis.[46] In one review of meningitis, 97 percent of patients had a temperature greater than 37.7°C, 66 percent complained of headache, 56 percent were confused, 55 percent had nausea or vomiting, and 51 percent had a decreased level of consciousness.[43] The classic features of meningitis, such as headache, fever, and nuchal rigidity, may not be present in the elderly.

Emergency Department Care and Disposition

An LP should be performed in all cases of suspected meningitis. The CSF findings of aseptic meningitis include a mild to moderate mononuclear pleocytosis with a normal or slightly decreased glucose concentration and a mild to slightly increased protein concentration. Culture may be negative in up to 22 percent of cases of bacterial meningitis.[43] Gram stain of the CSF is positive 75 to 90 percent of the time if no antibiotics have been administered, but sensitivity is highly dependent on the specific organism that is causing the infection. False-positive results are rare (0.1 percent).[47]

Empirical therapy for bacterial meningitis is selected on the basis of the patient's age and health status. Ampicillin plus a third-generation cephalosporin is recommended as empirical therapy for patients over age 50.[37] Some authorities also recommend adding vancomycin in order to cover for the possibility of penicillin-resistant streptococci or *Staphylococcus aureus* in neurosurgical patients. Antibiotics should be administered when the diagnosis is considered prior to LP and while the patient is awaiting head CT scan. Mortality increases with delays in antibiotic administration. Most cases of aseptic meningitis require supportive care only.[37]

GLAUCOMA

Glaucoma is caused by increased intraocular pressure. Acute-angle-closure glaucoma (AACG) is abrupt in onset, painful, and may result in severe visual impairment if not treated quickly—a true ocular emergency. The prevalence of angle-closure glaucoma increases with age and is more common in elderly women than in men (3:1).[48] The incidence of glaucoma in Caucasian patients is 0.1 percent.[49] Aqueous humor is produced by the ciliary process at the periphery of the posterior chamber and passes through the pupil (between the lens and iris) to the anterior chamber, where it is filtered through the trabeculae at the margin of the anterior chamber. The fluid then drains into the canal of Schlemm. Obstruction to aqueous humor outflow is the basic underlying problem in glaucoma. In angle-closure glaucoma, the peripheral iris blocks the trabecular meshwork, obstructing the outflow of aqueous humor. This occurs more easily in persons whose eyes have shallow anterior chambers because the angle between the cornea and iris is reduced. Angle-closure glaucoma is usually precipitated by pupillary dilatation, which further increases contact between the iris and lens as the iris becomes thicker. When the angle between the peripheral iris and cornea becomes acutely closed, a precipitous increase in intraocular pressure can result.[50]

As people age, the lens becomes less elastic and thicker, cataracts develop, and the iris has greater contact with the lens, increasing the degree of pupillary block. Anything causing pupillary dilatation can trigger an acute attack. The use of topical or systemic parasympatholytic agents (mydriatics, antihistamines) or sympathomimetics (epinephrine, pseudoephedrine), dim illumination and emotionally upsetting events have all been implicated.[50]

Clinical Features

Patients complain of sudden onset of severe pain in the affected eye, which may be described as a headache. Associated symptoms include blurred vision, nausea, and vomiting. Examination reveals a fixed midposition pupil and a hazy (cloudy/steamy) cornea with conjunctival injection prominent at the limbus. Palpation will reveal a rock-hard globe on the affected side.[50] AACG may be misdiagnosed as migraine, temporal arteritis, subarachnoid hemorrhage, intraabdominal emergency, and even the exacerbation of dementia.[51,52]

Emergency Department Care and Disposition

The intraocular pressure should be measured to establish the diagnosis, although the presence of the characteristic symptom complex is diagnostic—a cloudy cornea, a fixed midposition pupil, and a rock-hard globe. There are various devices to measure intraocular pressure, including Schiotz tonometry, the tonopen, air-puff tonometry, Goldman applination tonometry using a slit lamp, and pneumatonometry, listed from least to most accurate. Normal intraocular pressure is 20 mmHg or less, but it may exceed 60 to 80 mmHg in an acute attack.

Treatment of AACG involves lowering the intraocular pressure by blocking production of aqueous humor (topical beta blockers and acetazolamide), facilitating outflow of aqueous humor (parasympathomimetic miotic agents, e.g., pilocarpine), and reducing the volume of vitreous humor (hyperosmotic agents, e.g., mannitol, glycerin and isosorbide). Definitive treatment is laser iridectomy.

Treatment should be undertaken with ophthalmologic consultation.

TOXIC AND METABOLIC HEADACHE

Carbon Monoxide Poisoning

Carbon monoxide (CO) poisoning may cause headache, dizziness, nausea, and vomiting. Multiple members of the same family may be diagnosed with a viral syndrome or gastroenteritis. In fact, CO poisoning may be underdiagnosed in 30 to 50 percent of poisoned patients on their initial visit to the ED.[53] CO poisoning should be suspected in patients presenting with headache and dizziness if they use gas stoves for heating purposes or have cohabitants with similar symptoms.[54] Patients with headache also should be questioned about faulty furnaces and indoor use of generators or charcoal grills. Elders may be living marginally or be unaware of these dangers. The headache has no characteristic pattern or location and is moderate in intensity. Other symptoms may include nausea, vomiting, dizziness, weakness, lethargy, confusion, photophobia, phonophobia, dyspnea, and blurred vision.[55]

Hypoxia and Hypercapnia

Chronically reduced partial pressure of oxygen with resulting carbon dioxide retention may be seen in chronic obstructive and restrictive lung disease, sleep apnea, and other extrapulmonary disorders. During sleep, hypoventilation exacerbates carbon dioxide retention, causing cerebral vasodilatation and occasionally increased ICP and papilledema. Symptoms of chronic respiratory insufficiency include headache, motor disturbances, and impaired cognition. The headache is described as intense, aching, frontal or occipital in location, and maximal on awakening from sleep.[56] Treatment is directed at the underlying cause.

Other Metabolic Disorders

Sodium nitrite found in meats may cause a headache similar to that caused by nitroglycerin. Monosodium glutamate may cause headache, tightness of the face, diarrhea, and abdominal cramps.[57] Electrolyte disturbances (particularly a low serum sodium level), hypothyroidism, hypocalcemia, and hypercalcemia may cause headache in the elderly.[58] The astute emergency physician should be alert to these possibilities after ruling out other serious causes of headache.

MIGRAINE

The prevalence of migrane over age 70 is 5 percent in females and 2 percent in males.[59] A peak prevalence of migraine affecting 30 percent of females and 10 percent males occurs at age 40, declining with advancing age. Onset is unusual after age 60, with an annual incidence of 2 percent.[60,61] More than half of lifetime migraine sufferers still have active disease past the age of 65, but of those whose headaches cease, most stop in the sixth decade.[62]

The pathophysiology of migraine is complex and, despite more than 50 years of study, is not completely understood. There is no unifying theory that can explain all the distinct phases of migraine: prodrome, aura, headache, headache termination, and postdrome. Several different theories have been proposed. In the vascular theory, migraine develops because of vasospasm at the periphery of the vasculature.[63] The trigeminal system is a vasodilator pathway that responds to activation by neuropeptides.[63] Perivascular neurogenic inflammation is also linked to the production of pain in migraine. What activates the trigeminovascular sytem remains unknown.

Clinical Features

There are several types of migraines. Common migraine occurs in an estimated 90 percent of migraine patients and is not preceded by any aura. The headache tends to be unilateral, is pulsating or throbbing in nature, and often is accompanied by nausea, vomiting, and photophobia. Classic migraine is similar clinically to common migraine, except that it is preceded by an aura.

A migraine attack consists of several phases: prodrome, aura, headache, headache termination, and postdrome.[64] The prodrome (experienced by 88 percent) consists of subtle premonitory symptoms occurring 1 to 2 days prior to the aura or the headache. The symptoms may be general (e.g., fatigue, dizziness, and aching muscles), stiff neck, changes in mood or behavior, neurologic (e.g., phonophobia, photophobia, and hyperesthesia), or gastrointestinal (e.g., food cravings and hunger).[65,66]

Migraine auras most commonly consist of disturbances of vision, but they may have almost any neurologic symptom. The aura precedes the headache and lasts between 1 and 30 minutes, with 30 minutes between the end of the aura and the start of the headache.[67] The headache of migraine is gradual in onset and may last a few hours to several days. The intensity varies and tends to worsen with physical activity. The character is most often described as aching or pressure-like in the initial phase and only later develops a throbbing quality. Termination of migraine attacks can occur with sleep and occasionally after vomiting, but most often the headache diminishes gradually over hours to days. A postdromal phase of fatigue, lethargy, or depression lasting up to several days occurs in the majority of patients.[68]

Rarely, migraine aura can be accompanied by hemiparesis, disturbance of vision, ataxia, dysarthria, vertigo, tinnitus, peripheral parasthesias, hearing loss, paresis of one or more ocular cranial nerves, and blindness. These symptoms and signs must be differentiated from stroke.

Emergency Department Care and Disposition

The routine use of neuroimaging is not indicated in the patient with recurrent migraine.[69] The yield of potentially treatable lesions discovered on CT scan and MRI of patients with migraine headache is low (0.3 and 0.4 percent, respectively).[70] However, arteriovenous malformations (AVMs) or stroke could cause a migraine-like headache.[71,72]

Most migraine patients present to the ED after their usual home regimen has failed.[73] Pharmacologic treatment of migraines is the mainstay of ED care. The drugs used can be grouped as dopamine antagonists (antiemetics), serotonin receptor agonists, opioids, NSAIDs, and combination therapy. Therapeutic options in the elderly are no different from those in younger patients, although several considerations, unique to this age group must be kept in mind. Older patients are more likely to have coexisting medical illnesses such as coronary artery disease, hypertension, cerebovascular disease, and peripheral vascular disease, which may be complicated by the use of vasoconstricting agents.[74] The antiemetic agents, while not causing vasoconstriction, are associated with extrapyramidal side effects in the elderly, including akinesthesia.[75] The elderly are more likely to experience side effects such as sedation and confusion from narcotics or impaired renal function from NSAIDs. Considering the frequency of cerebrovascular and cardiovascular disease in the elderly, a reasonable choice of initial drug therapy would be prochlorperazine or metoclopramide. Drug-drug interactions always must be kept in mind.[76] If adequate relief is not obtained, one could consider the use of NSAIDs or narcotics. Rarely will patients require admission for pain control.[77]

CLUSTER HEADACHE

Cluster headache (CH) is the most painful primary headache disorder. Recurrent attacks of severe unilateral headache occur at the same time of the day for several days. Periods of complete freedom from pain occur in most patients with cluster headache.[78]

Epidemiology

The age-adjusted incidence of cluster headache is 15.6 per 100,000 person-years in males and 4.0 per 100,000 person-years in females.[79] CH can begin at any age up to around age 70, and 1.4 percent of patients have onset of CH after age 60.[80] Peak incidence in males is between 40 and 49 years of age and in females between 60 and 69 years.[81]

Clinical Features

As with migraine, the same mechanisms are theorized to explaine the pathophysiology of CH. Trigeminal pathways may be involved because the pain tends to be centered around the eye and forehead. Autonomic features such as miosis and ptosis suggest dysfunction of the sympathetic system, whereas lacrimation and rhinorrhea implicate activation of the parasympathetic system.

Episodes of CH occur at least once every 24 hours for weeks at a time, with remissions lasting from weeks to years. Headache occurs at the same time of day, with nocturnal attacks more common.[82] The cluster period averages 6 to 12 weeks.[78] The headache is described as boring, tearing, or burning, like "a hot poker in the eye," and the pain is the most severe of all headache syndromes. It is strictly unilateral but can switch sides in subsequent cluster period (15 percent).[78] The headache lasts 45 to 90 minutes and occurs one to three times a day.[83] The headache localizes to ocular, frontal, and temporal areas.[81] In contradistinction to migraine, aura is rare, and the headache comes on without warning. Nausea occurs in 40 percent of patients, but vomiting is rare.[78] Depression, resulting from sleep deprivation, can lead to suicidal ideation.[78] The diagnosis is clinical made on the characteristic description of periodic headaches associated with autonomic symptoms and signs.[81]

Emergency Department Care and Disposition

High-flow oxygen (100%) delivered by nonrebreather mask gives relief to 70 percent of patients within 15 minutes.[83] Sumitriptan 6 mg subcutaneously has been shown to be effective in 76 to 100 percent of patients within 15 minutes but may not be advisable in older patients. Intravenous, intramuscular, or intranasal dihydroergotamine (DHE) may be effective but again may not be advisable in older patients. Olanzipine, a serotonin dopamine receptor antagonist and atypical antipsychotic, has been shown to reduce pain by 80 percent within 20 minutes. Often narcotics must be given in the ED. Preventative medication can be started in the ED. Preventative treatments include corticosteroids, verapamil, lithium, methysergide, valproic acid, toprimate, and melatonin.

TENSION-TYPE HEADACHE

Tension-type headache (TTH) is the most common headache in both the general population and the elderly, with a prevalence rate of 44.5 percent in patients older than age 65.[5] On average, the frequency of TTH is six per month. Emotional and physical stress and lack of sleep may trigger TTH, but these features lessen in importance with advancing age. They do not differentiate TTH from other headache syndromes.[84] TTH may last from 30 minutes to 7 days, with an average duration of 3 to 11 hours.[85]

Clinical Features

Some experts propose a common pathopysiologic mechanism for TTH and migraine. Physical examination may demonstrate pericranial myofacial tenderness in patients with TTH, but this clinical finding is also present with migraine.[86] TTH lacks nausea and vomiting and photophobia. TTH has at least two of the following: steady pressing or tightening pain, mild or moderate pain (not preventing daily activities), and bilateral distribution. The diagnosis of TTH requires the exclusion of other headache disorders, such as head trauma, vascular disorders, intracranial lesions, substances or medication use, infection, and structural abnormalities of the head and neck. The neurologic examination is normal.

Emergency Department Care and Disposition

Treatment of TTH in the elderly includes nonpharmacologic means such as stress management therapy.[87] The drugs of choice for the ED treatment of TTH are acetaminophen and NSAIDs. Avoid narcotics in the treatment of TTH because it is a chronic pain syndrome.[86] Patients with chronic symptoms may benefit from antidepressant medication.

CERVICOGENIC HEADACHE

The association between disorders of the neck and headaches is well known. Despite the lack of diagnostic criteria for cervicogenic headache, some authors assert that clinical features allow for adequate differentiation.[88,89] One specific disorder especially pertinent in the elderly headache patient is the cervical disk disease spondylosis, a degenerative change in the spine that is nearly universal with aging. While some studies of patients with radiographically diagnosed cervical spondylosis find a low incidence of headache,[90] other investigators report that headache accounts for the chief complaint in 40 percent of patients with symptomatic cervical disk disease and a major symptom in 25 percent.[91] Treatment strategies are similar to those for TTH.

TRIGEMINAL NEURALGIA

Trigeminal neuralgia, the most common neuralgia in the elderly, causes severe facial pain that may lead to a complaint of unilateral headache. The typical age of onset is 50 years, with a higher incidence in women.[32] Various lesions may lead to demyelination of the trigeminal nerve, including tumors, plaques of multiple sclerosis, and most commonly, tortuous blood vessels, which may account for the increasing incidence of this disorder in the elderly.[92]

Clinical Features

Typically a disease of the elderly, trigeminal neuralgia is characterized by brief, unilateral paroxysms of electric shock–like pain in the distribution of one or more of the branches of the trigeminal nerve, typically the maxillay (V_2) and/or mandibular (V_3) divisions. Other than finding trigger zones at the medial face (nose, lips, and gingivae), the neurologic examination is normal.

Emergency Department Care and Disposition

Drugs of choice for the treatment of trigeminal neuralgia include anticonvulsants such as carbamazepine, ox-carbazepine, phenytoin, gabapentin, and lamotrigine, as well as the muscle relaxant baclofen. Approximately 70 percent of patients respond to medical management within 2 to 3 days. Carbamazepine at an initial dose of 200 to 300 mg in divided doses is followed by titration to a target dose of 600 to 800 mg. A study finding intracranial tumors (most commonly meningiomas and posterior fossa tumors) in 10 percent of patients with trigeminal neuralgia, coupled with a normal neurologic examination in the majority of these patients, emphasizes the importance of close follow-up and possible neuroimaging studies.[93]

MEDICATION-INDUCED HEADACHE

In many elderly patients, the increased use of medications, both prescription and over-the-counter medications, represents an important and often overlooked cause of headache. Medication-induced headache (MIH) includes both headaches triggered by the use of certain drugs and those associated with the chronic use of analgesics. The drugs most frequently associated with headaches in elders are indomethacin and other NSAIDs, nifedipine, cimetidine, atenolol, trimethoprim-sulfamethoxazole, isosorbide dinitrate, ranitidine, captopril, metoprolol, and methyldopa.[94] Medication-withdrawal headaches, or rebound headaches, occur most often when patients stop using drugs for a chronic headache disorder, such as TTH or migraine. The medications involved most commonly are barbiturate-analgesic-caffiene combinations, codeine, opioids, caffeine, ergotamine, acetaminophen, aspirin, and NSAIDs. *Medication-withdrawal headache* is defined as daily or near-daily headache associated with change in use of syptomatic medications after frequent use, development of tolerance, symptoms of withdrawal, and improvement of headache following complete discontinuation.

Emergency Department Care and Disposition

If a drug is identified as triggering the headache, the treatment, if possible, is simply to discontinue its use. For medication-withdrawal headache, the recommendation is discontinuing the offending analgesics (in a tapered regimen if the headache involves barbiturates, opioids, or benzodiazepines), coupled with the use of another agent such as an NSAID (if not already overused) for symptomatic relief of worsening headache.[95]

CONCLUSION

Headache in the elderly must be considered a serious symptom and approached with full consideration of emergent causes. Many headache disorders are more prominent in older patients, but neuroimaging yields more lesions than in a younger population. Treatment is specific to underlying cause, and full evaluation is usually required in the ED.

REFERENCES

1. Solomon GD, Kunkel RS Jr, Frame J: Demographics of headache in elderly patients. *Headache* 30(5):273, 1990.
2. Pascual J, Berciano J: Experience in the diagnosis of headaches that start in elderly people. *J Neurol Neurosurg Psychiatry* 57(10):1255, 1994.
3. Cook NR, Evans DA, Funkenstein HH, et al: Correlates of headache in a population-based cohort of elderly. *Arch Neurol* 46(12):1338, 1989.
4. Serratrice G, Serbanesco F, Sambuc R: Epidemiology of headache in elderly: Correlations with life conditions and socioprofessional environment. *Headache* 25(2):85, 1985.
5. Prencipe M, Casini AR, Ferretti C, et al: Prevalence of headache in an elderly population: Attack frequency, disability, and use of medication. *J Neurol Neurosurg Psychiatry.* 70(3):377, 2001.
6. Edlow JA, Caplan LR: Avoiding pitfalls in the diagnosis of subarachnoid hemorrhage. *New Engl J Med.* 342(1):29, 2000.
7. Linn FH, Wijdicks EF, van der Graaf Y, et al: Prospective study of sentinel headache in aneurysmal subarachnoid haemorrhage. *Lancet* 344(8922):590, 1994.
8. Inagawa T, Yamamoto M, Kamiya K, Ogasawara H: Management of elderly patients with aneurysmal subarachnoid hemorrhage. *J Neurosurg* 69(3):332, 1988.
9. Mayer PL, Awad IA, Todor R, et al: Misdiagnosis of symptomatic cerebral aneurysm: Prevalence and correlation with outcome at four institutions. *Stroke* 27(9):1558, 1996.
10. Becker KJ: Epidemiology and clinical presentation of aneurysmal subarachnoid hemorrhage. *Neurosurg Clin North Am* 9(3):435, 1998.
11. Longstreth WT, Nelson LM, Koepsell TD, van Belle G: Subarachnoid hemorrhage and hormonal factors in women: A population-based case-control study. *Ann Intern Med* 121(3):168, 1994.
12. van Gijn J, Rinkel GJ: Subarachnoid haemorrhage: Diagnosis, causes and management. *Brain* 124(pt 2):249, 2001.
13. Fontanarosa PB: Recognition of subarachnoid hemorrhage. *Ann Emerg Med* 18(11):1199, 1989.
14. Vermeulen M: Subarachnoid haemorrhage: Diagnosis and treatment. *J Neurol* 243(7):496, 1996.
15. Racz P, Bobest M, Szilvassy I: Significance of fundal hemorrhage in predicting the state of the patient with ruptured intracranial aneurysm. *Ophthalmologica* 175(2):61, 1977.
16. Seymour JJ, Moscati RM, Jehle DV: Response of headaches to nonnarcotic analgesics resulting in missed intracranial hemorrhage. *Am J Emerg Med* 13(1):43, 1995.
17. Vannemreddy P, Nanda A, Kelley R, Baskaya MK: Delayed diagnosis of intracranial aneurysms: Confounding factors in clinical presentation and the influence of misdiagnosis on outcome. *South Med J* 94(11):1108, 2001.
18. Mayberg MR, Batjer HH, Dacey R, et al: Guidelines for the management of aneurysmal subarachnoid hemorrhage: A statement for health care professionals from a special writing group of the Stroke Council, American Heart Association. *Circulation* 90(5):2592, 1994.
19. van der Wee N, Rinkel GJ, Hasan D, van Gijn J: Detection of subarachnoid haemorrhage on early CT: Is lumbar puncture still needed after a negative scan? *J Neurol Neurosurg Psychiatry* 58(3):357, 1995.
20. Eskey CJ, Ogilvy CS: Fluoroscopy-guided lumbar puncture: Decreased frequency of traumatic tap and implications for the assessment of CT-negative acute subarachnoid hemorrhage. *AJNR* 22(3):571, 2001.
21. Xanthochromia. *Lancet* 2(8664):658, 1989.
22. Ellis GL: Subdural hematoma in the elderly. *Emerg Med Clin North Am* 8(2):281, 1990.
23. Traynelis VC: Chronic subdural hematoma in the elderly. *Clin Geriatr Med* 7(3):583, 1991.
24. Iantosca MR, Simon RH: Chronic subdural hematoma in adult and elderly patients. *Neurosurg Clin North Am* 11(3):447, 2000.
25. Adhiyaman V, Asghar M, Ganeshram KN: Chronic subdural haematoma in the elderly. *Postgrad Med J* 78(916):71, 2002.
26. Levine SM, Hellmann DB: Giant cell arteritis. *Curr Opin Rheumatol* 14(1):3, 2002.
27. Solomon S, Cappa KG. The headache of temporal arteritis. *J Am Geriatr Soc* 35(2):163, 1987.
28. Salvarani C, Cantini F, Boiardi L, Hunder GG: Polymyalgia rheumatica and giant-cell arteritis. *New Engl J Med.* 347(4):261, 2002.
29. Smetana GW, Shmerling RH: Does this patient have temporal arteritis? *JAMA* 287(1):92, 2002.
30. Hunder GG, Bloch DA, Michel BA, et al: The American College of Rheumatology 1990 criteria for the classification of giant cell arteritis. *Arthritis Rheum* 33(8):1122, 1990.
31. Gorelick PB, Hier DB, Caplan LR, et al: Headache in acute cerebrovascular disease. *Neurology* 36(11):1445, 1986.
32. Dodick DW, Capobianco DJ: Headaches, In Sirven JI, malamut BL (eds): *Clinical Neurology of the Older Adult.* Philadelphia, Lippincott Williams & Wilkins, 2002, p 176.
33. Blumenthal DT, Posner JB: Intracranial neoplasms in the elderly, in Hazzard WR, Blass JP, Ettinger WH, Halter JB, Ouslander JG (eds): *Principles of Geriatric Medicine and Gerontology,* 4th ed. New York, McGraw-Hill, 1999, p 1323.

34. Forsyth PA, Posner JB: Headaches in patients with brain tumors: A study of 111 patients. *Neurology* 43(9):1678, 1993.

35. Ramirez-Lassepas M, Espinosa CE, Cicero JJ, et al: Predictors of intracranial pathologic findings in patients who seek emergency care because of headache. *Arch Neurol* 54(12):1506, 1997.

36. Falcone S, Post MJ: Encephalitis, cerebritis, and brain abscess: Pathophysiology and imaging findings. *Neuroimag Clin North Am* 10(2):333, 2000.

37. Townsend GC, Scheld WM: Infections of the central nervous system. *Adv Intern Med* 43:403, 1998.

38. Calfee DP, Wispelwey B: Brain abscess. *Semin Neurol* 20(3):353, 2000.

39. Mathisen GE, Johnson JP: Brain abscess. *Clin Infect Dis* 25(4):763, 1997.

40. Yoshikawa TT, Norman DC: Treatment of infections in elderly patients. *Med Clin North Am* 79(3):651, 1995.

41. Walling AD, Kallail KJ, Phillips D, Rice RB: The epidemiology of bacterial meningitis. *J Am Board Fam Pract* 4(5):307, 1991.

42. Coyle PK: Overview of acute and chronic meningitis. *Neurol Clin* 17(4):691, 1999.

43. Hussein AS, Shafran SD: Acute bacterial meningitis in adults: A 12-year review. *Medicine* 79(6):360, 2000.

44. Berk SL, Smith JK: Infectious diseases in the elderly. *Med Clin North Am* 67(2):273, 1983.

45. Thomas KE, Hasbun R, Jekel J, Quagliarello VJ: The diagnostic accuracy of Kernig's sign, Brudzinski's sign, and nuchal rigidity in adults with suspected meningitis. *Clin Infect Dis* 35(1):46, 2002.

46. Puxty JA, Fox RA, Horan MA: The frequency of physical signs usually attributed to meningeal irritation in elderly patients. *J Am Geriatr Soc* 31(10):590, 1983.

47. Thomson RB Jr, Bertram H: Laboratory diagnosis of central nervous system infections. *Infect Dis Clin North Am* 15(4):1047, 2001.

48. Morgan A, Hemphill RR: Acute visual change. *Emerg Med Clin North Am* 16(4):825, 1998.

49. Kranemann CF, Buys YM: Acute angle-closure glaucoma in giant cell arteritis. *Can J Ophthalmol* 32(6):389, 1997.

50. Bertolini J, Pelucio M: The red eye. *Emerg Med Clin North Am* 13(3):561, 1995.

51. Dayan M, Turner B, McGhee C: Acute angle closure glaucoma masquerading as systemic illness. *B Med J* 313(7054):413, 1996.

52. Siriwardena D, Arora AK, Fraser SG, et al: Misdiagnosis of acute angle closure glaucoma. *Age Ageing* 25(6):421, 1996.

53. Hampson NB: Emergency department visits for carbon monoxide poisoning in the Pacific Northwest. *J Emerg Med* 16(5):695, 1998.

54. Heckerling PS, Leikin JB, Maturen A, Perkins JT: Predictors of occult carbon monoxide poisoning in patients with headache and dizziness. *Ann Intern Med* 107(2):174, 1987.

55. Hampson NB, Hampson LA: Characteristics of headache associated with acute carbon monoxide poisoning. *Headache* 42(3):220, 2002.

56. Kirsch DB, Jozefowicz RF: Neurologic complications of respiratory disease. *Neurol Clin* 20(1):247, 2002.

57. Sands GH, Newman L, Lipton R: Cough, exertional, and other miscellaneous headaches. *Med Clin North Am* 75(3):733, 1991.

58. Poser CM: The types of headache that affect the elderly. *Geriatrics* 31(9):103, 1976.

59. Lipton RB, Pfeffer D, Newman LC, Solomon S: Headaches in the elderly. *J Pain Sympt Manag* 8(2):87, 1993.

60. Selby G, Lance J: Observations on 500 cases of migraine and allied vascular disease. *J Neurol Neurosurg Psychiatry* 23:23, 1960.

61. Stang PE, Yanagihara PA, Swanson JW, et al: Incidence of migraine headache: A population-based study in Olmsted County, Minnesota. *Neurology* 42(9):1657, 1992.

62. Wang SJ, Liu HC, Fuh JL, et al: Prevalence of headaches in a Chinese elderly population in Kinmen: Age and gender effect and cross-cultural comparisons. *Neurology* 49(1):195, 1997.

63. Edvinsson L: Aspects on the pathophysiology of migraine and cluster headache. *Pharmacol Toxicol* 89(2):65, 2001.

64. Blau J: *Migraine: Clinical and Research Aspects.* Baltimore, Johns Hopkins University Press, 1987.

65. Amery WK, Waelkens J, Vandenbergh V: Migraine warnings. *Headache* 26(2):60, 1986.

66. Blau JN: Migraine prodromes separated from the aura: complete migraine. *Br Med J* 281(6241):658, 1980.

67. Queiroz LP, Rapoport AM, Weeks RE, et al: Characteristics of migraine visual aura. *Headache* 37(3):137, 1997.

68. Davidoff RA: *Migraine: Manifestations, Pathogenesis and Management,* Vol 65, 2d ed. Contemporary Neurology Series 0069-9446. New York, Oxford University Press, 2002.

69. Practice parameter: The utility of neuroimaging in the evaluation of headache in patients with normal neurologic examinations (summary statement). Report of the Quality Standards Subcommittee of the American Academy of Neurology. *Neurology* 44(7):1353, 1994.

70. Evans RW: Diagnostic testing for headache. *Med Clin North Am* 85(4):865, 2001.

71. Frishberg BM: Neuroimaging in presumed primary headache disorders. *Semin Neurol* 17(4):373, 1997.

72. Kupersmith MJ, Vargas ME, Yashar A, et al: Occipital arteriovenous malformations: Visual disturbances and presentation. *Neurology* 46(4):953, 1996.

73. Edmeads J: Emergency management of headache. *Headache* 28(10):675, 1988.

74. Galer BS, Lipton RB, Solomon S, et al: Myocardial ischemia related to ergot alkaloids: A case report and literature review. *Headache* 31(7):446, 1991.

75. Bateman DN, Rawlins MD, Simpson JM: Extrapyramidal reactions with metoclopramide. *Br Med J* 291(6500):930, 1985.

76. Hohl CM, Dankoff J, Colacone A, Afilalo M: Polypharmacy, adverse drug-related events, and potential adverse drug interactions in elderly patients presenting to an emergency department. *Ann Emerg Med* 38(6):666, 2001.

77. Innes G, Macphail I, Dillon E, et al: Dexamethasone prevents relapse after emergency department treatment of acute

migraine: a randomized clinical trial. *Can J Emerg Med* 1(1):26, 1999.

78. Dodick DW, Rozen TD, Goadsby PJ, Silberstein SD: Cluster headache. *Cephalalgia* 20(9):787, 2000.

79. Swanson JW, Yanagihara T, Stang PE, et al: Incidence of cluster headaches: A population-based study in Olmsted County, Minnesota. *Neurology* 44(3 pt 1):433, 1994.

80. Ekbom K, Svensson DA, Träff H, Waldenlind E: Age at onset and sex ratio in cluster headache: Observations over three decades. *Cephalalgia* 22(2):94, 2002.

81. Zakrzewska JM: Cluster headache: Review of the literature. *Br J Oral Maxillofac Surg* 39(2):103, 2001.

82. Mathew NT: Cluster headache. *Neurology* 42(3 suppl 2):22, 1992.

83. Dodick DW, Capobianco DJ: Treatment and management of cluster headache. *Curr Pain Headache Rep* 5(1):83, 2001.

84. Smetana GW: The diagnostic value of historical features in primary headache syndromes: A comprehensive review. *Arch Intern Med* 160(18):2729, 2000.

85. Iversen HK, Langemark M, Andersson PG, et al: Clinical characteristics of migraine and episodic tension-type headache in relation to old and new diagnostic criteria. *Headache* 30(8):514, 1990.

86. Jensen R, Olesen J: Tension-type headache: An update on mechanisms and treatment. *Curr Opin Neurol* 13(3):285, 2000.

87. Holroyd KA, O'Donnell FJ, Stensland M, et al: Management of chronic tension-type headache with tricyclic antidepressant medication, stress management therapy, and their combination: A randomized controlled trial. *JAMA* 285(17):2208, 2001.

88. Headache Classification Committee of the International Headache Society: Classification and diagnostic criteria for headache disorders, cranial neuralgias and facial pain. *Cephalalgia* 8(suppl 7):1, 1988.

89. Vincent MB, Luna RA: Cervicogenic headache: A comparison with migraine and tension-type headache. *Cephalalgia* 19(suppl 25):11, 1999.

90. Iansek R, Heywood J, Karnaghan J, Balla JI: Cervical spondylosis and headaches. *Clin Exp Neurol* 23:175, 1987.

91. Edmeads J: The cervical spine and headache. *Neurology* 38(12):1874, 1988.

92. Love S, Coakham HB: Trigeminal neuralgia: Pathology and pathogenesis. *Brain* 124(pt 12):2347, 2001.

93. Cheng TM, Cascino TL, Onofrio BM: Comprehensive study of diagnosis and treatment of trigeminal neuralgia secondary to tumors. *Neurology* 43(11):2298, 1993.

94. Askmark H, Lundberg PO, Olsson S: Drug-related headache. *Headache* 29(7):441, 1989.

95. Zed PJ, Loewen PS, Robinson G: Medication-induced headache: Overview and systematic review of therapeutic approaches. *Ann Pharmacother* 33(1):61, 1999.

41

Stroke

Melissa Ann Eirich

HIGH-YIELD FACTS

- Subtle and varied symptoms occur during stroke, and these may not be reported by the patient. History from family and friends is often essential.
- Distinguishing an ischemic stroke from a hemorrhagic stroke is the primary determinant in forming a therapeutic plan and requires computed tomographic (CT) scanning or magnetic resonance imaging (MRI).
- Treating stroke with thrombolytic therapy requires adherence to strict inclusion and exclusion criteria with a relatively short window of time to intervene after the onset of symptoms.
- Controlling hypertension is important to allow thrombolytics therapy but remains controversial, especially in the management of hemorrhagic strokes.

Stroke is the third leading cause of death in the United States, killing almost 160,000 Americans yearly.[1,2] The impact of stroke is monumental in the United States. Approximately 750,000 strokes occur each year, costing an estimated $30 billion annually.[2] Stroke is one of the leading causes of disability in adults, and more than 4 million Americans are living with the effects of strokes.[1] With the aging of the U.S. population, these figures are expected to increase dramatically, making efforts to decrease the morbidity and mortality of strokes essential to the health of our population.

A twofold approach is underway to address stroke—risk reduction and acute intervention. Educating both health care practitioners and patients on the need to modify risk factors is one part of this effort. Smoking cessation, avoiding obesity, and exercise are being promoted to all age groups. Maximizing medical management of diabetes, atrial fibrillation, hypertension, coagulopathy,

atherosclerosis, and vascular disease is part of the effort to decrease the risk of strokes.[1,2] Prompt recognition and treatment of stroke are the second part of this approach. Public education is needed to prevent delays in seeking medical care after onset of stroke symptoms. Eventually, early treatment may have a tremendous impact, but there is a relatively narrow window of time for treatment.[2]

The medical management of stroke has been revolutionized in the last decade. The old "wait and see" attitude has been changed dramatically by the introduction of thrombolytic therapy. The American College of Emergency Physicians (ACEP), the American Heart Association (AHA), the National Stoke Association (NSA), and other agencies have all adopted similar guidelines for management of stroke.[1–5] These guidelines focus on rapid assessment, diagnosis, and management. The message has been codified into the maxim that "time is brain." This approach is being incorporated in many prehospital and emergency department (ED) care systems. The ultimate goal of early intervention is not only to prevent further insult to the cerebral tissue but to actually reverse ischemic damage by early reperfusion.

PATHOPHYSIOLOGY

Strokes are caused by one of many pathologic processes involving blood flow to the brain. The cause may be an intrinsic blood vessel problem, such as atherosclerosis, inflammation, or dissection. The cause can originate remotely and arrive as an embolus. Strokes also can be caused by a rupture of a cerebral vessel into the subarachnoid space or into tissue. They can be caused by decreased cerebral blood flow. A stroke can be caused by any vascular process that leads to acute neurologic injury, brain infarction, or hemorrhage. Ischemic cerebral infarction is responsible for approximately 80 percent of strokes, and the remaining 20 percent are hemorrhagic.[2,6]

Symptoms of stroke are myriad, including a sudden onset of any of the following: numbness or weakness of face, arm, or leg; confusion; trouble speaking or understanding; trouble seeing; difficulty walking; loss of balance or coordination; severe headache; or a sudden decline in the level of consciousness. Since the brain has specific functional areas, the location of the stroke usually can be correlated clinically with the presenting stroke syndrome (Table 41-1). Anterior strokes have findings limited to one side of the body, whereas posterior strokes can have crossed deficits. However, symptoms that cross the midline at the same central nervous system (CNS) level (e.g., a patient unable to move both legs only) or are inconsis-

Table 41-1. Common Major Stroke Syndromes

Anterior cerebral artery
- Paralysis of opposite lower limb and mild upper limb weakness
- Sensory deficits that parallel motor deficits
- Confusion/impaired judgment
- Gait apraxia
- Incontinence

Middle cerebral artery
- Paralysis of opposite side of body (arm and face worse than leg)
- Sensory deficits that parallel motor deficits
- Ipsilateral hemianopsia (blindness in half of visual field)
- Dysphagia
- Visual agnosia (unable to recognize objects)
- Aphasia

Posterior cerebral artery
- Homonymous hemianopsia
- CN III paralysis
- Visual agnosia
- Confusion and impaired memory
- Cortical blindness

Vertebrobasilar artery system
- Dysphagia and dysarthria
- Facial numbness
- Vertigo
- Syncope
- Contralateral loss of pain and temperature sensation
- Diplopia and visual field deficits

Table 41-2. Differential Diagnosis for Stroke

Ischemic stroke
Hemorrhagic stroke
Trauma (cranial, neck, or spinal)
Cerebral artery disection
Intracranial mass
    Subdural/epidural hematoma
    Brain abscess
    Tumor
Seizure with postictal paralyisis
Hypoglycemia
Complicated migraine
Hypertensive encephalopathy
Encephalitis/meningitis
Toxicologic
Myxedema coma
Shock and CNS hypoperfusion
Giant cell arteritis
Wernicke's encephalopathy
Meniere's/labyrinthitis
Dementia
Gullian-Barré syndrome
Psychiatric syndromes

tent with cerebral anatomy should raise the suspicion that a process other than stroke is involved (Table 41-2).

A transient ischemic attack (TIA) is a transient focal neurologic dysfunction due to ischemia. As with a stroke, the symptoms have a sudden onset and are myriad, but TIA symptoms resolve completely within 24 hours. Most patients with TIA have at least partial resolution of symptoms within 1 hour of onset. Once a patient has a TIA, his or her risk of a serious stroke within 1 year is approximately 10 to 20 percent, and the risk within 1 month is 2 to 5 percent.[2,7] Since a TIA is due to focal ischemia, the symptoms reflect the stroke syndromes. Three or more TIAs in 72 hours is termed *crescendo TIAs.* This presentation needs aggressive evaluation because of an even higher risk of a subsequent stroke.

There are multiple factors associated with an increased risk of ischemic stroke. Age, gender (male), race (African-American), and family history are all risk factors. Potentially modifiable risk factors include hypertension, diabetes, hyperlipidemia, coronary artery disease, atrial fibrillation, tobacco use, drug abuse, oral contraceptive use, pregnancy, and migraines.

The incidence of aneurysmal subarachnoid hemorrhage (SAH) increases with age from 1.5 to 2.5 per 100,000 person-years in the third decade of life to 40 to 78 per 100,000 person-years in the eighth decade of life.[8] SAH is more common in women than in men, with the age-adjusted rate 43 percent higher for women.[9] The incidence varies according to the geographic and ethnic group studied, with African-Americans having a twofold greater incidence than Caucasians.[10] SAH is the most common cause of sudden death due to stroke, with an overall mortality of 25 percent and significant morbidity among 50 percent of survivors.[11,12]

Diminished blood flow, ischemia, causes a time-dependent cellular cascade that is characterized by decreased energy production; overstimulation of glutamate receptors; increased intraneuronal sodium, calcium, and chloride ions; mitochondrial injury; and eventually, cell death[13] (Fig. 41-1). Studies have shown that a stroke pro-

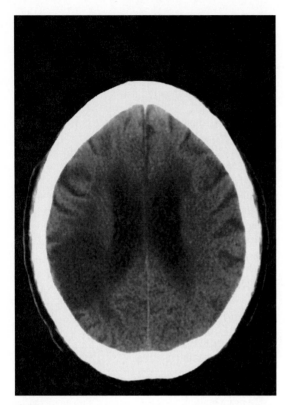

Fig. 41-1 Old CVA. Non-contrast-enhanced CT scan showing an old right-sided infract.

duces a core of infarcted brain tissue surrounded by a border zone of hypoxic but potentially salvageable tissue, the *ischemic penumbra*.[7,13] The goal of therapy is to restore normal blood flow as soon as possible, prevent damage in the ischemic penumbra, and reverse as much damage as possible in the infarct area.

The cause of SAH is a ruptured saccular aneurysm in 85 percent of patients. Other causes include arterial dissection, cerebral or cervical arteriovenous malformation, aneurysms of spinal arteries, cerebral artery metastasis of cardiac myxoma, septic aneurysm, and anticoagulant use.[14] The prevalence of intracranial aneurysms is greater than the incidence of SAH. The prevalence rate ranges from 1 to 6.5 percent, with an annual incidence of rupture from 1.4 to 2.3 percent. Risk of rupture increases with the size of an aneurysm and the presence of multiple aneurysms. The majority of aneurysms occur in the anterior circulation.[15] There is a genetic predisposition to aneurysmal rupture. Between 5 and 20 percent of patients with SAH have a positive family history. There are familial associations between aneurysms and polycystic

kidney disease, Marfan's syndrome, coarctation of the aorta, pseudoxanthoma elasticum, Ehler-Danlos syndrome, and other disorders of collagen.[15]

CLINICAL FEATURES

While time is of the essence, a thorough history and examination must be done on the patient with a suspected stroke. The National Institute of Neurological Disorders and Stroke (NINDS) has recommended a time line for ED evaluation of the stroke patient.[5] (Table 41-3). NINDS has set the goal of 10 minutes from ED arrival to physician contact and 25 minutes from arrival to completion of a computed tomographic (CT) scan. With this goal in mind, CT scans may need to be ordered before a complete assessment can be done.

History

Ischemic cerebral infarction usually presents as a sudden, well-defined focal deficit. However, strokes usually have an acute onset. While progression of symptoms does happen over the first few hours in approximately 10 to 20 percent of patients, a gradual onset of symptoms over days is unusual.[2] A common history is that of a patient waking with new neurologic symptoms.

The strict criteria for stroke therapy require a precise history, particularly of symptom onset. Since the symptoms may include confusion or difficulty communicating, witness accounts of the onset and progression of symptoms are important. When the time of onset is difficult to obtain, onset is defined as the last time the patient had a normal or baseline neurologic appearance. Thus a patient

Table 41-3. NINIDS Targets for Possible Fibrinolytic Therapy

ED Action	Time Target
Door to doctor	10 min
Door to CT completion	25 min
Door to CT read	45 min
Door to treatment	60 min
Access to neurologic consult*	15 min
Access to neurosurgical consult*	2 h
Admission to monitored bed	3 h

*In person or by phone.
Source: From Association AH: Guidelines 2000 for cardiopulmonary resuscitation and emergency cardiovascular care. *Circulation* 102 suppl (8):186–89, 2000.

who wakens with a neurologic deficit has an onset time of when he or she was last known to be asymptomatic.[16]

It is important to determine the baseline neurologic function of the patient in order to determine what symptoms are new. A routine past medical and surgical history, as well as a history of current medication use, should be obtained. Also important is any history of recent trauma, headache, seizures, infection, drug abuse, over-the-counter medication use, and use of herbal remedies. While many stroke patients complain of headache, a severe headache is more common with hemorrhagic stroke. Any history of previous stroke, particularly hemorrhagic stroke, seizure, recent major surgery, recent gastrointestinal or urinary tract hemorrhage, or recent arterial puncture (at a noncompressible site) may exclude patients from receiving thrombolytic therapy.

Physical Examination

Initial Assessment and General Examination

As with all ED patients, a primary survey is essential, and any immediately life-threatening problems should be addressed prior to obtaining a complete history or examination. Vital signs, including pulse oxigenation and Glasgow Coma Scale score, should be obtained and repeated frequently. The patient should be given oxygen by nasal prongs and placed on a cardiac monitor. Hyper- or hy-

potension should be monitored closely. Intravenous access and a bedside glucose determination should be obtained.

On secondary survey, the head and neck should be examined for any signs of trauma or meningismus. The cardiovascular examination should include auscultation of the carotids for bruits and the heart for arrhythmias or murmurs. The carotid and peripheral pulses should be evaluated. A routine examination of the lungs and abdomen should be done.

Neurologic Examination

The neurologic examination should be based on the National Institutes of Health Stroke Scale (Table 41-4). The Cincinnati Prehospital Stroke Scale (Table 41-5) can be used as a screening examination. However, a more complete emergency physician evaluation is necessary.

Mental Status

Since the term *mental status change* is nonspecific and nonmeasurable, the exact deficits should be described. Range of consciousness can vary from alert, somnolent (sleepy but easily aroused), stuporous (incomplete arousal but responds to noxious stimuli), to comatose (does not respond to noxious stimuli).[16] Most ischemic

Table 41-4. National Institutes of Health Stroke Scale

Level of consciousness	0–3 points	Normal to coma
Orientation:		
Two commands	0–2 points	Both to neither correct
Two questions	0–2 points	Both to neither correct
Eye movements	0–2 points	Normal to tonic gaze palsy
Visual fields	0–3 points	Normal to bilateral visual loss
Facial motor activity	0–3 points	Normal to bilateral weakness
Upper extremity motor:		
Right	0–4 points	Normal to no movement
Left	0–4 points	Normal to no movement
Lower extremity motor:		
Right	0–4 points	Normal to no movement
Left	0–4 points	Normal to no movement
Limb ataxia	0–2 points	Normal to two limbs ataxic
Sensory	0–2 points	Normal to severe sensory loss
Articulation	0–2 points	Normal to unintelligible speech
Language	0–3 points	Normal to none
Neglect	0–2 points	Absent to present (in two modalities)

Source: From Brott et al.[1]

Table 41-5. The Cincinnati Prehospital Stroke Scale

Facial droop (have patient smile or show teeth)
  Normal—symmetric movement
  Abnormal—asymmetric movement
Arm drift (patient closes eyes and holds both arms straight out with palms up for 10 seconds)
  Normal—both arms do not move *or* both arms move symmetrically
  Abnormal—one arm drifts down compared with other
Abnormal speech (have the patient say "you can't teach an old dog new tricks")
  Normal—uses correct words with no slurring
  Abnormal—slurring of words, uses wrong words, or is unable to speak
Interpretation: If any one of these three signs is abnormal, the probability of a stroke is 72 percent.

Source: From Kothari R, Hall K, Brott T et al: Early stroke recognition: developing an out-of-hospital NIH Stroke Scale. *Acad Emerg Med* 4(10):986-90, 1997.

stroke patients do not present with respiratory compromise or obtundation. A hemorrhagic event should be suspected when a patient presents with obtundation or respiratory compromise. The mental status examination may be difficult to assess in the presence of aphasia. However, it is important not to label an aphasic patient incorrectly as "confused."

Cranial Nerve Examination

Dysarthria (garbled speech or articulation) should be differentiated from aphasia, a language disorder affecting the reception, interpretation, generation, or content of speech, due to a dominant-hemisphere lesion. There are multiple classifications of aphasic disorders. It may be necessary to assess the ability to write, articulate, and comprehend. A patient should be assessed for the ability to follow simple commands and to name objects (e.g., watch, hand, etc.).

Visual loss may be monocular (usually due to disease anterior to the optic chiasm) or binocular (usually secondary to a parietal or occipital disease).[16] It is important to distinguish monocular blindness from visual field deficits. Spatial neglect may be found on visual field testing. Diplopia may be due to oculomotor dysfunction (of cranial nerve III, IV, or VI). Pupil size and reactivity should be assessed. Funduscopic examination should be completed. Approximately 20 percent of patients with cerebral hemorrhage will have retinal hemorrhages. In addition, the optic discs should be evaluated for papillary edema.

Facial weakness involving cranial nerve VII that is due to a stroke will spare the forehead because the stroke affects the descending motor tracts above the level of the facial nucleus (midpons). When nerve tracks from both sides cross. A lower motor neuron injury (e.g., Bell's palsy) will result in forehead and facial weakness. To evaluate the cranial nerves, the patient should be asked to raise the eyebrows, close the eyes, smile, and puff out the cheeks.

Sensory and Motor Examination

Individual muscle strength (quantitative and symmetry) should be assessed in all four extremities. Pronator drift will detect subtle upper extremity weakness. Have the patient hold out both arms (perpendicular to the chest) with palms up and close the eyes. An upper motor neuron lesion will produce a pronation of the affected arm due to forearm supinator weakness. A downward drift of the arm and pronation will be seen with a more severe weakness.

Performing both the finger-to-nose test and the heel-to-shin test can assess coordination. Ataxia can be difficult to assess in the presence of motor weakness. If the patient is able to stand, a Romberg test (ask the patient to stand with feet together and then close the eyes) can be done to examine position sense. A positive test is noted by any near-falling event.

Hypoactive reflexes usually are seen in the weak limb as a result of stroke or spinal cord injury. However, the lack symmetry is an important finding. Previous strokes cause increased reflexes on the affected side. A positive Babinski reflex (flexion and fanning of the toes after stroking the sole) is abnormal. Sensory examination includes the ability to detect pain (pinprick), light touch, and proprioception.

A complaint of dizziness should be further defined (see Chap. 43).

DIFFERENTIAL DIAGNOSIS

Few nonvascular diseases will cause a sudden and focal neurologic deficit. When a patient presents with a well-defined new neurologic deficit, the primary differential is ischemic or hemorrhagic stroke. However, pathologies such as hypoxia, hypotension, hypoglycemia, intracranial mass, Todd's paralysis, spinal cord trauma, and psychiatric symptoms all can exhibit focal symptoms (see Table 41-2). Patients who present with significant mental status changes have a much longer list of potential causes (see Chap. 39). A careful history and physical examination will allow the practitioner to significantly narrow the differential. Ancillary tests (especially CT scan and occasionally an abnormal routine laboratory test) assist in the diagnosis for most patients. If after a thorough evaluation the diagnosis is still in question, neurologic consultation is advised, and further imaging with magnetic resonance imaging (MRI) or arteriography may be indicated.

EMERGENCY DEPARTMENT CARE AND DISPOSITION

Diagnostic Tests

ED evaluation includes diagnostic tests to diagnose stroke and differentiate ischemic and hemorrhagic stroke. To determine if the patient qualifies for thrombolytic therapy, a thorough history and rapid CT scan are required. Tests to evaluate comorbid diseases (e.g., coronary artery disease), coagulopathies, and the acute complications of stroke can be undertaken in the ED. There have been multiple guidelines promulgated for diagnostic tests (Table 41-6).

The most important diagnostic test is the CT scan. The CT scan will differentiate an ischemic stroke from a hemorrhage or intracranial mass (Fig. 41-2). A non-contrast-enhanced CT scan will avoid mistaking contrast material for blood. If trauma is suspected, bone windows can be added to determine if skull fractures or subdural air or blood is present. Although CT scan is widely available,

Table 41-6. Tests Routinely Obtained on Suspected Stroke Patients

ECG
Chest x-ray
Complete blood count including platelets
PT/PTT
Electrolytes, BUN, Creatinine

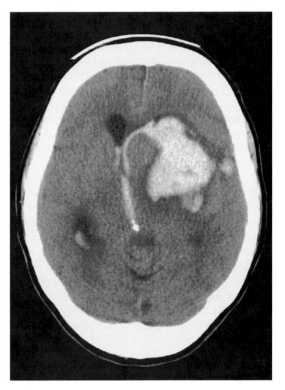

Fig. 41-2 Intracranial hemorrhage. Non-contrast-enhanced CT scan with left intraparenchymal blood, intraventricular blood, and midline shift with edema.

in smaller communities it may not be available at night. If a CT scan is not available and the patient meets criteria for thrombolytic therapy, rapid transport to an appropriate facility should be considered if it can be done to allow therapy within a 3-hour time frame. Patients should not be treated with anticoagulants or thrombolytics until an intracranial hemorrhage is ruled out.

CT scans of patients with an acute ischemic stroke are often normal. However, severe strokes can cause cerebral edema within 1 to 2 hours of the event.[2] Infarcts become more evident on CT scan over the next 2 days. The earliest sign of ischemic edema is a slight attenuation of the gray matter. Given the expertise required for interpretation, the CT scan should be interpreted by a radiologist or neurologist before thrombolytics are considered.[4,5]

Sensitivity of first-generation CT scans for intracranial hemorrhage varies over time, with 92 percent of scans positive on the day of rupture, declining to 50 percent positive at 1 week.[17] Studies of third-generation CT scanners show sensitivities for detection of SAH increasing to approach 100 percent.[17–20] The density of blood in a CT scan is related to hemoglobin concentration. Blood with a hemoglobin concentration of 10 g/dL may appear isodense.[21] Interpretation of CT scans by anyone other than a neuroradiologist may result in a lower sensitivity.[21]

After a negative CT scan, lumbar puncture (LP) is required to exclude SAH. A negative CT scan and cerebrospinal fluid (CSF) examination shortly after the onset of headache reliably excludes a ruptured aneurysm as the cause of a headache.[22] Traditional thinking holds that a traumatic tap will show a decreased red blood cell (RBC) count between the first and last tubes, whereas an SAH will not show this phenomenon. While this decreasing RBC count is most frequent in traumatic taps, it also has been observed in patients with SAH and, therefore, is unreliable.[22] The most reliable method to differentiate between the two is examination of the CSF for xanthochromia using a spectrophotometer or visual inspection. Xanthochromia, a yellow pigment appearing in CSF 12 hours after the bleeding episode, represents bilirubin formed from hemoglobin after the lysis of RBCs.[23] It persists for up to 2 weeks and may still be present in more than 40 percent of SAHs at 4 weeks.[22] CSF xanthochromia is 100 percent sensitive for SAH 12 hours after headache onset.[24] Some authors have suggested delaying LP for 12 hours after the onset of symptoms; however, the risk of rebleed within the first 24 hours makes such a delay inappropriate.[25]

MRI should not be used as the initial evaluation test in an acute stroke. MRI is more sensitive than CT scanning in detecting acute or small lesions.[1,2] However, MRI is not superior to CT scanning in detecting intracranial hemorrhage, is much more time-consuming, has less availability, and may prevent continuous monitoring. MRI and other imaging studies such as magnetic resonance angiography (MRA) and magnetic resonance venography (MRV), ultrasound, single-photon-emission computed tomographic (SPECT) scan, and angiography may have value in the ED assessment of selected patients.

Delineation of the location of an aneurysm or dissection (traditionally by four-vessel angiography) may be replaced by MRA and CT digital subtraction angiography,[14] which are increasingly available to EDs.[26]

Treatment of Ischemic Stroke

Intravenous fluids should be maintained at keep-vein-open or standard replacement levels. Fluid boluses should be avoided unless the patient is hypotensive. Fluid overload may increase intracerebral edema. Supplemental oxygen in a nonhypoxic patient may benefit patients with severe strokes.[5] Fever and vomiting should be treated. Avoid na-

sogastric tubes (or urinary catheters) unless needed. Headaches can be treated with analgesics, but avoid aspirin and nonsteroidal anti-inflammatory drugs (NSAIDs) until bleeding has been ruled out by CT scan. Until a full treatment plan has been established or if there is a risk of aspiration, it is better to withhold food and drink.

Hypertension

Treatment of hypertension usually is not required during an acute stroke. In many patients, the elevated blood pressure will decrease spontaneously over a few hours. The excessive use of antihypertensives may result in decreased cerebral perfusion. However, extreme hypertension should be treated because thrombolytic therapy cannot be given if the systolic blood pressure (SBP) is greater than 185 mmHg or the diastolic blood pressure (DBP) is greater than 110 mmHg. Treat secondary causes of hypertension (such as pain or vomiting) first. Blood pressure should be lowered slowly to avoid decreasing cerebral blood flow, which may worsen the stroke. If the SBP is 180 to 230 mmHg, or if the DBP is above 105 mmHg, 10 mg of intravenous labetolol can be given over 1 to 2 minutes. This dose can be repeated every 10 minutes to a maximum dose of 150 mg.[2] If the SBP is greater than 230 mmHg or the DBP is greater than 120 mmHg and labetolol is not working, sodium nitroprusside may be infused at 0.5 to 20 μg/kg/min. The aim of therapy is to reduce the mean arterial pressure by one-third. The use of calcium channel blockers in this setting is not recommended.[1,5]

Thrombolytic Therapy

Although thrombolytic therapy for stroke remains controversial, the NINDS study (parts I and II) demonstrated that intravenous administration of tissue plasminogen activator (tPA) is beneficial to carefully screened patients.[27] Very selective inclusion and exclusion criteria are needed to identify stroke patients who may benefit (see Table 41-3 and Table 41-7). Studies have shown that selected stroke patients treated within 3 hours of symptom onset have improved outcomes.[3,7–9] In the NINDS study, patients treated with tPA were at least 30 percent more likely to have minimal or no disability at 3 months than were patients treated with placebo.[27] However, the risk of fatal intracranial hemorrhage was 10 times greater in the treated group (3 versus 0.3 percent). The risk of symptomatic intracranial hemorrhage in the treated group also was increased from 0.6 to 6.4 percent.[27] Thrombolytics given after the 3-hour window were not beneficial.[13,27]

Table 41-7. Inclusion and Exclusion Criteria for Thrombolytic Therapy in Acute Stroke

Inclusion critera (must check yes for all)
1. Age $\geq$ 18 years
2. Clinical diagnosis of ischemic stroke causing a measurable neurologic deficit
3. Time of onset well established to be less than 180 minutes before treatment would begin

Exclusion criteria (do not administer thrombolytics if any of the following are true)
1. Evidence of intracranial hemorrhage on non-contrast-enhanced head CT
2. Only minor or rapidly improving stroke symptoms
3. High clinical suspicion of subarachnoid hemorrhage even with normal CT
4. Active internal bleeding (e.g., gastrointestinal or urinary tract) within last 21 days
5. Known bleeding diathesis, including but not limited to
   - Platelet count < 100,000/mm^3
   - Patient has received heparin within 48 hours and had an elevated activated partial thromboplastin time (greater than upper limit of normal of lab)
   - Elevated prothrombin time > 15 seconds
6. Intracranial surgery, serious head trauma, or previous stroke within the last 3 months
7. Major surgery or serious trauma within the last 14 days
8. Recent arterial puncture at a noncompressible site
9. Lumbar puncture within the last 7 days
10. History of intracranial hemorrhage, arteriovenous malformation, or aneurysm
11. Witnessed seizure at stroke onset
12. Recent myocardial infarction
13. Persistent systolic blood pressure > 185 mmHg or diastolic pressure > 110 mmHg at time of treatment, requiring aggressive treatment to bring pressure within these limits

Source: From Hazinski et al.[4]

Supportive Care

Approximately 5 percent of stroke patients have seizures.[2] Recurrent seizures should be controlled in order to avoid a worsening of the stroke. An acute seizure should be controlled with a short-acting benzodiazepine, and recurrent seizures should be treated with a longer-acting anticonvulsant such as phenytoin or phenobarbital. Prophylactic treatment to prevent seizure is not recommended.

Treatment of Hemorrhagic Stroke

Patients with SAH need skilled neurosurgical evaluation and treatment. Management requires localization of any aneurysm or arteriovenous molformation. Goals of treatment in the ED include resuscitation and stabilization, avoidance of secondary cerebral ischemia and vasospasm, and prevention of rebleeding. Close attention should be paid to the prevention of hypoxemia and hypercapnia, with early intubation for those patients with a significant change in or progressive deterioration of level of consciousness. Management of blood pressure is controversial and should be discussed with the consulting neurosurgeon. Most evidence supports the avoidance of antihypertensive drugs, except for those with "extreme elevation" of blood pressure (200/110 mmHg) and those with progressive end-organ dysfunction.[14] Seizures should be treated with standard anticonvulsant therapy. Hyovolemia may contribute to the development of secondary cerebral ischemia. Nimodipine 60 mg orally every 4 hours has been shown to improve outcome in SAH. It is unclear if this is on the basis of neuroprotection or reduction of vasospasm. Antifibrinolytic drugs (e.g., aminocaproic acid) should be used, if at all, in consultation with the neurosurgeon because they have been shown to prevent rebleeding but not to improve outcome.[14] The definitive treatment is surgical clip ligation of the aneurysmal neck or endovascular embolization using detachable coils. A small trial comparing surgical and endovascular treatment found no difference in outcome; timing of surgery, however, is controversial.[14] Treatment of the elderly patient is no different from that of other age group. Conservative therapy for SAH in patients over age

65 yields a 50 percent mortality rate. Advanced age, atherocslerosis, posterior aneurysms, and ischemic heart disease negatively affect mortality.[28]

CONCLUSION

Treating strokes is becoming a team effort, including prehospital personnel, the ED physician and nurse, the radiologist, and the neurologist or neurosurgeon. Some regional prehospital care systems triage suspected stroke patients to facilities that have defined stroke teams and the 24-hour ability to manage strokes with thrombolytics and surgical therapy.[10] This is similar to current regional trauma policies that triage serious trauma patients to designated trauma centers.

As technology and treatment options are developed, stroke care may progress much as cardiac care has done in the last two decades. Many of the acute interventions now available for coronary artery disease should be studied in stroke patients. MRIs likely will be used more in the evaluation of stroke. Research continues on cerebral angiography and direct arterial interventions such as infusion of thrombolytics into the clot. Several anticoagulant agents are being studied as well. Still, the largest hurdle to overcome at the moment is educating the public to recognize and seek help earlier so that more patients will be treated within the 3-hour window.

REFERENCES

1. Brott TG, Clark WM, Fagan SC, et al: *Stroke: The First Hours—Guidelines for Acute Treatment.* Consensus Statement, Vol 2002. Washington, National Stroke Association, 2000.
2. Adams HP, del Zoppo GJ, von Kummer R: *Management of Stroke: A Practical Guide for the Prevention, Evaluation, and Treatment of Acute Stroke.* Washington, Professional Communications, Inc., 1998, p 224.
3. Physicians ACEP: *Use of Intravenous tPA for the Management of Acute Stroke in the Emergency Department,* Vol 2002. Washington, ACEP Board of Directors, 2002.
4. Hazinski MF, Cummins RO, Field JM: *2000 Handbook of Emergency Cardiovascular Care for Healthcare Providers.* Chaiago, American Heart Association, 2000.
5. Association AH: Guidelines 2000 for cardiopulmonary resuscitation and emergency cardiovascular care. *Circulation* 102(suppl 8):1, 2000.
6. Kistler JP, Ropper AH, Martin JB: Cerebrovascular diseases, in Isselbacker KJ et al (eds): *Harrison's Principales of Internal Medicine,* 13th ed. New York, McGraw-Hill, 1999.
7. Barson WG, Bain M: Stroke, in Rosen P (ed): *Emergency Medicine,* Vol II. St Louis, Mosby–Year Book, 1992.
8. Elliott JP, Le Roux PD: Subarachnoid hemorrhage and cerebral aneurysms in the elderly. *Neurosurg Clin North Am* 9(3):587, 1998.
9. Bonita R, Thomson S: Subarachnoid hemorrhage: Epidemiology, diagnosis, management, and outcome. *Stroke* 16(4):591, 1985.
10. Broderick JP, Brott T, Tomsick T, et al: The risk of subarachnoid and intracerebral hemorrhages in blacks as compared with whites. *New Engl J Med* 326(11):733, 1992.
11. Phillips LH, Whisnant JP, Reagan TJ: Sudden death from stroke. *Stroke* 8(3):392, 1977.
12. Mayberg MR, Batjer HH, Dacey R, et al: Guidelines for the management of aneurysmal subarachnoid hemorrhage: A statement for healthcare professionals from a special writing group of the Stroke Council, American Heart Association. *Circulation* 90(5):2592, 1994.
13. Brott TG, Bogousslavsky J: Drug therapy: Treatment of acute ischemic stroke. *New Engl J Med* 343:710, 2000.
14. van Gijn J, Rinkel GJ: Subarachnoid hemorrhage: Diagnosis, causes and management. *Brain* 124(pt 2):249, 2001.
15. Becker KJ: Epidemiology and clinical presentation of aneurysmal subarachnoid hemorrhage. *Neurosurg Clin North Am* 9(3):435, 1998.
16. McDonagh DL, Goldstein LB: Assessing the patient with suspected stroke. *Emerg Med* 34:32, 2002.
17. Sidman R, Connolly E, Lemke T: Subarachnoid hemorrhage diagnosis: Lumbar puncture is still needed when the computed tomography scan is normal. *Acad Emerg Med* 3(9):827, 1996.
18. Morgenstern LB, Luna-Gonzales H, Huber JC Jr, et al: Worst headache and subarachnoid hemorrhage: Prospective, modern computed tomography and spinal fluid analysis. *Ann Emerg Med* 32(3 pt 1):297, 1998.
19. Sames TA, Storrow AB, Finkelstein JA, Magoon MR: Sensitivity of new-generation computed tomography in subarachnoid hemorrhage. *Acad Emerg Med* 3(1):16, 1996.
20. van der Wee N, Rinkel GJ, Hasan D, van Gijn J: Detection of subarachnoid hemorrhage on early CT: Is lumbar puncture still needed after a negative scan? *J Neurol Neurosurg Psychiatry* 58(3):357, 1995.
21. Edlow JA, Caplan LR: Avoiding pitfalls in the diagnosis of subarachnoid hemorrhage. *New Engl J Med* 342(1):29, 2000.
22. Vermeulen M: Subarachnoid hemorrhage: Diagnosis and treatment. *J Neurol* 243(7):496, 1996.
23. Roost KT, Pimstone NR, Diamond I, Schmid R: The formation of cerebrospinal fluid xanthochromia after subarachnoid hemorrhage: Enzymatic conversion of hemoglobin to bilirubin by the arachnoid and choroids plexus. *Neurology* 22(9):973, 1972.
24. Schull MJ: Lumbar puncture first: An alternative model for the investigation of lone acute sudden headache. *Acad Emerg Med* 6(2):131, 1999.
25. Eskey CJ, Ogilvy CS: Fluoroscopy-guided lumbar puncture: Decreased frequency of traumatic tap and implications for

the assessment of CT-negative acute subarachnoid hemorrhage. *AJNR* 22(3):571, 2001.

26. Jager HR, Mansmann U, Hausmann O: MRA versus digital subtraction angiography in acute subarachnoid haemorrhage: A blinded multireader study of prospectively recruited patients. *Neuroradiology* 42(5):313, 2000.

27. Group TnIoNDaSr-PSS. Tissue plasminogen activator for acute ischemic stroke. *New Engl J Med* 333:1581, 1995.

28. Rogg JM, Smeaton S, Doberstein C: Assessment of the value of MR imaging for examining patients with angiographically negative subarachnoid henmorrhage. *AJR* 172(1):201, 1999.

42

Seizures and Status Epilepticus in the Elderly

Gary Bubly

HIGH-YIELD FACTS

- The elderly have the highest incidence of acute seizures and epilepsy of any age group.
- The most commonly identified cause of seizures and status epilepticus in the elderly is cerebrovascular disease.
- The elderly have the highest mortality rate from status epilepticus.
- The most common seizure type in the elderly is partial complex.
- Treatment of seizures in the elderly is more complex due to comorbidities and concurrent medications.

In an older patient, prompt diagnosis and competent management of seizures can test the expertise and skills of the emergency physician. Recognizing the subtle presentations of partial seizure activity in an older patient challenges diagnostic acumen. The presentation of generalized seizures requires rapid intervention and critical care skills. The incidence of seizures and status epilepticus rises in old age.[1] As the population ages, emergency physicians should expect to see increasing numbers of older patient visits that are related to seizures. This chapter focuses on the unique features of emergency department (ED) management of older patients with new-onset seizures, recurrent seizures, and status epilepticus.

There is a higher incidence of epileptiform disorders in older adults. Different causes of seizures emerge as the body and brain age. A narrower spectrum of seizure types is seen in elders. The elderly are more likely to have co-existing medical problems that contribute to an increased morbidity and mortality. Altered pharmacokinetics should be considered when using antiepileptic drugs. In addition, multiple medications may complicate the se-lection of antiepileptic drugs as efforts are made to avoid harmful interactions.

Seizures are the manifestation of an abnormal discharge of neurons in the brain. Although the most obvious seizure is generalized tonic-clonic, the range of clinical manifestations is broad. Even a normal brain will seize if given an appropriate stimulus. Seizures provoked by such a stimulus, hypoglycemia, hypoxia, or ischemia are referred to as *acute symptomatic seizures*. Seizures attributable to a prior central nervous system (CNS) insult, such as trauma stroke or meningitis, are referred to as *remote symptomatic seizures*. Seizures without identifiable precipitants are labeled *idiopathic*. *Epilepsy* refers to a chronic condition characterized by recurrent seizures. *Serial seizures* are repetitive seizures separated by periods of a normal level of consciousness. *Status epilepticus* is a major threat to life and brain in which seizure activity continues uninterrupted, or seizures recur but are separated by periods of abnormal consciousness. The duration of seizure activity used to define status epilepticus should be shortened in the elderly, for whom prolonged seizures are particularly dangerous.[2,3]

EPIDEMIOLOGY

The prevalence and, more important, the incidence of seizures and epilepsy are highest in the elderly. The peak incidence of epilepsy occurs in those over age 75, exceeding the incidence of epilepsy in early childhood.[4] Some investigators estimate that more than 50,000 older Americans seize each year.[5] The majority of acute symptomatic seizures occur in those over age 60. Acute symptomatic seizures resulting from CNS insults are more common in men than in women and increase with advancing age.[1,5] In a U.S. study, the seizure incidence was 159 per 100,000 population for those over 80 years of age.[6] An epidemiologic study from France estimated an annual incidence for all seizures at 139.9 per 100,000 population in those over age 80.[7] When analyzed by seizure type, the incidence of partial complex seizures increased dramatically with age.[4] The elderly are also more likely to present initially in status epilepticus than are younger age groups.[8]

In addition to an increased incidence, the elderly also face higher mortality rates from status epilepticus than do younger patients, with death rates reported to exceed 50 percent in patients over 80 years of age.[9] Others have reported an age-related increase in mortality both for those in status epilepticus and those with acute symptomatic seizures.[10] Mortality rates are also increased in status epilepticus for patients with a seizure duration of greater than 1 hour and for those with anoxic brain injury.[3]

PATHOPHYSIOLOGY

The exact pathophysiology of seizure and status epilepticus is poorly understood. Given the diverse nature of associated causes, multiple mechanisms are likely. In simplistic terms, the neuronal hyperexcitation responsible for seizure is believed to result from an imbalance between excitatory and inhibitory neuronal activity in the brain. Mechanisms have been postulated that involve intracellular abnormalities, cellular membrane irregularities, and synaptic dysfunction. The consequences of seizure and status epilepticus are better understood. Prolonged seizure activity may result in cerebral injury, hyperthermia, lactic acidosis, rhabdomyolysis, aspiration, pulmonary edema, hypotension, myocardial infarction, lacerations, and fractures.[2]

The most common seizure type seen in the elderly was partial complex, found in 49 percent of patients with seizures. Twenty-seven percent of older patients had generalized tonic-clonic seizures, 13 percent had simple partial seizures, 6 percent had other partial seizures, 2 percent had myoclonic seizures, and 3 percent had multiple or unknown seizures.[4] This is a narrower clinical spectrum than is seen in the pediatric population. In patients over age 64, epilepsy was of unknown cause in 24 percent, cerebrovascular disease in 43 percent, degenerative diseases in 12 percent, trauma in 3 percent, and neoplasms in 18 percent.[4,7,11]

Seizures are common after hemorrhagic strokes involving cortical areas and more than one lobe of the brain.[12] Seizure after intracranial hemorrhage occurs in 4 to 25 percent of patients.[13] Most of these manifest initially as simple partial motor seizures, which subsequently generalize. Lobar hematomas and alcohol abuse increase the risk of seizure. Those occurring within 15 days of a stroke are most often motor sensory or visual.[14] Early seizures after stroke are associated with an increased risk of seizure recurrence.[15] Brain tumor is less frequently associated with seizures than is cerebrovascular disease. Seizures can be caused by metastic or primary tumor. Seizures associated with tumor are most frequently partial.[13] Neurodegenerative diseases may cause seizures. Some consider Alzheimer's disease alone to be the cause 7 percent of seizures. Cerebral amyloid angiopathy may be responsible for seizures as well.[16]

Many drugs are known to cause seizures in both ther-apeutic and toxic doses. In one review, the most common seizure-causing drugs were isoniazid, insulin, lidocaine, and psychotropic medications.[17] In some centers, isoniazid overdose is common enough to warrant routine treatment with pyridoxine for intractable seizures.[18] Other drugs that cause seizures include camphor, carbon monoxide, cyanide, imipenem, lithium, penicillins, propoxyphene, quinolones, theophylline, tricyclics, and salicylates. Withdrawal from benzodiazepines, alcohol, and barbiturates is also a well-known precipitants. Hypoglycemia, as a consequence of insulin or oral hypoglycemics, has been identified as a cause of seizures in ED patients.[19]

CNS infections are also associated with acute seizures and as antecedent precipitants in remote symptomatic seizures. The highest incidence occurs within 5 years of the CNS infection. Viral encephalitis is associated with an increased risk of remote symptomatic seizures, especially if associated with early acute seizures. Acute seizures caused by bacterial meningitis will increase the risk of future seizures as well. Viral meningitis does not appear to be associated with remote seizures.[20]

A number of metabolic abnormalities can cause seizures. Electrolyte disturbances, particularly hyponatremia and hypocalcemia, uremia, hepatic encephalopathy, hypothyroidism, and anoxia have been well documented as causes.[21] Hyperosmolar nonketotic hyperglycemia can cause focal seizures in up to 19 percent of patients.[22] Other conditions, such as thrombotic thrombocytopenia purpura, have been associated with acute seizures. Any global toxin, focal brain lesion, or combination of both factors can cause seizures. The brains of older patients may have accumulated small focal lesions over the years, and the blood flow to areas of the brain may be marginal due to vascular disease; thus hypovolemia, hypoglycemia, or hypoxia may manifest as a focal seizure originating from an area of the brain with less perfusion.

CLINICAL FEATURES

While the presentations of generalized tonic-clonic seizures, convulsive status epilepticus, and partial seizures are relatively easy to diagnose clinically, partial complex seizure activity and nonmotor syndromes may be difficult to recognize in the ED. Partial complex seizure activity may present with confusional episodes, memory loss, aphasia, or hallucinations and may be mistaken for transient ischemic attack or disorders that cause altered mental status.[23] Emergency physicians should consider seizure as a possibility for any patient presenting with "spells," episodic confusion, or variable alterations in mental status. Auras may be reported by patients experiencing partial seizures; they do not occur with generalized tonic-clonic seizures. Aura symptoms preceding generalized seizure activity suggest secondary generalization. In the elderly, ictal activity frequently originates in the frontal and parietal lobes rather than the temporal lobes. Hence auras present more commonly as dizziness rather than déjà vu. Unfortunately, these symptoms of seizure can be confused easily with other syndromes. Myoclonic seizures should prompt the search for anoxia, uremia, and other metabolic disturbances. Postictal confusion may be prolonged in the elderly, lasting days in some cases.[13]

DIAGNOSIS

History

Clinical diagnosis of seizure is based primarily on a thorough history and neurologic examination. A detailed history of the event should be obtained from the patient, caregiver, and witnesses. In addition to the patient's family members, nursing home staff and emergency medical services (EMS) personnel should be queried about the circumstances surrounding the episode, particularly with regard to motions or signs at the onset. The patient should be asked about any previous similar episodes and any prior precipitants such as remote trauma or CNS infections. The patient's medications should be reviewed thoroughly. Medication noncompliance should be ruled out in those on antiepileptic therapy. The possibility of withdrawal from alcohol, benzodiazepines, or barbiturates should be considered. Patients and families should be questioned about whether any new medications have been initiated because these may alter the pharmacokinetics of anticonvulsant medications. A social history should be obtained in order not only to investigate the patient's alcohol consumption but also to determine the level of independence and existing home support. Patients and caregivers should be questioned about the presence of fever or headache, as well as any new neurologic symptoms, including episodes of abnormal mental status.

Physical Examination

A complete examination should be performed after stabilization. This should include temperature with vital signs, pulse oximetry, a neurologic examination, and a funduscopic examination. Auscultation should include the carotid arteries. The examination should include a search for signs of trauma. Any seizure activity should be observed carefully, with attention to any focal motion or signs at onset.

Laboratory Tests

Laboratory tests should include a fingerstick blood sugar determination, electrolytes, calcium, creatinine, blood urea nitrogen (BUN), and liver function tests. A toxicology screen should be performed in patients presenting with first seizures. Not only are drugs of abuse a possibility, but inadvertent use of another patient's medication is possible. Patients presenting with recurrent seizures need to have anticonvulsant levels checked. Laboratory testing may reveal an elevated creatine phosphokinase level and acidosis following a seizure. Lumbar puncture is indicated when subarachnoid hemorrhage or CNS infection is suspected, such as meningitis or encephalitis

Neuroimaging

Neuroimaging is recommended in all elderly patients with new-onset seizures and status epilepticus. Magnetic resonance imaging (MRI) is preferred over computed tomographic (CT) scanning but may not be as readily available. Hence CT scanning is the study usually conducted during emergency evaluation.

Lumbar Puncture

Lumbar puncture should be performed in the ED for any patient with seizure and fever, those in whom CNS infection (such as meningitis or encephalitis) is suspected, or those in whom subarachnoid hemorrhage is considered. A mild pleocytosis, typically less than 30 nucleated cells/mL, is not unusual in patients with status epilepticus.[24] However, it is best to treat a presumed CNS infection when cerebrospinal fluid (CSF) white blood cell counts are elevated. Subsequent cultures and clinical course may allow discontinuance antibiotics started in the ED.

Electroencephalogram (EEG)

EEG generally is considered the single most helpful confirmatory test in establishing the diagnosis of seizure disorder. Unfortunately, EEG is rarely available in the ED. Often it is arranged on an outpatient basis after the ED visit. Important changes occur in the EEG with age, such as diffuse slowing and small, sharp spikes, rendering it less sensitive in the interictal period than with younger patients.[25] A normal interictal EEG does not rule out seizure activity. EEG is relatively insensitive to simple partial seizures. In some cases, patients need prolonged EEG monitoring to establish the diagnosis.[8] Occasionally, video and EEG monitoring may be necessary to correlate clinical activity with EEG abnormalities when psuedoseizure seems likely.[26]

DIFFERENTIAL DIAGNOSIS

The differential diagnosis of seizures in the elderly includes syncope, transient ischemic attacks, transient global amnesia, infections, and metabolic abnormalities. *Syncope* is a loss of consciousness occuring with cardiac arrhythmias, vasovagal episodes, orthostasis, and neurocardiogenic syncope, to name a few. Syncope may be associated with clonic muscular twitching and incontinence due to secondary cerebral hypoperfusion. Noncardiac syncope may be associated with postevent confusion and fatigue (see Chap. 11). These features may be difficult to distinguish from seizure activity and postictal symptoms. Transient ischemic attacks (TIAs) cause negative symptoms (e.g., inability to speak, walk, or use a limb) and are longer in duration than seizures. TIAs follow an identifiable cerebrovascular territory. Transient global amnesia causes short-term memory failure lasting generally 7 to 9 hours and may resemble complex partial seizure activity. The EEG typically is normal in transient global amnesia.[27] Neurology consultation may be helpful when the diagnosis is unclear. Infections and metabolic abnormalities should manifest with fever or abnormal laboratory tests.

EMERGENCY DEPARTMENT CARE AND DISPOSITION

Status Epilepticus

Prehospital management of status epilepticus with benzodiazepines has been shown to be safe and effective using lorazepam 2 mg or diazepam 5 mg intravenously.[28] Patients presenting in status epilepticus require multiple and simultaneous interventions. Initial ED efforts should be directed toward assessing the airway. Supplemental oxygen should be administered, preferably via bag-valve-mask setup, and an oral airway should be inserted, if possible. Vital signs should be obtained, as well as pulse oximetry and cardiac monitoring. Intravenous access should be established immediately, and a rapid test of

blood glucose should be done. If hypoglycemia is present or cannot be ruled out, thiamine should be administered followed by dextrose intravenously. In patients with infectious or metabolic causes, treatment should be aimed both at seizure abatement and at correction of the underlying cause. Lorazepam 4 to 8 mg or diazepam 10 to 20 mg should be administered intravenously. Preparation should begin for intubation if seizure activity continues despite repeated doses of benzodiazepines. Ideal induction agents are those with inherent anticonvulsant properties, such as thiopental and midazolam. Succinylcholine at 1.5 mg/kg intravenously is recommended when attempting to secure the airway in the shortest time possible. If concern exists about the possibility of increased intracranial pressure, premedication with a nondepolarizing agent is recommended, such as vecuronium 0.01 mg/kg. Lidocaine 1.5 mg/kg and fentanyl 3 μg/kg are recommended as well to avert further increasing intracranial pressure.[29] Although neuromuscular blockade will mask physical seizure activity, electrical status epilepticus may continue. This may result in cerebral cortical injury. Thus any patient with seizures who receives long-acting neuromuscular blockade should have EEG monitoring in order to rule out ongoing electrical status epilepticus.

If benzodiazepines fail to terminate seizure activity, phenytoin or fosphenytoin should be administered. Phenytoin should be given at a dose of 20 mg/kg at a rate not to exceed 50 mg/min. Hypotension and cardiac arrhythmias are common with this drug in the elderly, often necessitating slowing or stopping the phenytoin load. Fosphenytoin, the prodrug equivalent of phenytoin, can be delivered intramuscularly or intravenously and causes fewer local reactions than phenytoin. However, it is more expensive and no more effective than phenytoin. Care should be taken when ordering fosphenytoin so that the dose is expressed in phenytoin equivalents. The initial loading dose of phenytoin or fosphenytoin is 10 to 15 mg/kg or 10 to 15 mg/kg phenytoin equivalents.

If the previous measures are unsuccessful, phenobarbital can be used and administered intravenously at a dose of 20 mg/kg at a rate of 50 to 75 mg/min. If seizures are continuing, an additional 5 to 10 mg/kg may be administered. Prompt neurology consultation and admission to an intensive care unit are recommended for patients with prolonged or continuing seizures. Status epilepticus that is refractory to these three medications is usually treated either with propofol 1- to 2-mg intravenous bolus followed by an infusion at 2 to 10 mg/kg/h or with midazolam 0.2 mg/kg bolus followed by an infusion at 0.75 μg/kg/min. While some sources report using intravenous valproic acid in the treatment of status epilepticus, at this time there are no published trials establishing its efficacy, and it is not approved by the Food and Drug Administration (FDA) for this indication.[2] However, it is reasonable to consider its use when other measures fail.

Patients in whom seizures are successfully terminated, who regain a normal level of consciousness, and who have a low likelihood of prolonged seizing can be admitted to a medical floor. Given the high mortality rate of status epilepticus in the elderly, it seems prudent to admit patients with prolonged seizures for observation. Exceptions to this include seizure with a correctable precipitant, such as know seizure disorder and medication noncompliance. In patients with exacerbation of known seizure disorder, discussion with the patient's neurologist is recommended prior to discharge. A safe family or cargiver situation should be ensured prior to discharge.

First Seizure

Elderly patients presenting to the ED following a first seizure need a thorough evaluation to search for etiology, as well as an assessment of the likelihood of recurrence. This is critical when considering initiation of therapy. The history, physical examination, and laboratory workup, as described earlier, and neuroimaging are recommended in the ED. Although all patients with suspected seizures ultimately need MRI, a CT scan in the ED is typically more readily available and is recommended prior to disposition. Consultation with a neurologist is recommended. This allows coordination of MRI and EEG scheduling, as well as a discussion about possible initiation of antiepileptic medications. Most elderly patients with new-onset seizures should be admitted to the hospital for observation. It is often difficult to eliminate the possibility of syncope from the history. Patients with seizures related to metabolic, toxic, structural, or infectious causes, as well as those who fail to return to a baseline level of consciousness or who lack safe social environments, should be admitted to the hospital. Healthy elderly patients with a normal ED evaluation, close follow-up, and caregiver(s) who can observe them may be discharged.

Prior to discharging the patient, the emergency physician, and consultants need to decide whether to initiate antiepileptic medication. This is a complex decision based on etiology, likelihood of recurrence, confounding medical problems, current medications, and the patient's social situation. Thus the decision to treat a first seizure is then followed by a decision as to which drug to use. This also should be discussed with the neurology consultant and will be based on the suspected seizure type, cur-

rent medications, and tolerability of the expected side effects.

Drug Therapy

Emergency physicians should be familiar with both the standard and new antiepileptic medications. The standard agents are effective for both generalized and partial seizures yet have many drug interactions and side effects. The newer agents are approved by the FDA primarily for use in partial complex seizures and have several advantages over the standard antiepileptic medications. Generally, they have fewer side effects and fewer drug interactions and are well tolerated in the elderly. Most do not require blood levels. Despite these attractive features, their ED utility is limited. Unfortunately, none can be administered intravenously or even loaded orally. Instead, they require slow titration over days to weeks. In addition, the new drugs are all considerably more expensive than the standard antiepileptic drugs. Further, there is a dearth of literature available to help guide optimal drug therapy in the elderly at this time. Therefore, selection of an antiepileptic drug should be done in conjunction with the patient's neurologist (Tables 42-1 and 42-2).

CONCLUSION

Active elderly patients seen for seizure or status epilepticus will need to stop driving until they have been evaluated by a neurologist. Patients should be given appropriate discharge instructions that warn about medication side effects and drug interactions, as well as the potential hazards involved in activities such as swimming, operating machinery, or child care. More dependent patients may require home services and home safety assessments coordinated by a visiting nurse. In some EDs, case managers or social services can assist with this assessment. In one study, roughly two-thirds of elderly patients with seizures needed permanent help at home. The need for home services was related to the patient's martial status, cognitive function, and focal neurologic deficits.[30] Patients who cannot be discharged safely to home should be considered for an assisted-living setting or nursing home placement. Physicians should avoid using the label "epilepsy" with patients because of the negative connotations associated with it. The physician's reassurance will minimize the negative impact that seizures may have on the patient's self esteem. Physicians can sincerely inform patients that this is a common problem in their age group. Patients and families can obtain additional infor-

Table 42-1. Standard Anticonvulsants

Carbamazepine is indicated for the treatment of partial complex and secondarily generalized seizures and has the potential for many drug interactions. These include macrolide antibiotics, for example. It can only be administered orally. The side effects include ataxia, hyponatremia, diplopia, rash, and aplastic anemia.

Phenobarbital is indicated for the treatment of partial, partial complex, and secondary generalized seizures and generalized tonic-clonic seizures. It can be administered intravenously and orally. Dosages need to be reduced in the elderly, for whom it is a poor choice because of sedation, cognitive impairment, respiratory depression, and drug interactions.

Phenytoin is indicated for the treatment of generalized tonic-clonic seizures, complex partial seizures, and partial seizures. It may be administered intravenously and orally. Drawbacks for its use in the elderly include numerous drug interactions related to its high protein binding and hepatic metabolism. Side effects include cognitive impairment, ataxia, cardiac conduction problems, and gingival hyperplasia. Intravenous use complicated by extravasation may result in significant tissue loss, the "purple glove" syndrome.

Valproic acid is indicated for primary generalized tonic-clonic, myoclonic, and atonic seizures. It may be administered orally or intravenously, although, as mentioned previously, its intravenous efficacy remains unproven. Numerous drug interactions occur due to its high protein binding and hepatic metabolism. Side effects include weight gain, tremor, and hepatotoxicity.

Table 42-2. Newer Anticonvulsants

Gabapentin is indicated for the treatment of partial-onset and secondarily generalized seizures. It has few drug interactions and is not metabolized hepatically. Side effects are transient dizziness or sleepiness.

Lamotrigine is indicated for partial-onset seizures and primary generalized seizures, although there is little published evidence to support its efficacy in the elderly. Drug interactions occur with phenytoin and carbamazepine, which decrease its half-life. Valproic acid, on the other hand, will increase its half-life. A rash occurs in up to 10 percent of patients taking lamotrigine. This can be minimized by titrating the dose slowly.

Tiagabine is indicated as an adjunct for the treatment of partial-onset seizure. It interacts with phenytoin and carbamazepine, both of which decrease the level of tiagabine. Side effects include decreased cognitive function at higher doses.

Topiramate is also indicated as an adjunct for the treatment of complex partial seizures. It interacts with other antiepileptic drugs, including phenytoin and carbamazepine, which decrease topiramate levels. Side effects include cognitive impairment at higher doses.[29,32,33]

---

mation on the Internet from the International League Against Epilepsy Web site at *www.ilae.org.*[31]

REFERENCES

1. Hauser WA, Annegers JF, Kurland LT: Incidence of epilepsy and unprovoked seizures in Rochester, Minnesota: 1935–1984. *Epilepsia* 34(3):453, 1993.

2. Lowenstein DH, Alldredge BK: Status epilepticus. *New Engl J Med* 338:970, 1998.

3. Towne AR, Pellock JM, Ko D, et al: Determinants of mortality in status epilepticus. *Epilepsia* 35(1):27, 1994.

4. Hauser WA: Seizure disorders: The changes with age. *Epilepsia* 33(suppl 4):S6, 1992.

5. Annegers JF, Hauser WA, Lee JR, et al: Incidence of acute symptomatic seizures in Rochester, Minnesota, 1935–1984. *Epilepsia* 36(4):327, 1993.

6. Tallis R, Hall G, Craig I, et al: How common are epileptic seizures in old age?. *Age Ageing* 20(6):442,1991.

7. Loiseau J, Loiseau P, Duche B, et al: A survey of epileptic disorders in southwest France: Seizures in elderly patients. *Ann Neurol* 27(3):232, 1990.

8. Sirven JI: Acute and chronic seizures in patients older than 60 years. *Mayo Clin Proc* 76(2):175, 2001.

9. Delorenzo RJ, Pellock JM, Towne AR, et al: Epidemiology of status epilepticus. *J Clin Neurophysiol* 12:316, 1995.

10. Claassen J, Lokin JK, Fitzsimmons BF, et al: Predictors of functional disability and mortality after status epilepticus. *Neurology* 58:139, 2002.

11. Sander JW, Hart YM, Johnson AL, et al: National general practice study of epilepsy: Newly diagnosed epileptic seizures in a general population. *Lancet* 336(8726):1267, 1990.

12. Lancman ME, Golimstok A, Norscini J, Granillo R: Risk factors for developing seizures after a stroke. *Epilepsia* 34(1):141, 1993.

13. Thomas RJ: Seizures and epilepsy in the elderly. *Arch Intern Med* 157(6):605, 1997.

14. Giroud M, Gras P, Fayolle H, Andre N, et al: Early seizures after stroke: A study of 1640 cases. *Epilepsia* 35(5):959, 1994.

15. So EL, Annegers JF, Hauser WA, et al: Population-based study of seizure disorders after cerebral infarction. *Neurology* 46(2):350, 1996.

16. Forsgren L, Bucht G, Eriksson S, et al: Incidence and clinical characterization of unprovoked seizures in adults: A prospective population based study. *Epilepsia* 37(3):224, 1996.

17. Messing RO, Closson RG, Simon RP: Drug-induced seizures: A 10-year experience. *Neurology* 34(12):1582, 1984.

18. Nelson LS, Rella J, Hofman RS: Correspondence. *New Engl J Med* 339(6):409, 1998.

19. Malouf R, Brust JC: Hypoglycemia: Causes, neurological manifestations, and outcome. *Ann Neurol* 17(5):421, 1985.

20. Annegers JF, Hauser WA, Beghi E, et al: The risk of unprovoked seizures after encephalitis and meningitis. *Neurology* 38(9):1407, 1988.

21. Delanty N, Vaughan CJ, French JA: Medical causes of seizures. *Lancet* 352(9125):383, 1998.

22. Stephen LJ, Brodie MJ: Epilepsy in elderly people. *Lancet* 355:1441, 2000.

23. TatumWO, Ross J, Cole AJ: Epileptic pseudodementia. *Neurology* 50(5):1472, 1998.

24. Barry E, Hauser WA: Pleocytosis after status epilepticus. *Arch Neurol* 51:190, 1994.

25. Drury I, Beydoun A: Interictal epileptiform activity in elderly patients with epilepsy. *Electroencephalog Clin Neurophysiol* 106(4):369, 1998.

26. Drury I, Selwa LM, Schuh LA, et al: Value of inpatient diagnostic CCTV-EEG monitoring in the elderly. *Epilepsia* 40(8):1100, 1999.

27. Rowan AJ: Reflections on the treatment of seizures in the elderly population. *Neurology* 51(suppl 4):S28, 1998.

28. Alldredge BK, Gelb AM, Isaacs SM, et al: A comparison of lorazepam, diazepam, and placebo for the treatment of out-of-hospital status epilepticus. *New Engl J Med* 345(9):631, 2001.

29. Walls RM, Sagarin MJ: Correspondence. *New Engl J Med* 339(6):409, 1998.

30. Luhdorf K, Jensen LK, Plesner AM: Epilepsy in the elderly: Incidence, social functioning, and disability. *Epilepsia* 27(2):135, 1986.

31. Web site of the International League Against Epilepsy: *www.ilae.org*.

32. Rowan AJ: Epilepsy and seizures in the aged, in EttingerAB, Devinsky O (eds): *Managing Epilepsy and Co-Existing Disorders.* Boston, Butterworth-Heinemann, 2002, p 433.

33. Leppik IO: Treatment of epilepsy in the elderly, in Wylie E (ed): *The Treatment of Epilepsy: Principles and Practice,* 3d ed. Philadelphia, Lippincott Williams & Wilkins, 2001.

43

Dizziness, Weakness, and Vertigo

Melissa Ann Eirich

HIGH-YIELD FACTS

- Evaluation of dizziness, weakness, and vertigo relies on the history and physical examination, which guide subsequent cardiologic, neurologic, or other laboratory and ancillary studies.

- The first step to evaluating dizziness, weakness, and vertigo is to obtain enough history to define the symptom complex as cardiovascular, neurologic, or other.

- The causes of dizziness and weakness overlap with syncope significantly. Cardiovascular causes can be life-threatening.

- Most causes of dizziness and weakness are benign and self-limiting. Most vertigo is benign and peripheral.

An estimated 30 percent of elderly patients will suffer from dizziness at some time.[1] Dizziness is a common and confusing symptom with a list of causes that is lengthy. The symptom is often caused by multiple factors, but most etiologies are not life-threatening.[1] Although some patients suffer from chronic, even disabling dizziness, it resolves spontaneously in most.[2]

The first step in evaluating dizziness is to better define the patient's symptoms. Are the symptoms continuous or episodic? Patients and practitioners alike use the term *dizziness* to mean a variety of symptoms, such as light-headedness, confusion, blurred vision, gait disturbance, weakness, syncope, and vertigo. The complaint of dizziness is frequent, but it is essential to determine exactly what the patient means by feeling dizzy. Faintness or light-headedness may be a precursor to syncope, which may be life-threatening. Vertigo is a sensation that the room is spinning or tilting. Disequilibrium is a sense of imbalance that usually involves the trunk or legs, without

any sensations of the head moving.[1] Of course, there is a large group of patients with "dizziness" that will not fit into vertigo, disequilibrium, faintness, or light-headedness. Approximately half of all elderly patients complain of symptoms in two or more categories.[3] Continuous symptoms fit better with fixed lesion or a metabolic, toxic, or endocrine cause. Episodic symptoms, i.e., "spells," suggest cardiac rhythm disturbances or vertigo.

CLINICAL FEATURES

Cardiovascular Presentations

Syncope (fainting) is a loss of consciousness secondary to decreased blood flow to the brain. Light-headedness or faintness describes the prodromal symptoms of syncope, such as visual blurriness, a "swaying" of the floor, and diffuse weakness. During the faint, the patient often appears pale, ashen, and diaphoretic. Since the causes of syncope and presyncope are the same, a full investigation of any patient with these symptoms should be undertaken (see Chap. 11).

The differential for light-headedness and faintness is large (Table 43-1). It is important to ask about additional cardiac symptoms. Palpitations or chest pain can be caused by dysrhythmias or myocardial ischemia. What the patient was doing before and during the symptoms should be determined.

Vasovagal (or neurocardiogenic) syncope is the com-

Table 43-1. Causes of Presyncope

Reduced circulatory flow
Vasovagal
Postural hypotension
Primary autonomic insufficiency
Sympthectomy
Hypovolemia
Blood loss
Addison's disease
Decrease venous return
Valsalva
Cough/micturition
Reduced cardiac output
Ventricular outflow restriction (e.g., aortic stenosis)
Myocardial infarction/decreased ejection fraction
Arrhythmias
Bradyarrhythmias
Tachyarrhythmias

Source: Adapted with permission from Martin and Ruskin.[4]

mon faint and can be experienced by healthy individuals. It can occur under emotional stress, fear, pain, or injury. An overstimulation of the sympathetic nervous system results in peripheral vasodilatation and bradycardia, which causes hypotension. The hypotension causes decreased cerebral blood flow and symptoms of light-headedness or faintness. This mechanism is similar to the Valsalva maneuver, which can occur when vomiting, urinating, or coughing. The symptoms are often quickly reversed once the patient is supine.

Postural hypotension also may cause dizziness. Postural hypotension can be caused by a loss of vasoconstrictor reflexes that, on standing, results in hypotension. While there are primary causes (e.g., primary autonomic insufficiency, dysautonomias, etc.), medications are also a prime cause.[4] Many medications prescribed for hypertension, atrial fibrillation, and other cardiovascular conditions can cause postural hypotension. A thorough patient history should include current and new medications, as well as any recent dosage changes or lack of compliance. Postural hypotension also may be caused by hypovolemia, which can result from blood loss (e.g., gastrointestinal bleeding), dehydration, or sepsis. These patients will present with alterations of vital signs and other indications of an acute illness without resolution unless treated.

Vertigo

Vertigo is defined as a hallucination of movement. It is often described as a sense of spinning or tilting of either the room or the patient. Vertigo results from any imbalance of input and output signals exchanged between the vestibular organs (the semicircular canals, otolithic apparatus, and their central connections, the vestibular nuclei). This imbalance causes the hallucination of movement. Since the vestibular system affects other neural systems, multiple symptoms may result. Nausea, vomiting, and diaphoresis are common. Gait problems such as ataxia and falling are frequent symptoms. However, muscular weakness should not be present. Nystagmus is caused by an abnormality in the labyrinthine-vestibular system. Both nystagmus and vertigo can be a resulting side effect of many medications (Table 43-2).

Vertigo can originate centrally from stroke or neoplasm or peripherally from inner ear problems. Most causes of peripheral vertigo are benign, whereas central vertigo has more serious causes such as stroke and tumor (Table 43-3). Peripheral vertigo is usually sudden in onset, severe, and lasts for minutes to hours. However, it also

Table 43-2. Medications That Can Cause Vertigo and Nystagmus

Alcohol
Antibiotics
   Aminoglycosides
   Chloramphenicol
   Vancomycin
   Erythromycin
Barbiturates
Phenytoin
Diuretics
Quinine
Salicylates

Source: Adapted with permission from Olshaker.[5]

Table 43-3. Causes of Vertigo

Central	Peripheral
Infection	Otitis media
Brain abscess	Labyrinthitis
Meningitis	Serous otitis
Vertebral basilar insufficiency	Impacted cerumen
Subclavian steal	Foreign body in ear canal
Cerebellar ischemia or hemorrhage	Benign positional vertigo
Migraine	Meniere's disease
Tumor	Acoustic neuroma
Trauma (head or neck)	Motion sickness
Demyelinating disease	Vestibular neuronitis
Temporal lobe epilepsy	Vestibulotoxic drugs
Paraneoplastic syndromes	Perilymph fistula
	Third cranial nerve disease

can occur intermittently over days. Peripheral vertigo usually has horizontal nystagmus, and symptoms worsen with changes in head position. Occasionally, hearing loss or tinnitus is present. Positional vertigo can be stimulated by laying the head back (to the right or left). Benign positional vertigo (BPV) is common, but it is a diagnosis of exclusion. Head trauma has been found to be a precipitating factor for BPV. Sudden and severe vertigo often occurs several seconds after moving, but if the patient remains still, it usually lasts less than a minute. The patient also can reduce symptoms by rapidly reproducing the sudden head movement and fatiguing the symptoms of vertigo. BPV usually disappears over a few weeks.

Labyrinthitis is caused by an inflammation of the inner ear, with hearing loss. Serious labyrinthitis is secondary to a nearby infection of the ears, nose, throat, or meninges. Acute suppurative labyrinthitis is a bacterial infection of the inner ear often due either to chronic otitis media or to meningitis. Medications can cause toxic labyrinthitis (see Table 43-2). Chronic labyrinthitis can occur secondary to a fistula from the middle to the inner ear.

Central vertigo has a more gradual onset of less severe symptoms. It usually lasts for weeks or months and is constantly present. Nystagmus may be horizontal, vertical, or rotary. Also, central vertigo is less sensitive to changes in head position. While acute hearing loss is usually not present, gradual unilateral loss can be due to an acoustic neurinoma. Additional associated neurologic symptoms are often present. Vertebrobasilar insufficiency (VBI) is a common cause of vertigo; however, most patients with VBI also have visual disturbances, weakness, dysarthria, or other focal neurologic findings.

In addition to other neurologic abnormalities, ischemia, hemorrhage, or infarction of the brain stem or cerebellum may cause vertigo. Transient ischemic attacks can cause vertigo, but other neurologic findings are usually present.[5] Cerebellopontine angle tumors (e.g., meningioma, acoustic neuroma) grow slowly and often create auditory symptoms (i.e., tinnitus, hearing loss). A sense of being pushed or pulled while walking is common with acoustic neuroma. Vertigo may be the first symptom noted in patients with multiple sclerosis or Guillain-Barré syndrome. Illnesses affecting the eighth cranial nerve, such as the Ramsay Hunt syndrome, also can result in vertigo. The emergency physician should seek a history of head or neck trauma because disruption of otoliths in the semicircular canals or dissection of the posterior cerebral arteries may cause vertigo.

Other Causes of Dizziness and Weakness

Psychogenic causes of dizziness, such as hyperventilation and anxiety, are common. Hyperventilation causes hypocapnia, alkalosis, and a decreased cerebral blood flow. Patients who hyperventilate often complain of perioral and bilateral fingertip and hand numbness or tingling. The symptoms often can be reproduced by asking the patient to hyperventilate. In addition, dizziness can be part of an anxiety attack with chest pain (or tightness), agoraphobia, and feelings of terror or apprehension. Of course, persistent weakness should suggest toxic, metabolic, or endocrine causes. The astute clinician should seek other signs or symptoms. For example, a noxious odor or headache may indicate carbon monoxide poisoning.

Physical Examination

A cardiovascular examination should include listening for bruits (suggesting atherosclerosis) and any signs of subclavian steal (suggesting vertebrobasilar insuffiency). Orthostatic vital signs should be obtained. The ears should be examined for impacted cerumen, a foreign body, or fluid behind the tympanic membrane. Hearing should be tested informally.

Extraocular movement should be examined carefully. Nystagmus is present when the patient is unable to maintain conjugate deviation of the eyes. Jerk nystagmus involves a slow phasing away from the object followed by a quick jerk back toward midline. Fine horizontal nystagmus at the extremes of gaze is common and usually not significant.

Any other cranial nerve abnormalities should be noted because they may indicate a central cause of vertigo. Motor strength should be evaluated while the patient is supine or sitting in order to differentiate true muscular weakness from weakness secondary to vertigo. Cerebellar function should be checked, including finger-to-nose pointing and rapid alternating movements. The gait should be evaluated if the patient can tolerate standing.

Dizzy patients often note weakness when they stand or walk. Consistent falling to one side raises suspicion of a central process. A "cerebellar gait" is characterized by a wide base, irregular steps, unsteadiness, and a lurching from side to side. A patient's inability to ambulate prohibits safe discharge from the emergency department (ED) regardless of cause. Patients with severe, persistent symptoms of vertigo must be hospitalized.

EMERGENCY DEPARTMENT CARE AND DISPOSITION

Diagnostic Tests

Results of the history and physical examination will guide laboratory testing and ancillary studies. In patients who are light-headed or faint, suggesting cardiac causes, orthostatic symptoms should be elicited, a 12-lead electrocardiogram (ECG) should be done, and the patient should be placed on a cardiac monitor to detect any cardiac dysrhythmias. When cardiac ischemia or infarction are considered, cardiac enzymes should be obtained. If there is any suspicion of intracranial ischemia, hemorrhage, or mass, a computed tomographic (CT) scan should be done.

Hypoglycemia and hypoxia are metabolic causes of persistent dizziness that should be easily diagnosed by bedside testing and treated. When other specific metabolic and toxic causes are suspected, blood levels can be obtained for sodium, carboxy hemoglobin, aspirin, alcohol, phenytoin, etc.

Treatment and Disposition

It is clear that treatment and disposition vary widely depending on the underlying cause. Cardiac presyncope requires aspirin and admission to a monitored unit. Intracranial ischemia, hemorrhage, or a mass may require neurologic or neurosurgical consultation and admission. Hypovolemia can be resolved easily with intravenous fluids. Bacterial labyrinthitis requires intravenous antibiotics and admission. Vertigo can be treated with meclizine (25 mg every 8 hours) or diazepam (2–10 mg orally or intravenously). Antihistamines (e.g., diphenhydramine) and antiemetics also may be useful.[5] After a trial of medications for vertigo in the ED, patients who are unable to walk or who persist with severe symptoms such as vomiting should be admitted for intravenous fluids and continued intravenous medication.

CONCLUSION

Dizziness and weakness are common complaints in the geriatric population. Their evaluation and diagnosis should be based primarily on a thorough history and physical examination. Vertigo is distinct symptom often described as dizziness or weakness. Vertigo has specific causes and treatment. While most causes of dizziness, weakness, and vertigo are benign, it is important to consider and identify cardiac, central nervous system, and other causes that have significant associated morbidity.

REFERENCES

1. Sloane PD, Coeytaux RR, Beck RS, Dallara J: Dizziness: State of the science. *Ann Intern Med* 134:823, 2001.
2. Sloane PD, Blazer D, George L: Which primary care patients with dizziness will develop persistent impairment? *Arch Fam Med* 2:847, 1993.
3. Sloane PD, Baloh RW: Persistent dizziness in geriatric patients. *J Am Geriatric Soc* 37:1031, 1989.
4. Martin JB, Ruskin J: Faintness, syncope, and seizures, in Isselbacher KJ et al (eds): *Harrison's Principles of Internal Medicine,* 13th ed. New York, McGraw-Hill, 1994 p 90.
5. Olshaker JS: Vertigo, in Rosen P (ed): *Emergency Medicine: Concepts and Clinical Practice,* Vol II. St Louis, Mosby-Year Book, 1992, p 1806.

44

Geriatric Trauma Overview

O. John Ma
Stephen W. Meldon

HIGH-YIELD FACTS

- Falls are the most common accidental injury in persons over 75 years of age and the second most common injury in the 65- to 74-year age group.

- A normal tachycardic response to pain, hypovolemia, or anxiety may be absent or blunted in the elderly trauma patient.

- Prior to contrast-enhanced computed tomographic (CT) scanning, ensure adequate hydration and baseline assessment of renal function.

- Elder patients with underlying coronary artery disease and cerebrovascular disease are at a greater risk of suffering the consequences of ischemia when they become hypotensive after sustaining trauma.

- Detection of unrecognized shock may be difficult in the older trauma patient. Early invasive monitoring may provide important hemodynamic information, limit hypoperfusion, help prevent multiple organ failure, and improve survival.

With the rapid growth in the size of the elderly population, the incidence of geriatric trauma is expected to increase as well. Although the elderly experience the same types of injuries that younger individuals do, there are significant differences in injury mechanisms, patterns of injury, and outcomes. Emergency physicians need to be aware of the unique injury mechanisms and patterns associated with geriatric trauma. Elderly patients also respond differently to traumatic injuries because age-related changes may produce a diminished physiologic reserve. Therefore, special management principles should be considered when caring for geriatric trauma victims.

In trauma, defining the term *elderly* is a difficult task because it involves both chronologic and physiologic components. The literature has divided the elderly population into two groups: the *young old* (65–80 years of age) and the *old old* (80 years of age and older).[1,2] Although this is a somewhat arbitrary division, it is helpful in interpreting the geriatric trauma literature.

One of the difficulties in describing the elderly population is the potential discrepancy between chronologic age and physiologic age. *Chronologic age* is the actual number of years the individual has lived. *Physiologic age* describes the functional capacity of the patient's organ systems. Comorbid disease states such as diabetes mellitus, coronary artery disease, renal disease, arthritis, and pulmonary disease can decrease the physiologic reserve of certain patients, which makes it more difficult for them to recover from a traumatic injury.[3,4] *Physiologic reserve* describes the various levels of functioning of the patient's organ systems that allows the patient to compensate for traumatic derangement. For example, a 65-year-old patient with diabetes, arthritis, and chronic obstructive pulmonary disease may have less physiologic reserve and, hence, an older physiologic age than an 80-year-old without any comorbid conditions.

EPIDEMIOLOGY

Geriatric trauma patients represent between 8 and 12 percent of the general trauma population. While male trauma victims are predominant in the younger age groups, males and females are equally represented in the geriatric trauma population.[5]

Persons over age 65 represent 12 percent of the general population; however, they account for 36 percent of all ambulance transports, 25 percent of hospitalizations, and 25 percent of total trauma costs.[1] Although the elderly are less likely to be involved in trauma compared with other age groups, they are more likely to have fatal outcomes when they are injured. Approximately 28 percent of deaths due to accidental causes involve persons age 65 and older, and the elderly have the highest population-based trauma mortality rate of any age group.[1]

PATHOPHYSIOLOGY

Common Mechanisms of Injury

The elderly experience similar types of injuries as younger individuals do. There are differences, however, in the mechanisms and the incidence and patterns of injury between older and younger persons.

Falls

Falls are the most common accidental injury in patients over age 75 and the second most common injury in the group aged 65 to 74 years (see Chap. 5). Fifty percent of elderly persons who fall will do so repeatedly. Most individuals who fall will do so on a level surface, and most will suffer an isolated orthopedic injury.[1,6] Falls are reported as the underlying cause of 9500 deaths each year in patients over age 65. Many falls in the elderly population occur in residential institutions such as nursing homes. In the over-85 age group, 20 percent of fatal falls occur in nursing homes.[6]

Age-related changes in postural stability, balance, motor strength, and coordination make the elderly more prone to tripping and falling and contribute to the increased incidence of falls in this population. Decreased visual acuity and increased memory loss in older persons also can cause difficulty in recognizing and avoiding environmental hazards. Acute illness and preexisting chronic diseases also may lead to falling. Syncope has been implicated in approximately 10 percent falls and often is due to defective blood pressure control, primary cardiac dysfunction, diminished cerebral blood flow, and metabolic or respiratory derangement. Other contributing factors include alcohol use and medications, most notably sedative, antihypertensive, antidepressant, diuretic, and hypoglycemic agents.[6]

Motor Vehicle Crashes

Motor vehicle–related injuries rank as the leading mechanism of injury that brings elderly patients to a trauma center in the United States. Motor vehicle crashes are the most common mechanism for fatal incidents in elderly persons through age 80.[1] Emergency physicians should anticipate an increase in motor vehicle trauma involving the elderly due to the growth in this subset of the population and the increase in elderly drivers and occupants. Recent data have shown that the crash fatality rate among the elderly is considerably higher than for younger age groups.[7] As noted earlier, similar effects of acute and chronic medical conditions can influence the incidence of motor vehicle crashes (MVCs). Older persons may have decreased cerebral and motor skills and memory and judgment losses that can compound the difficulty in operating a motor vehicle. Older drivers also are more likely to have decreased auditory or visual acuity, which may make it more difficult to recognize dangerous traffic situations. Furthermore, decreased strength and slower reaction times may hinder an individual's ability to respond to a hazardous traffic situation.[1] One study reported the number of MVCs per driver's license increased with age in elderly drivers.[8] Older drivers are more likely to be involved in crashes during daylight hours, in good weather, at intersections, and involving two vehicles.

Pedestrian-Automobile Accidents

When elderly patients are struck by automobiles, devastating injuries may result. Elders are second only to children as victims of automobile-pedestrian accidents. The 65 and older age group accounts for 22 percent of pedestrian-automobile fatalities in the United States.[1] Elderly pedestrians struck by a motor vehicle are much more likely to die compared with younger pedestrians.[9] Pedestrian-vehicle collisions are one of the most lethal mechanisms of injury in this age group, with a greater then 50 percent case-fatality rate. A number of factors contribute to the increased risk of older persons becoming pedestrian-vehicle collision victims. Reduced peripheral vision and decreased hearing may limit access to information needed to make rational decisions about crossing the street. Cognitive, memory, and judgment skills often are diminished and may increase the risk of older pedestrians being struck by automobiles. Postural changes due to musculoskeletal decline may lead to kyphosis, which results in difficulty in lifting the head to see and obey traffic signals. Traffic signals, which operate at a crossing rate of 4 ft/s, may not account for slower walking speeds.[1] Thus elderly individuals may not have enough time to safely cross an intersection.

Burns

Thermal injuries are another significant mechanism of injury. Most burn injuries in this age group are a result of careless activity in the home setting and are due to either flame injuries from smoking or cooking or tub scald injuries. The elderly constitute between 13 and 20 percent of admissions to burn units but have the highest case-fatality rate of any age group. The elderly have a higher fatality rate than younger adults with the same extent of burn, and even nonmajor burns (<20 percent of body surface area) may be significant injuries in this age group. Increasing age, male gender, burn size, presence of third-degree burn, and presence of inhalation injury contribute to mortality.[10,11] The relationship between higher age and increased burn mortality has been long recognized, and geriatric patients with burns of 70 percent or greater usually do not survive, even with aggressive management. The Baux index, a simple addition of age and percentage body surface area burned, has continuing prognostic value. A Baux index of 75 represents a severe burn, and an index of 100 is usually fatal.

Violence

The overall increase in violent crimes in the United States has not spared the elderly. Violent assaults account for 4 to 14 percent of trauma admissions in this age group. Elderly persons are often seen as ideal targets for robberies because they may possess various age-related physical deficiencies.[1] While blunt trauma to date has been the most frequent injury mechanism, penetrating injuries are on the rise.[1] Emergency physicians should have a heightened suspicion for elder or parental abuse in the geriatric trauma patient (see Chap. 6).

Prehospital Considerations

Following injury, older patients have higher admission rates, longer hospital stays, increased long-term morbidity, and higher mortality rates despite lower injury severity.[12] Emergency medical services (EMS) providers should recognize that seemingly minor trauma mechanisms, such as low-level falls and low-speed MVCs, may result in significant injury to older persons. For these reasons, it has been recommended that the threshold for scene triage or transfer to a trauma center be lower for elderly patients than for younger patients.

Despite these recommendations, there is evidence that elderly patients are disproportionately underrepresented at trauma centers.[2,13] Whether this is secondary to minor injury mechanisms, an initial assessment that underestimates the severity of their trauma, existing prehospital triage protocols, or a bias against aggressively treating elderly patients is not clear. Most trauma protocols typically rely on anatomic and physiologic criteria to mandate transfer to a trauma center, and patient age greater than 55 years is often listed as one of several comorbid conditions for which transport to a trauma center should be considered. Phillips and colleagues[14] documented that among patients who were judged to require trauma care, only 29 percent of those age 55 or older were identified by their trauma criteria, in contrast to 64 percent of patients 15 to 54 years of age. In addition to the inadequacy of triage protocols for this age group, a lower compliance with triage protocols for elderly trauma patients also has been reported.[15] Given these findings, consideration of patient age should be a component of prehospital trauma protocols that direct the triage and transport of injured patients.

CLINICAL FEATURES

History

Since elderly patients may have a significant past medical history that has an impact on their trauma care, obtaining a precise history is vital. Often the time frame for obtaining information about the traumatic event, past medical history, medications, and allergies is quite short. Medical records and consultation with the patient's family physician may be helpful. Family members also may be able to provide information regarding the traumatic event and the patient's previous level of function.

Vital Signs

Early assessment and frequent monitoring of vital signs are essential in the geriatric trauma patient. The clinician, however, should not be led into a false sense of security by "normal" vital signs. In a study by Scalea and colleagues,[16] 8 of 15 patients initially considered to be hemodynamically "stable" had cardiac outputs less than 3.5 L/min, and none had an adequate response to volume loading. Of 7 patients with a normal cardiac output, 5 had inadequate oxygen delivery.

There is progressive stiffening of the myocardium with age that results in a decreased effectiveness of the pumping mechanism. An 80-year-old will have approximately 50 percent of the cardiac output of a 20-year-old even without significant atherosclerotic coronary artery disease. The myocardium also becomes less sensitive to endogenous and exogenous catecholamines. Conduction defects may be exacerbated by the stress of illness or trauma. A normal tachycardic response to pain, hypovolemia, or anxiety may be absent or blunted in the elderly trauma patient.[17] Medications such as beta blockers may mask tachycardia and hinder evaluation of the elderly patient. Blood pressures also may be misleading because the prevalence of preexisting hypertension in this age group approaches 70 percent. Emergency physicians should be wary of a "normal" heart rate and blood pressure in the geriatric trauma victim.

DIAGNOSIS AND DIFFERENTIAL

As in all trauma patients, the primary survey should be assessed expeditiously. Special attention should be paid to anatomic variation that may make airway management more difficult. These include the presence of dentures (which may occlude the airway), cervical arthritis (which adds danger to extending the neck), or temporomandibular joint arthritis (which may hinder mouth opening).

A thorough secondary survey is essential to uncover less serious injuries. These injuries, which include various orthopedic injuries and "minor" head trauma, may not be severe enough to cause problems during the initial resuscitation but cumulatively may cause significant morbidity and mortality. Significant head and spine fractures, such as subdural hematomas and upper cervical spine fractures, may occur from seemingly minor trauma and will be discussed in Chaps. 45 and 47. An important point to note is that patients with no apparent life-threatening injuries actually can have potentially fatal injuries if there is some degree of limited physiologic reserve. Seemingly stable geriatric trauma patients can deteriorate rapidly and without warning.

EMERGENCY DEPARTMENT CARE AND DISPOSITION

Special Management Principles

Emergency physicians often are faced with the challenging task of assessing elderly trauma patients' cardiovascular status and reserve. The work by Scalea and colleagues[16] demonstrated that trauma physicians frequently fail to recognize the severity of hemodynamic instability in geriatric patients. Therefore, early invasive monitoring has been advocated to help assess hemodynamic status.

Scalea and coworkers showed that by reducing the time to invasive monitoring in elderly trauma patients from 5.5 to 2.2 hours and thus recognizing and appropriately treating occult shock, the survival rate of their patients increased from 7 to 53 percent. Survival was improved because of enhanced oxygen delivery through the use of adequate volume loading and inotropic support. They concluded that urgent invasive monitoring provides important hemodynamic information early, aids in identifying occult shock, limits hypoperfusion, helps prevent multiple organ failure, and improves survival.[16]

The insertion of invasive monitoring catheters occurs infrequently in the emergency department (ED) because of institutional practice, availability of equipment, and time constraints. Thus every effort should be made by emergency physicians to expedite ED care of elderly trauma patients and prevent unnecessary delays. In the ED evaluation of blunt trauma patients, the chest radiograph, cervical spine series, and pelvic radiographs are necessary diagnostic tests during the secondary survey. After ordering this set of plain radiographs, emergency physicians must resist the temptation of trying to appease consultants by immediately obtaining plain films of every other body region that may have sustained minor trauma. While it is vital to be thorough in the diagnosis of occult orthopedic injuries, expending a great deal of time in the radiology suite may compromise patient care. Only a few radiographic studies, such as emergent head and abdominal computed tomographic (CT) scans, should take precedence over obtaining vital information from invasive monitoring. Elderly trauma patients will benefit most from an expeditious transfer to the intensive care unit for invasive monitoring so that their hemodynamic status can be further assessed. Invasive monitoring in the intensive care environment may provide clues to subtle hemodynamic changes that may compromise geriatric patients with limited physiologic reserve. After being assured that their hemodynamic status has been stabilized, patients can be transported back to the radiology suite for further plain radiographic studies.

In the ED, critical management decisions regarding volume resuscitation often must be made without the benefit of sophisticated invasive monitoring devices. Elderly patients with underlying coronary artery disease and cerebrovascular disease are at a much greater risk of suffering the consequences of ischemia to vital organs if they become hypotensive after sustaining trauma. Monitoring acid-base status, lactate levels, and base deficit may aid in recognizing shock. Base deficits have been correlated with significant injury and a significant increase in mortality in the elderly.[18] Importantly, while the positive predictive value of base deficit for significant injury was similar between young and old patients, the negative predictive value was significantly better in younger patients. Therefore, a normal base deficit is older patients should not always confer reassurance and lack of significant injury. During the initial resuscitative phase, crystalloid, while the primary option, should be administered judiciously because elderly patients with diminished cardiac compliance are more susceptible to volume overload. Geriatric trauma patients can decompensate with overresuscitation just as quickly as they can with inadequate resuscitation.[17] Strong consideration should be given to early and more liberal use of red blood cell transfusion. This practice early in the resuscitation enhances oxygen delivery and helps minimize tissue ischemia.

Emergency physicians also must recognize that older trauma patients have a significantly higher prevalence of preexisting comorbid conditions. The most common comorbidities include cardiovascular disease, pulmonary disease, and diabetes. Since the presence of these comorbidities may contribute to poor outcome, management of these preexisting conditions becomes important. Another pitfall in geriatric trauma is not recognizing that these comorbidities may be a precipitating factor in the trauma. Syncope, acute myocardial infarction, and stroke may predispose to and result in trauma. In addition, adverse drug reactions and medication side effects are important considerations in this population. The importance of the patient's medical history cannot be overemphasized. Medication lists, prior electrocardiograms, and contacting the primary care physician can be extremely helpful.

Prevention, Prognosis, and Outcome

For elderly patients who are discharged home after sustaining an injury from a fall, it is appropriate for emergency physicians to encourage them to work with their primary care physicians in conducting a home safety assessment to help prevent future falls. Chronic medications that may adversely affect the vestibular system, cause profound sedation, or produce postural hypotension should be identified; patients can then discuss alternative therapies or dosages with their primary care physicians.[6] When discharging to home a patient with a new medication prescription, emergency physicians should select drugs that are least centrally acting, least associated with postural hypotension, and have the shortest duration.

Among geriatric trauma patients who are hospitalized,

the mortality rate has been reported to be between 15 and 30 percent. These figures far exceed the mortality rate of 4 to 8 percent found in younger patients.[1] In general, late deaths due to complications, multiple organ failure, and sepsis are more common in elderly patients than in younger trauma victims.[19] Geriatric patients also are more likely to die following minor traumatic events.[20]

Several markers for poor outcome in elderly trauma victims have been determined. Age greater than 75 years, Glasgow Coma Scale score less than 7, presence of shock on admission, severe head injury, and the development of sepsis are associated with worse outcome and higher mortality figures.[21] Although several series have shown a correlation between Injury Severity Score (ISS) and mortality in the elderly,[2,12,22] this has not been a universal finding,[23,24] and an anatomic injury scale, such as the ISS, may not be the most sensitive tool to predict mortality in this age group.

The ultimate goal in the care of elderly trauma patients is to return them to their preinjury state of independent function. Public debate has raised questions about the ethics and cost benefits of trauma care for the elderly. There are conflicting data on the ability of elderly patients to return to independent living. One early study showed a mortality rate of 15 percent among geriatric trauma patients and a dismal 12 percent of patients returning to their baseline independent state.[24] However, subsequent work has demonstrated that following discharge, one-third of older trauma survivors return to independent living, one-third return to dependent status living at home, and one-third require nursing home facilities. At long-term follow-up, 89 percent returned home after trauma, and 57 percent returned to independent living.[25,26] These findings are supported by the investigation of van Aalst and colleagues,[21] who also showed that the majority of their elderly trauma patients regained an independent level of function.

Many questions regarding the ultimate outcome of geriatric trauma patients remain unanswered. In light of these investigations showing that elderly patients can return to independent living after trauma and demonstration of the beneficial effect of early invasive monitoring and trauma center care, it appears that aggressive resuscitation efforts for geriatric trauma patients are warranted.

ADDITIONAL ASPECTS

The following are pitfalls in the management of geriatric trauma:

- Failure to recognize that patients may have limited physiologic reserve. Seemingly minor injuries actually may be life-threatening in the face of limited physiologic reserve.

- Assuming that some patients are "stable" based solely on their vital signs. These patients may become unstable quickly and with little warning. Early invasive hemodynamic monitoring often will provide valuable diagnostic and resuscitation information.

- Overresuscitation with intravenous fluids is as detrimental as inadequate resuscitation. Blood transfusion for volume replacement early in the resuscitation phase will improve oxygen delivery in hypovolemic patients.

REFERENCES

1. Schwab CW, Kauder DR: Trauma in the geriatric patient. *Arch Surg* 127:701, 1992.
2. Meldon SW, Reilly M, Drew BL, et al: Trauma in the very elderly: A community-based study of outcomes at trauma and non-trauma centers. *J Trauma* 52:79, 2002.
3. MacKenzie EJ, Morris JA, Edelstein SL: Effect of pre-existing disease on length of hospital stay in trauma patients. *J Trauma* 29:757, 1989.
4. Morris JA, MacKenzie EJ, Edelstein SL: The effect of pre-existing conditions on mortality in trauma patients. *JAMA* 263:1942, 1990.
5. Schiller WR, Knox R, Chleborad W: A five-year experience with severe injuries in elderly patients. *Accid Anal Prev* 27:167, 1995.
6. Tinetti ME, Speechley M: Prevention of falls among the elderly. *New Engl J Med* 320:1055, 1989.
7. Li G, Baker SP, Longlois JA, et al: Are female drivers safer? An application of the decompression method. *Epidemiology* 9:379, 1998.
8. Hakamies-Blomqvist LE: Fatal accidents of older drivers. *Accid Anal Prev* 25:19, 1993.
9. Sklar DP, Demarest GB, McFeeley P: Increased pedestrian mortality among the elderly. *Am J Emerg Med* 7:387, 1989.
10. Tobiasen J, Hiebert JH, Edlich RF: Prediction of burn mortality. *Surg Gynecol Obstet* 154:711, 1982.
11. Hammond J, Ward CG: Burns in octogenarians. *South Med J* 84:1316, 1991.
12. Finelli FC, Johnsson J, Champion HR, et al: A case control study for major trauma in geriatric patients. *J Trauma* 29:541, 1989.
13. Zimmer-Gembeck ML, Southard PA, Hedges JR, et al: Triage in an established trauma system. *J Trauma* 39:922, 1995.
14. Phillips S, Rond PC III, Kelly SM, et al: The failure of triage criteria to identify geriatric patients with trauma: Results from the Florida Trauma Triage Study. *J Trauma* 40:278, 1996.
15. Ma MH, MacKenzie EJ, Alcorta R, et al: Compliance with prehospital triage protocols for major trauma patients. *J Trauma* 46:168, 1999.
16. Scalea TM, Simon HM, Duncan AO, et al: Geriatric blunt trauma: Improved survival with early invasive monitoring. *J Trauma* 30:129, 1990.
17. Demarest GB, Osler TM, Clevenger FW: Injuries in the elderly: Evaluation and initial response. *Geriatrics* 45:36, 1990.
18. Davis JW, Kaups KL: Base deficit in the elderly: A marker of severe injury and death. *J Trauma* 45:873, 1998.
19. Perdue PW, Watts DD, Kaufmann CR, Trask AL: Differences in mortality between elderly and younger adult trauma patients: Geriatric status increases risk of delayed death. *J Trauma* 45:805, 1998.
20. Smith DP, Enderson BL, Maull KI: Trauma in the elderly: Determinants of outcome. *South Med J* 83:171, 1990.
21. van Aalst JA, Morris JA, Yates HK, et al: Severely injured geriatric patients return to independent living: A study of factors influencing function and independence. *J Trauma* 31:1096, 1991.
22. Knudson MM, Lieberman J, Morris JA, et al: Mortality factors in geriatric blunt trauma patients. *Arch Surg* 129:448, 1994.
23. Osler T, Hales K, Baack B, et al: Trauma in the elderly. *Am J Surg* 156:537, 1988.
24. Oreskovich MR, Howard JD, Copass MK, et al: Geriatric trauma: Injury patterns and outcome. *J Trauma* 24:565, 1984.
25. DeMaria EJ, Kenney PR, Merriam MA, et al: Survival after trauma in geriatric patients. *Ann Surg* 206:738, 1987.
26. DeMaria EJ, Kenney PR, Merriam MA, et al: Aggressive trauma care benefits the elderly. *J Trauma* 27:1200, 1987.

45

Head Trauma

David F. E. Stuhlmiller

HIGH-YIELD FACTS

- Even seemingly minor trauma, such as a fall from a standing position, can result in a significant head injury in the elderly.
- Elderly individuals are predisposed to falls due to a variety of physiologic and pathophysiologic conditions, making falls the most common cause of head trauma.
- Subdural hematomas account for the majority of findings on head computed tomographic (CT) scanning and remain the primary neurosurgical indication in this patient population.
- Elderly patients have a worse prognosis and higher mortality rate than younger patients with the same head injury.
- Elderly individuals have an increased incidence of dementia and have persistent cognitive and functional deficits following severe head trauma.

Cases of head trauma in the geriatric population will present more commonly to the emergency department (ED) as elderly individuals continue to stay active. Due to interplay between the normal aging process and preexisting medical conditions, elderly individuals are more prone to injury than their younger counterparts. Head trauma is one of the most challenging injuries to evaluate in the geriatric population because both the consequences and the cause of the trauma are crucial to identify. Early involvement of the family is an important component of the ED evaluation because family members may notice subtle changes in the patient's baseline neurologic status before they become apparent to the emergency physician. Moreover, some elderly patients may be noncommunicative and cannot participate in their own evaluation.

EPIDEMIOLOGY

Trauma was the seventh leading cause of death for people 65 years of age and older in the United States in 1995.[1] Many studies have found the primary cause of death in these patients to be head trauma.[2-4] Head trauma in geriatric individuals carries a higher mortality rate than in younger individuals.[5,6] Unlike the younger trauma population, where men predominate, trauma in the geriatric population shows no gender bias.[3,4,7,8,18]

PATHOPHYSIOLOGY

As the body ages, elderly individuals become predisposed to injury for a variety of interrelated reasons. Vision, hearing, balance, and coordination deteriorate, and reaction time decreases, even more so in individuals with cerebrovascular or degenerative joint disease. Cardiovascular disease leads to dysrhythmia or syncope, and prescribed medications can alter the normal cardiac compensation that occurs with a change in position. As a result, elderly individuals are more susceptible to falls than younger individuals. Falls cause the majority of head injuries in elderly patients,[3,4,7-9,18] nearly three times more often than motor vehicle crashes.[9] Motor vehicle crashes, pedestrians struck, and assaults account for nearly all the remaining head injuries. Penetrating head trauma in the elderly is uncommon.

The changes in brain anatomy that occur with the natural aging process lead to a unique pattern of intracranial injuries in elderly patients who suffer blunt head trauma. Consistent with all mechanisms of injury is an acceleration-deceleration force on the brain. In elderly individuals, the dura mater is firmly adherent to the calvaria; thus epidural hematomas are extremely uncommon in the elderly. Cerebral atrophy leads to tension on the short bridging veins that connect the skull to the arachnoid and pia mater. With a significant acceleration-deceleration force, these fragile bridging veins tear, causing an acute subdural hematoma (Fig. 45-1). Brain atrophy also leads to increased mobility of the brain within the skull. As a result, contusions due to coup or contrecoup impact of the brain with the skull are more common in elderly victims of blunt head trauma. Acute subdural hematomas and cerebral contusions represent the majority of intracranial injuries, and they commonly occur together.[10-13] Acute subdural hematomas become symptomatic when blood rapidly accumulates in the subdural space, which applies pressure on the brain and causes neurologic dysfunction. Most acute sub-

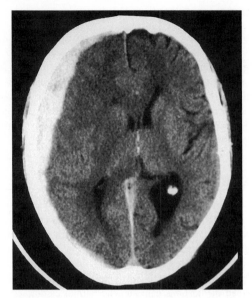

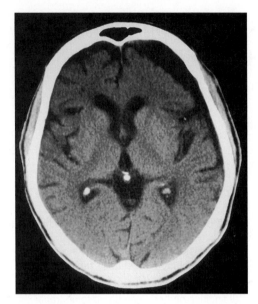

Fig. 45-1 Acute subdural hematoma. Right-sided hyperdense collection of blood crossing calvaria suture lines with compression of the sulci and lateral ventricles and some midline shift. *(Courtesy of David Effron, M.D., Department of Emergency Medicine, MetroHealth Medical Center.)*

Fig. 45-2 Subdural hygroma. Bifrontal collections of hypodense fluid associated with brain atrophy. Note suggestion of a vascular membrane and mixed attenuation on the left associated with some compression of the sulci. Some institutions may term this a chronic subdural hematoma on the left or even bilateral chronic subdural hematomas. *(Courtesy of David Effron, M.D., Department of Emergency Medicine, MetroHealth Medical Center.)*

dural hematomas require surgical intervention; it is extremely uncommon for acute subdural hematomas to progress to chronic subdural hematomas despite the terminology.[14]

With less severe head trauma, fluid can accumulate slowly in the subdural space and form a subdural hygroma (Fig. 45-2). This entity is most often bilateral, located anterior to the frontal lobes, asymptomatic due to brain atrophy, and associated with previous subacute trauma. The hygroma fluid is composed of protein-rich cerebrospinal fluid mixed with a small amount of blood. These lesions may remain asymptomatic for the life of the individual; a vascular membrane may surround the fluid collection over time (see Fig. 45-2). The fibrinolytic properties of the subdural hygroma fluid can lead to the accumulation of blood within the subdural space, which converts this entity into a chronic subdural hematoma[13,14] (Fig. 45-3). As a result, long after a seemingly minor head trauma event, a chronic subdural hematoma can become symptomatic from pressure on the adjacent brain by this delayed collection of blood. In addition, subsequent head trauma can convert a chronic subdural hematoma into an acute subdural hematoma (Fig. 45-4).

CLINICAL FEATURES

The evaluation of an elderly patient with a head injury can be challenging. Not only may elderly patients possess a baseline mental status that does not allow for active participation with their history or physical examination, but these patients also may have an abnormal baseline neurologic examination from prior cerebrovascular disease or head injury. While changes in memory, thought process, and personality may go unnoticed by those unfamiliar with the patient, these subtle changes may portend a significant head injury. In addition, significant time delays between time of injury and presentation may occur in this age group.

Prehospital Considerations

Since elderly patients can suffer significant intracranial, spinal, and orthopedic injuries from what may be considered minor trauma, prudent use of spinal immobilization by out-of-hospital personnel is warranted. Paramedics are an invaluable source of information and should be interviewed in the ED prior to their departure.

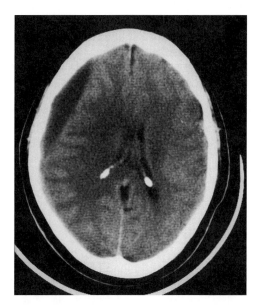

Fig. 45-3 Chronic subdural hematoma. Right-sided collection of hypodense fluid with slight compression of sulci and midline shift. *(Courtesy of David Effron, M.D., Department of Emergency Medicine, MetroHealth Medical Center.)*

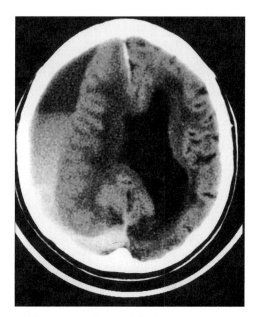

Fig. 45-4 Acute on chronic subdural hematoma. Large right-sided collection of chronic hypodense fluid with layering of acute hyperdense hemorrhage associated with complete effacement of sulci and lateral ventricles and some midline shift. *(Courtesy of David Effron, M.D., Department of Emergency Medicine, MetroHealth Medical Center.)*

They can describe the events surrounding the trauma, describe the home status or scene, and relay the statements of witnesses and family members.

History

Most patients with a head injury will complain of headache. Nausea is also a common complaint. Historical elements of importance relate to the circumstances surrounding the traumatic event. Key elements of the history that should be obtained include recollection of the traumatic event and the events immediately preceding the trauma, distance of fall, and the presence of headache, neck pain, back pain, limitation of movements of any extremity, any symptoms that are consistent with stroke syndromes, and any prior neurologic deficits. Other important historical elements include the presence or absence of diabetes, hypertension, heart disease, prior stroke, hematochezia, melena, and the use of alcohol. Special attention should be paid to the medication regimen, including any recent change in medications.

Physical Examination

Special consideration must be given to the interpretation of vital signs in elderly individuals. Elderly patients com-

monly take beta blockers that may blunt the expected tachycardia associated with trauma. Inadequately or untreated hypertension is common in elderly patients; thus a low-normal blood pressure may indicate shock. Tachypnea may indicate acidemia from shock, pain, or an intracranial injury. Pulse oximetry should be used to ensure adequate oxygenation throughout the evaluation.

A detailed neurologic examination is crucial to establish a baseline on which serial examinations are founded. Level of consciousness, orientation, speech pattern and quality, and the ability to follow commands should be noted. Pupillary size and reactivity are equally important to note. The Glasgow Coma Scale (GCS) must be recorded because this provides a consistent tool to assess neurologic status between multiple physicians and has been shown to be prognostic[3,6,15–18] (Table 45-1). However, clinical evidence of increased intracranial pressure may be delayed in older patients with underlying brain atrophy.

DIAGNOSIS AND DIFFERENTIAL

Patients with head trauma may present to the ED with only a history of altered mental status or level of functioning.

Table 45-1. Glasgow Coma Scale (GCS)

Response	Score
Eyes	
Open spontaneously	4
Open to voice command	3
Open to noxious stimulus	2
Do not open	1
Verbal	
Normal speech and communication	5
Confused speech	4
Inappropriate words	3
Incomprehensible sounds	2
No verbal communication	1
Motor	
Follows commands	6
Localizes noxious stimulus	5
Withdraws from noxious stimulus	4
Abnormal flexion to noxious stimulus (decorticate)	3
Abnormal extension to noxious stimulus (decerebrate)	2
No movement to noxious stimulus	1

The cause and effect of the trauma are intimately related. Since a syncopal episode may have precipitated the fall that caused the head injury, emergency physicians should be cautioned that the cause of the trauma may be more of a threat to the elderly patient's health than the injury itself. This differential diagnosis is broad and important to pursue because each diagnosis carries a different management priority and plan. Fever, dehydration, sepsis, dysrhythmia, myocardial infarction, syncope, vertigo, gastrointestinal bleeding, ruptured abdominal aortic aneurysm, stroke syndrome, medication interaction or adverse effect, hypoglycemia, hypoventilation, progressive dementia (cerebrovascular or degenerative), sundowning, depression, alcoholism, carbon monoxide and other poisonings, and elder abuse or neglect are all important to consider.

A non-contrast-enhanced computed tomographic (CT) scan of the head should be a standard part of the ED evaluation of an elderly patient with a head injury. Head CT scans are more likely to be positive in elderly individuals who suffer head trauma than in younger patients.[9,19] Even with a GCS of 15 in the ED, 28 percent of patients older than age 60 with a history of loss of consciousness or amnesia following blunt head trauma had an abnormality on head CT in one study.[19]

Acute subdural hematoma is the most common indication for neurosurgical intervention.[9,10,13] Acute subdural hematomas appear hyperdense on head CT scan and do not respect calvaria suture lines, differentiating these entities from epidural hematomas (see Fig. 45-1). Reabsorption of the blood causes the subdural fluid to become isodense with the adjacent brain, making identification challenging.[20] Subdural hygromas are hypodense collections of subdural fluid that are most often bilateral and located in the frontal lobes (see Fig. 45-2). Chronic subdural hematomas are hypodense collections of blood that also may have mixed attenuation from new bleeding or with additional head trauma even may transform into an acute subdural hematoma[20] (Figs. 45-3 and 45-4).

The use of ancillary studies often provides useful information. The electrocardiogram evaluates for dysrhythmia or acute cardiac ischemia, either of which can cause a fall. The complete blood count establishes a baseline hemoglobin level and hematocrit and evaluates for anemia. A basic metabolic panel provides information on electrolyte disturbances, renal function, and glycemic control. A urinalysis screens for genitourinary tract hemorrhage, provides information regarding hydration status, and evaluates for urinary tract infection. An ethanol level is important to obtain because ethanol intoxication has a prevalence of 10 to 34 percent in geriatric trauma patients.[6–10,21] An arterial blood gas determination may reveal inadequate resuscitation with either a low pH or a large base deficit (negative base excess) and also guides management of mechanical ventilation. Coagulation studies play a limited role in the initial ED evaluation, with the exception of patients on oral anticoagulants or with advanced liver disease.

EMERGENCY DEPARTMENT CARE AND DISPOSITION

As with every ED patient, immediate attention to airway, breathing, and circulation is critical. Even patients who are talking on arrival to the ED can deteriorate rapidly; constant reassessment is needed.[15,22] If there is any question regarding airway patency, endotracheal intubation is warranted. Special attention should be paid to maintaining cervical spine immobilization. Etomidate is an ideal induction agent because it has minimal adverse hemodynamic consequences. Adequate oxygenation and intravascular volume maintenance are crucial to prevent secondary brain injury from hypoxia and hypoperfusion. If at all possible, a thorough neurologic examination should be performed before using sedation and induction agents for intubation. The need for hyperventilation to maintain an arterial partial pressure of carbon dioxide ($Paco_2$) of 35 mmHg remains controversial; most authorities recommend its use only as a last resort to treat high intracranial pressure (ICP).

The use of short-acting analgesics (such as fentanyl) may be warranted for pain control. In a combative patient, short-acting benzodiazepines may be needed to help prevent further injury. Involvement of the family in the medical decision making is crucial. Open discussion regarding the need for intubation and restraints will alleviate tension.

The precise prognosis of an elderly patient following head injury is difficult to predict. Various studies have come to different conclusions regarding the important factors that predict morbidity and mortality, indicating that the response to traumatic brain injury is multifactorial. The most commonly identified factors that contribute to morbidity and mortality are absolute age,[5,6,11,16–19] lower presenting GCS,[3,5,6,11,12,15,16] presence of unreactive pupils,[6,11,16] a focal abnormality on neurologic examination,[9,10] the need for neurosurgery,[11,16–18] and host factors regardless of injury type or severity.[23] The patient's baseline use of anticoagulation agents has not been reported to be a risk factor for morbidity or mortality in these patients.[10,18]

For acute subdural hematomas in the elderly, mortality rates vary from 31 to 82 percent,[13,15,18,24,25] again suggesting that many factors contribute to injury response. The older the patient is, the less likely the patient is to survive[15–18]; patients over age 80 with an acute subdural hematoma had an 88 percent mortality rate in one study.[15] Studies suggest that patients undergoing early surgical intervention have a more favorable outcome.[16,24] However, patients who have a lower presenting GCS have a worse outcome regardless of timing of surgery.[15–17] Moreover, these patients rarely return to their preinjury level of functioning, as measured by the Glasgow Outcome Scale[16,17] (Table 45-2). In general, early neurosurgical consultation appears to optimize the potential outcome of geriatric patients with an acute subdural hematoma.

Not every acute subdural hematoma, however, requires neurosurgical evacuation.[17,25] One study concluded that nonoperative management is preferred if the subdural hematoma is smaller than 10 mm, there is less than 5 mm of midline shift, the patient has an ICP of less than 20 mmHg, and the cerebral perfusion pressure can be maintained at greater than 75 mmHg.[25] The decision to operate on a chronic subdural hematoma is more individualized. If there is progressive neurologic deterioration, then surgical intervention is indicated; however, overall this entity carries a lower mortality, so nonoperative management is often chosen.[26] In one case report, evacuation of a chronic

Table 45-2. Glasgow Outcome Scale (GOS)

Score	Outcome
5	Mild or no disability—able to resume normal occupational and social activities
4	Moderate disability—independent but disabled
3	Severe disability—requiring assistance with activities of daily living (ADLs)
2	Persistent vegetative state
1	Death

subdural hematoma proved to be fatal due to the development of a contralateral acute subdural hematoma.[27]

ADDITIONAL ASPECTS

All traumatic brain injuries in the elderly lead to some amount of cognitive, functional, and neuropsychiatric decline.[28] This effect is more pronounced in severe head injuries, where elderly patients fare worse than younger patients.[28,29] The effect of age plays a smaller role in minor head injuries, where elderly patients recover equally as well as younger patients.[30,31] Whether head injury is a risk factor for developing Alzheimer's disease remains controversial.[32–34] Some studies have concluded that head injury patients are at risk to develop all forms of dementia, not only Alzheimer's disease.[35,36]

The financial impact of caring for elderly head-injured patients is staggering. Elderly trauma patients use more health care dollars than their younger counterparts,[37] a fact that is most pronounced for moderately severe head injuries because these patients are hospitalized for longer periods and have a slower recovery.[6,38]

REFERENCES

1. Desai MM, Zhang P, Hennessy CH: Surveillance for morbidity and mortality among older adults—United States 1995–1996. *MMWR* 48(SS08):7, 1999.
2. Shapiro MB, Dechert RE, Colwell C, et al: Geriatric trauma: Aggressive intensive care unit management is justified. *Am Surg* 60:695, 1994.
3. Zietlow SP, Capizzi PJ, Bannon MP, et al: Multisystem geriatric trauma. *J Trauma* 37:985, 1994.
4. Ferrera PC, Bartfield JM, D'Andrea CC: Outcomes of admitted geriatric trauma victims. *Am J Emerg Med* 18:575, 2000.
5. Pennings JL, Bachulis BL, Simons CT, et al: Survival after

severe brain injury in the aged. *Arch Surg* 128:787, 1993.

6. Schiller WR, Knox R, Chleborad W: A five-year experience with severe injuries in elderly patients. *Accid Anal Prev* 27:167, 1995.

7. Sasser HC, Hammond FM, Lincourt AE: To fall or not to fall: Brain injury in the elderly. *North Carolina Med J* 62(6):364, 2001.

8. Roy CW, Pentland B, Miller JD: The causes and consequences of minor head injury in the elderly. *Injury* 17:220, 1986.

9. Nagurney JT, Borczuk P, Thomas SH: Elder patients with closed head trauma: A comparison with nonelder patients. *Acad Emerg Med* 5:678, 1998.

10. Nagurney JT, Borczuk P, Thomas SH: Elderly patients with closed head trauma after a fall: Mechanisms and outcomes. *J Emerg Med* 16:709, 1998.

11. Ritchie PD, Cameron PA, Ugoni AM, et al: A study of the functional outcome and mortality in elderly patients with head injuries. *J Clin Neurosci* 7:301, 2000.

12. Kilaru S, Garb J, Emhoff T, et al: Long-term functional status and mortality of elderly patients with severe closed head injuries. *J Trauma* 41:957, 1996.

13. Meldon SW, Delaney-Rowland S: Subdural hematomas in the elderly: The great neurological imitator. *Geriatric Emerg Med Rep* 1:21, 2000.

14. Lee KS, Bae WK, Doh JW, et al: Origin of chronic subdural haematoma and relation to traumatic subdural lesions. *Brain Injury* 12:901, 1998.

15. Cagetti B, Cossu M, Pau A, et al: The outcome from acute subdural and epidural intracranial haematomas in very elderly patients. *Br J Neurosurg* 6:227, 1992.

16. Dent DL, Croce MA, Menke PG, et al: Prognostic factors after acute subdural hematoma. *J Trauma* 39:36, 1995.

17. Croce MA, Dent DL, Menke PG, et al: Acute subdural hematoma: Nonsurgical management of selected patients. *J Trauma* 36:820, 1994.

18. Rozzelle CJ, Wofford JL, Branch CL: Predictors of hospital mortality in older patients with subdural hematoma. *J Am Geriatr Soc* 43:240, 1995.

19. Jeret JS, Mandell M, Anziska B, et al: Clinical predictors of abnormality disclosed by computed tomography after mild head trauma. *Neurosurgery* 32:9, 1993.

20. Scotti G, Terbrugge K, Melancon D, et al: Evaluation of the age of subdural hematomas by computerized tomography. *J Neurosurg* 47:311, 1977.

21. Higgins JP, Wright SW, Wrenn KD: Alcohol, the elderly, and motor vehicle crashes. *Am J Emerg Med* 14:265, 1996.

22. Lobato RD, Rivas JJ, Gomez PA, et al: Head-injured patients who talk and deteriorate into coma: Analysis of 211 cases studied with computerized tomography. *J Neurosurg* 75:256, 1991.

23. van der Sluis CK, Timmer HW, Eisma WH, et al: Outcome in elderly injured patients: Injury severity versus host factors. *Injury* 28:588, 1997.

24. Wilberger JE Jr, Harris M, Diamond DL: Acute subdural hematoma: Morbidity and mortality related to timing of operative intervention. *J Trauma* 30:733, 1990.

25. Servadei F, Nasi MT, Cremonini AM, et al: Importance of a reliable admission Glasgow Coma Scale score for determining the need for evacuation of posttraumatic subdural hematomas: A prospective study of 65 patients. *J Trauma* 44:868, 1998.

26. Jones S, Kafetz K: A prospective study of chronic subdural haematomas in elderly patients. *Age Ageing* 28:519, 1999.

27. Turgut M, Akalan N, Saglam S: A fatal acute subdural hematoma occurring after evacuation of "contralateral" chronic subdural hematoma. *J Neurosurg Sci* 42:61, 1998.

28. Rapoport MJ, Feinstein A: Outcome following traumatic brain injury in the elderly: A critical review. *Brain Injury* 14:749, 2000.

29. Rothweiler B, Temkin NR, Dikmen SS: Aging effect on psychosocial outcome in traumatic brain injury. *Arch Phy Med Rehabil* 79:881, 1988.

30. Klein M, Houx PJ, Jolles J: Long-term persisting cognitive sequelae of traumatic brain injury and the effect OF Age. *J Nerv Ment Dis* 184:459, 1996.

31. Luukinen H, Viramo P, Koski K, et al: Head injuries and cognitive decline among older adults: A population-based study. *Neurology* 52:557, 1999.

32. Mortimer JA, van Duijn CM, Chandra V, et al: Head trauma as a risk factor for Alzheimer's disease: A collaborative re-Analysis of case-control studies. *Int J Epidemiol* 20:S28, 1991.

33. Mehta KM, Ott A, Kalmijn S, et al: Head trauma and risk of dementia and Alzheimer's disease: The Rotterdam Study. *Neurology* 53:1959, 1999.

34. Nemetz PN, Leibson C, Naessens JM, et al: Traumatic brain injury and time to onset of Alzheimer's disease: A population-based study. *Am J Epidemiol* 149:32, 1999.

35. Salib E, Hillier V: Head injury and the risk of Alzheimer's disease: A case control study. *Int J Geriatr Psychiatry* 12:363, 1997.

36. Plassman BL, Havlik RJ, Steffens DC, et al: Documented head injury in early adulthood and risk of Alzheimer's disease and other dementias. *Neurology* 55:1158, 2000.

37. Sartorelli KH, Rogers FB, Osler TM, et al: Financial aspects of providing trauma care at the extremes of life. *J Trauma* 46:483, 1999.

38. Saywell RM Jr, Woods JR, Rappaport SA, et al: The value of age and severity as predictors of costs in geriatric head trauma patients. *J Am Geriatr Soc* 37:625, 1989.

46

Chest and Abdominal Trauma

Liudvikas Jagminas
Jeremiah Schuur

HIGH-YIELD FACTS

- With aging, there is an increase in the anteroposterior diameter of the thoracic cage; combined with kyphosis, this can cause a severe loss of intrathoracic volume and thoracic cage compliance.

- At the outset of trauma resuscitation, cardiac output is the physiologic variable that has been shown to differ most between elderly and young trauma patients and carries the most clinical significance.

- Elderly patients sustaining major chest trauma are at high risk for rib fractures or pulmonary contusion, even if not evident on the initial chest radiograph.

- Unstable vital signs following thoracoabdominal trauma can be the result of tension pneumothorax, cardiac tamponade, cardiac contusion, hemothorax, thoracic aortic rupture, intraabdominal solid-organ hemorrhage, or other associated pathology. A rapid assessment for these etiologies is essential.

The elderly are less likely to suffer a traumatic injury than those in younger age groups[1]; however, their morbidity and mortality for given levels of injury are higher.[2] Even though patients over 65 years of age constitute only 12 percent of the population of the United States, they consume one-fourth of all trauma health care dollars.[3] Among those who survive the initial hemodynamic stress of trauma, deaths are more likely related to impaired pulmonary or immunologic reserves.[4]

Thoracoabdominal trauma is a significant source of this morbidity and mortality. Expeditious decisions about which patients require surgical consultation and explo-

ration are critical for preventing morbidity and mortality. Despite decreased physiologic reserve and significant comorbidity, geriatric trauma patients often respond to aggressive resuscitation.

The division of thoracoabdominal trauma patients into "stable" and "unstable" may be quite challenging in the elderly. This division is made frequently based on vital signs and clinical appearance. Early invasive monitoring has been shown to identify a subset of elderly blunt trauma patients with normal vital signs and diminished cardiac output. A prolonged emergency department (ED) evaluation of hemodynamically "stable" elderly patients for occult injuries is probably less beneficial than early transfer to an intensive care unit (ICU) for invasive monitoring and data-driven resuscitation.[5,6]

EPIDEMIOLOGY

The prevalence of thoracoabdominal trauma in the elderly is unknown in comparison with that in the general population. Blunt trauma predominates in the elderly, accounting for greater than 90 percent of elderly trauma patients.[7] Significant abdominal injury requiring an operative procedure occurs in up to one-third of injured geriatric patients presenting to a trauma center.[3,8] One study reported that 14 percent of 852 geriatric blunt trauma patients had significant abdominal injuries identified.[9] Abdominal trauma carries a 4.7-fold higher mortality in the elderly than in younger patients with similar injuries.[10] In a study of 85 elderly penetrating trauma victims, mortality was found to be significantly higher in the elderly than in younger patients (9 versus 0 percent).[11]

PATHOPHYSIOLOGY

The three most common mechanisms of trauma in the elderly—falls, motor vehicle crashes (MVCs), and pedestrian–motor vehicle accidents—all harbor the risk for significant thoracoabdominal injury; however, MVCs and pedestrian–motor vehicle accidents involve much greater transfers of energy and are associated with a higher potential for serious injury. Elderly persons are also affected by violent crime but rarely are victims of penetrating trauma. While penetrating trauma accounts for between 5 and 10 percent of all elderly trauma patients,[12] there is evidence that it is increasing in frequency. Specific information about the mechanisms of trauma can be obtained from Chap. 44.

Several anatomic and physiologic changes occur with

aging. This is due in part to the aging process but is greatly accelerated by comorbid diseases such as diabetes, atherosclerosis, osteoporosis, and emphysema. There is an increase in the anteroposterior (AP) diameter of the thoracic cage; combined with kyphosis, this can cause a severe loss of intrathoracic volume and thoracic cage compliance.[13] With aging, the lung loses much of its elasticity because of decreased elastin and continued cross-linkage between subunits of collagen. Although total lung capacity essentially remains constant with age, the residual volume tends to increase from a normal of 25 percent in young adults to 45 percent of the total lung capacity in the elderly, with a concomitant decrease in expiratory and inspiratory reserve volumes and vital capacity.[14] Owing to these changes and a decreased diffusion capacity, there is an almost linear decline in the Pa_{O_2} of 2 to 3 mmHg per decade after age 20. Little change is noted in the P_{CO_2} in normal subjects as a result of the aging process; however, if the patient suffers from emphysema, the P_{CO_2} may rise to levels exceeding 55 to 60 mmHg. At these levels, hypoxia is the main ventilatory drive mechanism. The arterial pH in patients with emphysema and hypercarbia is usually maintained at approximately 7.35 by a compensatory rise in plasma bicarbonate levels.[14] Should the bicarbonate–carbonic acid ratio change abruptly due to mechanical ventilation, pH will rise, thereby reducing ionized calcium levels, which may lead to dangerous arrhythmias.

Cardiac output is the physiologic variable that differs the most between elderly and younger trauma patients, and it carries the most clinical significance during trauma resuscitation. Older patients have a significantly lower cardiac index, which is due to multiple factors.[6] Foremost, there is an age-dependent decline in cardiac output in the general population. In addition, the elderly patient's myocardium is more resistant to the effect of circulating catecholamines, and elderly patients are frequently on multiple medications (beta blockers, calcium channel antagonists) that can blunt normal physiologic responses to injury.[15] Vital signs are thus less responsive to hypovolemia and less predictive of serious injury in the elderly.

This directly affects resuscitation of geriatric patients with thoracoabdominal trauma. They are at greater risk from hypovolemia, hypotension, and poor perfusion. They are also less able to mount a normal physiologic response to these insults. Shock in the elderly is less likely to reflect only hemorrhage. Cardiac insufficiency is a likely factor. Noncavitary hemorrhage (caused by bleeding at fracture sites or lacerations) is more likely to be a significant contributor to shock in the elderly.[16]

Renal changes that are physiologic with aging include decreased renal blood flow and corollary lower glomerular filtration rate, tubular dysfunction, and decreased creatinine clearance. These should be taken into account when evaluating urine output, administering contrast material, and initiating antibiotic therapy.

CLINICAL FEATURES

Out-of-hospital reports should be examined for mechanism of injury, initial mental status, loss of consciousness, and initial vital signs. The history should help in identifying patients with high-risk injuries. (Specific information about out-of-hospital considerations and the history can be obtained from Chap. 44.) In their study of invasive monitoring in elderly patients with blunt trauma, Scalea and coworkers[5] identified six high-risk injuries: (1) pedestrian versus motor vehicle trauma, (2) diffuse trauma such as being "beaten," (3) initial systolic blood pressure less than 130 mmHg, (4) systemic acidosis, (5) multiple fractures, and (6) head injuries.

Chest Trauma

One of the roles of the primary and secondary surveys is to stratify patients who need (1) emergent invasive procedures or operative intervention, (2) diagnostic studies, or (3) serial clinical examinations. Penetrating thoracic trauma patients need a thorough search for all wounds; those in the posterior thorax and axilla may be easily overlooked. The emergency physician should inspect for ecchymosis, sucking chest wounds, flail segments, or paradoxical motions of the hemithorax. The chest should be auscultated for quality and symmetry of breath sounds. The chest wall should be palpated for crepitus and localizing tenderness. After the patient has been log-rolled (with maintenance of cervical spine precautions), the posterior thorax should be carefully examined as well. Heart sounds should be auscultated for murmurs or rubs. Distal pulses should be assessed for symmetry.

Abdominal Trauma

In blunt abdominal trauma, the physical examination has a low sensitivity for determining the need for laparotomy, with accuracy rates between 35 and 65 percent.[17] Palpation of the abdomen should evaluate for evidence of lower rib fracture because up to 20 percent of left-sided fractures are associated with splenic injury and up to 10 percent of right lower rib fractures are associated with hepatic injury.[18] Kehr's sign (shoulder pain not related to shoulder motion or palpation) is associated with blood irritating the diaphragm and frequently is related to splenic or hepatic injury. Pelvic stability should be assessed because up to 50 percent of patients with a major pelvic fracture have a concomitant intraabdominal injury. The rectal examination should examine for a superiorly displaced or "high riding" prostate. Frank rectal blood may indicate gastrointestinal disruption.

Penetrating abdominal trauma patients need a thorough search for all wounds. In addition, the zone of injury should be identified because this is indicative of potential underlying injuries. There are four anatomic zones of the abdomen:

1. *Anterior abdomen.* The area between the costal margins and the inguinal ligaments bordered laterally by the anterior axillary lines. Approximately one-third of injuries in this zone will result in injury to peritoneal structures. If there is evidence of peritoneal entrance, it must be assumed that there has been an intraabdominal injury.

2. *Thoracoabdominal.* The area from the nipple line to the costal margin anteriorly and the scapular tips to the costal margins posteriorly. There is high risk of intrathoracic injury with penetrating wounds in this area, but there is also risk of diaphragmatic and intraabdominal injuries. All penetrating thoracoabdominal wounds require surgical consultation.

3. *Flank.* The costal margins to the iliac crests from anterior to posterior axillary lines. These injuries carry an increased risk of retroperitoneal and colonic injuries and often need evaluation by computed tomographic (CT) scanning with rectal contrast material added if there is suspicion of colonic injury.

4. *Back.* The costal margins to the iliac crests between the posterior axillary lines. These injuries also carry a high risk of retroperitoneal injury and thus often require CT evaluation.

DIAGNOSIS AND DIFFERENTIAL

Unstable vital signs following thoracoabdominal trauma can be the result of tension pneumothorax, cardiac tamponade, cardiac contusion, hemothorax, thoracic aortic rupture, intraabdominal solid-organ hemorrhage, and other associated pathology. The emergency physician also should be cognizant of the fact that concomitant medical problems may have precipitated the traumatic event (e.g., myocardial infarction, arrhythmia, stroke, or hypoglycemia secondary to diabetes therapy).

Multiple diagnostic tests are available to assist emergency physicians with the evaluation of the geriatric patient who has sustained thoracoabdominal trauma.

Radiographs

The initial plain radiographs that should be obtained include chest, cervical spine, and AP pelvis films. Chest radiographs are of paramount importance in the evaluation of thoracic trauma, and only attention to life-threatening problems should delay obtaining one. A systematic review of the bony thorax, including ribs, clavicles, scapulae, and vertebrae, should be made. The lung fields should be examined for pneumothorax, hemothorax, or pulmonary contusion. Abnormalities of the mediastinum (Fig. 46-1) are suggestive of several injuries. Pneumomediastinum suggests airway rupture; widening of the mediastinum, loss of the aortic knob contour, shift of the nasogastric tube to the right, and an apical cap suggest aortic disruption; and shift of the mediastinum suggests tension pneumothorax. Diaphragmatic injury is often missed acutely. Initial chest radiograph findings of intrathoracic bowel gas or a nasogastric tube in the chest are seen in only 44 percent of patients.[19] Other findings suggestive of diaphragmatic injury are air-fluid levels in the lower thorax, indistinct hemidiaphragm, mediastinal shift, and lower rib fractures (Fig. 46-2). Finally, assessment of the cardiac silhouette may help in the diagnosis of myocardial injury, such as pneumopericardium.

Computed Tomography

CT angiography has essentially replaced aortography for the evaluation of aortic disruption. A normal spiral CT scan of the chest virtually excludes traumatic aortic injury. It has a sensitivity and specificity of 100 and 83 percent, respectively, for detecting aortic injury.[20] In addition, CT scan is able to evaluate other mediastinal structures and identify pneumothorax not readily apparent on plain chest radiographs. It also has been used for the evaluation of stable patients with penetrating thoracic trauma to determine the trajectory of the bullet in an effort to reduce exploratory surgery.[21] Helical CT scanning of the chest may be useful for detecting diaphragmatic injury.[22,23] Some centers report that magnetic resonance imaging (MRI) may be even better at detecting diaphragmatic injury.[24] The drawback with MRI is that it is not suitable for unstable trauma patients and may not be readily available.

CT remains the "gold standard" in the evaluation of blunt abdominal trauma patients, particularly those who

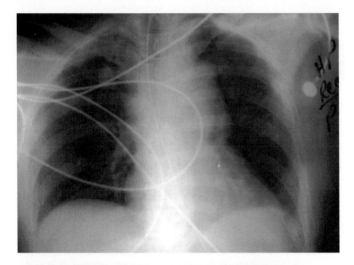

Fig. 46-1 Chest radiograph showing a wide mediastinum. *(Courtesy of David Effron, M.D., Metro-Health Medical Center, Cleveland, OH.)*

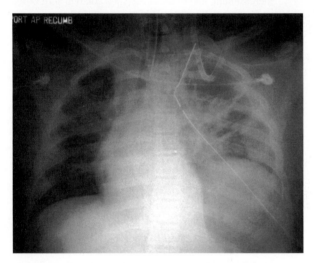

Fig. 46-2 Chest radiograph with diaphragmatic rupture. Note mediastinal shift, indistinct left hemidiaphragm, and left lower rib fractures. *(Courtesy of David Effron, M.D., MetroHealth Medical Center, Cleveland, OH.)*

are hemodynamically stable. It also can be helpful in defining peritoneal penetration in the penetrating trauma patient with equivocal findings. The problem arises in deciding which geriatric trauma patients are hemodynamically "stable" for CT scanning. Geriatric trauma patients with normal vital signs but with high-risk injuries or multiple comorbid diseases should be considered "unstable."

Disadvantages of CT scanning are its expense, time needed to perform the study, location outside the ED, and risk of allergic reaction and nephrotoxicity to the contrast material. Geriatric patients, who are often initially volume contracted, are at highest risk from the nephrotoxic effects of contrast material.[25]

Diagnostic Peritoneal Lavage

Diagnostic peritoneal lavage (DPL) is a rapid, simple, and accurate test for determining the presence or absence of intraperitoneal blood. DPL is highly sensitive for identifying intraperitoneal hemorrhage, but it lacks specificity in determining the organ(s) injured. It has a complication rate below 1 percent[26]; however, since many in the elderly population have had multiple previous abdominal surgeries, the complication rate is likely to be higher in this subgroup of patients.

Disadvantages of DPL include its lack of specificity for identifying injury, poor sensitivity for bowel and diaphragmatic injuries, and inability to detect retroperitoneal injuries. Up to 30 percent of patients with a positive DPL may be candidates for nonoperative management.[27] The only absolute contraindication to DPL is the need for emergent laparotomy.

Ultrasonography

Emergency physicians and surgeons have reported the focused assessment with sonography for trauma (FAST) examination to have a sensitivity ranging from 85 to 99 percent and a specificity ranging from 88 to 100 percent for detecting hemoperitoneum in blunt trauma patients.[28–30] The FAST examination is a bedside screening tool that aids clinicians in identifying free intraperitoneal or intrathoracic fluid. The underlying premise behind the use of the FAST examination is that clinically significant injuries will be associated with the presence of free fluid accumulating in dependent areas.

The subxiphoid view of the FAST scan is useful for identifying the presence of pericardial fluid. If there is a high index of suspicion for blunt myocardial injury or thoracic aortic injury, transesophageal echocardiography (TEE) is helpful in evaluating cardiac valve and wall motion and the presence and extent of aortic disruption. TEE offers several advantages. It can be performed at the bedside, does not require contrast material, is rapid, provides data on other cardiovascular structures, and is minimally invasive. Sensitivity and specificity of TEE for detecting aortic injury are 100 and 98 percent, respectively.[31] The disadvantages of TEE are that it is limited by the experience of the operator, may not be as readily available, requires that the airway be protected, is contraindicated in patients with cervical spine and esophageal injuries, and is limited in the evaluation of other aortic branch injuries.[31]

Laboratory Testing

Laboratory results should not delay time to invasive monitoring in elderly patients with high-risk injuries. The type and crossmatch is often the single most important blood test to obtain for patients with thoracoabdominal trauma. The hemoglobin level and hematocrit are affected by many factors and are insensitive indicators of acute hemorrhage. Serial arterial blood gas (ABG) measurements can be helpful in evaluating the severity of shock, respiratory acidosis, and response to resuscitation. A base deficit of −6 or less is an indicator of shock and a marker of severe injury and potential poorer outcome, and it can be an indication for further evaluation in a patient without an identified bleeding source.[32]

Electrolyte measurement is helpful when evaluating renal function and before administering contrast material. Coagulation studies are important in elderly patients who are taking oral anticoagulant therapy or who have medical coagulopathies. Although preinjury warfarin use has not been shown to affect outcome in trauma,[33] reversal of anticoagulation is frequently indicated. Urine should be checked for blood.

EMERGENCY DEPARTMENT CARE AND DISPOSITION

Geriatric patients who have sustained thoracoabdominal trauma require immediate attention to airway, breathing, and circulation. Even patients who are talking on arrival to the ED can deteriorate rapidly; constant reassessment is needed. If there is any question regarding airway patency, endotracheal intubation is warranted. Special attention should be paid to maintaining cervical spine immobilization. Lack of mobility of the cervical spine, specifically at the atlanto-occipital joint, may limit visualization of the vocal cords. Due to the likelihood of underlying cardiac or respiratory disease, initial application of supplemental oxygen is indicated.

Evaluation of circulation in the elderly trauma patient is different from that in younger patients because there is a high likelihood of myocardial dysfunction. Vital signs alone are not sufficient for identifying patients at risk from poor perfusion. Cardiac monitoring and intravenous access should be secured in all patients, with administration of crystalloid to hypotensive or tachycardic patients. It remains controversial how rapidly to administer intravenous fluids in the elderly patient with presumed myocardial dysfunction. It has been recommend that 1 to 2 L of crystalloid be administered in discrete boluses.[34] Older patients are extremely intolerant of shock and hypoperfusion. Mortality is increased in those who experience shock even transiently.[3] The emergency physician should monitor the patient closely for signs of fluid overload because overresuscitation can be as detrimental to the elderly as underresuscitation. In addition, early transfusion of packed red blood cells is likely to be beneficial. Initially, O-negative packed red blood cells should be transfused. Type-specific blood is often available within 10 minutes and is preferable to waiting for full crossmatch.

Chest Trauma

For geriatric patients who sustain significant penetrating or blunt chest trauma, management principles are similar to those for younger victims of trauma. Hemodynamically unstable patients with a penetrating injury to the thorax, especially those to the "box" described as the area located within the confines of the nipples laterally, clavicles superiorly, and costal margin inferiorly, require rapid transport to the operating room for definitive repair. Only lifesaving interventions should occur prior to transfer to the operating room (e.g., intubation, needle decompression of tension pneumothorax, pericardiocentesis, ED thoracotomy). Candidates for ED thoracotomy are patients in profound shock who do not respond to fluid administration and those who are agonal and appear to be in impending cardiac arrest on arrival or who suffered loss of vital signs en route to the hospital. Penetrating thoracic stab wounds have a better prognosis for survival (70–80 percent) than gunshot wounds (30–40 percent).[35] If pulseless electrical activity (PEA) is present, then the emergency physician needs to expeditiously identify and treat tension pneumothorax, cardiac tamponade, massive hemothorax, or cardiac rupture.

Geriatric patients sustaining blunt thoracic trauma generally have suffered multisystem injury. Osteoporosis and increased chest wall rigidity contribute to a higher incidence of rib and sternal fractures in elderly patients. These injuries, combined with reductions in lung function due to aging, result in an increased mortality associated with thoracic trauma.[16] As the number of rib fractures increase, so does the likelihood of associated injuries. The emergency physician should evaluate for flail chest, pneumothorax, and hemothorax if multiple rib fractures are present. Lower rib fractures of the ninth through twelfth ribs are associated with liver, kidney, and spleen injuries. First rib fractures may be associated with brachial plexus injuries, heart and great vessel injuries, and pneumothorax.[36] Sternal fractures may be associated with myocardial contusion and great vessel injury.[37] There should be a low threshold for admission and monitoring of patients with chest wall pain after trauma.

Segmental fractures of three or more adjacent ribs produce a flail segment of the chest, which can increase the work of breathing. Flail chest is recognized by paradoxical movement of the segment during the respiratory cycle (outward during expiration, inward during inspiration). Hypoxia results from primary underlying lung injury but also can be caused by paradoxical chest wall movement and pain that restricts deep breathing. Treatment includes supplemental oxygen, pain control, and intubation and ventilation as clinically indicated.

Pulmonary contusion is less common in geriatric trauma patients because their stiffer rib cage fractures rather than compresses to bruise the lung. When pulmonary contusion does occur, greater intraalveolar and interstitial edema is produced, leading to decreased pulmonary compliance and ventilation-perfusion mismatch. On chest radiograph, the contusion will appear as patchy or diffuse airspace disease. CT scan is more sensitive and specific than chest radiographs[38]; management, however, should be based on clinical findings.

Hemothorax is a common finding in major trauma victims and is associated with a pneumothorax in 25 percent of cases.[39] The blood should be evacuated with a large-bore (38 F or larger) chest tube. If more than 1 L of blood drains initially or more than 200 mL/h for 2 to 4 hours, a surgeon should be consulted for a decision to perform a thoracotomy.

In a simple pneumothorax, air enters the pleural space through a rent in the parietal pleura that acts as a one-way valve allowing air to enter but not completely exit the pleural space. If more air accumulates, the ipsilateral lung will collapse and begin to compress mediastinal structures, causing a tension pneumothorax. When this occurs, signs of neck vein distension, tracheal deviation, hypoxia, diminished lung sounds, and hypotension develop, and treatment must be rapid to prevent cardiovascular collapse. If a tension pneumothorax is suspected, a large-bore needle or intravenous catheter (14 G) should be inserted in the second intercostal space at the midclavicular line for needle decompression. Simple pneumothoraces are readily seen on expiratory chest radiographs. An *occult pneumothorax* (one seen on CT scan but not on plain radiographs) does not require chest tube insertion unless the patient is on a ventilator. Insertion of a small (24 or 28 F) chest tube is adequate if no hemothorax is present.

Tracheobronchial injuries occur in 1 to 2 percent of blunt thoracic trauma victims and 2 to 9 percent of penetrating trauma victims. Symptoms include dyspnea, dysphonia, hoarseness, and hemoptysis. Signs may include subcutaneous emphysema, hypoxia, or a persistent air leak from a chest tube. Massive subcutaneous emphysema and pneumomediastinum are often seen on chest radiograph, although up to 10 percent of patients with this injury will have a normal chest radiograph.[40] Respiratory distress and hypoxia will prompt intubation; however, there is a risk of extratracheal placement of the endotracheal tube. Whenever possible, endotracheal intubation should be performed with flexible bronchoscopy, preferably in the operating suite. Repair of these injuries is surgical.

Blunt trauma is responsible for 75 percent of diaphragmatic injuries. Approximately 70 percent will be right-sided, and 1.5 percent will be bilateral. Signs and symptoms depend on whether the bowel has herniated into the chest cavity. Patients without herniation are often asymptomatic or experience only mild pain. If, on the other hand, herniation has occurred, compression of the lung will cause dyspnea and tachypnea. If the bowel strangulates, the patient will exhibit signs of bowel obstruction. On chest radiograph, bowel loops or a nasogastric tube in the chest cavity are classic signs, yet few patients demonstrate these acutely. Other radiographic findings include an irregular, elevated, or indistinct outline of the hemidiaphragm or atelectasis of the lower lobe.[41] CT scan will diagnose the injury initially if herniation is present. If there is rupture without herniation, CT scan is unreliable for diagnosis,[41] and MRI should be considered. Treatment is surgical repair.

Esophageal injuries can result from either blunt or penetrating trauma. Penetrating trauma leads to immediate perforation in most cases, but high-velocity missiles can lead to late necrosis and delayed perforation.[42] The symptoms are chest, throat, or neck pain. Signs may include fever, subcutaneous emphysema, swelling, and shock. Cervical and thoracic spine radiographs may reveal air in the deep cervical tissue or air in the mediastinum. Gastrografin swallow is the initial test of choice; if it is nondiagnostic, a barium swallow should follow. This will identify up to 62 percent of esophageal injuries.[42] Endoscopy remains the "gold standard" for evaluating these injuries but is riskier than esophagography in the acute setting.[42] Surgical repair is required.

Diagnosis and management of cardiac contusion in blunt trauma remain controversial. Cardiac markers, echocardiography, cardiac scintigraphy, and gated blood pool scanning all have been studied, and none of them has been found to be highly sensitive or specific for the diagnosis. Elderly patients should be monitored for up to 6 hours, but no further testing is needed unless they become symptomatic or there is a change from their baseline electrocardiogram (ECG).[35]

Cardiac tamponade's classic findings of hypotension, muffled heart tones, and distended neck veins are present is less than 10 percent of patients. Any evidence of an entry wound in the epigastrium or the precordium within 3 cm of the sternum carries a risk for penetrating cardiac injury. The FAST examination has a sensitivity and specificity of 100 and 97.3 percent, respectively, for pericardial fluid.[43] Pericardiocentesis may serve as a temporizing measure in the treatment of cardial tamponade; most often the patient will require a pericardial window or thoracotomy for definitive repair of the underlying injury.

Cardiac rupture is documented to occur in 15 percent of MVC fatalities.[44] The mechanism for rupture is the same as for traumatic aortic injury, with 20 percent of these patients suffering a simultaneous aortic rupture.[44] Signs on presentation may include a precordial murmur that sounds like a "splashing mill wheel." ECG may show a bundle-branch block or, if herniation occurs, axis deviation. FAST may confirm pericardial fluid. Treatment is immediate operative repair.

High-speed deceleration injuries to the thorax may damage the thoracic aorta. In geriatric trauma patients, the aorta's inelasticity due to atherosclerotic disease and changes in elastin makes it particularly vulnerable to transection. Aortic transection is a common cause of immediate death following blunt trauma. With a history of deceleration or high-speed impact, the emergency physician should consider diagnostic CT scan or aortography, even without a widened mediastinum or other abnormalities on the chest radiograph. Treatment is immediate operative repair.

Abdominal Trauma

Emergent laparotomy is indicated for geriatric trauma patients who have sustained a high-velocity penetrating injury to the abdomen. Other clear indications for laparotomy include evisceration, signs of peritoneal irritation on physical examination, signs of acute gastrointestinal hemorrhage, or a positive FAST examination or DPL in the hypotensive blunt trauma patient.

The role of nonoperative management of traumatic abdominal injuries has become more popular among the surgical community. Nonoperative management of blunt splenic injury has been studied extensively regarding the effect of age on outcome. Studies disagree about whether elderly patients have a higher rate of failure of nonoperative management. One study retrospectively reviewed 1488 patients with blunt splenic injury, in whom 15 percent were older than 55 years. It found that patients 55 years of age or older failed nonoperative management at a higher rate (19 versus 10 percent) than younger patients. In addition, failed nonoperative management in patients 55 years of age or greater was associated with a higher mortality rate than operative management.[45] Other studies have not demonstrated a difference in the nonoperative management failure rate for patients older than age 55.[46,47]

For low-velocity penetrating trauma, local wound exploration can be performed safely only on the anterior abdomen. An exploration that ends anterior to the rectus fascia is negative, and the patient requires only local wound care.[48] An indeterminate exploration must be considered positive for peritoneal perforation.[49] CT scans are helpful in defining extent of injury, especially in the flank and back. Violation of the transversus abdominis or hematoma near the colon is an indication for consultation.

Disposition

Although CT scanning is not 100 percent sensitive, several studies have shown that in stable patients with blunt abdominal trauma and a negative CT scan, discharge after a period of several hours of observation can be safe.[50] There is a subset of elderly trauma patients that may be discharged safely from the ED, but it is not clearly defined. It may be prudent to admit most elderly trauma patients for observation because they likely have multiple comorbidities.

ADDITIONAL ASPECTS

Pitfalls in the management of geriatric chest and abdominal trauma include

- Overreliance on vital signs or urine output to determine elderly patients at risk of shock.
- Ordering multiple diagnostic tests prior to invasive hemodynamic monitoring in elderly patients with high-risk injuries.
- Failure to factor in all the comorbid disease entities associated with geriatric trauma patients when establishing an initial management plan.

REFERENCES

 1. Hogue CC: Injury in late life: I. Epidemiology. *J Am Geriatr Soc* 30:183, 1982.
 2. Demaria EJ: Evaluation and treatment of the elderly trauma victim. *Clin Geriatr Med* 9:461, 1993.
 3. Oreskovich MR, Howard JD, Copass MK, et al: Geriatric trauma: Injury patterns and outcome. *J Trauma* 24:565, 1984.
 4. Osler T, Hales K, Baack B, et al: Trauma in the elderly. *Am J Surg* 156:537, 1988.
 5. Scalea TM, Simon HM, Duncan AO et al: Geriatric blunt multiple trauma: Improved survival with early invasive monitoring. *J Trauma* 30:129, 1990.
 6. McKinley BA, Marvin RG, Cocanour CS, et al: Blunt trauma resuscitation: The old can respond. *Arch Surg* 135: 688, 2000.
 7. Osler T, Hales K, Baack B, et al: Trauma in the elderly. *Am J Surg* 156: 537, 1988.
 8. Morris JAJ, MacKenzie EJ, Damiano AM, Bass SM: Mortality in trauma patients: The interaction between host factors and severity. *J Trauma* 30:1476, 1990.
 9. Knudson MM, Lieberman J, Morris JA, et al: Mortality factors in geriatric blunt trauma patients. *Arch Surg* 129:448, 1994.
10. Finelli FC, Johnsson J, Champion HR, et al: A case-control study for major trauma in geriatric patients. *J Trauma* 29:541, 1989.
11. Nagy KK, Smith RF, Roberts RR, et al: Prognosis of penetrating trauma in elderly patients: A comparison with younger patients. *J Trauma* 49:190, 2000.
12. Champion HR, Copes WS, Buyer D, et al: Major trauma in geriatric patients. *Am J Public Health* 79:1278, 1989.
13. Brandstetter RD, Kazemi H: Aging and the respiratory stytem. *Med Clin North Am* 67:419, 1983.
14. Pontoppidan H, Geffins B, Lowenstein A: Acute respiratory failure in the adult. *New Engl J Med* 287:690, 1972.
15. Cheitlin MD, Zipes DP: Cardiovascular disease in the elderly, in Braunwald E, Zipes DP, Libby P (eds): *Heart Disease: A Textbook of Cardiovascular Medicine,* 6th ed. Philadelphia, Saunders, 2001, p 2019.
16. Martin RE, Teberian G: Multiple trauma and the elderly patient. *Emerg Med Clin North Am* 8:411, 1990.
17. Olsen WR, Hildreth DH: Abdominal paracentesis and peritoneal lavage. *J Trauma* 11:824, 1971.
18. Lee RB, Bass SM, Morris JA, et al: Three or more rib fractures as an indication for transfer to a level I trauma center: a population based study. *J Trauma* 30:689, 1990.
19. Gelman R, Mirvis SE, Gens D: Diaphragmatic rupture due to blunt trauma: Sensitivity of plain chest radiographs. *AJR* 156:51, 1991.
20. Fabian TC, Davis KA, Gavant ML, et al: Prospective study of blunt aortic injury: Helical CT is diagnostic and antihypertensive therapy reduces rupture. *Ann Surg* 227:666, 1998.
21. Grossman MD, May AK, Schwab CW, et al: Determining anatomic injury in selected torso gunshot wounds. *J Trauma* 45(3):446–56, 1998.
22. Marts B, Durham R, Shapiro M, et al: Computed tomography in the diagnosis of blunt thoracic injury. *Am J Surg* 168:688, 1994.
23. Demos TC, Solomon C, Posniak HV, et al: Computed tomography in traumatic defects of the diaphragm. *Clin Imag* 13:62, 1989.
24. Mirvis SE, Keramati B, Buckman R, et al: MR imaging of traumatic diaphragmatic rupture. *J Comput Assist Tomogr* 12:147, 1988.
25. Schwab CW, Kauder DR: Trauma in the geriatric patient. *Arch Surg* 27:701, 1992.
26. Gomez GA, Alvarez R, Plasencia G, et al: Diagnostic peritoneal lavage in the management of blunt abdominal trauma: A reassessment. *J Trauma* 27:1, 1987.
27. Thal ER, May RA, Beesinger D: Peritoneal lavage: Its unreliability in gunshot wounds of the lower chest and abdomen. *Arch Surg* 115:430, 1980.
28. Rozycki GS, Ochsner MG, Schmidt JA, et al: A prospective

study of surgeon-performed ultrasound as the primary adjunct modality for injured patient assessment. *J Trauma* 39:492, 1995.

29. Ma OJ, Mateer JR, Ogata M, Kefer MP, et al: Prospective analysis of a rapid trauma ultrasound examination performed by emergency physicians. *J Trauma* 38:879, 1995.

30. Tso P, Rodriquez A, Cooper C, et al: Sonography in blunt abdominal trauma: A preliminary progress report. *J Trauma* 33:39, 1992.

31. Buckmaster MJ, Kearney PA, Johnson SB, et al: Further experience with transesophageal echocardiography in the evaluation of thoracic aortic injury. *J Trauma* 37:989, 1994.

32. Davis JW, Shackford SR, Holbrook TL: Base deficit as a sensitive indicator of compensated shock and tissue oxygen utilization. *Surg Gynecol Obstet* 173:473, 1991.

33. Wojcik RW, Cipolle MD, Seislove E, et al: Preinjury warfarin does not impact outcome in trauma patients. *J Trauma* 51:1147, 2001.

34. Santora TA, Schinco MA, Trooskin SZ: Management of trauma in the elderly patient. *Surg Clin North Am* 74:163, 1994.

35. Brown B, Grover FL: Trauma to the heart. *Chest Surg Clin North Am* 7:325, 1997.

36. Trinkle JK: Management of major thoracic wall trauma. *Curr Probl Surg* 22:181, 1985.

37. Brookes JG, Dunn RJ, Roger IR: Sternal fractures: A retrospective analysis of 272 cases. *J Trauma* 35:45, 1995.

38. Rhea JT, Novelline RA, Lawrason J, et al: The frequency and significance of thoracic injuries detected on abdominal CT scans of multiple trauma patients. *J Trauma* 29:502, 1989.

39. Sturm JT, Points BJ, Perry JF Jr: Hemothorax following blunt trauma of the thorax. *Surg Gynecol Obstet* 141:539, 1975.

40. Huh J, Milliken JC, Chen JC: Management of tracheobronchial injuries following blunt and penetrating trauma. *Am Surg* 63:896, 1997.

41. Singh N, Narasimhan KL, Rao KL, et al: Bronchial disruption after blunt trauma chest. *J Trauma* 46:962, 1999.

42. Reber PU, Schmied B, Seiler CA, et al: Missed diaphragmatic injuries and their long-term sequelae. *J Trauma* 44:183, 1998.

43. Bastos RBN, Graeber GM: Esophageal injuries. *Chest Surg Clin North Am* 7:357, 1997.

44. Parmley LF, Manion WC, Mattingly TW: Nonpenetrating traumatic injury to the heart. *Circulation* 18:371, 1958.

45. Harbrecht BG, Peitzman AB, Rivera L, et al: Contribution of age and gender to outcome of blunt splenic injury in adults: Multicenter study of the eastern association for the surgery of trauma. *J Trauma* 51:887, 2001.

46. Cocanour CS, Moore FA, Ware DN, et al: Age should not be a consideration for nonoperative management of blunt splenic injury. *J Trauma* 48:606, 2000.

47. Myers JG, Dent DL, Stewart RM, et al: Blunt splenic injuries: dedicated trauma surgeons can achieve a high rate of nonoperative success in patients of all ages. *J Trauma* 48:801, 2000.

48. Henneman PL, Marx JA, Moore EE: Diagnostic peritoneal lavage: Accuracy in predicting necessary laparotomy following blunt and penetrating trauma. *J Trauma* 30:1345, 1990.

49. Rosenthal RE, Smith J, Walls RM, et al: Stab wounds to the abdomen: Failure of blunt probing to detect peritoneal penetration. *Ann Emerg Med* 16:172, 1987.

50. Liningston DH, Lavery RF, Passannante MR, et al: Admission or observation is not necessary after negative abdominal CT scan in patients with suspected blunt abdominal trauma: Results of a prospective multi-institutional trial. *J Trauma* 44:273, 1998.

47

Orthopedic and Spinal Injuries

Jason Wilkins

HIGH-YIELD FACTS

- Osteoporosis is the most common bone disease in the United States and a significant factor for morbidity in the geriatric population.
- Hip fractures have a 15 to 20 percent mortality rate within the first year. Between 25 and 50 percent of patients will not regain their ability to ambulate.
- Morbidity and mortality associated with hip fractures are related to the development of a deep venous thrombus or pulmonary embolus.
- Wrist fractures account for 15 percent of all fractures requiring emergency department (ED) care. Wrist fractures are more common than hip fractures until age 70.

Physiologic and metabolic changes make the geriatric patient more susceptible to orthopedic injury. While geriatric patients can have injuries similar to younger patients, emergency physicians should be able to recognize orthopedic injuries specific to the geriatric population. Emergency physicians also should identify the importance of early intervention and treatment of geriatric orthopedic injuries. Comorbid diseases and diminished physiologic reserve affect the rehabilitation and long-term treatment of elderly patients. A multidisciplinary approach is needed to reduce morbidity, mortality, and health care costs and facilitate return to preinjury function.

EPIDEMIOLOGY

The U.S. Census Bureau predicts that by the year 2020, 52 million people will be over the age of 65 and 6.7 million people will be over the age of 85.[1] Orthopedic injuries in this age group have a major impact on the lifestyle and independence of these people.[2] Women have a 40 percent lifetime risk of a hip fracture, wrist fracture, or vertebral body fracture.[3] Men have a 25 percent risk of experiencing fracture during their lifetime.[4] Approximately 20 percent of patients with hip fractures die within the first year of injury.[5] Half of them become partially dependent for care, and one-third are totally dependent.

PATHOPHYSIOLOGY

Osteoporosis

Osteoporosis is the most common musculoskeletal disease in the United States. It plays a significant role in the morbidity and mortality of the geriatric population. Aging, activity level, genetic predisposition, hormonal factors, and nutrition influence the effect it has on the human body. Hip fractures, wrist fractures, and vertebral body fractures are attributed most commonly to osteoporosis.

Osteoporosis is described as a process in which simultaneous reduction in bone mass and deterioration of bone microstructure result in defects in bone integrity. Homeostasis between osteoclasts and osteoblasts is disrupted with subsequent loss of bone mass and density. Due to the weakened state of the bone, it cannot withstand the normal physiologic forces placed on it.

Osteoporosis in women is highest within the first 5 years after menopause. Both age-related loss and loss of hormonal influences contribute to bone loss. An annual rate of 2 to 4 percent of density can be lost during this time.[6] Bone mass and density loss then continues with aging at a rate of 1 percent per year. Alcohol abuse, glucocorticoid excess, and hypogonadism contribute to 50 percent of cases of male osteoporosis.[3]

Pathologic Fractures

Pathologic fractures result from a focal disease process within the bone. Fractures may result from minor trauma or normal activities. Metastatic bone disease from breast, lung, prostate, kidney, or ovarian cancer is the most common causes of malignant pathologic fractures. Multiple myeloma is the most common primary bone malignancy resulting in fracture. Paget's disease, lymphoma, leukemia, and other hematopoietic malignancies can precipitate fractures and also must be considered.[7]

Comorbid Disease

Preexisting disease states play a large role in injury, treatment, and rehabilitation. Gait disorders from stroke or Parkinson's disease predispose elderly people to falls and household accidents. Cardiovascular disease, peripheral vascular disease, and diabetes cause weaknesses in gait, function, and healing and also limit rehabilitation. Depression, resulting from loss of function and independence, is common and has a significant impact on outcome. As a result, a multidisciplinary approach is essential for treating the geriatric patient.

Common Mechanisms of Injury

The geriatric population sustains unique injuries from similar mechanisms as the younger population. However, the incidence and prevalence of injury increase following minor trauma or falls in elders. It is important to evaluate the cause of the orthopedic injury because it may be an indicator of more severe health problems such as cerebrovascular accidents, myocardial infarction, arrhythmias, hypoglycemia, or sepsis. Appropriate tests should be ordered to exclude any other exacerbating problems. The emergency physician must be vigilant for possible elder neglect and abuse. Careful evaluation of all these factors may help to refine a treatment strategy for the patient.

Motor Vehicle Crashes

Motor vehicle crashes are the leading cause of fatal traumatic injuries through age 80 and the leading mechanism of injury for the geriatric patient.[1] Crash fatality rates are higher for the geriatric group than for younger groups.[8] Deteriorating cerebral function and motor skills impair the ability to operate an automobile. Decreased visual acuity and hearing impair identification and avoidance of dangerous traffic situations. Diminished reaction times and weakness impair the ability to control the automobile to avoid collisions.[1]

Falls

Falls are the leading cause of accidental injury over 75 years of age (see Chap. 5). Twenty percent of patients over age 65 and 40 percent of patients over age 85 require assistance to ambulate.[9] People over age 85 have a 50 percent chance of falling.[10] Half of all those who fall do so repeatedly.[1]

Most of these patients will fall on a level surface and sustain an isolated orthopedic injury.[11] It is imperative to evaluate the cause of the fall. Visual impairments, gait disturbances, changes in medication, loss of balance, postural changes, and environmental hazards predispose the geriatric patient to falls.

Elder Abuse

Elder abuse may include physical abuse, emotional abuse, financial abuse, and neglect (see Chap. 6). Neglect can be either active or passive by the caretaker. Physical examination findings of various aged contusions or abrasions should raise suspicion. Dehydration, malnutrition, poor hygiene, fecal impaction, or decubitus ulcers should raise suspicion of neglect. As with children, physical abuse or neglect may result in orthopedic injuries.

CLINICAL FEATURES

Elderly patients typically have contributing factors to their injuries that need to be addressed. The history of preceding events often dictates evaluation and treatment protocols. History taking should be directed at what caused the incident. Patients who report a fall should be questioned for tripping hazards, visual problems, problems with balance or strength, and syncope. Caretakers, family members, and medical records should be used to fill in any gaps in the history and to confirm any changes in mental status. Time of injury, mechanism of injury, postinjury care, and any prehospital medications for pain control are all important factors to consider. Past medical history, current medication lists, and allergies should be noted.

The initial management should be performed in the same manner as in a younger patient. Degenerative changes and osteoporosis increase the chances of occult fractures of the cervical spine. Cervical spine immobilization should be maintained at all times until a thorough evaluation can be performed. Emergency physicians should have a low threshold for imaging any area of discomfort in the elderly.

PELVIC INJURIES

Geriatric patients who have sustained serious trauma should be presumed to have a pelvic injury until proven otherwise. Elderly patients with osteoporosis are also at risk for pelvic injuries after minor trauma. Standard anteroposterior (AP) pelvis radiographs should be obtained on every geriatric or comatose patient with a history of multiple trauma.

Classification of Pelvic Fractures

Pelvic fractures include isolated single-bone fractures, complex fractures "breaking the ring," and acetabulum

Table 47-1. Injury Classification Keys According to the Young System

Category	Distinguishing Characteristics
LC	Transverse fracture of pubic rami, ipsilateral or contralateral to posterior injury
	I—Sacral compression on side of impact
	II—Crescent (iliac wing) fracture on side of impact
	III—LC-I or LC-II injury on side of impact; contralateral open-book (APC) injury
APC	Symphyseal diastasis and/or longitudinal rami fractures
	I—*Slight* widening of pubic symphysis and/or anterior SI joint; stretched but intact anterior SI, sacrotuberous, and sacrospinous ligaments; intact posterior SI ligaments
	II—Widened anterior SI joint; disrupted anterior SI, sacrotuberous, and sacrospinous ligaments; intact posterior SI ligaments
	III—Complete SI joint disruption with lateral displacement; disrupted anterior SI, sacrotuberous, and sacrospinous ligaments; disrupted posterior SI ligaments
VS	Symphyseal diastasis or vertical displacement anteriorly and posteriorly, usually through the SI joint, occasionally through the iliac wing and/or sacrum
CM	Combination of other injury patterns, LC/VS being the most common

Abbreviations: APC = anteroposterior compression; CM = combination; LC = lateral compression; VS = vertical shear.

fractures. Pelvic injuries are difficult to classify, and multiple classification systems exist. Young and Burgess[12] developed a system of classification based on mechanism of injury and causative directional force loads (Table 47-1). It is the most useful system for classifying pelvic injuries involving the pelvic ring because it correlates complications with the fracture pattern, making it clinically useful in evaluating patients. Three patterns of injury have been recognized. Lateral compression, anteroposterior compression, and vertical shear injuries are suggested by history and confirmed radiographically. As a general rule, horizontal fractures result from lateral compressive forces, and vertical fractures result from AP compression. Vertical displacement is usually from a shearing injury. Combinations of these injuries are not uncommon. Isolated single-bone fractures such as pubic rami fractures or acetabular fractures are not included in the Young and Burgess system.

Specific Pelvic Injuries

Fractures of the Pelvic Ring

Lateral compression injuries account for half of all pelvic fractures. Side-impact MVCs and pedestrians struck by automobile are primary mechanisms of injury. Lateral compression injury is characterized by transverse fractures through the pubic rami and is graded by the amount of sacral involvement. Type I injuries show signs of sacral compression on the affected side (Fig. 47-1). Type II in-

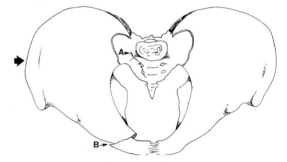

Fig. 47-1   Type I—lateral compression fracture. The lateral force is applied posteriorly (*arrow*). This causes a crush effect on the SI joint; this may be visible radiographically as a sacral fracture (*A*). The characteristic fracture pattern of the pubic rami will be seen (*B*). No ligamentous injury is seen.

juries involve an iliac wing fracture on the side of impact (Fig. 47-2). Type III injuries involve a type I or II injury and an open-book sacral injury on the contralateral side (Fig. 47-3). Complex pelvic fractures or "a break in the ring" can cause significant blood loss and neurologic injuries.

AP compression accounts for 25 percent of pelvic injuries and is most commonly associated with head-on motor vehicle crashes. AP compression is graded by the amount of sacroiliac (SI) joint disruption. Type I injury is characterized by slight widening of the pubic symphysis and stretching of the anterior SI ligaments (Fig. 47-

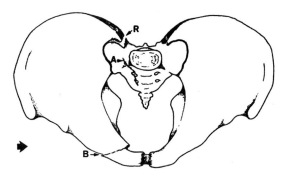

Fig. 47-2   Type II—lateral compression fracture. The force is applied anteriorly (*arrow*), causing the typical anterior pubic rami fractures (*B*). In this case, however, rotation of the pelvis around the anterior sacral margin may occur, causing rupture of the posterior SI ligaments (R). A crush fracture of the sacrum also may be seen (*A*).

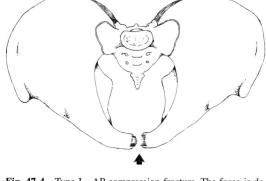

Fig. 47-4   Type I—AP compression fracture. The force is delivered in an AP direction (*large arrow*), tending to "open" the pelvis. This gives rise to mild splaying of the symphysis due to rupture of the anterior sacroiliac ligaments.

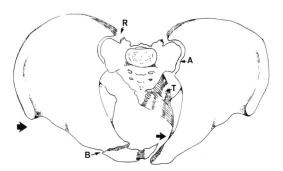

Fig. 47-3   Type III—lateral compression fracture. The force is applied anteriorly (*arrow*), causing internal rotation of the anterior hemipelvis. Continuing through to the contralateral hemipelvis (*arrow*), the force causes it to rotate externally. The result is a pattern of lateral compression on the ipsilateral side, with apparent AP compression on the contralateral side. This results in rupture of the posterior sacroiliac ligaments on the ipsilateral side (R) and sacrospinous/sacrotuberous complex (T) and anterior ligaments (A) on the contralateral side. Typical public rami fractures (*B*) are to be expected.

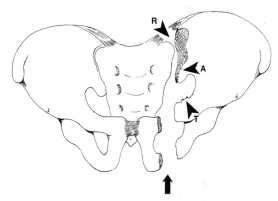

Fig. 47-5   Vertical shear vector. The injury force vector is delivered in a vertical plane (*large arrow*), causing disruption along this line. Fractures of the pubic rami usually are seen anteriorly, whereas fractures of the sacrum, SI joint, or iliac wing usually are seen posteriorly. The fractures are vertical and are associated with vertical displacement of fragments. Ligamentous injury to the posterior (R) and anterior (A) sacroiliac ligaments may be seen, as well to sacrospinous/sacrotuberous (T), and (possibly) symphysis ligaments.

4). Type II injury involves widening of the pubic symphysis with disruption of the anterior ligaments. Type III injury involves disruption of all ligaments and lateral displacement of the iliac bones.

Vertical shear injuries are associated with falls from height (Fig. 47-5). They account for approximately 5 percent of pelvic injuries. They are characterized by pubic symphysis diastasis or vertical displacement usually through the SI joint or iliac wing.

Isolated Fractures and Avulsions

Isolated bony fractures include avulsions of the anterior iliac spines, avulsions of the ischial tuberosities, pubic rami fractures, iliac wing fractures, ischial body fractures, and sacral and coccygeal fractures. Avulsions are seen most commonly in the adolescent population. Pubic rami and iliac wing fractures are very common in the elderly. Pubic ramus fractures are seen most often after falls or direct trauma. Patients with pubic rami fractures frequently complain of perineal pain, especially with standing or walking. Iliac wing fractures are a result of direct trauma to the lateral pelvis. Localized pain and swelling are common. Severe pain with ambulation and a waddling gait (Trendelenburg's sign) are often present with these injuries. Abdominal injuries are infrequent, but patients frequently will have lower quadrant tenderness and ileus.

Acetabulum Fractures

Acetabulum fractures generally are seen when forces are transmitted from the knee through the femur and into the hip. MVCs account for most of these injuries, but they can be seen from falls as well. Acetabular fractures present with hip or gluteal pain and are commonly associated with hip dislocations and subluxations. There are four general classifications of acetabulum fractures. Posterior fractures, ilioischial column fracture, transverse fractures, and iliopubic column fractures are defined by their anatomic involvement. Posterior fractures usually result from injuries with a flexed knee. Radiographs will reveal both the posterior fracture and a dislocation of the femoral head. Sciatic nerve injuries are common with this mechanism.

Diagnosis and Differential

The standard AP pelvis view should be obtained in any patient with a suspected pelvic fracture. Lateral, obturator oblique, inlet, and outlet views of the pelvis may be ordered to further evaluate the pelvis. The inlet view shows anterior or posterior displacement of pelvic ring fractures. The outlet view shows any superior or inferior displacement of fractures. Oblique views of the hemipelvis are true AP and lateral views of the acetabulum.

Computed tomographic (CT) scanning is most helpful in evaluating acetabular and sacral fractures. It is also helpful in evaluating for free fragments in the joint space and in identifying the presence of hemorrhage. Angiography and embolization are useful for the evaluation and treatment of hemorrhage from pelvis injuries.

Emergency Department Care and Disposition

Complex Pelvic Fractures

The emergency department (ED) care of complex pelvic fractures should focus on resuscitation and stabilization. A multidisciplinary approach should be taken because patients with these injuries have a high risk of other potentially fatal injuries. Complications from hemorrhage, rectal or urogenital injuries, diaphragm rupture, and potential nerve root injuries must be addressed. One study found that an average of 6 units of blood was needed in the resuscitation phase.[13] External fixators can help control hemorrhage from vascular injuries. A circumferential splint fashioned from a sheet can be used as a temporary measure to control bleeding. Angiography and embolization can be lifesaving for exsanguinating patients.

Pubic Ramus Fractures

The treatment of isolated pubic rami fractures focuses solely on pain control. Injuries usually can be differentiated from hip fractures by inspection of the pelvic bones. AP pelvis radiographs most likely will show nondisplaced fractures. Symptomatic treatment of pain with nonsteroidal anti-inflammatory drugs (NSAIDs) or opioid analgesics is recommended. Crutches or walkers may be necessary to aid in ambulation. Follow-up in 1 to 2 weeks with an orthopedic surgeon or the primary physician should be arranged. Intractable pain or an inability to ambulate should warrant admission and observation.

Iliac Wing Fractures

Treatment of iliac wing fractures is symptomatic with NSAIDs or opioid medications. Crutches or a walker will aid in ambulation. Open fractures or uncontrolled pain warrant admission and antibiotics. Follow-up should be arranged in 1 to 2 weeks with an orthopedic surgeon or the primary physician.

Acetabular Fractures

Early orthopedic consultation and hospital admission are indicated for all acetabulum fractures. Nondisplaced fractures may be treated with analgesics, bed rest, and non-weight bearing on the affected side. Displaced or fragmented fractures require surgical intervention. CT scanning of the pelvis can be beneficial for operative planning and evaluation of intraarticular bony fragments. Traction should be applied to displaced fractures that involve dislocation of the femoral head to reduce sciatic nerve compression.

HIP FRACTURES

Clinical Features

Ninety percent of these fractures occur in the elderly secondary to falls or torsion injuries.[14] Half of all 90-year-old women will have suffered a hip fracture. The physical examination should begin with a visual inspection of the hip and leg. Any scars, bruising, deformities, shortening, or rotation should be noted. Palpation of the femoral and pelvic bones should localize the area of injury. The stability of the ligament structure should be tested by compression of the pelvis. Range of motion should then be tested cautiously, with attention paid to any pain with internal or external rotation. A neurovascular examination should document any signs of sciatic nerve injury. Examination of the knee should be performed because knee and distal femur injuries may present with hip pain. Displaced fractures are diagnosed clinically by a shortened, externally rotated leg on the involved side. Nondisplaced fractures may present only with pain on ambulation and have a normal range of motion.

Diagnosis and Differential

Radiographic evaluation should consist of an AP pelvis view and AP and lateral views of the hip. The AP view should be taken with maximal internal rotation to obtain the best view of the neck. The trabecular lines in the femoral neck should be evaluated for any discontinuity or disruption, which may be the only evidence of a nondisplaced fracture. A line drawn from the inferior margin of the superior pubic ramus to the medial margin of the femoral neck should be a smooth, continuous arc (Shenton's line). A disruption of this line is indicative of hip pathology and is most often due to a femoral neck fracture.

Degenerative changes can make occult fractures difficult to diagnose. Any patient with severe pain with weight bearing needs further study. CT scanning and magnetic resonance imaging (MRI) are both helpful in further evaluating hip pain. MRI is capable of detecting fractures within 24 hours of injury.[15]

Emergency Department Care and Disposition

Femoral Head Fractures

Isolated femoral head fractures are commonly associated with hip dislocations. Superior shearing fractures are common with anterior dislocations, whereas inferior head fractures are common with posterior dislocations.

Comminuted fractures and dislocations are associated with high-energy injuries, which also place patients at higher risk for associated injuries.

Orthopedic consultation for reduction of the dislocation and fracture segment should be obtained in an expeditious manner. Delays in reduction and anatomic realignment increase the likelihood of avascular necrosis. Repeated attempts at reduction also increase morbidity. Posttraumatic arthritis is seen in two-thirds of all patients with these injuries. Avascular necrosis occurs in 10 to 20 percent of patients.[16]

Femoral Neck Fractures

The femoral neck is very susceptible to injury in the elderly population. The mean age for femoral neck fractures is 74 to 78 years. Classification of femoral neck fractures is based on anatomic area of involvement and displacement of pieces. All these fractures are intracapsular. Subcapital femoral fractures are the most common type of femoral neck fractures. The Garden classification system is the most widely used system for grading femoral subcapital neck fractures. Types 1 and 2 are nondisplaced, and types 3 and 4 are displaced. Midcervical and basocervical fractures are less common. AP and cross-table lateral radiographs are most useful in evaluating these fractures.

Orthopedic consultation should be initiated in the ED. Due to the tenuous blood supply across the femoral neck, these fractures are associated with a high rate of avascular necrosis. Early reduction and fixation are needed for nondisplaced fractures. Treatment commonly involves in situ fixation with cannulated screws. Displaced fractures have a high rate of nonunion and require primary prosthetic replacement. Traction decreases blood flow to the femoral head and increases the chance of avascular necrosis. Pain can be controlled adequately with rest and opioid analgesics until definitive treatment.

Intertrochanteric Fractures

Intertrochanteric fractures are seen more commonly in elderly women and usually are associated with falls. Torsion or rotational injuries also play a role in causing these injuries. Significant leg shortening and external rotation usually are observed on physical examination. Intertrochanteric fractures are identified most easily on the AP view of the hip. Intertrochanteric fractures are extracapsular and are defined as being in the line from the greater trochanter to the lesser trochanter. The fracture can be classified as stable or unstable, with alignment of the medial cortex of the neck and femoral component defining a stable fracture.

Orthopedic consultation should be initiated in the ED. Operative management usually involves a sliding hip screw or intramedullary nail and screw. Avascular necrosis is less of a concern. Buck's traction and opioid analgesics may help alleviate pain.

Subtrochanteric Fractures

Subtrochanteric fractures can be an extension of an intertrochanteric fracture or an isolated fracture below the level of the lesser trochanter. Physical examination findings of pain and swelling are similar to those of intertrochanteric fractures. Subtrochanteric fractures have the potential for significant hemorrhage. Stable fractures are defined as having an intact medial and posterior cortex.

Orthopedic consultation should be initiated in the ED. Traction with a Hare or Sager splint and opioid analgesics will help to alleviate pain until definitive treatment.

HIP DISLOCATIONS

Clinical Features

Most hip dislocations result from MVCs, but they may occur following a fall. Elderly patients with hip prostheses may sustain dislocations from simple tasks such as tying shoelaces or crossing their legs. Dislocations can be classified as anterior, posterior, or central. Posterior dislocations are the most common and result from the application of posterior force on a knee that is flexed or adducted and flexed. On examination, the leg is usually shortened, internally rotated, and adducted. Sciatic nerve injuries are seen in approximately 10 percent of these dislocations. Avascular necrosis is a common complication, and its likelihood increases with the duration of the dislocation. Anterior dislocations account for 10 to 15 percent of hip dislocations. A combination of abduction and flexion of the hip may result in an anterior dislocation. On examination, the leg is usually held in abduction and external rotation. The hip may be flexed (if the femoral head is inferior) or either extended or slightly flexed (if the femoral head is dislocated superiorly). Neurovascular injuries are uncommon. Central dislocations are associated with acetabular fractures, as discussed earlier.

Diagnosis and Differential

Standard AP and lateral hip films will reveal the dislocation (Fig. 47-6). Acetabular fractures, periprosthetic frac-

tures, or prosthetic dislocations must be excluded prior to manipulation. The femoral head must be examined for any signs of fracture. Hip dislocations are difficult to detect clinically when associated with femoral shaft fractures; in these cases, both pelvic and femur radiographs should be obtained.

Emergency Department Care and Disposition

Closed reduction of the isolated hip dislocation should be performed as soon as possible. Traction is best achieved with assistants exerting downward force countertraction on the pelvis with inline traction pulled tangentially. Anterior dislocations can be reduced with traction, flexion, and internal rotation. Once the femoral head clears the rim of the acetabulum, the hip is then abducted. Posterior dislocations are reduced with traction, flexion to 90 degrees, and gentle internal-external rotation (Allis maneuver) (Fig. 47-7). Reduction also may be achieved with the Stimson maneuver in certain situations (Fig. 47-8). Postreduction radiographs should be obtained to confirm reduction and exclude occult or iatrogenic fractures. General anesthesia or open reduction may be required to achieve reduction in difficult cases. Orthopedic consultation should be obtained for follow-up care. Fracture dislocations or complicated prosthetic failures require immediate orthopedic consultation.

HUMERUS FRACTURES

Clinical Features

Proximal humerus fractures account for 5 percent of all fractures presenting to the ED. They are seen most commonly in the geriatric population after a fall on an outstretched hand or a direct blow.[2] Proximal fractures present with pain, swelling, and ecchymosis of the shoulder. The arm is usually cradled next to the body with the elbow in flexion. A thorough neurovascular examination must be performed. Neurovascular injuries are a common complication of humeral shaft fractures but are rare with proximal humeral fractures. Brachial, radial, and ulnar pulses should be palpated. Axillary nerve function should be documented by deltoid firing and sensation over the deltoid area. Radial nerve function and distal pulses must be documented for humeral shaft fractures. Radial nerve palsies can be seen in 10 to 20 percent of humeral shaft fractures. Humeral shaft fractures are also a common initial presentation of metastatic breast cancer.

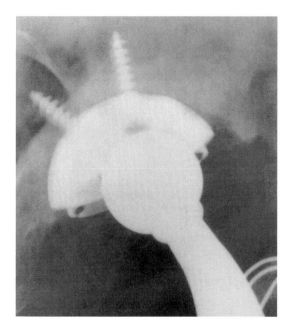
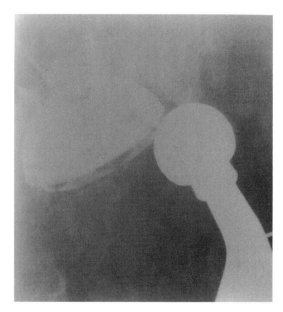

Fig. 47-6 This patient's total hip arthroplasty is dislocated. The slight asymmetry on the first view was not detected, and further radiographs were needed to diagnose the dislocation.

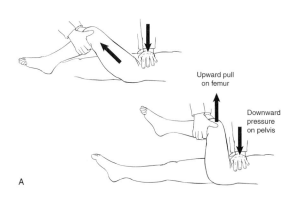
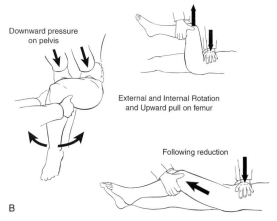

Fig. 47-7 Allis maneuver.

Diagnosis and Differential

Standard AP, lateral, and axillary views of the shoulder are adequate to evaluate for fractures and dislocations. Humeral head fractures involving articular surface may have a pseudosubluxation inferiorly due to accumulation of clot. Transthoracic views, scapular Y-views, CT scanning, or MRI also may be of use in complicated cases.

AP and lateral views of the humerus are adequate to evaluate humeral shaft injuries.

Emergency Department Care and Disposition

Most injuries can be treated with immobilization and pain management. Proximal humerus fractures are classified

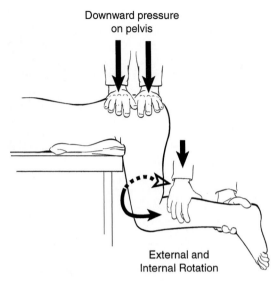

Downward pressure
on pelvis

External and
Internal Rotation

Fig. 47-8   Stimson maneuver.

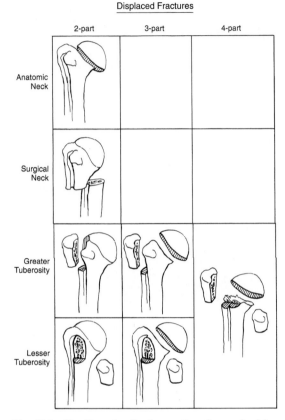

Displaced Fractures

2-part   3-part   4-part

Anatomic
Neck

Surgical
Neck

Greater
Tuberosity

Lesser
Tuberosity

Fig. 47-9   The Neer classification systems for proximal humerus fractures.

by the Neer classification system (Fig. 47-9). It uses the relationship between the anatomic neck, surgical neck, greater tuberosity, and lesser tuberosity to direct the management of fractures. Significant displacement is defined as greater than 45 degrees of angulation or 1 cm of separation.

One-part fractures account for 80 percent of proximal fractures. Soft tissues and periosteum support the fracture fragments and limit displacement. Treatment involves ice, analgesics, sling and swathe or shoulder immobilizer, and orthopedic referral. Early motion generally is desired to avoid adhesive capsulitis.

Two- and three-part fractures of the proximal humerus are more difficult to manage. Neurovascular and rotator cuff injuries are common. Analgesia and early orthopedic consultation are required. Closed reduction and possible surgical intervention may be needed. Fractures involving the anatomic neck or articular surface are at high risk for avascular necrosis. Greater tuberosity fractures are seen in approximately 15 percent of shoulder dislocations.

Humeral shaft fractures without evidence of neurovascular injury usually can be treated with closed management, ice, and analgesics. Sarmiento braces, coaptation (sugar tong) splints, hanging casts, or shoulder immobilizers all can used for closed treatment. Orthopedic follow-up should be arranged.

DISTAL RADIUS FRACTURES

Clinical Features

Fractures of the distal radius are very common. Women over age 50 account for almost 85 percent of all distal radius fractures.[17] These fractures are seen most frequently with falls on outstretched hands.[2] Muscular attachments, point of impact, degree of force, and age factor into the amount of angulation and displacement of these fractures.

Patients with complaints of pain at the distal radius should be evaluated for fractures. Displaced fractures generally show some degree of deformity. Examination of the joint above and below the injury is mandatory. Careful assessment of the neurovascular status of the hand is important. Median nerve compression is common with displaced fractures. Colles' fractures have the characteristic "dinner fork deformity" of the extensor surface of the wrist. Smith's fracture (or a reverse Colles' fracture) has deformity of the flexor surface of the wrist. Barton's fractures are fractures of the dorsal or volar rim and are associated with displacement of the carpus.

Diagnosis and Differential

Standard AP and lateral views of the wrist generally are sufficient to evaluate the wrist for fractures. Coned-down images may be ordered for specific areas of injury.

Emergency Department Care and Disposition

Nondisplaced fractures can be managed effectively on an outpatient basis with a sugar tong or volar splint. Short-arm casts can be placed at a later time. Analgesics, ice, and elevation will alleviate most pain and swelling. Orthopedic follow-up should be arranged within the week.

Complex or displaced fractures need closed or open reduction. Although elderly patients tolerate higher degrees of postreduction displacement, orthopedic consultation should be sought for the management of these fractures. Highly comminuted fractures have a high rate of failure with closed treatment and may need internal or external fixation. Attempts at reduction in the ED should be performed with care. Conscious sedation or local pain control with a hematoma block should be used to provide pain control. Care of soft tissues and adequate splint padding are imperative to prevent skin breakdown. Postreduction splinting with a sugar tong splint is adequate, and follow-up within 1 week for radiographic reevaluation is recommended. Reduction failure will need operative treatment. External fixation is generally the treatment of choice for elderly patients. Open fractures generally require antibiotics, evaluation of tetanus status, and operative debridement.

SPINE FRACTURES

Clinical Features

Geriatric patients commonly sustain spinal fractures due to osteoporotic and degenerative changes of the spine. Vertebral fractures are the most common fracture over age 65. An estimated 90 percent of all patients over age 75 have vertebral compression fractures.[18] Compression fractures can even occur from common events, such as coughing or picking up a basket of laundry. Most frac-

tures occur below the T6 level. Patients will complain of pain at the localized area. A meticulous neurologic examination must be performed.

A high index of suspicion for cervical spine fractures should be maintained in the older trauma patient. One study found the incidence of cervical spine injury to be twice as great in geriatric patients as it was in a younger cohort of blunt trauma patients. Odontoid fractures were particularly common in geriatric patients, accounting for 20 percent of geriatric cervical spine fractures compared with 5 percent of nongeriatric fractures.[19]

Diagnosis and Differential

Lateral cervical spine radiographs will detect 70 to 80 percent of cervical spine fractures. AP and odontoid views are needed to complete the series. Oblique views may be of limited benefit. Owing to degenerative changes, fracture lines may be obscured and hidden within the masses of degenerative bone. Persistent neck pain with "normal" radiographs warrants further study. CT scanning is helpful in evaluating for fractures or fracture/dislocations of the spine. MRI is helpful in evaluating soft tissue injuries or cord compression and contusions.

Thoracic and lumbar radiographs are sufficient for evaluating most cases of suspected compression fractures. Radiographs should be evaluated thoroughly for any signs of destructive bone loss from metastatic diseases. MRI is useful in facilitating a diagnosis of metastatic disease.

Emergency Department Care and Disposition

Cervical spine injuries require meticulous spinal immobilization and prompt neurosurgical or orthopedic evaluation. Documentation of neurologic deficits and their time of onset is necessary. Standard methylprednisolone therapy for neurologic deficits associated with blunt spinal cord injuries should be initiated.

Severe depression and limitations of activity can result from vertebral compression fractures. Patients with central fractures are at a much higher risk for peripheral fractures in the future. Multiple compression fractures lead to deformity of the chest and abdomen causing respiratory and potential gastrointestinal problems. Vertebral compression fractures require aggressive pain management for resumption of activities. Patients with intractable pain should be admitted for pain control.

ADDITIONAL ASPECTS

The following are pitfalls in the management of geriatric orthopedic injuries:

- Failure to advise elderly patients that they need further education on strategies to impede the progression of bone loss and reduce the risk of fracture from osteoporosis. Smoking cessation, reducing alcohol consumption, and regular weight-bearing exercises will significantly reduce this risk. Physical activity may be the most important method to reduce bone loss and improve bone mass. Regular weight-bearing exercises can reduce the risk of fracture by 50 percent.[20] Calcium supplementation of 1500 mg/day with 800 units of vitamin D is recommended by the National Institutes of Health and has been shown to decrease hip fractures by 43 percent and vertebral fractures by 32 percent in patients over age 68.[21]

- Failure to properly arrange investigation of the cause of the fall and correct any precipitating factors. Environmental hazards contribute to 44 percent of falls.[22] Stairs, uneven or wet floors, electrical cords, and inadequate lighting are potentially preventable causes of falls. Assist devices such as walkers or lifts can aid patients in self-care and provide them with a certain level of security. Footwear should be well fitted and be able to provide good traction. A home inspection can be arranged through the patient's primary physician and social worker.

REFERENCES

1. Schwab CW, Kauder DR: Trauma in the geriatric patient. *Arch Surg* 127:701, 1992.
2. Demarest GB, Osler TM, Clevenger FW: Injuries in the elderly: Evaluation and initial response. *Geriatrics* 45:36, 1990.
3. Melton LJ, Atkinson EJ, O'Fallon WM, et al: Long-term fracture risk prediction with bone mineral measurements made at various skeletal sites. *J Bone Miner Res* 6:S136, 1991.
4. Looker AC, Orwoll ES, Johnston CC Jr, et al: Prevalence of low femoral bone sensitivity in older US adults from NHANES III. *J Bone Res* 12:1761, 1997.
5. Bredahl C, Nyholm B, Hindsholm KB: Mortality after hip fracture: Results of operation with 12 hours of admission. *Injury* 23:83, 1992.
6. Ross PD: Risk factors for osteoporotic fracture. *Endocr Metab Clin* 27:289, 1998.
7. Higinbotham NL, Marcove RC: The management of pathological fractures. *J Trauma* 5:792, 1985.
8. Li G, Baker SP, Longlois JA, et al: Are female drivers safer? An application of the decompression method. *Epidemiology* 9:379, 1998.
9. Close J, Ellis M, Hooper R, et al: Prevention of falls in the elderly trial: A randomized controlled trial. *Lancet* 353:93, 1999.
10. Nelson RC, Amin MA: Falls in the elderly. *Emerg Med Clin North Am* 8:309, 1990.
11. Tinetti ME, Speechley M: Prevention of falls among the elderly. *New Engl J Med* 320:1055, 1989.
12. Young JWR, Burgess AR: Radiologic management of pelvic ring fractures, in Urban T, Schwarzenberg E (eds): *Systematic Radiologic Diagnosis.* Baltimore, Williams & Wilkins, 1987.
13. Burgess AR, Eastridge BJ, Young JW, Ellison TS: Pelvic ring disruptions: Effective classification and treatment protocols. *J Trauma* 30:848, 1990.
14. Grisso JA, Kelsey JL, Strom BL, et al: Risk factors for falls as a cause of hip fracture in women. *New Engl J Med* 324:1326, 1991.
15. Pandey R, McNally E, Ali A, Bulstrode C: The role of MRI in the diagnosis of occult hip fractures. *Injury* 29:61, 1998.
16. Rosenthal RE, Coker WL: Posterior fracture dislocation of the hip. *J Trauma* 19:572, 1979.
17. Dinowitz MI, Koval KJ, Meadows S: Distal radius, in Koval KJ, Zuckerman JD (eds): *Fractures in the Elderly.* Philadelphia, Lippincott-Raven, 1998, p 127.
18. Cohen LD: Fractures of the osteoporotic spine. *Orthop Clin North Am* 21:143, 1990.
19. Touger M, Gennis P, Nathanson N, et al: Validity of a decision rule to reduce cervical spine radiography in elderly patients with blunt trauma. *Ann Emerg Med* 40:287, 2002.
20. Law MR, Wald NJ, Meade TW: Strategies for the prevention of osteoporosis and hip fracture. *Br Med J* 303:453, 1991.
21. Optimal calcium intake. *NIH Consensus Statement* 12:1, 1994.
22. Tinetti ME, Speechley M, Ginter SF: Risk factors for falls among the elderly persons living in the community. *New Engl J Med* 319:1701, 1988.

48

Dehydration and Electrolyte Disorders

Ethan Heit
Stephen W. Meldon

HIGH-YIELD FACTS

- Dehydration is the most common fluid and electrolyte disorder in both nursing home and community-dwelling elders.

- Between 1 and 2 percent of elders will be hospitalized due to dehydration each year.

- Physical findings and vital signs are not always reliable when assessing older persons for dehydration.

- Electrolyte disorders are also common in this age group, especially alterations in sodium and potassium; the prevalence of hyponatremia, for example, is approximately 8 percent in ambulatory geriatric patients.

- Risk factors for electrolyte disorders include renal insufficiency and medications such a diuretics and angiotensin-converting enzyme (ACE) inhibitors.

- Severity of symptoms for electrolyte disorders depends on both the amount and rate of decline of serum electrolyte levels.

The average total-body water content in healthy 30- to 40-year-olds is approximately 55 to 60 percent. This declines with aging and reaches 50 percent by age 75 to 80 years. The total-body water is divided into three compartments: the intracellular, the interstitial, and the in-travascular. The intracellular compartment is approximately two-thirds of the total-body water, with the remaining one-third divided between the interstitial compartment (approximately three-quarters) and the intravascular or plasma volume (one-quarter).

OSMOLALITY

Biochemically, 1 osmole is defined as the molecular weight of of a substance divided by the number of individual disassociated particles in solution. The osmolarity is the number of osmoles per liter of solution, whereas the osmolality is the number of osmoles per kilogram of solution. Osmolality has the benefit of not being affected by the temperature, nor by the volume resulting from other particles in the solution. Since plasma is approximately 92 percent water, which has a density of 1 kg/L, osmolality can be expressed in osmoles per liter, which will more closely approximate osmotic pressure.

The effective osmolality, or tonicity, is made of the solutes that do not freely diffuse across biologic membranes. These solutes affect the distribution of water in the fluid compartments of the body because water does freely cross biologic membranes.

Plasma osmolality ranges from 280 to 295 mmol/kg in the general population and is fairly constant for each individual. Osmolality can be measured directly from the freezing point, where 1 mol/L of ideal solute lowers the freezing point 1.86°C (1°F). In clinical practice, the osmolality can be estimated by adding the serum electrolyte, glucose, and blood urea nitrogen (BUN) values. Nonelectrolytes can be converted to molar equivalents by dividing by one-tenth the molecular weight. Since electrolytes are more or less electrically neutral, the sodium, chloride, potassium, and bicarbonate can be estimated by simply twice the sodium concentration, yielding a final formula of

$$\text{Osmolality (mOsm/L)} = 2 \times [\text{Na}^+] + \text{glucose}/18 + \text{BUN}/2.8$$

THIRST

Thirst is regulated by the organum vasculosum of the lamina terminalis, which is located in the anterior wall of the third ventricle. Thirst begins to increase when the serum osmolality increases beyond 290 mmol/kg. It is also increased by hypotension and hypovolemia, starting when volume changes more than 10 percent.

Thirst sensation declines with age. In addition, the ability of thirst to regulate body water depends on the ability to act on it. Patients who are unable to obtain or drink water lose the ability for thirst to help regulate free body water. This makes patients with gastrostomy or jejunostomy tubes, who do not control their own feedings, at risk.

WATER EXCRETION

Water loss occurs by three principal methods. The first is insensible loss, via the skin and respiratory system. These losses average 0.6 mL/kg/h but can be increased by many factors, including changes in ambient temperatures and humidity, fever and other states of increased heat production, and loss of skin integrity, such as burns. These losses are not physiologically regulated.

The second method is via the gastrointestinal tract. This loss is usually less than 150 mL/day but will be increased with increased fluid losses, including vomiting, diarrhea, gastric suction, and other forms of drainage from gastrointestinal organs. These losses are also not physiologically regulated.

The third method of water loss is via the kidney and urinary system. This is the method of physiologically regulated water loss that is responsive to changes in serum osmolality and effective arterial volume. Urine volume can range from 500 mL to 20 L in a healthy person, but the range will be restricted in the elderly because they have a decreased ability to excrete a water load. This is due to a combination of decreased renal mass, cortical blood flow, and glomerular filtration rate, as well as a decreased responsiveness to the sodium balance. Renal water excretion is controlled directly by vasopressin [antidiuretic hormone (ADH)], which is synthesized in the supraoptic and paraventricular nuclei of the hypothalamus and is stored in the posterior pituitary. The release is stimulated by an increase in plasma osmolality.

DEHYDRATION

Dehydration is a common problem in the elderly patient, accounting for significant morbidity and hospitalization. Assessing hydration status in older patients can be difficult because physical examination findings may be absent or nonspecific, and laboratory analysis must take the patient's baseline status into account.

No absolute definition of dehydration exists. One useful definition is rapid weight loss of greater than 3 percent of body weight.[1] Serum osmolality can be quantitated and is useful for both defining and categorizing dehydration. Different types of dehydration occur and should be distinguished because the type dictates treatment.[1] Isotonic dehydration results from a balanced loss of water and sodium. Vomiting and diarrhea typically result in isotonic dehydration. Hypertonic dehydration occurs when water losses are greater than sodium losses. Fever, which increases insensible water loss, combined with an inability to increase oral fluid intake is a common cause of this type of dehydration. Hypernatremia (serum sodium levels >145 mEq/L) and hyperosmolality (serum osmolality > 300 mmol/kg) are characterisitic. Hypotonic dehydration occurs when sodium loss exceeds water loss. Serum sodium levels (<135 mEq/L) and serum osmolality (<280 mmol/kg) are decreased. This type of dehydration occurs commonly with diuretic overuse. Additionally, the term *volume depletion* needs to be distinguished from *dehydration*.[2] Volume depletion describes loss of sodium from the extracellular space (intravascular and interstitial fluid) that occurs after gastrointestinal hemorrhage, vomiting, diarrhea, and diuresis. Dehydration refers to losses of intracellular water that elevate the serum sodium levels and osmolality. Volume depletion should be referred to as *extracellular* volume depletion to avoid confusion. This distinction is important to clinicians because patients with volume depletion exhibit circulatory instability and need prompt infusions of normal saline (0.9% NS) solution, whereas those with pure dehydration often lack this finding and should receive 5% dextrose and water more slowly. Most patients presenting with dehydration, however, also have volume depletion. The term *hypovolemia* may be used to collectively refer to both conditions.[2]

Epidemiology and Impact

Dehydration is the most common fluid and electrolyte disorder in both the nursing home setting and among at-risk community-dwelling elders.[3] In 1991, it was estimated that 189,000 elders were discharged from acute care hospitals with a primary diagnosis of dehydration, at a cost of $1.16 billion.[1] Approximately 1.5 percent of community-dwelling elderly will be hospitalized with dehydration annually.[4] Dehydration was one of the six most frequent discharge diagnoses in older patients who developed progressive disability, with a cumulative percentage similar to those of pneumonia and diabetes.[5]

Two general factors place older persons at risk for dehydration: decreased fluid intake and increased fluid loss. Underlying physiologic changes that increase the risk of dehydration include decreased ability of the aged kidney to concentrate urine and altered thirst sensation in the elderly. The total-body water requirement for older persons is 1500 to 2500 mL/day, which can be provided by a variety of fluids and foods high in water content.[1] In general, it is recommended that adults drink six to eight 8-oz cups of water or liquid per day to maintain adequate hydration.[22] In addition, solid food consumption can add an additional 2 to 4 cups of water. For example, fruits and vegetables can contain up to 95 percent water by weight.[22] Elderly patients should be advised that the best sources of fluid replacement are water, fruit and vegetable juices, milk, and caffeine-free beverages. The sensation of thirst already means that the body has lost between 1 and 2 cups of water.

Specific risk factors for dehydration in the elderly include female gender, age older than 85 years, having more than four chronic medical conditions, taking more than four medications, and being confined to bed.[3] Confusion and dementia may cause or contribute to decreased fluid intake because of impaired communication and

Table 48-1. Dehydration Triggers and Risk Factors

Change in cognitive status or functional abilities
Diarrhea or vomiting
Fever
Weight loss (> 5 percent in last 30 days)
Insufficient fluid intake
Diuretic use
Uncontrolled diabetes mellitus
Swallowing difficulties
Purposeful fluid restriction
Need for enteral feeding
Previous history of dehydration

Source: Adapted with permission from Weinberg AD, Minaker KL: Dehydration: Evaluation and management in older adults. *JAMA* 274:1552, 1995.

feeding disorders. Depression also may result in poor fluid and food intake. Immobility, including the use of patient restraints, also may contribute to decreased fluid intake and dehydration. Because of these multiple factors, many long-term institutionalized elders are potentially mildly dehydrated at baseline. Acute illness, such as infection, then results in more significant hypovolemia. Additional conditions and risk factors that should trigger an assessment for dehydration are shown in Table 48-1. In the community setting, risks for dehydration include medication use (diuretics, laxatives), poor dietary and fluid intake because of the lack of a caregiver, limited or absent air conditioning during periods of hot weather, and poor or no access to regular medical care.[1]

Clinical Features

Signs and symptoms of dehydration and volume depletion in geriatric patients may be absent, misleading, or nonspecific. Constipation, weakness, and acute functional impairment [change in the activities of daily living (ADLs), for example] may be manifestations of dehydration in this age group. An acute confusional state (delirium) also may be a presentation of dehydration. Acute confusional state represents a transient dysfunction precipitated by physiologic, psychological, or environmental factors and increases morbidity, mortality, and length of hospitalization.[1,6] Risk factors for developing an acute confusional state include fluid/electrolyte imbalance, infection, hypoxia, kidney dysfunction, and multiple medication use.[1]

Abnormal declines in orthostatic blood pressure (BP) may be a sign of dehydration. Orthostatic hypotension (OH) is considered significant if the systolic BP declines 20 mmHg or more after standing from a supine or sitting position for 1 to 3 minutes. Orthostatic pulse rate increases of 10 to 20 beats per minute are also suggestive of hypovolemia. OH, however, is not specific for volume depletion. Prevalence of OH in the elderly ranges from 5 to 30 percent and is even higher in nursing home residents, occurring in more than half.[7–9] Ooi and colleagues[9] also demonstrated that OH was highly variable over time and most prevalent in the morning and in those on antihypertensive agents. Caution should be used in interpreting supine and sitting vital signs because the sensitivity of the test is greatly diminished if the patient cannot or does not stand.[2] In addition, the general decrease in sensitivity to adrenergic stimulation and hypotension, use of beta blockers, and pacemaker dependence limit the utility of pulse rate changes in assessing volume depletion in this age group. Finally, the presence of mild or moderate postural dizziness is a poor predictor of OH.[2]

Diagnosis

The bedside diagnosis of hypovolemia also can be misleading in the elderly. Physical examination findings most consistent with dehydration include a dry axilla, dry mucous membranes, and a dry, furrowed tongue.[10,11] A combination of the physical signs of confusion, weakness, nonfluent speech, sunken eyes, and dry mucous membranes and tongue is more helpful than individual signs alone.[11] The most predictive negative signs indicating absence of dehydration are moist mucous membranes and lack of sunken eyes or tongue furrows. Capillary refill time and skin turgor appear to have limited diagnostic value for hydration status.[2]

Laboratory parameters that are used frequently to determine hydration status include electrolytes, osmolality, creatinine, blood urea nitrogen (BUN) and BUN-creatinine ratio, urinalysis, and hematocrit. A BUN-creatinine ratio of 25 or greater, in the absence of known renal disease or gastrointestinal hemorrhage, is highly suggestive of dehydration. Serum osmolality should be measured if hypertonic or hypotonic dehydration is suspected. Measured osmolality is affected by azotemia (elevated BUN), glucose, mannitol, and ethanol and must be adjusted accordingly.[1] Serum osmolalities greater than 295 mmol/kg indicate that a significant percentage of body water has been lost.

The presence of hypernatremia (>148 mmol/L) is indicative of hypertonic dehydration. In older adults this is frequently encountered in febrile illnesses and is secondary to increased insensible water losses and an inability to increase fluid intake.[1] In the setting of isotonic or hypotonic dehydration, however, significant hypovolemia may be present with normal or low serum sodium levels.

Hematocrit does not provide a direct measure of water deficit, *but* an elevated hematocrit in conjunction with hypernatremia or hyperosmolality is strong evidence of sodium deficit.[12] Urine specific gravity, although commonly measured, is a poor correlate with other laboratory measurements of dehydration.[1]

These simple serum chemistries are useful and readily available in the emergency department (ED) setting. Although absolute values are helpful (i.e., a serum osmolality > 300 mmol/kg), interpretation also should consider any changes in value from the patient's baseline.

Emergency Department Care

Initial ED treatment should be based on the degree and type of dehydration present. In mild cases, supplemental oral hydration may be all that is necessary. Patients with circulatory instability, alterations in serum chemistries, acute confusional states, or an inability to take oral fluids require intravenous fluids.

Patients with hypertonic dehydration often have osmolalities greater than 300 mmol/kg and hypernatremia. Serum sodium values greater than 160 mEq/L often result in central nervous system (CNS) disturbances. A goal should be to correct one-half the free-water deficit in the first 24 hours.[13] Most cases are due to loss of salt and water; therefore, appropriate replacement choices initially should be normal saline or Ringer's lactate; both will be hypotonic relative to the patient's serum.

Hypotonic dehydration can occur when sodium loss exceeds water loss.[1] CNS symptoms also occur with significant hyponatremia (serum sodium levels < 120 mEq/L). ED management must be tailored to each individual patient. If the hyponatremia is mild and asymptomatic, water restriction may correct the problem. If the patient has evidence of hypovolemia, the appropriate fluid choice is normal saline. Patients with significant clinical manifestations of hyponatremia, such as seizures, should have their sodium deficit corrected more rapidly at a rate of 2 mEq/L/h. 3% NaCl at a rate of 75 to 100 mL/h plus addition of a loop diuretic such as furosemide (1 mg/kg) can be used.[13] Caution should be used with aggressive correction of sodium levels because circulatory overload and central pontine myelinolysis can occur.

Isotonic dehydration reflects a balanced loss of water and sodium and is usually accompanied by significant volume loss.[1] Replacement should be made with isotonic saline. The aggressiveness of replacement and the extent of monitoring this replacement should be tailored to each patient depending on the patient's circulatory instability. Overly aggressive replacement can result in congestive heart failure and even death in elderly patients.[1]

Additional Aspects

Dehydration is a common finding in elderly patients, and making the diagnosis of dehydration/volume depletion in the elderly can be a difficult proposition. Clinical signs and symptoms of increased thirst or postural hypotension can be misleading or nonexistent. Laboratory values with the measurement of blood urea nitrogen, osmolality, and sodium concentration are the most reliable indicators, and ordering these tests should be common practice on admission.

The lack of recognition and treatment results in significant morbidity, increased mortality, and additional costs and duration of hospital stays. Clinicians should assess hydration status in nursing home residents and older patients who present with acute changes in mental status, fever, new functional impairments, or the complaint of weakness or dizziness. Each ED should adopt guidelines for fluid assessment of their elderly patients based on geriatric ED volume and resources.

ELECTROLYTE ABNORMALITIES

Electrolyte abnormalities are common in older adults because of the prevalence of dehydration, renal insufficiency, and the use of medications that can alter electrolyte levels, such as diuretics and angiotensin-converting enzyme (ACE) inhibitors. This section will review the most common and significant of these disorders. Clinical features and ED treatment will be emphasized.

Sodium

Sodium is the most prevalent ion in the plasma and is found predominantly in the extracellular space. Total-body sodium content is approximately 40 to 50 mg/kg.

Sodium status is determined by the water homeostasis. It is regulated by the reabsorption and loss of free water through the renal system, mainly through the activity of vasopressin (ADH).

Hyponatremia

Prevalence of laboratory-indicated hyponatremia (<137 mEq/L) is approximately 8 percent in ambulatory geriatric patients. One-sixth of patients in chronic care facilities may be hyponatremic, with more then half having at least one clinical episode in a year. Since sodium level is determined by water homeostasis, hyponatremia can be seen as a syndrome of excess water in relation to extracellular sodium. Hyponatremia can be divided into categories based on the tonicity and total-body sodium level.

Hyponatremia with a normal tonicity is considered fictitious (*pseudohyponatremia*). It is seen in presence of increased lipids or protein and is a result of the method used in most laboratories to determine serum sodium. This is becoming less common with improved laboratory techniques. Hypertonic hyponatremia, on the other hand, is due to the presence of nonelectrolyte solutes that are osmotically active, drawing water out of the intracellular compartment. The most common clinical example of this is glucose. The amount of plasma sodium is diluted by the extra water drawn out due to the osmotic effect of the glucose. The actual serum sodium level can be estimated by assuming a 1.6 mEq/L fall in serum sodium concentration for each 100 mg/dL rise in serum glucose concentration. A similar effect can be seen with other osmotically active solutes such as mannitol, sorbitol, maltose, and radiocontrast material. The hyponatremia usually does not require correction beyond correction of the underlying disorder.

Hypotonic hyponatremia can be further divided into categories based on the extracellular fluid volume. Noneuvolemic hyponatremia can be caused by a loss of volume overall or by a loss of effective arterial volume. The hypovolemic form can be caused by an increase in losses, resulting in decreased total-body sodium. These losses can be from the gastrointestinal system, excretory system, or skin. The hypervolemic form is a result of a decrease in the effective arterial volume, resulting from increased sequestration of fluid into a "third space." This results from a relative decrease in plasma oncotic pressure, producing the clinical finding of edema, peripheral or central.

Hyponatremia that is euvolemic is usually the result of an increase in free water without a commensurate increase in body sodium. This can be caused by certain medications, glucocorticoid deficiency, hypothyroidism, psychogenic polydipsia, reset osmostat syndrome, or the syndrome of inappropriate antidiuretic hormone secretion (SIADH) (Table 48-2).

SIADH is a syndrome characterized by the continued release of vasopressin in a state of increased extracellular volume and dilution of body fluids. The diagnostic criteria for SIADH are

1. Hypotonic hyponatremia
2. Urine osmolality of greater than 100 mosmol/kg, with elevated urinary sodium
3. Clinical euvolemia
4. Normal cardiac, hepatic, renal, adrenal, and thyroid function

Also included in the definition of SIADH is that correction occurs with water restriction.

ADH will be released from nonosmotic stimulation, from low intravascular volume, so as to attempt to preserve circulating volume at the expense of sodium bal-

Table 48-2. Hypotonic Hyponatremia

Euvolemic	Hypervolemic	Hypovolemic
SIADH	Chronic heart failure	Gastrointestinal losses
CNS—meningitis	Chronic liver disease	Renal losses
Drugs	Chronic renal disease	Diuretics
Ectopic ADH secretion	Hypoalbuminemia	Mineralocorticoid deficiency
Lung disease		Salt-wasting nephropathies
Compulsive water drinking		Skin losses
Hypothyroidism		

ance. This is a physiologic compensatory method and is not part of SIADH.

Clinical Features

The symptoms of hyponatremia occur in proportion to both the severity and speed of the decrease in sodium, with the rapidity being the dominant factor. While the neurologic changes may be most pronounced, many other systems are affected as well. Patients with hyponatremia usually have normal muscle tone and function but may develop weakness and cramping with acute changes.

The neurologic symptoms of hyponatremia range from mild confusion to coma. Seizures may occur, typically with a sodium level below 115 mEq/L, and have a mortality rate as high as 50 percent. Focal signs such as hemiparesis, monoparesis, ataxia, nystagmus, tremor, rigidity, aphasia, and corticospinal tract signs also may be seen.

As a compensatory mechanism, the brain will attempt to lower the osmotic cellular pressure in response to the lower extracellular osmotic pressure. If the change in serum sodium is sufficiently slow, since the process requires 48 to 72 hours for completion, brain swelling will be minimal.

Emergency Department Treatment

The treatment of hyponatremia is also based on both the severity and rapidity of the insult. As noted previously, given sufficient time, the body, and more specifically the brain, will adapt to the decreased serum tone. The first priority for correction is the volume status of the patient. With hyponatremia secondary to low extracellular volume, normal saline should be used for volume expansion prior to correction of the serum sodium concentration. In patients who are hypotonic and hypervolemic, correction of the underlying mechanism is the key because it will discontinue the compensatory release of vasopressin. In

a euvolemic patient, fluid restriction generally is sufficient to correct the hyponatremia, with the discontinuation of medications that affect free-water excretion and correction of underlying causes. In the elderly patient, this would require a total fluid intake of less than 500 to 800 mL/day.

Overall, it is generally considered safe to raise the serum sodium concentration at a rate of no more than 12 meq/L over the first 24 hours. This should be done in patients who are symptomatic from their hyponatremia. Normal saline may be used to correct the deficit, or 3% saline at a rate of 1 to 2 mL/kg/h may be used. Hyponatremic seizures can be controlled by raising the serum sodium concentration by 3 to 5 meq/L using 3% saline, using 4 to 6 mL/kg. In the setting of congestive heart failure, a loop diuretic may be used to prevent worsening volume overload when using normal saline.

With rapid increase in the serum tonicity, the relative decrease in intracellular tone will cause the shift of intracellular fluids out of cells. In the brain, this can cause an osmotic myelinolysis. While this process diffusely affects the entire brain, the pons is a preferred site for disruption of the blood-brain barrier, producing symptoms such as spastic quadriparesis, psuedobulbar palsy, swallowing dysfunction, and mutism.

SIADH is treated primarily with water restriction pending treatment of the underlying cause. Demeclocycline (Declomycin), a medication causing a nephrogenic diabetes insipidus, has been used with some success in patients. Dosage is 600 to 1200 mg/day, but it is contraindicated in patients with renal or hepatic disease.

Hypernatremia

Just as hyponatremia represents a syndrome of excess extracellular water, hypernatremia can be viewed as a syndrome of insufficient extracellular water. Hypernatremia can be divided into categories based on the mechanism of water imbalance; however, more than one can coexist.

Hypernatremia due to excess sodium is unusual. It requires the administration of sodium beyond which the kidneys can excrete. The most common method in patients is iatrogenic, from administration of hypertonic sodium-containing fluid. The same effect can be seen with ingestion of seawater exclusively.

On the other hand, hypernatremia due to decreased water intake is far more common. In the elderly, it is the seen from inadequate fluid intake in the setting of increased losses, in which a decreased thirst mechanism and ability to obtain fluids play a role. Decreased access to fluids plays a key role in the nursing home setting, especially with patients who no longer regulate their own intake.

Increased loss of free body water is the third cause of hypernatremia. This may result from the kidney's inability to further concentrate urine, whether due to a large solute load causing an osmotic diuresis or due to the kidney no longer being regulated by vasopressin. Diabetes insipidus is due to a defect in the regulation of water by vasopressin. Central diabetes insipidus is due to a lack of production of vasopressin by the hypothalamus; the kidneys are normal. Nephrogenic diabetes insipidus, on the other hand, is due to a lack of renal response to the normal release of vasopressin. In both cases, there is polyuria and polydipsia in the setting of dilute urine (Table 48-3).

Table 48-3. Causes of Diabetes Insipidus

Central	Nephrogenic
Primary	Primary
Congenital/familial	Genetic
Nonfamilial	
Secondary	Secondary
Granulomatous disease	Electrolyte imbalance
Head trauma or surgery	Obstructive uropathy
Infection	Renal disease
Supra- and intrasellar tumor	
Thrombosis	
Vascular lesions and	
hemorrhage	
Medications	Medications
Carbon monoxide	Amphotericin B
Clonidine	Cisplatin
Diphenylhydantoin	Demeclocycline
Ethanol	Lithium
	Osmotic agents
	Propoxyphene

Clinical Features

The primary effects of hypernatremia are neurologic, from the decreased water content of brain cells. Initial effects include anorexia, nausea, and vomiting. Symptoms such as irritability, restlessness, lethargy, muscle twitching, spasticity, and hyperreflexia can be seen later on. In severe cases, a decrease in brain size can lead to increased traction on blood vessels, making hemorrhage more likely to occur.

Emergency Department Treatment

The treatment of hypernatremia is also based on the severity and rapidity of the insult. As with a decreased tone, the body and brain will adapt to an increased tonicity, and a rapid decrease in serum tonicity may result in the rapid movement of fluid into cells, causing a cerebral edema. As always, the first priority should be to restore extracellular volume if the patient is hypovolemic.

In general, the first step to the correction of hypernatremia, after volume correction, is the estimation of the free water deficit. Free water deficit can be estimated by

$$\text{Water deficit} = (\text{plasma sodium} - 140)/140 \times \text{total-body water.}$$

Approximately half the water deficit should be corrected over the first 12 to 24 hours, with the remainder over the next 1 to 2 days. Frequent measurement of electrolytes will be required to guide treatment. If neurologic symptoms develop during the correction, this may indicate cerebral edema, and the correction should be stopped while the patient is reevaluated. In the setting of acute solute excess, a diuretic may be required along with fluid replacement. Dialysis may be required in the setting of volume overload.

For diabetes insipidus, the same corrective measures should be applied. Medications should be reevaluated with regard to possible etiologies. With central diabetes insipidus, exogenous vasopressin can be used. Pitressin, a short-acting agent, can be given as 5 units every 3 to 4 hours based on urine volume and specific gravity. Nephrogenic diabetes insipidus, on the other hand, often requires the use of thiazide diuretics and a low-salt diet.

Potassium

Potassium is found predominantly in the intracellular space, with 98 percent being intracellular. Total-body stores contain 3500 mEq on average, or approximately 50 mEq/kg.

The minimum daily requirement of potassium is approximately 1.6 to 2 g. Since 1 mEq is 40 mg, this requirement is about 40 to 50 mEq/day. Approximately 80 to 90 percent of potassium is excreted in the kidneys, where its reabsorption is regulated by serum potassium levels and partly by aldosterone. A normal kidney may excrete up to 6 mEq/kg/day. The remainder of potassium is lost in the gastrointestinal tract, with a small portion lost in sweat.

Hypokalemia

Hypokalemia can be caused by multiple mechanisms but can be viewed as either a shift in relative concentrations of potassium or as a decrease in the total-body stores, although most cases involve multiple elements. One form of hypokalemia to be aware of is psuedohypokalemia, which is a due to the absorption of potassium by white blood cells at room temperature after a blood sample has been taken. This effect is exaggerated by high numbers of white blood cells, such as in acute myelogenous leukemia, and can be avoided by either storing blood at 4°C or rapid separation of the plasma.

Hypokalemia secondary to redistribution of potassium is based on a change in activity of Na$^+$,K$^+$-ATPase used to maintain normal cellular electrolyte gradients. Insulin is a potent activator, but only in settings of acutely increased insulin levels. Chronically high levels of insulin do not cause hypokalemia. Aldosterone is another, slower activator of Na$^+$,K$^+$-ATPase, as are all beta-agonist agents (Table 48-4).

Total-body decrease in potassium thus can be viewed from an intake or loss perspective. Decrease intake is difficult with a regular diet because the average Western diet contains approximately 70 mEq of potassium. It is contained in large amounts in fruits and vegetables. The elderly are at risk due to poorly balanced means, especially if disabled or living alone. Inability to absorb or removal of potassium by substances that bind potassium from dietary sources also play a role.

Because potassium has three routes of excretion, an increase in any one of these can cause a decrease in total-body potassium. The gastrointestinal losses of potassium are not regulated, and while relatively small under normal conditions, large amounts of potassium can be lost in pathologic states. Prolonged loss of gastric contents will cause hypokalemia not only from the direct removal, which is relatively small at 5 to 8 mEq/L, but also from the resulting volume loss and metabolic alkalosis. The alkalosis may cause a transcellular shift in potassium and a bicarbonaturia. Diarrhea will cause a hypokalemia, es-

Table 48-4. Causes of Hypokalemia

Inadequate potassium intake	Sympathomimetics
Clay ingestion	Hypokalemic periodic paralysis
Decreased dietary potassium	Acute anabolic states
Impared absorption	Alkalosis
Kayexalate	Increased renal losses
Increase gastrointestinal losses	Bicarbonaturia
Diarrhea	Defects of intrinsic renal transport
Emesis	Drugs
Ileostomy	Diuretics
Inflammatory bowel disease	Carbonic anhydrase inhibitors
Laxitive abuse	Antibiotics
Malabsorption	Aminoglycosides
Nasogastric suction	Amphotericin B
Villous adenoma	Penicillin and analogues
Increased skin losses	Hormones
Burns	Aldosterone
Excessive sweating	Glucocorticoid-remediable hypertension
Heat stroke	
Fever	Glucocorticoid excess
Intracellular shifts	
Hormones	Magnesium deficiency
Aldosterone	
Insulin	

pecially in the setting of a secretory diarrhea or laxative abuse, primarily through the direct loss of potassium.

Since the majority of potassium is excreted in the kidney, the most common cause of hypokalemia is increased renal loss. A defect in renal potassium transport will prevent its adequate reabsorption, leading to a chronic hypokalemic state. All diuretics will cause hypokalemia to some degree, although thiazide diuretics are more potent, partly due to their longer duration of action. Certain antibiotics cause hypokalemia either as a result of direct inhibition of reabsorption or by increasing the delivery of a nonreabsorbable anion to the distal tubular, causing increased unrinary excretion. Hormonal effects, most notably aldosterone, also play a large role in causes of hypokalemia. Aldosterone increases the reabsorption of sodium and the excretion of potassium; thus any excess aldosteronism, primary or secondary, frequently leads to hypokalemia. Glucocorticoids with mineralocorticoid action will have a similar effect. Glycyrrhizic acid, found in certain chewing tobaccos and licorice, have mineralocorticoid properties and also may cause hypokalemia. A deficiency of magnesium also will lead to hypokalemia, although the mechanism is not certain.

Clinical Features

Since potassium is one of the principal determinants of resting cell membrane potential, the primary effect of hypokalemia is a hyperpolarization of cell membranes. In the cardiovascular system, this is seen primarily as either hypokalemia-induced ventricular arrhythmias or hypokalemia-related hypertension. The exact mechanism for the hypertension is not clear but may be related to increased salt retention resulting in an increased intravascular volume.

Electrocardiographic findings commonly associated with hypokalemia include diffuse ST- and T-wave changes, PR prolongation, T-wave flattening, and U waves. Reentrant atrial and ventricular tachycardias, atrioventricular dissociation, and ventricular fibrillation may occur due to prolongation of the action potential and refractory period.

Most other systems are affected by hypokalemia as well. Hypokalemia, by hyperpolarizing cells, impairs the ability of muscle cells to depolarize, preventing contraction. It also can reduce the blood flow to muscles, which may lead to cramping, fatiguability, myalgias, and ultimately, rhabdomyolysis. Hypokalemia impairs the ability of the kidney to concentrate urine, causing polyuria, partially from a nephrogenic diabetes insipidus. As a result of hyperaldosteronism causing hypokalemia, renal cystic disease can occur. Hypokalemia is also associated with a metabolic alkalosis, both in direct effect on the renal reabsorption of bicarbonate and in transcellular shifts of potassium for hydrogen ions. Hypokalemia also has been seen to worsen the symptoms of hepatic encephalopathy because it favors the production of renal ammonia.

Emergency Department Treatment

The primary treatment of hypokalemia is the correction of the serum potassium concentration, followed by correction of the underlying causes. The risks of correction are associated with the cardiovascular effects of potassium and are related to the speed of the correction. The method of correction, parenteral or oral, depends on the ability of the gastrointestinal tract to absorb potassium, the ability of the patient to take oral medication, and the acuity of the need for correction. Potassium chloride is the preferred form used for oral therapy, with the exception of patients with a metabolic acidosis, in whom the bicarbonate or citrate form is preferred.

Intravenous potassium is usually safe at a rate of 10 mEq/h and can be given through peripheral access. Under more urgent settings, up to 40 mEq/h can by given through a central catheter, with cardiac monitoring required. Serum potassium concentration will increase, on average, at 0.25 mEq/L/h for an infusion rate of 20 mEq KCl per hour. The fluid used should be isotonic; use normal saline for small amounts, but this may be administered in half-normal strengths if larger concentrations are used to prevent hypertonic infusion. Dextrose in the solution should be avoided because it will stimulate the production of insulin in nondiabetic patients and may lead to a paradoxical worsening of the hypokalemia.

In emergent conditions, a rapid increase in potassium may be required. These setting may include patients with hypokalemia in the setting of acute myocardial infarction or with hypokalemia in the setting of emergent surgery. In these patients, 5 to 10 mEq of KCl over 15 to 20 minutes can be used to increase the serum potassium concentration to 3.0 mEq/L. Cardiac monitoring in this setting is highly recommended.

Hyperkalemia

Hyperkalemia, like all other electrolyte disorders, also can be caused by several mechanisms and can be viewed as either a shift in transcellular potassium or a total-body increase in potassium. One of the more commonly seen forms of hyperkalemia in the ED is psuedohyperkalemia. This is commonly caused by hemolysis of a blood sample after collection. Psuedohyperkalemia also may be seen in the setting of leukocytosis or thrombocytosis. Hyperkalemia very uncommonly is associated with otherwise normal electrolytes, so an isolated hyperkalemia should be viewed with suspicion. Management should include obtaining an electrocardiogram, if not previously preformed, to look for signs of changes associated with hyperkalemia and verification of the test on a new sample (Table 48-5).

Hyperkalemia from an increased potassium intake is very rare in people with normal renal function. This also depends on the ability to maintain urine output. Potassium-rich food includes most fruit and vegetables and related products. Other sources of increased potassium include intravenous fluids, as well as many medications that are delivered associated with potassium. These should be recognized when used in patients with decreased renal function.

Extracellular shifts of potassium can cause hyper-

Table 48-5. Causes of Hyperkalemia

Extracellular shifts	Decreased excretion
Hyperosmolarity	Renal failure
Metabolic acidosis	Medication induced
Insulin deficiency	Hypoaldosteronism
Rhabdomyolysis	Increased intake
Transfusion of aged	Potassium-rich foods
blood	Potassium supplements
Tumor lysis syndrome	Potassium-containing
	medications

Table 48-6. Medications Associated with Hyperkalemia

Potassium-sparing diuretics
  Spironolactone
  Triamterene
  Amiloride
Heparin
Digitalis
Nonsteroidal anti-inflammatory agents
Antibiotics
  Bactrim
  Pentamidine
Antihypertensives
  Beta blockers
  Alpha and beta blockers
Angiotensin-converting enzyme inhibitors

kalemia with a normal total-body potassium level or may be found in addition to other forms of hyperkalemia. Hemolysis and other cell breakdown, such as rhabdomyolysis or tumor lysis syndrome, will cause the release of the contained potassium into the serum. A metabolic acidosis, such as diabetic ketoacidosis or lactic acidosis, will cause the exchange of hydrogen ions with potassium. Overdose of digitalis will prevent the uptake of potassium into cells, as will beta blockers to some extent. The hyperkalemic form of periodic paralysis is due to an efflux of potassium from the intracellular space.

Failure of the ability to excrete potassium is one of the cornerstones of hyperkalemia. With normal excretion, it is very difficult to obtain high levels of potassium. However, in a large number of medical conditions, the original insult producing the initial hyperkalemia also causes a decrease in the ability to excrete. The loss of this ability can be due to an overall decrease in the glomerular filtration rate, a deficiency of or insensitivity to aldosterone, or a drug-related inhibition (Table 48-6). Hyperkalemia is seen more commonly in acute rather than chronic renal failure. This is in great part due to the original insult causing both the hyperkalemia and the acute renal failure, as well as a compensatory increase in the gastrointestinal excretion of potassium seen in chronic renal failure patients.

Addison's disease, or adrenocortical insufficiency, is characterized by lack of aldosterone and produces a hyperkalemia accompanied by hyponatremia, hypovolemia, hypotension, and renal insufficiency. The underlying mechanism of the hyperkalemia is the inhibition of potassium secretion in the kidneys. Hypoaldosteronism can be either idiopathic or secondary to hyporeninemia, and the associated hyperkalemia is seen with a three- to fivefold higher frequency in diabetics and people over age 60. Heparin may cause a suppression of aldosterone release (Table 48-6).

Clinical Features

A patient with hyperkalemia may first present with chest pain similar to a myocardial infarction or even cardiac arrest because the initial clinical manifestations can be more subtle than hypokalemia. Other complaints, such as general weakness or parethesias, may be seen.

Electrocardiographic features of hyperkalemia are fairly typical but may vary in patients with chronic hyperkalemia. Typically, at a serum level of 6 to 7 mEq/L, T waves will become peaked, usually greater than 5 mm, or greater than one-third the height of the R wave. At levels of 7 to 8 mEq/L, the QRS complex will widen and P waves will flatten. At levels of 8 to 9 mEq/L, fusion of the QRS complex with the T wave will occur, producing the classic sine-wave appearance. Serum levels over 9 mEq/L are associated with ventricular tachycardia or fibrillation, or atrioventricular dissociation, and may be lethal. However, the electrocardiogram alone should not be used to diagnose hyperkalemia independently because findings are not specific and may lead to mistreatment in at least 15 percent of patients.

Emergency Department Treatment

Management of hyperkalemia should depend on the effect of the level of potassium, especially with respect to cardiac response. In the absence of cardiac irritation or instability, the first step should be confirmation of the hyperkalemia.

The treatment is divided into three main goals. The first is stabilization of cell membranes, most significantly cardiac cell membranes. This can be achieved with the use of intravenous calcium. Either 5 mL of 10% calcium chloride or 10 to 20 mL of 10% calcium gluconate may be used and should be given over 3 to 5 minutes to prevent other side effects. Calcium should be used with caution in the setting of digitalis use, and if used, it should be given over a period of at least 30 minutes; the use of digitalis antibodies should be the primary treatment of digitalis-induced symptomatic hyperkalemia. One important thing to remember is that while the effects of calcium may last up to 1 hour, the level of potassium in the blood has not been corrected.

The second phase of the treatment of hyperkalemia is the intracellular shifting of potassium. This will lower the serum levels but will have no effect on the total-body potassium concentration. The most rapid method is the administration of glucose and insulin, using 10 to 20 units of intravenous regular insulin and 50 g of glucose. The glucose may be withheld in patients who are hyperglycemic, but close monitoring of the glucose level is advisable. Under normal conditions, this will maintain the intracellular shift for approximately 4 to 6 hours; however, it should be remembered that insulin is cleared primarily by the kidneys, and the duration will be extended and the dose may need to be modified in renal failure patients. Beta agonists such as salbutamol or albuterol also will cause the intracellular shift of potassium, and albuterol is readily available in the ED. Sodium bicarbonate also may be used; however, this has shown less than ideal results in patients without a concomitant metabolic acidosis.

The final phase of treatment is the elimination of potassium. Since the predominant excretion of potassium occurs via the renal and gastrointestinal systems, these can be used to facilitate excretion. In patients with normal renal function, loop diuretics can be used to promote potassium loss. The speed of this method depends on the responsiveness of the kidney to the diuretic and may be relatively rapid. Elimination via the gastrointestinal tract requires the use of binding resins, usually sodium polystyrene. The mechanism for this is the exchange of sodium for potassium, and 1 g will remove approximately 1 mEq of potassium. The time of onset of this is approximately 1 to 2 hours, and treatment may be repeated every 4 to 6 hours as necessary. It should be remembered that sodium polystyrene is commonly used with sorbitol and usually causes diarrhea. When used without sorbitol, it may cause anorexia, nausea, vomiting, and constipation.

The other method for removal of potassium is direct removal from the blood using dialysis, either peritoneal or hemodialysis. This should be considered promptly in patients with acute renal failure as a secondary cause of the hyperkalemia.

Calcium

About 40 percent of extracellular calcium is protein-bound, mostly to albumin.

Hypocalcemia

Hypocalcemia also can be caused by several different mechanisms. It may result from an intracellular shift or conjugation in the bone or other mineral formation. Hungry bone syndrome, which is caused by the rapid remineralization of bone after surgical correction of hyperparathyroidism, results in the accretion of calcium into bone. Precipitation of calcium is another cause of hypocalcemia, with the total-body content remaining unchanged. Organic anions, including phosphorous in hyperphosphotemic states, citrate from blood transfusions, or free fatty acids liberated in acute pancreatitis, will complex with ionic calcium, causing a hypocalcemia. This also will occur in fluoride poisoning.

Changes in the absorption or elimination of calcium also may result in hypocalcemia. In primary vitamin D deficiency, there will be a decrease in gastrointestinal absorption of calcium. The elderly are susceptible to this due to a decreased exposure to sunlight, especially in the chronically ill or debilitated. Hypoparathyroidism will cause hypocalcemia from decreased release from bone and increased renal excretion, as well as a secondary deficiency in vitamin D. This can result from the surgical removal of the parathyroid glands or infiltrative disorders causing loss of tissue. Both hypomagnesemia and hypermagnesemia may impair parathyroid hormone release, causing hypocalcemia.

Owing to the high percentage of calcium being protein-bound, a decrease in serum albumin will cause a low serum calcium level; however, since the level of ionized calcium is not changed, the patient is asymptomatic, and no intervention is required. Hyperventilation syndrome causes a transient hypocalcemia through rapidly occurring respiratory alkalosis, resulting in dissociation of the hydrogen ions normally associated with albumin and thus increasing the amount of bound calcium (Table 48-7).

Clinical Features

The effects of hypocalcemia are usually not seen until the ionized serum level falls below approximately 1.5 mEq/L (or < 7.0 mg/dl). Severity usually depends on both the magnitude and rapidity of the deficiency (Table 48-8).

Table 48-7. Causes of Hypocalcemia

Normal Total-Body Calcium	Low Total-Body Calcium
Increased sequestration	Low serum ionized calcium
Pancreatitis	Hyperphosphatemia
Rhabdomyolysis	Hypomagnesemia
Tumor lysis syndrome	Hypoparathyroidism
Hungry bone syndrome	Vitamin D deficiency
Hyperventilation	Low serum bound calcium
syndrome	Gastrointestinal mal-
	absorption
	Hepatic cirrhosis
	Hypoalbuminemia
	Nephrotic syndrome

Table 48-8. Effects of Hypocalcemia

General	Cardiovascular
Fatigue	Bradycardia
Weakness	Heart failure
Neurologic	Vasoconstriction
Hyperreflexia	Pulmonary
Parethesias	Brochospasm
Seizures	Laryngeal spasm
Tetany	Muscular
Chovostek sign	Cramping
Trousseau sign	Spasm
Dermatologic	Weakness
Coarse, brittle hair	Skeletal
Dry, scaly skin	Osteodystrophy
Hyperpigmentation	Rickets
Psychiatric	Osteomalacia
Anxiety	Miscellaneous
Confusion	Cataracts
Dementia	Decreased insulin secretion
Hallucinations	Dental hypoplasia
Impaired memory	

Emergency Department Treatment

The first step in the treatment of hypocalcemia is verification of the status, with measurement of ionized calcium levels. As always, definitive treatment requires correction of the underlying disorder. In the presence of symptoms of hypocalcemia, treatment should not be withheld pending laboratory confirmation. Calcium is commonly found in two preparations: 10% calcium chloride is available in 10-mL ampules, which contain 360 mg elemental calcium, and 10% calcium gluconate, also available in 10-mL ampules and containing 93 mg elemental calcium. The recommended initial dose for symptomatic hypocalcemia in adult patients is 100 to 300 mg elemental calcium, which should be given over 10 to 20 minutes and will have a duration of action of approximately 1 to 2 hours. The initial bolus can be followed by repeat boluses or by a calcium infusion at a rate of 0.5 to 2 mg/kg/h, preferably diluted using D_5W. Less symptomatic patients may be given 20 mg/kg elemental calcium over 4 to 8 hours.

Common side effects of intravenous administration are hypertension, nausea, vomiting, and flushing, and are rate-dependant. Heart blocks and bradycardias also may occur, so cardiac monitoring is recommended. This effect is amplified in patients on digoxin, and calcium administration may result in a digoxin-induced cardiotoxicity. Calcium administration also may be required with rapid transfusions of large volumes of blood, especially in the setting of shock. Oral calcium supplementation can be used for asymptomatic patients requiring 1 to 4 g elemental calcium in divided doses daily.

Hypercalcemia

Hypercalcemia has many causes, but over 90 percent of cases result from either malignancy or primary hyperparathyroidism. Hypercalcemia can be looked at from the standpoint of increased absorption, decreased excretion, extracellular shifting, or a combination of the three. Most cases of hypercalcemia are a combination.

Parathyroid hormone is one of the prime regulating factors of serum calcium concentration and has effects on the skeletal, gastrointestinal, and renal systems both directly and indirectly. In the bone, parathyroid hormone prevents bone resorption and has the net effect of increasing bone turnover. In the kidney, parathyroid hormone acts to increase the reabsorption of calcium and to increase the formation of active vitamin D. Vitamin D acts on the intestine to increase the absorption of calcium. Parathyroid adenomas are the most frequent tumors causing hyperparathyroidism, but many other tumors may secrete a similarly acting substance (Table 48-9).

Clinical Features

Symptoms of hypercalcemia usually are not seen at levels below 12 mg/dL (3 mEq/L). One mnemonic used to remember the symptoms of hypercalcemia is *stones* (nephrolithiasis), *bones* (osteolysis), *groans* (gastroin-

Table 48-9. Causes of Hypercalcemia

Increased gastrointestinal intake
   Milk-alkali syndromes
   Increased vitamin D
Decreased renal excretion
   Thiazide diuretics
Extracellular shift
   Increased bone resorption
   Decreased bone formation
      Paget's disease
      Bedfast patients
   Metastases to bone
   Multiple myeloma
Multifactorial
   Hyperparathyroidism
   Increased PTHrP secretion
   Hyperthyroidism

Table 48-10. Effects of Hypercalcemia

General	Neurologic
Fatigue	Ataxia
Malaise	Coma
Cardiovascular	Hypotonia
Atrioventricular block	Headache
Bundle branch blocks	Lethargy
ECG abnormalities	Weakness
Hypertension	Psychiatric
Potentiation of digoxin	Confusion
toxicity	Decreased memory
Sinus bradycardia	Hallucinations
Ventricular dysrhyth-	Renal
mias	Dehydration
Gastrointestinal	Electrolyte disorders
Anorexia	Nephrolithiasis
Constipation	Polyuria
Ileus	Polydipsia
Peptic ulcer disease	Prerenal azotemia
Pancreatitis	Skeletal
Vomiting	Bone pain
Nausea	Deformities
	Fractures
	Nephrocalcinosis

testinal pain), and *psychic moans*. A more complete list of symptoms is given in the Table 48-10.

Electrocardiographic changes associated with hypercalcemia are shortened and depressed ST segments, widened T waves, and shortened QT intervals. As levels increase, bradyarrhythmias and bundle-branch blocks may occur, followed by second-degree heart block, complete heart block, and ultimately, cardiac arrest.

Emergency Department Treatment

Treatment of hypercalcemia is basically directed at correction of the serum calcium concentration by either excretion or resorption from bone. In most emergent cases, this will be done without knowing the underlying cause; however, definitive treatment requires correction of the underlying cause. The initial treatment is to correct the loss of volume associated with hypercalcemia, primarily using normal saline. Excretion of calcium is enhanced with the use of furosemide, but this should only be used once adequate hydration has been achieved.

Mithramycin and calcitonin both inhibit osteoclastic activity, suppressing calcium release from bone. Mithramycin is cytotoxic, although resistance to calcitonin may occur. Bisphosphonates also may be used to prevent bone resorption and can be highly effective in inhibiting osteoclasts. Etidronate and pamidronate are available, and side effects may include increased in serum creatinine and phosphate. Glucocorticoids act by inhibiting gut absorption of calcium and inhibiting bone resorption. It is also used to decrease formation of resistance to calcitonin. These medications should be used in severe cases.

Magnesium

Magnesium is found predominantly in the intracellular space, with only 1 to 2 percent in the extracellular fluid. The adult human body contains approximately 2000 mEq of magnesium, half contained in the mineral component of bone and the remainder in the intracellular space. In the serum, 30 percent of magnesium is bound to albumin, 15 percent is chelated with various anions, and the remainder is present as the biologically active ion.

The minimum daily intake of magnesium is 20 to 28 mEq, or 240 to 336 mg. Excretion is approximately 40 percent renal and 60 percent gastrointestinal.

Hypomagnesemia

Hypomagnesemia has been estimated to occur in up to 12 percent of all hospitalized patients. The mechanisms by which it occurs can be divided into categories based on intracellular shifting, insufficient intake, or increased loss and further divided by the source of the loss. Magnesium is absorbed in the jejunum and ileum by both active and passive transport. Under normal conditions, the gastrointestinal system absorbs approximately half the daily intake. Deficiency occurs with severe malnutrition, insufficient dietary formulas, or the setting of total parenteral nutrition (Table 48-11).

Intracellular shift of magnesium will result from metabolic acidosis, as well as from increased stimulus from catecholamines and infusions of glucose, insulin, or amino acids. Magnesium will be chelated by citrate found in blood products and can be diluted by large volumes of hypotonic intravenous solutions. Resumption of bone mineralization, as occurs after surgical treatment of hyperparathyroidism or hyperthyroidism, will cause a depletion of magnesium through reuptake. Hypomagnesemia is also seen in pregnancy, with decline seen in the third trimester; it is seen most commonly in patients with preterm labor.

Losses of magnesium from the gastrointestinal tract can be severe. Diarrhea, as a primary cause or secondary to malabsorption or a short bowel syndrome, can produce large losses of magnesium. This also can occur through nasogastric suctioning. Pancreatitis can cause hypomagnesemia due to sequestration of fluids rich in magnesium, as well as any accompanying diarrhea or nasogastric suctioning.

Table 48-11. Causes of Hypomagnesemia

Increased renal loss	Increased gastrointestinal loss
Alcohol	
Diabetes	Diarrhea
Drugs	Emesis
Beta agonists	Malabsorption
Diuretics	Nasogastric suction
Digoxin	Pancreatitis
Amphotericin B	Short bowel syndrome
Aminoglycosides	Miscellaneous
cis-Platinum	Total parenteral nutrition
Cyclosporine	
Pentamidine	Malnutrition
Osmotic agents	Alcohol abuse
Renal tubular injury	Phosphorus depletion
Acute intracellular shift	Hungry bone syndrome
Amino acid infusions	Citrated blood products
Catecholamines	Hyperthyroidism
Glucose infusion	Hypercalcemia
Insulin	Cardiopulmonary bypass
Metabolic acidosis	Intravascular volume expansion
Refeeding syndromes	

Loss of magnesium via the kidneys can occur in the form of magnesium wasting characterized by inappropriate excretion of magnesium in the urine in the setting of hypomagnesemia. This can be induced by loop or thiazide diuretics, as well as by many other medications. Ethanol has been shown to induce a tubular dysfunction causing a defect in urinary excretion of magnesium; this process is reversible with cessation of ethanol ingestion. This also will occur in other forms of renal tubular dysfunction. Hypercalcemia will cause an inappropriate excretion of magnesium through competitive inhibition in the loop of Henle.

Clinical Features

Magnesium appears to play many roles. It is required for proper functioning of the Na^+,K^+-ATPase and other ion channels on cell membranes; thus low levels of magnesium may favor the transport of potassium out of cells. Hypokalemia commonly coexists with hypomagnesemia and may in part be due to an underlying disorder that causes loss of both potassium and magnesium or due to an increased secretion of potassium that has been seen in low-magnesium states.

Hypocalcemia is considered a classic sign of severe hypomagnesemia, which may be due to an increased resistance to parathyroid hormone seen with a low-magnesium state. Magnesium also acts as a calcium channel blocker, inhibiting flux of calcium into cells; thus low levels of magnesium may favor a rise in intracellular calcium.

The electrocardiographic changes with hypomagnesemia progress with the magnitude of loss. Moderate magnesium losses may produce a widened QRS complex with a peaking of T waves, whereas more severe losses may produce a prolongation of the PR interval, diminution of the T wave, and progressive widening of the QRS complex. Hypomagnesemia has been associated with increased ventricular arrhythmias in acute myocardial infarction and other cardiac disease.

Emergency Department Treatment

Treatment of hypomagnesemia can be by either the oral or the intravenous route and should be based on the severity of the clinical manifestations and on the underlying cause. With more severe symptoms, magnesium should be given as 50 mEq, or 600 mg, over 8 to 24 hours, which may be repeated to maintain a serum concentration greater than 1.0 mg/dL. In life-threatening conditions, 2 to 4 g over 30 to 60 minutes can be used, diluted in intravenous fluid. Since the reabsorption of magnesium is based on the serum level, an abrupt elevation will remove the stimulus to reabsorb magnesium, causing the excretion of up to half the infused magnesium. Oral replacement is preferred in the asymptomatic patient and is available in magnesium chloride and magnesium lactate forms. For severe magnesium depletion, approximately 500 mg magnesium should be given orally in divided does; 250 mg may be sufficient for more mild disease.

Hypermagnesemia

Hypermagnesemia is usually a multifactorial event, requiring more than one underlying process to occur. A healthy adult can excrete more the 6 g of magnesium daily; thus hypermagnesemia is rarely seen in the ED. It is seen most commonly in patents with renal insufficiency, and although it is possible for that alone to be the cause, it usually requires an increased load of magnesium. This can be produced in several ways. First, oral administration of magnesium, which is commonly found in cathartics, can provide a sufficiently large load to produce hypermagnesemia. Intravenous loading will have a similar effect. Second, prevention of elimination in the bowel, which is usually accompanied by increased absorption, will occur from nearly any disorder causing a decrease in gastrointestinal motility. Finally, disorders causing an extracellular shift of magnesium, whether from cellular stores or bone, also may produce a hypermagnesemia (Table 48-12).

Clinical Features

Magnesium suppresses the transmission of neurotransmitter messages, acting as a CNS and neuromuscular depressant. The manifestations of hypermagnesemia correlate well with the serum level. Initial symptoms, including nausea, may begin to appear at serum levels as low as 2 mg/dL. At serum levels of 3 mg/dL, signs and symptoms include weakness and cutaneous flushing. At levels above 4 mg/dL, hyporeflexia will begin and will continue to progress as the level increases. Between levels of 5 and 6 mg/dL, hypotension and electrocardiographic changes are seen, including widening of the QRS complex, prolongation of the QT and PR segments, and conduction abnormalities. Levels above 9 mg/dL have been associated with respiratory depression, complete heart block, and coma, and cardiac arrest has been reported with serum levels greater than 10 mg/dL.

Table 48-12. Causes of Hypermagnesemia

Impaired excretion
  Acute renal failure
  Chronic renal failure
Exogenous administration
  Antacids
  Cathartics
  Dialysate
  Laxatives
  Parenteral
Impaired elimination
  Anticholinergics
  Bowel obstruction
  Chronic constipation
  Colitis
  Gastric dilation
  Narcotics
Miscellaneous
  Adrenal insufficiency
  Familial hypocalciuric hypercalcemia
  Hyperparathyroidism
  Hypothyroidism
  Lithium
  Rhabdomyolysis

Emergency Department Treatment

The treatment of hypermagnesemia can be divided into two goals. First, the effects of hypermagnesemia can be eliminated through the direct antagonist effect of calcium at the cell membrane. For life-threatening manifestation, 100 to 200 mg calcium should be used as a starting dose and can be maintained with an infusion at 2 to 4 mg/kg/h.

The second goal of treatment is the removal of magnesium from the serum. This depends on the patient's renal function. With normal renal function, hydration alone may be sufficient, although furosemide will accelerate magnesium elimination. In patients with renal failure, dialysis may be the only option. Dialysis also should be considered in patients with severe and life-threatening manifestations, such as respiratory failure, hemodynamic instability, or coma.

Phosphorus

Total-body stores of phosphorous are estimated at 10 g/kg total body weight, with approximately 80 percent in bone, 9 percent in skeletal muscle, and the remainder distributed in extracellular fluid and viscera. Less than 1 percent is present in plasma. Inorganic phosphate is the form measured in most laboratories.

Average daily intake of phosphorous ranges from 10 to 12 mmol, and because it is ubiquitous in regular diets, it is very unusual to have a selective dietary deficiency. Absorption in the duodenum and jejunum is 70 percent passive, with the remainder regulated by vitamin D and indirectly by parathyroid hormone. Renal excretion is the primary means of regulation, with 80 to 90 percent being reabsorbed in the renal tubules.

Hypophosphatemia

There are two main mechanisms of hypophosphatemia, which can be looked at from the standpoint of total-body depletion of phosphorus versus a decrease in serum phosphate levels. With decreased total levels, the total-body phosphorous level can be low, normal, or high. The cause is usually a transcellular shift in phosphorous, which can have a number of underlying mechanisms. Hypophosphatemia in hospitalized patients is most commonly due to transcellular shifts, as a result of carbohydrate infusions or respiratory alkalosis (Table 48-13).

The other mechanism of hypophosphatemia, total-body depletion, can be viewed as a relative decrease in the gastrointestinal absorption of phosphorous or a relative increase in excretion. Other causes of loss of phosphorous include skin loss from burns or sequestration from pancreatitis (Table 48-14).

Clinical Features

Like other electrolytes abnormalities, hypophosphatemia affects multiple organ systems. Part of this is the role that phosphorous plays in the formation of many macromol-

Table 48-13. Factors for Transcellular Phosphorus Shifts

Carbohydrate infusions	Respiratory alkalosis
Fructose	Gout
Glucose	Heat stroke
Glycerol	Hyperventilation
Lactate	Salicylate overdose
Hormonal effects	Sepsis
Calcitonin	Increased cellular uptake
Catecholamines	Erythropoietin therapy
Glucagon	Hungry bone syndrome
Insulin	Leukemia blast crisis

Table 48-14. Factors for Total-Body Phosphorous Loss

Decreased absorption	Increased Excretion
Dietary insufficiency	Alcoholism
Hyperalimentation	Alkaluria
Refeeding syndrome	Diuretics
Malabsorption	Fanconi syndrome
Steatorrhea	Hypercalcemia
Phosphate-binding	Hyperparathyroidism
antacids	PTH-related protein
Vitamin D deficiency or	Metabolic acidosis
resistance	Renal transplant
	Steroid therapy
	Volume expansion

ecules used in metabolism. It is one of the main components of adenosine triphosphate (ATP), as well as 2,3-diphosphoplycerate (2,3-DPG). Depletion of phosphate may result in loss of cellular structural integrity and cell membrane function.

Hypophosphatemia can cause complaints of weakness and bone pain in a chronic setting. Osteopenia and osteomalacia also may occur. Acute decreases in patients who are chronically hypophosphatemic may result in rhabdomyolysis. Cardiomyopathy may occur in the chronic setting, with acute changes resulting in arrhythmias. Respiratory insufficiency, which may be due to a decrease in diaphragmatic strength, also has been seen. This can result in difficulties in ventilator weaning. Patients have been shown to have a wide range of neurologic manifestations, including irritability, apathy, delirium, hallucinations, delusions, obtundation, and seizures. Hypophosphatemia has been shown to affect leukocyte activity, causing a decrease in immune function; and has been associated with an increase in hemolysis. It also may increase tissue insulin resistance and decrease insulin release. In the kidney, reduced phosphate excretion leads to an overall decrease in excretion of titratable acids, leading to an overall metabolic acidosis.

Emergency Department Treatment

The treatment of hypophosphatemia can be accomplished by both oral and intravenous methods, which should be determined based on clinical status, severity of symptoms, and potential complications. Intravenous supplementation is usually reserved for patients who are both severely symptomatic and have a serum phosphate level less than 1 mg/dL. In an emergency setting, 2.5 to 5 mg/kg of body weight may be infused over a period of 6 hours, with the amount based on the severity of symptoms. Oral phosphorous supplementation is usually done over 7 to 10 days using approximately 60 mmol of phosphate in three or four divided doses daily. Other forms of dietary supplementation with phosphorous-rich foods, such as cow's milk, also may be used.

Both oral and intravenous supplements are found as potassium or sodium salts, which should be remembered when they are used in the context of other electrolyte disorders. Phosphorus will conjugate with calcium, which may lead to hypocalcemia or to metastatic calcification in the setting of hypercalcemia. In addition, the oral supplements have a dose-related diarrhea that is reduced by dividing into smaller doses.

Hyperphosphatemia

Like hypophosphatemia, hyperphosphatemia can be a result of changes in absorption, excretion, or transcellular shifts. Absorption will be increased either by a increase in the total phosphorous intake or by excessive intake of vitamin D. Renal failure is a common cause, resulting in an inability to excrete. It will be released from cells in rhabdomyolysis and tumor lysis syndrome. It is also seen commonly coexisting with hypocalcemia or hypomagnesemia.

Clinical Features

Unlike hypophosphatemia, the symptoms of hyperphosphatemia are usually not seen because the associated hypocalcemia, hypomagnesemia, or renal failure overshadows them.

Emergency Department Treatment

The primary treatment for hyperphosphatemia is the removal of phosphate, which can be done via the renal or gastrointestinal system. Renal excretion can be increased in patients with normal renal function through saline diuresis and acetazolamide; diuresis using mannitol also may be an option. Phosphate is removed from the gastrointestinal system through the use of binding resins, which can remove phosphate that is normally excreted and reabsorbed passively in the intestines. Both aluminum- and calcium-based treatments exist, but the former should be avoided in patients with renal failure to prevent aluminum toxicity. Hemodialysis is also a treatment option. Hypocalcemia coexisting with hyperphosphatemia should be treated cautiously because a similar metastatic calcification can occur.

REFERENCES

1. Weinberg AD, Minaker KL: Dehydration: Evaluation and management in older adults. *JAMA* 274:1552, 1995.
2. McGee S, Abernathy WB, Simel DL: Is this patent hypovolemic? *JAMA* 281:1022, 1999.
3. Lavizzo-Mourey R, Johnson J, Stolley P: Risk factors for dehydration among elderly nursing home residents. *J Am Geriatr Soc* 36:213, 1988.
4. Warren JL, Harris T, Phillips C: Dehydration in older patients. *JAMA* 275:912, 1996.
5. Ferrucci L, Guralnik JM, Pahor M, et al: Hospital diagnoses, Medicare charges, and nursing home admissions in the year when older persons become severely disabled. *JAMA* 277:728, 1977.
6. Mentes J, Buckwalter K: Getting back to basics: Maintaining hydration to prevent confusion in frail elderly. *J Gerontol Nurs* 23:48, 1997.
7. Mader SL, Josepheson KR, Rubenstein LZ: Low prevalence of postural hypotension among community-dwelling elderly. *JAMA* 258:1511, 1987.
8. Tilvis RS, Hakala SM, Valvanne J, et al: Postural hypotension and dizziness in a general aged population: A four year follow-up of the Helsinki Aging study. *J Am Geriatr Soc* 44:809, 1996.
9. Ooi WL, Barrett S, Hossain M, et al: Patterns of orthostatic blood pressure change and their clinical correlates in a frail, elderly population. *JAMA* 277:1299, 1997.
10. Eaton D, Bannister P, Mulley GP, et al: Axillary sweating in clinical assessment of dehydration in elderly patients. *Br Med J* 308:1271, 1994.
11. Gross CR, Lindquist RD, Woolley AC, et al: Clinical indicators of dehydration severity in elderly patients. *J Emerg Med* 10:267, 1992.
12. Walker WG, Mitch WE: Disturbances of water and sodium metabolism, in Harvey AM, et al (eds): *The Principles and Practice of Medicine,* 22 ed. Norwalk, CT, Appleton and Lange; 1998, p 668.
13. Janson CL, Marx JA: Fluid and electrolyte balance, in Rosen P, et al (eds): *Emergency Medicine: Concepts and Clinical Practice,* 3d ed. St Louis, Mosby–Year Book, 1992, p 2132.

49

Hypothermia and Hyperthermia

Alexander Rachmiel
Mark D. Levine

HIGH-YIELD FACTS

- Disorders of temperature regulation are more common and cause greater morbidity and mortality in older patients.
- Accurate measurement of temperature is essential.
- Hypo- and hyperthermia may be due to environmental exposure or may accompany other illnesses (e.g., trauma, sepsis, endocrine diseases, or stroke).

HYPOTHERMIA

Hypothermia is defined as a core temperature of less than 35°C and may be divided into mild, moderate, and severe categories. Classification schemes vary slightly among authors, but most consider a temperature of less than 32°C to constitute moderate hypothermia, and a temperature below 28°C is usually considered severe hypothermia. *Accidental hypothermia,* defined as the unintentional decline in core temperature to below 35°C in the absence of primary disease in the brain's thermoregulatory center,[1] is a major source of preventable morbidity and mortality, particularly among the elderly. This discussion will focus on accidental hypothermia because this is the type of hypothermia that will be seen most often in the emergency department (ED).

While accidental hypothermia is often associated with cold climates and severe winter weather, the only absolute requirement for its development is an environment cooler than that of the human body, and cases may occur in susceptible persons under a wide range of climatic conditions. Furthermore, elderly patients suffering from hypothermia may present with subtle or nonspecific symptoms, and hypothermia may complicate other illnesses or

injuries in this population. Every physician who treats older patients therefore should maintain an awareness of the signs and symptoms of hypothermia and be familiar with its management.

Epidemiology

During the period of 1979 through 1995, Centers for Disease Control and Prevention (CDC) data showed an average of 723 deaths per year in the United States attributed to hypothermia, for a rate of 0.3 deaths per 100,000 population. About half (49 percent) these deaths occurred among persons 65 years of age or older, and the death rate among this age group was 1.2 per 100,000, with age-adjusted death rates much higher in men than in women.[2] In addition to age and sex, risk of death from hypothermia is linked to preexisting disease, nutritional status, alcohol and drug intoxication, and socioeconomic factors such as social isolation or homelessness. Hypothermia is also a frequent complication in patients with serious injury, particularly with advanced age, and contributes to morbidity and mortality in this setting.[3]

Pathophysiology

The human body produces heat as a by-product of cellular metabolism, and heat is lost continually as a result of radiation, evaporation, conduction, and convection. Under normal environmental conditions, radiation accounts for the greatest part of heat loss, with evaporation via the skin and respiratory tract second in importance. Conduction becomes more important in a victim of submersion because water is many times more conductive than air. Convection via cooling air currents moving over the body surface is a relatively minor source of heat loss except in very cold and windy environments.

Under normal conditions, body temperature is maintained in a narrow range (36–37.5°C rectal) by a complex system of neuroendocrine and metabolic mechanisms. The brain's thermoregulatory center resides in the preoptic area of the anterior hypothalamus. Input is received from temperature sensors in the skin and other remote sites such as the abdominal viscera, spinal cord, and great vessels.

Under cold conditions, efferent nerves from the hypothalamus mediate increased cardiac output and peripheral vasoconstriction, as well as shunting of blood to striated muscles, where the blood can be warmed through shivering. A slower neuroendocrine response via the anterior pituitary gland results in increased thyroid and adrenocortical output to promote increased cellular metabolism and heat production. Behavioral changes such as leaving the cold environment or putting on more clothing are also important in reversing mild hypothermia among patients who are capable of sensing cold and responding to it.

Any or all of these compensatory responses may be impaired in the elderly. Studies have shown that older people have a diminished ability to sense cold.[4] Aging limits the ability to increase basal metabolism and heat production, and older people have lower ratios of basal metabolic rate to body surface area under both resting and active conditions. Many older individuals have some degree of autonomic dysfunction, resulting in decreased ability to compensate with increased cardiac output or peripheral vasoconstriction. Immobility, socioeconomic factors, or neuropsychiatric disease may impair the ability to make behavioral changes, including removing oneself from a cold environment.

Multiple other factors may predispose the elderly to hypothermia. Malnutrition results in decreased subcutaneous tissue for insulation and decreased availability of metabolic substrates. Central nervous system (CNS) pathology such as cerebrovascular disease, trauma, malignancy, and Wernicke's encephalopathy may damage the brain's temperature control centers, whereas peripheral nerve disease from diabetes or spinal cord pathology also may disrupt thermoregulatory response. Cardiovascular disease and drugs limit the ability to increase cardiac output in response to cold. While many medications, including sedatives, hypnotics, antidepressants, and phenothiazines, predispose patients to hypothermia, the drug most closely linked to hypothermia is alcohol. Acute intoxication often leads indirectly to environmental exposure and has multiple pathophysiologic effects such as peripheral vasodilatation and impairment of the shivering response. Chronic alcohol abuse leads to Wernicke's disease and its associated hypothalamic damage and dysfunction.

Cardiovascular changes in hypothermia follow a predictable pattern. Mild hypothermia results in tachycardia and a physiologic increase in cardiac output. With progressively lower core temperatures, bradycardia occurs as a result of decreased spontaneous depolarization of cardiac pacemaker cells, and cardiac output falls. In moderate hypothermia, cardiac irritability produces arrhythmias; atrial fibrillation with slow ventricular response is common.[5] The threshold for ventricular arrhythmias is also lowered, producing ventricular ectopy. With core temperatures below 28°C, ventricular fibrillation becomes much more likely, and for this reason, most authors advise against unnecessary movement of patients or procedures that may irritate the myocardium, such as internal jugular or subclavian vein cannulation. Ultimately, severe hypothermia results in asystole.

Renal pathophysiology follows changes in cardiac output. The initial increase in cardiac output results in increased renal blood flow, and a "cold diuresis" occurs. Later, renal blood flow drops with progressive oliguria. Likewise, endocrine and metabolic functions rise and fall with changes in perfusion; for example, the pancreas stops producing insulin as hypothermia worsens, but glucose levels are likely to remain normal due to increased use of glucose stores.

Progressive depression of the CNS occurs with hypothermia. Mild hypothermia may result in subtle alterations in speech or behavior. With lower temperatures there is progressive depression of consciousness culminating in coma. The peripheral nervous system is also depressed, and with severe hypothermia, deep tendon reflexes are lost.

Hypothermia's effects on the respiratory system include initial tachypnea, producing a mixed respiratory alkalosis and metabolic acidosis.[6] Later, respiratory depression occurs, causing respiratory acidosis. As CNS depression occurs, airway protective reflexes are lost. With worsening hypothermia, cold-induced bronchorrhea and pulmonary edema may be seen.

Clinical Features

In patients who have obviously been exposed to a cold environment for a prolonged period of time, the diagnosis of hypothermia will be obvious. However, hypothermia may go unrecognized initially by prehospital or triage personnel. Therefore, emergency physicians should consider the possibility of hypothermia in older patients who present with altered mental status, diminished level of consciousness, or other nonspecific symptoms. It also should be considered in trauma patients, patients presenting with signs of intoxication, and patients presenting in cardiac arrest. A core temperature should be obtained early in the workup of all such patients. While some reports have suggested that infrared tympanic thermometry may be useful in the hypothermic patient,[7] most authorities recommend that a rectal, bladder, or esophageal temperature be obtained. One should ensure that the thermometer used is capable of measuring temperatures below 30°C; otherwise, the degree of hypothermia may be underestimated.

Diagnosis and Differential

In addition to an accurate determination of core temperature, the initial workup of the hypothermic patient should include cardiac monitoring (this may require needle electrodes through the skin in the severely hypothermic patient). In addition to any of the arrhythmias discussed earlier, the electrocardiogram (ECG) may show Osborn (J) waves at the conjunction of the QRS complex and ST segment. These occur commonly with temperatures below 32°C, and their size correlates inversely with temperature.[8] They do not appear to have any prognostic value. One should keep in mind that ECG changes of hypokalemia may be masked in hypothermia.

When interpreting laboratory data in the setting of hypothermia, some characteristic alterations should be expected. For example, blood gas analyzers typically warm blood to 37°C, increasing the partial pressure of dissolved gases and thereby increasing oxygen and carbon dioxide levels and decreasing pH. Traditionally, these results have been "corrected" to account for temperature differences; however, recent literature suggests that uncorrected pH and Pco_2 values are more useful in guiding therapy.[9] The exception is Po_2; one should keep in mind that a borderline "normal" Po_2 in the setting of hypothermia may represent hypoxemia. A complete blood count should be reviewed, keeping in mind that hematocrit tends to be misleadingly high due to decreased plasma volume. If coagulation studies are obtained, one should keep in mind that they may be normal even in the presence of hypothermic coagulopathy. This is so because clotting factor function is temperature-dependent, and in vivo activity may differ from that in the warmer laboratory environment. Although there is no predictable pattern of electrolyte changes in hypothermia, serum chemistries should be followed closely.

While accidental hypothermia is invariably related to some degree of cold exposure, there may be other medical conditions that contribute to its development. The emergency physician therefore must consider several diagnostic possibilities when confronted with a hypothermic patient. The possibility of sepsis should be pursued in the hypothermic elderly patient, and appropriate cultures and empirical antibiotics should be strongly considered. Hypoglycemia is associated with hypothermia, and a blood glucose level always should be obtained. Drug overdose also can lead to hypothermia, and toxicologic screening should be considered. If there is any question of chronic alcohol abuse and Wernicke's encephalopathy contributing to the patient's presentation, intravenous thiamine should be administered. Other diagnostic possibilities to be considered in the elderly patient with hypothermia and altered mental status include hypothyroidism with myxedema coma and, less commonly, acute adrenal insufficiency. Laboratory evaluation of thyroid function, including thyroid-stimulating hormone (TSH), and adrenal function should be obtained if these diagnoses are considered. Given the frequent association of hypothermia and trauma, every hypothermic patient should have a thorough evaluation for signs of injury, particularly head trauma, and indications for radiography should be liberalized.

Emergency Department Care and Disposition

Along with initial efforts to support airway, breathing, and circulation, an immediate priority in the hypothermic patient is rewarming. Rewarming techniques may be divided into passive rewarming, active external rewarming, and active core rewarming. Any or all of these modalities may be used in the hypothermic patient depending on the clinical setting and the resources available to emergency medical staff. In practice, multiple techniques are often combined.

Passive rewarming includes removal from the cold environment, drying the patient and removing wet clothing, and providing insulation (i.e., simple blankets) to minimize further heat loss, thereby allowing the body's own thermoregulatory mechanisms to recover gradually. Passive measures alone usually will suffice for otherwise healthy patients with mild hypothermia.

Active external rewarming involves exposing the patient to exogenous heat sources such as radiant heat, forced warm air (i.e., "bair hugger" devices), and hot water bottles or other local heat sources. Immersion in warm water also has been used, but this technique makes resuscitation and monitoring difficult and therefore is not recommended. One concern often raised regarding active external rewarming is that of *core temperature afterdrop*, a decline in core temperature after the initiation of rewarming that has been associated with cardiovascular collapse.[10] This phenomenon is thought to be due to heat loss across temperature gradients as peripheral vasodilatation increases blood flow to cold tissues. To avoid this complication, most authors recommend that active external rewarming in moderately or severely hypothermic patients should be confined to truncal areas or used in conjunction with active core rewarming. A combination of passive and active external warming may be used for mild or moderate hypothermia in patients without signs of hemodynamic compromise.

Active core rewarming techniques, which tend to be more invasive, should be considered in hypothermic patients with signs of hemodynamic compromise or in any patient with severe hypothermia. Most hypothermic patients will require intravenous fluid administration, and crystalloids may be warmed to 40 to 42°C prior to administration, whereas crystalloids or colloids may be given through countercurrent heat exchanger devices. Warmed intravenous fluids serve mainly to prevent further heat loss because, by themselves, they effect only minimal changes in core temperature. Administration of warmed (up to 45°C) and humidified air or oxygen by mask or endotracheal tube prevents further respiratory heat losses and can raise core temperature by 1 to 2°C per hour.[11] Gastric and bladder irrigation with warmed fluids has been advocated in the past but appears to have limited benefit due to relatively small surface areas available for heat exchange. Peritoneal lavage with warmed fluids, on the other hand, has been shown to be effective in experienced hands, with demonstrated core rewarming rates of 2 to 4°C per hour. Some authors have reported on the use of pleural or thoracic cavity lavage via thoracostomy tubes[12] to achieve rapid elevation of core temperature.

In critically ill patients, extracorporeal rewarming by means of cardiopulmonary bypass appears to be the most effective way to raise core temperature quickly.[13,14] However, this requires specialized equipment and personnel, and it may be contraindicated in patients with significant trauma because of the need for anticoagulation. Depending on the resources and expertise available locally, other options for extracorporeal rewarming include standard hemodiaysis and continuous arteriovenous or venovenous rewarming. If any of these techniques are used, vascular access should be by the femoral vessels because attempts at internal jugular or subclavian vein cannulation may induce ventricular fibrillation in the irritable hypothermic heart.

Immediate drug therapy in the hypothermic patient may include intravenous dextrose administration if the blood glucose level is low or unknown and intravenous thiamine if Wernicke's encephalopathy is a possibility. Given the possibility of sepsis, empirical antibiotics should be strongly considered in the elderly patient with hypothermia. Levothyroxine should be given only if the history or physical examination findings suggest thyroid disease. Likewise, high-dose corticosteroids should be given only if there is a history of adrenocortical insufficiency or chronic steroid use or if a patient fails to respond to rewarming.

Patients who have been brought to the hospital for hypothermia should be admitted for further workup and follow-up of any cardiac, neurologic, or laboratory abnormalities. On hospital discharge, social services should be involved in the further care of the patient as an outpatient to ensure that there is adequate heat in the patient's residence, drug regimens are accessible and followed appropriately, medical follow-up is accessible and available, and any substance abuse issues are dealt with appropriately.

HYPERTHERMIA

Hyperthermia is defined as a core temperature greater than 37.5°C.[15] The term *fever* refers to a specific subtype of hyperthermia in which there a controlled increase in temperature under the control of an intact thermoregulatory system. Thus, while all patients with a fever are hyperthermic, not all hyperthermic patients can be said to have a fever. This discussion will concern itself mainly with nonfever types of hyperthermia and particularly with those related to environmental heat stress. Of illnesses related to heat stress, the most serious is *heat stroke,* which is defined as uncontrolled hyperthermia with neurologic changes. For a variety of reasons that will be discussed below, the elderly are particularly susceptible to hyperthermic illnesses, especially under conditions of extreme environmental heat. The emergency physician should maintain a high awareness of heat-related illnesses and hyperthermia in all elderly patients and be familiar with their diagnosis and treatment.

Epidemiology

While exact numbers of patients affected by heat stroke and hyperthermia are unavailable, the CDC keeps statistics on deaths related to "excessive heat exposure." During the 19-year period from 1979 through 1996, there were, on average, 381 such deaths per year in the United States. The number of deaths per year varied widely (from a low of 148 in 1979 to a high of 1700 in 1980), with higher numbers of deaths corresponding to "heat waves." Among those deaths related to extreme hot weather conditions, 44 percent occurred among persons 65 years of age or older, and death rates correlated with increasing age, with those 65 years of age and older at highest risk. Death rates also were found to be higher in males than in females, and among racial groups, blacks had a higher death rate than whites.[16]

Pathophysiology

As with hypothermia, the body's response to hyperthermia is mediated by the brain's thermoregulatory center in the anterior preoptic hypothalamus. Input is received from temperature sensors in the skin, great vessels, abdominal viscera, and spinal cord and efferent nerves to multiple sites effect physiologic adaptations. Under warm conditions, these include peripheral vasodilatation, sweating, decreased heat production, and behavioral modification. As with the response to hypothermia, any or all of these responses may be impaired in the older patient.

Age- or disease-related changes in the cardiovascular system result in a limited ability to increase cardiac output, and this in turn limits the ability to achieve shunt blood flow to the skin surface. The sweating response is also diminished with age, due to a decrease in the number and efficiency of sweat glands, as well as a higher core temperature needed to elicit sweating, and this further limits heat dissipation.[17] Dehydration is more common among older individuals for a variety of reasons, and this limits both sweating and changes in vasomotor tone. As is the case with extreme cold conditions, elderly patients may have limited ability to effect behavioral responses (moving to a cooler environment, removing clothing) because of immobility, neuropsychiatric illness, or socioeconomic factors.

Drugs, either in overdose or with therapeutic dosing, also may play a part in the development of hyperthermia in the elderly patient. Salicylates or thyroid hormone may increase metabolic rate and heat production. Cardiovascular medications such as beta blockers or calcium channel blockers limit the ability to increase cardiac output in response to heat stress. Anticholinergic agents, antidepressants, antidopaminergic agents, and antipsychotics impair heat dissipation and thermoregulation. Multiple drugs, including anticholinergic and serotonergic agents, sympathomimetics, lithium, theophylline, and dopaminergic agents, may result in muscular hyperactivity. Alcohol does not directly increase core temperature, but its abuse often contributes to the development of hyperthermia by causing malnutrition and hypothalamic dysfunction, and intoxication may lead to the combination of dehydration, environmental exposure, altered sensorium, and immobility.

When core temperature exceeds approximately 42°C, normal temperature control mechanisms fail, and hyperthermia can accelerate, causing the denaturing of proteins and cellular necrosis. This leads to end-organ damage and failure. The combination of hyperthermia with signs of CNS dysfunction such as altered level of consciousness, focal neurologic deficits, seizures, or coma, is known as *heat stroke*. This is a true medical emergency and requires immediate treatment to decrease the risk of morbidity and mortality. An elderly patient who presents with significant hyperthermia and neurologic changes should be assumed to have heat stroke and treated as such until proven otherwise.

Clinical Features

Heat-related illnesses occupy a spectrum from mild to life-threatening. Mild forms of heat illness include heat cramps, heat edema, heat syncope, and heat exhaustion. In contrast to heat stroke, these are all characterized by essentially normal neurologic status and normal or only mildly elevated (<39°C) body temperature. Heat cramps are involuntary muscle spasms after cessation of exercise in the heat; treatment consists of rest and fluid replacement. Heat edema usually occurs in the lower extremities when unacclimitized individuals are exposed to heat. It is usually minor and usually improves with elevation of the extremities. Heat syncope is related to vasodilatation in individuals who are unable to mount a compensatory tachycardia and occurs commonly in older individuals who take beta blockers. Treatment includes rest, elevation of the legs, and removal from the heat stress.[18] Heat exhaustion is a poorly defined constellation of symptoms that may include headache, nausea, vomiting, lightheadedness, fatigue, malaise, and myalgias. Treatment is generally supportive, including rest and fluid supplementation. Elderly patients and those with serious comorbidities usually will require hospitalization, particularly if there is a question of heat stroke.[19]

With true heat stroke, there is always some alteration of neurologic status, such as altered level of consciousness or coma, seizures, or focal neurologic deficit. Core temperature often will be markedly elevated (>40.6°C), but this is not always the case. If cooling measures have been started prior to arrival in the ED, patients may present with mildly elevated or even normal core temperatures, and improvement of neurologic status may have occurred. In such cases, the diagnosis of heat stroke may be made based on the history combined with a characteristic setting and consistent laboratory data (see below).

Heat stroke is also characterized by tachycardia, normal or low blood pressure, and tachypnea. Physical examination may reveal warm and dry skin or diaphoresis. Neurologic examination may show almost any type of abnormality, including delirium, focal neurologic deficits, and obtundation. If toxic effects of drugs contributed to the patient's hyperthermia, signs of anticholinergic or sympathomimetic toxidromes may be seen on physical examination.

Diagnosis and Differential

Hyperthermia may occur due to environmental factors alone, but more often in the elderly patient other medical problems contribute to its development. Therefore, hyperthermia in an older individual should prompt consideration of a wide variety of possible diagnoses. Even in patients found in a hot environment, hyperthermia may represent sepsis, and a thorough search for sources of infection should be undertaken. One infectious syndrome that should be kept in mind in the older patient with hyperthermia and signs of increased muscular activity is tetanus. Though rare in overall terms among the U.S. population, it has a much greater incidence in patients older than 60 years of age than in younger adults and carries a higher risk of mortality in this age group.[20]

Hyperthermia is a well-recognized complication of CNS pathology, including stroke or trauma to the region of the hypothalamus or anterior pituitary. Prolonged seizures may cause hyperthermia (as may other disorders characterized by increased muscular activity) or be caused by it. Endocrine causes of hyperthermia include thyroid storm and pheochromocytoma. Almost any medication can cause a drug fever, although certain types of drugs such as anticholinergics, sympathomimetics, neuroleptics, and others discussed earlier are more likely to cause temperature elevations, and toxicologic etiologies of hyperthermia should be considered.

Neuromuscular rigidity is not normally seen in cases of environmental hyperthermia, and the presence of rigidity and an elevated creatine phosphokinase (CPK) level in an elderly patient who has taken any neuroleptic medication should prompt suspicion of neuroleptic malignant syndrome.

While the immediate priorities in the truly hyperthermic patient include stabilization of the airway, breathing, and circulation in conjunction with rapid cooling, initial laboratory tests should include a complete blood count and coagulation studies with fibrinogen and fibrin degradation products because of the possibility of disseminated intravascular coagulation. Given the possibility of renal failure, electrolytes, blood urea nitrogen, creatinine, and a urinalysis should be checked. Liver and muscle enzymes (AST, ALT, CPK) almost always will

be elevated in heat stroke and appear to have prognostic value.[21] In borderline cases where it is unclear whether a patient's diagnosis is heat exhaustion or true heat stroke, liver enzyme levels can be helpful in making the distinction.

An ECG and cardiac enzymes should be followed to look for signs of myocardial ischemia. Toxicologic screening should be considered, and if the patient is known to take lithium, theophylline, or salicylates, drug levels may be useful. In patients with hyperthermia and altered mental status, a head computed tomographic (CT) scan may show signs of CNS pathology such as intracranial hemorrhage or infection. Some form of septic workup (e.g., blood, urine, and cerebrospinal fluid cultures, along with chest radiograph and thorough physical examination) should be a part of the workup of every hyperthermic patient, and empirical antibiotic administration should be strongly considered in the elderly patient with hyperthermia.

Emergency Department Care and Disposition

In the patient with suspected heat stroke, rapid cooling should be an immediate priority and should proceed simultaneously with initial evaluation and stabilization of airway, breathing, and circulation. Outcomes are directly related to the amount of time tissues are exposed to heat stress, and therefore, cooling must be accomplished as quickly as possible. Most authors recommend that cooling proceed at a rate of 0.1°C per minute or more, with a goal temperature of less than 39°C.[22] Core temperature should be monitored continuously during the cooling process with a rectal or esophageal probe, and cooling measures should be discontinued on reaching 39°C in order to avoid overcorrection.

In true hyperthermia, as opposed to fever, antipyretics are not effective, and they should not be used. Instead, physical cooling modalities such as immersion and evaporation are recommended. Ice-water immersion has been widely advocated in the past and has been demonstrated to be effective in achieving rapid reduction in core temperature.[23] However, there are some practical difficulties associated with this method, and monitoring and resuscitation are rendered nearly impossible. With evaporative cooling, currently the most widely used method, the patient is placed naked on a stretcher and sprayed with lukewarm water while fans blow room-temperature air across the body surface. While some studies demonstrating the effectiveness of evaporative cooling have employed specialized equipment such as specially constructed body cooling units or helicopter blades,[24,25] others have shown effectiveness with equipment comparable with that found in the average ED.[26] Given its practical and patient comfort advantages and comparable effectiveness, many authors now recommend evaporative cooling over immersion. Whatever method is used, the most important thing is that emergency medical staff recognize the need for cooling and begin it as quickly as possible. Because most EDs will not encounter this situation frequently, predetermined protocols may be useful in guiding the cooling process.

Several other techniques have been used to aid in cooling. Iced peritoneal lavage has been used successfully in animal models,[27] but experience in humans is limited.[28] Iced gastric lavage also has shown effectiveness in animals,[29] and while not recommended as a primary cooling technique, it may be useful as an adjunctive measure in patients who have a nasogastric tube in place. Packing the patient's groin, neck, and axillae with ice is also not sufficient by itself but may help in conjunction with evaporative cooling.[22] Cooled air or oxygen and intravenous fluid contribute little to heat transfer. Cardiopulmonary bypass has been used for treatment of malignant hyperthermia,[30] but because of the need for specialized equipment and personnel and the time required to set it up, it probably has no place in the ED care of hyperthermia.

In addition to rapid cooling, another consideration in the ED treatment of the hyperthermic patient is to minimize heat production through relaxation or paralysis. This is particularly important in conditions that produce increased muscular tone (including various toxidromes, neuroleptic malignant syndrome, and tetanus) but should be considered in any patient with heat stroke.

The major determinants of morbidity and mortality in acute hyperthermia due to heat stroke are the degree of temperature elevation and the duration of time that temperature elevation persists.[31] Other poor prognostic factors include prolonged coma and marked elevation of liver enzymes (AST > 1000 IU/L).[21]

Patients who present with mild hyperthemic changes such as heat cramps or heat edema can be discharged safely following a full evaluation, fluid supplementation, and correction of any electrolyte abnormalities. They also should have follow-up arranged through a social services entity to ensure that their living conditions are appropriate (air conditioning, ability to easily ambulate or relocate themselves from heated areas, easy access to hydration). Patients who have profound laboratory value

irregularities, altered mental status, syncopal episodes, or any indications of heat stroke should be admitted to the hospital for further evaluation and treatment.

REFERENCES

1. Manning B, Stollerman GH: Hypothermia in the elderly. *Hosp Pract* 28:53, 1993.
2. Centers for Disease Control and Prevention: Hypothermia-related deaths—Georgia, January 1996–December 1997, and United States, 1979–1995. *JAMA* 281:124, 1999.
3. Luna GK, Maier RV, Pavlin EG, et al: Incidence and effect of hypothermia in seriously injured patients. *J Trauma* 27:1014, 1987.
4. Collins KJ, Exton-Smith AN, Dore C: Urban hypothermia: Preferred temperature and thermal perception in old age. *Br Med J* 282:175, 1981.
5. Vassallo SU, Delaney KA, Hoffman RS, et al: A prospective evaluation of the electrocardiographic manifestations of hypothermia. *Acad Emerg Med* 6:1121, 1999.
6. Jolly BT, Ghezzi KT: Accidental hypothermia. *Emerg Med Clin North Am* 10:311, 1992.
7. Zehner WJ, Terndrup TE: Ear temperatures during rewarming from hypothermia. *Ann Emerg Med.* 23:901, 1994.
8. Vassallo SU, Delaney KA, Hoffman RS, et al: A prospective evaluation of the electrocardiographic manifestations of hypothermia. *Acad Emerg Med* 6:1121, 1999.
9. Danzl DF: Accidental hypothermia, in Marx JA, Hockberger RS, Walls RM, et al (eds): *Rosen's Emergency Medicine: Concepts and Clinical Practice.* St Louis, Mosby, 2002, p 1979.
10. Hayward JS, Eckerson JD, Kemna D: Thermal and cardiovascular changes during three methods of resuscitation from mild hypothermia. *Resuscitation* 11:21, 1984.
11. Danzl DF, Pozos RS: Accidental hypothermia. *New Engl J Med* 331:1756, 1994.
12. Hall KN, Syverud SA: Closed thoracic cavity lavage in the treatment of severe hypothermia in human beings. *Ann Emerg Med* 19:204, 1990.
13. Splittgerber FH, Talbert JG., Sweezer WP, et al: Partial cardiopulmonary bypass for core rewarming in profound accidental hypothermia. *Am Surg* 52:407, 1986.
14. Vretenar DF, Urshel JD, Parrott JC, et al: Cardiopulmonary bypass resuscitation for accidental hypothermia. *Ann Thorac Surg* 58:895, 1994.
15. Harchelroad F: Acute thermoregulatory disorders. *Clin Geriatr Med* 9:621, 1993.
16. Centers for Disease Control and Prevention: Heat-related illnesses, deaths, and risk factors—Cincinnati and Dayton, Ohio, 1999, and United States, 1979–1997. *JAMA* 284:34, 2000.
17. Ballester JM, Harchelroad FP: Hyperthermia: How to recognize and prevent heat-related illnesses. *Geriatrics* 54:20, 1999.

18. Harchelroad F: Acute thermoregulatory disorders. *Clin Geriatr Med* 9:621, 1993.

19. Tek D, Olshaker J: Heat illness. *Emerg Med Clin North Am* 10:299, 1992.

20. Bardenheier B, Prevots DR, Khetsuriani N, et al: Tetanus surveillance—United States, 1995–1997. *MMWR* 47:1, 1998.

21. Kew M, Bershas I, Sefteh H: The diagnostic and prognostic significance of the serum enzyme changes in heatstroke. *Trans R Soc Trop Med Hyg* 65:325, 1971.

22. Tek D, Olshaker J: Heat illness. *Emerg Med Clin North Am* 10:299, 1992.

23. Costrini A: Emergency treatment of exertional heat stroke and comparison of whole body cooling techniques. *Med Sci Sport Exerc* 22:15, 1990.

24. Weiner JS. Khogali M: A physiological body-cooling unit for treatment of heat stroke. *Lancet* 1:507, 1980.

25. Poulton TJ, Walker RA: Helicopter cooling of heatstroke victims. *Aviat Space Environ Med* 58:358, 1987.

26. Graham BS, Lichtenstein MJ, Hinson JM, et al: Nonexertional heat stroke: Physiologic management and cooling in 14 patients. *Arch Intern Med* 146:87, 1986.

27. Bynum G, Patton J, Bowers W, et al: Peritoneal lavage cooling in an anesthetized dog heatstroke model. *Aviat Space Environ Med* 49:779, 1978.

28. Horowitz Z: The golden hour in heat stroke: Use of iced peritoneal lavage. *Am J Emerg Med* 7:616, 1989.

29. Syverud SA, Barker WJ, Amsterdam JT, et al: Iced gastric lavage for treatment of heat stroke: Efficacy in a canine model. *Ann Emerg Med* 14:424, 1985.

30. Ryan JF, Donlon JV, Malt RA, et al: Cardiopulmonary bypass in the treatment of malignant hyperthermia. *New Engl J Med* 290:1121, 1974.

31. O'Donnell TF: Acute heat stroke: Epidemiologic, biochemical, renal and coagulation studies. *JAMA* 234:824, 1975.

50

Diabetes and Diabetic Emergencies

Micheal D. Rush

HIGH-YIELD FACTS

- It is estimated that 7 million people in the United States are 65 years of age or older, and about 20.1 percent of the people in this age group have physician-diagnosed diabetes. This is nearly quadruple the prevalence of diagnosed diabetes in all other adults.

- Rates of undiagnosed diabetes and prediabetes in the people aged 60 to 74 years in the United States are more than double that of all other adults.

- About 1 million new cases of diabetes are diagnosed each year in U.S. adults. The overwhelming majority, 90 to 95 percent, are diagnosed with type 2 diabetes.

- Ischemic heart disease is the most frequent cause of death in patients with diabetes. Risk of heart disease in those with diabetes is two to four times that of those without the disease.

- Common emergency department (ED) presentations of the complications of diabetes include hypoglycemia, diabetic ketoacidosis, and hyperglycemic, hyperosmolar, nonketotic syndrome.

Diabetes mellitus represents a group of diseases in which there is a defect in insulin secretion, an inability of the body to respond to insulin, or a combination of these two problems. Type 2 diabetes is the most common form overall, accounting for 90 to 95 percent of all cases. It is by far the most common manifestation in the elderly patient population. Type 2 diabetes usually begins as insulin resistance often resulting from obesity, poor dietary habits, and lack of exercise and ultimately leads to beta cell failure and partial or even absolute insulin defi-

ciency. There is believed to be a genetic predisposition to type 2 diabetes in the form of a "scavenger" gene that allowed for efficient use of food when humans were primarily hunter gatherers. In modern times when food is plentiful for most adults in the United States, the gene predisposes to obesity and insulin resistance. The American diet, which is high in fat and low in complex carbohydrates and dietary fiber, coupled with an increasingly sedentary lifestyle, also has contributed to the increasing prevalence of diabetes. Obesity is epidemic in the United States, with 17.9 percent of the combined adult population reported to have a body mass index of 30 kg/m^2 or greater in 1998 compared with only 12.0 percent in 1991. Approximately 36 percent of people in the United States over age 60 were considered obese in 1998 versus only 26 percent in 1991.[3]

Common diabetic emergencies include diabetic ketoacidosis (DKA); hyperglycemic, hyperosmolar, nonketotic syndrome (HHNS); and hypoglycemia.

EPIDEMIOLOGY

It is estimated that 7 million people in the United States are aged 65 years or older, and about 20.1 percent of people in this age group have physician-diagnosed diabetes. This is nearly quadruple the prevalence of diagnosed diabetes in all adults 20 years of age and older (5.1 percent).[1] According to data from the Third National Health and Nutrition Examination Survey (NHANES III), prevalence of physician diagnosed type 2 diabetes increases with age from 1.1 percent in people 20 to 29 years of age to 13.2 percent in those 75 years of age and older. Type 2 diabetes occurs relatively equally in men and women when age is standardized. Type 2 diabetes is more prevalent in African-Americans (8.2 percent) and Hispanic/Mexican-Americans (9.3 percent) than in their non-Hispanic white counterparts (4.8 percent). Prevalence of undiagnosed diabetes and impaired fasting glucose (IFG) or prediabetes is also high at 2.8 and 6.9 percent, respectively, when standardized for race, age, and sex. Rates of undiagnosed diabetes in the population 60 to 74 years of age in the United States are more than double those of the age- and sex-standardized population of all adults 20 years of age and older (6.2 versus 2.8 percent).[2]

In the 60- to 74-year age group, 6.2 percent have undiagnosed diabetes, and 14 percent have prediabetes. Given that 12.6 percent of patients in this age group have physician-diagnosed diabetes, this means that nearly half the people in this age group do not know that they have diabetes.[1] The relative risk of death in patients with diabetes aged 65 to 74 years is about 1.5 times that of an age-matched nondiabetic cohort. Median life expectancy is approximately 4 years less in this age group and 8 years less in the 55- to 64-year age group.[4]

Risk factors for type 2 diabetes also increase with age. Other risk factors include family history in first-degree relatives; being overweight (body mass index $\geq$ 25 kg/m^2); no regular physical activity; African, Mexican, Asian/Pacific Island, or Native American ethnicity; blood pressure of 140/90 mmHg or greater; dyslipidemia (low high-density lipoprotein, high triglycerides); history of gestational diabetes or having a baby weighing 9 lb or greater at birth; IFG or impaired glucose tolerance (IGT); and polycystic ovary disease.

PATHOPHYSIOLOGY

The ability of the body to respond to the actions of insulin declines with age due to decreases in skeketal muscle mass and the natural tendency toward glucose intolerance as one ages. Depending on body habitus, there may be defects in glucose-induced insulin secretion, which are observed more commonly in lean elderly patients with diabetes, or in the insulin-mediated peripheral uptake/disposal of glucose, which are seen primarily in obese elderly patients with diabetes. An increase in fasting hepatic glucose production secondary to increased levels of insulin is less often observed in elderly patients.[5] In older patients, fasting blood sugar levels may be normal secondary to this absence of increased fasting hepatic glucose production. In many elderly patients, glucose tolerance is impaired secondary to a loss of skeletal muscle mass and the resulting effect of diminished use of glucose peripherally. Consequently, the oral glucose tolerance test may still have a role in screening for type 2 diabetes in elderly patients because it independently predicts increased mortality in the elderly even in the presence of a normal fasting glucose level.[6] Elevated blood glucose levels are related, in a dose-response fashion, to risk for microvascular complications of diabetes such as retinopathy, nephropathy, and neuropathy. Diabetes is a leading cause of blindness (from proliferative retinopathy), renal failure (basement membrane damage in the glomeruli of the kidneys), and lower extremity amputations (resulting from foot ulcers secondary to diabetes-related peripheral neuropathy). Hyperglycemia also contributes to, but is not directly causal of, the macrovascular complications of diabetes: heart disease, peripheral vascular disease, and stroke.

Hyperglycemia and insulin resistance, together with hypertension, dyslipidemia, and obesity, are known as the *dysmetabolic syndrome,* an important and emerging concept in understanding the pathophysiology of the accelerated atherogenesis associated with diabetes. The dysmetabolic syndrome and a sedentary lifestyle are essential cofactors in the pathogenesis of the accelerated atherogenesis and resulting macrosvascular complications of diabetes, primarily through endothelial damage, oxidative stress, hypercoagulability, and abnormal inflammatory responses.

CLINICAL FEATURES

The clinical presentation of diabetes in elderly patients is most often insidious. Traditional symptoms of hyperglycemia such as polydipsia and polyuria may not be as prominent in an elderly population because of age-related decreases in the thirst responses and increases in the renal threshold for spilling glucose in the urine. Unexplained weight loss, fatigue, and nocturia are more typical symptoms in this population. All these symptoms may be attributed to aging by the patient or their clinician and further delay the diagnosis. Often the diagnosis of diabetes is made in conjunction with one or more of the complications of diabetes, most commonly ischemic heart disease. Microvascular complications such as neuropathy may present as an increasing inability to get up from chairs or climb stairs secondary to polyneuropathy or as isolated cranial mononeuropathies, most commonly oculomotor and abducens palsies, which present clinically as blurred vision and/or diplopia. Proteinuria in the absence of infection should prompt investigation for diabetes. Proliferative retinopathy or glaucoma, common complications of diabetes, may be diagnosed during routine ophthalmologic examinations. Certain infections that are commonly associated with diabetes occur more frequently in elderly patients, such as malignant otitis externa, rhinocerebral mucormycosis, and candidal urogenital infections.

Patients also may present in the metabolic decompensation states of diabetic ketoacidosis (DKA) and hyperglycemic, hyperosmolar, nonketotic syndrome (HHNS). Last, patients may present with hypoglycemia secondary to diabetes medications. Hypoglycemic episodes typically present with mental status changes and neurologic symptoms, including seizures and focal findings. Diaphoresis or bradycardia may be present.

DIAGNOSIS

Many older patients presenting to the ED will have a known history of diabetes. However, the diagnosis is often made on routine laboratory evaulation, which reveals an elevated serum glucose level, or during an ED evaluation for mental status changes, infection, or other acute complaint.

Fasting plasma glucose determination is the American Diabetes Association (ADA)–recommended preferred screening test for diabetes in deference to its sensitivity, relatively low cost, and ease of performance. Screening in asymptomatic individuals should begin at age 45, and negative tests should be repeated every 3 years. A value of 7 mmol/L or 126 mg/dL or greater is considered diagnostic of diabetes. Patients with values of 6.1 mmol/L (110 mg/dL) or greater but less than 7 mmol/L (126 mg/dL) are considered to have IFG or prediabetes. The oral glucose tolerance test, in which a 75-g load of anhydrous glucose is given orally and a plasma glucose level is determined 2 hours after administration, may still have a role in diagnosing high-risk individuals, especially elderly patients. Values of 11.1 mmol/L or 200 mg/dL or greater at 2 hours are diagnostic of diabetes, while values of 7.8 mmol/L or 140 mg/dL or greater but less than 200 mg/dL are indicative of impaired glucose tolerance (IGT), another prediabetes state.[7]

The diagnosis of diabetes also may be first discovered when the the patient presents with the metabolic complications of DKA or HHNS. Table 50-1 illustrates the diagnostic features of DKA versus HHNS.

The diagnosis of hypoglycemia is confirmed by finding a low serum glucose level. Although the actual level that defines hypoglycemia is somewhat arbitrary, most patients will be symptomatic when levels fall below 40 to 50 mg/dL. A rapid dextrose determination should be obtained routinely on all patients who present with mental status changes or neurologic symptoms.

EMERGENCY DEPARTMENT CARE AND DISPOSITION

Emergency Therapy: DKA, HHNS, Hypoglycemia

If the patient is obtunded or comatose, the airway should be controlled with rapid-sequence endotracheal intubation. Basic laboratory studies such as a complete blood count and electrolyte, blood urea nitrogen (BUN), creatinine, and serum glucose determinations are indicated in all patients suspected of having DKA or HHNS. Arterial blood gas analysis may be helpful in obtunded, unconscious patients to assess ventilatory status and overall acid-base status; otherwise, a venous pH correlates well with arterial pH and is usually adequate in making the diagnosis and for following therapy in DKA. Serum ketone analysis is still done commonly but is seldom useful in assessing DKA because the common nitroprusside reaction assay measures only acetoacetate, whereas the primary ketone body in DKA is beta-hydroxybutyrate. Ultimately, beta-hydroxybutyrate is broken down to acetoacetate in the presence of insulin, and so, paradoxically, serum ketone levels often will increase as the patient improves with treatment.

DKA is most commonly associated with infection. Myocardial infarction and stroke, in addition to infection, are also commonly associated with both DKA and HHNS in the elderly population. Infection as a comorbid diagnosis should be high in the differential, and appropriate cultures of blood, urine, sputum, and cerebrospinal fluid should be obtained and broad-spectrum parenteral antibiotics initiated. The electrocardiogram may be especially useful in the elderly population to diagnose myocardial ischemia and severe electrolyte disorders. Computed tomographic (CT) scanning of the head is indicated in all stable obtunded and comatose patients to assess for stroke or cerebral edema.

Table 50-1. Diagnostic Features of DKA versus HHNS

	DKA	HHNS
Plasma glucose, mg/dL	> 250	> 600
Arterial pH	< 7.30	> 7.30
Serum bicarbonate, meq/L	< 15	> 15
Urine ketones	Positive	Small to negative
Serum ketones	Positive	Small to negative
Serum osmolality mosm/kg	Variable from normal to high	> 320
Anion gap	> 12	< 12
Mental status	Alert to comatose	Lethargic to comatose

Further laboratory and diagnostic imaging workup should be dictated by the history and physical examination and should be very broad in the comatose/unresponsive patient. Noncompliance with insulin or oral antidiabetic medications always should be a diagnosis of exclusion.

Principles of therapy for DKA and HHNS are similar and involve intravenous fluid therapy, insulin therapy, and repletion of electrolytes, most importantly potassium.

Intravenous fluid therapy should begin with an assessment of patient's hydration status and clinical condition. Presence of cardiogenic shock should prompt hemodynamic monitoring prior to aggressive fluid resuscitation. For most other patients, hydration should begin with normal saline (NS) (0.9% NaCl) at a rate of 1 L/h until the chemistry panel (electrolytes, BUN, creatinine, glucose) is available. Bewteen 500 mL and 1 L of NS may be given as a bolus if the patient is hypotensive. Based on the corrected serum sodium (add 1.6 meq/L Na$^+$ to measured value for each 100 mg/dL of glucose > 100 mg/dL), NS should be continued if the corrected sodium is low or the patient is extremely dehydrated clinically, or one-half NS (0.45% NaCl) may be used if the corrected sodium is high or normal. Rates of fluid administration after the first 1 to 2 L should be decreased to 4 to 14 mL/kg/h unless the patients remains in hypovolemic shock. When serum glucose level reaches 250 to 300 mg/dL, intravenous fluids should be changed to one-half NS with 5% dextrose. Once the serum glucose reaches these levels, it is possible to use urine output, ideally 50 mL/h or greater, as a measure of adequate volume repletion.

Insulin therapy is accomplished primarily as intravenous regular human insulin infused at a constant rate of 0.1 unit/kg/h. If the serum potassium level is not less than 3.3 meq/L, an initial intravenous bolus of 0.1 to 0.15 unit/kg/h may halt the further production of ketone bodies and initiate ketone metabolism in DKA and will speed reduction of the serum glucose level in HHNS. Capillary blood glucose level should be measured hourly to monitor insulin therapy. The insulin dose may be doubled if the glucose level is not falling by 50 to 75 mg/dL in the first hour of therapy.

Total-body potassium deficits are usually in the range of 3 to 5 meq/kg in DKA or HHNS. Potassium repletion is based on the initial measured value at presentation. If it is less than 3.3 meq/L, insulin is held, and up to 40 meq KCl is given per hour intravenously until measured potassium level exceeds 3.3 meq/L. If the serum potassium level is in the normal range of 3.3 to 5.0 meq/L then 20 to 40 meq KCl may be added to each liter of intravenous fluid being given. If the patient is alert and not vomiting,

consider oral potassium repletion of 20 to 40 meq KCL every 2 to 4 hours. If the serum potassium level is greater than 5.0 meq/L, then potassium repletion is held until values are below this level. Aggressive therapy to lower potassium is generally not necessary unless there is associated electrocardiographic changes (QRS widening or loss of P waves), the patient is on digoxin, or the patient is in acute renal falure. Potassium level should be monitored every 2 hours for at least the first 8 hours of therapy.

Sodium bicarbonate administration is not indicated for pH values of 6.9 or greater in DKA and may even be harmful, delaying ketone body metabolism and causing paradoxical acidosis in the central nervous system.[8] The sodium load in a dose of sodium bicarbonate also may contribute to the development of cerebral edema, a frequently deadly complication of DKA. Sodium bicarbonate should be given slowly (100 mmol in 500 mL of D$_5$W infused over 2 hours) only if the pH is below 6.9 or the clinical situation warrants its use (e.g., severe hyperkalemia). Routine phosphorus repletion has not been shown to be beneficial and may be harmful, causing severe hypocalcemia.[9] Phosphorus levels less than 1.0 meq/L, which may be associated with skeletal and respiratory muscle weakness, can be treated with 20 to 30 meq potassium phosphate added to 1 L of intravenous fluid.

Therapy for hypoglycemia consists of glucose administration, either orally or intravenously. Diabetics with insulin reactions may require a continuous infusion of a 5% or 10% glucose solution to maintain a serum glucose level greater than 100 mg/dL. Glucagon, 0.5 to 2.0 mg intravenously, intramuscularly, or subcutaneously, may be used in select patients, such as those who lack intravenous access or if there is not a prompt response to the glucose infusion. Most patients with insulin reactions respond rapidly. Patients with long-acting insulin or sulfonylureas overdoses are at risk for recurrent hypoglycemia.

Therapeutic recommendations in this section, except where specifically referenced, were taken from an ADA position statement.[10] As with all practice guidelines, they should be adapted to the individual clinical situation by an experienced clinician.

Long-Term Therapy for Diabetes

The goals of long-term therapy are focused on preventing complications. Until recently, it was believed that aggressive blood glucose control was not warranted in the elderly population secondary to the risks of hypoglycemia associated with oral sulfonylurea therapy and the tendency for the elderly to not recognize the autonomic signs and symptoms of hypoglycemia (e.g., sweating, tachycardia) as readily as younger patients. However, life expectancies have now increased over the last several decades (with an average person living at least 10 to 15 years after retirement), and appropriate glucose, blood pressure, and lipid control can have a tremendous impact on the quality and quantity of life in older patients with newly diagnosed diabetes. Furthermore, data from the United Kingdom Prospective Diabetes Study (UKPDS) demonstrate that severe oral agent–related hypoglycemia is a relatively uncommon event.[11]

Clearly, not all elderly patients are candidates for aggressive glycemic control. The glucagon counterregulatory response to hypoglycemia is less functional in the elderly, leading to increased release of epinephrine to raise blood glucose level and release lipids. This can lead to a potential increase in cardiovascular events in association with hypoglycemia. Elderly patients with severe macrovascular complications, significant cognitive impairment from dementia or other psychiatric reasons, malignancy, or who are unable or unwilling to comply with an intensive regimen may not benefit from and may even be harmed by aggressive diabetes management. The most effective diabetes management plan is an individualized regimen of blood glucose control that takes into account the individual's overall health, life expectancy, presence of complications, ability to tolerate hypoglycemia physiologically, and the ability to comply with an intensive regimen including medical therapy, diet, and exercise. Intensive management regimens have been proven to significantly lessen the risk of microvascular complications in both type 1 and type 2 diabetes.[11,12] For type 2 diabetes, an intensive glucose control scheme may include one or more oral medications, insulin injection(s), and frequent self-monitoring of blood glucose. Management of hypertension (≤130/80 mmHg) and control of dyslipidemia (LDL ≤ 100 mg/dL, high-density lipoprotein ≥ 45 mg/dL in men and ≥ 55 mg/dL in women, and triglycerides ≤ 150 mg/dL) are also essential. Intensive glycemic control, blood pressure control, and control of blood lipid levels have been shown not only to be effective at reducing the micro- and macrovascular complications of diabetes but also to be cost-effective when compared with other major disease interventions.[13]

Glycemic therapy generally is initiated on a stepwise basis, with diet and exercise being the first step. This may be difficult for some seniors who may have significant physical limitations and comorbidities that limit the ability to exercise effectively. Shopping for and preparing regular, healthy meals also may be extremely difficult for many older patients. Problems with diminished vision,

smell, and taste, as well as poor dentition/poorly fitting dentures, may lead to irregular eating habits. Many assisted living and nursing care homes now offer exercise programs designed for elders, and meals are often part of the benefits of these living arrangements.

The next stage of therapy is oral agents, which act through a variety of physiologic mechanisms to decrease glucose levels. Table 50-2 details the various classes of oral antidiabetic agents available, their mechanisms of action, and their important side effects and cautions. Hepatic and renal function diminishes with age, so care should be taken when adding medications to avoid both adverse drug reactions and interactions. Many oral antidiabetic agents are very expensive, and clinicians should consider costs when choosing among agents.

Many patients ultimately will require insulin as part of their therapeutic regimens. The risk of severe hypoglycemia with insulin increases with age, and the elderly are more prone to the adverse effects of hypoglycemia, such as falling. Older patients may not exhibit classic signs of hypoglycemia other than mental status impairment secondary to diminished counterregulatory hormone (epinephrine, glucagon, and growth hormone) axes with aging.[14]

Compliance also may be more difficult for the elderly patient because the syringes are small with small print and may be difficult to handle and read. Prefilled insulin delivery devices may make insulin administration easier for the elderly patient. Insulin therapy has become more attractive with the availability of shorter-acting insulin analogues, such as lispro and aspart, and true nonpeaking basal insulin, insulin glargine. Table 50-3 presents types of insulin along with their pharmacologic properties. Starting an insulin regimen in an elderly patient should be done in conjunction with the primary care physician and an endocrinologist. Effective regimens may include premeal injections with short-acting lispro or aspart to supplement sulfonylureas, evening injections of intermediate-acting insulin such as NPH, and bedtime injections of insulin glargine. There are few problems with hypoglycemia due to insulin glargine because it has virtually no peak of action and delivers a steady basal insulin activity.

Hypertension therapy in diabetes should include angiotensin-converting enzyme inhibitors because they have renal protective effects and also have been shown to reduce cardiovascular mortality independent of blood pressure, an effect that was most pronounced in the elderly subgroup.[15] Thiazide diuretics should be avoided because they can elevate blood glucose and lipid levels. Beta-blocking agents should be considered only if their

Table 50-2. Oral Antidiabetic Agents

Class	Typical Agent(s)	Mechanism	Side Effects/Cautions
Sulfonylureas	Glyburide, glipizide	Increase insulin secretion by beta cells	Hypoglycemia, use with caution with hepatic/renal disease, weight gain
Thiazolidinediones	Rosiglitazone, pioglitazone	Increase glucose uptake by skeletal muscle, decrease insulin resistance	Hypoglycemia in combination with insulin, rare liver injury
Biguanides	Metformin	Reduces hepatic glucose production in presence of insulin	Lactic acidosis, weight loss, caution with serum creatinine >1.4 mg/dL
Alpha glucosidase inhibitors	Acarbose, miglitol	Inhibit carbohydrate absorption in small intestine	Bloating, flatulence, diarrhea, seldom lowers A1C enough to use as monotherapy
Nonsulfonylurea secretatgogues	Repaglinide, nateglinide	Increase insulin secretion by beta cells	Hypoglycemia, use with caution with hepatic/renal disease, weight gain

benefits, as in congestive heart failure and ischemic heart disease, outweigh the risks of orthostasis and diminished perception of the autonomic symptoms of hypoglycemia.

Therapy for hyperlipidemia generally should include a drug from the statin class of cholesterol-lowering agents. In older patients with a history of myocardial infarction (MI), aggressive therapy with statins to lower even modestly high cholesterol levels (to 200 mg/dL or less of low-density lipoprotein cholesterol) significantly reduced the risk of recurrent MI and stroke over a 5-year follow-up period.[16]

Antiplatelet therapy, aspirin or clopidogrel, has been shown to be effective both as primary and secondary preventive agents in reducing risk for a first or recurrent MI or stroke and, in the absence of contraindications, is indicated for all diabetes patients who have other risk factors for cardiovascular disease.[17]

Immunizations for influenza (annually) and pneumococcal pneumonia (one-time administration) should be considered for all elderly diabetic patients. There is substantial evidence that patients with diabetes, particularly those with complications of cardiac and renal disease, are at substantially increased risk for death from these illnesses. Revaccination with polyvalent pneumococcal vaccine is indicated in elderly patients 64 years of age or older if the initial immunization was more than 5 years ago.[18]

Smoking should be discouraged in all diabetic patients because it has been shown to accelerate progression of both the macro- and microvascular complications of diabetes. Patients should be informed of the increased health risks and provided with information on smoking cessation.

Table 50-3. Commonly Used Insulin Preparations

Preparation	Onset of Action	Peak	Duration
Lispro/aspart	5–15 min	1–2 h	4–6 h
Regular human	30–60 min	2–4 h	6–10 h
NPH/lente	1–2 h	4–8 h	10–20 h
Ultralente	2–4 h	Variable	16–20 h
Glargine	1–2 h	No peak/flat	Approx. 24 h

DISPOSITION

Complications of diabetes, which are numerous and especially important to recognize in older patients, often warrant a hospital admission. Indications for hospital admission[19] include

- DKA or HHNS
- Sulfonylurea-related hypoglycemia
- Hypoglycemia that does not respond rapidly with prompt recovery of sensorium
- Persistent or recurrent hypoglycemia with neuroglycopenia, insulin- or oral agent–related, despite intervention
- Hypoglycemic episode resulting in coma, seizures, paresis, dysphasia, loss of motor coordination, or ataxia
- Lack of a responsible adult to be with a successfully treated patient with hypoglycemia for the next 12 hours
- Hyperglycemia associated with severe extracellular volume depletion
- When diabetes is a complicating factor in the treatment of other medical conditions and rigorous control of hyperglycemia can improve outcome, e.g., infections, or if treatment of the concurrent illness can adversely impact diabetes control, e.g., large doses of corticosteroids for asthma/chronic obstructive pulmonary disease exacerbations
- Acute onset or worsening of macrovascular (heart disease, peripheral vascular disease, cerebrovascular disease) or microvascular (renal, opthalmologic, neurologic) complications of diabetes

ADDITIONAL ASPECTS

Complications of diabetes can be especially devastating to the elderly patient. Because of the insidious presentation of diabetes in the elderly patient, complications may already be present and even advanced in stage at the time diabetes is recognized.

The macrovascular complications of diabetes—ischemic heart disease, peripheral vascular disease, and cerebrovascular disease—frequently can shorten and devastate the quality of life of any diabetes patient. This is especially true for the older patient whose physiologic reserves may already be depleted by the aging process. Patients with advanced macrovascular disease often have difficulty complying with an exercise regimen, a key component in controlling type 2 diabetes. Patients also may find it logistically and financially difficult to comply with a multidrug regimen designed to treat hyperglycemia, hypertension, and hyperlipidemia and reduce the risk of progression of macrovascular complications or further coronary or cerebrovascular events.

The microvascular complications of diabetes—proliferative retinopathy, nephropathy, and autonomic and peripheral neuropathy—each present unique challenges in the elderly patient both diagnostically and therapeutically. Retinopathy may be masked by cataracts and the errant belief that visual acuity declines solely as a result of age. Routine urine dipstick analysis may not detect microalbuminuria associated with early nephropathy. Poor eating and early satiety associated with the autonomic neuropathy presentation of gastroparesis may be attributed to age-related decline in appetite. Gait disturbances and falls associated with diminished proprioception as a consequence of peripheral neuropathy may be attributed to age-related sensory decline or arthritis.

Whenever an elderly patient is discharged from the ED after being evaluated and treated for a diabetes-related problem, consider the following issues:

- Is adequate follow-up care available from a primary physician or endocrinologist?
- Does the patient have transportation/mobility to get to a follow-up appointment?
- Does the patient have the cognitive ability to comply with an outpatient treatment regimen?
- Can the patient afford the medications/treatments prescribed?
- If changes are made in the antidiabetic regimen, can the patient adequately monitor his or her blood glucose?
- Does the patient have a friend or relative living with him or her or nearby who can check on him or her frequently in the hours/days following treatment?

REFERENCES

1. Harris MI, Flegal KM, Cowie CC, et al: Prevalence of diabetes, impaired fasting glucose, and impaired glucose tolerance in U.S. adults. *Diabetes Care* 21:518, 1998.
2. National Diabetes Statistics: *General Information and National Statistics on Diabetes in the United States, 2000.* NIH Publication No. 02-3892, March 2002; accessed online 4/03/02 at *http://www.niddk.nih.gov/health/diabetes/pubs/dmstats/htm.*

3. Mokdad AH, Serdua MK, Dietz WH, et al: The spread of the obesity epidemic in the United States, 1991–1998. *JAMA* 282:1519, 1999.

4. Go K, Cowie CC, Harris MI: Mortality in adults with and without diabetes in a national cohort of the U.S. population, 1971–1993. *Diabetes Care* 21:1138, 1998.

5. Meneilly GS, Elliott T: Metabolic alterations in middle-aged and elderly obese patients with type 2 diabetes. *Diabetes Care* 22:112, 1999.

6. European Diabetes Epidemiology Group: Glucose tolerance and mortality: Comparison of WHO and American Diabetes Association diagnostic criteria. The DECODE study. *Lancet* 354:282, 1999.

7. Expert Committee on the Diagnosis and Classification of Diabetes Mellitus: Report of the Expert Committee on the Diagnosis and Classification of Diabetes Mellitus. *Diabetes Care* 25(suppl 1):S5, 2002.

8. Okuda Y, Androgue HJ, Field JB, et al: Counterproductive effects of sodium bicarbonate in diabetic ketoacidosis. *J Clin Endocrinol Metab* 81:314, 1996.

9. Fisher JN, Kitabchi AE: A randomized study of phosphate therapy in the treatment of diabetic ketoacidosis. *J Clin Endocrinol Metab* 57:177, 1983.

10. American Diabetes Association: Hyperglycemic crises in patients with diabetes mellitus (position statement). *Diabetes Care* 25(suppl 1):S100, 2002.

11. UK Prospective Diabetes Study Group: Intensive blood-glucose control with sulphonylureas or insulin compared with conventional treatment and risk of complications in patients with type 2 diabetes. *Lancet* 352:837, 1998.

12. Diabetes Control and Complications Trial (DCCT) Research Group: The effect of intensive treatment of diabetes on the development and progression of long-term complications in insulin-dependent diabetes mellitus. *New Engl J Med* 329:977, 1993.

13. The CDC Diabetes Cost Effectiveness Group: Cost effectiveness of intensive glycemic control, intensified hypertension control, and serum cholesterol level reduction for type 2 diabetes *JAMA* 287:2542, 2002.

14. Meneilly GS, Cheung E, Tuokko H: Altered responses to hypoglycemia of healthy elderly people. *J Clin Endocrinol Metab* 78:1341, 1994.

15. Heart Outcomes Prevention Evaluation Study Investigators: Effects of an angiotensin-converting-enzyme inhibitor, ramipril, on cardiovascular events in high-risk patients. *New Engl J Med* 342:145, 2000.

16. Lewis SJ, Moye LA, Sacks FM, et al: Effect of pravastatin on cardiovascular events in older patients with myocardial infarction and cholesterol levels in the average range: Results of the Cholesterol and Recurrent Events (CARE) trial. *Ann Intern Med* 129:681, 1998

17. CAPRIE Steering Committee: A randomized, blinded trial of clopidogrel vs aspirini in patients at risk of ischaemic events (CAPRIE). *Lancet* 348:1329, 1996.

18. American Diabetes Association: Position statement: Immunization and the prevention of influenza and pneumococcal disease in people with diabetes. *Diabetes Care* 25(suppl 1):S117, 2002.

19. American Diabetes Association: Hospital admission guidelines for diabetes mellitus (position statement). *Diabetes Care* 25(suppl 1):S109, 2002.

51

Thyroid Emergencies

Jonathan Glauser

HIGH-YIELD FACTS

- Thyroid disease may have protean manifestations and in the elderly typically presents with less specific findings.

- Although thyroid disease is quite common, thyroid-related emergencies are rare and require a high index of suspicion in order to address their high mortality rate.

- In general, serum thyroid-stimulating hormone (TSH) and free thyroxine (FT_4) determinations will suffice in the emergency department (ED) to make the diagnosis of thyroid emergencies.

- In hypothyroid patients, a precipitating illness, altered mental status, and hypothermia are characteristic of myxedema coma.

- Suppressed TSH levels and increased FT_4 occur in 95 percent of patients with clinically evident thyrotoxicosis.

HYPOTHYROIDISM

Despite the relative high prevalence of hypothyroidism, true emergencies, including myxedema coma, are rare. There is little objective evidence on which to base diagnosis and triage disposition of thyroid emergencies because no comparative studies have been done. Suggested therapies are based on the practice guidelines and recommendations of experts. Until 1996, only approximately 200 cases of myxedema coma were reported in the literature.[1]

Hypothyroidism mimics a great number of other disease entities in medicine, presenting in many possible ways, including fatigue, anemia, cold intolerance, change in mental status, and a variety of other symptoms. With rapid thyroid hormone assays now available, the diagnosis of hypothyroidism can be made promptly. True emergencies, however, continue to be evident clinically and require laboratory tests mainly to confirm the diagnosis. Hypothyroid coma, or myxedema coma, requires prompt recognition and treatment because it carries a mortality rate approaching 60 percent. Cases of hypothyroidism that require laboratory testing to make the diagnosis generally will not be emergencies and as a rule can be referred for initiation of treatment.

Epidemiology

The annual incidence for hypothyroidism is 0.08 to 0.2 percent, with higher incidence cited in the elderly female population. Subclinical hypothyroidism as defined by elevated thyroid-stimulating hormone (TSH) exists in 6 to 8 percent of adult women and 3 percent of adult men, with a slightly greater prevalence in whites (versus blacks), in women, and in subjects over 75 years of age.[2,3] In one report, the prevalence of hypothyroidism was 10.3 percent in the elderly.[4] In another, hypothyroidism was found to affect approximately 8 percent of women and 2 percent of men over the age of 50 years.[5] The elderly may be prone to thyroid dysfunction for several reasons. The incidences of autoimmune thyroiditis and nodular goiter rise with age. These predispose to hypothyroidism and hyperthyroidism, respectively.

Pathophysiology

Thyroid hormones are secreted in response to stimulation from TSH, which is secreted from the anterior pituitary gland. TSH release is promoted by thyroid-releasing hormone (TRH) from the hypothalamus. Sensitive biologic feedback mechanisms generally control excretion of these neuroendocrine hormones.

The actions of thyroid hormone are mediated by nuclear receptors. A major effect is to stimulate the sodium pump via the cell membrane enzyme Na^+, K^+-ATPase. Mitochondrial metabolism is also influenced by thyroid hormone, which is therefore involved intimately in calorigenesis. Many of the symptoms of the hypothyroid state stem from this hormonal action.[6]

Free thyroxine is actually a prohormone, converted by deiodination in peripheral tissues, largely liver and kidney, to T_3, the more active form. The thyroid gland is the sole source of T_4, normally the predominant circulating hormone. FT_4 measures the non-protein-bound circulating T_4.

Patients with previous thyroid ablation or a history of elevated thyroid autoantibodies have been shown to progress to overt clinical hypothyroidism. A history of prior thyroid surgery, autoimmune thyroiditis, or use of medications containing lithium or iodine is suggestive. The most common cause of hypothyroidism is autoimmune or Hashimoto's thyroiditis.

Clinical Features

The hypothyroid state may present in myriad ways, many of which are nonspecific (Table 51-1). The patient may be less active than usual, with loss of interest in things previously enjoyed. Lethargy may be a prominent complaint, as is decreased mobility and misdiagnosis as depression is common. Fatigue and dry skin may be prominent complaints. Caregivers may report that the patient has been acting confused, with memory problems. The usual clinical findings in the elderly population are apathy and psychomotor retardation, which may develop over a long period of time. Patients also may present with weakness, arthralgias, and myalgias. Coarsening of the voice may have been noted. Lethargy, dry skin, constipation, edema, and weight gain may be elicited in the history. A history of cold intolerance is typical.

There is a diminished ventilatory drive, possibly leading to alveolar hypoventilation, carbon dioxide (CO_2) retention, and coma in a hypothyroid patient. An impaired ventilatory drive leads to increased sensitivity to sedative

Table 51-1. Sign and Symptoms of Hypothyroidism

Paresthesias	Tiredness	Deafness (in elderly)
Loss of energy	Weakness	Macroglossia
Cold intolerance	Constipation	Intestinal ileus
Pseudomyotonic reflexes	Joint pains	Gastric atony
Hypothermia	Muscle pains	Nonpitting edema of the hands, feet
Dry, coarse, scaly skin	Depression	Cognitive impairment
Puffy eyelids	Weight gain	Delayed deep tendon reflexes
Hoarse voice	Ataxia	Psychosis
Carotenemic pallor	Hair loss	Bradycardia
		Diastolic hypertension

drugs. Obesity and sleep apnea may contribute to respiratory alterations.

Vital signs suggestive of the hypothyroid state include hypotension or diastolic hypertension. Body temperature is below normal in 80 percent,[7] and bradycardia may be present.[8] Classically, patients who are hypothyroid have facial features that are puffy and coarse. The skin may be dry and cold. An orange or yellow tint without scleral icterus indicates carotenemia. Most patients have varying degrees of brittle nails and hair. The skin may exhibit pallor, induration, and thickening. Periorbital edema and macroglossia may be present. Myxedema is a peculiar nonpitting edema of the skin, classically of the lower extremities. Neurologic findings may include mental status changes. Delayed relaxation time of deep tendon reflexes is variably present. Physical evidence of effusions into the pleural, peritoneal, or pericardial cavities may be detectable. Delirium and psychosis may be present, characteristic of "myxedema madness."

Inotropic and chronotropic alterations of hypothyroidism may be manifested by decreased stroke volume, bradycardia, and decreased cardiac output. Peripheral vasoconstriction shunts blood away from the skin and muscle to maintain core body temperature. Diminished beta-receptor responsiveness leads to unopposed alpha activity and contributes to the diastolic hypertension seen in hypothyroidism.[6]

The electrocardiogram (ECG) may show a variety of abnormalities. Sinus bradycardia and prolonged PR and QT intervals may be present. Low voltage as evidence of a pericardial effusion may be present. Heart block and T-wave flattening or inversion may be present, but ST-segment abnormalities are nonspecific. Torsades de pointes with marked QT prolongation[8] and sudden death[9] have been reported in association with the hypothyroid state.

Echocardiography may be useful to show regional wall-motion abnormalities and to verify infiltrative cardiomyopathy. It also will diagnose a pericardial effusion, which may occur in 30 to 80 percent of severely hypothyroid patients.[10] Pericardial tamponade is rare, so a pulsus paradoxus and distended neck veins are not common findings.

Diagnosis

TSH and FT_4 levels are needed to confirm the diagnosis of hypothyroidism. The normal range for TSH is 0.4 to 5.5 IU/L, and levels are invariably high. TSH generally will be elevated in the great majority of cases but rarely may be decreased if there is a central (hypothalamic or pituitary) cause. In unselected populations, TSH has a sensitivity of 89 to 95 percent and a specificity of 90 to 96 percent for overt thyroid dysfunction.[11] Subtle abnormalities in these tests can be found but do not warrant further workup in the emergency department (ED) because these can be referred. The normal range for FT_4 is 0.7 to 1.8 ng/dL and will be decreased in hypothyroidism.

A macrocytic anemia due to vitamin B_{12} deficiency may be present. Erythropoietin levels are also low, leading to a fall in hematocrit, typically to approximately 30 percent. Hyponatremia with low serum osmolality is characteristic of hypothyroidism and should respond to thyroid hormone replacement. Hyponatremia may be due to reduced free water clearance, reduced renal blood flow and glomerular filtration, and elevated plasma vasopressin levels. Hypoglycemia occurs because of increased insulin sensitivity, along with decreased gluconeogenesis and glycogenolysis.[6,12]

Cardiac enzymes such as aspartate aminotransferase (AST/SGOT) or creatine kinase (CK) may be elevated as a result of increased muscle membrane permeability and reduced metabolic clearance.[13] However, in severe hypothyroidism without acute myocardial infarction, the troponin I level remains normal.[14]

Adrenal hypofunction is important to consider following a diagnosis of severe hypothyroidism. Central hypothyroidism may be associated with adrenocorticotropic hormone deficiency, and primary hypothyroidism may be associated with primary adrenal insufficiency (Schmidt syndrome). Serum prolactin levels, growth hormone levels, and luteinizing hormone (LH) and follicle-stimulating hormone (FSH) levels may help delineate this but are of little value in the emergency setting.[12]

MYXEDEMA COMA

The hypothyroid crisis of myxedema coma is a life-threatening manifestation of the hypothyroid state. *Myxedema* coma can be defined as severe thyroid hormone deficiency contributing to a decreased level of consciousness.[15] In severe decompensated hypothyroidism, respiratory depression is characteristic as a result of respiratory muscle weakness and upper airway obstruction due to an enlarged tongue and myxedematous infiltration of the upper airway. Defective thermoregulation is characteristic of myxedema coma. It is encountered most frequently in patients with a known history of hypothyroidism in the winter months, often after cold exposure. Thyroid hormone exerts its action by stimulating calorigenesis via Na^+, K^+-ATPase, and most of the clinical fea-

Table 51-2. Common Precipitating Events for Hypothyroid Crisis

Infection
Trauma
Burns
Surgery
Stroke
Hypoglycemia
Hyponatremia
Hypercapnea
Acidosis
Hypothermia/cold exposure
Drug overdose
Diuretic therapy
Rifampin, diphenylhydantoin therapy

tures of myxedema coma are related to failure of this action. The diagnosis of myxedema coma is largely a clinical one. Abnormal TSH and FT_4 values in the presence of nonpitting edema, hypothermia, hypoventilation, and stupor confirm the diagnosis.[13] Hyponatremia, hypoglycemia, and associated infection are confirmatory.

The typical presentation is that of elderly women in the winter. Approximately 80 percent of myxedema coma cases occur in females.[16] There is usually a history of hypothyroidism, hypopituitarism, or use of antithyroid medications.[6] True myxedema coma is rare and to a certain extent depends on one's definition. One report covering a 2-year period noted only 24 cases in all of Germany, of which 12 were reclassified by the authors as severe hypothyroidism without coma.[17]

Potential precipitating events for myxedema coma are numerous and include surgery, severe infection, and trauma. Some medications, including sedatives, narcotics, and tranquilizers, as well as missed doses of thyroxine, may be implicated. (Table 51-2)

Clinical Features

Myxedema coma may present with many features of the hypothyroid state. (Table 51-3). Recognition may be hampered by its insidious onset and rarity. The characteristic four features facilitating the diagnosis include alteration in mental status, presence of a precipitating factor, hypothermia, and increased serum creatine phosphokinase levels.[18]

The patient typically appears pale and edematous. Periorbital edema is common. The lateral eyebrows may be

Table 51-3. Major Clinical Features of Myxedema Coma

Decreased mental status	Paralytic ileus
Hypoventilation	Macroglossia
Hypothermia	Facial or periorbital edema
Bradycardia	Pallor
Hyponatremia	Sparse body hair, alopecia
Hypoglycemia	Thyroidectomy scar
Associated infection (pneumonia, UTI)	Nonpitting edema of the extremities
Toxic drug levels secondary to decreased drug clearance	Bladder dystonia and distension
Delayed reflex relaxation	Dry, cool, doughy skin

missing. A neck scar may be a clue to a previous thyroidectomy.

Respiratory symptoms may be related to stupor, obesity, and to the large myxedematous tongue, which, along with aspiration, may cause obstruction of the upper airway. Myxedematous patients exhibit decreased respiratory drive in response to carbon dioxide. Ascites, pericardial effusions, and pleural effusions related to the hypothyroid state may impede effective ventilation. Defective cough reflex, inability to clear secretions, and sleep apnea all may contribute to respiratory acidosis. Cardiac sounds may be distant. Usually bradycardia is present along with low voltage on the ECG. With long-standing hypothyroidism, patients may develop various cardiac manifestations. Dyspnea on exertion, fatigue, and edema may be a result of pericardial effusion or congestive heart failure. Patients have an increased incidence of hypercholesterolemia and hypertriglyceridemia. The decreased metabolic demands on the heart may be protective from myocardial infarction and angina.

Gastrointestinal findings include signs of decreased motility. The abdomen is distended, and paralytic ileus and fecal impaction may be present. Myxedema megacolon is an unusual and late finding appearing as pseudomembranous colitis and intestinal ischemia.

All patients with myxedema coma display deterioration of their mental status. Central nervous system (CNS) findings may include disturbances in consciousness ranging from delirium to stupor and coma. Some of the depressed levels of consciousness as well as seizures have been attributed to hyponatremia. Hallucinations ("myxedema madness"), cerebellar signs, or somnolence

may be present. Muscle relaxation times of the deep tendon reflexes are markedly delayed.

Diagnosis

Three findings are required to make the diagnosis of myxedema coma:

1. A precipitating illness or event
2. Defective thermoregulation (hypothermia)
3. Altered mental status

Confirmatory TSH and FT_4 levels should be obtained. Since treatment includes corticosteroid replacement, the serum cortisol level should be determined in a patient suspected of having myxedema coma. Chest films, urinalysis, and blood cultures should be obtained to look for evidence of infection, which may be masked by the hypothermic state. Creatine kinase (CK-MM fraction) and serum glutamic oxaloacetic transaminase (SGOT/AST) elevations may demonstrate enzyme leakage or evidence of rhabdomyolysis. Arterial blood gas determinations may need to be repeated at intervals due to insensitivity of the respiratory centers in the brain stem to hypoxia and hypercapnea and to weakness of the intercostal and diaphragmatic muscles. Serum electrolytes, creatinine, blood urea nitrogen (BUN), and glucose should be monitored. Hyponatremia occurs in approximately 50 percent of severely hypothyroid patients,[7] possibly related to decreased delivery of sodium and volume to the distal renal tubules as a result of decreased renal blood flow.[15] Serum concentrations of atrial natriuretic peptide have been noted to be low and may contribute to the hyponatremia.[19]

Emergency Department Care and Disposition

Thyroid hormone replacement is the definitive treatment for myxedema coma. Because this condition is rare and prospective, randomized, controlled clinical trials are lacking, and there is not uniform agreement as to the optimal dosage or form of replacement of thyroid hormone that is most effective. Since hypotension and intestinal ileus are common, intravenous therapy is preferred. Levothyroxine has been given via nasogastric tube, but its bioavailability (50–80 percent) is unpredictable.[13] Initiation of ED treatment for myxedema coma is shown in Table 51-4.

Liothyronine (T_3) is the biologically active form, and levothyroxine (T_4) is converted to T_3 in vivo. Liothyronine is ideal for immediate thyroid hormone action be-

Table 51-4. Initiation of Treatment in ED for Myxedema Coma

1. 200–300 μg (4 μg/kg) IV bolus thyroxine, followed by 50–100 μg/day
2. T_3 20 μg IV bolus (loading dose 10–25 μg), then 10 μg every 8–12 hours for 24–48 hours until the patient is conscious and taking maintenance T_4
3. Hydrocortisone 100 mg every 8 hours
4. Broad-spectrum antibiotics pending culture results recommended if there is evidence of infection
5. Supportive care for underlying illness
6. Consider elective intubation for myxedema coma
7. Consider hypertonic saline for severe hyponatremia
8. Consider appropriate rewarming techniques

cause it binds serum proteins to a lesser extent than levothyroxine, has a larger volume of distribution, and has a shorter half-life. Both levothyroxine and liothyronine can be given alone or in combination,[18] but levothyroxine alone is often recommended.[6,13,15] Intravenous liothyronine, marketed for parenteral administration as Triostat, is expensive and may be associated with increased mortality.[20] Oral T_3 is well absorbed even in a severely hypothyroid state.[6] Thyroxine-binding proteins have a large binding capacity, and it is necessary to saturate these proteins to provide an effective circulating level of T_4. Conversely, rapid thyroid replacement runs a risk of inducing cardiac dysrhythmias, ischemia, and death. As discussed earlier, due to the adrenal hypofunction that accompanies severe hypothyroidism, it is important to give steroids when starting thyroid replacement therapy to avoid precipitating adrenal crisis.

Treatment guidelines are summarized in Table 51-4. There is evidence that high-dose thyroid replacement of more than 500 μg/day of levothyroxine or more than 75 μg/day of T_3 may be associated with a high incidence of fatal outcome.[21] Treatment adjuncts include passive rewarming for hypothermia and maintenance of appropriate hydration status to address hyponatremia. Transfusion with packed cells is appropriate if the hematocrit is below 20 percent. The pathogenesis of hypotension may be multifactorial. Possible adrenal insufficiency should be addressed. Infectious sources should be sought and treated. Echocardiography should be performed to evaluate for evidence of pericardial effusion and global versus regional hypokinesis.

If sodium values are below 120 meq/L and there are significant mental status changes, isotonic or even hypertonic saline may be needed to raise levels to above 120

meq/L. Asymptomatic hyponatremia can be monitored and usually resolves with L-thyroxine therapy. After establishment of adequate respiratory ventilation, thyroid hormone replacement, and care for the precipitating illness, patients should begin to show clinical improvement within the following 24 to 48 hours. Animal studies indicate that the earliest metabolic effects of T_3 can be seen after 12 to 24 hours.[18]

General Treatment Recommendations in Myxedema Coma

1. Confirm diagnosis of hypothyroidism in the ED with highly sensitive TSH and FT_4 tests if rapidly available.

2. Consider endocrinology consult prior to initiation of therapy in the elderly hypothyroid patient or those with medical complexity. Full thyroid replacement can precipitate a myocardial infarction.[13]

3. Initiate treatment promptly if there is clinical evidence of myxedema coma; treatment should not await laboratory confirmation unless results are available rapidly. Aggressively address ventilatory, chemical, and vital-sign abnormalities. Treatment of myxedema coma takes precedence over possible cardiac complications of therapy.

4. Hypotension should prompt a search for associated illness, including myocardial infarction or sepsis. Prophylactic antibiotics generally are not recommended. Cautious volume expansion should be tried initially. Dopamine may be preferable to other pressors because it better maintains coronary perfusion.[6] Amrinone, an inovasodilator, may improve myocardial contractility because its mechanism of action does not depend on beta receptors.[26]

5. Starting thyroid hormone replacement without also giving steroids (hydrocortisone) may precipitate adrenal crisis. Appropriate use of steroids is also important because thyroxine increases cortisol clearance.

Factors associated with poor outcome include advanced age, body temperature less than 93°F, hypothermia persisting over 3 days, bradycardia of less than 44 beats/min, hypotension, myocardial infarction, and sepsis[6,22]

Clinical diagnosis of myxedema coma warrants intensive care unit (ICU) admission. Initiate treatment in the ED. Body temperature of less than 93°F or bradycardia of less than 44 beats per minute warrants ICU admission. Admissions decisions for other presentations of hypothyroidism should consider comorbidities such as congestive heart failure (CHF), cachexia, COPD, pneumonia, or other pulmonary problem. Underlying disorders that would warrant admission include aspiration pneumonia, urosepsis, myocardial infarction, and evidence of CNS dysfunction (including seizures, ataxia, somnolence, lethargy, confusion, coma; or behavioral disorders) such as disorientation, paranoia, hallucination ("myxedema madness"). Other considerations include hypoglycemia suggesting hypopituitarism or adrenal insufficiency, hyponatremia of less than 128 meq/dL, and social factors that jeopardize patient outcomes.

HYPERTHYROIDISM

In older patients, the clinical expression of the hyperthyroid hypermetabolic state becomes blunted. Some have proposed routine screening for thyroid disease in the elderly because the medical history and findings on physical examination become less sensitive and less specific for thyrotoxicosis. In addition, treatment with medications such as beta-adrenergic blocking drugs and antianxiety medications also may blunt symptoms and signs of the hypermetabolic state. Many of the signs and symptoms of thyroid hormone excess described may have different manifestations in patients older than age 60.[23] Symptoms can be masked in apathetic hyperthyroidism.

Similarly to hypothyroidism, given the paucity of true hyperthyroid emergencies in the literature and in clinical practice, no objective studies are in existence as to admission criteria or as to what constitutes thyroid storm. Recommendations are based on literature review and expert opinion.

Epidemiology

The incidence of clinical and subclinical hyperthyroidism has been estimated to be 0.05 to 0.1 percent. Subclinical hyperthyroidism, as recognized by a subnormal TSH level, is seen in 0.2 to 5 percent of the elderly population, with less than 1 percent progression per year to overt disease.[24,25]

Historically, thyroid storm was associated with surgery. Now, with pretreatment of hyperthyroidism prior to surgery, surgically related storm is rare; the majority of episodes are triggered by the stresses of medical illnesses. Graves' disease accounts for the great majority of hyperthyroidism currently, followed by functionally au-

tonomous (TSH-independent) multiple or solitary nodules.[26] The exacerbation can be secondary to a known hyperthyroid state that is being treated or an exacerbation of unknown, or apathetic, hyperthyroidism.

Pathophysiology

Hyperthyroidism is an illness that can present a diagnostic challenge. For all practical purposes, the disease can be broken down into three categories: (1) subclinical, (2) clinical hyperthyroid state, and (3) storm. Subclinical hyperthyroidism represents a pathologic state not yet clinically evident with corresponding abnormal thyroid function. Clinical hyperthyroidism and thyroid storm, however, have signs and symptoms that may make the diagnosis evident clinically and which can then be confirmed with laboratory tests. Now that high-sensitivity TSH assays are commonly available to emergency physicians, it is possible to make or confirm the diagnosis of hyperthyroidism in less obvious cases. In individuals without signs or symptoms, emergency treatment or admission generally is not required. The diagnosis of storm or hyperthyroid crisis, however, is critical because these patients invariably die without treatment.

Clinical Features

Thyrotoxicosis is a hypermetabolic state, and one of the common findings is excessive weight loss despite an unchanged or even increased caloric intake. It is notable that hyperthyroidism may present with a paucity of symptoms in the elderly, especially those past age 75. In older patients, weight loss may be the most common presenting complaint, along with palpitations, weakness, dizziness, and syncope.[27] Alteration in mental status may be a presenting sign in the elderly. The American College of Emergency Physicians lists thyroid screening tests in its guidelines for the workup of the elderly patient with lethargy, agitation, or any alteration in level of consciousness.[28] Weight loss results in depletion of fat stores and a decrease in muscle mass. Patients may complain of heat intolerance, with hyperhidrosis and flushing. They may have nonspecific symptoms of generalized weakness and a sense of fatigue resulting from changes both in their cardiorespiratory and neuromuscular systems. They may report nervousness or restlessness.

Weakness in respiratory and skeletal muscles may be factors in decreased exercise tolerance and dyspnea. Tracheal compression from an enlarged thyroid gland may cause shortness of breath, hoarseness, wheezing, and stridor. Pemberton's sign is defined as inducing these dyspneic symptoms when patients are asked to raise their arms above their heads. Thyromegaly may cause wheezing, hoarseness, stridor, or dysphagia.

Vital signs classically include fever with tachycardia out of proportion to the fever. However, these findings may be muted in the elderly, especially in patients on beta blockers.

Gastrointestinal symptoms may be prominent. Dysphagia may be related to an enlarged thyroid gland that compresses the esophagus. Rapid intestinal transit time may cause increased bowel movement frequency. Nausea and vomiting occur frequently. Jaundice may be present but is unusual.

Most patients with thyrotoxicosis have myopathy that affects the proximal muscle groups of the shoulder and pelvic girdles more than distal muscles. Patients most often complain of difficulty standing up from a squatting position or difficulty in climbing stairs.[29] Muscle weakness resolves with therapy.

Many thyrotoxic patients complain of memory loss, confusional states, and short attention span. Unusual CNS presentations include chorea, delirium, convulsions, stroke, coma, and cerebral venous thrombosis.[30–32] Some psychiatric conditions may be mistaken for thyrotoxicosis. Patients may exhibit anxiety and restlessness. They may be emotionally labile or irritable. Speech and thought processing may be rapid. Dysphoric moods may be manifested by insomnia, phobias, delusions, vivid dreams, psychosis, or nightmares.

Thyrotoxic patients typically have a warm, smooth, velvety skin texture. The skin may be flushed, with hyperhidrosis of the palms and soles. Fever and tachycardia may be prominent. Hair may be fine and brittle; alopecia is common, and vitiligo may be present.

The orbitopathy of thyrotoxicosis is the result of contraction of the levator palpebrae superioris because of sympathetic hyperactivity. Measurable proptosis in Graves' disease is caused by enlargement of the extraocular muscles. There may be lid lag, chemosis, exophthalmos, and vasodilatation of the conjunctiva with edema of the lids. Visual acuity may be compromised by compressive optic neuropathy.

Myxedema of the pretibial areas, feet, and toes is associated with autoimmune thyroid disease and affects women more frequently than men. Raised pink or purple plaques are characteristic, with nonpitting edema.

Diffuse enlargement of the thyroid gland is characteristic of thyrotoxicosis from Graves' disease, but it is infrequently palpable in patients over 75 years of age.[27] Elderly patients frequently have shrinking of the gland with age; alternatively, the thyroid may be substernal in older persons. A bruit may be audible over the thyroid gland and is virtually diagnostic of Graves' disease.[23] One or more nodules palpable over the thyroid gland is suggestive of toxic adenoma or toxic multinodular goiter (Plummer's disease). Patients with subacute thyroiditis may have tender thyroid glands.

The resting heart rate is typically fast. There is a brisk and rapid upstroke of the carotid arteries. There may be systolic murmurs heard as the result of increased blood flow across the aortic outflow tract. Regurgitant flow across the mitral valve may be from mitral valve prolapse, left ventricular dilatation, or functional changes of the mitral valve apparatus.

Thyrotoxicosis increases the work of the heart. Thyroid hormone can increase myocardial inotropy and heart rate and dilate peripheral arteries to increase cardiac output, causing diminished systemic vascular resistance and diastolic blood pressure.[33,34] Overall, thyroid hormone increases ATP use, with more heat and less contractile energy production. This inefficiency may explain heart failure after prolonged hyperthyroidism.[35] Most thyrotoxic patients report palpitations. A sense of irregular or rapid heart beat becomes more apparent with increases in activity or exercise, eventually leading to decreased exercise tolerance. Dyspnea on exertion is common. Decreased lung compliance, an engorged pulmonary capillary bed, and high-output left ventricular failure all may be factors in producing dyspnea.

Hyperthyroidism may be associated with varying degrees of chest pain. An increased myocardial oxygen demand as a result of the increased cardiac work of thyrotoxicosis may unmask previously unsuspected coronary artery disease. Sinus tachycardia and atrial fibrillation are common. Atrial arrhythmias frequently are accompanied by high-output failure.[36] In hyperthyroid patients over age of 75, atrial fibrillation has been reported in 32 to 39 percent of cases.[27,37] Anginal pain in the absence of coronary atherosclerosis may occur secondary to coronary artery spasm.[38]

ECG changes generally are nonspecific and may include shortening of the PR interval or ST-segment changes suggestive of myocardial ischemia or coronary spasm. Atrial fibrillation may be present.

Apathetic thyrotoxicosis in the elderly is characterized by extreme fatigue, weakness, decreased activity, and emotional apathy.[39] Tachycardia and thyromegaly may be absent. The patient is mentally slow and withdrawn. The skin is dry, coarse, cool, and wrinkled. There may be muscle wasting and proximal myopathy. Apathetic hyperthyroidism occurs frequently in advanced age, making the clinical diagnosis of hyperthyroidism in the elderly difficult. Symptoms such as tachycardia, weight loss, weakness, nervousness, palpitations, and heat intolerance, which make the diagnosis easier in younger patients, may be present in a minority of older individuals.[27] The diagnosis of apathetic hyperthyroidism frequently is made only during the workup for atrial fibrillation, unexplained weight loss, or worsening cardiovascular disease in the elderly. Dementia and severe psychomotor retardation may be the most prominent findings.[40]

Diagnosis

The diagnosis of hyperthyroidism generally requires testing for T_4 and TSH. However, other tests may be applicable in the workup of thyrotoxicosis and are worthy of mention.

Free thyroid hormone determinations are recommended for the assessment of thyroidal state. Since the FT_4 level correlates best with the thyroidal state, it is most significant clinically. It is notable that FT_4 may be elevated with a normal TSH in patients taking levothyroxine for primary hypothyroidism, as well as in patients taking amiodarone.

TSH is also required to diagnose hyperthyroidism. Rarely, hyperthyroidism results from a TSH-secreting pituitary tumor. Suppressed TSH levels ($<0.05 \mu U/mL$) and increased serum FT_4 estimates occur in approximately 95 percent of patients with clinically evident thyrotoxicosis.

While FT_4 and TSH will suffice in the diagnostic workup from the ED, a note on further testing is in order. The erythrocyte sedimentation rate (ESR) may be markedly elevated in patients with subacute (viral) thyroiditis. Since treatment of thyroid storm includes corticosteroids, a serum cortisol level prior to treatment should be obtained to document adrenal function.

THYROID STORM

Thyroid storm is a life-threatening crisis of the hyperthyroid state characterized by decompensation of one or more organ systems. Exaggerated signs and symptoms of hyperthyroidism are present, characterized by fever, altered mental status, and cardiovascular dysfunction, usually with precipitating medical or surgical illness. Estimated mortality historically has been 20 to 30 percent.[41] Historically, thyroid storm was mainly the result of thyroid surgery, although with preoperative treatment, thyrotoxic crisis has been caused more often by antecedent Graves' disease, frequently with an identifiable precipitating event. Toxic multinodular goiter or toxic adenomas are less frequent causes of the hyperthyroid state.

Precipitants include surgery, radioiodine therapy, iodinated contrast dyes, thyroid hormone ingestion, and a variety of medical emergencies, including diabetic ketoacidosis, cerebrovascular accident, pulmonary embolism, and congestive heart failure (Table 51-5). Events that decompensate the hyperthyroid patient into thyroid storm must be identified and treated. Withdrawal or discontinuation of antithyroid medications may be causative as well.

The specific mechanism by which thyroid storm occur remains uncertain, and many theories have been proposed for the development of thyroid storm. The effects of acidosis or medical illness on thyroid hormone binding to carrier proteins has been proposed. While levels of circulating thyroid hormone consistently have not been found to be significantly different from those in uncomplicated thyrotoxicosis, some authors have found higher levels of free hormone, possibly due to an acute decrease in thyroxine-binding globulin.[18] This theory has credence because a variety of systemic illnesses may cause alteration of binding proteins, causing a sudden change in functioning hormone levels.

Another theory proposes a role for enhanced adrenergic activity. There appears to be an exaggerated response to adrenergic stimuli, although levels of catecholamines do not seem to be higher in hospitalized patients with thyroid storm compared with other medically ill patients. While plasma levels of norepinephrine and epinephrine

Table 51-5. Precipitants of Thyroid Storm

Infection
Surgery (thyroid and nonthyroid)
Trauma
Hypoglycemia
Vigorous palpation of the thyroid
Withdrawal of antithyroid drug therapy
Diabetic ketoacidosis
Pulmonary thromboembolism
Cerebrovascular accident
Congestive heart failure
Lithium treatment
Amiodarone treatment
Thyroid hormone ingestion
Iodine, iodinated contrast dyes, or ingestion of other iodides (expectorants, kelp)
Phenylephrine
Severe emotional stress
Bowel infarction

have not been shown to be elevated in thyroid storm, thyroid hormone has been shown to increase the density of beta-adrenergic receptors and appears to alter responsiveness to catecholamines at a postreceptor level.[41]

Diagnosis

Thyroid storm is largely a clinical diagnosis. On physical examination, many of the stigmata of the hyperthyroid state may be present, e.g., the exophthalmos, goiter, and widened pulse pressure of Graves' disease. Thyrotoxic myopathy, with weakness of the proximal muscles, may occur. Fever, tachycardia, diaphoresis, and emotional lability may be present.

Anorexia and crampy abdominal pain may be other gastrointestinal manifestations. Jaundice is a poor prognostic sign. CNS disturbances occur in 90 percent of patients and range from restlessness, agitation, emotional lability, psychosis, and manic behavior to obtundation and coma. Staus epilepticus and stroke may be presenting signs. Nausea, vomiting, and diarrhea may contribute to dehydration. Atrial arrhythmias and ventricular tachyarrhythmias may complicate high-output congestive heart failure. Thyroid storm involves multiple systems and may be associated with lactic acidosis, evidence of liver dysfunction, rhabdomyolysis, and reversible cardiomyopathy.[42]

It is critical for the emergency physician to diagnose storm or impending storm. Mortality untreated is nearly 100 percent[43] but treated has been reported to be 20 to 50 percent.[44] Recently published data listed in-hospital mortality at 1.8 percent with aggressive therapy.[45] While no uniform diagnostic criteria have been established to differentiate uncomplicated thyrotoxicosis from impending thyroid storm and established thyroid storm, Burch and Wartofsky[46] have authored diagnostic criteria to diagnose impending thyroid storm (Table 51-6). Using these criteria, a score of greater than 45 is highly suggestive of thyroid storm; 25 to 44 is suggestive of impending storm, and less than 25 is unlikely to represent thyroid storm.

Current recommendations include obtaining TSH and FT_4 levels. FT_4 is elevated in 95 percent of hyperthyroid patients.[47] FT_4 has been shown to differentiate simple thyrotoxicosis from thyroid storm.[48] TSH is highly sensitive, but its use alone is not recommended at this time. A combination of low TSH and elevated FT_4 makes the diagnosis. If TSH is lower than normal and FT_4 is normal, FT_3 testing is recommended. FT_3 will confirm the diagnosis of hyperthyroidism that results mostly from T_3 secretion as well as providing a quantitative assessment of the hyperthyroid state, since T_3 is the metabolically more active hormone.

Table 51-6. Diagnostic Criteria for Thyroid Storm

Temperature, °F	Rating	Cardiovascular Dysfunction	Rating
99–99.9	5	Tachycardia, bpm	
100–100.9	10	90–109	5
101–101.9	15	110–119	10
102–102.9	20	120–129	15
103–103.9	25	130–139	20
>104	30	>140	25

Source: Adapted from Burch and Wartofsky.[46]

Levels of circulating hormone may not be significantly different in thyroid storm from those seen in uncomplicated thyrotoxicosis. The clinical state may relate more to the rapidity with which thyroid hormone levels rise rather than absolute levels measured.

Emergency Department Care and Disposition

Treatment should address the following broad categories: supportive care, correction of the hyperthyroid state, managing the end-organ effects of the syndrome, and diagnosis and treatment of the precipitating event. Specifically, thyroid hormone formation should be inhibited, release of hormone from the thyroid gland should be accomplished, and beta-adrenergic blockade should be provided.[49] Dehydration and electrolyte imbalances should be addressed aggressively. Fever should be controlled with acetaminophen and additional cooling measures as needed. Since aspirin decreases protein binding and theoretically may increase free levels of T_3 and T_4, it should be avoided. Since thyrotoxic patients have accelerated degradation of cortisol, glucocorticoids should be administered to treat relative adrenal insufficiency.

Propylthiouracil (PTU) and methimazole (MMI) are thioamides that block synthesis of thyroid hormone. The onset of action is within 1 hour and peaks within weeks. These drugs inhibit synthesis of new thyroid hormone but do not affect the release of stored hormone. PTU has the additional benefit of inhibiting T_4 to T_3 conversion at high doses.[50] It can be administered rectally (by retention enema) when abdominal distension and hyperemesis are present.[51]

Iodide or lithium carbonate block release of preformed hormone within the gland. They should be given at least 1 hour after the loading dose of PTU or MMI. The iodinated medications used include the oral contrast agents iopanoic acid (Telepaque) and ipodate (Oragrafin), Lugol's iodine, and a saturated solution of potassium iodide (SSKI). Iopanoic acid and ipodate inhibit T_4 to T_3 conversion and have been considered the iodide preparations of choice.[18] SSKI 5 drops every 6 hours and Lugol's solution 30 drops each day in three to four divided doses are acceptable alternatives.[52] Therapy with iodides may preclude future therapy with radioiodine for several months. SSKI has been administered sublingually,[51] and potassium iodide has been administered rectally when emesis or small bowel obstruction has been present.[51] When iodide is used in conjunction with the thionamides, serum T_4 levels approach normal within 4 to 5 days.[41]

Glucocorticoids at high doses may reduce conversion of T_4 to T_3. Use of glucocorticoids in thyroid storm is associated with improved survival rates. Administration of stress doses of corticosteroids, typically 100 mg hydrocortisone every 6 to 8 hours, is now routine. There is a higher incidence of concomitant adrenal insufficiency in patients with Graves' disease.

Blockade of peripheral thyroid hormone effects with beta-adrenergic blocking agents is the mainstay of treatment for thyroid storm. Oral propranolol has onset of action within 1 hour. For patients with contraindications to beta-blocker use, such as bronchospastic disease or heart block, a short-acting beta blocker such as esmolol has been used safely.[53] If beta blockers are absolutely contraindicated, guanethidine 1 to 2 mg/kg/day in divided doses (30–40 mg orally every 6 hours) or reserpine 2.5 to 5 mg every 6 hours may be considered.[41,54]

The treatment of thyroid storm is summarized in Table 51-7. Degradation of the circulating thyroid hormones must occur for complete resolution of the illness. The average duration of thyroid storm is 3 days, although the disease may take 1 week to resolve. Improvement in clinical status occurs over several days, although it may be 7 to 8 days before full recovery occurs, and a euthyroid state may not be achieved for 6 to 8 weeks. Mental status is a good clinical marker to monitor response to therapy.

Adjunctive therapies for thyroid storm are listed in Table 51-8. Blood cultures, urinalysis, urine cultures, and chest radiography are recommended to look for infection in thyroid storm.

In thyrotoxicosis without storm, beta blockers such as propranolol are considered the drugs of choice to reverse the tachycardia, widened pulse pressure, palpitations, and increased stroke volume that are present. Beta-adrenergic blockade is accompanied by improvement in tremulousness and heat intolerance and is the treatment of choice for rate control for patients with atrial fibrillation. Cal-

Table 51-7. Treatment of Thyroid Storm

1. Block hormone synthesis with either
   a. Propylthiouracil 100–600 mg load, PO or NG 200–250 mg every 4 hours for total daily dose of 1200–1500 mg
      Also stops peripheral conversion of T_4 to T_3
      or
   b. Methimazole 20 mg PO (10–40 mg range) every 4 hours
2. Inhibit hormone release (at least 1 hour after 1):
   Iodides: Potassium iodide (SSKI) 5 drops PO every 6–8 hours *or*
      Lugol's solution 7–8 drops to 1 mL PO every 6 hours *or* ipodate (Orografin) 1–3 g daily as 1 g every 8 hours for 24 hours, then 500 mg twice daily
   If severe iodide allergy: Lithium carbonate 300 mg every 6 hours
3. Glucocorticoids:
   Hydrocortisone 300 mg IV, then 100 mg IV every 8 hours
   Dexamethasone 2 mg IV every 6 hours
4. Adrenergic blockade:
   Propranolol 0.5–3 mg IV over 15 minutes slow IV, then 60–80 mg PO every 4 hours
   Esmolol 0.25–0.5 µg/kg loading, infusion of 0.05 to 0.1 µg/kg/min
   If propanolol is contraindicated because of congestive heart failure of reactive airway disease, use reserpine 2.5 to 5 mg IM every 4 hours following a test dose of 1 mg.

cium channel blockers have been used successfully to decrease the heart rate in patients with contraindications to beta-blocker use.[55] Verapamil has been cited as the drug of choice.

The presentations of thyroid crisis and malignant hyperthermia may be similar in the setting of anesthesia induction. Dantrolene has been proposed as a safe agent to use to treat either entity when the precise etiology is unclear.[56] Central thermal regulation, especially shivering, may be controlled with chlorpromazine 25 to 50 mg intravenously every 4 to 6 hours.

Definitive ways to reduce thyroid hormone secretion include radioiodine and surgical ablation. The latter entails subtotal thyroidectomy and has fallen out of favor.[26] Radioactive iodine, when it is trapped by hyperactive thyroid tissue, causes an intense radiation thyroiditis that leads to progressive fibrosis and glandular atrophy. The resulting

Table 51-8. Therapies Addressing Systemic Decompensation

1. Treat fever aggressively with acetaminophen, not aspirin (which releases bound hormone).
2. Intravenous fluids containing 10% dextrose are recommended because patients have depleted glycogen stores.
3. Vitamin supplements including thiamine should be administered.
4. Treat CHF using conventional methods (digitalis, diuretics).
5. Identify the precipitating event, including infection. Fever and leukocytosis alone are not indications for initiating antibiotic therapy in hyperthyroid disorders. Panculture and observation are recommended.

destruction of the gland's synthetic activity often causes hypothyroidism. Thionamides are prescribed to make the patient euthyroid prior to administration of radioiodine.

Admission recommendations for the hyperthyroid states in the elderly include admission of any patient with impending or clinical thyroid storm by Burch and Wartofsky criteria (see Table 51-6). In addition, admit patients with clinical hyperthyroidism *and*

1. CNS effects, including agitation, chorea, delirium, psychosis, seizures, or coma
2. GI effects, including frank diarrhea, vomiting, jaundice, dehydration, or abdominal pain
3. Cardiovascular dysfunction, including congestive heart failure, sinus tachycardia unresponsive to oral beta blockade in the ED, new-onset atrial fibrillation, or angina pectoris
4. Persistent fever greater than 38°C after rest, without source or without easily treatable source
5. Syncopal episode (suggestive of hypovolemia or cardiovascular disorder)
6. History of recent radioiodine therapy
7. Thyrotoxic periodic paralysis (address hypokalemia)

Further, admit patients if the underlying precipitating cause warrants hospitalization.

ADDITIONAL ASPECTS

Euthyroid Sick Syndrome

In patients with severe systemic illness and after major surgical procedures, patients may have normal or decreased levels of T_4 with normal levels of TSH. FT_3 and total T_3 levels are diminished. This syndrome may be an adaptive response to systemic illness that will revert to normal without hormone supplementation as the illness subsides. There is no firm evidence that thyroid hormone in these situations is beneficial.

Thyrotoxic Periodic Paralysis

Thyrotoxic periodic paralysis (TPP) is the most common acquired form of periodic paralysis and can be fatal. The most common age of onset is 20 to 40 years, affecting males more often than females and occurring more frequently in Asian populations.

Patients with TPP experience sporadic episodes of symmetric muscle weakness that may progress to paralysis. Episodes usually begin in the early morning after sleep and frequently are preceded by muscle pain and tightness. Lower extremities are affected typically more than the upper. The motor-sensory peripheral neuropathy and paresis may be asymmetric.[57] This syndrome has been reported in association with a variety of hyperthyroid states. The characteristic laboratory abnormality is hypokalemia, and the syndrome is alleviated with administration of potassium salts. Attacks last from 3 to 36 hours and usually are self-limited.[58] Definitive treatment is control of the thyrotoxicosis.[30,59] Precipitating factors include strenuous exercise, high-carbohydrate load, and insulin administration. The mechanism may be related to sensitivity of cell membrane Na^+-K^+ pumps, causing intracellular potassium sequestration.

Subclinical Hypothyroidism

This is characterized by an increase in serum TSH concentration in individuals who have either normal or decreased serum T_4 and T_3 and are asymptomatic. The overall prevalence is up to 16 to 20 percent in women over age 60.[2,5] It may represent the earliest detectable stage of hypothyroidism. Goiter is common, and 50 to 80 percent of patients have antibodies against thyroperoxidase.[60] The usual causes of subclinical hypothyroidism are thyroid autoimmunity and inadequately treated hypothyroidism. Treatment with iodine, lithium, or amiodarone and a history of neck radiation are potential iatrogenic causes.

Treatment of subclinical hypothyroidism has been reported to decrease systolic time intervals, increase nerve conduction, and restore abnormalities of serum lipid concentrations toward normal.[61] While the benefits of therapy in patients who have no symptoms have not been established in prospective clinical trials, potential benefits to treatment might include preventing progression to overt hypothyroidism, decreasing the risk of death from cardiovascular causes, or reversal of cognitive and psychiatric abnormalities. Factors favoring treatment include symptoms consistent with mild hypothyroidism, hypercholesterolemia, and goiter. Some clinicians feel that this entity should not be treated unless severe hyperlipidemia not previously diagnosed is present or serum TSH is markedly elevated (>10 mU/L).[62]

For these potential benefits of therapy, the College of American Pathologists,[63] the American Academy of Family Physicians,[64] and the American Thyroid Association[65] recommend screening of asymptomatic adults for thyroid dysfunction, generally every 5 years, at years greater than 50, greater than 60, and greater than 35 years of age, respectively.

Subclinical Hyperthyroidism

This is defined by normal serum levels of T_4 and T_3 with suppressed TSH. These patients have predictable changes in the cardiovascular system, most notably resting tachycardia and episodes of atrial fibrillation. Patients have enhanced cardiac contractility and left ventricular mass. The presence of a decreased TSH level in these patients was associated with a threefold greater risk for development of atrial fibrillation over a 10-year interval.[61] Reasons for treatment of subclinical hyperthyroidism might include the following: prevention of osteoporosis, which is associated with the hyperthyroid state; prevention of atrial fibrillation; and prevention of the development of overt hyperthyroidism.[66] There is only limited evidence that normalization of the serum thyrotropin level might cause atrial fibrillation to revert spontaneously.[67] There is more evidence that treatment that restores serum thyrotropin levels to the normal range reverses loss of bone mineral density in postmenopausal women.[68]

Thyroid Surgery

Surgery is performed much less frequently now than in the past, although subtotal thyroidectomy is felt by some to be underused today in the treatment of Graves' disease.[69,70] Abnormalities associated with unresolved thyromegaly, dysphagia, or tracheal compression may require surgical intervention. In general, surgery is recommended only for very large, symptomatic goiters (>100 g).[26]

If suspicion exists that the gland is cancerous, surgery is warranted. Patients with Graves' disease and a "cold"

nodule on scan may fall into this category. Rarely, surgery may be indicated for patients who refuse or who do not have success with iodine-131 ablative therapy for Graves' disease. Operations for solitary toxic adenoma have met with success.[71] It is recommended that nonpalpable nodules found incidentally via ultrasound, computed tomography, or magnetic resonance imaging, termed *thyroid incidentalomas,* be biopsied if they are larger than 1 cm.[72] Complications of surgery include hypocalcemia from inadvertent removal of the parathyroids and damage to the recurrent laryngeal nerve.

REFERENCES

1. Wartofsky L: Myxedema coma, in Braverman LE, Utiger RD (eds): *The Thyroid.* Philadelphia, Lippincott, 1996, p 871.
2. Tunbridge WMG, Evered DC, Hall R, et al: The spectrum of thyroid disease in a community: The Whickham survey. *Clin Endocrinol (Oxf)* 7:481, 1977.
3. Bagchi N, Brown TR, Parish RF: Thyroid dysfunction in adults over 55 years. *Arch Intern Med* 150:785, 1990.
4. Sawin CT, Castelli WP, Hershman JM, et al: The aging thyroid: Thyroid deficiency in the Framingham study. *Arch Intern Med* 145:1386, 1985.
5. Canaris GJ, Manowitz N, Mayor G, et al: The Colorado Thyroid Disease Prevalence Study. *Arch Intern Med* 160:526, 2000.
6. Jordan RM: Myxedema coma. *Med Clin North Am* 79:185, 1995.
7. Olsen CG: Myxedema coma in the elderly. *J Am Fam Pract* 8:376, 1995.
8. Kumar A, Bhandari AK, Rahimtoola SH: Torsades de pointes and marked QT prolongation in association with hypothyroidism. *Ann Intern Med* 106:712, 1987.
9. Guthrie GP Jr, Hunsaker JC III, O'Connor WN: Sudden death in hypothyroidism. *New Engl J Med* 317:1291, 1987.
10. Khaleeli AA, Memon N: Factors affecting resolution of pericardial effusions in primary hypothyroidism: A clinical, biochemical and echocardiographic study. *Postgrad Med* 58:473, 1982.
11. US Preventive Services Task Force: *Guidelines from Guide to Clinical Preventive Services,* 2d ed. Baltimore, Williams & Wilkins, 1996, p 1.
12. Nicoloff JT, LoPresti JS: Myexedema coma: Myxedema coma. *Endocrinol Metab Clin North Am* 22:279, 1993.
13. Pittman CS, Zayed AA: Myxedema coma. *Curr Ther Endocrinol Metab* 6:98, 1997.
14. Cohen LF, Mohabeer AJ, Keffer JH, Jialal I: Troponin I in hypothyroidism. *Clin Chem* 42:1494, 1996.
15. Myers L, Hays J: Myxedema coma. *Crit Care Clin* 7:43, 1991.
16. Davis PJ, Davis FB: Hypothyroidism in the elderly. *Compr Ther* 10:17, 1984.

17. Reinhardt W, Mann K: Incidence, clinical picture and treatment of hypothyroid coma. *Med Klin* 92:521, 1997.

18. Burger AG, Philippe J: Thyroid emergencies. *Baillieres Clin Endocrinol Metab* 6:77, 1992.

19. Zimmerman RS, Gharib H, Zimmerman D, et al: Atrial natriuretic peptide in hypothyroidism. *J Clin Endocrinol Metab* 64:353, 1987.

20. Hylander B, Rosenquist U: Treatment of myxedema coma: Factors associated with a fatal outcome. *Acta Endocrinol* 180:65, 1985.

21. Yamamoto T, Fukuyama J, Fujiyoshi A: Factors associated with mortality of myxedema coma: Report of eight cases and literature survey. *Thyroid* 9:1167, 1999.

22. Senior RM, Birge SJ, Wessler S, et al: The recognition and management of myxedema coma. *JAMA* 217:61, 1971.

23. Dabon-Almirante CL, Surks MI: Clinical and laboratory diagnosis of thyrotoxicosis. *Endocrinol Metabol Clin* 27:26, 1998.

24. Sawin CT, Geller A, Kaplan MM, et al: Low serum thyrotropin (TSH) in older persons without hyperthyroidism. *Arch Intern Med* 151:165, 1991.

25. Sundbeck G, Lundberg P-A, Lindstendt G, et al: Incidence and prevalence of thyroid disease in elderly women: Results from the longitudinal population study of elderly people in Gothenburg, Sweden. *Age Ageing* 20:291, 1991.

26. Wartofsky L: Treatment options for hyperthyroidism. *Hosp Pract* 31:69, 1996.

27. Tibaldi JM, Barzel U, Albin J, Surks M: Thyrotoxicosis in the very old. *Am J Med* 81:619, 1986.

28. American College of Emergency Physicians: Clinical policy for the initial approach to patients presenting with altered mental status. *Ann Emerg Med* 33:251, 1999.

29. Engel A: Neuromuscular manifestations of Graves' disease. *Mayo Clin Proc* 47:919, 1972.

30. Logothetic L: Neurologic and muscular manifestations of hyperthyroidism. *Arch Neurol* 5:533, 1961.

31. Verberne HJ, Fliers E, Prummel MF, et al: Thyrotoxicosis as a predisposing factor for cerebral venous thrombosis. *Thyroid* 10:607, 2000.

32. Lee TG, Ha CK, Lim BH: Thyroid storm presenting as status epilepticus and stroke (letter). *Postgrad Med* 73:61, 1997.

33. Gomberg-Maitland M, Frishman WH: Thyroid hormone and cardiovascular disease. *Am Heart J* 135:187, 1998.

34. Klein I, Ojamaa K: Thyrotoxicosis and the heart. *Endocrinol Metab Clin* 27:51, 1998.

35. Alpert NR, Nulieri LA: Thermomechanical energy of hypertrophied hearts, in Alpert NR (ed): *Perspectives in Cardiovascular Research: Myocardial Hypertrophy and Failure.* New York, Raven Press, 1983, p 619.

36. Woeber KA: Thyrotoxicosis and the heart. *New Engl J Med* 327:94, 1992.

37. Davis PJ, Davis FB: Hyperthyroidism in patients over the age of 60 years. *Medicine* 53:161, 1974.

38. Moliterno D, DeBold CR, Robertson RM: Case report: Coronary vasospasm: Relation to the hyperthyroid state. *Am J Med Sci* 304:38, 1992.

39. Thomas F, Mazzaferri EL, Skillman TG: Apathetic thyrotoxicosis: A distinctive clinical and laboratory entity. *Ann Intern Med* 72:679, 1970.

40. Talbot-Stern JK, Green T, Royle TJ: Psychiatric manifestations of systemic illness. *Emerg Med Clin North Am* 18:199, 2000.

41. Tietgens ST, Leinung MC: Thyroid storm. *Med Clin North Am* 79:169, 1995.

42. Jiang YZ, Hutchinson KA, Bartelloni P, Manthous CA: Thyroid storm presenting as multiple organ dysfunction syndrome. *Chest* 118:877, 2000.

43. Lahey FH: The crisis of exophthalmic goiter. *New Engl J Med* 199:255, 1928.

44. Mazzaferri EL, Skillman TG: Thyroid storm: A review of 22 episodes with special emphasis on the use of guanethidine. *Arch Intern Med* 124:684, 1969.

45. Sherman SI, Simons L, Ladenson PW: Clinical and socioeconomic predispositions to complicated thyrotoxicosis: A predictable and preventable outcome? *Am J Med* 101:192, 1996.

46. Burch HB, Wartofsky L: Life-threatening thyrotoxicosis: Thyroid storm. *Endocrinol Metab Clin North Am* 22:263, 1993.

47. Surks M, Chopra IJ, Mariash CN, et al: American Thyroid Association guidelines for use of laboratory tests in thyroid disorders. *JAMA* 263:1529, 1990.

48. Brooks MH, Waldstein SS: Free thyroxine concentrations in thyroid storm. *Ann Intern Med* 93:694, 1980.

49. Dillman WH: Thyroid storm. *Curr Ther Endocrinol Metab* 6:81, 1997.

50. Geffner DL, Azukizawa M, Hershman JM: Propylthiouracil blocks extrathyroidal conversion of thyroxine to triiodothyronine and augments thyrotropin secretion in man. *J Clin Invest* 55:224, 1975.

51. Yeung SC, Go R, Balasubramanyam A: Rectal administration of iodide and propylthiouracil in the treatment of thyroid storm. *Thyroid* 5:403, 1995.

52. Hurley DL, Gharib H: Detection and treatment of hypothyroidism and Graves' disease. *Geriatrics* 50:41, 1995.

53. Brunette DD, Rothong C: Emergency department management of thyrotoxic crisis with esmolol. *Am J Emerg Med* 9:232, 1991.

54. Anaissie E, Tohme JF: Reserpine in propranolol resistant thyroid storm. *Arch Intern Med* 145:2248, 1985.

55. Valcavi R, Menozi C, Roti E, et al: Sinus node function in hyperthyroid patients. *J Clin Endocrinol Metab* 75:239, 1992.

56. Ebert RJ: Dantrolene and thyroid crisis. *Anesthesia* 49:924, 1994.

57. Pandit L, Shankar SK, Gayathri N, Pandit A: Acute thyrotoxic neuropathy: Basedow's paraplegia revisited. *J Neurol Sci* 155:211, 1998.

58. Ober KP: Thyrotoxic periodic paralysis in the United States:

Report of 7 cases and review of the literature. *Medicine* 71:109, 1992.

59. Shayne P, Hart A, et al: Thyrotoxic periodic paralysis terminated with intravenous propranolol. *Ann Emerg Med* 24:736, 1994.

60. Cooper DS: Subclinical hypothyroidism. *New Engl J Med* 345:260, 2001.

61. Surks MI, Ocampo E: Subclinical thyroid disease. *Am J Med* 100:217, 1996.

62. Chu JW, Crapo LM: The treatment of subclinical hypothyroidism is seldom necessary. *J Clin Endocrinol Metab* 86:4591, 2001.

63. Glenn GC: Laboratory Task Force of the College of American Pathologists: Practice parameter on laboratory testing for screening and case finding in asymptomatic adults. *Arch Pathol Lab Med* 120:929, 1996.

64. *Periodic Health Examination: Summary of AAFP Policy Recommendations and Age Charts,* revision 4.0. Kansas City, MO, American Academy of Family Physicians, 2000.

65. Ladenson PW, Singer PA, Ain KB, et al: American Thyroid Association guidelines for detection of thyroid dysfunction.

Arch Intern Med 160:1573, 2000.

66. Toft AD: Subclinical hyperthyroidism. *New Engl J Med* 345:512, 2001.

67. Forfar JC, Feek CM, Miller HC, Toft AD: Atrial fibrillation and isolated suppression of the pituitary-thyroid axis: Response to specific antithyroid therapy. *Int J Cardiol* 1:43, 1981.

68. Faber J, Jensen IW, Petersen L, et al: Normalization of serum thyrotropin by means of radioiodine treatment in subclinical hyperthyroidism: Effect on bone loss in postmenopausal women. *Clin Endocrinol (Oxf)* 48:285, 1998.

69. Alsanea O, Clark OH: Treatment of Graves' disease: The advantages of surgery. *Endocrinol Metab Clin North Am* 29:321, 2000.

70. Weber C, Scholz GH, Lamesch P, Paschke R: Thyroidectomy in iodine induced thyroid storm. *Exp Clin Endocrinol Diabetes* 107:468, 1999.

71. Gittoes NJ, Franklyn JA: Hyperthyroidism: Current treatment guidelines. *Drugs* 55:543, 1998.

72. Fatourechi V: Subclinical thyroid disease. *Mayo Clin Proc* 76:413, 2001.

52

Nutritional Issues

David C. Lee
Christopher C. Raio

HIGH-YIELD FACTS

- The elderly represent the most diverse physiologic subset of any age group.
- Thorough dietary guidelines have not been established in the elderly.
- The elderly are more vulnerable to malnutrition when compared with other age groups.
- Malnutrition has been reported in up to 50 percent of all hospitalized adults.
- Malnutrition is a multifactorial disease, and malnutrition and suboptimal nutrition are underrecognized chronic diseases.
- There are few studies in the areas of assessments and interventions in the emergency department (ED).

The area of geriatric nutrition is a growing field. Recent efforts and studies over the past decade focusing on optimal dietary and food supplement regimens have revolutionized the approach to geriatric nutrition. Yet there are still relatively few large-scale studies that focus on nutrition, assessment, interventions, and outcomes in the elderly.[1,2] Addressing the nutritional needs of elderly patients is compounded by further difficulties:

1. *There is a wide spectrum of nutritional needs in the elderly.* This reflects the wide spectrum of individual health of the elderly. The elderly represent the most diverse physiologic subset of any other age group.[1] The nutritional requirements of an invalid nursing home patient are quite different from those of a healthy active elderly patient. The nutritional requirements of a 65-year-old man and 95-year-old women may be very different. Yet all the aforementioned patients are lumped together as elderly.

The most common standard used in the United States for recommended dietary allowances and tolerances is the Recommended Dietary Allowances (RDAs). The RDAs were developed for healthy adults and do not reflect the nutritional needs of sick individuals, who may be under a stress state or in a hypermetabolic state. Furthermore, the RDA does not specifically address the elderly. The RDAs group all patients 50 years of age and over into one group. Thus the RDAs for a healthy 51-year-old are the same as for an institutionalized 90-year-old. Other commonly used benchmarks include estimated average requirement (EAR), the adequate intake (AI), and the safe upper level (UL). The most comprehensive of these (which actually includes all the aforementioned values) is the dietary reference intakes (DRIs).

2. *Geriatric nutritional issues are multifactorial.* An appropriate assessment of the nutritional state of geriatric patients is complex, time-consuming, and expensive. These are not the characteristics that typify an emergency department (ED) workup.[3] Furthermore, there is scant literature addressing malnutrition as a primary or secondary issue. For instance, dementia is closely associated with malnutrition. Although folate deficiency can be the primary cause of dementia in a select group of elderly patients,[4,5] it is unclear if this is true for the general elderly population. Yet a comprehensive workup of malnutrition will reveal a primary cause in 93 percent of malnourished elderly.[6]

3. *Nutritional issues are usually low-priority issues in the ED.* Geriatric nutritional deficiencies are chronic conditions that often are overlooked and underdiagnosed. By themselves, these conditions rarely present with life-threatening emergencies. The most pressing needs of the patients are addressed first in the ED. For instance, an elderly patient who presents with congestive heart failure is at high risk for thiamine deficiency. Such a patient often will be treated for the complaints of dyspnea or weight gain, overlooking or not addressing the nutritional deficiencies.

4. *There is a difference between malnutrition and hypovitaminosis.* Often these terms are used synonymously. *Malnutrition* is an inclusive term referring to the lack of one or more of the over 40 nutrients required physiologically.[3] *Hypovitaminosis* refers to a condition in which there are suboptimal levels of a particular vitamin that is associated with inadequate or abnormal metabolic function. It has been reported that over 20 percent of the U.S. population suffers from some form of hypovitaminosis.[7] Hypovitaminosis is a condition that can be corrected with supplementation of the particular vitamin that is deficient.[8,9]

EPIDEMIOLOGY

Studies on the prevalence of malnutrition in the elderly in industrialized nations vary greatly. One of the difficulties interpreting these studies is the lack of uniform standards. Another difficulty is that the majority of these studies are done by surveys.[10] Surveys questioning dietary food records, food recall, and food frequency may not be appropriate for elderly subjects with difficulties with memory.[11] Elderly patients often are inaccurate in their self-assessments.[12] There are only a handful of large-scale prevalence studies that use biochemical markers to assess nutritional status and fewer that actually measure intervention and outcomes.[13] Finally, the clinical diagnosis of malnutrition can be difficult. There is no specific validated instrument to detect malnutrition in the elderly.[14,15] Thus the prevalence of reported malnutrition ranges from 0.7 to12 percent of community-dwelling elderly, 30 to 60 percent of hospitalized elderly, and 40 to 85 percent of long-term institutionalized elderly. Malnutrition is associated with decreased activities of daily living (ADL) function, higher rates of ED visits, and increased mortality.[14,16–22]

There are multiple studies on hypovitaminosis in the elderly. Folic acid and vitamin D have been studied most extensively. In a population-based cohort study in Framingham, Selhub and colleagues[23] studied 1160 elderly subjects. The authors noted that approximately 20 percent of their study subjects had low levels of one or more B complex vitamin that contributed to high homocysteine levels. Studies on vitamin D deficiencies in the elderly report prevalence rates from 6 to 79 percent.[9,24–27] There are multiple smaller studies on each individual vitamin.

PATHOPHYSIOLOGY

Protein-Calorie Deficiencies

Malnutrition includes a number of conditions that reflect over- or undernutrition of protein, energy, or nutrient status. In general, most clinicians associate malnutrition with dietary deficiencies. The two classic extremes of protein-energy malnutrition—marasmus, a deficiency of calories resulting in poor growth and loss of adipose and lean mass, and kwashiorker, a primary deficiency of protein manifested by edema and ascites—are observed rarely in this country. Many individuals who are malnourished have elements of both protein and calorie deficiencies.

Risk factors for poor nutrition in older adults include low income, social isolation, loneliness, chronic and acute disease states, compromised functional status, and polypharmacy.

These common etiologies of malnutrition in the elderly are remembered most easily by the pneumonic DETERMINE: *d*iseases that affect appetite and gastrointestinal function; *e*ating poorly (lack of fruits and vegetables and excess alcohol consumption are common problems); *t*ooth loss/pain (poor dentition reduces food intake); *eco*nomic hardship (40 percent of the elderly have poverty-level incomes); *r*educed social contacts (people who live alone do not eat properly); *m*ultiple medications (these can cause gastrointestinal upset with reduced food intake); *in*voluntary weight loss/gain (such loss or gain of greater than 10 pounds in 6 months is highly significant); *e*lder (age over 80 years increases the risk of the preceding and is associated with impairments in independent IADLs, such as shopping and cooking). Malnutrition in institutionalized elders has been associated with dysphagia, slow eating, low protein intake, poor appetite, presence of a feeding tube, and increasing age

Caloric requirements decrease progressively with age. This is mainly due to a combination of decreased physical activity, decreased metabolically active skeletal muscle mass, and decreased metabolic rate. In contrast, protein requirements actually increase with age.[1,28] Cederholm and colleagues[29] reported that noncancer medical patients who suffer from protein-calorie deficiencies have a significantly higher mortality rate than their well-nourished counterparts.

Vitamin Deficiencies

Elderly patients are highly susceptible to hypovitaminosis and suboptimal vitamin intake. This usually occurs with more than one vitamin. The diets of the elderly tend to be frequently deficient in the B complex vitamins and vitamin D.[28]

Vitamin A

Vitamin A deficiency is one of the more common deficiency syndromes and is a significant public health issue in developing countries. Vitamin A is a high-molecular-weight alcohol found in pigmented vegetables. It plays a key role in wound healing and is essential for retinal function, cell growth, and differentiation. Daily requirements have been found to decrease with age. In the United States, clinical deficiency may result secondary to fat malabsorption syndromes or mineral oil laxative abuse, and it is seen most commonly in the elderly and urban poor.

Clinically, night blindness is the earliest symptom. In patients presenting with dark maladaptation, vitamin A deficiency should be considered. Xerosis and Bitot's spots (small white conjunctival spots) also can be seen early in the course of the disease. As the deficiency state progresses, keratomalacia, perforated cornea, endophthalmitis, and blindness can result.

Early deficiency can be treated with 30,000 IU of vitamin A daily for 1 week. The prognosis for treated night blindness is excellent. More advanced deficiency (corneal damage) should be treated with 20,000 IU for a minimum of 5 days. Beta-carotene toxicity resulting from excess intake can result in a yellow-orange skin tone clinically distinguishable from jaundice in that in concentrates in the palms and soles with conjunctival sparing.

Vitamin B$_1$/Thiamine

Thiamine plays an important role in several of the body's biochemical reactions of carbohydrate metabolism. It also plays a separate role in peripheral nerve conduction. During deficiency states, the relatively small amounts of thiamine stored by the body are depleted rapidly. Most deficiency states seen in industrialized nations are secondary to alcoholism, although clinical deficiency also may be seen in patients with malabsorptive problems, patients on dialysis, and patients with other causes of protein-energy malnutrition. Chronic alcoholics tend to have prolonged poor dietary intake along with impaired absorption, metabolism, and storage of thiamine. Thiamine deficiency actually can be precipitated in patients with marginal stores with the administration of dextrose. There are multiple reports suggesting that the elderly are at significant risk for thiamine deficiency. This is probably due to the combination of medication effect (especially diuretic use), diet, and age-associated decreases in the physiologic efficiency of thiamine-dependent cellular functions.[30–32] The prevalence of low thiamine stores in the elderly ranges from 14 to 37 percent.[33–36]

As with most deficiencies of water-soluble vitamins, the diagnosis of thiamine deficiency usually is made on presumptive clinical grounds. A wide range of tests are available to assess thiamine stores and function, including the most commonly used measurements of plasma thiamine levels, erythrocyte transketolase activity, or urinary thiamine excretion. The response to thiamine administration also can be used to support the diagnosis of thiamine deficiency.

Patients with early thiamine deficiency often will present with anorexia, muscle wasting, paresthesias, and general irritability. As the deficiency state worsens, one of two clinical syndromes may develop. *Wet beriberi* occurs in patients with high carbohydrate intake and is associated with physical exertion. High-output heart failure with resulting dyspnea, tachycardia, cardiomegaly, and pulmonary/peripheral edema is seen. Peripheral vasodilation gives rise to warm extremities that often can be misdiagnosed as cellulitis.

Dry beriberi, conversely, occurs in inactive patients with low-calorie intake. Patients develop neurologic sequelae involving both the peripheral and central nervous systems. Peripherally, a symmetric combined sensorimotor neuropathy may be seen. Pain, paresthesias, and areflexia are seen more commonly, and they are worse in the lower extremities. Centrally, Wernicke's encephalopathy with nystagmus progressing to ophthalmoplegia, truncal ataxia, and confusion develops. Korsakoff's syndrome of amnesia, confabulation, and impaired learning also may be apparent.

Thiamine-deficient patients should be treated with 50 to 100 mg/day of parenteral thiamine for 3 days followed by 5 to 10 mg/day of oral thiamine. Fifty percent of patients will see no resolution of symptoms, whereas 25 percent will experience almost immediate improvement. The question has been raised as to whether or not empirical treatment of elderly patients seen in the ED is appropriate. Although it has been shown that the acutely ill elderly patient is at greater risk for thiamine deficiency, it has not been proven that empirical administration of thiamine results in any significant improvement in outcome for these patients.[33]

Vitamin B$_2$/Riboflavin

Riboflavin functions in the body as a coenzyme and as a component of other processes involved in oxidation-reduction reactions. It is found abundantly in many foods. Like many other vitamin deficiencies, riboflavin deficiency is seen rarely as an isolated entity. Most reported cases have been secondary to decreased dietary intake, medication interactions, alcoholism, and other causes of protein-calorie malnutrition. Jamieson and colleagues[37] have reported a 2.7 percent prevalence rate of riboflavin deficiency in patients admitted to the hospital through the ED.

The clinical effects of riboflavin deficiency can be appreciated as generalized weakness, cheilosis, angular stomatitis, glossitis, seborrheic dermatitis, corneal vascularization, and anemia. When clinical suspicion for a deficiency exists, empirical therapy is usually begun. Several diagnostic tests are available, including erythrocyte glutathione reductase levels, urinary riboflavin excretion, and serum levels of plasma and erythrocyte flavins.

Vitamin B_2 deficiency is readily treated with the appropriate intake of certain foods, including meat, fish, and dairy. In addition, oral preparations and intravenous formulation are also available.

Vitamin B_6/Pyridoxine

Pyridoxal-5-phosphate is the major coenzyme involved in the metabolism of amino acids and is also required in the synthesis of heme. Pyridoxine deficiency is seen most commonly secondary to interaction with various medications, including isoniazid, cycloserine, penicillamine, and birth control pills. It also is seen more commonly in alcoholics. A number of inborn errors of metabolism and B_6-responsive syndromes (such as B_6-responsive anemia) also exist and usually are responsive to high doses of the vitamin (up to 600 mg/day). Pyridoxine hypovitaminosis is common among the elderly, with rates as high as 67 percent in institutionalized elderly females.[35,38]

Vitamin B_6 deficiency presents clinically in patients with mouth soreness, glossitis, cheilosis, weakness, and irritability. These symptoms can progress to a more serious peripheral neuropathy, anemia, and seizures. The deficiency is diagnosed based on clinical findings and can be confirmed by measuring pyridoxal phosphate in the blood.

Pyridoxine deficiency is treated with oral replacement of 10 to 20 mg/day, although patients taking medications interfering with B_6 metabolism may require up to 100 mg/day. Pyridoxine should be prescribed routinely with certain medications, especially in susceptible populations, including the elderly, urban poor, and alcoholics. Certain authors encourage higher daily doses of vitamin B_6 for the elderly than suggested by the RDAs.[1,23] Vitamin B_6 toxicity has been reported to cause an irreversible peripheral neuropathy in high doses.[38]

Vitamin B_{12}/Cyanocobalamin

Vitamin B_{12} is present in all foods of animal origin and is supplied only through dietary intake. It belongs to the cobalamin family and plays an important role in many of the body's reactions. After ingestion, B_{12} is bound to intrinsic factor (secreted by the parietal cells), is absorbed in the terminal ileum, and is then stored in the liver. Deficiency states may take up to 3 years to develop. Dietary deficiency is rare and usually is seen in certain at-risk groups: vegans, patients with gastrectomies, patients with blind loop syndrome (competition for B_{12} by bacterial overgrowth), and those who have had surgical resection of the ileum. Rarer causes of B_{12} deficiency include patients with fish tapeworm infection, pancreatic insufficiency, or severe Crohn's disease. The most common cause is pernicious anemia, which is rarely seen clinically before the age of 35. However, vitamin B_{12} deficiency can occur in the general elderly population with a reported prevalence of from 7 to 16 percent.[39]

Patients with vitamin B_{12} deficiency develop characteristic megaloblastic anemia, which can be severe. This megaloblastic state also produces changes in the mucosal cells that can lead to glossitis, anorexia, and diarrhea. The classic peripheral neuropathy (paresthesias) can progress to affect the posterior columns, producing balance disturbances. In severe forms, cerebral function may be impaired, and dementia may develop. Patients often present appearing pale and icteric, with decreased position/vibratory sense.

Laboratory data can aid in diagnosing deficiency states. Although mean corpuscular volumes are usually high, they can be surprisingly normal. Peripheral blood smears may reveal anisocytosis and poikilocytosis. The characteristic macroovalocyte as well as hypersegmented neutrophils will be demonstrated. In severe cases, pancytopenia is seen. Bone marrow morphology is abnormal, and increases in lactate dehydrogenase (LDH) and indirect bilirubin are common. The Schilling test is used to document the decreased absorption characteristic of pernicious anemia. Undiagnosed pernicious anemia can be a common finding in the elderly, especially in females.[40]

The treatment for vitamin B_{12} deficiency is repletion via intramuscular injection or oral cobalamin. Patients usually recover rapidly; however, neurologic sequelae may persist if symptoms have been present for greater than 6 months.

Folate

Folate is found abundantly in citrus fruits and green leafy vegetables. It is a mediator of many biochemical reactions. Folate is absorbed from the entire gastrointestinal tract, and body stores of folate can last up to 3 months. Certain drugs (phenytoin, trimethoprim-sulfamethoxazole, sulfasalazine) may interfere with absorption. Patients experience deficiency states primarily from inadequate dietary intake. Patients at risk are chronic alcoholics, anorectics, those who do not eat fruits and vegetables, and those who overcook their food. Folate deficiency in adults may lead to an increased risk of coronary artery disease, cerebrovascular accidents, and cancer.[9]

Folate deficiency classically presents as a megaloblastic anemia. Erythrocyte folate levels of less than 150 ng/mL are diagnostic. Plasma homocysteine also has been found to be a sensitive biomarker of folate deficiency.[41] Serum B_{12} levels will be normal, and a peripheral blood smear will show macroovalocytes with hypersegmented neutrophils. In adults with folate deficiency–induced megaloblastic anemia, two-thirds also will have neuropsychiatric disorders, with the highest incidence of folate deficiency in psychiatric elderly patients.[4]

Folate deficiency is treated with 1 mg/day of oral folic acid. Improvement is usually rapid, with reticulocytosis occurring at 5 to 7 days and total correction of hematologic abnormalities within 2 months. If a patient is actually B_{12} deficient and treated with folate only, the anemia may resolve with persistent neurologic sequelae.[39]

Niacin

Niacin is found in various protein-rich foods containing tryptophan (cereals, vegetables, and dairy). Niacin is a unique vitamin in that it can be manufactured from an amino acid precursor (tryptophan). Historically, niacin deficiency was seen in areas where corn was the major source of calories. Today, deficiency states are associated with alcoholism, certain inborn errors of metabolism, and nutrient-drug interactions. Niacin is an essential component of both nicotinamide adenine dinucleotide (NAD) and nicotinamide adenine dinucleotide phosphate (NADP), which are involved in many oxidation-reduction reactions. It is also used in the treatment of hypercholesterolemia and hypertriglyceridemia.

Niacin deficiency is diagnosed primarily on clinical grounds. Patients may present with generalized weakness, irritability, anorexia, mouth soreness, glossitis, stomatitis, and weight loss. As the deficiency state progresses, the classic triad of pellagra (dermatitis, dementia, diarrhea) can develop and may be fatal. The dermatitis occurs as dark, dry, scaling skin seen in sun-exposed areas. The diarrhea can be severe, and the dementia may progress from insomnia, irritability, and apathy to confusion, memory loss, hallucinations, and frank psychosis. Niacin metabolites (N-methylnicotinamide) can be measured in the urine, and serum and erythrocyte NAD/NADP also can be measured. Abnormal results from these tests may not be specific for niacin deficiency and may reflect overall malnutrition.

Niacin deficiency is treated with oral supplementation of 10 to 150 mg/day. Toxicity can develop and is seen commonly in patients taking niacin for medical benefit. Cutaneous flushing, partially prevented by pretreatment with aspirin, and gastric irritation are the most common untoward effects.

Vitamin C/Ascorbic Acid

Vitamin C can be found abundantly in certain fruits and vegetables. It acts as an antioxidant and is also required for the synthesis of collagen. Vitamin C functions to increase the absorption of nonheme iron, is involved in wound healing, and also plays a role in tyrosine and drug metabolism. High intake and plasma levels of vitamin C may be protective against mortality from heart disease.[42] Groups at risk for clinical deficiency states include the isolated elderly, the urban poor, the mentally ill, food faddists, smokers, and chronic alcoholics.[43]

Scurvy should be suspected when evaluating certain skin lesions and in patients presenting with spontaneous bleeding such as atraumatic hemarthroses or gingival bleeding.[44,45] Vitamin C stores can be depleted within 30 days, and clinical symptoms can arise in this time period. Patients also may present with malaise or generalized weakness. More severe forms classically present with impaired wound healing and associated anemia. Other manifestations include perifollicular hemorrhages, hyperkeratotic papules, petechiae, purpura, and splinter hemorrhages. Late findings include edema, oliguria, neuropathy, intracerebral hemorrhage, and eventual death.

Vitamin C deficiency can be treated with 300 to 1000 mg/day of ascorbic acid. Symptoms usually will improve dramatically within days. Vitamin C toxicity has a theoretical risk of increased formation of oxalate kidney stones, and there is no evidence that supplementation is helpful in general healthy elderly people.[9]

Vitamin D and Calcium

Although Vitamin D is naturally present in few foods, it is not considered a true vitamin because the human body can synthesize this compound. With adequate sunlight exposure, 7-dehydrocholesterol is metabolized to previtamin D_3 in the skin. This in turn is metabolized to 25-hydroxyvitamin D_3 in the liver and then to the active 1,25-dihydroxyvitamin D_3 in the kidneys.[9]

Vitamin D deficiency is associated with rickets in the younger population. It can cause secondary hyperparathyroidism, bone loss, and increased risks for bone fracture. Vitamin D and calcium deficiencies are very common in the elderly. Three-quarters of elderly have inadequate intake of vitamin D and calcium.[1] Over 50 percent of elderly medical inpatients have been shown to have biochemical evidence of vitamin D and calcium deficiencies.[25] The elderly are susceptible to vitamin D and calcium deficiencies for multiple reasons. Gastrointestinal absorption and skin-mediated production of vitamin D become inefficient during the aging process.[1,27] Second, the institutionalized and homebound elderly have less exposure to sunlight. Finally, the elderly may have higher requirements for vitamin D and calcium than younger patients.[9,26]

Laboratory documentation of deficiency can be ascertained by measuring serum 25-hydroxyvitamin D, parathyroid hormone, and calcium concentrations.[25] Vitamin D and calcium supplementations in the elderly have been shown to reduce the incidence of fracture and its accompanying morbidity and mortality in the elderly. Typical supplemental doses are 400 IU of vitamin D and 1500 mg of calcium.

Vitamin E/α-Tocopherol

Vitamin E is found abundantly in the diet, and clinical deficiency states are rare. It is involved in free-radical scavenging, and it has been found to mediate age-associated increases in membrane viscosity and immune function. There is little evidence to suggest that supplementation provides any beneficial effects in patients of any age.

Deficiency states have been reported secondary to severe malabsorption and genetic abetalipoproteinemia, as well as in children with chronic cholestatic liver disease, biliary atresia, and cystic fibrosis. Clinically, patients may present with areflexia, gait disturbances, decreased proprioception/vibratory sense, or ophthalmoplegia.

Vitamin K

Vitamin K is contained in leafy vegetables and is also synthesized by intestinal bacteria. It is an essential component of both the intrinsic and extrinsic clotting cascades. Deficiency states usually result from the administration of medications that interfere with absorption of the vitamin or interfere with the bacterial milieu of the intestine. The geriatric population is inherently at risk for clinical deficiency because elderly persons are more likely to be exposed to multiple medications. The body stores only small amounts of vitamin K, and deficiency states may develop in as few as 5 to 7 days. Bleeding from any site may result. This bleeding can be treated with either oral or subcutaneous supplementation.

CLINICAL FEATURES OF MALNUTRITION

One of the most important interventions of an ED visit for a geriatric patient is further assessment of the patient's life situation and identification of additional medical evaluations. Certain subsets of the elderly are at a much higher risk for malnutrition. Health care providers should be aware of the association between malnutrition and underlying illness (especially malignancy), depression, dementia, advanced chronic disease states, polypharmacy, alcohol use, and decreased functional levels (low ADL scores).

A nutritional history should include several elements. First, any history of weight loss/anorexia should be determined. A weight loss of 5 lb is significant and a loss of 10 lb in 6 months is highly correlated with malnutrition. An involuntary weight loss should be confirmed by caregivers or significant others. At least half the time the patients' history is not accurate. In the majority of these cases, a treatable etiology will be found. Second, difficulty in chewing and swallowing should be assessed; chewing and swallowing difficulties are most commonly due to decayed or absent teeth or broken or ill-fitting dentures. Dysphagia also can be due to neurologic, physiologic, and anatomic etiologies, the most significant being tumors of the esophagus and mediastinum. Next, the number of meals consumed per day should be assessed; many elders who live alone skip meals or are unable to prepare them. Chronic illnesses, such as prior known malignancy, gastrointestinal dysfunction, and depression, are significant causes of malnourishment and should be documented. Gastrointestinal dysfunction, including anorexia, pain, diarrhea, and constipation, should be particularly assessed. The patient's living arrangements and functional status should be addressed: Does the patient live alone? Is the patient able to live independently? Last, a history of consumption of alcoholic beverages should be obtained.

The physical examination should include the following elements: general appearance, examination of the mouth and dentition, pulmonary examination for signs of consolidation or effusion, abdominal examination including palpatation for masses and hepatomegaly and performance of a rectal examination to check for occult blood and neoplasms, and a height and weight determination to calculate body mass index (BMI). BMI can be calculated by using the formula BMI (kg/m^2) = weight (kg)/height^2 (m). A general rule is that a BMI of less than 22 is consistent with nutritional impairment and over 27 is excessive. Another important item of the physical ex-

Table 52-1. Physical Findings of Malnutrition

Finding	Deficiency/Interpretation
General appearance	
Weight loss	Malnutrition < 90% of ideal body weight
	Severe < 70% of ideal body weight
Decreased temporal and proximal extremity muscle mass	Decreased skeletal protein
Decreased skin-fold thickness by "pinch test"	Decreased body fat stores
Skin, nails, and hair	
Easily plucked hair	Protein
Easy bruising, perifollicular hemorrhages	Vitamin C
"Flaky paint" rash of lower extremities	Zinc
Coarse skin, "goose bumps"	Vitamin A
Hyperpigmentation of sun-exposed areas	Niacin, tryptophan
Spooning of nails	Iron
Eyes	
Conjunctival pallor	Anemia (nonspecific)
Bitot spot	Vitamin A
Ophthalmoplegia	Thiamine
Mouth and mucus membranes	
Nasolabial seborrhea	Essential fatty acids
Glossitis (smooth, red tongue) and/or cheilosis	Riboflavin, niacin, vitamin B_{12}, pyridoxine, folate
Diminished taste	Zinc
Neurologic system	
Disorientation	Niacin, phosphorus
Confabulation	Thiamine
Cerebellar gait, past pointing	Thiamine
Peripheral neuropathy	Thiamine, pyridoxine, vitamin B_{12}
Lost vibratory, position sense	Vitamin B_{12}

Source: Adapted from Halsted CH: Malnutrition and nutritional assessment, in Braunwald E, et al (eds): *Harrisons's Principles of Internal Medicine,* 15th. New York, McGraw-Hill, 2001. Used with permission.

amination is anthropometric measurements, such as midarm and midthigh circumference, which are most useful in the elderly. Unfortunately, nomograms are not available past 75 years of age, but these measurements are useful to establish trends for follow-up.

It is important to note that the physical signs of malnutrition (Table 52-1) can be quite varied.

DIAGNOSIS AND DIFFERENTIAL

Malnutrition and undernutrition can be a difficult clinical diagnosis. There are many potential biochemical indicators of nutritional status, but few markers have clearly established associations with malnutrition in older persons, and criteria for their interpretation in this age group are not always clear. Preliminary studies investigating the utility of biochemical levels and surrogate markers have been inconclusive.[46] Tests for specific vitamin levels are available commercially, but test results are rarely available to influence clinical decision making in the ED.[8] Some authors have recommended albumin levels as a readily available screening tool in the ED for malnutrition.[18,29,47] However, other authors report that this is neither a sensitive nor a specific test for malnutrition.[3,48]

Despite these limitations, several commonly available laboratory tests can heighten suspicion for possible malnutrition. Complete blood counts (CBCs) are useful for detecting anemia, which can be associated with vitamin deficiencies, and leukopenia. Total lymphocyte counts of less than 1500 cells/mL are associated with a higher risk of mortality. It has been observed that the lymphocyte count is reduced with age, but it is unclear if these studies accounted for nutritional states. A comprehensive metabolic profile is useful to evaluate for electrolyte imbalance, diabetes, renal insufficiency, liver disease, and dehydration. Thyroid function studies are useful to rule out occult hyperthyroidism, especially in the older patient who may manifest weight loss and otherwise lack typical signs of thyrotoxicosis. The most useful serum indicator as a screen for chronic protein-energy malnutrition is the serum albumin level. However, cardiac, hepatic, and renal diseases; trauma; sepsis; and autoinflammatory processes can alter albumin concentrations. These diseases usually cause a fall in albumin levels, and in settings of acute inflammatory states, a low serum albumin level may be regarded as a negative acute-phase reactant. An albumin level of less than 3.5g/dL is abnormal, and protein deficiency may be categorized as follows: mild protein deficiency, albumin 2.9 to 3.2 g/dL; moderate, 2.6 to 2.8 g/dL; and severe, less than 2.5 g/dL. Albumin has a half-life of 21 days and is not reliable in the evaluation of acute changes in nutritional status. Prealbumin is a better indicator of short-term nutritional status changes. It has a half-life of only 2 days, and increasing levels are associated with nutritional repletion. As a marker of malnutrition it also has limited utility in the presence of acute inflammation and hepatic or renal disease. Prealbumin is measured in milligrams per deciliter, and generally accepted levels are as follows: mild nutritional impairment, 14 to 16 mg/dL; moderate, 14 to 13 mg/dL; and severe impairment, less than 11 mg/dL. Prealbumin determinations often are not immediately available and generally have high costs, both of which limit their utility in the ED setting.

A simple combination of functional ability, low albumin level, and subjective assessment has been found to be accurate for malnutrition and is more applicable in the ED setting. In a study published 25 years ago, investigators found that an inability to perform the ADLs, subjective assessment that the patient was malnourished by the physician, and a serum albumin level of less than 3.5 g/dL identified 75 percent of malnourished geriatric patients at risk for death.[49] This study suggests that general clinical assessment is a reproducible and valid technique for evaluating nutritional status.

EMERGENCY DEPARTMENT CARE AND DISPOSITION

Prehospital Considerations

The routine and liberal administration of intravenous glucose and thiamine by trained prehospital and health care providers for patients who present with altered mental status should be encouraged. Some authors have suggested a broader range of indications for aggressive thiamine supplementation, e.g., patients who present with congestive heart failure.[31–33] Although the clinical science to support these recommendations has not been thoroughly validated, the administration of thiamine is relatively cheap and has few side effects.[50]

Prevention, Prognosis, and Outcome

Prevention

In the ED, the health care practitioner must recognize the prevalence and manifestations of malnutrition in the elderly. Multivitamin supplementation has been shown to be an effective therapy in certain populations, e.g., pregnant patients. Elderly patients, especially those who have poor ADLs, can be considered an at-risk population. Elderly patients should receive nutritional consultations and/or dietary advice. Dietary and vitamin supplementation should be considered and encouraged.[8,9,41,51–53]

Prognosis

Malnourishment is clearly linked with higher morbidity and mortality. In a Swedish study, Cederholm and colleagues[29] reported a 44 percent mortality rate at 9 months in hospitalized malnourished patients admitted through the ED versus 18 percent in hospitalized well-nourished elderly admitted through the ED. Malnourished patients with congestive heart failure had the highest 9-month mortality rate (80 percent).

Outcome

Although there have been no large studies investigating outcomes of ED interventions in nutritional deficiencies in the elderly, there have been several studies that investigated nutritional supplementation in the hospitalized patients. In an English study, Vlaming and colleagues[54] reported that 18 percent of hospitalized patients admitted through the ED were undernourished. In their randomized, placebo-controlled study of 1561 patients admitted through the ED, they reported that 18 percent were undernourished. Implementing vitamin supplementation was associated with a decreased length of stay. In a Scottish study, Potter and colleagues[55] performed a prospective, randomized, controlled study investigating protein supplementation in elderly patients admitted through the ED. They reported a prevention of weight loss while hospitalized. The authors believed that in-hospital nutritional supplementation would reduce mortality. Milne and colleagues[2] performed a meta-analysis of 22 randomized and quasi-randomized, controlled trials of protein and energy supplementation in elderly patients. These authors reported that supplementation was associated with decreasing mortality rates and shorter length of hospital stays.

ADDITIONAL ASPECTS

Most important, physicians and nursing staff should incorporate some aspect of nutritional screening into the ED care of the older person. In one study of geriatric ED care, investigators were able to perform a nutritional assessment to screen older ED patients (using BMI, midarm circumference, and history of weight loss) in less than 3 minutes.[56] A geriatric nurse-practitioner program would be especially helpful in departments with a large geriatric population. Social services, dietary services, and home care nurses can be used to follow up at-risk patients who are discharged to ensure appropriate intervention and monitoring of the patients' status.

REFERENCES

1. Ausman LM, Russell RM: Nutrition in the elderly, in Shils ME, Olson JA, Shike M, Ross AC (eds): *Modern Nutrition in Health and Disease.* Baltimore, Williams & Wilkins, 1999, p 869.
2. Milne AC, Potter J, Avenell A: Protein and energy supplementation in elderly people at risk from malnutrition. *Cochrane Database Syst Rev* 3, 2002.
3. McCall PL: Nutritional emergencies, in Judd RL, Warner CG, Shaffer MA (eds): *Geriatric Emergencies.* Rockville, MD, Aspen, 1986, p 221.
4. Reynolds EH: Folic acid, ageing, depression, and dementia. *Br Med J* 324:1512, 2002.
5. Passeri M, Cucinotta D, Abate G, et al: Oral 5'-methyltetrahydrofolic acid in senile organic mental disorders with depression: Results of a double-blind multicenter study. *Aging (Milano)* 5:63, 1993.
6. Wilson MM, Vaswani S, Liu D, et al: Prevalence and causes of undernutrition in medical outpatients. *Am J Med* 104:56, 1998.
7. Flood A, Schatzkin A: Colorectal cancer: Does it matter if you eat your fruits and vegetables? *J Natl Cancer Inst* 92:1706, 2000.
8. Fletcher RH, Fairfield KM: Vitamins for chronic disease prevention in adults: Clinical applications. *JAMA* 287:3127, 2002.
9. Fairfield KM, Fletcher RH: Vitamins for chronic disease prevention in adults: Scientific review. *JAMA* 287:3116, 2002.
10. Briefel RR: Assessment of the US diet in national nutrition surveys: National collaborative efforts and NHANES. *Am J Clin Nutr* 59:164S, 1994.
11. Briefel RR, Flegal KM, Winn DM, et al: Assessing the nation's diet: Limitations of the food frequency questionnaire. *J Am Diet Assoc* 92:959, 1992.
12. Brown EL: Factors influencing food choices and intake. *Geriatrics* 31:89, 1976.
13. Cederholm T, Arner P, Palmblad J: Low circulating leptin levels in protein-energy malnourished chronically ill elderly patients. *J Intern Med* 242:377, 1997.
14. Thomas DR, Morley JE: Nutritional assessment and indicators of undernutrition in the elderly. *Res Staff Phys* 48:47, 2002.
15. Vellas B, Guigoz Y, Garry PJ, et al: The Mini Nutritional Assessment (MNA) and its use in grading the nutritional state of elderly patients. *Nutrition* 15:116, 1999.
16. Edington J, Boorman J, Durrant ER, et al: Prevalence of malnutrition on admission to four hospitals in England. The Malnutrition Prevalence Group. *Clin Nutr* 19:191, 2000.
17. Coe RM, Romeis JC, Miller DK, et al: Nutritional risk and survival in elderly veterans: A five-year follow-up. *J Commun Health* 18:327, 1993.
18. Incalzi RA, Gemma A, Capparella O, et al: Energy intake and in-hospital starvation: A clinically relevant relationship. *Arch Intern Med* 156:425, 1996.
19. Maaravi Y, Berry EM, Ginsberg G, et al: Nutrition and quality of life in the aged: The Jerusalem 70-year olds longitudinal study. *Aging (Milano)* 12:173, 2000.
20. Irving GF, Olsson BA, Cederholm T: Nutritional and cognitive status in elderly subjects living in service flats, and the effect of nutrition education on personnel. *Gerontology* 45:187, 1999.
21. Cederholm T, Hellstrom K: Nutritional status in recently hospitalized and free-living elderly subjects. *Gerontology* 38:105, 1992.
22. Thomas DR, Zdrowski CD, Wilson MM, et al: Malnutrition in subacute care. *Am J Clin Nutr* 75:308, 2002.
23. Selhub J, Jacques PF, Wilson PW, et al: Vitamin status and intake as primary determinants of homocysteinemia in an elderly population. *JAMA* 270:2693, 1993.
24. McKenna MJ: Differences in vitamin D status between countries in young adults and the elderly. *Am J Med* 93:69, 1992.
25. Thomas MK, Lloyd-Jones DM, Thadhani RI, et al: Hypovi-

taminosis D in medical inpatients. *New Engl J Med* 338:777, 1998.

26. Gloth FM 3d, Tobin JD, Sherman SS, Hollis BW: Is the recommended daily allowance for vitamin D too low for the homebound elderly? *J Am Geriatr Soc* 39:137, 1991.

27. Gloth FM 3d, Gundberg CM, Hollis BW, et al: Vitamin D deficiency in homebound elderly persons. *JAMA* 274:1683, 1995.

28. Katz PR, Grossberg GT, Potter JF, Solomon DH: Malnutrition, in Katz PR (ed): *Geriatrics Syllabus for Specialists.* New York, American Geriatrics Society, 2002, p 10.1.

29. Cederholm T, Jagren C, Hellstrom K: Outcome of protein-energy malnutrition in elderly medical patients. *Am J Med* 98:67, 1995.

30. Hardig L, Daae C, Dellborg M, et al: Reduced thiamine phosphate, but not thiamine diphosphate, in erythrocytes in elderly patients with congestive heart failure treated with furosemide. *J Intern Med* 247:597, 2000.

31. Shimon I, Almog S, Vered Z, et al: Improved left ventricular function after thiamine supplementation in patients with congestive heart failure receiving long-term furosemide therapy. *Am J Med* 98:485, 1995.

32. Suter PM, Haller J, Hany A, Vetter W: Diuretic use: A risk for subclinical thiamine deficiency in elderly patients. *J Nutr Health Aging* 4:69, 2000.

33. Lee DC, Chu J, Satz W, Silbergleit R: Low plasma thiamine levels in elder patients admitted through the emergency department. *Acad Emerg Med* 7:1156, 2000.

34. Brady JA, Rock CL, Horneffer MR: Thiamine status, diuretic medications, and the management of congestive heart failure. *J Am Diet Assoc* 95:541, 1995.

35. Mantero-Atienza E, Beach RS, Sotomayor MG, et al: Nutritional status of institutionalized elderly in south Florida. *Arch Latinoam Nutr* 42:242, 1992.

36. Iber FL, Blass JP, Brin M, Leevy CM: Thiamine in the elderly: Relation to alcoholism and to neurological degenerative disease. *Am J Clin Nutr* 36:1067, 1982.

37. Jamieson CP, Obeid OA, Powell-Tuck J: The thiamine, riboflavin and pyridoxine status of patients on emergency admission to hospital. *Clin Nutr* 18:87, 1999.

38. Bender DA: Vitamin B_6 requirements and recommendations. *Eur J Clin Nutr* 43:289, 1989.

39. Green R, Kinsella LJ: Current concepts in the diagnosis of cobalamin deficiency. *Neurology* 45:1435, 1995.

40. Carmel R: Prevalence of undiagnosed pernicious anemia in the elderly. *Arch Intern Med* 156:1097, 1996.

41. Oakley GP Jr: Eat right and take a multivitamin. *New Engl J Med* 338:1060, 1998.

42. Sahyoun NR, Jacques PF, Russell RM: Carotenoids, vitamins C and E, and mortality in an elderly population. *Am J Epidemiol* 144:501, 1996.

43. Weinstein M, Babyn P, Zlotkin S: An orange a day keeps the doctor away: Scurvy in the year 2000. *Pediatrics* 108:E55, 2001.

44. Stephen R, Utecht T: Scurvy identified in the emergency department: A case report. *J Emerg Med* 21:235, 2001.

45. Blee TH, Cogbill TH, Lambert PJ: Hemorrhage associated with vitamin C deficiency in surgical patients. *Surgery* 131:408, 2002.

46. Lumbers M, New SA, Gibson S, Murphy MC: Nutritional status in elderly female hip fracture patients: Comparison with an age-matched home living group attending day centres. *Br J Nutr* 85:733, 2001.

47. Potter MA, Luxton G: Prealbumin measurement as a screening tool for protein calorie malnutrition in emergency hospital admissions: A pilot study. *Clin Invest Med* 22:44, 1999.

48. Liu L, Bopp MM, Roberson PK, Sullivan DH: Undernutrition and risk of mortality in elderly patients within 1 year of hospital discharge. *J Gerontol* 57:M741, 2002.

49. Incalzi RA, Landi F, Ciprianin L, et al: Nutritional assessment: A primary component of multidimensional geriatric assessment in the acute care setting. *J Am Geriatr Soc* 44:166, 1966.

50. Wrenn KD, Murphy F, Slovis CM: A toxicity study of parenteral thiamine hydrochloride. *Ann Emerg Med* 18:867, 1989.

51. Tice JA, Ross E, Coxson PG, et al: Cost-effectiveness of vitamin therapy to lower plasma homocysteine levels for the prevention of coronary heart disease: Effect of grain fortification and beyond. *JAMA* 286:936, 2001.

52. Utiger RD: The need for more vitamin D. *New Engl J Med* 338:828, 1998.

53. Potter JM: Oral supplements in the elderly. *Curr Opin Clin Nutr Metab Care* 4:21, 2001.

54. Vlaming S, Biehler A, Hennessey EM, et al: Should the food intake of patients admitted to acute hospital services be routinely supplemented? A randomized placebo controlled trial. *Clin Nutr* 20:517, 2001.

55. Potter JM, Roberts MA, McColl JH, Reilly JJ: Protein energy supplements in unwell elderly patients: A randomized controlled trial. JPEN 25:323, 2001.

56. Miller DK, Lewis LM, Nork MJ, et al: Controlled trial of a geriatric case-finding and liaison service in an emergency department. *J Am Geriatr Soc* 44:513, 1996.

53

Toxic Epidermal Necrolysis and Stevens-Johnson Syndrome

Victor A. Pinkes

HIGH-YIELD FACTS

- Stevens Johnson syndrome (SJS) and toxic epidermal necrolysis (TEN) are gradations of the same disease process that results in severe desquamation of the skin.

- The Nikolsky sign, described as easily disrupting the epidermis in erythematous areas between bullae with pressure, is positive in SJS-TEN.

- The usual cause of SJS-TEN is a medication, in particular an antibiotic, anticonvulsant, or nonsteroidal anti-inflammatory drug (NSAID).

- Elderly patients with SJS-TEN are twice as likely to die from the disease as younger patients.

- Patients with SJS-TEN die from multiorgan failure secondary to sepsis.

- Poor prognostic indicators for SJS-TEN are delay in referral to a burn unit, larger total body surface area involvement (TBSA), and older age.

Emergency physicians and the emergency department (ED) team form an important portal to health care. Often the first line in the chain of care, the team is frequently faced with perplexing and demanding challenges of di-agnosis and treatment, and nowhere is that more apparent than in life-threatening dermatologic conditions, especially as related to the elderly population. Although rare, toxic epidermal necrolysis (TEN), also known as *Lyell's syndrome,* and Stevens-Johnson syndrome (SJS) are destructive, most often medication-induced autoimmune responses that lead to large areas of denuded skin and a subsequent high mortality. The number of ED presentations of SJS-TEN will increase with the increasing elderly population and their use of multiple medications.

It is first important to recognize this disease, which until recently has not been well distinguished from other disorders, such as erythema multiforme (EM), also known as *erythema exudativum multiforme* and *hypersensitivity syndrome.* In a series of case-controlled studies, distinct patterns have been identified, and improved classification has emerged. EM is now thought to be entirely caused by the herpes simplex virus (HSV). It occurs rarely after age 40 and is histopathologically distinct from SJS-TEN. Hypersensitivity syndrome, although clinically related, is also histopathologically distinct.[1,2]

SJS and TEN are gradations of a syndrome in which an autoimmune response to medication causes a disruption of the dermal-epidermal junction; however, less frequently, SJS can have an infectious cause.[2] In patients with this disease there is extensive cutaneous and mucocutaneous involvement. SJS-TEN begins as a flat, irregular macular rash and quickly progresses to large coalescing bullae with a positive Nikolsky sign.[1] This leads to sloughing of large areas of epidermis. The current classification considers 10 percent or less involvement of the body surface area (BSA) to be SJS. A 30 percent or greater involvement of the BSA is considered TEN. With between 10 and 30 percent BSA involvement, there is SJS-TEN overlap.[2,3] For the purpose of this chapter, SJS-TEN will be discussed as one entity. Since EM is extremely rare over age 40, it will not be discussed. Other bullous diseases, e.g., bullous pemphigoid and pemhigus vulgaris, are discussed in Chap. 54.

EPIDEMIOLOGY

Difficulties exist in studying the epidemiology of SJS-TEN. First, the disease entity is rare, and thus any large case-series, case-control, or population-based studies had to be conducted in large geographic areas and over long periods. A limited amount of clinical data are available. Second, during the time of many studies of SJS-TEN, the classification of the disease was still being defined. SJS-TEN occurs in all races and in all parts of the world. The incidence ranges between 0.4 and 1.89 per 1 million people, and the disease has been studied extensively in the United States,[5] France,[6] Germany,[4] and Asia.[7]

There seems to be a distinct preponderance of SJS-TEN in older patients. Two studies show a higher incidence of TEN in the elderly, with one study demonstrating an increased risk among females as well.[8] A 5-year retrospective study found that the incidence of TEN was 2.7 times higher among the elderly, and the mortality rate for the this population was twice as high as that in younger patients (51 versus 25 percent).[9] The mean age of patients who died from TEN was 64.5 years versus a mean age of 47.5 years for those who survived.[10] The incidence is also increased in patients with immunodeficiency syndromes.[11,12] This may become a factor in the elderly population as patients with HIV infection live longer.

PATHOPHYSIOLOGY

The exact pathophsysiologic process for SJS-TEN is not known. There are multiple etiologies for this disease complex, but the two main concepts are a defect in the metabolism of patients who develop the syndrome and that medications induce an immune cytotoxic response that results in cell death.[13] The pathogenic factors of SJS and TEN include medications, infections, immunizations, graft-versus-host disease, and even herbal remedies. In some cases there is no identifiable cause. The leading contributing feature is medications in over 95 percent of cases of TEN and in 50 percent of cases of SJS.[14] There are many factors that impede identification of the causative agent, including multiple use of medications, delay in diagnosis, and lack of an in vitro or clinical test. In many cases the diagnosis represents a consultant's best guess and the coincidence of an etiologic agent with the syndrome. The inventory of offending drugs has grown to greater then 100. Case-control studies have elucidated the relative risk of certain medication groups and some specific drugs. The three primary classes that have an increased risk for inducing SJS-TEN are antibiotics, anticonvulsants, and nonsteroidal anti-inflammatory drugs (NSAIDs). For short-course medications, the prolonged-half-life sulfa-containing antibiotics, specifi-

cally trimethoprim-sulfamethoxazole, are at the top of the list of offending agents.[15] Other antibiotics found to be of higher risk are quinolones, cephalosporins, and aminopenicillins. Anticonvulsants such as phenytoin, carbamazipine, and valproic acid also have a increased relative risk.[15] The most recent class of drugs implicated is the oxicam NSAIDs. Potentially offending drugs are allopurinol and corticosteroids. It is surprising that corticosteroids are implicated in SJS-TEN. This is important in that systemic corticosteroids are useful early in the treatment of hypersensitivity syndrome but can, in fact, worsen TEN if they are given late in the course of the disease.[2] Infectious causes are rare, but multiple case reports have been cited, with the most common infectious agent being *Mycoplasma pneumoniae.*[16]

The most pressing predisposition for developing SJS-TEN in the elderly population is increased medication use. With the increasing population of elders, more cases of SJS-TEN will be seen. It has been suggested that affected patients may have a defective metabolism of the offending drug. A link between sulfonamide-induced TEN and patients who are slow acetylators has been shown.[17] However, it is not clear if this defect is familial, but there have been associations with HLA gene expression.[15] It also has been shown that there is an increased risk for those patients with HIV-1 infection.[12,18]

SJS-TEN is thought to be a cytotoxic immune response that results in the destruction and apoptosis of keratinocytes.[19] These keratinocytes become necrotic intermittently along the dermal-epidermal junction. There is a release of multiple cytokines that contributes to fever and other metabolic derangements, such as anemia and leukopenia.[20] The necrotic keratinocytes coalesce and lead to disruption of the dermal-epidermal junction, which in turn leads to the distinctive clinical feature of large areas of sloughing skin up to or greater than 50 percent of the total body surface area (TBSA).[20] The mechanism by which drugs induce this cytotoxic attack is not clear. It is postulated that the drugs and/or their metabolites induce an antigenic response of the keratinocytes by acting as haptens.[21]

While the skin is the primary organ system involved with extensive cutaneous and mucocutaneous blistering and desquamating, other organ systems are often involved. All organs with epithelium are susceptible, such as the eye and organs of the gastrointestinal, respiratory, and genitourinary systems. SJS-TEN is thus a multisystem entity. It can involve the gastrointestinal and esophageal mucosae, leading to dysphagia and an inability to eat. The respiratory system can be involved with traceobronchial erosions and respiratory compromise.

There are also renal effects, including acute tubular necrosis and glomerulonephritis.[22] Ophthamologic consequences can be moderate (with conjunctival irritation) to severe, resulting in blindness.[22]

After a few initial lesions appear, the full appearance of the disease occurs 4 to 6 days later. The hospital course can last from 6 to 67 days. Hospitalization is often prolonged, averaging 31 days for elderly survivors.[23] The mortality ranges between 30 and 60 percent, with most studies reporting a higher mortality for older patients.[9,10] The predictors of poor prognosis are age and extent and rapidity of body surface involvement. Referral to a burn unit has been recommended and reported to improve survival.[10,24] However, one study found that there was no significant improvement in mortality with early as opposed to delayed referral.[23]

CLINICAL FEATURES

Most SJS-TEN patients present without ambulance transport. For the few patients who present with extensive disease requiring critical-care transport to a burn unit, most of the considerations that apply to burn transports will be applicable. These patients may require supplemental oxygen for airway involvement, temperature regulation, intravenous fluid replacement, medications for pain control, aseptic technique, and careful avoidance of adhesives. Most patients will present with a chief complaint of a rash that begins as a painful and burning cutaneous eruption. The rash begins on the face, neck, and shoulders and eventually extends to the entire body, particularly the trunk and proximal extremities. The early lesions are described as atypical targets. They are irregular macules with purpuric centers. These lesions extend over 4 to 5 days but sometimes quicker, within hours. There is formation of large bullae that coalesce, leading to the large areas of sloughing skin and desquamation. The Nikolsky sign is present, and skin is dislodged easily by pressure in the erythematous areas in between bullae. The examiner wiping a finger over the reddened area will dislodge a thin pile of epidermis. TBSA involvement varies and can be up to 100 percent in some patients, with a mean of 70 percent.[13] There is erosive mucosal involvement starting with the oropharynx, followed by ocular and then by anogenital involvement in that order of frequency. Patients complain of dry, burning, painful eyes and photophobia. Ocular consequences range in intensity and can be severe, including fibrous band formation and symblepharon. Severe corneal involvement can lead to scarring and epithealization of the cornea and even blindness.

The problems experienced by elderly patients with SJS-TEN are linked to their underlying comorbitites. For patients who already may have sensory impairment from decreased vision and hearing, severe skin pain and increased anxiety can lead to difficult management issues. Secondary to pervasive skin loss, there is extensive fluid loss and electrolyte imbalance that can lead to prerenal azotemia, as seen in extensive burns. This is a particularly difficult management issue in elderly patients who have preexisting renal or cardiac dysfunction. Persistent cough and shortness of breath can herald involvement of the respiratory system. Sloughing in the trachea and brochi may progress to adult respiratory distress syndrome. Involvement of the respiratory system is a poor prognostic sign, in particular in elder patients who may have COPD or restrictive lung disease and a decreased vital capacity and forced expiratory volume in 1 second (FEV_1).[13] Respiratory involvement may be devastating, and an emergent oral tracheal or surgical airway may be an ED imperative in patients with delayed presentations. Diarrhea, melena, and abdominal pain may be an indication of involvement of the gastrointestinal system. Gastrointestinal bleeding can occur but is rarely the initial presentation. Loss of protective barriers leaves patients vulnerable to infection. However, fever is a common associated symptom, and it may develop without an underlying infection.

The key historical points to consider are medications, especially those which have been started within the month prior to presentation. Particular attention should be paid to antibiotics (specifically long-acting sulfonamides), anticonvulsants, and NSAIDs. It is also important to time the onset of disease because delay in presentation can be an indication of poor prognosis. SJS-TEN is a clinical diagnosis that is relatively distinct on initial presentation.

Early SJS, in which there is less skin involvement, may be confused with other drug eruptions, but for the most part, SJS-TEN is a clinically discrete entity. The early syndrome can be identified by two components: (1) the severe skin pain and tenderness of the early macular lesions and (2) a positive Nikolsky sign. Once SJS-TEN reaches maximum desquamation, there are only a few other syndromes that need to be considered. Staphylococcal scalded skin syndrome is clinically similar to TEN but occurs almost entirely in children.[1] There is a more superficial sloughing, and the separation occurs at the subcorneal layer of the epidermis.[22] The diagnosis can be confirmed by biopsy. The differential diagnosis of SJS-TEN also includes EM with mucous membrane involvement. This entity can be differentiated by the Nikolsky sign. The Nikolsky sign is not present in EM, and this dis-

Table 53-1. Differential Diagnosis of SJS-TEN

Burns
Exfoliate dermatitis
Hypersensitivity syndrome
Bullous pemphigoid
Paraneoplastic pemphigus
Bullous fixed drug eruption
Staphyloccal scalded skin syndrome
Erythema multiforme

ease is extremely rare past age 40. When mucocutaneous and cutaneous lesions are present, the differential diagnosis includes hypersensitivity syndrome, bullous pemphigoid, paraneoplastic pemphigus, and pemphigus vulgaris. These disease entities can be difficult to differentiate from SJS-TEN because the Nikolsky sign is positive. Early dermatologic consultation and biopsy with immunofluorescence straining of tissue samples will make diagnosis. When seeking the cause in patients with a syndrome compatible with SJS-TEN, the emergency physicians also must considered burns and caustic ingestions such as boric acid (Table 53-1). Fortunately, scarring is rare with this disorder as opposed to other bullous diseases of the elderly.

EMERGENCY DEPARTMENT CARE AND DISPOSITION

ED care of SJS-TEN can be equated to burn care in the elderly, with some differences in fluid management. Diagnosis and appropriate referral of early SJS-TEN to a burn care or intensive care unit are essential. Although controversy exists, rapid referral to a specialized unit that can manage this dermatologic emergency can lead to improved mortality.[10,24]

The initial priorities with SJS-TEN in the elderly should include pain management and determination of major fluid and electrolyte imbalances. Fluids should be replaced intravenously, and peripheral access is recommended. These intravenous sites should be away from the affected areas. SJS-TEN is equivalent to deep partial-thickness burns and may not require the same fluid replacement as third-degree burns. Prevention of hypothermia should be a consideration as well. If one is available in the ED, an isolation room with temperature control should be used for the patient so that an increased room temperature can be maintained.

Routinely advised laboratory tests include a complete blood count (CBC), a chemistry profile, a chest x-ray, and a coagulation profile. Although routine laboratory tests aid in the confirmation, there are associated laboratory abnormalities with this syndrome. Almost all patients are found to be anemic. Neutropenia is present in up to 30 percent of patients. Thombocytopenia also may be present. Both neutropenia and thombocytopenia have been found to indicate poor prognosis.[10,13] SJS-TEN usually results in an elevated erythrocyte sedimentation rate and an increased white blood cell (WBC) count. There also may be elevations in the liver transaminases and electrolyte imbalances similar to burns. Blood cultures are also important, particularly in patients with delayed presentation or fever. Sepsis is the primary cause of death in these patients, and blood cultures are important tools in determining antibiotic use. Most patients have fever and leukocytosis, so these tests cannot be used as evidence of infection.

Early determination of airway involvement is crucial. A controlled intubation is preferred before there is bleeding and glottic or pharyngeal edema.[10] Tools and techniques for management of a difficult airway should be available. Preparation for conversion to a surgical airway should be undertaken prior to standard elective intubation.

Ideal disposition should be to a burn unit, which has distinct advantages over other types of units, for the treatment of SJS-TEN. These units have experience with skin care, aseptic technique, and prevention of bacterial contamination. No definitive treatment exists for SJS-TEN, only supportive care. There is also significant disagreement concerning the use of specific dressings and the use of porcine and artificial grafts. The most important factor appears to be the removal of all possible offending medications. Early withdrawal of the culprit drug decreases mortality.[25] Fluid and electrolyte replacement and timely disposition to a burn unit also may improve outcome.[10] Early dermatologic consultation may be required to avoid misdiagnosis and to initiate appropriate therapy.

Intravenous immunoglobulin (IVIG), plasmopheresis, intravenous cyclosporin A, and intravenous *N*-acetyl-cyctein (NAC) are therapies under study as treatments for SJS-TEN. These treatments have been advocated in order to limit the extent of epidermal detachment and show promise, but they must be studied further to confirm their usefulness.[26] The use of systemic steroids is not without consequence and has not proven useful. Further study is necessary before they can be recommended.[13,27] Plasmopheresis also shows promise but remains experimental until trials are completed.

REFERENCES

1. Freedberg IM, Fitzpatrick TB: *Fitzpatrick's Dermatology in General Medicine,* 5th ed. New York: McGraw-Hill, 1999.

2. Roujeau JC: Stevens-Johnson syndrome and toxic epidermal necrolysis are severity variants of the same disease which differs from erythema multiforme. *J Dermatol* 24(11):726, 1997.

3. Kelly JP, Auquier A, Rzany B, et al: An international collaborative case-control study of severe cutaneous adverse reactions (SCAR): Design and methods. *J Clin Epidemiol* 48(9):1099, 1995.

4. Rzany B, Mockenhaupt M, Baur S, et al: Epidemiology of erythema exsudativum multiforme majus, Stevens-Johnson syndrome, and toxic epidermal necrolysis in Germany (1990–1992): Structure and results of a population-based registry. *J Clin Epidemiol* 49(7):769, 1996.

5. Chan HL, Stern RS, Arndt KA, et al: The incidence of erythema multiforme, Stevens-Johnson syndrome, and toxic epidermal necrolysis: A population-based study with particular reference to reactions caused by drugs among outpatients. *Arch Dermatol* 126(1):43, 1990.

6. Roujeau JC, Guillaume JC, Fabre JP, et al: Toxic epidermal necrolysis (Lyell syndrome) : Incidence and drug etiology in France, 1981–1985. *Arch Dermatol* 126(1):37, 1990.

7. Chan HL: Toxic epidermal necrolysis in Singapore, 1989 through 1993: Incidence and antecedent drug exposure. *Arch Dermatol* 131(10):1212, 1995.

8. Schopf E, Stuhmer A, Rzany B, et al: Toxic epidermal necrolysis and Stevens-Johnson syndrome: An epidemiologic study from West Germany. *Arch Dermatol* 127(6):839, 1991.

9. Bastuji-Garin S, Zahedi M, Guillaume JC, et al: Toxic epidermal necrolysis (Lyell syndrome) in 77 elderly patients. *Age Ageing* 22(6):450, 1993.

10. Schulz JT, Sheridan RL, Ryan CM, et al: A 10-year experience with toxic epidermal necrolysis. *J Burn Care Rehabil* 21(3):199, 2000.

11. Bayard PJ, Berger TG, Jacobson MA: Drug hypersensitivity reactions and human immunodeficiency virus disease. *J Acquir Immune Defic Syndr* 5(12):1237, 1992.

12. Saiag P, Caumes E, Chosidow O, et al: Drug-induced toxic epidermal necrolysis (Lyell syndrome) in patients infected with the human immunodeficiency virus. *J Am Acad Dermatol* 26(4):567, 1992.

13. Wolkenstein P Revuz J: Toxic epidermal necrolysis. *Dermatol Clin* 18(3):485, 2000.

14. Revuz J: New advances in severe adverse drug reactions. *Dermatol Clin* 19(4):697, 2001.

15. Roujeau JC, Kelly JP, Naldi L, et al: Medication use and the risk of Stevens-Johnson syndrome or toxic epidermal necrolysis. *New Engl J Med* 333(24):1600, 1995.

16. Tay YK, Huff JC, Weston WL: *Mycoplasma pneumoniae* infection is associated with Stevens-Johnson syndrome, not erythema multiforme (von Hebra). *J Am Acad Dermatol* 35(5 pt 1):757, 1996.

17. Wolkenstein P, Revuz J: Drug-induced severe skin reactions: Incidence, management and prevention. *Drug Saf* 13(1):56, 1995.

18. Rzany B, Mockenhaupt M, Stocker U, et al: Incidence of Stevens-Johnson syndrome and toxic epidermal necrolysis in patients with the acquired immunodeficiency syndrome in Germany. *Arch Dermatol* 129(8):1059, 1993.

19. Paul C, Wolkenstein P, Adle H, et al: Apoptosis as a mechanism of keratinocyte death in toxic epidermal necrolysis. *Br J Dermatol* 134(4):710, 1996.

20. Roujeau JC: Treatment of severe drug eruptions. *J Dermatol* 26(11):718, 1999.

21. Revuz JE, Roujeau JC: Advances in toxic epidermal necrolysis. *Semin Cutan Med Surg* 15(4):258, 1996.

22. Becker DS: Toxic epidermal necrolysis. *Lancet* 351(9113):1417, 1998.

23. Honari S, Gibran NS, Heimbach DM, et al: Toxic epidermal necrolysis (TEN) in elderly patients. *J Burn Care Rehabil* 22(2):132, 2001.

24. McGee T, Munster A: Toxic epidermal necrolysis syndrome: Mortality rate reduced with early referral to regional burn center. *Plast Reconstr Surg* 102(4):1018, 1998.

25. Garcia-Doval I, LeCleach L, Bocquet H, et al: Toxic epidermal necrolysis and Stevens-Johnson syndrome: Does early withdrawal of causative drugs decrease the risk of death? *Arch Dermatol* 136(3):323, 2000.

26. Viard I, Wehrli P, Bullani R, et al: Inhibition of toxic epidermal necrolysis by blockade of CD95 with human intravenous immunoglobulin. *Science* 282(5388):490, 1998.

27. Stern RS: Improving the outcome of patients with toxic epidermal necrolysis and Stevens-Johnson syndrome. *Arch Dermatol* 136(3):410, 2000.

54

Autoimmune Bullous Diseases

Paula F. Moskowitz

HIGH-YIELD FACTS

- Autoantibodies produced in pemphigus induce flaccid blistering of skin and mucosal surfaces with resulting erosions and denuded skin leading to severe morbidity and, potentially death.
- Nikolsky's sign is positive in pemphigus.
- The pemphigus vulgaris antigen has been identified as a 130-kDa glycoprotein.
- Desmoglein-3 is a desmosomal component important in cell-cell adhesion.
- Paraneoplastic pemphigus is associated most commonly with non-Hodgkin's lymphoma and chronic lymphocytic leukemia.
- Treatment of pemphigus includes use of systemic steroids and immunosuppressive agents.

PEMPHIGUS

Pemphigus refers to a group of autoimmune blistering diseases of skin and mucous membranes. The most common form is pemphigus vulgaris. There are several variants: vegetans foliaceus, erythematosus, herpetiformis, paraneoplastic, and (in Brazil) fogo selvagem. These disorders are characterized by the development of blisters and erosions on skin and mucous membranes caused by acantholysis (cell-cell detachment) of epidermal and mucosal epithelial cells. In vivo bound and circulating IgG directed against cell surface antigens of epithelial cells[1-3] causes this epidermal acantholysis. Each type of pemphigus has distinct clinical and immunopathologic features. This chapter will discuss pemphigus vulgaris and paraneoplastic pemphigus because they are the most severe and the most likely to bring elders to the emergency department (ED).

Pemphigus vulgaris (PV), the most common form of pemphigus, predominates in middle-aged and elderly Jews, as well as in persons of Mediterranean origin. It is characterized by flaccid blisters and/or erosions in the oral cavity and on the skin. Patients with extensive disease often appear very ill. Before the advent of glucocorticoids, PV was associated with high morbidity and mortality.

Paraneoplastic pemphigus (PNP) is associated with an underlying neoplasia, most commonly of lymphoproliferative origin.[4,5] It is characterized by painful mucosal ulcerations and polymorphous skin lesions. The clinical course of PNP depends on the behavior of the underlying neoplasia. However, with few exceptions, the disorder tends to progress rapidly and become fatal despite aggressive supportive and immunosuppressive therapy.

Epidemiology

Pemphigus Vulgaris

Several retrospective studies of patients with PV have allowed some general conclusions to be drawn regarding epidemiology.[6-8] The prevalence in men and women appears to be equal, and the mean age of onset is approximately 50 to 60 years. PV is a rare disorder (0.1 to 0.5 cases per 100,000). However, the incidence of the disease depends on the population studied. As stated, PV is more common in Jewish persons and persons of Mediterranean origin, in whom the incidence can be as high as 1.6 per 100,000. Jewish patients with PV have an increased incidence of the HLA-DR4 haplotype.[9] PV is a sporadic disease, but there have been isolated reports of PV occurring in families. Mortality due to PV is approximately 10 percent in the United States.[10]

Paraneoplastic Pemphigus

Since the original description of paraneoplastic pemphigus by Anhalt and colleagues in 1990,[5] more than 70 cases of PNP have been described in the literature.[4] Reported cases include persons of Polish, Japanese, Dutch, Iranian, Hispanic, Bosnian, and American origin. The age of onset is variable and ranges from 7 to 77 years, with a mean age of 51 years. No gender predominance has been noted, and most patients have lymphoproliferative disorders. In the United States, mortality due to paraneoplastic pemphigus approaches 95 percent.

Pathophysiology

Pemphigus Vulgaris

The characteristic histopathologic finding of PV is a split in the epidermis above the basal cell layer with loss of keratinocyte cell-to-cell adhesion, acantholysis. Suprabasal acantholysis leads to blister formation. Direct immunofluorescence demonstrates the hallmark of pemphigus, IgG autoantibodies against the cell surface of keratinocytes in a network-like pattern.[11] In addition, indirect immunofluorescence demonstrates circulating antiepithelial cell surface IgG in 75 percent of patients with PV. Pemphigus antigens are complexes of desmosomal molecules, important in cell-cell adhesion. The PV antigen has been identified as a 130-kDa glycoprotein, desmoglein-3.[3,12] The events that induce autoantibody production are unknown, but suspected culprits are drugs such as D-penicillamine[13] and captopril.[14] In some cases the disease disappears when the drug is withdrawn, but usually it continues even after removal of the initiating agent.[15]

Paraneoplastic Pemphigus

The histopathologic findings in paraneoplastic pemphigus show a unique combination of pemphigus vulgaris–like and erythema multiforme–like histology[16] Direct immunofluorescence reveals IgG and complement deposition along the cell surfaces of epidermal keratinocytes, often with linear/granular deposition along the dermal-epidermal basement membrane zone. Indirect immunofluorescence demonstrates circulating IgG antibodies that bind the cell surface of skin and mucosa in a pattern similar to that of pemphigus but in addition bind to simple columnar and transitional epithelia. Circulating autoantibodies recognize a unique set of epidermal antigens including desmoglein-3 and other cell proteins.[4]

Most patients presenting with PNP have lymphoproliferative disorders. Approximately 80 percent of all cases are linked to just three neoplasms: non-Hodgkin's lymphoma, chronic lymphocytic leukemia, and Castleman's disease.[17] In most cases the malignancy is identified before onset of the mucocutaneous eruption, which may occur during or after treatment. However, the eruption may be a symptom of an occult neoplasm. Thus examination for an occult neoplasm is important in suspected cases of PNP. Computed tomographic (CT) scanning of the chest, abdomen, and pelvis may be undertaken in the hospital. The actual cause of PNP is unclear. Multiple theories have been postulated and include an antitumor immune response that cross-reacts with normal epithelial proteins and dysregulated cytokine production by tumor cells.[17]

Clinical Features

Pemphigus Vulgaris

The primary lesion of PV is a flaccid blister that may occur anywhere on normal or erythematous skin. The blisters are fragile, and intact blisters are not seen commonly because of their tendency to spread by peripheral extension; ruptured blisters leave erosions that are often painful and large. This characteristic finding in pemphigus patients can be elicited by applying lateral pressure to normal-appearing skin at the periphery of an active lesion. The resulting shearing away of the epidermis, known as the *Nikolsky sign,* is characteristic but not diagnostic of pemphigus. Nikolsky's sign can be seen in other active blistering diseases, including bullous pemphigoid, erythema multiforme, Stevens-Johnson syndrome, and toxic epidermal necrolysis. Substantial portions of the body surface may be denuded in severe cases of PV. Lesions usually heal without scarring, except at sites complicated by secondary infection or mechanically induced dermal wounds. The skin lesions in PV typically appear on the scalp, face, neck, axilla, trunk, and oral cavity. In approximately 50 to 70 percent of patients, oral lesions are the initial presenting sign and may precede the skin lesions by an average of 5 months.[6–8] If oral involvement is not present initially, most patients will develop oral lesions during the course of the disease. Painful erosions are seen commonly on the oral mucosa, causing an inability to eat or drink and contributing to malnutrition and severe debilitation, as seen in untreated patients. Erosions may spread to involve the larynx and pharynx with subsequent hoarseness. Involvement of other mucous membranes has been reported, including conjunctivae, rectum, urethra, cervix, labia, and esophagus.[8,18–20]

Paraneoplastic Pemphigus

This disease is unique and clinically, histologically, and immunopathologically different from other forms of pemphigus. Clinically, PNP patients are ill-appearing and present with painful erosions and ulcerations involving oral, genital, and conjunctival mucosal surfaces. The most constant clinical feature is the presence of intractable stomatitis, which is usually the earliest presenting sign. The stomatitis consists of painful erosions and ulcerations of the vermilion borders of the lips and oropharynx. Cutaneous lesions are polymorphous and often pruritic, seen as confluent erythema on the chest and back, with vesicles, bullae, and erosions. Nikolsky's sign may be positive. Erythematous papules on the trunk and extremities often ensue, forming targetoid lesions with central bullae resembling erythema multiforme. Palmar and plantar surface involvement is encountered commonly as well. Ocular involvement includes conjunctival hyperemia, diffuse papillary tarsal conjunctival reaction, and pseudomembranous conjunctivitis, often resulting in scarring and synblepharon formation.[5,21] Involvement of esophageal, gastrointestinal, tracheal, and bronchial mucosa has been reported.[21,22]

Diagnosis and Differential

Pemphigus Vulgaris

A diagnosis of pemphigus should be based on a combination of the following clinical, histologic, and immunopathologic findings: (1) clinical findings of flaccid blisters and erosions on the skin and/or oral mucosa, (2) histologic examination of affected skin revealing characteristic intraepidermal clefting and acantholysis (cell-cell separation), and (3) direct immunoflurescence of perilesional skin demonstrating IgG deposition in a characteristic network-like pattern on keratinocyte cell surfaces.

In the ED, the clinical findings of erosions and/or flaccid blisters in an older patient should prompt dermatologist consultation. When only oral lesions are present, the differential diagnosis includes apthous stomatitis, herpes simplex, erosive lichen planus, erythema multiforme, Behçet's disease, and cicatricial pemphigoid. When both oral and cutaneous lesions are present, the differential diagnosis includes Stevens-Johnson syndrome, toxic epidermal necrolysis. drug hypersensitivity syndrome, paraneoplasic pemphigus, and other autoimmune blistering diseases such as bullous pemphigoid.

Paraneoplastic Pemphigus

Diagnostic criteria were proposed initially by Anhalt and colleagues[5] based on clinical, histopathologic, and immuno logic data and modified by Camisa and Helm.[23] The major criteria include polymorphous mucocutaneous eruption, concurrent internal neoplasia, and characteristic serum immunoprecipitation findings. The differential diagnosis of PNP includes blistering disorders of the skin and mucous membranes, including Stevens-Johnson syndrome, toxic epidermal necrolysis, drug hypersensitivity syndrome, pemphigus vulgaris, and other autoimmune blistering diseases, such as bullous pemphigoid, linear IgA bullous dermatosis, and epidermolysis bullosa acquisita.

Emergency Department Care and Disposition

Pemphigus Vulgaris

Acute treatment in the ED consists of supportive care with intravenous fluids, correction of electrolyte disturbance, correction of hypothermia by passive warming, and pain control. In a febrile, seriously ill patient, skin lesions may be a manifestation of sepsis. A lesion should be opened and its contents Gram stained and cultured. Appropriate antibiotics for skin pathogens such as *Staphylococcus* and *Streptococcus* should be used when secondary skin infection is suspected. Early consultation with a dermatologist may be necessary to avoid misdiagnosis and inappropriate treatment. The goal of therapy in pemphigus is directed toward reducing synthesis of pathogenic autoantibodies. This is accomplished by the use of systemic corticosteroids as the first-line therapy—usually prednisone (1–2 mg/kg/day)—and later immunosuppressive agents. Combination therapy includes the use of oral immunosuppressive agents, such as azathioprine, mycophenylate mofetil,[24,25] and cyclophosphamide as steroid-sparing agents, and is advised for long-term control.[26] These agents are especially useful in elderly patients who are at high risk for osteoporosis and other corticosteroid-induced adverse effects. Other immunomodulatory agents (such as methotrexate, cyclosporine, intravenous immunoglobulin, and gold) have shown inconsistent results in PV patients.[27]

Pemphigus vulgaris is a chronic, severely debilitating disease that can be life-threatening. Prior to the availability of glucocorticoids, the mortality ranged from 60 to 90 percent. The use of systemic glucocorticoids and immunosuppressive therapy has improved the prognosis of pemphigus dramatically; however, significant morbidity and mortality still exist. Sepsis is often the cause of death. Immunosuppressive therapy is often a contributing factor. Poor prognostic factors include advanced age, widespread involvement, and the requirement for high doses of glucocorticoids to control the disease process.[8,28] Most deaths occur during the first few years of the disease. If the patient survives 5 years, the prognosis is excellent. With glucocorticoid and immunosuppressive therapy, the mortality is 10 percent or less.[10,29]

Paraneoplastic Pemphigus

The initial ED management is similar to that of pemphigus vulgaris. Supportive care with intravenous fluids, correction of electrolyte disturbances, airway evaluation, correction of hypothermia by passive warming, and pain control are the mainstay of treatment. If PNP is suspected, physicians should obtain a history and perform a physical examination directed at detecting the underlying malignancy. Additional studies such as CT scanning of the chest, abdomen, and pelvis may be indicated subsequently. Again, early consultation with a dermatologist may be necessary.

Once a diagnosis of PNP is made, treatment is very difficult. Removal of a benign neoplasm, such as Castleman's tumor, leads to substantial improvement or clearance of the skin disease.[30] There is no consensus on a standard, effective therapeutic regimen. Treatment of the underlying malignancy and the use of systemic corticosteroids, cyclophosphamide, azathioprine, cyclosporine, gold, dapsone, plasmaphoresis, and photophoresis have met with limited success. Although the skin lesions may improve with therapy, the mucosal lesions are especially resistant. With its associated malignancy, PNP is progressive and almost always fatal within 2 years. Respiratory failure, clinically resembling bronchiolitis obliterans, is often the cause of death.[31]

BULLOUS PEMPHIGOID

Bullous pemphigoid (BP) is one of a group of autoimmune blistering disorders characterized clinically by thick-walled, tense blisters and histologically by a separation between the epidermis and dermis at the basement membrane zone. BP is the most common autoimmune blistering skin disease. Clinical features include tense blisters on the trunk and extremities with predilection for intertriginous areas. In general, patients have a benign course with low morbidity and mortality. BP is highly responsive to oral corticosteroids.

Epidemiology

BP is mainly a disease of the elderly, with the majority of patients past 60 years of age at presentation.[18,32] The incidence is approximately 7 cases per 1 million population,[33] and the prevalence of BP is increasing with the aging population in the United States. There is no known racial, ethnic, or gender predominance.[34]

Pathophysiology

The characteristic histopathologic finding is a subepidermal blister with an eosinophil-rich inflammatory infil-

trate. Direct immunofluorescence of perilesional skin reveals linear IgG and C3 at the basement membrane.[35] Indirect immunofluorescence demonstrates circulating autoantibodies in 70 to 80 percent of patients' sera.[36] Autoantibodies in BP target proteins in the hemidesmosome, an organelle thought to be important in anchoring the basal cell to the basement membrane. The target antigen proteins are BPAg1 (230 kDa) and BPAg2 (180 kDa) and have been well characterized at the molecular level.[37,38]

Clinical Features

Clinically, BP is characterized by large, tense blisters rising on erythematous or normal-appearing skin. The blisters may occur anywhere on the skin but with a predilection for the lower abdomen, flexor surfaces of the extremities, and anterior or inner thighs.[34] Unlike pemphigus, blisters do not expand peripherally, and Nikolsky's sign is negative. Blisters and erosions heal with hyperpigmentation but without scarring. Patients often complain of pruritus, and urticaria-like lesions may be the cutaneous finding early in the course of the disease.

Mucous membrane lesions are uncommon and occur in approximately 10 to 35 percent of patients.[18,32] Any mucosal lesions usually are limited to oral cavity, especially the buccal mucosa. Erosions, not intact blisters, are seen commonly. Unlike erythema multiforme and PNP, the vermilion border of the lips is rarely involved.

BP is often a self-limited disease lasting from months to years. Approximately half of treated patients will go into remission within 2.5 to 6 years of onset of disease. However, for some individuals the disease may continue for 10 or more years.

Diagnosis and Differential

A diagnosis of BP should be based on a combination of the following clinical, histologic, and immunopathologic findings: (1) clinical findings of tense blisters arising on erythematous or normal-appearing skin, (2) histologic examination of affected skin revealing a subepidermal blister with an eosinophil-rich inflammatory infiltrate, and (3) direct immunoflurescence of perilesional skin demonstrating linear IgG and C3 along the basement membrane. The differential diagnosis of BP includes several subepidermal blistering diseases, including cicatricial pemphigoid, epidermolysis bullosa acquisita, bullous drug eruption, bullous lupus erythematosus, dermatitis herpetiformis, and linear IgA bullous dermatosis. Based on histology and immunofluorescence, BP can be distinguished readily from most other bullous eruptions. The most difficult diseases to differentiate from BP are cicatricial pemphigoid and epidermolysis bullosa acquisita; both these disorders have characteristic distributions of lesions. Unlike BP, cicatricial pemphigoid affects mucous membranes almost exclusively. Cicatricial pemphigoid often presents in the elderly and is characterized by desquamative gingivitis and inflammation and scarring of the conjunctiva. Large, tense blisters are not usually seen. Epidermolysis bullosa acquisita is a scarring disease of skin primarily affecting trauma-prone extensor surfaces such as the knuckles, dorsal hands, elbows, knees, and ankles.

Emergency Department Care and Disposition

Dermatologic consultation may be helpful in the differential diagnosis of a patient presenting with tense blisters in the ED setting. A careful drug history should be obtained. Laboratory testing may be helpful if the diagnosis of bullous systemic lupus erythematosus is being considered. Appropriate tests, such as skin biopsy, should be performed but usually can wait until referral is completed as an outpatient. If conjunctival involvement is present, a diagnosis of cicatricial pemphigoid should be considered, and early opthamological consultation is advised. Once the diagnosis is established, the mainstay of therapy for BP is corticosteroids. Localized BP often can be treated successfully with potent topical glucocorticoids alone. More extensive disease responds rapidly to oral prednisone.[39] However, in elderly patients the complications of systemic glucocorticoid therapy (such as osteoporosis, diabetes, and immunosupression) may be severe. Thus limiting the total dose and duration of therapy is paramount. Immunosupressive agents such as azathioprine may be used for steroid-sparing effects. Recent studies have described successful treatment of BP with a regimen of tetracycline (2 g/day) alone or in conjunction with niacinamide (1.5–2.5 g/day).[40–42]

REFERENCES

1. Nousari H Anhalt G: Pemphigus and bullous pemphigoid. *Lancet* 354(9179):667, 1999.
2. Stanley J: Pemphigus, in Freedberg I, et al (eds): *Fitzpatrick's Dermatology in General Medicine*. New York, McGraw-Hill, 1999, p 654.
3. Udey MC Stanley JR: Pemphigus: Diseases of antidesmosomal autoimmunity. *JAMA* 282(6):572, 1999.
4. Robinson N, Hashimoto T, Amagai M, et al: The new pemphigus variants. *J Am Acad Dermatol* 40(5 pt 1):649, 1999.
5. Anhalt G, Kim S, Stanley J, et al: Paraneoplastic pemphigus: An autoimmune mucocutanoeus disease associated with neoplasia. *New Engl J Med* 323(25):1729, 1990.
6. Krain L: Pemphigus: Epidemiologic and survival characteristics of 59 patients. *Arch Dermatol* 110:862, 1974.
7. Pisanti S, Sharav Y, Kaufman E, et al: Pemphigus vulgaris: Incidence in Jews of different ethnic groups, according to age, sex, and initial lesion. *Oral Surg Oral Med Oral Pathol* 38:382, 1974.
8. Rosenberg F, Sanders S, Nelson C: Pemphigus: A 20-year review of 107 patients treated with corticosteroids. *Arch Dermatil*, 112:962, 1976.
9. Ahmed A, Yunis E, Khatri K, et al: Major histocompatibility complex haplotype studies in Ashkenazi Jewish patients with pemphigus vulgaris. *Proc Natl Acad Sci USA* 87(19):7658, 1991.
10. Carson P: Influence of treatment on the clinical course of pemphigus vulgaris. *J Am Acad Dermatol* 34:645, 1996.
11. Beutner E, Lever W, Witebsky E: Autoantibodies in pemphigus vulgaris: Response to an intercellular substance of epidermis. *JAMA* 192:682, 1965.
12. Amagai M, Klaus-Kovtun V, Stanley J: Autoantibodies against a novel epithelial cadherin in pemphigus vulgaris: A disease of cell adhesion. *Cell* 67:869, 1991.
13. Korman N, Eyre R, Zone J: Drug-induced pemphigus. *J Invest Dermatol* 96:273, 1991.
14. Katz R, Hood A, Anhalt G: Pemphigus-like eruption from captopril. *Arch Dermatol* 123:20, 1987.
15. Anhalt G, Diaz L: Prospects for autoimmune disease: Research advances in pemphigus. *JAMA* 285(5):652, 2001.
16. Horn T, Anhalt G: Histologic features of paraneoplastic pemphigus. *Arch Dermatol* 128:1091, 1992.
17. Anhalt G: Paraneoplastic pemphigus, in *Advances in Dermatology*, St Louis, Mosby-Year Book, 1997, p 77.
18. Lever W: *Pemphigus and Pemphigoid.* Springfield, IL, Charles C. Thomas, 1965.
19. Hodak E, Kremmer L, David M, et al: Conjunctival involvement in pemphigus vulgaris: A clinical, histopathological and immunofluorescence studt. *Br J Dermatol* 123:615, 1990.
20. Trattner A, Lurie R, Leiser A, et al: Esophageal involvement in pemphigus vulgaris: A clinical, histologic, and immunopathologic study. *J Am Acad Dermatol* 24:223, 1991.
21. Lam S, Stone M, Goeken J, et al: Paraneoplastic pemphigus, cicatricial conjunctivitis, and acanthosis nigracans with patchy dermatoglyphy in a parient with bronchogenic squamous cell carcinoma. *Ophthalmology* 99:108, 1992.
22. Fullerton S, Woodley D, Smoller B, et al: Paraneoplastic pemphigus with autoantibody deposition in bronchial epithelium after autologous bone marrow transplantation. *JAMA* 267:1500, 1992.

23. Camisa C Helm T: Paraneoplastic pemphigus is a distinct neoplasia-induced autoimmune disease. *Arch Dermatol* 129:883, 1993.

24. Nousari H, Sragovich A, Kimyai-Asadi A: Mycophenylate mofetil in autoimmune and inflammatory skin disorders. *J Am Acad Dermatol* 40:265, 1999.

25. Enk A, Knop J: Mycophenylate is effective in the treatment of prmphigus vulgaris. *Arch Dermatol* 135:54, 1999.

26. Stanley J: Therapy of pemphigus vulgaris. *Arch Dermatol* 135:76, 1999.

27. Nousari HC, Anhalt GJ: Autoimmune bullous diseases. *Curr Probl Dermatol* (January-February):17, 2000.

28. Lever W, White H: Treatment of pemphigus with corticosteroids: Results obtained in 46 patients over a period of 11 years. *Arch Dermatol* 87:12, 1963.

29. Bystryn J, Steinman N: The adjuvant therapy of pemphigus. *Arch Dermatol* 132:203, 1996.

30. Mutasim D, Pelc N, Anhalt G: Paraneoplastic pemphigus. *Dermatol Clin* 11(3):473, 1993.

31. Nousari H, Deterding R,Wojtczack H: The mechanisms of respiratory failure in paraneoplasic pemphigus. *New Engl J Med* 340:1406, 1999.

32. Rook A, Waddington E: Pemphigus and pemphigoid. *Br J Dermatol* 65:425, 1953.

33. Yancey K, Egan C: Pemphigoid: Clinical, histologic, immunopathologic, and therapeutic considerations. *JAMA* 284(3):350, 2000.

34. Stanley J: Bullous pemphigoid, in Freedberg I, et al (eds): *Fitzpatrick's Dermatology in General Medicine*, Vol I. New York, McGraw-Hill, 1999, p 666.

35. Jordan R, Beutner E, Witebsky E: Basement zone antibodies in bullous pemphigoid. *JAMA* 200:751, 1967.

36. Beutner E, Jordan R, Chorzelski T: The immunopathology of pemphigus and bullous pemphigoid. *J Invest Dermatol* 51(2):63, 1968.

37. Mutasim D, Morrison L, Takahashi Y, et al: Definition of bullous pemphigoid antibody binding to intracellular and extracellular antigen associated with hemidesmosomes. *J Invest Dermatol* 92(2):225, 1989.

38. Stanley J, Hawley-Nelson P, Yuspa S, et al: Characterization of bullous pemphigoid antigen: A unique basement membrane protein of stratifies squamous epithelia. *Cell* 24(3):897, 1981.

39. Fine J-D: Management of acquired bullous skin diseases. *New Engl J Med* 333(22):1475, 1995.

40. Berk M, Lorincz A: The treatment of bullous pemphigoid with tetracycline and niacinamide: A preliminary report. *Arch Dermatol* 122:670, 1986.

41. Fivenson D, Breneman D, Rosen G, et al: Nicotinamide and tetracycline therapy of bullous pemphigoid. *Arch Dermatol* 130(6):753, 1994.

42. Thomas I, Khorenian S, Arbesfeld D: Treatment of generalized bullous pemphigoid with oral tetracycline. *J Am Acad Dermatol* 28(1):74, 1993.

55

Zoster

Matthew A. Kopp

HIGH-YIELD FACTS

- Pain usually precedes the lesions by 1 to 3 days and is the most common reason patients seek medical attention.[1]
- Pain preceding herpes can be misdiagnosed as cardiac ischemia, renal colic, or another malady.[2]
- Pain that lasts longer than 1 month after resolution of the rash is considered postherpetic neuralgia.[2,3]
- Antiviral medications given within 72 hours of the onset of rash decrease the duration of postherpetic neuralgia.[4,5]
- Postherpetic neuralgia occurs in up to 75 percent of patients who develop herpes zoster and who are 70 years of age and older.[6]
- The role of steroids in the treatment of postherpetic neuralgia remains controversial in the literature.[6,7]
- Patients are contagious 1 to 2 days prior to the onset of the rash and until all the lesions have crusted over.[8]

As the population continues to mature, approximately 17 percent of the U.S. population will be over age 65 by the year 2003.[6] As a result of several physiologic changes that occur with aging, elders are more susceptible to infection than are their younger counterparts.[9,10] Several factors play a role in placing the geriatric population at higher risk for infection. As an individual ages, the immune system becomes less effective[2] (see Chap. 9). In addition, changes in both behavior and choice of climate contribute to an increased susceptibility to various infections. Sun exposure, which is typical of the warmer climates, increases the risk of viral stimulation.[11] Older patients may develop herpes zoster (HZ, or "shingles") as a result of their diminished cellular immunity. The HZ virus initially causes chickenpox and then becomes latent in cranial nerves and dorsal root ganglia. HZ reactivates decades later, resulting in shingles.[11,12] Both the acute and chronic sequelae of this disorder can have a profound effect on quality of life.

EPIDEMIOLOGY

In the United States there are approximately 1 million new cases of chicken pox each year.[13] Currently, humans are the only known reservoir for the virus.[8,14] HZ virus has no seasonal, gender, or racial predilection, and by age 18, approximately 95 percent of people in the United States have had contact with the virus.[14] Interestingly, while only 5 percent of chicken pox occurs in adults, 55 percent of varicella-related mortality is seen in the adult group.[15] The lifetime incidence of developing shingles is approximately 10 to 20 percent.[11] This number, however, is likely to change because of introduction of the HZ virus vaccine. Of those affected by shingles, one in five will experience postherpetic neuralgia.

PATHOPHYSIOLOGY

HZ virus belongs to the alphaherpesvirus subfamily, along with herpes simplex viruses 1 and 2. It has a double-stranded DNA core and elicits both a humeral and a cell-mediated immune response.[14] Chicken pox, which is the initial infection caused by HZ virus, usually resolves within 2 weeks. While the rash disappears, the virus migrates to the dorsal root ganglia of multiple dermatomes. The HZ virus genome has been identified in the trigeminal ganglia of nearly all seropositive patients.[2] Herpes zoster is caused by reactivation of the virus previously dormant in the dorsal root ganglia. Person-to-person transmission by individuals infected with herpes zoster occurs via direct contact and rarely through respiratory droplets.[8]

CLINICAL FEATURES

The natural progression of the disease involves a rash with discrete groups of vesicles on an erythematous base in a dermatomal distribution. While any dermatome may be affected, the thoracic nerves are affected most often, followed by the cranial nerves[13] (Fig. 55-1). Initially, the blisters may be described as "dew drops on a rose pedal." The vesicles progress to pustules within 3 days and be-

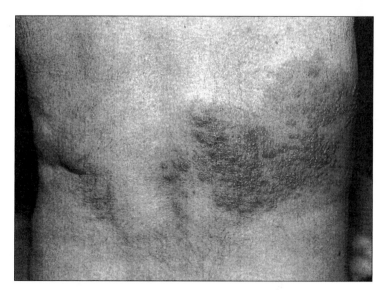

Fig. 55-1 Varicella-zoster virus infection: herpes zoster in T2 dermatome. Grouped and confluent papules, vesicles, and crusted erosions arising in the fourth left cervical dermatome in a healthy 41-year-old female. Pruritus and a burning sensation accompanied the clinical findings. The involvement is relatively mild and can be mistaken for other dermatoses, such as allergic contact dermatitis.

gin to crust over by the fifth day. By 7 to 10 days, all the lesions will have crusted over, and the skin will begin to heal.[11] A burning pain may precede the rash by several days. This condition, known as *prezoster neuralgia,* may not involve the same dermatome as the rash.[12] During the acute reaction, it is common for the patient to experience flulike symptoms. A history of a prodromal phase is more likely to result in a patient who will develop postherpetic neuralgia.[2]

DIAGNOSIS AND DIFFERENTIAL

The diagnosis of shingles generally is made presumptively by recognition of the rash and can be confirmed by performing a Tzanck smear when clinical diagnosis is uncertain. This involves scraping the base of an early lesion and then staining, using hematoxylin and eosin. The Tzanck smear will show multinucleated cells containing acidophilic inclusion bodies. Unfortunately, the Tzanc smear cannot distinguish the varicella-zoster virus from the herpes simplex virus. Direct immunofluorescence of scrapings from a skin lesion is the diagnostic test of choice used to distinguish between viruses.[16] Polymerase chain reaction was used initially to determine if thoracic and trigeminal nerves contain HZ.[12] The rash of the HZ virus can be confused with scabies, erythema multiforme, papular uriticaria, drug eruptions, dermatitis herpetiformis, insect bites, and other viral exanthems.[16]

The prodromal phase is often misdiagnosed as a vari-

ety of common painful disorders. The most common include cardiac ischemia, cholycystitis, muscle strain, cervical spine injury, herniated disk, appendicitis, renal colic, ovarian cysts, and other pathologies.[7,16] In 98 percent of patients, the rash is unilateral, and lesions do not cross the midline. Simultaneous involvement of more than one noncontiguous dermatome is suggestive of an immunocomprimised patient.[11] Unlike herpes simplex, varicella-zoster cannot be cultured from infected dorsal root ganglia.

EMERGENCY DEPARTMENT CARE AND DISPOSITION

When considering treatment options in the elderly, one must consider the convenience of dosing as well as the bioavailability of any medication. Acyclovir, which has been shown to be slightly less effective than valacyclovir and famcyclovir, has to be taken five times per day. It is an analogue of 2'-deoxyguionosine and is converted to acyclovir triphosphate by the enzyme thymidine kinase.[4] It has only 15 percent bioavailability. Famcyclovir and valacyclovir can be taken three times daily due to improved bioavailability.[5,16] Valacyclovir is converted to acyclovir. Famcycovir is a prodrug to pencyclovir, which has a prolonged half-life in infected cells.[17] Headache and gastrointestinal upset are the most common side effects of the three aforementioned antiviral medications. Fortunately, most adverse side effects are mild and well tolerated.[18] For acyclovir-resistant varicella-zoster virus, foscarnet is the drug of choice.[4,8] Foscarnet does not require phosphorolyation to become active. Since most resistance to antivirals involves phosphorylation via thymidine kinase, it remains a true alternative for treating resistant strains of herpes. Currently, it is only available in intravenous or intravitreal form, and its use must be limited in patients with suboptimal kidney function.[14] In patients over age 50 with shingles, administration of antivirals within 72 hours of onset of the rash decreases the duration of the acute pain and rash by approximately 1 to 2 days. It also may decrease the duration of postherpetic neuralgia, but it does not reduce its incidence.[5] The addition of prednisone to antiviral treatment may hasten rash healing and reduce the severity of pain in the first few weeks of illness but has no significant effect on the long-term duration and incidence of postherpetic neuralgia.[7,12]

Disseminated Varicella

When more than 20 HZ lesions are noted outside a particular dermatomal distribution, the illness is considered to be *disseminated varicella*. The mortality rate when this occurs is approximately 15 percent; therefore, these patients require admission and intravenous acyclovir.[2,16] Disseminated varicella is more common in immunocompromised patients.

Herpes Ophthalmicus

Facial lesions present most commonly in the ophthalmic region of the trigeminal nerve[13] (Fig. 55-2). Herpetic keratitis is a common sequela when the eye is involved and may lead to loss of vision if not treated properly. Any patient with facial involvement needs to undergo an immediate examination by an ophthamologist.[16] Direct ocular treatment may be indicated. Fifty percent of those affected in the ophthalmic branch of the trigeminal nerve will experience ocular complications such as iritis, uveitis, conjunctivitis, episcleritis, keratitis, and ocular muscle palsies.[2,16]

Postherpetic Neuralgia

Pain that lasts longer than 1 month after resolution of the rash is considered to be postherpetic neuralgia.[6] This condition is due to a disturbance in nerve function or structure in which there is selective loss of the larger fibers that inhibit pain transmission.[6] Postherpetic neuralgia occurs in up to 70 percent of patients with herpes zoster and is not associated with the severity of pain of the preceding rash. Patients over age 50 are affected most commonly. Both acute zoster and postherpetic neuralgia can result in impaired sleep, poor appetite, diminished libido, and depression.[1] The initiation of antiviral medications within 72 hours can reduce the duration of the rash, acute pain, and viral shedding by 1 to 2 days.[9,11] Fifty percent of those who develop postherpetic neuralgia will experience complete relief of pain within 3 months.[6] Historically, prednisone has been thought to be the treatment for shingles and postherpetic neuralgia. No studies have supported this treatment.[11,16] Treatment with acyclovir for longer than 21 days confers a slight benefit over the traditional 7-day treatment, but this results in an increased incidence of adverse reactions. Acyclovir treatment with or without steroids does not reduce the frequency of postherpetic neuralgia. The 5% topical lidocaine patch is the only medication approved for the treatment of postherpetic neuralgia.[3] Narcotics generally should be avoided because they have been found to be ineffective in long-term pain control. Narcotics have side effects in the elderly, such as lethargy, confusion, unsteadiness, falls, and constipation.[19,20] Tricyclic antidepressants are among the first-line treatments for the neuropathic pain associated with postherpetic neuralgia. Amitryptyline has been shown to relieve neuropathic pain independent of mood elevation. In the elderly, the side effects of the drug make it difficult to use. With its significant anticholinergic properties, it often causes sedation, urinary retention, constipation, othostasis, and cognitive impairment. The initial dose should be 10 mg 2 hours prior to bedtime.[6] gabapentin, an anticonvulsant, has been used in doses up to 3600 mg/day without side effects. In addition to gabapentin's analgesic properties, it also improves sleep, mood, and several quality-of-life measures. With the exception of gabapentin, no other antidepressant, including the selective serotonin reuptake inhibitors (SSRIs), has been shown to be beneficial in the management of pain.[13] Capsaicin, which works by depleting substance p, is applied as a 0.075% cream for several weeks. It can reduce the pain of postherpetic neuralgia by 40 percent compared with placebo. It is frequently associated with a burning sensation; hence it is not well tolerated. Surgery and nerve blocks have been discouraged.[16] While the true pathophysiology of postherpetic neuralgia remains a mystery, it has been demonstrated that in the affected dermatomes the sensory nerves, dorsal root ganglia, and dorsal horns are damaged.[2]

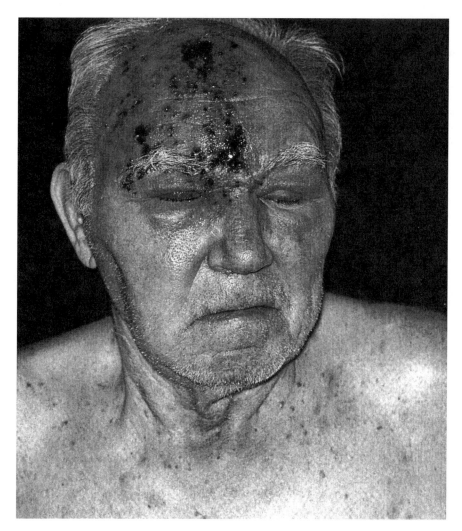

Fig. 55-2 Varicella-zoster virus infection: necrotizing ophthalmic herpes zoster with cutaneous dissemination. Hemorrhagic, crusted ulcerations and vesicles on the right forehead and periorbital area in the ophthalmic branch of the trigeminal nerve; note the bilateral facial edema and erythema. Hematogenous cutaneous dissemination has occured with hundreds of vesicles and erythematous papules on the trunk. In spite of the extensive cutaneous infection, this immunocompetent patient was relatively pain free.

Central Nervous System Involvement

One of the most serious central nervous system (CNS) complications of herpes zoster is ophthalmic zoster granulomatous cerebral angiitis. This condition occurs weeks to months following resolution of the virus and may present with strokelike symptoms.[12,21] Myelitis, which involves muscle weakness and cerebral spinal fluid pleocystosis, may complicate herpes zoster when it involves the CNS. In immunocomprimised patients, the course is more insidious and progressive, often leading to death. Aseptic meningitis and meningioencephalitis can occur with varicella-zoster virus infection. Bell's palsy has long been believed to be a sequela of varicella-zoster virus infection. It occurs when the geniculate ganglion is involved and frequently will present without a rash.[12] It has been postulated that Guillian-Barré syndrome may be a complication of reactivated HZ virus, but the association may be coincidental.[22]

Prevention

A live, attenuated varicella vaccine was approved for use in the United States in March of 1995 and is now recommended for all susceptible persons 12 months of age and older. The vaccine has an 85 percent efficacy rate in preventing herpes zoster, and those who develop the disease tend to experience a much milder case.[23] The widespread use of a live vaccine could increase prevalence of the disease among adults who never experienced chicken pox, but this has not occurred. [24] In February 1999 the Advisory Committee on Immunization Practices recommended use of the varicella vaccine for all adults at high risk for exposure, such as health care professionals, teachers, nonpregnant women of child-bearing age, day-care workers, and travelers.[25,26] Since the inception of the vaccine, the incidence of herpes zoster has decreased in every age group.[27] Despite this recommendation, geriatric patients frequently choose not to receive the vaccine because of doubts about safety and efficacy.[25] Prior to the availability of the vaccine there were 4 million cases of infections caused by varicella-zoster virus in the United States annually; 11,000 of those infected required hospitalization, with 100 resulting in death.[28] Where vaccination is indicated, adults should receive two doses 4 to 8 weeks apart.[25] The vaccine is effective for postexposure prophylaxis when given within 3 days of exposure.[29] Suppressive therapy with acyclovir has been used in patients who are chronically immunocompromised and therefore at increased risk for developing the infection.

Prognosis

In patients with a competent immune system, the rash usually will resolve within 2 to 3 weeks. Approximately 50 percent of patients will be pain-free within 2 months, and by 6 months, 95 percent of patients have no residual symptoms. Less than 5 percent of patients will experience complications that persist longer than 6 months.[13]

ADDITIONAL ASPECTS

Zoster Sine Herpete

Zoster sine herpete is defined as a dermatomal distribution of pain similar to that found with herpes zoster but without the antecedent rash.[1,12]

Ramsey Hunt Syndrome

When the seventh cranial nerve is involved, it is common to see ipsilateral facial muscle weakness and lesions in the external auditory canal and the anterior two-thirds of the tongue. Tinnitus, vertigo, deafness, otalgia, and loss of taste may result.[16] Facial weakness is a common complication that frequently does not recover fully.[12]

Hutchinson's Sign

Vesicular lesions that are noted on the side or top of the nose suggest involvement of the nasociliary branch of the ophthalmic division of the trigeminal nerve.[16]

Bacterial Superinfection

As with chickenpox, bacterial superinfection is not uncommon. The same holds true for patients with herpes zoster. When superinfection occurs, the bacteria are generally gram-positive skin flora, and the infection should be treated with systemic antibiotics.[1]

REFERENCES

1. O'Donnell JA, Hofmann MT: Skin and soft tissues: Management of four common infections in the nursing home patient. *Geriatrics* 56:33, 2001.
2. Stankus SJ, Dlugopolski M, Packer D: Practical therapeutics management of herpes zoster (shingles) and postherpetic neuralgia. *Am Fam Phys* 61:1, 2000.
3. Kost RG, Straus SE: Postherpetic neuralgia: Pathogenesis, treatment, and prevention. *New Engl J Med* 335:32, 1996.
4. Balfour HH: Antiviral drugs. *New Engl J Med* 340:1255, 1999.
5. Abramowicz M: Drugs for non-HIV viral infections. *Med Lett Drugs Ther* 44:9, 2002.
6. Freedman GM, Peruvemba R: Geriatric anesthesia geriatric pain management the anesthesiologist's perspective. *Anesthesiol Clin North Am* 18:123, 2000.
7. Rosencrance G: Herpes zoster. *New Engl J Med* 330:906, 1994.

8. American Academy of Pediatrics: Varicella-zoster infection. *AAP 2000 Red Book: Report of the Committee on Infectious Diseases* 25:625, 2000.

9. Mouton CP, Bazaldua OV, Pierce B, et al: Common infections in older adults. *Am Fam Phys* 63:8, 2001.

10. Elgart ML: Geriatric dermatology: II. Skin infections and infestations in geriatric patients. *Clin Geriatr Med* 18:1, 2002.

11. Gnann JW, Whitley RJ: Herpes zoster. *New Engl J Med* 347:340, 2002.

12. Gilden DH, Kleinschmidt-DeMasters BK, LaGuardia JJ, et al: Neurologic complications of the reactivation of varicella-zoster virus. *New Engl J Med* 342:635, 2000.

13. Fitzpatrick TB, Johnson RA, Wolf K: *Color Atlas and Synopsis of Clinical Dermatology.* McGraw Hill 2001, 805.

14. Miedziak AI, O'Brien TP: Ocular infections: Update on therapy of varicella-zoster virus ocular infections. *Ophthalmol Clin North Am* 12:51, 1999.

15. Seidman D, Pont E: Risks and benefits of varicella vaccine. *JAMA* 279:1, 1998.

16. McCrary ML, Severson J, Tyring SK: Continuing medical education varicella-zoster virus. *J Am Acad Dermatol* 41:1, 1999.

17. Brisson M, Edmunds WJ, Gay NJ, et al: Varicella vaccine and shingles. *JAMA* 287:1, 2002.

18. Tyring SK, Beutner KR, Tucker BA, et al: Antiviral therapy for herpes zoster: Randomized, controlled clinical trial of valacyclovir and famciclovir therapy in immunocompetent patients 50 years and older. *Arch Fam Med* 9:863, 2000.

19. Carver A, Payne R, Foley K: Herpes zoster. *New Engl J Med* 343:221, 2000.

20. Zenz T, Zenz M, Tyrba M: Treatment of postherpetic neuralgia. *New Engl J Med* 335:1768, 1996.

21. Nogueira RG, Sheen VL: Images in clinical medicine: Herpes zoster ophthalmicus followed by contralateral hemiparesis. *New Engl J Med* 346(15):1127, 2002.

22. Roccatagliata L, Uccelli A, Murialdo A: Guillian-Barré syndrome after reactivation of varicella-zoster virus. *New Engl J Med* 344:65, 2001.

23. Vazquez M, LaRussa PS, Gershon AA, et al: The effectiveness of the varicella vaccine in clinical practice. *New Engl J Med* 344:955, 2001.

24. Lowe L: Diagnosis: Herpes zoster without vesicles. *Arch Dermatol* 134:1, 1998.

25. Zimmerman RK, Ball JA: Immunizations: Adult vaccinations. *Primary Care* 28:4, 2001.

26. Prevention of varicella: Updated recommendations of the Advisory Committee on Immunization Practices (AICP). *MMWR* 48:1, 1999.

27. Seward JF, Watson BM, Peterson CL, et al: Varicella disease after introduction of varicella vaccine in the United States, 1995–2000. *JAMA* 287:606, 2002.

28. Galil K, Mootrey GP, Seward J, et al: Prevention of varicella: Updated recommendations of the Advisory Committee on Immunization Practices (ACIP). *MMWR* 48(RR-6):1, 1999.

29. Bajwa ZH, Ho CC: Herpetic neuralgia: Use of combination therapy for pain relief in acute and chronic herpes zoster. *Geriatrics* 56:18, 2001.

56

Wound Care Issues

Jonathan H. Valente
Mark C. Muetterties

HIGH-YIELD FACTS

- Skin tears are common, preventable injuries often best closed by conservative measures with skin tapes.

- Burns in elderly patients have a lower incidence and higher mortality rate relative to younger patients with similar burns.

- Pressure ulcers are a common and easily overlooked wound in the emergency department (ED) evaluation of the elderly. Ulcers require initation of care, especially diabetic foot ulcers.

- Elderly patients often have unknown tetanus immunization status or low serologic levels of tetanus antibodies and may need to receive tetanus immune globulin.

- Factors that improve healing and prevent acute and chronic wounds include modification of the home environment, proper patient positioning and handling, nutritional support, and appropriate local topical wound care.

- Simple wound care can require additional duties from a caregiver at home.

Wounds are a frequently encountered problem in the emergency department (ED). This chapter will review the epidemiology, pathophysiology, assessment, and treatment of acute and chronic wounds encountered most frequently in the elderly. Covered topics will include skin tears, pretibial lacerations, burns, ulcerations, and tetanus prophylaxis. Risk factors and preventative strategies will be discussed.

EPIDEMIOLOGY

Elderly patients are at an increased risk of injury secondary to declining physical and mental abilities. Their declining abilities may include gait or balance difficulties, visual impairment, changes in sensory perception, postural hypotension, and impaired cognitive function from Alzheimer's disease.[1] These factors significantly increase the risk of sustaining injuries such as abrasions, lacerations, and skin tears from bumps or falls. Additionally, declining agility puts elders at risk for burn injuries. Elderly patients who have sustained minor injury have been shown to be at risk for short-term functional decline,[2] thus requiring more home support and increasing their risk for further injury.

Comorbid disease and certain medications, such as steroids, place the elderly at an increased risk for poor wound healing and the development of chronic wounds. Such wounds include pressure ulcers, diabetic ulcers, and vascular ulcers. Pressure ulcers and diabetic ulcers often occur as a result of immobility, diabetes-associated neuropathy, and soft tissue trauma caused by improperly fitted shoes, orthopedic devices, or chronic foot deformities.

PATHOPHYSIOLOGY

Skin changes occur with the aging process. With aging there is thinning of the epidermis and a loss of subcutaneous tissue. The result is a flattening of the dermal-epidermal junction. There is a loss of the rete pegs that fasten the dermis to the subcutaneous tissue. The skin is far less cellular with a loss of keratinocytes. Over time, the skin loses tensile strength, and blood vessels become fragile and thinner. In addition, the skin appears more dry, wrinkled, thin, and transparent.[3–6] Wound epithelialization and noncollagenous protein accumulation are both necessary for wound healing and are delayed in elderly patients. Holt and colleagues[7] showed that healthy elderly human volunteers older than 65 years of age have delayed epithelialization of wounds compared with healthy young volunteers. Minor shearing forces may lead to separation of the epidermis from the dermis, resulting in a skin tear or partial-thickness wound.[4,8] Each of these changes makes the skin of the elderly much more susceptible to injury.

The elderly have more dermatologic breakdown than the young. There are other causes of skin breakdown, such as ischemia, edema, trauma (both occult and obvious), primary diseases of the skin, diabetes, peripheral vascular disease, chronic venous insufficiency, and dependent edema. In addition, patients with any disease that causes chronic pruritus will have an increased risk of skin infection. Lastly, the presence of incontinence or maceration has been shown to hasten the breakdown of the skin. A 30 percent decrease in Langerhans' cells due to a slower replacement of cells in the stratum corneum impairs immune function of the skin. In addition to having fewer Langerhans' cells, the function of these cells is impeded. Pathologic studies have shown a decrease in interleukin 1 (IL-1) secretions and activity in Langerhans' cells, as well as a decreased response to cytokines. These changes allow easier entry of bacteria.

In the elderly, chronic wounds such as pressure ulcers heal slowly and poorly due to a variety of factors. In chronic ulcers, there is no local hemorrhage. This prevents the body's intrinsic wound-healing factors from contacting the surrounding tissues, resulting in decreased fibrinolytic activity and decreased platelet release at the wound site. In addition, chronic wounds are susceptible to complex polymicrobial colonization. All these factors lead to a reduced healing rate.[9]

The most likely organisms in an elderly person with cellulitis are the gram-positive organisms such as group A *Streptococcus* and *Staphylococcus aureus*. However, patients with pressure sores or systemic infection are more likely to harbor polymicrobial infections including anaerobes, *Enterobacter, Pseudomonas, Bacteriodes,* or *Streptococcus.*

Diabetes, cardiovascular disease, and malnutrition are some comorbid conditions that decrease the body's ability to heal wounds. Certain medications also inhibit wound healing (Table 56-1). These factors make wounds in the elderly more susceptible to complications such as delayed healing, infection, and dehiscence.[7,10,11]

Table 56-1. Medications Inhibiting Wound Healing

Steroids
Nonsteroidal anti-inflammatory drugs
Colchicine
Chemotherapy agents
Penicillamine
Anticoagulants

Source: Pollack S: Systemic medications and wound healing. *Int J Dermatol* 21:491, 1982.

Acute Wounds

In 1996, approximately 11 million traumatic wounds were treated and evaluated in EDs across the country.[12] While most traumatic wounds occur in young males, EDs are seeing an increased frequency of these wounds in elderly patients. This is due in part to the dramatic increase in the population of people older than age 65.[1] While many of these wounds can be treated in standard fashion, certain acute wounds in the elderly deserve special attention.

Skin Tears

Minor trauma in elderly patients, especially nursing home patients, often results in a skin tear. Upper extremity skin tears are encountered more frequently among dependent patients needing assistance with activities of daily living (ADLs).[8] In studies of patients in long-term-care facilities, nearly 80 percent of all skin tears were located on the upper extremities.[4,10] Ambulatory patients more frequently sustain these injuries on the lower extremities. Visually impaired patients are at risk for skin tears as a result of bumping into unseen objects.[8]

Skin tears occur most often secondary to minor shearing or friction forces.[3,8] Even seemingly benign mechanisms, such as being lifted and transferred from a wheelchair, may result in a skin tear.[4] According to one study, risk factors associated with skin tears include the following: age, history of prior skin tears, senile purpura, cognitive impairment, dependency on others for assistance with movement, and impaired mobility.[10]

Wound Assessment

Skin tears often appear as wedge-shaped, crescent-shaped, or jagged flaps of skin.[4] A categorized system to classify skin tears was first developed by Payne and Martin[6,10] (Table 56-2).

Treatment

Standard wound care practices for preparation of the skin tear include gentle irrigation with normal saline and debridement of devitalized tissue. The next step is to approximate the epidermal flap, if still present, and apply a skin adhesive such as benzoin with Steri-Strips (3M, St. Paul, MN) to secure the wound. Occlusive dressings, such as Tegaderm or Opsite, have been shown to adhere tightly to the surrounding skin and, on removal, may traumatize

Table 56-2. Payne-Martin Classification System for Skin Tears

---

Category 1: Skin tear without tissue loss
  a. Linear skin tear: Full-thickness, incision-like wound, typically occurs over a wrinkle of skin often in an area of ecchymosis
  b. Flap-type skin tear: Epidermal flap wrinkled back exposing dermal layer, easily pulled back and "grafted" to cover dermis to within 1 mm of wound margin

Category 2: Skin tear with partial-thickness tissue loss
  a. Scant tissue loss type: 25 percent or less of the epidermal flap lost
  b. Moderate tissue loss type: More than 25 percent of epidermal flap lost

Category 3: Skin tears with complete tissue loss: Epidermal flap absent due to original trauma, necrosis, cleansing, may even have loss of dermal layer

---

Source: Payne RL, Martin MLC: Skin Tears- The epidemiology and management of skin tears in older adults. *Ostomy Wound Manage* 1990; 26: 26–37.[6]

the healing wound and the surrounding tissue.[3,8] Edwards and colleagues[13] showed improved healing rates with Steri-Strips covered by a nonadherent dressing compared with an occlusive dressing. Dressings with a high-moisture vapor-transmission rate have been shown to improve rates of healing. Applying a hydrogel dressing over the Steri-Strips and covering with a nonadherent dressing, such as Telfa, may further improve wound healing.[8] Twice-daily dressing changes are recommended. If a hydrocolloid dressing is used instead of hydrogel, the dressing changes can be done weekly.[8]

Skin tapes may not work well for wounds located on flexible surfaces, such as joints, or poorly adhesive surfaces, such as oily or hairy skin. An alternative to wound tape closures is opposing the edges with a horizontal mattress suture. This type of suture provides more anchor points, allowing less tension to be applied to the viable tissue. However, the skin is often very friable and thin, making this type of repair difficult.

Pretibial lacerations, a form of skin tear, are even more problematic. Repair of these wounds with sutures has been shown to be associated with increased necrosis and slower healing rates than repair with adhesive tapes. This is especially evident in patients with skin flaps.[14] In addition, the jagged edges of skin tears make skin glue difficult to use.[3] Frequently, these flap injuries will slough and require skin grafting later.[15]

One approach developed specifically for the treatment of pretibial skin lacerations includes the use of sutures in combination with Steri-Strips. This technique may be especially beneficial in the care of superficial flap wounds in the ED[16] (Figs. 56-1 through 56-5). Sutures are anchored through the skin tapes in order to immobilize the skin flap and relieve tension on the fragile skin. Silk[16] reported a much shorter healing time compared with previ-

ously reported healing times in patients treated conservatively with debridement and skin tapes or simple sutures. In this prospective case series involving 147 patients, none of the patients required skin grafting.

Prevention

Preventative strategies for skin tears include proper positioning and transfer techniques to avoid shearing or friction injuries, padded rails and supports for extremities, avoidance of pulling fragile skin with gentle handling of patients, use of nonadherent dressings, and gentle removal of tapes and dressings. Bathing every other day instead of every day and the use of moisturizers and emollient soaps every other day are also recommended for keeping the skin soft and well hydrated.[3] One recent study reported a 34.8 percent lower incidence of skin tears with the use of emollient soaps versus nonemollient soaps.[5]

Burns

Burn injuries are one of the leading causes of death in the geriatric population despite a lower incidence in this age group.[17] A number of retrospective studies of elderly burn patients have been published.[18–21] Burns from a flame source are most common, followed by hot water scalds, flammable liquids, and contact with hot surfaces.[19,21,22]

Several reasons for the increased mortality are a direct result of the skin's aging process. This includes thinning of the skin, loss of dermal thickness, and loss of elastin.[18] These skin changes make the elderly more susceptible to a burn. Coexisting diseases, such as hypertension, cardiovascular disease, and diabetes, also contribute to the increased mortality in the elderly. Improved survival from burns has been noted over recent years, but this has only

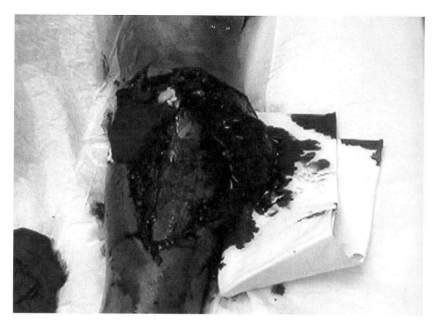

Fig. 56-1   A severe pretibial laceration.

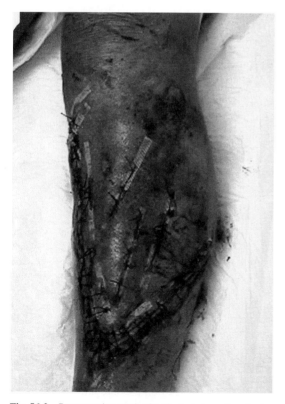

Fig. 56-2   Postoperative result after the technique described.

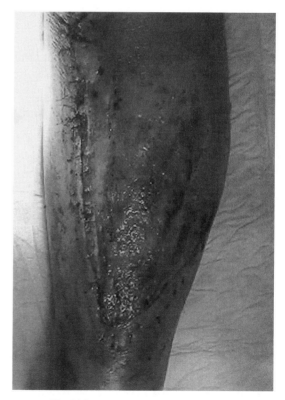

Fig. 56-3   Pretibial flap 19 days after repair.

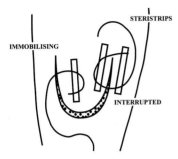

Fig. 56-4 Skin flap laceration. Types of deep reinforced sutures (through Steri-Strips).

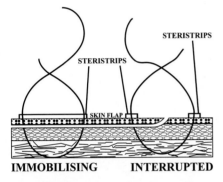

Fig. 56-5 Technique for deep reinforced suturing of skin flap laceration (see text).

been achieved in the younger segment of the geriatric population.[22]

The LA_{50} (burn area resulting in 50 percent mortality) offers insight into the relative burn mortality of the elderly. A retrospective review at one burn center during the period of 1977–1996 reported an LA_{50} of 43.1 percent for patients aged 60 to 69, 25.9 percent for those aged 70 to 79, and 13.1 percent for those over age 80.[22] Elderly burn patients with significant inhalation injuries have reported mortality rates as high as 100 percent.[23]

Several methods have been proposed to predict the associated mortality of burn patients.[24] The Abbreviated Burn Severity Index (ABSI) is a scoring system by which points are added based on age, sex, presence of inhalation injury, presence of full-thickness burn, and total of burn surface area. A simpler method of predicting mortality is with the Baux rule. The patient's age is added to the total burn surface area. Several retrospective studies have found the Baux system to accurately predict mortality in elderly burn patients.[18,22]

Treatment

Burn management for the elderly in the prehospital setting and ED differs little from that of any other patient. Standard airway, breathing, and circulation assessment is critical. Oxygen, intravenous fluid resuscitation, cervical spine precautions, tetanus prophylaxis, and surgical consultation should occur following standard protocols. Emergency physicians should have a low threshold for admission and/or transfer of elderly to a regional burn center. Swan-Gantz catheters may be needed to guide fluid resuscitation depending on both the extent of the burn and comorbidity.[25] Early excision and grafting have been shown to decrease mortality in younger patients, but their ability to reduce mortality in the elderly patient is not generally accepted.[19,26,27] Donor grafts are limited due to the slow healing of elderly patients, necessitating homologous grafts from skin banks.

Prevention

Many hot water scald or immersion burns are preventable. However, the reduced mobility and decreased reaction times in the geriatric population put them at a higher risk. These burns tend to involve larger surface areas than flame burns. Lowering the set temperature of hot water heaters to 120°F (49°C) from the usual 140°F (60°C) or higher would result in a significant reduction in the incidence of scald burns. Large hot water delivery systems in hospitals and nursing homes, however, are potential sources of *Legionella pneumophilia* and should be kept at 140°F or higher to prevent colonization. In these cases, thermostatic mixing devices can be installed to prevent scald burns.[28–30]

Chronic Wounds

Chronic skin wounds such as ulcerations are common in the geriatric population and may lead to increased patient morbidity and cost to society. The three basic types of ulcers include pressure, diabetic, and vascular ulcers. The estimated cost of care for pressure ulcers alone in 1992 was more than $1.3 billion,[31,32] with the prevalence of chronic skin ulcerations in patients older than age 75 estimated at more than 800 wounds per 100,000 persons.[33] One inpatient study found vascular leg ulcers or pressure ulcers in 22 percent of 360 patients. Eleven percent had a leg ulcer, and 11 percent had a pressure ulcer. Interestingly, many of these went unrecognized. Fewer than half the patients with pressure ulcers had nursing documentation of the ulcer.[31] A recent study evaluating home-care patients for the presence of chronic wounds found that they were present in 36.3 percent of all patients. In addition, 41.7 percent of these patients had multiple wounds, and 47.1 percent of all the wounds were classified as either pressure ulcers or vascular leg ulcers.[33]

Pressure Ulcers

Pressure ulcers have been defined by the Agency for Health Care Policy and Research (AHCPR) as any lesion caused by unrelieved pressure resulting in damage of underlying tissue[34,40,41,8,34] (Table 56-3). Ulcers located on the sacrum often have been referred to as *decubitus ulcers*. Pressure ulcers are the most common chronic wound in the elderly. Greater than half of all patients with pressure ulcers are older than age 70.[35,36] Elderly women are affected more frequently than are elderly men, which may only reflect the greater number of women in the geriatric population.[34] It is estimated that 2.7 to 29.9 percent of patients in acute care facilities and 2.4 to 23 percent of patients in long-term care facilities develop pressure ulcers.[8,37] Others report the prevalence of significant pressure ulcers to be from 3.0 to 11 percent in hospitalized and 1.2 to 11.2 percent in nursing home patients.[34] Risk factors implicated in causing pressure ulcers include immobility, incontinence, diabetes mellitus, increasing age, decreased dietary protein intake, impaired nutrition, lymphopenia, decreased body weight, dry skin, and altered level of consciousness.[34,35,38,39]

Treatment and Prevention

Major goals in ulcer treatment are maintaining a moist environment, avoiding wound dehydration, and protecting the area from further damage and infection. Moist wounds resurface and heal faster than do air-exposed wounds.[9,42–45] The application of occlusive dressings over the wound creates a moist environment. This may allow certain wound fluid factors such as IL-1, epidermal growth factor, and platelet-derived growth factor to remain active, enhancing wound healing.[9,46]

Occlusive dressings include moist saline gauze, polymer films, polymer foams, hydrogels, hydrocolloids, alginates, and biomembranes.[8,9,43] These dressings are most useful with granulating wounds, necrotizing wounds with low exudate levels, or as secondary dressings combined with an absorbent material in wounds with higher exudate levels.[47] Each occlusive dressing has its own advantages and disadvantages. Wet-to-dry gauze dressings are cost-effective, readily available, and support autolytic wound debridement. However, moisture from the dressing may cause maceration of the surrounding skin. Preventive techniques include application of petroleum jelly to the area surrounding the wound and application of the wet-gauze dressing into the wound itself.[44] Polyvinyl dressings such as Tegaderm or Opsite provide a transparent membrane that is semipermeable to oxygen and moisture but impermeable to bacteria. Polyvinyl dressings are recommended for noninfected partial-thickness wounds.[44] Hydrocolloid dressings provide a moist wound environment and are nonadherent to the wound tissue.

Table 56-3. Wound Assessment: Staging of Pressure Ulcers I–IV

Stage I:	Area of nonblanchable, intact, erythematous skin
	Skin discoloration, edema, induration
	May be more difficult to recognize in patients with darker skin tones
	May be painful or itchy
Stage II:	Partial-thickness skin loss; extends through epidermal and dermal layers
	Extends to, but not through, subcutaneous layer
	Pink, wet, shallow crater, abrasion, or blister
	Painful
Stage III:	Full-thickness skin loss; extends through subcutaneous tissue
	Extends to, but not through, fascia
	Deep crater with or without tissue necrosis and/or undermining of surrounding tissue
	Painless
Stage IV:	Full-thickness skin loss; extends through fascia
	May involve muscle, bone, tendons, or other deep structures
	Painless

Source: Allman, RM: Dressore ulcer prevalence, incidence, risk factors, and impact. *Clin Geriatr Med* 13(3):421, 1997.[8,40,41]

This prevents damage to wound epithelialization. Another advantage of polyvinyl and hydrocolloid dressings is that the dressings can be left in place for several days.[9,44] Alginates are highly absorbent, nonadherent dressings that are most useful in highly exudative wounds. However, if these dressings are allowed to dry, they may adhere to the wound surface and damage epithelial tissue during removal.[9,44] Occlusive dressings should be applied and remain in place until the accumulating wound fluid is seen leaking out or disrupting the dressing. This period of time may range from one to several days depending on the wound and the selected dressing. Autolyzed nonviable tissue should be removed during the dressing changes.[9,43] Occlusive dressings used for chronic wounds can reduce infection, reduce wound pain, improve autolytic debridement, and promote the development of granulation tissue.[9,43]

Debridement of ulcers may be necessary for prevention of bacterial infection and promotion of wound healing. Necrotic debris has been shown to increase the risk of infection and delay wound healing.[9,48] However, the value and the best method of debridement are controversial.[9,43] There are several different approaches to wound debridement, including mechanical debridement with wet-to-dry gauze dressings, surgical debridement by scalpel, autolytic debridement with occlusive dressings, or application of exogenous enzymes. Wet-to-dry dressing changes are controversial, especially after the formation of granulation tissue within the wound, because granulation tissue also adheres to the dry gauze, leading to a disruption of the healing process.[44,45] However, remoistening the gauze dressings prior to removal will minimize disruption of the granulation tissue.[44] Occlusive dressings promote fluid retention within the wound that in turn facilitates autolysis.[47] Surgical debridement is indicated most often in the presence of infection.[9,43,44] For pressure ulcers that do not respond to conservative management, operative repair may be necessary, especially for stage III or IV wounds. Reconstructive procedures can vary from skin grafts to muscle flaps as required.[41]

Factors that improve healing and prevent pressure ulcers include providing topical wound care, improving nutrition, using support surfaces, improving mobility, and protecting the skin from fecal and urine exposure in patients with a history of incontinence and diaper use. High-protein diets have been shown to prevent and improve healing of pressure ulcers.[8,44] Specialty beds, cushions, and simple positioning maneuvers such as elevating the heels from the surface of the bed decrease contact time over pressure-sensitive areas of the skin. Optimally, regular positioning changes should be scheduled every 2 hours. Application of moisture barriers, such as petroleum jelly products, to skin areas will help decrease maceration and breakdown of the skin secondary to exposure to stool and urine. Enzymes in stool promote a chemical breakdown of skin. It is recommended that moisture barriers be applied with each diaper change.[8,9,43,44] Sheepskins, foam or rubber ring devices, and massage are not recommended. These devices or measures may make pressure ulcers worse.[41]

Diabetic Ulcers

The majority of diabetic ulcers are located on the foot. These wounds have a high morbidity, since 14 to 24 percent of patients with a foot ulcer will require an amputation.[43,49] Most diabetic ulcers are secondary to peripheral neuropathy. The failure of the patient to recognize pressure or trauma at insensate sites results in cronic wounds. Large-vessel arterial disease may contribute either primarily or secondarily. Nonocclusive small-vessel disease also may play a role.[43]

Treatment

The Wound Healing Society's treatment standards for diabetic ulcers include pressure off-loading, debridement of necrotic tissue and moist wound dressings (see "Pressure Ulcers" above for a discussion of dressings and debridement).[43] Pressure off-loading treatments include total contact casts, castboots, sandals, and felted-foam dressings. Blood glucose regulation, nutritional support, and treatment of lower extremity edema and comorbid medical conditions serve as adjunctive treatments.[49] In addition, platelet-derived growth factor has been studied and shown to be an effective agent that may become an adjunct to ulcer treatment in the future.[43] For more severe conditions, amputation and vascular reconstructive procedures may be necessary.

Vascular Ulcers

Venous ulcers account for approximately 65 to 90 percent of all leg ulcers.[43,50] Approximately 3.5 percent of patients older than age 65 have a venous ulcer, with women three times more likely than men. In addition, venous ulcers have a recurrence rate of about 70 percent.[51]

Venous hypertension, or high venous pressure, leads to poor venous blood flow through the lower extremities. Patients with venous insufficiency have either underlying damage to the leg veins or a decreased ability of the calf muscle to act as a pump and return blood to the central circulation. Factors that increase the risk of developing venous hypertension include congestive heart failure, muscle weakness, immobility, obesity, pregnancy, deep vein thrombosis, and venous valvular incompetence.[51]

Ulcers caused by arterial insufficiency are less common than those caused by venous hypertension.[8] Arterial insufficiency ulcers account for approximately 5 percent of all lower extremity ulcers.[52,53] These ulcers are found most often in men between the ages of 50 and 70 years and diabetics.[54] Risk factors are the same as those risks for coronary artery disease.[8]

Wound Assessment

Venous ulcers typically are located on the medial aspect of the lower leg above the medial malleolus along the saphenous vein. The skin surrounding the wound appears hyperpigmented, brownish, and edematous. The wound itself has irregular margins with a "beefy red," granular base and exudates.[50,51,53] The ankle-brachial index should be measured to rule out arterial disease, especially in patients with poor peripheral pulses.

Arterial ulcers typically are located distal to the ankle, involving the digits, metatarsal heads, heel, and malleoli. Arterial insufficiency ulcers are painful, but they are often less painful when placed in a more dependent position. In addition, patients with these ulcers often have a history of intermittent claudication.[50] Other physical findings include localized hair loss, skin atrophy, poor or absent pulses, skin pallor or grayness, and nail deformity. The ulcer edges are often sharp and well demarcated with a base that is necrotic gray, yellow, or black.[8,50,53] Physical assessment should include evaluation of peripheral pulses, capillary refill, and bruits; skin temperature determination; and determination of the ankle-brachial index (ABI). The ABI is a noninvasive screening test used to determine the need for further testing and referral to a vascular surgeon. However, the ABI is an indirect measure of perfusion and is not accurate in patients such as diabetics with noncompressable arteries.[8,50] The ability to heal wounds is usually maintained with venus insufficiencies. However, with severe arterial insufficiency, wound healing is unlikely unless a revascularization procedure is done. An ABI of less than 0.5 is an indication of severe arterial insufficiency.

Treatment

The Wound Healing Society's treatment standards for venous ulcers include compression therapy, debridement of necrotic tissue, and moist wound dressings (see "Pressure Ulcers" above for a discussion of dressings and debridement).[43] Compression therapy includes either the traditional Unna's boot or gradient compression hose. A large selection of gradient compression hose is available from a variety of manufacturers. The Unna's boot is a nonelastic compression bandage impregnated with zinc oxide. This bandage is used frequently either alone or in combination with a primary wound dressing for the treatment of venous ulcers. It is applied from the midfoot to below the knee and forms a semirigid structure as it dries. The calf muscles press against the Unna's boot during ambulation. This action creates a compressive effect, assisting the return of blood from the extremity to the central circulation.[43,51] However, some authors believe that the Unna's boot may not be as effective as other true compression bandages in nonambulatory or minimally active patients such as the elderly.[43] In addition, disadvantages of the Unna's boot include the inability to conform to changes in the volume of the lower extremity (i.e., reduced edema in the extremity), the inability to absorb large amounts of wound drainage, and an unpleasant smell.[51] Newer therapies include systemic medications such as high-dose pentoxifylline (which has been reported to improve the rate of healing for venous ulcers), bioengineered skin, and topical growth factors.[50,55] Indicators of poor healing include an ABI of less than 0.8, a history of venous ligation, a history of hip or knee replacement, and the presence of fibrin in the wound.[50]

The primary therapy for severe arterial insufficiency is revascularization. Referral for vascular surgery is recommended in patients with an ABI of less than 0.5.[8] More palliative therapies would include lifestyle changes, such as smoking cessation, weight reduction, proper foot care, and exercise. General treatment includes wound debridement, prevention of infection, and maintenance of a moist wound environment for other ulcers.[8] Among other treatment modalities are hyperbaric oxygen therapy, platelet-derived growth factor, pentoxifylline, clopidogrel, and cilostazol.[50]

Complications of Chronic Wounds

Increased mortality has been associated with the development of chronic wounds. In one study, patients in long-term facilities who developed pressure ulcers within 3 months of admission had a 92 percent mortality rate as compared with only 4 percent among patients without pressure ulcers. The reason for this association between increased death and pressure ulcers is unclear.[9] Other complications include bacteremia, localized infection, osteomyelitis, and amputation. In addition, it is important to remember that ulcers that fail to heal occasionally may represent a rare neoplasm or infectious organism.[50]

Infection is a very important and common complication of all ulcers. Approximately 25 percent of diabetic foot ulcers become infected,[9,56,57] and 38 percent of patients with infected pressure ulcers develop osteomyelitis.[9,58] Plain radiographs have been shown to be a poor method for the diagnosis of osteomyelitis in patients with pressure sores, and radionuclide scans have been reported to have false-positive rates of 41 percent.[9,58] Needle biopsy is considered the most useful single test for the diagnosis of osteomyelitis.[9]

TETANUS PROPHYLAXIS

Tetanus remains a rare but often fatal disease, with fewer than 50 total U.S. cases having been reported each year from 1995 through 1997 based on the most recent Centers for Disease Control and Prevention (CDC) survey. Elderly patients age 60 and older had the highest incidence, 0.33 per 1 million population, roughly twice that of the 20- to 59-years age group. They also had the highest case-fatality rate at 18 percent. No deaths were reported in patients of any age who had completed the primary series of three tetanus vaccinations. Nearly two-thirds of the patients who sought medical care in this survey did not receive prophylaxis according to current recommendations.[59]

The elderly are at a higher risk for tetanus primarily because of low rates of immunity. In a large population-based serologic survey of 10,618 persons, the percentage of Americans with protective levels of antibodies (>0.15 IU/mL) dropped from more than 80 percent for 6- to 39-year olds to 27.8 percent for age 70 and older.[60] A smaller sample from an urban comprehensive care geriatric center found inadequate tetanus antibody levels in 50 percent of 129 patients. In this group, they were only able to obtain accurate immunization history in 36 percent of the 129 patients.[61] Thirty-five of the patients with inadequate levels were then tested for a response to a single dose of tetanus toxoid. At 2 months, 86 percent had achieved protective levels, whereas at one year, 82 percent continued to have protective levels.[62] Another study that followed patients with inadequate antibody titers found that only 56 percent seroconverted by day 14 after a tetanus booster was given.[63]

Current wound management guidelines from the Advisory Committee on Immunization Practice of the CDC divide patients into two groups depending on prior immunization status. Patients who have completed their primary tetanus series (three or more prior tetanus toxoid doses) should receive tetanus and diptheria toxoids (Td) for clean, minor wounds if their last booster was more than 10 years prior. Td should be given for larger wounds and for tetanus-prone wounds if their last booster was more than 5 years prior. Those with unknown immunization history or less than three prior tetanus toxoid doses also should receive tetanus immune globulin (TIG) in addition to the Td.[64] Elderly patients presenting to the ED may be unaware of their immunization history or unable to provide that information because of dementia, aphasia, or other medical problems. In these cases, if the primary physician is unable to confirm the patient's tetanus immunization status, it is imperative that the patient also receive TIG for tetanus-prone wounds.

PREVENTION

The occurrence of many of the wounds discussed in this chapter could be decreased or eliminated by preventive measures. One particular home-visit program was successful in decreasing the incidence of falls, scalds, and burns by removing clutter, securing rugs and electrical cords, and installing assistance devices such as hand rails, grab bars, and nonskid strips. They were able to reduce falls by 60 percent (0.81 to 0.33 falls per person per year). Scalds were reduced from 9 to 0 cases and burns from 7 to 0 cases over a 6-month period.[65] These interventions and others discussed throughout this chapter can reduce the incidence of injuries in the elderly population significantly.

REFERENCES

1. Miller KE, Zylstra RG, Standridge JB: The geriatric patient: A systematic approach to maintaining health. *Am Fam Phys* 61(4);1089, 2000.
2. Shapiro MJ, Partridge RA, Jenouri I, et al: Functional decline in independent elders after minor traumatic injury. *Acad Emerg Med* 8(1):78, 2001.
3. Pearson AS, Wolford RW: Management of skin trauma. *Primary Care* 27(2):475, 2000.
4. Malone ML, Rozario N, Gavinski M, et al: The epidemiology of skin tears in the institutionalized elderly. *J Am Geriatr Soc* 39:591, 1991.
5. Mason SR: Type of soap and the incidence of skin tears among residents of a long-care facility. *Ostomy Wound Manage* 43(8):26, 1997.
6. Payne RL, Martin MLC: Defining and classifying skin tears: Need for a common language. *Ostomy Wound Manage* 39:16, 1993.

7. Holt DR, Kirk SJ, Regan MC, et al: Effect of age on wound healing in healthy human beings. *Surgery* 112(2):293, 1992.

8. Wooten MK: Management of chronic wounds in the elderly. *Clin Fam Pract* 3(3):599, 2001.

9. Thomas DR, Kamel HK: Wound management in postacute care. *Clin Geriatr Med* 16(4):783, 2000.

10. Payne RL, Martin MLC: Skin tears: The epidemiology and management of skin tears in older adults. *Ostomy Wound Manage* 26:26, 1990.

11. Neuberger G, Recking J: Wound care: What's clear, what's not. *Nursing* 17:34, 1987.

12. Hollander JE, Singer AJ: Laceration management. *Ann Emerg Med* 34:356, 1999.

13. Edwards H, Gaskill D, Nash R: Treating skin tears in nursing home residents: A pilot study comparing four types of dressings. *Int J Nurs Pract* 4(1):25, 1998.

14. Sutton R, Pritty P: Use of sutures or adhesive tapes for primary closure of pretibial lacerations. *Br Med J* 290:1627, 1985.

15. Crawford BS, Gipson M: The conservative management of pretibial lacerations in elderly patients. *Br J Plast Surg* 30:174, 1977.

16. Silk J: A new approach to the management of pretibial lacerations. *Injury Int J Care Injured* 32:373, 2001.

17. Jerrard AJ, Cappadoro K: Burns in the elderly. *Emerg Med Clin North Am* 8(2):421, 1990.

18. Stassen NA, Lukan JK, Mizuguchi, NN et al: Thermal injury in the elderly: When is comfort care the right choice? *Am Surg* 67(7):704, 2001.

19. Covington DS, Wainwright DJ, Parks DH: Prognostic indicators in the elderly patient with burns. *J Burn Care Rehabil* 17(3):222, 1996.

20. Wibbenmeyer LA, Amelon MJ, Morgan, LJ et al: Predicting survival in an elderly burn patient population. *Burns* 27:583, 2001.

21. Ho WS, Ying SY, Chan HH: A study of burns in the elderly in a regional burn center. *Burns* 27:382, 2001.

22. Hammond J, Ward CG: Burns in octogenarians. *South Med J* 84(11):1316, 1991.

23. Hunt JL, Purdue, GF: The elderly burn patient. *Am J Surg* 164:472, 1992.

24. Tobiasen J, Hiebert JH, Edlich RF: Prediction of burn mortality. *Surg Gynecol Obstet* 154:711, 1982.

25. Schiller WR, Bay RC: Hemodynamic and oxygen transport monitoring in management of burns. *New Horizons* 4(4):475, 1996.

26. Kirn DS, Luce EA: Early excision and grafting versus conservative management of burns in the elderly. *Plast Reconst Surg* 102(4):1013, 1998.

27. Mann R, Heimbach D: Prognosis and treatment of burns. *West J Med* 165(4):215, 1996.

28. Stone M, Ahmed J, Evans J: The continuing risk of domestic hot water scalds to the elderly. *Burns* 26:347, 2000.

29. Huyer D, Corkum S: Reducing the incidence of tap-water scalds: Strategies for physicians. *Can Med Assoc J* 156(6):841, 1997.

30. Weaver AM, Himel HN, Edlich RF: Immersion scald burns: Strategies for prevention. *J Emerg Med* 11:397, 1993.

31. Gruen RL, Chang S, MacLellan DG: The point prevalence of wounds in a teaching hospital. *Aust NZ J Surg* 67:686, 1997.

32. Miller H, Delozier J. *Cost Implications of the Pressure Ulcer Treatment Guideline.* AHCPR Pub No 282-91-0070. Columbia, MD, Center for Health Policy Studies, Agency for Health Care Policy and Research, 1994.

33. Pieper B, Templin TN, Dobal M, et al: Wound prevalence, types, and treatments in home care. *Adv Wound Care* 12:117, 1999.

34. Allman RM: Pressure ulcer prevalence, incidence, risk factors, and impact. *Clin Geriatr Med* 13(3):421, 1997.

35. Goode PS, Allman RM: Pressure ulcers, in Duthie EH, Katz PR (eds): *Duthie: Practice of Geriatrics.* Philadelphia, Saunders, 1998, p 228.

36. Petersen MC, Bittmann S: The epidemiology of pressure sores. *Scand J Plast Reconstr Surg* 5(1):62, 1971.

37. Bergstrom N, Allman RM, Carlson CE, et al: *Pressure Ulcers in Adults: Prediction and Prevalence.* Clinical Practice Guideline No 3, AHCPR Pub No 92-0047. Rockville, MD, US Department of Health and Human Services, Public Health Service, Agency for Health Care Policy and Research, 1992.

38. Bergstrom N, Braden B: A prospective study of pressure sore risk factors among institutionalized elderly. *J Am Geriatr Soc* 40(8):747, 1992.

39. Allman RM, Goode PS, Patrick MM, et al: Pressure ulcer risk factors among hospitalized patients with activity limitation. *JAMA* 273(11):865, 1995.

40. Johnson CS, Preuss HS, Eriksson E: Plastic surgery, in Townsend CM (ed): *Sabiston Textbook of Surgery.* Philadelphia, Saunders, 2001, p 1550.

41. Peerless JR, Davies A, Klein D, et al: Skin complications in the intensive care unit. *Clin Chest Med* 20(2):453, 1999.

42. Eaglstein WH, Mertz PM: New methods for assessing epidermal wound healing: The effects of triamcinolone acetonide and polyethylene film occlusion. *J Invest Dermatol* 71(6):382, 1978.

43. Eaglestein WH, Falanga V: Chronic wounds. *Surg Clin North Am* 77(3):689, 1997.

44. Frantz RA, Gardner S: Elderly skin care: Principles of chronic wound care. *J Gerontal Nurs* 20(9):35, 1994.

45. Alvarez OM, Mertz PM, Eaglestein WH: The effect of occlusive dressings on collagen synthesis and re-epithelialization in superficial wounds. *J Surg Res* 35(2):142, 1983.

46. Lawrence WT, Diegelmann RF: Growth factors in wound healing. *Clin Dermatol* 12(1):157, 1994.

47. Tong A: Back to basics wound care. *Nurs Times Nurs Homes* 1(3):21, 1999.

48. Constantine BE, Bolton LL: A wound model for ischemic ulcers in the guinea pig. *Arch Dermatol Res* 278(5):429, 1986.

49. Lee A: Management of elderly diabetic patients in the sub-acute care setting. *Clin Geriatr Med* 16(4):833, 2000.

50. Paquette D, Falanga V: Geriatric dermatology: II. Leg ulcers. *Clin Geriatr Med* 18(1):77, 2002.

51. Hess CT: Management of the patient with a venous ulcer. *Adv Skin Wound Care* 13(2):79, 2000.

52. Litchfield R, Wolfson P, Haspel L, et al: Differential diagnosis of leg ulcers. *J Am Osteopath Assoc* 78(5):364, 1979.

53. Aufderheide TP: Peripheral arteriovascular disease, in Rosen P, Barkin R (eds): *Emergency Medicine: Concepts and Clinical Practice.* St Louis, Mosby–Year Book, 1998, p 1826.

54. Choucair MM, Fivenson DP: Leg ulcer diagnosis and management. *Dermatol Clin* 19(4):659, 2001.

55. Falanga V, Fujitani RM, Diaz C, et al: Systemic treatment of venous leg ulcers with high doses of pentoxifylline: Efficacy in a randomized, placebo-controlled trial. *Wound Repair Regen* 7(4):208, 1999.

56. Lipsky BA, Pecoraro RE, Wheat LJ: The diabetic foot: Soft tissue and bone infection. *Infect Dis Clin North Am* 4(3):409, 1990.

57. Most RS, Sinnock P: The epidemiology of lower extremity amputations in diabetic individuals. *Diabetes Care* 6(1):87, 1983.

58. Sugarman B, Hawes S, Musher DM, et al: Osteomyelitis beneath pressure sores.*Arch Intern Med* 143(4):683, 1983.

59. Centers for Disease Control and Prevention: Tetanus surveillance—United States, 1995–1997. *MMWR* 47:1, 1998.

60. Gergen PJ, McQuillan GM, Kiely M, et al: A population-based serologic survey of immunity to tetanus in the United States. *New Engl J Med* 332(12):761, 1995.

61. Alagappan K, Rennie W, Kwiatkowski T, et al: Seroprevalence of tetanus antibodies among adults older than 65 years. *Ann Emerg Med* 28(1):18, 1996.

62. Alagappan K, Rennie W, Lin D, Auerbach C: Immunologic response to tetanus toxoid in the elderly. *Ann Emerg Med* 32(2):155, 1998.

63. Gareau AB, Elby RJ, MeLellan BA, Williams DR: Tetanus immunization status and immunologic response to a booster in an emergency department geriatric population. *Ann Emerg Med* 19(12):1377, 1990.

64. Centers for Disease Control and Prevention: Diphtheria, tetanus, and pertussis. *MMWR* 40:1, 1991.

65. Plautz B, Beck DE, Selmar C, Radetsky M: Modifying the environment: A community-based injury-reduction program for elderly residents. *Am J Prevent Med* 12(4S):33, 1996.

57

Approach to Ocular Complaints

Steven Go
Anne L. Clevenger

HIGH-YIELD FACTS

- Many eye complaints of the elderly are due to the physiologic changes that occur in the aged eye.

- The emergency physician should strive to take a thorough history and perform a detailed physical examination on all elderly patients with eye complaints—with particular attention to sight-threatening causes of eye complaints.

- The emergency physician should have a low threshold for appropriate referral to an ophthalmologist whenever a sight-threatening condition is suspected.

As patients age, the rates of eye disease and blindness increase.[1] The physiologic changes that occur in aged eye over time are primarily responsible. Most of these changes are inevitable and pervasive. Consequently, as the proportion of aged patients in the emergency department (ED) increases over time, it is reasonable to expect that the prevalence of these ocular diseases presenting in the ED will increase as well. In addition, it has been suggested that there are large deficits in the public's knowledge and understanding of geriatric eye disease[2] that might lead to delayed presentations of serious eye disease. The emergency physician must be conversant with the most common eye emergencies, recognize those which are sight-threatening, and diagnose, manage, and

refer appropriately. This chapter will outline an overview strategy to deal with geriatric eye complaints in the ED. Subsequent chapters will explore various disease entities in detail.

EPIDEMIOLOGY AND PATHOPHYSIOLOGY

There have been numerous population-based studies examining the prevalence of eye disease in the elderly.[1,3,4] Most of these studies have found that the most common sight-threatening conditions are (listed in order of prevalence) senile cataract, age-related macular degeneration, open-angle glaucoma, and diabetic retinopathy. However, although these are the most common, they are not the most emergent. We generally will confine our discussion in this and subsequent chapters to the most emergent conditions. However, it is important to realize that since patients often will present with other, less acute ophthalmic conditions, the emergency physician must be conversant with them as well.

As the eye ages, a plethora of physiologic changes take place.[5,6] Those most relevant to the emergency physician are listed below.

Eyelids

The skin of the eyelids loses elasticity, and the surrounding muscles also lose some of their strength. In addition, fat also infiltrates the tissues. The result of these changes is a laxity of the eyelids, which can disrupt the former relationship between the lids and globe. For example, the lower lid may turn out (senile ectropion), which can cause degeneration of the conjunctiva and cornea, along with chronic tearing. Senile entropion, a turning in of the eyelid, can lead to severe inflammation and ulceration of the cornea.

Lacrimal System

The amount (and often the quality) of the tear film diminishes (15 percent of patients over age 80 have a dry conjunctivitis, which can lead to corneal lesions). Excessive mucus production also can result, which may be confused with eye infections.

Conjunctiva

As the conjunctiva ages, it also loses elasticity as altered tissue trophism takes place. Probably as a result of years of ultraviolet (UV) light exposure, ptergygia (a raised conjunctival lesion extending onto the cornea), pinguecula (a raised conjunctival lesion extending only to the limbus), pemphigus, and pemphigoid can result.

Cornea

Various degenerative changes occur in the cornea with age. Arcus senilis, a fatty generation visible as a white concentric lesion at the limbus, is considered by some experts to be a risk factor for ischemic heart disease in males 60 years of age and older.[7]

Anterior Chamber

Over time, the anterior chamber becomes shallower, thus increasing the likelihood of angle-closure glaucoma. In addition, patients are at increased risk for open-angle glaucoma secondary to the relative incompetence of the trabecular network.

Iris

The iris becomes thickened and more rigid. This change, coupled with weakening of the cilliary muscle, leads to smaller papillary diameters (senile miosis). This can be mistaken for a true physical finding or may limit examination of the posterior structures. The situation may be exacerbated by various medications.

Lens

The most familiar senile change is the development of cataracts, which can impair vision (especially while driving at night) and may be perceived as a "new change" by the elderly. In addition, the increased rigidity and thickening of the lens contribute to depth reduction of the anterior chamber, as well as reduction in the ability to accommodate—thus leading to presbyopia.

Vitreous

Degenerative condensations form that present as black spots noticed by the patient (muscae volitantes). They may appear suddenly, which may herald a posterior peeling off of the vitreous. As the vitreous pulls away, a retinal tear may result, possibly associated with a small vitreous bleed.

Retina

Senile vascular disease can lead to retinal central artery occlusion or retinal central vein thrombosis (see Chap. 59). In addition, ischemic optic retinopathy in association with temporal arteritis may occur. It should be remembered that arteriosclerotic changes in the retina are associated with arteriosclerosis elsewhere in the vascular tree, especially the cerebral vasculature. Evidence of systemic hypertension may be indicated by the presence of arterial narrowing or compression of veins by crossing arterioles (A-V nicking). Other senile changes include mixed areas of increased and decreased pigment proliferation in the macula or a detachment of the macular epithelium from the underlying layer. These mechanisms are thought to lead to age-related macular degeneration (ARMD), the primary cause of blindness in the aged.

It should be noted that despite these seemingly inevitable changes with age, the eye is an extremely adaptable organ and in many cases continues to function well even to an advanced age.

CLINICAL FEATURES AND HISTORY AND DIFFERENTIAL

As in most disease entities, diagnosis begins with taking an accurate and relevant history. Even if the emergency physician must resort to consultation with an ophthalmologist, being able to describe the exact symptoms in a comprehensive, succinct way will facilitate patient care. At a minimum, the following aspects of the patient's history should be obtained.[8]

Specific Nature of the Problem

However, very often the patient's chief complaint is documented by nursing staff as "blurry vision" or "I can't see." It is imperative to aggressively induce the patient to specify the exact nature of the complaint as precisely as possible. For example, is the problem diplopia or a decrease in acuity? If it is diplopia, is it monocular or binocular, horizontal or vertical? Is the lack of acuity due to pain with bright lights, or does it occur only while driving at night?

Onset and Chronicity

Was the onset sudden or gradual? As in most cases, sudden onset suggests an acutely ominous etiology. Sudden processes include an ophthalmic vascular event (retinal central artery occlusion or retinal central vein thrombosis), hemorrhage, retinal detachment, optic neuritis, acute-angle-closure glaucoma, amaurosis fugax, vertebrobasilar artery insufficiency, or migraine variant. On the other hand, a gradual onset (weeks or longer) might suggest slowly evolving events such as cataracts, refractive errors, open-angle glaucoma, or ARMD.

Pain

The presence or absence and degree of severity of pain can help discriminate between various etiologies of vision loss. Classic causes of mild to moderate pain include conjunctivitis, blepharitis, superficial punctate keratitis, and foreign bodies. Moderate to severe pain causes include acute-angle-closure glaucoma, optic neuritis, uveitis, and herpes keratitis. Painless vision loss causes include vascular occlusions, vitreous hemorrhages, retinal detachments, ischemic optic neuropathy.

Associated Symptoms

Various possible associated symptoms should be inquired about. They include photophobia (corneal abnormality), consensual pain (uveal tract involvement), pruritus (conjunctivitis, allergic reactions, contact lens–related problems), foreign-body sensation (trichiasis, corneal abnormality), tearing (dry-eye syndrome, blepharitis, ectropion), discharge (conjunctivitis, allergic reaction), night blindness (refractive error, advanced glaucoma), spots in front of the eyes (vitreous detachment, vitreous hemorrhage, cataract), and headache (temporal arteritis, acute-angle-closure glaucoma, migraine).

The past medical and ocular history, medications, and allergies should be documented for all patients.

PHYSICAL EXAMINATION

A complete description of the ocular examination is beyond the scope of this chapter, but it is imperative that a systematic approach be taken to maximize the diagnostic efficacy of the examination.

Initial Examination

Visual Acuity

Visual acuity is truly the "vital sign" for the eyes. Ideally, the test should be performed by a trained operator in good light and with appropriate standardized equipment. Unfortunately, in many EDs these are often in short supply. Since many elderly patients have difficulty with accommodation, a standard Snellen chart at 20 ft may be most useful. The visual acuity should be recorded for each eye. Because it is important to document the *best* acuity, corrective lenses should be used whenever possible. A pinhole device may be useful for correcting refractive errors if corrective lenses are not available (or optimal). In addition, patients should be strenuously urged to attempt to read the smallest line possible. Much in the way patients' Wright peak flows increase when effort is vigorously encouraged by staff, patients' visual acuities often "improve" with spirited encouragement from ED staff. Visual acuity should be checked prior to placing medications in the eye, except in cases where topical pain relief would facilitate the examination (e.g., corneal abrasion).

Pupillary Examination

The size, shape, and reactivity of the pupils should be recorded. Remember that small pupils can be caused by senile miosis, medications, or pathology. The presence of consensual pain (pain in one eye caused by shining light in the other eye) and afferent papillary defect should be noted.

Extraocular Movements

These movements may be limited by age-related changes, but the patient should still have gaze in the six cardinal directions. Asymmetric limitation of these movements should be noted. The presence of pain with these maneuvers is also an important finding.

Visual Fields

If a visual field examination is indicated, allowances should be made for the natural diminution of the visual field.[5] Simple confrontational checks of visual fields are appropriate in the ED setting.

Surrounding Structures

Evaluation of the supporting structures of the eye is important, and the geriatric eye may demonstrate some unique findings, as well as clue the examiner in to underlying systemic pathology. For example, inspection of the eyebrows might signal a hypothyroid state if they appear very coarse or do not extend past the lateral canthus. The presence of xanthelasma, yellowish lipid deposits commonly found in the nasal portion of the superior or inferior lids, is usually indicative of hyperlipidemia. Any degree of exophthalmos should be noted. A finding of unilateral exophthalmos should alert the physician to the possibility of a retrobulbar process such as tumor.[10]

Slit Lamp Examination

If available, a slit lamp always should be used to perform a thorough examination of the geriatric eye. The slit lamp examination is often crucial when there is a suspected foreign body, corneal injury, or anterior segment pathology. The examination requires that a patient is physically able to sit up and maintain proper head position in the chin rest. It is beyond the scope of this text to review how to use a slit lamp. If the reader finds himself or herself unfamiliar, it would be a good idea to review this topic. The examination should begin with the external eye and move in an anterior to posterior direction.[9]

Lids and Lashes

While examining the lids, one should note symmetry and any presence of redness or swelling of the lid margins. Ptosis should be recognized if the superior lid covers any portion of the pupil when the eye is open. Ptosis may be congenital, may herald a third cranial nerve palsy, or be indicative of Horner's syndrome.

Ectropion is present if the lower lid turns away or is everted from the eye. The most common cause of senile ectropion is horizontal tarsal plate laxity, and it can be demonstrated by easily pulling the central portion of the lower lid away from the eye as much as 1 cm.[11] This condition leads to chronic watering of the eye and eventually drying out of the conjunctiva because the lower lid is unable to hold moisture close to the eye. The conjunctiva will appear inflamed or injected without the presence of discharge or a follicular appearance as with infectious conjunctivitis.

Entropion is present when the lower lid inverts or turns in chronically. Examination will reveal injection of the bulbar conjunctiva, and the eye should be examined with flourescein to rule out the presence of abrasion. Chronic irritation from lower lashes is termed *trichiasis.*[12]

Examination of the tarsal margins may reveal entities such as hordeolum or blepharitis or the presence of carcinoma. Hordeolum or stye appears as a focal, painful swelling of the anterior lid margin and represents an acute staphylococcal infection. A chalazion or meibomian cyst is seen in the posterior margin of the lid. It is usually painless and appears as a hardened granulomatous lesion seen when the lid is everted.

Blepharitis is present when the lid margin appears chronically irritated or inflamed, and the patient relates chronic itching and soreness. The cause is thought to be staphylococcal infection or chronic inflammation of the meibomian glands. Examination will reveal dilated marginal vessels and thus redness. Collarettes, or dry scales at the base of the lashes, may be present.[12]

Any lesion of the lid should be considered for malignancy. Basal cell carcinoma is the most common eyelid malignancy, and appearance may vary widely from a pearly nodule to the characteristic rodent ulcer. Squamous cell and sebaceous gland carcinomas are possible, although less common, comprising less than 5 percent of lid tumors.[12]

Conjunctiva

The conjunctiva normally appears as a clear mucous membrane covering the anterior sclera and the inner surfaces of the lids. Any inflammatory reaction of this layer is termed *conjunctivitis* and usually presents as a red eye. In general, conjunctivitis will demonstrate chemosis (edema of the conjunctiva), copious tearing, and a normal pupillary response to light. Key physical examination findings with the slit lamp will aid in differentiating the various types. Care always should be taken to prevent spread of an infectious cause by wearing gloves during the examination.

Viral conjunctivitis classically will display a watery discharge. The inflammation of the conjunctiva may display a follicular response with scattered white structures. Often viral conjunctivitis is unilateral. Epidemic keratoconjunctivitis (EKC) typically will show intense inflammation and erythema.[13]

Bacterial conjunctivitis may be distinguished by the presence of mucopurulent discharge. Involvement may be bilateral (see Chap. 60). Examination of the tarsal conjunctiva typically will reveal deep erythema and papillae. If the amount of discharge is copious and especially purulent, a Gram stain and culture should be obtained for *Neisseria gonorrhoeae.*[14,15]

Conjunctivitis is not always a result of an infection and may be a feature of seasonal allergies or environmental irritants. Allergic conjunctivitis may demonstrate a stringy white discharge, and chemosis often will have a pale appearance.[14]

The presence of pterygia will be evident as scarring or overgrowth of conjunctival epithelium typically extending from the medial canthus to the cornea.

Cornea

The cornea should be examined with tangentially oriented light for clarity. The presence of arcus senilis is a common finding in the geriatric examination. This appears as a pale concentric deposition of lipids at the periphery of the cornea, the limbus.

Inflammation or irritation of the cornea is termed *keratitis.* Etiologies vary as with conjunctivitis. Flourescein staining must be performed to thoroughly evaluate the cornea for the presence of ulceration. Bacterial or fungal ulcers appear gray with a surrounding infiltrate and have increased fluorescein uptake. Ulcers typically are painful, and an associated iritis is not uncommon.

Herpes simplex keratitis will demonstrate a classic dendriform ulcer. There is no surrounding infiltrate as with bacterial organisms. There is usually an accompanying conjunctivitis. Herpes zoster keratitis also will display a dendritric pattern, but usually the presence of classic zoster lesions of the lid and V_1 dermatome will distinguish it from herpes simplex[14] (see Chap. 60).

Sclera

The sclera normally should appear white. Any presence of pigment changes should be noted. Senile hyaline plaques are not uncommon in this setting and are a benign finding. They appear as a dark, rust-colored pigment of the medial sclera.[10]

Inflammation of the sclera, or *scleritis,* is often associated with collagen-vascular diseases. It is typically painful and appears as a deep purplish injection of the anterior sclera, usually occurring on the medial side.[10,14]

Anterior Chamber

Evaluation of the anterior chamber should be performed in all examinations. Depth may be estimated by shining the light source in a tangential direction from lateral to medial across the cornea. With normal chamber depth, the light will pass through the cornea, and the entire iris will be illuminated. Light deflected by the iris (seen if the nasal portion of the iris is not well lighted) represents a shallow anterior chamber. Iatrogenic mydriasis should be avoided so as not to precipitate an acute onset of glaucoma.[10,13]

Acute closed-angle glaucoma presents with sudden onset of pain and blurred vision. Examination will reveal a shallow anterior chamber. The conjunctiva may be injected. The pupil usually will be poorly reactive and moderately dilated. The cornea appears hazy and edematous. The hallmark of acute-angle glaucoma is increased intraocular pressure.[15]

Uveitis is inflammation of any portion of the uveal tract (iris, choroid, and ciliary body). Usually involvement is confined to the iris and is termed *iritis.* This condition may be spontaneous but often is a related to trauma or may accompany severe cases of conjunctivitis. Slit lamp examination will reveal classic "cell and flare" in the anterior chamber. Cells are seen floating in the aqueous of the anterior chamber, and flare appears as a fog secondary to protein leakage from damaged blood vessels of the iris.[14,15]

White blood cells or red blood cells that layer out in the anterior chamber are termed *hypopyon* and *hyphema,* respectively.

Lens

The lens should be transparent. Any clouding or opacification should be noted and represents cataract formation. The presence of a large, central cataract will inhibit the examiner from an effective funduscopic examination. Almost every patient over age 65 will have some degree of cataract on examination.[10]

Retina

The retina or fundus generally should be uniform in background color. Color will vary depending on the amount of melanin present. Vessels should appear distinct. The optic disc should have sharp margins. Examination of the fundus is invaluable in the diagnosis of acute retinal vessel disease.

Central retinal artery occlusion is a sight-threatening emergency. Visual inspection of the retina on funduscopic examination reveals a pale, gray-white edematous retina. The macula will appear "cherry red." If examination is performed early in the course, "boxcarring," or segmentation of red blood cells due to slow flow through the arterioles, may by seen.[16,17]

Central retinal vein occlusion demonstrates dilated and tortuous veins in all four quadrants. There may be multiple areas of retinal hemorrhage and retinal or macular edema. "Cotton wool spots" or nerve layer infarcts may be present.[16,17]

The possibility of branch retinal vein occlusion exists

and demonstrates the preceding findings limited to the distribution of a branch vessel and not the entire fundus.[14]

Retinal detachment may be spontaneous or a result of trauma. Inspection of the fundus will reveal an area of gray elevation secondary to separation of the retina from the pigmented layer.[16]

Ischemic optic neuropathy occurs when ciliary vessels supplying the optic nerve are occluded leading to ischemia. Examination of the retina demonstrates a pale, edematous optic disc. Small nerve layer flame hemorrhages may be present at or close to the disc margins. Palpation of the temporal artery should be performed to help distinguish temporal arteritis as a source for ischemia, which is a relatively common vasculitis in the elderly population of Western countries[14,18,19] (see Chaps. 59 and 69).

Retinal findings in ARMD are generally one of two forms. "Dry" ARMD may demonstrate an atrophic macula. "Wet" ARMD is thought to be a result of "leaky" neovascularization of the submacular layer. The macula will appear edematous.[19]

Over time, the systemic effects of hypertension will be evident in the retina. The classic finding of arteriovenous cross-changes or AV nicking is present. As hypertensive effects progress, "cotton wool spots" representing nerve layer infarctions become evident. There also may be areas of hemorrhage. Finally, the presence of papilledema may occur in advanced, long-standing hypertension. These findings should be evident in both fundi because they are a result of systemic disease.[10,14]

Diabetic patients often will demonstrate retinal changes over time. Changes generally are divided into two types. Background diabetic retinopathy is represented by the presence of small microaneurysms. Hard or soft exudates may be appreciated. Hard exudates are thought to be deposition of lipid through leaking capillaries and appear as bright yellow and distinct. Soft exudates are a result of nerve layer infarction.[10]

Proliferative diabetic retinopathy is a result of neovascularization secondary to relative anoxia. The new, fragile vessels are prone to hemorrhage or leaking and may lead to macular degeneration. Retinal findings are similar to ARMD along with the presence of many small vessels of the background retina.[10]

EMERGENCY DEPARTMENT CARE AND DISPOSITION

The appropriate ED care and disposition of patients depends on the conditions diagnosed. Emergency care for glaucoma (see Chap. 58), vascular occlusions (see Chap.

59), and eye infections (see Chap. 60) are discussed elsewhere. The emergency physician should have a low threshold for appropriate referral to an ophthalmologist whenever a sight-threatening condition is suspected.

PREVENTION, PROGNOSIS, AND OUTCOME

Even if the emergency physician is able to quickly diagnose sight-threatening causes of eye complaints and make the appropriate referral to a specialist, the prognosis is variable, depending on the condition diagnosed. For example, a large traumatic retinal detachment in a poorly controlled myopic diabetic likely will have a poor outcome. In contrast, a healthy patient with a rapidly diagnosed acute-angle-closure glaucoma after an inhaled anticholinergic exposure probably will do well. Nevertheless, the emergency physician should strive to take a thorough history and perform a detailed physical examination on all elderly patients with eye complaints—with particular attention to sight-threatening causes of eye complaints. The emergency physician should take pains to look for signs of systemic illness during the eye examination and refer or work up the patient appropriately.

REFERENCES

1. Kahn HA, Leibowitz HM, Ganley JP, et al: The Framingham Eye Study: Outline and major prevalence findings. *Am J Epidermiol* 106:17, 1997.
2. Livingston PM, McCarty CA, Taylor HR: Knowledge, attitudes, and self care practices associated with age related eye disease in Australia. *Br J Ophthalmol* 82:780, 1998.
3. Ganely JP, Roberts J: *Eye Conditions and Related Need for Medical Care Among Persons 1–74 Years, United States 1971–1972.* National Center for Health Statistics, Vital and Health Statistics Series 11, No 2228, USPS Pub No 82-1678. Washington, US Government Printing Office, 1983.
4. Tielsch JM, Sommer A, Witt K, et al: Blindness and visual impairment in an American urban population: The Baltimore Eye Survey. *Arch Ophthalmol* 108:286, 1990.
5. Nuzzi N, Schiavino R: Geriatric ophthalmology. *Panminerva Med* 35:36, 1993.
6. Chatterjee PR, Dutta H, Mukherjee K, Nath S: The eye in old age. J Indian Med Assoc 97:136-7, 1999.
7. Luff A, Elkington A: The eye in systemic disease. *Practitioner* 236:186, 1992.
8. Rhee DJ, Pyfer MF (eds): *The Wills Eye Manual,* 3d ed. Philadelphia, Lippincott Williams & Wilkins, 1999.
9. Knoop K, Trott A: Ophthalmologic procedures in the emergency department: III. Slit lamp use and foreign bodies. *Acad Emerg Med* 2(3):224, 1995.

10. Seidel HM, Ball JW, Dains JE (eds): *Mosby's Guide to Physical Examination,* 3d ed. St Louis, Mosby, 1995.

11. Frueh BR, Schoengarth LD: Evaluation and treatment of patient with ectropion. *Ophthalmology* 89(9):1049, 1982.

12. Wishart K: Diagnosing the most frequent eyelid conditions. *Practitioner* 242:844, 1998.

13. Stock EL: External eye diseases. *Postgrad Med* 78(8):102, 1985.

14. Janda AM. Ocular emergencies, in Tintinalli JE, Ruiz E, Krome RL (eds): *Emergency Medicine: A Comprehensive Study Guide,* 4th ed. New York, McGraw-Hill, 1996; p1059.

15. Bertolini J, Pelucio M: The red eye. *Emerg Med Clin North Am* 13(3):561, 1995.

16. Morgan A, Hemphill RR: Acute visual change. *Emerg Med Clin North Am* 16(4):825, 1998.

17. Weinstock FJ, Weinstock MB: Common eye disorders: Six patients to refer. *Postgrad Med* 99(4):107, 1996.

18. Gonzalez-Gay MA, Garcia-Porrua C, Llorca J, et al: Visual manifestations of giant cell arteritis. *Medicine* 79(5):283, 2000.

19. Cormack G, Dhillon B: Sudden loss of vision. *Practitioner* 242(1593):851, 1998.

58

Narrow-Angle-Closure Glaucoma

MaryAnn E. Smith

HIGH-YIELD FACTS

- Narrow-angle-closure glaucoma represents an immediate threat to the patient's vision. Rapid recognition and treatment can reduce the risk of permanent visual loss.
- Measurement of intraocular pressure using the Schiotz tonometer or Tono-pen is an essential component of the eye examination.
- Geriatric patients may experience significant side effects from the antiglaucoma medications. Prudent therapy selection and careful monitoring for medication reactions are essential.

Aging produces physiologic changes in the anatomy of the eye that increase the risk for a number of ophthalmologic problems. While many of these ocular diseases are characterized by slow and subtle progression, acute narrow-angle-closure glaucoma is an exception. Typically, narrow angle closure glaucoma presents as a sudden, painful loss of vision in one eye. If left untreated, permanent visual loss will result. The precipitous, painful nature of this disease makes it likely that affected individuals will present to an emergency department (ED).

EPIDEMIOLOGY

Glaucoma, in all forms, is a common disease and a leading cause of blindness worldwide. For the year 2000, it is estimated that 66.8 million people worldwide will have some form of glaucoma, and over 6 million of those people will be blind secondary to the disease.[1] In the United States alone, approximately 80,000 Americans over age 65 are blind due to glaucoma.[2] There are many types of glaucoma; in fact, the term refers to multiple pathologic processes that result in irreversible damage to the optic nerve producing vision loss. Narrow-angle-

closure glaucoma makes up about 10 percent of all the glaucomas.[3]

PATHOPHYSIOLOGY

There are approximately 60 different forms of glaucoma. Open-angle glaucoma, the most common type, is a slow and insidious disease that, in the early stages, is usually asymptomatic. Narrow-angle-closure glaucoma is a rapid event with sudden symptomology of both vision impairment and pain. The two types of glaucoma have in common an underlying pathologic problem of increased intraocular pressure (IOP) due to aqueous flow obstruction and resulting retinal or optic nerve ischemia.

The pathologic mechanisms that produce increased IOP occur in the anterior part of the eye. This area is anterior to the lens, bounded by the cornea, and divided by the iris. The anterior and posterior chambers are connected through the pupillary opening. Aqueous humor, a clear, low-viscosity fluid, is produced by the epithelium of the ciliary body, a peripheral structure of the posterior chamber. The ciliary epithelium filters fluid from the systemic circulation using the enzyme carbonic anhydrase. Entering from its peripheral production site, aqueous humor flows behind the iris toward the pupil, through the pupillary opening, and into the anterior chamber. At the most peripheral aspect of the anterior chamber, where iris meets cornea, the aqueous exits via the trabecular network. Final disposition of the aqueous is accomplished by reabsorption into the systemic circulation via the episcleral vessels. Aqueous humor turnover is brisk, with complete volume replacement every 60 minutes. If at any point along the pathway aqueous flow is blocked, the continual production of fluid will lead to a precipitous rise in anterior and posterior chamber pressure. This pressure is transmitted rapidly to the rest of the eye and can inhibit retinal and optic nerve blood flow. Ischemia results, and if not treated promptly, retinal cell death and necrosis occur.

In narrow-angle-closure glaucoma, the obstruction takes place at the iris-cornea angle. Normally, the iris is not in contact with the cornea, which allows the aqueous humor unimpeded exit from the anterior chamber. Any force that pushes the iris forward closes the angle, blocking off the trabecular network. There are two predominant causes of narrow-angle-closure glaucoma: pupillary block and plateau iris.

Pupillary block occurs secondary to aging changes of the lens. In a normal eye, the lens is positioned posterior to the iris. As the eye ages, the lens enlarges and assumes a more forward position. If the lens comes in contact with the iris, it effectively seals off the posterior chamber, trapping aqueous humor and causing an elevation of IOP. Subsequently, the iris bows forward, closing the iris-cornea angle and preventing the egress of residual anterior chamber aqueous. Plateau iris is a congenital condition in which the iris has an unusual curved shape at the periphery, placing it close to the cornea and creating a narrow angle. Patients with this condition are at risk for angle closure with even slight changes of iris position. In either situation, the increased anteroposterior chamber pressure affects the entire eye, and retinal circulation is threatened.

CLINICAL FEATURES

Older patients are at increased risk for narrow-angle-closure glaucoma. Presentation occurs more frequently in the 50- to 69-year age range.[4] Women, farsighted individuals, and persons of Caucasian, Inuit, Chinese, or Asian origin are at increased risk. Typical symptoms are sudden onset of unilateral eye pain, perception of colored halos around lights, blurred vision, and headache. The headache is often severe, may be accompanied by nausea or vomiting, and can be the patient's chief complaint. Painless attacks have been reported but are rare.[5] The attack may be unprovoked or triggered by anything that produces pupil dilatation such as walking into a dark room or topical mydriatics. Many medicines can precipitate an attack, including anticholinergics, oral and inhaled beta agonists,[6] and serotoninergic psychoactive agents.[7,8] The patient may recall similar, less severe episodes in the past.

Physical examination reveals a reddened eye with diffuse conjunctivitis and ciliary flush. The cornea becomes edematous, clouded, and hazy. Small blisters may appear on the surface. Due to iris ischemia, the pupil is not reactive and usually mid-dilated. If examined carefully, the lens may show small gray-white opacities (glaukomflecken) that indicate previous episodes of high pressure. Gentle palpation of the eye will reveal a rock-hard globe. Slit lamp examination or oblique flashlight examination will demonstrate a shallow anterior chamber and iris bowing. Applied tonometry (Schiotz or Tono-pen) will demonstrate increased IOP. Any reading over 22 mmHg is abnormal, and in the setting of narrow-angle-closure glaucoma, pressures may be over 70 mmHg.

EMERGENCY DEPARTMENT CARE AND DISPOSITION

Initial control of increased IOP is attempted with topical ophthalmologic and/or oral and parenteral medications.

These agents temporarily affect IOP by decreasing aqueous production or volume, facilitating reabsorption, or constricting the pupil. Topical medications should be considered first-line therapy because these agents are fast-acting, readily available, and relatively well tolerated. Multiple topical agents should be used simultaneously to lower IOP in the affected eye. Topical beta blockers, such as timolol 0.5%, lower IOP directly by constricting the blood vessels supplying the ciliary body, thereby decreasing aqueous production, and may facilitate the effect of cholinergics agents. Alpha agonists, such as apraclonidine 1%, increase trabecular outflow by dilating episcleral vessels. A relatively new option, a topical prostaglandin agonist (latanoprost), increases uveoscleral outflow.[9,10] Steroid drops may be used to provide an anti-inflammatory effect. Cholinergic or miotic compounds, such as pilocarpine 2%, work by constricting the pupil but may be ineffective due to iris ischemia and generally should not be used with pressures over 40 mmHg. Miotic agents are also not indicated if the patient has had a lens implant or cataract surgery. Oral or parenteral osmotic diuretics, such as glycerol 50%, isosorbide 45%, and mannitol 20%, decrease IOP by drawing water out of the systemic circulation and decreasing the volume of the vitreous and aqueous humor and may be given intravenously if topical medications are ineffective. Carbonic anhydrase inhibitors, such as acetazolamide, decrease aqueous production by inhibiting synthesis within the ciliary epithelium and also may be given intravenously. Nonmedicinal therapy includes having the patient lie supine, which may allow gravity to pull the lens and/or iris away from the cornea. Definitive treatment is surgical. Laser iridectomy, where a hole is created through the iris, provides a permanent alternative pathway for aqueous humor flow.

ADDITIONAL ASPECTS

Geriatric patients who may have recognized or subclinical comorbid medical conditions must be monitored carefully for medication side effects. While effective, all the antiglaucoma medications, including topicals, can precipitate serious neurologic, cardiac, or pulmonary problems.[11–14] Table 58-1 summarizes a number of common glaucoma medications and potential side effects. Topical medications are the least systemically absorbed. Absorption can be further limited by applying nasolacrimal pressure (fingers pressed against the inner corners of lower eyelids) for a minute after drops are administered.[15] After each topical medication is applied to the patient, an

Table 58-1. Glaucoma Medications and Side Effects

Drug	Route	Examples	Mechanism	Side Effects
Beta blocker	T	Timolol Levobunolol Betaxolol	↓Aqueous production	Myocardial depression Bronchospasm Bradyarrhythmia Depression
Alpha-adrenergic	T	Apraclonidine Brimonidine	↓Aqueous production ↑Trabecular outflow	Hypertension Tachyarrhythmia Tremor Allergic conjunctivitis Headache
Carbonic anhdrase inhibitor	T O	Dorzolamide Brinzolamide Acetozolamide	↑Aqueous production	Corneal irritation Keratitis Headache Vertigo Blood dyscrasia Renal calculi
Miotics	T	Pilocarpine	Iris constriction ↑Aqueous outflow	Headache Ocular pain Hypotension Dyspnea
Prostaglandin analogue	T	Latanoprost	↑Uveoscleral outflow	Iris pigmentation Corneal irritation Myalgias Arthralgias
Osmotic diuretic	O IV	Glycerine Mannitol	↓Vitreous volume	Hypotension CHF

T = topical; O = oral; IV = intravenous.
Sources: Quillen DA: Common causes of vision loss in elderly patients. *Am Fam Physician* 60:99, 1999; Singh K, Bautista RD: Advances in glaucoma therapy. *Int Ophthalomol Clin* 39:1, 1999.

assessment for change in symptoms or examination will determine if any further therapy is needed. Repeat tonometry is helpful in monitoring for improvement. Most patients can have their IOP lowered without using systemic therapy. In one study, 44 percent of patients had their glaucoma pressures controlled without osmotic diuretics.[16] Osmotic diuretics have the most potential for serious side effects and should be reserved for the patient who does not respond to more conservative therapies. If the antiglaucoma medications are not effective or if intolerable side effects occur, the patient requires immediate ophthalmologic consultation for possible emergent laser iridectomy. In all cases, timely consultation and follow-up with an ophthalmologist are essential.

REFERENCES

1. Quigley HA: Number of people with glaucoma worldwide. *Br J Ophthalmol* 80:389, 1996.
2. Pizzarello LD: The dimensions of the problem of eye disease among the elderly. *Ophthalmology* 94:1191, 1987.
3. Erie JC, Hodge DO, Gray DT: The incidence of primary angle-closure glaucoma in Olmsted County, Minnesota. *Arch Ophthalmol* 115:177, 1997.
4. Congdon N, Wang F, Tielsch JM: Issues in the epidemiology and population-based screening of primary angle closure glaucoma. *Surv Ophthalmol* 36:411, 1992.
5. Rosenberg CA, Adams SL: Narrow-angle glaucoma presenting as acute, painless visual impairment. *Ann Emerg Med* 20:1020, 1991.

6. Hall SK: Acute angle-closure glaucoma as a complication of combined beta-agonist and ipratropium bromide therapy in the emergency department. *Ann Emerg Med* 4:844, 1994.

7. Denis P, Charpentier D, Berros P, et al: Bilateral acute angle-closure glaucoma after dexfenfluramine treatment. *Ophthalmologica* 209:223, 1995.

8. Aragona M, Inghilleri M: Increased ocular pressure in two patients with narrow angle glaucoma treated with venlafaxine. *Clin Neuropharmacol* 21:130, 1998.

9. Palmberg P: A topical carbonic anhydrase inhibitor finally arrives. *Arch Ophthalmol* 113:985, 1995.

10. Georgopoulos GT, Diestelhorst M, Fisher R, et al: The short term effect of latanoprost on intraocular pressure and pulsatile ocular blood flow. *Acta Ophthalmol Scand* 80:54, 2002.

11. Diamond JP: Systemic adverse effects of topical ophthalmic agents: Implications for older patients. *Drugs Aging* 11:352, 1997.

12. Nygaard HA, Hording G: Adverse effects of local use of beta-blocker in glaucoma: A literature review and a survey of reports and the adverse drug reaction authority 1985–1995. *Tidsskr Nor Laegeforen* 117:2019, 1997.

13. Johns MD, Ponte CD: Acute pulmonary edema associated with ocular metipranolol use. *Ann Pharmacother* 29:370, 1995.

14. Diggory P, Heyworth P, Chau G, McKenzie S: Unsuspected bronchospasm in association with topical timolol: A common problem in elderly people. Can we easily identify those affected and do cardioselective agents lead to improvement? *Age Aging* 1:17, 1994.

15. Zimmerman TJ, Kooner KS, Kandarakis AS, Ziegler LP: Improving the therapeutic index of topically applied ocular drugs. *Ann Ophthalmol* 102:551, 1984.

16. Choong YF, Irfan S, Menage MJ: Acute angle closure glaucoma: An evaluation of a protocol for acute treatment. *Eye* 13:613, 1999.

59

Retinal Vascular Occlusions and Ischemic Optic Neuropathy

MaryAnn E. Smith

HIGH-YIELD FACTS

- Retinal vascular occlusions are a devastating visual event that can lead to complete and irreversible vision loss
- Current treatment options for retinal vascular occlusions are limited; intraarterial thrombolytics may represent a promising future intervention
- Recognition of underlying medical conditions may be essential in preventing subsequent loss of sight in the unaffected eye
- Ischemic optic neuropathy is a common cause of vision loss in the elderly population.
- Giant cell (temporal) arteritis is a potentially treatable cause of optic neuropathy; it should be included in the differential diagnosis of any older person with unexplained vision loss.

RETINAL VASCULAR OCCLUSIONS

Epidemiology

Vascular disease of the retina is a relatively rare event, but it can have a devastating permanent effect on a patient's vision. Victims of either embolic or thrombotic events, the persons at risk for retinal artery or vein occlusions are those already at risk for systemic atherosclerotic disease. Retinal vascular occlusions are almost unheard of in young patients; they are most common in the fifth and sixth decades of life. Carotid vascular disease, hypertension, and hyperlipidemia are associated with arterial occlusions. Diabetes, collagen-vascular disease, and hypercoagulable states are additional risk factors for venous events.

Pathophysiology

Visual impairment results when blood flow to the retina is interrupted. Retinal arterial occlusive disease is a reflection of arteriosclerosis of the carotid vessels. Central retinal artery occlusion can be a thrombotic or, more commonly, embolic event. Emboli typically come from the common or internal carotid arteries but also can originate from a fibrillating atria or rheumatic heart disease. Occlusion of the central artery produces rapid retinal ischemia, and complete loss of vision results. The occlusion may resolve spontaneously, and the patient will recover his or her vision (amaurosis fugax). In some cases, a small embolus may lodge in a more distant arteriole, causing only partial retinal ischemia and less severe vision impairment. Irreversible retinal damage occurs in approximately 60 minutes, with permanent blindness as a result.

Central retinal vein occlusions usually are thrombotic in nature. Retinal vessels are subject to the same atherosclerotic changes seen in the rest of the circulatory system, and sufficient plaque can impede blood flow. When occlusion occurs, venous congestion produces retina and optic disc edema, hemorrhages, and nerve fiber infarcts ("cotton wool spots"). Branch retinal vein occlusions may occur at arteriovenous crossings or where vessels turn or bend, producing ischemia in only a section of the retina. Eventually, there is permanent nerve damage, and blindness in the affected eye is the final outcome.

Clinical Features

Retinal vascular occlusions cause sudden, painless monocular vision loss. The patient may describe a graying out or "a shade pulling down." There is usually no specific precipitating event. For both types of occlusion, the external eye examination is unremarkable. Visual acuity is markedly decreased. Light (swinging flashlight) testing can demonstrate an afferent pupillary defect. Funduscopic examination allows differentiation of the type of occlusion. In the case of retinal artery occlusion, there is little or no retinal blood flow, and the retina is pale gray or white. The fovea appears cherry red where the underlying choroid vasculature is visible through the underperfused retina. If any arteries can be visualized, there may be observed segmentalization or "boxcarring," an indication of slow-moving blood flow. When a venous occlusion occurs, the retina is congested and dark red in color; engorged vessels, "cotton wool spots," and flame hemorrhages can be observed. The optic disc may appear edematous. If a branch vessel is affected, then these changes may be seen in only one area of the retina.

Tonometry will demonstrate normal or low intraocular pressure.

Emergency Department Care and Disposition

Unfortunately, no effective therapy exists to treat retinal vascular occlusions. In the case of arterial occlusions, treatments such as ocular massage, carbon dioxide inhalation, and anterior chamber paracentesis have been recommended, but these interventions have demonstrated little or no benefit.[1,2] At best, these treatments produce sporadic results.[3] In the absence of other treatment options, however, they should be attempted expeditiously, and an ophthalmologist consulted immediately. Intraarterial thrombolytics may emerge as a new therapeutic intervention; preliminary reports show some efficacy for both arterial[4–7] and venous occlusions.[8,9] Currently, definitive trials are lacking, and the potential for serious side effects makes this a controversial therapy. At this time, no specific acute treatment exists for venous occlusions, but evaluation and follow-up with an ophthalmologist are necessary.

The patient who presents with visual loss due to retinal vascular occlusion may be exhibiting the first signs of a systemic disease, and while sight-preserving treatment for the affected eye may not be effective, recognition and management of any underlying medical conditions are essential to preserve the function of the fellow eye as well as the patient's general health. Giant cell (temporal) arteritis is a potentially treatable cause of arterial blockages. Timely diagnosis and treatment of this condition can decrease the risk of bilateral blindness significantly. Appropriate referral for management of hypertension, hyperlipidemia, or other contributing problems is also important. While the loss of vision is a catastrophic event for any person, elderly individuals with limited hearing, balance, or motor skills are at increased risk for a poor long-term outcome.[10–12] Assessment of the patient's ability to cope with a new visual impairment may prompt the practitioner to involve social services or other means to ensure the individual's safety.

ISCHEMIC OPTIC NEUROPATHY

Epidemiology

Ischemic optic neuropathy (ION) is the eye's version of a stroke—sudden cessation of blood flow to the optic nerve resulting in infarction and vision loss. ION is divided into two categories, arteritic or nonarteritic, in reference to the cause of the interrupted blood flow. If the optic nerve vascular insufficiency is associated with giant cell (temporal) arteritis, then the condition is termed *arteritic* ION. Giant cell arteritis has a causal role in a number of visual conditions; it is seen more commonly in aged persons and women. *Nonarteritic* ION has no known cause but is the most common type of optic neuropathy in persons over age 50.[13] Optic neuropathies usually strike in the sixth or seventh decades of life and represent a relatively common cause of visual loss in the elderly population.

Pathophysiology

The posterior ciliary arteries supply the optic nerve. An infarction may occur close to the optic disk and thus produce observable optic disk swelling (anterior ION) or, less commonly, may occur in the retrobulbar structures with no detectable disk changes (posterior ION). Anterior ION is most commonly arteritic in nature. Arteritic ION is a manifestation of giant cell arteritis, when the posterior ciliary arteries become involved in the generalized vasculitis. In nonarteric ION, the exact pathophysiology remains unknown, but the obstruction is not due to inflammation, compression, or demyelinization disease. There is an association with hypertension, heart disease, hypercholesterolemia, tobacco use, and diabetes, and there may be a familial predisposition.[14] Thromboembolism does not appear to be a factor. Individuals with a small optic cup may be at increased risk. Whatever the etiology, sudden interruption of blood supply to the optic nerve head produces vision loss, and if flow does not return spontaneously, edema and nerve cell death lead to permanent blindness.

Clinical Features

ION usually presents with sudden, painless loss of visual acuity. The vision loss is often described as altitudinal (upper or lower half of the visual field is missing), with inferior loss more common. A large central scotoma (black dot) may be reported. There is usually no precipitating event, and there are rarely any associated ocular symptoms. Physical examination will show an unremarkable external eye. Afferent pupillary defect may be present. If the anterior aspect of the optic nerve is involved, a swollen optic disc will be seen on funduscopic examination. However, the disk and retina may appear completely normal.

Giant cell arteritis (see Chap. 69) should be in the differential diagnosis of any older patient presenting with a visual loss. The patient interview should include questions about headache, jaw claudication, myalgias, or malaise. A complete examination with attention to palpation of the temporal arteries and measurement of the sedimentation rate is appropriate and helpful in identifying this potentially treatable disease. Definitive diagnosis of giant cell arteritis is made with temporal artery biopsy, but a presumptive diagnosis can be made based on clinical findings and/or an elevated sedimentation rate.

Emergency Department Care and Disposition

Once the optic nerve infarction has occurred, there is little that can be done to rescue the affected eye. Unfortunately, in the case of nonarteric ION, up to 10 percent of patients will develop symptoms in the fellow eye. Aspirin may decrease the frequency of second eye involvement, and if the patient does not have any contraindications, this is an appropriate recommendation.[15,16] Any associated comorbid medical conditions, such as hypertension or hypercholesterolemia, should be managed diligently. About one-third of patients will experience spontaneous improvement of their vision.[17] Of paramount importance, giant cell arteritis must be considered as a possible etiology. If suspected as the cause of a patient's vision loss, high-dose steroid therapy should be initiated as soon as possible because this may help restore vision in the affected eye and also protect the fellow eye.[18] Consultation with an ophthalmologist and early follow-up are necessary to preserve as much of the patient's sight as possible.

REFERENCES

1. Atebara NH, Brown GC, Cater J: Efficacy of anterior chamber paracentesis and Carbogen in treating acute nonarteritic central retinal artery occlusion. *Ophthalmology* 102:2029, 1995.
2. Beatty S, Au Eong KG: Acute occlusion of the retinal arteries: Current concepts and recent advances in diagnosis and management. *J Accid Emerg Med* 17:324, 2000.
3. Neubauer AS, Mueller AJ, Schriever S, et al: Minimally invasive therapy for clinically complete central retinal artery occlusion-results and meta-analysis of literature. *Klin Monatsbl Augenheilkd* 217:30, 2000.
4. Beatty S, Au Eong KG: Local intra-arterial fibrinolysis for acute occlusion of the central retinal artery: A meta-analysis of the published data. *Br J Ophthalmol* 84:914, 2000.
5. Padolecchia R, Puglioli M, Ragone MC, et al: Superselective intraarterial fibrinolysis in central retinal artery occlusion. *Am J Neuroradiol* 20(4):565, 1999.
6. Weber J, Remonda L, Mattle HP, et al: Selective intra-arterial fibrinolysis of acute central retinal artery occlusion. *Stroke* 29(10):2076, 1998.
7. Richard G, Lerche RC, Knospe V, et al: Treatment of retinal arterial occlusion with local fibrinloysis using recombinant tissue plasminogen activator. *Ophthalmology* 106(4):768, 1999.
8. Glacet-Bernard A, Kuhn D, Vine AK, et al: Treatment of recent onset central retinal vein occlusion with intravitreal tissue plasminogen activator: A pilot study. *Br J Ophthalmol* 84(6):609, 2000.
9. Vallee JN, Masin P, Aymard A, et al: Superselective ophthalmic arterial fibrinolysis with urokinase for recent severe central retinal venous occlusion: Initial experience. *Radiology* 216(1):47, 2000.
10. Glynn RJ, Seddon JM, Krug JH, et al: Falls in elderly patients with glaucoma. *Arch Ophthalmol* 109:205, 1991.
11. Owsley C, McGwin G, Ball K: Vision impairment, eye disease, and injurious motor vehicle crashes in the elderly. *Ophthalmic Epidemiol* 5:101, 1998.
12. Parrish RK, Gedde JJ, Scott IU, et al: Visual function and quality of life among patients with glaucoma. *Arch Ophthalmol* 115:1447, 1997.
13. Johnson LN, Arnold AC: Incidence of nonarteritic and arteritic anterior ischemic neuropathy: Population based study in the state of Missouri and Los Angeles county. *J Neuroophthalmol* 14:38, 1994.
14. Salomon O, Huna-baron R, Kurtz S, et al: Analysis of prothrombic and vascular risk factors in patients with nonarteritic anterior ischemic neuropathy. *Ophthalmology* 106:739, 1999.
15. Salomon O, Huna-baron R, Steinberg DM, et al: Role of aspirin in reducing the frequency of second eye involvement in patients with nonartertic anterior ischemic optic neuropathy. *Eye* 13:357, 1999.
16. Beck RW, Hayreh SS, Podhajsky PA, et al: Aspirin therapy in nonarteritic anterior ischemic optic neuropathy. *Am J Ophthalmol* 123:212, 1997.
17. Ischemic Optic Neuropathy Decompression Trial: Twenty-four month update. *Arch Ophthalmol* 118:793, 2000.
18. Hayreh SS: Ophthalmic features of giant cell arteritis. *Baillieres Clin Rheumatol* 5:431, 1991.

60

Eye Infections

Steven Go
Craig T. Florea

HIGH-YIELD FACTS

- Hyperacute conjunctivitis and herpes keratitis are potentially devastating ophthalmologic emergencies that must be suspected, diagnosed rapidly, and treated aggressively
- Before the diagnosis of preseptal cellulitis can be safely made, orbital cellulitis must be ruled out.
- The emergency physician should have no hesitation in obtaining a timely consult with an ophthalmologist when a dangerous eye condition cannot be excluded.

From birth, the conjunctiva is rapidly colonized by bacteria. During most of life, these bacteria exist in a symbiotic relationship with their surroundings—they prevent the proliferation of more virulent pathogens, and the host provides a place for them to survive.[1] However, in the elderly, physiologic changes take place that alter this normally mutually beneficial balance. Specifically, the thinning and decrease in quality of the tear layer that occurs with age[2] causes a gradual degradation of the surface defenses of the eye. In addition, as other systemic immunocompromising conditions afflict the elderly, they also may predispose these patients to particular eye infections. For the purposes of this chapter, we will confine our discussion to three of the most common infections encountered by the emergency physician: conjunctivitis, herpes infections, and periorbital infections.

EPIDEMIOLOGY AND PATHOPHYSIOLOGY

Conjunctivitis

Conjunctivitis can be caused by a variety of organisms, most commonly bacteria and viruses. Severe, rapidly progressing (hyperacute) conjunctivitis is generally caused by

Neisseria gonorrhoeae or *N. meningitides*,[3] whereas acute conjunctivitis pathogens most commonly include *Staphylococcus aureus* and *Streptococcus pneumoniae*. Chronic conjunctivitis (duration > 4 weeks) is typically caused by *Staphylococcus* species, *Chlamydia*, *Bartonella* species, *Moraxella*,[4] or miscellaneous bacteria. Other less common etiologies include tularemia, tuberculosis, and syphilis. Viral conjunctivitis is usually caused by adenovirus.

Herpes Infections

Herpes infections of the eye are caused by herpes simplex and herpes zoster (which usually has a much more benign course).[5] Herpes simplex virus (HSV) is one of the most common causes of corneal blindness in the industrial world, with an estimated 50,000 new and recurrent cases in the United Sates per year. It is a large DNA virus with two distinct antigenic forms: type 1 (nongenital) and type 2 (genital). It is important to remember that much overlap can occur. Primary HSV infection is usually subclinical, with the virus having a latent stage in the trigeminal ganglion. Reactivation occurs in response to stress, sunlight, or immunodeficiency, and the virus travels down the nerve distribution causing an infection. In the United States, an estimated 0.15 percent of the population has a history of ocular HSV infection.[6]

Herpes zoster represents reactivation of varicella; it can occur at any age but is seen primarily in the elderly.[7] The primary infection usually occurs in childhood with chickenpox. After the initial infection, the virus enters a latent stage in the nearest sensory ganglion. In the case of herpes zoster ophthalmicus, it is the trigeminal ganglion. It is estimated that up to 90 percent of healthy individuals have latent varicella-zoster virus (VZV) infection in their trigeminal ganglia.[8] As with herpes simplex, reactivation occurs in times of stress or immunodeficiency, and the elderly are especially predisposed.

Preseptal and Orbital Cellulitis

S. pneumoniae and *S. aureus* are the typical culprits in orbital and preseptal cellulitis, although anaerobes also can play a role in cellulitis secondary to puncture wounds.[6] In immunocompromised hosts, polymicrobial infections should be considered.

The primary pathophysiology of these infections is the breaching of host defenses discussed earlier. The epithelial glycocalyx normally prevents adhesion (and thus infection) by bacteria in the eye.[9] However, a breakdown in this barrier can allow bacterial invasion and a keratitis. Some bacteria, notably *Pseudomonas*, have the ability to infiltrate the intact epithelium. In addition, penetrating injury can seed bacteria in formerly sterile spaces, leading to orbital or periorbital cellulitis. Local spread from adjacent structures and hematologic spread of bacteria are two alternate mechanisms for these disease entities.

CLINICAL FEATURES

Conjunctivitis

The various types of conjunctivitis presentations may be classified as hyperacute (12–24 hours onset), acute (1–4 weeks of symptom duration), and chronic (>4 weeks of symptom duration).

Hyperacute gonococcal conjunctivitis presents with a rapid onset of severe purulent discharge. Associated features include marked hyperemia and swelling of the conjunctiva (chemosis), preauricular adenopathy, eyelid swelling, and nonspecific red spots on the conjunctiva (papillae).[10,11] Patients may admit to sexual activity and exposure.

Acute bacterial conjunctivitis generally has a much less severe presentation than gonococcal conjunctivitis, with conjunctival hyperemia and a foreign-body sensation being most prominent. Mild to moderate purulent discharge is present, but preauricular adenopathy is usually absent. Chemosis can be present but is less marked than that seen in hyperacute conjunctivitis.[10] Superficial punctate keratitis can be seen early in the course of infection, but it usually resolves spontaneously.[1]

Chronic conjunctivitis presents as patients who complain of a month or more of waking up in the mornings with their eyelids stuck together and a foreign-body sensation. Conjunctival hyperemia generally is mild, and any discharge is scant.[6]

Viral conjunctivitis often occurs in the wake of a recent viral upper respiratory infection, with a predominance of itching, burning, and a foreign-body sensation. Watery discharge is typical, and preauricular adenopathy may be present. Small, pale elevated nodules, prominent in the lower tarsal conjunctiva (follicles), can be present.[11] Small, punctate epithelial erosions may be seen as well.[6] It is highly contagious and spreads frequently from one eye to the other.

Herpes Infections

Patients with ocular HSV infection complain of eye pain, photophobia, blurred vision, tearing, and eye redness. Important historical information to gather includes the use of contact lenses, vesicular eruption (in the nasal, oral, or genital regions), and any history of corneal ulcer. The physician should look for the characteristic vesicular lesions of the skin. Unilateral blepharoconjunctivitis is present, and preauricular adenopathy may be present. The key to physical examination is the slit lamp evaluation with fluorescein. HSV classically presents with a dendritic ulcer in a linear branching pattern. In more serious forms, the dendritic ulcer widens, forming a geographic ulcer; this occurs more frequently in the immunosuppressed and following the use of topical steroids.[7] The ulcer also can appear near the corneal margins where leukocytic infiltration can occur, giving the appearance of a staphylococcal ulcer.

The symptoms of herpes zoster ophthalmicus (HZO) include eye pain and red eye, which is usually unilateral. Tearing and visual alterations also can occur. The most serious ocular complications occur when reactivation involves the nasocillary branch of the ophthalmic division of the fifth cranial nerve.[12] The physical examination should include observation of the characteristic vesicular rash in the distribution of the ophthalmic branch of the fifth cranial nerve, typically involving the tip of the nose. The intraocular pressure should be measured, and the corneal reflex should be tested in all patients suspected of having HZO. As in HSV infection, the key to diagnosis is the slit lamp examination with fluorescein, which typically shows corneal ulceration.

Preseptal and Orbital Cellulitis

Patients with preseptal cellulitis complain of eyelid erythema, pain, and swelling but have no eye pain. They may have fever as well. If the patient has any of the following signs: pain with extraocular movements, proptosis, diplopia secondary to limited ocular motility, decreased acuity, afferent pupillary defect, decreased color vision,[6], cranial nerve deficits, or eye pain, then the possibility of orbital cellulitis must be entertained. Necrotizing fasciitis of the eyelids, a rare condition with significant morbidity, has been described in the literature.[13] The characteristic defining feature of this disorder is a rapidly progressive, extensive necrosis of the subcutaneous tissues of the eyelid that is readily apparent on physical examination.

DIAGNOSIS AND DIFFERENTIAL

Conjunctivitis

The key initial question in the diagnosis of conjunctivitis is whether or not the red eye with discharge represents hyperacute conjunctivitis instead of other more benign entities. This is not always an inherently obvious distinction. Therefore, even in older patients, gonococcal conjunctivitis should be considered in cases of severe purulent conjunctivitis with rapid onset. A potentially useful test is a stat Gram stain of conjunctival scrapings looking for gram-negative intracellular diplococci.[14] However, it should be noted that Gram stains can be falsely negative, so clinical suspicion is paramount. Cultures for *N. gonorrhoeae* also should be done. Corneal lesions should be excluded because their presence most likely will affect treatment and disposition.

Once hyperacute conjunctivitis has been excluded, the differentiation between acute bacterial and viral conjunctivitis can be attempted on clinical grounds, as noted earlier; however, it is important to realize that significant overlap of signs and symptoms occurs frequently. Although some experts recommend routine cultures in these cases,[10] in common emergency medicine practice, treatment is often empirical and clinically based. In any case, special attention should be paid to making sure the patient does not have corneal involvement (keratitis or abrasions), which sometimes can be confused with conjunctivitis if a careful slit lamp examination is not done.

The diagnosis of chronic conjunctivitis is made largely based on the extended duration. Cultures for *Staphylococcus* species and *Chlamydia* should be done. A history of a recent incidence of a cat scratch (*Bartonella*) should be sought. Again, corneal involvement should be excluded.

Herpes Infections

The diagnosis of herpes simplex keratitis is made primarily on clinical grounds based on characteristic skin and corneal lesions. Laboratory confirmation is available with Giemsa stain looking for multinucleated giant cells, viral cultures, and polymerase chain reaction (PCR). The differential diagnosis includes corneal abrasion; bacterial, fungal, or interstitial keratitis; and all causes of conjunctivitis.

The diagnosis of VZO is also made on clinical grounds with the characteristic skin rash and corneal findings on slit lamp examination. Laboratory confirmation is available in the form of a Tzank smear, immunologic testing, PCR, or enzyme-linked immunoabsorbent assay (ELISA). The differential diagnosis is the same as for HSV keratitis.

Preseptal and Orbital Cellulitis

The primary task in these patients is to determine whether or not the infection has spread past the orbital septum. If there are clinical indications that this has occurred, then emergent orbital computed tomographic (CT) scanning (with axial reconstruction and coronal views) is indicated. Complete blood count, blood cultures, and wound cultures (if present) should be considered. Other entities that should be differentiated from preseptal and orbital cellulitis by history, appearance, or presence of other findings include allergies (eyelid swelling with allergic exposure and lack of pain), viral conjunctivitis (conjunctival follicles, eyelid matting, and discharge), and cavernous sinus thrombosis (cranial nerve paresis out of proportion to the amount of swelling).[10]

EMERGENCY DEPARTMENT CARE AND DISPOSITION

Conjunctivitis

If gonococcal conjunctivitis is suspected and there is no evidence of corneal involvement, treatment should begin immediately with ceftriaxone 1 g intramuscularly (penicillin-allergic patients may be treated with ciprofloxacin 500 mg orally) *plus* empirical treatment for possible coinfection with *Chlamydia* (doxycycline 100 mg orally twice daily or clarithromycin 250 to 500 mg orally twice daily). Topical bacitracin ointment four times daily or ciprofloxacin drops every 2 hours should be used. The eye should be irrigated with saline four times daily until discharge is removed.

If corneal involvement is detected (or if it cannot be ruled out), then treatment with ceftriaxone 1 g intravenously should begin, along with treatment for *Chlamydia*. In addition, topical treatment for the corneal lesions should begin with tobramycin drops every hour for the corneal lesions. Eye irrigation as described earlier also should occur.

If there is no corneal involvement, then patients may be discharged from the emergency department (ED) with daily follow-up with an ophthalmologist. However, if the possibility of corneal involvement exists, then admission is indicated. Emergent consultation with an ophthalmologist is mandatory for anyone suspicious for gonococcal conjunctivitis, and treatment and disposition decisions should be made in concert with them.

Routine antibiotic treatment for all cases of nongonococcal conjunctivitis is controversial because authors disagree on how precise a distinction can be made between bacterial and viral etiologies.[15] Given the occasional difficulty of discriminating between these two etiologies, some experts recommend empirical antibiotics for all conjunctivitis, whereas others recommend culture diagnosis.[10] There does not seem to be an evidenced-based consensus in the literature on this topic. However, it seems reasonable that classic cases of bacterial and viral conjunctivitis probably should be treated accordingly, with antibiotics used only when bacterial conjunctivitis is strongly suspected.[16] Nongonococcal bacterial conjunctivitis may be treated with a variety of topical agents. Ciprofloxacin, tobramycin, and sulfacetamide (drops or ointment) are commonly used agents. Classic viral conjunctivitis should receive supportive care and infection precautions, and antibiotics should be reserved only for cases of bacterial superinfection.

Because the number of possible causative agents can be very extensive, the treatment of chronic conjunctivitis should be done in consultation with an ophthalmologist. As long as corneal involvement is absent, treatment can be deferred safely until the appropriate specialized cultures can be done.

Herpes Infections

The primary ocular herpes infection is a self-limited infection that lasts approximately 3 weeks. The rationale for treatment is to reduce stromal damage. Topical treatment options include trifluridine 1% drops nine times per day or virabine 3% ointment five times per day. In addition, oral acyclovir 400 mg five times per day for 10 days is the preferred treatment in those patients who are unable to tolerate topical treatments and have good renal function. A cycloplegic agent may be added to this regimen to give comfort from ciliary body spasm. The use of topical steroids is absolutely contraindicated early in treatment but may be added after several days of topical antiviral. Surgical debridement of dendritic, geographic, or marginal ulcers may be indicated but should be performed by an ophthalmologist. If intraocular pressure is found to be elevated, timolol drops and acetazolamide should be added. All patients suspected of HSV keratitis require consultation with an ophthalmologist.

The treatment of HZO is with antiviral medications such as acyclovir 800 mg five times daily, famciclovir 500 mg three times daily, or valcyclovir 1 g three times daily. All treatment regimens are for 7 days. A large randomized trial showed that ocular complications occurred in 29 percent of treated patients versus 71 percent of untreated payients.[7] Strong analgesia is also indicated. If severe symptoms are present, inpatient treatment should be considered. Outpatient management should be under close supervision of an ophthalmologist.

Preseptal and Orbital Cellulitis

Simple preseptal cellulitis with no signs or symptoms of systemic illness may be treated safely on an outpatient basis. Treatment should include broad coverage with agents such as amoxicllin-clavulanate 500 mg orally every 8 hours or cefaclor 250 to 500 mg orally every 8 hours. In the penicillin-allergic patient, erythromycin 250 mg orally every 6 hours may be used. A consult with an ophthalmologist should be obtained to direct treatment and follow-up

If the patient with preseptal cellulitis has signs or symptoms of systemic illness, abnormal vital signs, significant comorbidities (e.g. diabetes, AIDS), a history of medication noncompliance, or has failed outpatient therapy, then he or she should be admitted for broad-spectrum intravenous antibiotics and consultation with an ophthalmologist. Typical regimens include ampicillin-sulbactam or ceftriaxone and vancomycin.

The presence of orbital cellulitis should provoke an emergent consultation with an ophthalmologist for admission, broad-spectrum intravenous antibiotics, and possibly surgical drainage of any associated abscess.

ADDITIONAL ASPECTS

Conjunctivitis

If gonococcal conjunctivitis is diagnosed and treated promptly, prognosis is excellent. The converse is also true.[17] Uncomplicated acute bacterial and viral conjunctivitis generally is self-limited, without significant sequelae. The outcome of chronic conjunctivitis depends on the specific etiology.

Herpes Infections

The prognosis of HSV keratitis is generally favorable with aggressive treatment. The complication of corneal scarring may occur. If the resulting scar is located centrally, permanent loss of visual acuity may result. It is imperative to educate the patient on medication compliance and need for follow-up. The patient also should be educated on early recognition of symptoms in recurrence. Patients should be urged to seek emergent care if such symptoms appear. Acyclovir 400 mg twice daily has been shown to be an effective agent to prevent recurrence.[18]

The overall prognosis of HZO is quite good with treatment, but serious ocular and neurologic complications may occur. The abrupt cessation of topical steroids has been related to more serious ocular complications.[8] The patient should be educated on diligent medication compliance and follow-up. Patients should be informed of the risk of spreading the infection to uninfected individuals. Patients with HSV keratitis or HZO also should be taught to avoid any known precipitating factors.

Preseptal and Orbital Cellulitis

Much like hyperacute conjunctivitis, favorable outcomes largely depend on the rapidity of an accurate diagnosis and aggressive treatment.

REFERENCES

1. Limbert, MB: A review of bacterial keratitis and bacterial conjunctivitis. *Am J Ophthalmol* 112:2S, 1991.
2. Nuzzi N, Schiavino R: Geriatric ophthalmology. *Panminerva Med* 35:36, 1993.
3. Ullman S, Roussel TJ, Culbertson WW, et al: *Neisseria gonorrhoeae* conjunctivitis. *Ophthalmology* 94:525, 1987.
4. Kowalski RP, Harwick JC: Incidence of moraxella conjunctival infection. *Am J Ophthalmol* 101:437, 1986.
5. Garcia GE: Management of ocular emergencies and urgent eye proglems. *Am Fam Phys* 53:565, 1996.
6. Donahue SP, Khoury JM, Kowalski RP: Common ocular infections: A prescriber's guide. *Drugs* 52:526, 1996.
7. Liesegang TJ: Varicella-zoster viral disease. *Mayo Clinc Proc* 74:983, 1999.
8. Liesegang TJ: Ophthalmic herpes zoster diagnosis and antiviral treatment. *J Geriatr* 46:64, 1997.
9. Reed WP, Williams RC: Bacterial adherence: First step in pathogenesis of certain infections. *J Chron Dis* 31:67, 1978.
10. Conjunctiva/Sclera/External Disease in Rhee DJ, Pyfer MF (eds): *The Wills Eye Manual,* 3d ed. Philadelphia, Lippincott Williams & Wilkins, 119, 1999.
11. Auckland Allergy Clinic: *Allergic Conjunctivitis.* Retrieved June 7, 2002 from *http://www.allergyclinic.co.nz/guides/9.html.*
12. McGill JI, White JE: Acyclovir and post-herpetic neuralgia and ocular involvement. *Br Med J* 309:1124, 1994.
13. Overholt EM, Flint PW, Overholt EL, Murakami CS: Necrotizing fasciitis of the eyelids. *Otolaryngol Head Neck Surg* 106:339, 1992.
14. Benton B, Ocular Emergencies in Cline DM, Ma OJ, et al (eds): *Emergency Medicine: A Comprehensive Study Guide, Companion Handbook,* 5th ed. New York, McGraw-Hill, 761, 2000.
15. Rees MK: The red eye. *New Engl J Med* 343:1577, 2000.
16. Sheikh A, Hurwitz B: Topical antibiotics for acute bacterial conjunctivitis: A systematic review. *Br J Gen Pract* 51:473, 2001.
17. Bashour M: *Gonococcus.* Retrieved June 11, 2002 from *http://www.emedicine.com/oph/topic497.htm.*
18. Jabs DA: Acyclovir for HSV ocular disease. *New Engl J Med* 339:300, 1998.

61

Epistaxis

Thomas K. Swoboda

HIGH-YIELD FACTS

- Anterior epistaxis accounts for 90 percent of all nosebleeds and is often self-limited.

- Older patients on aspirin or other anticoagulant therapies are at a higher risk for epistaxis.

- Hypertension seen in older patients with epistaxis is usually due to anxiety and resolves after control of bleeding is achieved.

- Patients discharged home with anterior nasal packing require pain medication and antibiotics to prevent sinusitis and toxic shock syndrome.

- Patients with posterior nasal packing should be admitted to the hospital and may require supplemental oxygen and sedation.

Epistaxis is a commonly seen condition among elderly patients presenting to the emergency department (ED). Most people have had at least one nosebleed during their lives. Patients often present to the ED after attempts to control the bleeding on their own by direct pressure have failed. For patients with chronic medical problems, such as chronic obstructive pulmonary disease (COPD) and atherosclerotic heart disease, prolonged bleeding from epistaxis can worsen the patient's underlying condition. In these patients, prompt recognition of the severity of bleeding must occur. The emergency physician should develop a strategy that can be relied on to both identify and control the source of bleeding.

EPIDEMIOLOGY

Epistaxis affects people of all ages but is seen most often in young children and the elderly. The elderly frequently present with sustained bleeding that cannot be controlled at home. It is a common condition, with 15 people per 10,000 annually requiring physician care and 1.6 in 10,000 requiring hospital admission.[1] Of these hospitalized patients, 29 percent require transfusion, and 5.6 percent require surgical intervention.[2] It occurs more frequently in northern climates during the winter months because of decreased relative humidity that dries nasal mucosa.

PATHOPHYSIOLOGY

Numerous causes exist for epistaxis. Local disruption of the nasal mucosa can predispose that area to bleeding. Trauma, commonly caused by nose picking, is the most common local etiology. Inducers of inflammation and friability of the nasal mucosa, such as sinusitis, viral rhinitis, use of nasal sprays, and dry air, will increase the likelihood of substantial nasal hemorrhage.

Prolonged epistaxis in the elderly that is difficult to control with direct pressure is commonly secondary to atherosclerosis and anticoagulant therapy. Atherosclerosis causes fibrous tissue and collagen to be deposited in the muscular tunica media layer of vessels. These deposits can calcify and reduce the vessel's elasticity, preventing vessel contraction. Anticoagulant therapy requires application of direct pressure for longer periods of time to achieve hemostasis. Many elderly patients take a daily aspirin or anticoagulant medications such as warfarin or subcutaneous heparin. These patients frequently cannot control their nasal bleeding by direct pressure.

Hypertension, a common condition among elderly patients, has not definitively been shown to cause an increase in the occurrence of epistaxis.[3] Patients with epistaxis have a higher prevalence of elevated blood pressure.[4] However, this is likely due to patient anxiety that frequently occurs at time of presentation. Resolution of the bleeding or administration of mild anxiolytic medication frequently results in a lowering of the blood pressure.

Approximately 90 percent of epistaxis cases occur in

the anterior nasal septum region known as *Kiesselbach's plexus.* Kiesselbach's plexus is supplied by branches of both the internal and external carotid arteries. From the internal carotid artery, the ophthalmic artery branches off the anterior ethmoidal artery that supplies the superior portion of the anterior third of the nasal septum via small branches into Kiesselbach's plexus. One branch of the external carotid artery, the superior labial artery, supplies the anterior nasal spine and also has branches in Kiesselbach's plexus.

Posterior nasal blood supply comes from the posterior ethmoid artery, a branch of the internal carotid artery, and the internal maxillary artery, which is a major branch of the external carotid artery. The posterior ethmoid artery directly supplies blood to the posterior third of the septum. The terminal branch of the internal maxillary artery, the sphenopalatine artery, supplies blood to the lateral wall and septum.

CLINICAL FEATURES

Patients with epistaxis typically present with a history of intermittent bleeding that may be either active or temporarily controlled at the time of presentation to the ED. Rapid assessment of the amount and severity of bleeding determines the need for immediate attention. Patients with stable vital signs should attempt to control their bleeding by pinching the nares just below the nasal bridge for 10 to 15 minutes. Pressure also can be applied by use of a commercially available nose clip. If the patient appears unstable, priority should be placed on the ABCs. Intravenous access, cardiac monitoring, and supplemental oxygen should be set up prior to obtaining the history or doing the physical examination. After stabilization, if the patient is still bleeding heavily, the physician's attention should be directed at controlling the hemorrhage.

Patients presenting without active bleeding require a complete history and ear, nose, and throat (ENT) examination. The history obtained from all patients with epistaxis should include the following:

- Duration of the most recent episode of bleeding
- Quantity of bleeding
- Nostril from which bleeding was first noted
- Attempts made to control bleeding by the patient
- Results of pressure on nose (stop bleeding or drainage posteriorly)
- History of any trauma as a cause to bleeding
- Medications, including over-the-counter medications

- Medical conditions that predispose to persistent bleeding (e.g., liver failure, hemophilia)
- Illicit drug use
- Prior episodes of epistaxis and how they were controlled
- Any bleeding from gums or blood in stool or urine
- History of easy bruising, recent chemotherapy, prior neoplasm, or prior nasal surgery

Examination of the patient requires several essential pieces of equipment. A light source that provides direct illumination of the nasal cavities while leaving both hands free for examination is vital. A battery-operated headlamp or overhead surgical lamp should be used. A nasal speculum, several cotton-tipped applicators, bayonet forceps, cotton pledgets, and medication for vasoconstriction and anesthesia are also essential for proper examination. Prior to examining a patient with epistaxis, the physician should wear protective eyewear, mask, gloves, and gown because blood particles can easily become aerosolized when patients sneeze or cough.

Examination should be geared toward determining the source of bleeding. If bleeding is active, the physician will need both hands to thoroughly examine the nasal cavity. While holding the nasal speculum in one hand, a cotton-tipped applicator in the other hand should be used to remove blood to examine for any active bleeding. If bleeding is brisk, Frazier tip suction can remove clots and continuously clear sources of bleeding.

To slow or stop the bleeding, a topical combination of local anesthetic and vasoconstrictive agent can be applied. A mixture of 4% lidocaine with 1% phenylephrine on a cotton-tipped applicator is often effective. A 4% solution of cocaine has both anesthetic and vasoconstrictive properties but is not used commonly due to logistic problems associated with storing this agent. Oxymetazoline (Afrin) is a vasoconstrictive agent with no anesthetic properties that can be used to gain control of bleeding. If bleeding is profuse and the cotton-tipped applicator is ineffective, the preceding agents can be applied to cotton pledgets or a compressed nasal tampon (e.g., Merocel) to slow the bleeding.

Once the site of bleeding becomes apparent, definitive control of the bleeding should occur. If the site of bleeding is not visualized, the bleeding is likely to be from a posterior source, and posterior packing should be considered. If the patient has severe hemorrhaging that does not allow visualization of any source or the patient shows signs of impending exsanguination, both nostrils should receive anterior packing. If bleeding persists, then posterior packing is necessary.

DIAGNOSIS AND DIFFERENTIAL

A type and cross-match, hemoglobin, and hematocrit should be ordered if there is significant bleeding. An international normalization ratio (INR), prothrombin time (PT), activated partial thromboplastin time (aPTT), platelet count, and liver function tests should be ordered as the first step in working up a possible coagulopathy.

In older patients who have a history of repeated epistaxis or are severely ill, it is important not to mistake hemoptysis or hematemesis for epistaxis. Patients with coagulopathies or severe liver disease may present with any of these conditions concurrently.

EMERGENCY DEPARTMENT CARE AND DISPOSITION

Anterior Epistaxis

If a source of bleeding is visualized during examination, it is likely to be from Kiesselbach's plexus. Cauterization is the initial maneuver for controlling visible hemorrhage. If slight oozing is noted, silver nitrate may be used as a first-line cauterizing agent. A cotton-tipped applicator or Frazier tip suction can be used to minimize the amount of fresh blood in the area. The silver nitrate stick can be rolled over the area of bleeding for 5 to 10 seconds to cauterize the bleeding. Application of silver nitrate in the same area for more than 20 seconds will devitalize the nasal mucosa on the opposite side of the nasal septum, possibly causing septal perforation; thus silver nitrate should not be applied blindly. Disposable electrocautery units also can be used but are bulky in comparison with silver nitrate applicators. They may not safely access the site of bleeding.

If anterior bleeding is not stopped by administration of vasoconstrictive agents or cauterization, nasal packing must be used. Commercially available pressed tampons, such as Merocel, are easy to use and well tolerated by patients. The tampons expand on any contact with fluid, exerting pressure onto the nasal mucosa. After the tampon is covered with an antibiotic ointment, it is inserted until the proximal end is flush with the nasal opening. Saline drops or vasoconstrictive agents are then added to the end of the tampon, causing expansion. Some tampons have a suture attached to one end that should be left outside the nasal cavity. It can be taped to the cheek and used to facilitate removal of the tampon 2 to 3 days later. In all cases of anterior packing with persistent bleeding, the nonbleeding nostril also should be packed to achieve hemostasis by keeping the septum in the midline and main-taining pressure on the actively bleeding side. If this fails, posterior packing should be performed.

An intranasal single-balloon catheter also can be used for anterior packing. After applying antibiotic ointment to the catheter and balloon, they are inserted into the nasal cavity, and the balloon is inflated with saline or sterile water. This method generally is well tolerated by patients.

For patients with coagulopathies or friable nasal mucosa, subsequent rebleeding is likely to occur when anterior packing is removed; as a result, an absorbable packing should be used. Absorbable packing made from materials such as Gelfoam can be soaked in a vasoconstrictive agent and gently inserted up against the bleeding area. Eventually, this packing falls out or is blown out of the nose by the patient.

Failure of these methods will require the use of the more "traditional" method of applying petroleum ribbon gauze in the nasal cavity. With the free end of the gauze protruding from the nares, the ribbon is folded on itself inferiorly to superiorly using nasal forceps until the entire cavity is filled. Between 3 and 6 ft of gauze generally is required. The second end also should protrude from the nares. Both the bleeding and nonbleeding cavities are filled using the same method.

For all patients with anterior epistaxis, discharge instructions should be given to refrain from blowing the nose, avoid digital trauma, and use a room humidifier. Patients should be instructed to pinch their nares for 15 to 20 minutes if bleeding recurs. Saline nasal spray also can be given to maintain the moisture of mucosal membranes. Patients discharged with any type of nasal packing should be prescribed prophylactic oral antibiotics (amoxicillin-clavulanate, cephalosporins, or fluoroquinolones) to prevent development of sinusitis and toxic shock syndrome.[5] Analgesic medication also should be prescribed to patients with anterior packing.

All patients with anterior packing should receive follow-up within 2 to 3 days for packing removal. They should be instructed to return for fever, nausea, vomiting, or recurrent bleeding that cannot be controlled with self-applied pressure.

Posterior Epistaxis

Epistaxis that is not controlled with adequate anterior packing requires placement of a posterior pack and consultation with an otolaryngologist. All patients with posterior packing require hospital admission after the pack is placed. Bleeding not controlled with anterior and posterior packing will require surgical intervention such as embolization or arterial ligation.

Posterior packing does not exert direct pressure on the site of bleeding. When placed with anterior packing, it allows the entire nasal cavity to be occluded, enhancing clot formation within the entire cavity. It also prevents blood from being aspirated and swallowed. To achieve these results, posterior packing should occlude the distal nasopharynx.

The most common type of posterior packing uses a no. 14F Foley catheter with a 30-mL balloon. The tip of the Foley catheter should be cut off as close to the balloon as possible, and the balloon should be tested with saline for leaks. The Foley catheter should be lubricated with a water-soluble ointment and inserted in the side of the nose with active bleeding. With the distal end of the Foley catheter visible in the posterior pharynx, the balloon should be inflated slowly with water until the patient feels discomfort. Only 10 to 15 mL of water is usually required. Gentle traction should be applied to the proximal end of the Foley catheter at the nasal opening until resistance is felt. The Foley catheter should be anchored in place with an umbilical clamp or similar device. Placement of anterior packing, either petrolatum gauze or nasal tampons, around the Foley catheter will prevent blood from oozing out anteriorly. Placement of gauze between the anterior surface of the nasal opening and the clamp prevents necrosis of the nasal tissues over the next 24 to 36 hours.

Commercial posterior nasal balloon catheters are also available. They consist of two balloons that can be filled with saline or sterile water, with the smaller balloon acting as the posterior pack. The catheter should be lubricated with antibiotic or water-soluble gel and then placed in the nasal cavity and slid down until its distal portion is in contact with the posterior pharynx. The posterior balloon is filled with sterile water or saline, and traction is applied to the catheter anteriorly until the posterior balloon seals the posterior nasopharynx. The anterior balloon is then filled. Anterior packing should be placed in the opposite nasal cavity to prevent deviation of the nasal septum that would allow continued bleeding.

The "traditional" method of constructing a posterior nasal pack with gauze rolls and either silk ties or rubber catheters is time-consuming and difficult to perform in patients with severe bleeding. Methods using the Foley catheter or commercial balloon devices are more favorable because of their effectiveness and ease of use. Long nasal tampons that cover both anterior and posterior parts of the nasal cavity also can be used to stop posterior bleeding using the same methods as discussed previously for anterior packing.

Complications secondary to posterior packing are not uncommon. These include sinusitis, aspiration, otitis media, eustachian tube dysfunction, cardiac dysrhythmias, stroke, myocardial infarction, and death. Elderly patients, particularly those with COPD or congestive heart failure, are at increased risk for hypoxia secondary to a hypothesized nasopulmonary reflex.[6]

Posterior packing should be left in place for 3 to 5 days because removal within 48 hours is associated with an increased incidence of rebleeding.[7] All patients with posterior packing require cardiac monitoring and pulse oxymetry. Empirical antibiotic therapy (amoxicillin-clavulanate, cephalosporins, or fluoroquinolones) should be initiated to prevent the development of sinusitis and toxic shock syndrome. Patients should be admitted to a monitored setting with otolaryngologic consultation.

REFERENCES

1. Josephson GD, Godley FA, Stierna P: Practical management of epistaxis. *Med Clin North Am* 75:1311, 1991.
2. Levin WJ: Epistaxis: New ticks for an old dog. Presentation, ACEP Scientific Assembly, Las Vegas, NV 1999.
3. Lubianca-Neto JF, Bredemeier M, Carvalhal EF, et al: A study of the association between epistaxis and the severity of hypertension. *Am J Rhinol* 12:269, 1998.
4. Herkner H, Laggner AN, Mullner M, et al: Hypertension in patients presenting with epistaxis. *Ann Emerg Med* 35:126, 2000.
5. Tag AR, Mitchell FB, Harell M, et al: Toxic shock syndrome: Otolaryngologic presentations. *Laryngoscope* 92:1070, 1982.
6. Loftus BC, Blitzer A, Cozine K: Epistaxis, medical history, and the nasopulmonary reflex: What is clinically relevant? *Otolaryngol Head Neck Surg* 110:363, 1994.
7. Viducich RA, Blanda MP, Gerson LW: Posterior epistaxis: Clinical features and acute complications. *Ann Emerg Med* 25:592, 1995.

62

ENT Infections

Jason Graham
Michael Polka

HIGH-YIELD FACTS

- Sinusitis is responsible for 17 percent of office and emergency department visits in the elderly.
- Malignant otitis externa is a potentially life-threatening illness occurring most often in diabetic and immunocompromised patients.
- Complications of ear, nose, and throat (ENT) infections in the elderly have increased morbidity and mortality when compared with younger population groups.
- Airway control is the first priority in the management of serious ENT infections such as Ludwig's angina and epiglottitis.

One of the most common complaints in the elderly is that of ear, nose, and throat (ENT) symptomatology. Sinusitis alone is one of the most frequent infections in the geriatric population and is responsible for 17 percent of office and emergency department (ED) visits in the elderly.[1] ENT infections also may carry significant morbidity in the geriatric patient.

EPIDEMIOLOGY

ENT infections are the etiology of fever in fewer then 5 percent of patients.[2] In general, the incidence of ENT infection in the elderly parallels that in younger population groups. However, sequelae of ENT infections in the elderly are associated with increased morbidity and mortality when compared with younger population groups. For example, bacterial meningitis carries a threefold increased mortality rate in the elderly.[2]

PATHOPHYSIOLOGY

Physiologic changes contribute to ENT infections in the elderly. Barrier protection of the skin and mucosa decreases with aging. Impaired circulation, decreased cough reflex, and immune dysregulation lead to delayed healing and an increase in opportunistic infections.

The external auditory canal, middle ear, cochlear system, and vestibular system all undergo structural and functional changes with aging. The skin of the external auditory canal becomes atrophic and dry. There is a decrease in both the function and number of apocrine sweat glands and cerumen glands that occupy the outer half of the auditory canal. The cerumen becomes thicker, dryer, and more adherent to the skin of the external canal. Bony growths, such as benign osteophytes and osteomas, cause narrowing of the external auditory canal and further predispose the geriatric patient to cerumen impaction. These changes lead to pruritus and irritation of the external auditory canal. There is not an increase in the incidence of otitis externa in the elderly compared with the younger age groups.[3] When disease of the external ear does occur, these changes lead to an increased amount of otalgia.

Atrophic and sclerotic changes of the tympanic membrane are common. Age-related changes in the middle ear include degenerative changes of the ossicular articulations and calcification of the articular cartilage and joint capsule. These changes do not affect conductive hearing.

Myelinated nerve fibers of the vestibular system are decreased by up to 40 percent in the elderly.[3] Fibrosis of tissue between the bony vestibular aqueduct and the endolymphatic duct occurs. Saccular membrane rupture in the elderly is a common event. Dense deposits of insoluble particles in the semicircular canal can lead to postural vertigo.

With aging, there is a decrease in adipose tissue of the nose. Atrophy of the muscular structure also occurs. The cartilage of the nasal alae thins and softens. There is a decrease in mucus production, and a lessening of internal moisture leads to a thickening of mucus secretions. Sclerosis and fragility of the venous plexus contribute to epistaxis. These changes coupled with years of gravitational effects cause the nose to gradually elongate and narrow with a drooping at the tip. Nasal obstruction may result from these changes. Obstruction occurs when drooping of the nose is pronounced as the walls of the softened alae close against the septum with inspiration.

Several changes occur within the oral cavity of the aging patient. The mucosa has a thinned epithelium with a reduced functional vascular bed. Salivary ductal adhesions and acinar hyalinization lead to a decrease in salivary gland production of up to 25 percent.[4] These changes lead to an increase in tissue injury and dental caries. Taste bud sensitivity also decreases with aging.

In the throat, muscle atrophy occurs, and the false vocal cords produce less mucus. Joint capsule relaxation or fixation of the cricothyroid joint and cricoarytenoid joint may occur. These changes result in bowing of the vocal cords, dryness of the mucosa, and vocal changes.

CLINICAL FEATURES AND EMERGENCY DEPARTMENT CARE

Otitis Externa

Diffuse bacterial otitis externa presents with otalgia and a sensation of fullness in the auditory canal. Erythema and swelling of the external canal are usually present. A foul-smelling watery otorrhea and desquamated debris also may be present. Swelling may completely occlude the external auditory canal, leading to reversible conductive hearing loss.

Infection arises in humid conditions in which there has been damage to the skin of the external auditory canal. The disease process is often precipitated by immersion in water, hence the name swimmer's ear. Otitis externa also may result from attempts to remove wax from the external canal, hearing aid use, or seborrheic dermatitis. Intense pruritus often leads the patient to scratch the irritated tissue with objects such as pen caps and bobby pins. This leads to further compromise of the epithelium and a worsening of the infection. Common pathogens include *Staphylococcus aureus, Pseudomonas aeruginosa, Streptococcus* species, and *Proteus* species.[5,6]

Treatment of otitis externa consists of leaving the external canal open to air. During bathing, the ear should be kept dry. A cotton ball impregnated with petroleum jelly can be used to prevent water from entering the external canal while bathing. A 1:1 mixture of rubbing alcohol and white vinegar may be used to irrigate the external ear after bathing. Alcohol helps dry the ear, and vinegar acidifies the ear, which may prevent superinfection. Use of this solution is contraindicated if the tympanic membrane has been ruptured. Both components of the mixture are irritating to the middle ear.

Otitis externa is best treated with topical antibiotics. Effective choices include neomycin, polymyxin, fluoroquinolone, and Cortisporin.[5,6] Cortisporin contains hydrocortisone, which helps decrease inflammation. In cases of tympanic membrane rupture, a nonototoxic drug should be used. Quinolone solutions should be reserved for more severe infections. Neomycin is present in many topical preparations because of its effectiveness in treating gram-positive infections. Preparations containing neomycin can be a cause of skin irritation and localized allergic reaction.[5] If sensitivity occurs, the topical antibiotic should be changed to a compound free of neomycin. Treatment should continue for 5 to 7 days.

If swelling and inflammation have resulted in occlusion of the external auditory canal, an otic sponge or an ear wick should be inserted. Topical antibiotic drops can be placed directly on the wick, causing it to expand. The expanding wick reduces edema, allowing the antibiotic to reach all portions of the external canal. Sponges and wicks should be removed after 5 to 7 days.

In cases where there is cervical lymphadenopathy, severe otalgia, infection beyond the pinna, or fever, dicloxacillin 500 mg four times daily should be prescribed. Hearing aids should not be used until the infection resolves.

Malignant Otitis Externa

Malignant otitis externa is a form of necrotizing infection of the external auditory canal. This is a potentially life-threatening infection occurring almost exclusively in diabetic and immunocompromised patients.[5] Initially, only acute otitis externa may be present. Severe deep ear pain and granulation tissue in the posterior inferior auditory canal then develop. Granulation tissue may be absent in AIDS patients. With penetration of the epithelium, the infection advances along facial and vascular planes, leading to complications such as temporal bone osteitis, chondritis, cellulites, lateral venous sinus thrombosis, paralysis of the seventh through twelfth cranial nerves, and extension through the clivus to the contralateral temporal bone.

P. aeruginosa is the most common pathogen.[5,6] Culture and sensitivity of the infected tissue should be ordered. Technetium-99m bone scanning and computed tomographic (CT) scanning can be used to detect osteo-myelitis.

Patients should be admitted and treated with both intravenous and topical antibiotics. Appropriate antibiotic choices include third- and fourth-generation cephalosporins, aminoglycosides, and fluoroquinolones. Several weeks of intravenous antibiotics may be required for effective treatment. ENT consultation should be initiated because local debridement of tissue is often needed.

Otomycosis

Otomycosis is a fungal infection of the external auditory canal. It presents most commonly following prolonged use of topical antibiotic drops or in immunocompromised patients. A moist environment within the external canal is conducive to fungal growth. Pruritus is usually severe. Pain and swelling of the external canal are typical but not commonly as severe as the pain and swelling associated with otitis externa. Fluffy white hyphae with a velvety appearance are characteristic of otomycosis. The hyphae are sometimes mistaken for cotton strands. *Aspergillus niger* causes a grayish black mass to form in the canal. Other common fungal pathogens are *Candida albicans, A. flavus,* and *A. fumigatus.*[5]

Treatment includes meticulous cleaning of the auditory canal and tympanic membrane followed by a 7- to 10-day treatment with an antimycotic solution such as clotrimazole.[5]

Furunculosis

Furunculosis is an infection of the hair follicles at the lateral aspect of the external canal. Severe pain is present with manipulation of the auricle. Cellulitis and fluctuant swelling close to the external meatus may be present. Spontaneous drainage of pus and regional lymphadenopathy also may occur. Infection is commonly the result of *Staphylococcus* species.[5]

Treatment includes incision and drainage of any formed abscess. An ear wick should be inserted into the external canal. A commercial acetic acid solution such as VoSol should be placed on the wick to acidify the canal and decrease bacterial growth. If cellulitis is noted, oral antibiotics with proven gram-positive coverage should be used. Antibiotic choices include dicloxacillin, amoxicillin-clavulanate, and levofloxacin.[5] Narcotic analgesics may be needed for pain control.

Bullous Myringitis

Bullous myringitis presents with otalgia, a sense of fullness in the ear, and blebs on the lateral surface of the tympanic membrane. A reversible sensorineural hearing loss is present in up to one-third of patients with this disease.[7] The cause remains unknown; however, several viruses and *Mycoplasma pneumoniae* have been implicated.[7]

The disease is usually self-limited. Rupturing the bullae does not decrease the pain or duration of the illness.[7] Pain is treated with Auralgan and oral analgesics. If hearing loss is present, the patient should be started on a 7- to 10-day course of oral steroids and referred to their primary physician for follow-up of the hearing loss.

Acute Otitis Media

Acute otitis media is a middle ear infection that is characterized by otalgia that may radiate to the jaw. This pain may intensify with opening and closing of the mouth. An effusion may be present, causing bulging of the tympanic membrane and tension of the middle ear space. An air-fluid level may be present posterior to the tympanic membrane. Erythema of the tympanic membrane is common.

Hemophilus influenzae, Pneumococcus, Staphylococcus, and *Moraxella* are the pathogens most commonly cultured from acute otitis media infections.[8]

First-line oral antibiotic therapy includes amoxicillin and trimethoprim-sulfamethoxazole.[8] Second-line therapy covers β-lactamase–producing stains of common pathogens and includes amoxicillin-clavulanate, cefaclor, and cefuroxime. Decongestants and antihistamines may help to reduce nasopharyngeal edema. Auralgan is often helpful for pain control. In adults, myringotomy may be preformed to relieve pain, but this is usually not preformed in the ED.

Mastoiditis, sepsis, meningitis, and intracranial abscess are serious complications of acute otitis media.

Chronic Otitis Media

Chronic otitis media is a persistent infection of the middle ear. Painless otorrhea also may be associated with this process. Chronic tympanic membrane perforation often is present and causes conductive hearing loss. Hypertrophic, inflamed polypoid tissue may develop in the middle ear. The resulting polyps may protrude into the external canal. Labyrinthine bone erosion is suggested by dizziness and facial nerve paralysis.

Common pathogens include *S. aureus* and *P. aeruginosa.*[8] Culture and sensitivity of otic discharge should be preformed. CT scanning may be required in advanced cases to evaluate the damage to the middle ear and surrounding structures.

Patients who are discharged home should be instructed to irrigate the auditory canal three times daily with a dilute acidic solution, such as a 1:1 mix of vinegar and water. This technique helps remove any loose debris. A topical fluoroquinolone should be applied following irrigation. Aminoglycoside preparations should be avoided because they are toxic to the middle ear. Oral antibiotics that cover *S. aureus* and *P. aeruginosa* should be prescribed. Hospitalization and intravenous antibiotics may be required.

Complications of chronic otitis media include mastoiditis, sepsis, meningitis, and intracranial abscess.[8] Surgical treatment is often required for resolution of complications.

Serous Otitis Media

Serous otitis media is an effusion in the middle ear. Patients may experience painless conductive hearing loss and a sensation of aural fullness. On otoscopy, there is little or no movement of the tympanic membrane with pneumatoscopy. An air-fluid level or air bubbles behind the tympanic membrane often are present on otoscopic examination. Autoinflation of the ear (by pinching and blowing the nose) leads to a bubbling or squealing sound with transient improvement in hearing.

Serous otitis media usually is due to Eustachian tube obstruction.[8] The cause of dysfunction is usually secondary to an acute upper respiratory infection. Unilateral serous otitis media in the elderly patient may be caused by an underlying nasopharyngeal mass. In such cases, CT scan, magnetic resonance imaging (MRI), or direct visualization with a mirror or fiberoptic scope should be performed.

Topical corticosteroid nasal sprays and local nasal vasoconstrictive agents may relieve symptoms. Patients who have had a nasopharyngeal mass ruled out may require myringotomy with insertion of a ventilation tube.

Cholesteatoma

A cholesteatoma is a collection of keratin debris located within a sac of squamous epithelium. Poor ventilation of the superior portion of the tympanic membrane leads to retraction. A sac in which keratin debris forms then develops. Cholesteatoma leads to recurrent ear infections with purulent drainage; however, an abnormal-appearing tympanic membrane and conductive hearing loss may be the only symptoms. Occasionally, erosion of the cochlea and semicircular canals leads to sensorineural hearing loss and vertigo.

In advanced disease, a CT scan should be preformed to evaluate the middle ear and surrounding structures. Topical and oral antibiotics as used in chronic suppurative otitis media should be administered if purulent drainage is present. Surgical removal is almost always recommended.

Sinusitis

Sinusitis is an infection of the paranasal sinuses. Sinusitis may result from an allergic component or bacterial, viral, or fungal infection. Fungal sinusitis is a potentially life-threatening disease that occurs in patients with impaired immune function or comorbidities, such as diabetes, cancer, chronic renal insufficiency, or AIDS. The most common bacteria causing acute sinusitis are *S.* *pneumoniae*, *S. pyogenes*, *S. aureus*, *M. catarrhalis*, and anaerobic flora.[2] Preexisting conditions, such as dental infection, nasal polyps, secondary infection from nasal packing after epistaxis, or upper respiratory infection, may predispose a patient to sinus infections.

Patients most commonly complain of fullness or pain of the paranasal sinuses. Purulent rhinorrhea is common. Fever may be present if infection has spread past the sinus system.

The mainstay of treatment of sinusitis is the facilitation of clearing of the sinuses. Treatment with antibiotics such as amoxicillin, fluoroquinolone, or cephalosporin is indicated if acute bacterial sinusitis is suspected. Duration of antibiotic treatment should be for 14 days. Systemic vasoconstrictors should be avoided in the elderly. Topical vasoconstrictors should be used less than 7 days due to the risk of rebound edema. If resolution does not occur with antibiotic treatment, then surgical sinus drainage should be considered.

Nasopharyngitis

Elderly patients have a greater susceptibility to infections than children and young adults.[8] Exposure to small children may increase their likelihood of contracting pharyngitis.

Sore throat, dysphagia, fever, malaise, tonsillar exudates, and tender anterior cervical lymphadenopathy of abrupt onset are common presenting symptoms and signs of acute pharyngitis. The most common etiologic agent is group A *Streptococcus pyogenes*. Viruses also cause pharyngitis and should be considered in patients who present with sore throat in addition to rhinitis, laryngitis, or bronchitis.

Although a rapid antigen test for *Streptococcus* is available, the diagnosis is often made clinically. Treatment consists of a 10-day course of oral penicillin G 500 mg four times daily or 1 g twice daily. A single dose of bicillin LA 1.2 million units intramuscularly is also a suitable treatment. Penicillin-allergic patients should be prescribed erythromycin.

Ludwig's Angina

Ludwig's angina is a progressive gangrenous infection of the submandibular or submaxillary space that may produce rapid airway obstruction. Due to the anatomic planes of the neck, spread of the infection inferiorly is limited. The forming mass thus pushes upward, displacing the tongue and floor of the mouth superiorly, further worsening airway obstruction. A recent dental infection may be the initial inciting infection in this disease.

Presenting signs consist of a distressed patient with trismus, swelling of the neck, and tongue displacement. Woody edema may be present in the submandibular space, as well as swelling of the floor of the mouth.

Ensuring a patent and secure airway is the initial priority in the management of patients with Ludwig's angina. If the airway is unstable, endotracheal intubation should be performed, although it may be difficult secondary to anatomic changes. Blind nasotracheal intubation is dangerous for this subset of patients and should not be attempted. Fiberoptic intubation is an optimal airway adjunct for this subset of patients. Some patients may require a tracheostomy.

Since the infection is polymicrobic in nature, it is recommended to administer penicillin G 4 million units every 4 hours along with metronidazole 1.0 g intravenously. Surgical intervention may be required.

Peritonsillar Abscess

While peritonsillar abscess is seen more often in young patients, it also can occur in the elderly. Peritonsillar abscess is most common in people between the ages of 20 to 40 years of age.[9]

Patients with peritonsillar abscess complain of fever, severe sore throat, dysphagia, and trismus. A "hot potato voice" may be present. Physical examination findings consist of enlarged, erythematous tonsils that are asymmetric in size. A shift of the uvula away from the affected tonsil is a classic sign. Edema of the soft palate also may be present.

Laboratory and radiographic testing are rarely indicated in the diagnosis of this disease. CT scan of the neck may be indicated in patients with unilateral swelling in the absence of fever.[9] CT of the neck also may be considered in a patient who undergoes aspiration of a possible peritonsillar abscess with no return of pus.

Definitive treatment of a peritonsillar abscess consists of surgical drainage and antibiotics. Incision and drainage are preferred, although three-point needle aspiration also may be performed.[9] Although drainage will resolve the abscess, a 7-day course of penicillin, clindamycin, or third-generation cephalosporin should be prescribed to cover β-hemolytic *Streptococcus, S. aureus,* and anaerobes. Patients who undergo incision and drainage should be followed up within 24 hours.

Epiglottitis

Epiglottitis is a potentially life-threatening infection of the epiglottis and surrounding tissues. Progression to complete airway obstruction may occur. With the widespread availability of the *H. influenzae* vaccine, the incidence of epiglottitis in adults is approximately 2 cases per 100,000 people per year.[10]

The presentation of epiglottitis in adults is frequently more indolent than that of children. Patients will commonly complain of a viral illness approximately 2 to 4 days prior to the onset of distinguishing symptoms such as a "hot potato voice," sore throat, stridor, and fever. Drooling or the inability to swallow secretions also may be present.

When the diagnosis of epiglottitis is entertained, equipment needed to secure the airway, including a cricothyrotomy tray, should be moved to the patient's bedside. Ideally, if an airway appears to be unstable, the patient should be transferred to the operating room, where an ENT surgeon can perform a formal tracheotomy.

Most adult patients with epiglottitis will have a stable airway; in these patients, flexible nasopharyngoscopy can be performed to make the diagnosis. A soft tissue lateral radiograph of the neck may demonstrate the classic "thumbprint" of the edematous epiglottis.

A second- or third-generation cephalosporin, such as cefuroxime or ceftriaxone, is the antibiotic of choice in epiglottitis.[10] All patients should be admitted to a monitored bed. A surgical airway kit should be at the bedside at all times.

Cricoarytenoiditis

Cricoarytenoiditis is a rare condition that may present in the elderly afflicted with severe arthritis. Patients may complain of pain with swallowing or with speech. Fiberoptic laryngoscopy may demonstrate erythema or edema of the arytenoid cartilage. If chronically inflamed, the cricoarytenoid joint may become rigid, thus causing speech and respiratory difficulty. Treatment consists of endotracheal intubation for patients in severe respiratory distress.

REFERENCES

1. Slavin RG: Management of sinusitis. *J Am Geriatric Soc* 39:212, 1991.
2. Sokol W: Epidemiology of sinusitis in the primary care setting: Results from the 1999–2000 respiratory surveillance program. *Am J Med* 111:19, 2001.
3. Anderson RG, Meyerhoff WL: Otologic manifestations of aging. *Otolaryngol Clin North Am* 15:353, 1982.
4. Koopmann CF Jr, Coulthard SW: The oral cavity and aging. *Otolaryngol Clin North Am* 15:293, 1982.

5. Bojrab DI, Braderly T, Abdurazzak Y: Otitis externa. *Otolaryngol Clin North Am* 29:761, 1996.

6. Brook I, Frazier EH, Thompson DH: Aerobic and anaerobic microbiology of external otitis. *Clin Infect Dis* 16:955, 1992.

7. Marais J, Dale BAB: Bullous myringitis: A review. *Clin Otolaryngol* 22:497, 1997.

8. Yoshikawa T: Epidemiology and unique aspects of aging and infectious disease. *Clin Infect Dis* 30:931, 2000.

9. Steyer T: Peritonsillar abscess: Diagnosis and treatment. *Am Fam Phys* 65:93, 2002.

10. Khanna D, Ost D: How to identify and manage life-threatening infections of the upper airway, part 1. *J Crit Illness* 65:10, 2002.

63

Tracheostomy Issues

Robert J. Vissers

HIGH-YIELD FACTS

- Tracheostomy patients presenting with respiratory distress should be assumed to have a complete or partial obstruction of their tracheostomy tube.
- The most important factor in maintaining tracheostomy function is keeping the tube clean and clear of secretions.
- Tracheoinnominate fistula is a rare but life-threatening complication that may be preceded by small sentinel bleed.
- Increased secretions, cough, and dyspnea after feeding may indicate the presence of a tracheoesophageal fistula.
- False passages can be created during tube replacement; this complication may be reduced by using a Seldinger technique over a catheter.

Tracheostomy is one of the earliest surgical procedures performed, possibly dating back 5000 years. In 1909, Chevalier Jackson defined the procedure that most resembles how tracheostomies are performed today.[1] Patients with a tracheostomy can present with acute life-threatening conditions, such as airway obstruction, infection, and arterial bleeding, or the delayed complications of stenoses and fistulas.

Most tracheostomies are placed for airway obstruction, prolonged respiratory insufficiency, and pulmonary toilet. Since these indications are more frequent in the geriatric population, tracheostomy issues most commonly present in the older patient. Traditionally performed in the operating room, tracheostomies are now frequently done bedside in the intensive care unit, either open or using percutaneous devices. There continues to be debate regarding the timing of tracheostomies, the relative merits of prolonged endotracheal intubation versus tracheostomy, and traditional tracheostomy versus percutaneous tracheostomy.[2] Most of the controversy involves

the associated complications, and it is these delayed complications that typically precipitate an emergency evaluation.

PATHOPHYSIOLOGY

Tracheostomies reduce the anatomic dead space by 50 percent, which is advantageous to patients with poor pulmonary reserve. Many of the issues associated with tracheostomies involve the physiologic consequences that come with also bypassing the airway's defense mechanisms.[3] The loss of humidification that ordinarily takes place in the upper airways causes thick, dry secretions to accumulate. The ability to cough up and clear secretions is also reduced.[4] The inability to close the glottis and create a physiologic positive end-expiratory pressure (PEEP) weakens the cough and reduces alveolar gas mixture.

CLINICAL FEATURES

A common tracheostomy problem is obstruction of the tube secondary to the accumulation of secretions. A patient with respiratory distress and a tracheostomy should be assumed to have occlusion of the tracheostomy tube.[5] Inability to replace the tube after accidental or intentional removal for cleaning may represent the most common tracheostomy issue presenting to the emergency department (ED).[6] Occasionally, patients will present requesting to have their tracheostomy tube changed.

Less commonly, patients present with hemorrhage from the tube. Bleeding from local trauma and granulation tissue may occur; however, copious arterial bleeding may be due to a tracheoinnominate artery fistula. This may present with airway obstruction or shock and is associated with a high mortality rate.[3] Infections can occur at the stoma and present with local pain, erythema, and tenderness. Respiratory distress associated with altered mental status, fever, cough, or increased sputum production may be due to aspiration pneumonia. Increased cough and dyspnea, particularly in association with feeding, may indicate a tracheoesophageal fistula.[4]

Tracheostomy Tubes

Tracheostomy tubes are made in a variety of designs and materials.[7] They may have a single lumen, although many have a removable inner cannula that can be removed easily to allow for routine cleaning and prevention of mucus

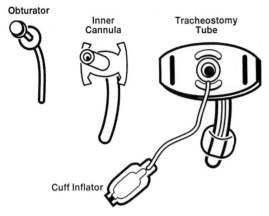

Fig. 63-1 Contents of a tracheostomy tube.

obstruction (Fig. 63-1). Many tubes come with a blunt-tipped obturator that is used to facilitate insertion and reduce trauma. The tubes also may be rigid or flexible and kink-resistant and of variable curves, angles and sizes depending on the anatomic needs of the patient. Tracheostomy tubes are secured with twill or a padded fastener that goes around the neck and attaches to the neck plate of the tube.

Tubes may be cuffed or uncuffed. Cuff pressures should be kept at inflation pressures of 20 to 25 mmHg.[4] Underinflation can increase aspiration, whereas high cuff pressures can cause mucosal ischemia and subsequent tracheal stenosis or tissue necrosis. In general, cuffed tubes are used initially and then replaced by cuffless tubes once the patient is no longer ventilator-dependent. This reduces the incidence of stenosis but places these patients at a higher risk for aspiration.[2]

Speech

Tracheostomies can present barriers to normal speech, particularly if associated with laryngectomies. Commonly, patients have learned alternative methods of communication via hands, writing, or artificial voice devices. In patients with a larynx, fenestrated cuffs or use of the Passy-Muir valve (a one-way valve that fits directly on the tracheostomy tube externally) allows forcefully exhaled air to pass through to the vocal cords and mouth to allow for speech.[7] Patients presenting with obstruction and a Passy-Muir valve should have the valve removed to allow air to move freely during both inhalation and exhalation. If there is no improvement, the tracheostomy tube should be assessed for obstruction.

In postlaryngectomy patients, speech is possible using

a Blom-Singer voice prosthesis.[8] This is a surgically placed one-valve between the trachea and the cervical esophagus. While occluding the tracheal airway with a thumb, exhaled air is forced into the upper esophagus, causing vibrations much like a belch, which allows speech. Patients may present with aspiration of the device. The device is visible by radiograph and requires bronchoscopic removal. Dislodgement of the device requires recannulation of the tracheoesophageal fistula as soon as possible, which is ideally performed by an otolaryngologist. The fistula can be stented temporarily with a lubricated Foley or red rubber catheter, which is taped to the chest wall until the device is replaced. Forceful attempts should be avoided because false passages may be created.

EMERGENCY DEPARTMENT CARE AND DISPOSITION

General Tracheostomy Care and Suctioning

The most important aspect of tracheostomy care is the control of secretions and maintaining tube patency. Humidification of inhaled air keeps mucus liquid and allows expulsion through ciliary function and cough.[4] The intermittent use of a humidifier in the home may help in reducing secretion buildup and obstruction. Humidified air or aerosol should be used when ventilating through a tracheostomy in the ED.[9] Frequent cleaning of the inner cannula is important to reduce the occurrence of contamination or obstruction. It is unclear how often a tracheostomy tube should be changed, beyond the obvious indications of gross contamination, malfunction, or persistent obstruction.

When excessive mucus causes obstruction, suctioning becomes necessary. Routine suctioning is not warranted due to its discomfort and potential for complications. Cardiac instability may be exacerbated by the procedure and represents a relative contraindication; however, suctioning should be performed with the appropriate precautions when the obstruction is significantly contributing to the underlying problem.[9]

Patients should be preoxygenated with 100% oxygen prior to suctioning. The largest catheter that easily fits in the lumen should be used at about 120 to 150 mmHg suction.[9] The catheter should be inserted until resistance is met and then pulled back slightly before suction is applied through occlusion of the vacuum vent. Suctioning should not exceed 15 seconds and should be followed by oxygenation. Excessive coughing can be suppressed with nebulized lidocaine.[3] Sterile saline may be instilled to loosen secretions. Mucosal irritation can cause vagal and sympathetic stimulation, leading to bradydysrhythmias and tachydysrhythmias, respectively. Prolonged suctioning can cause hypoxemia, which also may precipitate dysrhythmias.[9]

Changing a Tracheostomy Tube

It is common practice to change the tracheostomy tube for cleaning, and this is often performed by the patient or family. The first tube replacement after the creation of the stoma should be performed by the surgeon and is usually delayed for at least 1 week after surgery. The emergency physician may be required to change the tube in the event of partial or complete obstruction, tube malfunction (such as breakage or cuff rupture), or accidental expulsion of the tube.[6]

Ideally, the same type and size of tracheostomy tube should be used when a change is required. Consultation with otolaryngology or respiratory therapy, if circumstances and time allow, may assist in identifying and obtaining the correct device. Sizing can be identified on the tube or neck plate and usually represents the internal diameter in millimeters. In instances where a tracheostomy tube is not available and an airway is needed, an endotracheal tube can be substituted. These should only be used as a temporizing measure because they are prone to kinking, and their length creates higher airway resistance.

Before removing the existing tube, the emergency physician should ensure that the replacement tube is assembled properly with the obturator in place and is lubricated and that the cuff has been checked. The patient may be sitting or lying with the neck hyperextended. A roll under the shoulders of the prone patient may be required to achieve this. The patient should receive preoxygenation prior to the procedure. In a smooth, circular motion in the curve of the device, the tube is removed. The new tube is placed during inspiration using the same technique (Fig. 63-2). Forceful placement should be avoided because this may create a false passage. If resistance is met, even with the neck fully extended, switching to a smaller-sized tube is prudent. The cuff, if present, is then inflated, and placement is confirmed with auscultation during respiration. There is usually an inner cannula, which must be inserted before a bag-valve mask or ventilator may be attached. In an unresponsive or hypoxic patient, a bag-valve mask should be used to ventilate and oxygenate, and a colorimetric CO_2 detector should be used for tube confirmation. Once placement is confirmed, the tube should be secured with the provided tracheostomy tape snugly around the neck while the neck is in a flexed position.[9]

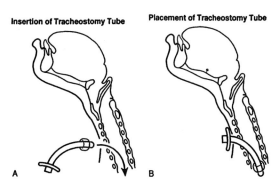

Fig. 63-2 Insertion and placement of the tracheostomy tube.

Complications of tube changing include failure to insert the replacement tube, creation of a false passage, and bleeding.[4] If difficulty finding the passage is encountered, increasing neck extension can assist in aligning the tissues. False passages are identified by inability to ventilate the lungs and the development of subcutaneous emphysema in the neck. If time allows, the tube can be placed over a flexible fiberoptic laryngoscope. In circumstances where the tube cannot be placed and the patient has respiratory compromise, an endotracheal tube often can be placed orally. There may be subglottic stenosis present, so a smaller tube size should be employed if resistance is encountered.

The tracheostomy tube also may be exchanged using a Seldinger technique over a catheter.[9] This method greatly reduces the chance of creating a false passage and should be considered in patients in whom difficulty is anticipated (obese patients, short and thick neck, anatomic anomalies, recent stoma creation).[4]

Complications of Tracheostomy

Obstruction

Obstruction is one of the most common complications associated with tracheostomy tubes.[5] In patients with tracheostomies presenting in respiratory distress, patency of the airway must take priority.[3] Oxygenation through the tracheostomy tube should be initiated. Cardiac monitoring and intravenous access should be established. Preparation of emergency bedside equipment should be done early in the course of managing a possible tube obstruction and must be done before removal of the tube. Recommended equipment includes tracheostomy tubes in several sizes, lubricant, suction catheters, endotracheal tubes, a bag-valve mask, a laryngoscope, and a catheter or tube exchanger. A tracheal hook and dilator may be helpful if available and often can be found in cricothyrotomy kits. Often, manual removal of dried crusts, secretions, or blood from the opening can relieve the obstruction. If this is not successful, careful suctioning after oxygenation may remove intraluminal secretions or mucus plugs. If there is no improvement to flow, the inner cannula should be removed for inspection and cleaning.[7]

Persistent obstruction or the absence of an inner cannula requires removal of the tracheostomy tube. This should only be performed once the equipment is available. Replacement of the tube should then be performed. If respiratory distress continues after tube replacement, other etiologies such as mucus plugs, pneumonia, pneumothorax, pulmonary embolus, and cardiac disease must be considered.

Tracheal and Stomal Stenosis

Patients with tracheal stenosis may present to the ED with dyspnea, wheezing, stridor, or inability to handle secretions. Treatment includes humidified oxygen, nebulized racemic epinephrine, and steroids. Consultation with an ear, nose, and throat (ENT) or thoracic surgeon is required for treatment. Radiographs may be helpful, but flexible fiberoptic evaluation is required.[3]

The stoma can begin to close over within days after removal of the tube, making reinsertion difficult. A smaller replacement tracheostomy tube is often required if the tube has been out for any period of time.

Bleeding

Bleeding usually comes from the tracheostomy skin edges, most frequently in the first 3 weeks following the procedure. Minor bleeding can be controlled by light packing of the stomal edges with petrolatum gauze or with the use of silver nitrate. Cautery is required occasionally, particularly if the bleeding is associated with granulation tissue.[6] If a patient presents with stomal bleeding and the source is not easily visualized, then the stoma should be examined with a nasopharyngeal scope to assess the amount of bleeding and examine for the presence of a tracheoinnominate artery fistula.

Tracheoinnominate artery fistulas are rare, occurring in less than 1 percent of tracheostomies; however, the associated mortality is 75 percent.[10] More than 10 mL of bleeding should raise suspicion for this complication.[6] Some patients can present with a herald episode of minimal bleeding that precedes the sudden hemorrhage. Therefore, any bleeding in which the source is not visu-

alized should prompt removal of the tube and evaluation of the trachea with a scope. The fistula results from direct pressure of the tube against the innominate artery and is visualized on the anterior tracheal wall, inferior to the sternal notch.

When the patient presents with significant bleeding, immediate control of the hemorrhage and maintenance of the airway must take place; death from airway obstruction or hemorrhagic shock can occur rapidly. Hyperinflation of the cuff at the site of the fistula has been reported to temporarily control bleeding.[3] An endotracheal tube also can be used and allows for manipulation over the stenosis or tracheal protection and ventilation distal to the fistula. The bleeding can then be controlled with digital pressure through the stoma. The pressure should be applied anteriorly, compressing the innominate artery against the posterior aspect of the sternum until the patient reaches the operating room. A vertical incision of the stoma may be required to allow entry of the compressing digit.

Infection

Infection is the second most common reason for tracheostomy patients to present to the ED, accounting for 30 percent of the complications.[6] Although bacterial contamination is present in most stomas, the exposure to infected secretions and the trauma of frequent tube manipulation predispose the patient to local cellulitis. The organisms cultured most frequently are *Staphylococcus aureus*, *Pseudomonas aeruginosa*, Enterobacteriaceae, and *Candida albicans*. Local cellulitis is treated with oral antibiotics, topical antibiotic ointment, frequent dressing changes and tube cleaning, and good wound care. Mediastinitis is a rare but potentially fatal complication of untreated cellulitis.

Tracheitis presents with a purulent discharge that requires frequent suctioning, intravenous antibiotics, possible debridement, and frequently, the creation of an alternative airway. A weakened cough and poor ciliary function may lead to recurrent purulent bronchitis and pneumonia.[11] Patients with tracheostomies are at particular risk for aspiration pneumonia. Admission for broadspectrum intravenous antibiotics is often indicated due to their impaired ability to clear secretions.

Tracheoesophageal Fistula

Tracheoesophageal fistula may be created surgically to allow for esophageal speech. In less than 1 percent of patients this can occur from posterior erosion into the esophagus. Increased secretions, coughing after feedings, and aspiration pneumonia or pneumonitis suggest the presence of this complication.[9] Risk factors include high airway pressures, cuffed tubes, presence of a nasogastric tube, and diabetes mellitus.[4] Diagnosis is made by endoscopy or the presence of swallowed methylene blue in the trachea. Surgical repair is required because these lesions will not heal spontaneously.

REFERENCES

1. Jackson C: Tracheotomy. *Laryngoscope* 19:285, 1990.
2. Pryor JP, Reilly PM, Shapiro MB: Surgical airway management in the intensive care unit. *Crit Care Clin* 16:473, 2000.
3. Tayal VS: Tracheostomies. *Emerg Med Clin North Am* 12:707, 1994.
4. Heffner JE, Hess D: Tracheostomy management in the chronically ventilated patient. *Clin Chest Med* 22:1, 2001.
5. Rowe BH, Rampton J, Bota GW: Life-threatening luminal obstruction due to mucous plugging in chronic tracheostomies: Three case reports and a review of the literature. *J Emerg Med* 14:565, 1996.
6. Hackeling T, Triana R, Ma OJ, Shockley W: Emergency care of patients with tracheostomies: A 7-year review. *Am J Emerg Med* 16:681, 1998.
7. Triana RJ, Hackeling TA: Complications of airway devices, in Tintinalli JE, Kelen GD, Stapczynski JS (eds): *Emergency Medicine: A Comprehensive Study Guide,* 5th ed. New York, McGraw-Hill, 1999, p 1565.
8. Singer MI, Blom ED: An endoscopic technique for voice restoration after total laryngectomy. *Ann Otol Rhinol Laryngol* 89:529, 1980.
9. Joyce SM: Tracheostomy care and tracheal suctioning, in Roberts J (ed): *Clinical Procedures in Emergency Medicine,* 3d ed. Philadelphia, Saunders, 1998, p 74.
10. Yang FY, Criado E, Schwartz JA, et al: Trachea-innominate artery fistula: Retrospective comparison of treatment methods. *South Med J* 81:701, 1988.
11. Niederman MS, Ferranti RD, Zeigler A, et al: Respiratory infection complicating long-term tracheostomy. *Chest* 85:1, 1984.

64

Bleeding and Coagulation

Lance H. Hoffman

HIGH-YIELD FACTS

- Quantitative and qualitative platelet disorders tend to produce atraumatic mucocutaneous bleeding, whereas coagulation factor disorders tend to produce delayed traumatic bleeding and bleeding into potential spaces.

- Elderly patients receiving blood product transfusions are at risk of volume overload, warranting close monitoring of volume status during transfusions.

- Major bleeding emergencies in patients with hemophilia that require coagulation factor replacement prior to confirmatory testing include bleeding into the central nervous system, retroperitoneum, oropharynx, and neck.

- Indications for platelet transfusion include a platelet count less than 50,000 platelets/dL and active bleeding or a platelet count less than 10,000 platelets/dL, which places the patient at an increased risk of spontaneous life-threatening hemorrhage.

- Heparin or low-molecular-weight heparin (LMWH) needs to be administered concurrently at the beginning of warfarin therapy to prevent precipitating thromboembolic disease secondary to the early depletion of proteins C and S.

Disorders of coagulation include those diseases which impair hemostasis, resulting in hemorrhage, as well as those which promote inappropriate clot formation, resulting in vascular occlusion. Both are detrimental and require prompt recognition and treatment. Most bleeding encountered in the emergency department (ED) is the result of traumatic compromise of blood vessel integrity. This type of bleeding usually is controlled using solely mechanical means, such as direct pressure and sutures. In most patients, the coagulation mechanism functions normally, allowing simple mechanical means of controlling hemorrhage to be effective. However, on occasion, patients may present with bleeding directly related to or complicated by a coagulation disorder that requires medical therapy to control the bleeding.

These disorders may include derangements in the function of connective tissue, platelets, coagulation factors, or combinations of these. In the elderly population, hemostasis may be impaired by a variety of mechanisms, most commonly related to comorbid diseases and medications. Congenital and acquired coagulopathies need to be considered in the care of the elderly patient.

Within the realm of coagulation also lies the opposite extreme of inappropriate thrombus formation. This mechanism underlies a multitude of diseases commonly encountered by the emergency physician. Thromboembolic phenomena may be the underlying etiology of acute myocardial infarction, ischemic stroke, deep venous thrombosis, mesenteric ischemia, and other disease entities. Both hereditary and acquired factors, including comorbid disorders, may play a causative role.

EPIDEMIOLOGY

Coagulopathies may be precipitated by a variety of etiologies. For this reason, it is difficult to accurately estimate the prevalence of many of these coagulopathies. However, given the number of elderly individuals taking oral anticoagulants, as well as those with comorbid diseases affecting coagulation, the potential for encountering a coagulopathic disorder is common.

The prevalence of elders prescribed platelet inhibitors, such as aspirin and clopidogrel, and warfarin, plays a role in the emergency physician's care of the elderly patient with bleeding. More than a million patients are treated with warfarin each year in the United States for thromboembolic diseases such as ischemic cerebral vascular disease, coronary artery disease, prosthetic heart valves, atrial fibrillation, cardiomyopathy, and deep venous thrombosis.[1] Of patients taking warfarin for atrial fibrillation, the incidence of major warfarin-related bleeding was 1.7 percent in those younger than 75 years of age, whereas it was 4.2 percent in those older than 75 years of age.[2] Fihn and colleagues[1] also demonstrated that individuals taking warfarin with more than three additional chronic diseases were at a significantly greater risk of having a bleeding complication. This finding underscores the importance of the role concurrent illnesses may play in coagulopathies. Multiple chronic illnesses are known to contribute to bleeding disorders. Two commonly implicated processes involve hepatic and renal dysfunction.

Furthermore, hereditary bleeding disorders also must be considered. Von Willebrand's disease is the most common hereditary bleeding disorder, with an estimated prevalence of approximately 1 percent of the population.[3] Additionally, hemophilia A, factor VIII deficiency, affects 1 in 5000 to 10,000 live male births.

Much less common are acquired bleeding disorders, such as spontaneously acquired factor VIII inhibitors. In nonhemophiliacs, this disease occurs almost exclusively in people over age 60 at a rate of 1 in 1 million per year, and approximately 50 percent of these patients have a concurrent autoimmune disorder or malignancy.[4] Finally, advanced age may contribute to a worse prognosis for a given acquired bleeding disorder. For example, the incidence of adult idiopathic thrombocytopenic purpura (ITP) is approximately 38 in 1 million new cases annually; however, patients over age 60 have more hemorrhagic complications, specifically intracranial hemorrhage, compared with patients younger than 60 years of age with equivalent platelet counts.[5]

At the other end of the spectrum, thromboembolic disease results in the morbidity and mortality of acute myocardial infarction, ischemic stroke, and deep venous thrombosis, with or without pulmonary embolus. Over 745,000 deaths in individuals 65 years of age and older were attributed to heart disease and cerebrovascular disease in 1997, according to the Centers for Disease Control and Prevention (CDC).[6] Over 200,000 new cases of venous thromboembolism occur in the United States each year, with approximately 28 percent of those individuals developing venous stasis syndrome within 20 years.[7] The incidence of venous thromboembolism has been demonstrated to increase with age. In hospitalized patients, Anderson and colleagues[8] found an incidence of 0.03 percent at age 40, 0.09 percent at age 60, and 0.26 percent at age 80. Goldhaber and colleagues[9] reported the crude mortality rate of pulmonary embolism at 3 months to be as high as 17.4 percent.

PATHOPHYSIOLOGY

Hemostasis is a complex process with components acting simultaneously to preserve vascular integrity when a blood vessel has been compromised mechanically. These components work to form a blood clot at the site of injury while also preventing the propagation of that blood clot beyond the site of injury. In the most basic of terms, the prevention of bleeding begins by depending on blood vessels with normal architecture that can sustain normal stresses of daily life. If the integrity of the vessel should be breached, then the platelets form an initial plug at the site of injury through the process of primary hemostasis. Coagulation proteins then reinforce the platelet plug to form a stable clot through secondary hemostasis. At the same time, the fibrinolytic system acts to prevent extension of the clot beyond the site of vessel injury, which potentially could occlude the injured blood vessel. Derangements have been described in each of these processes that, in turn, predispose to hyper- and hypocoagulable disorders.

Primary hemostasis begins with the expression of von Willebrand factor (vWF) by damaged endothelium. Circulating platelets then adhere to vWF. Additional platelets are recruited and adhere to each other via the interaction of glycoprotein IIb-IIIa and fibrinogen. This process is represented in Fig. 64-1 and is responsible for the formation of the initial "platelet plug" at the site of injury.

Secondary hemostasis is the process through which fibrin is generated to add stability to the platelet plug. These interactions are illustrated in Fig. 64-2. Once again, damaged endothelium triggers a cascade of events leading to thrombus formation. A series of zymogens interacts, producing the active form of the coagulation factor, which activates the next step in the process. Ultimately, thrombin is generated and converts fibrinogen to fibrin, leading to a cross-linked fibrin structure that has incorporated circulating erythrocytes and platelets into the architecture to form a thrombus. Antithrombin interacting with endothelial heparan, thrombomodulin, protein C, and protein S plays a key role in limiting extension of the thrombus past the site of injury.

Fibrinolysis, diagrammed in Fig. 64-3, is the process by which a thrombus is dissolved. The liver synthesizes circulating plasminogen. Tissue plasminogen activator

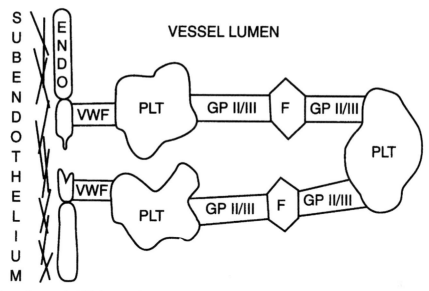

Fig. 64-1   Primary hemostasis. ENDO = endothelium; vWF = von Willebrand factor; PLT = platelet; F = fibrinogen; GP II/III = glycoprotein IIb-IIIa.

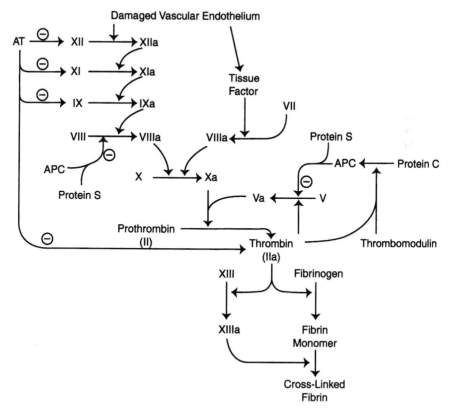

Fig. 64-2   Secondary hemostasis. Coagulation factors denoted with Roman numerals; AT = antithrombin; APC = activated protein C. AT inhibits factors XII, XI, IX, and II. APC with cofactor protein S inhibits factors V and VII.

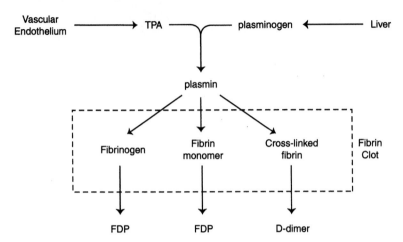

Fig. 64-3 Fibrinolysis. tPA = tissue plasminogen activator; FDP = fibrin degradation products.

(tPA) synthesized by intact vascular endothelium converts plasminogen to plasmin. The plasmin then dissolves the fibrin clot into fibrin degradation products (FDPs) and D-dimers, which are both measurable in the serum.

Bleeding disorders may be the result of dysfunction at any one of many levels of this tightly regulated process. For example, structural defects in blood vessels may produce bleeding, as well as quantitative and qualitative disorders of platelets or coagulation factors. Acquired and inherited factors may be etiologic.

The triad of factors first described by Virchow promotes inappropriate thrombosis. These include vascular endothelial injury, stasis of blood, and a hypercoagulable state. Vascular endothelial injury triggers both the primary and secondary hemostatic systems and is a reason why atherosclerosis and surgical procedures promote thrombus formation. Stasis of blood is postulated to promote thrombus formation by preventing activated coagulation factors from being mixed with nonactivated blood components.[10] Finally, a hypercoagulable state may be produced by acquired and inherited factors, such as malignancy, hormone-replacement therapy (HRT), autoimmune disease, deficiencies of hemostatic counterregulatory enzymes, and resistance of coagulation factors to those counterregulatory enzymes.

CLINICAL FEATURES

Hypocoagulability

Obtaining an accurate medical history from the patient may be complicated by dementia, delirium, or other base-line medical conditions. As a result, reviewing medical records and contacting the patient's primary care provider for further information are essential. Important historical facts include the site, timing, quantity, and circumstances of the bleeding episode. Consideration should be given to a bleeding diathesis in the event of bleeding without prior trauma or delayed after trauma, at multiple sites, and into joint and potential spaces. Mucocutaneous bleeding tends to signal a platelet disorder, whereas atraumatic hemarthrosis, bleeding into a potential space, or delayed traumatic bleeding may indicate a disorder involving the coagulation factors.

The past medical history and current medications of older individuals may be complex. An inquiry should be made regarding inherited bleeding diatheses, hepatic or renal disease, bone marrow or rheumatologic disorders, and chronic alcoholism. The patient also should be questioned about medications that may affect coagulation. Long-term glucocorticoid therapy may weaken blood vessel walls. Aspirin and nonsteroidal anti-inflammatory drugs (NSAIDs) inhibit platelet function to varying degrees and can prolong bleeding times. Ticlopidine and clopidogrel also impair platelet aggregation. Vitamin K antagonists such as warfarin impair the synthesis of coagulation factors II, VII, IX, and X, as well as proteins C and S. Additionally, several other medications have been shown to potentiate the action of warfarin. These include antiarrhythmics such as amiodarone; antibiotics such as the macrolides, fluoroquinolones, cephalosporins, and penicillins; antifungals such as itraconazole; and proton pump inhibitors such as omeprazole, to name a few.

Special attention should be given to the vital signs early

in the evaluation, recognizing that tachycardia may be attenuated and hypotension may be exacerbated by antihypertensive medications. Tachypnea also may signal impending airway obstruction secondary to a pharyngeal hematoma. The head and neck examination should focus on cranial trauma, epistaxis, and hematomas that may lead to airway obstruction. Neurologic abnormalities may herald an intracranial hemorrhage. Hepatosplenomegaly may be a sign that liver disease or hematologic malignancy is the cause of abnormal bleeding. The presence of blood in the stool needs to be determined because gastrointestinal bleeding can be rapidly fatal. Bleeding disorders also may lead to a spontaneous hemarthrosis or tissue hematoma, causing an acute compartment syndrome. Finally, the skin may show petechiae, purpura, or ecchymoses in bleeding disorders.

Hypercoagulability

Thromboembolic phenomena are etiologic in a multitude of diseases primarily affecting the older population. Consequently, the chief complaint will vary according to the involved site and level of tissue ischemia. Medical records, family members, friends, and the patient's primary care physician are resources that should be used. Particular attention should be given to the timing and acuity of the event because thromboembolism results in vascular occlusion with resulting tissue ischemia. Additionally, a history of prior episodes is extremely helpful because thromboembolic disease at one site frequently recurs and may present atypically in the elderly population. Elderly patients with a hereditary thrombophilia nearly always will have had similar events in the past.

Pertinent past medical history would include stroke, myocardial infarction, cardiac dysrhythmias such as atrial fibrillation, cardiomyopathy, deep venous thrombosis with or without pulmonary embolus, and hereditary thrombophilias. If the patient's medications are readily obtainable, then the presence of cardiovascular medications, warfarin, and HRT should prompt thromboembolic diseases to be considered in the differential diagnosis.

Multiple risk factors for venous thrombotic disease have been described, and an inquiry about each should be made. The incidence of venous thrombosis and pulmonary embolus has been shown to increase markedly with age, especially in individuals over age 65.[7] The mechanism through which malignancy promotes a hypercoagulable state is complex and incompletely understood. However, tumor cells have been demonstrated to activate platelets and express a procoagulant substance that activates factor X.[11,12] Immobilization from a variety

of causes also predisposes to thromboembolism through venous stasis.[10] Pain or casting from surgery, deconditioning from cardiac or pulmonary disease, and paralysis from neurologic disease all may impair mobility. Vascular trauma may cause endothelial injury. Orthopedic and pelvic surgery, extremity trauma, and central venous instrumentation all predispose to thrombosis through this mechanism.[13] In the elderly, HRT with estrogens in postmenopausal women increases the risk of venous thrombosis.[14]

Tachycardia, tachypnea, hypotension, and oxygen desaturation all may be associated with acute myocardial infarction and pulmonary embolus. An irregular cardiac rhythm and murmur should be identified. Asymmetric pulses can indicate an acute arterial occlusion, whereas asymmetric peripheral edema may be present with deep venous thrombosis. Mesenteric ischemia causes abdominal pain out of proportion to abdominal tenderness. Stroke causes a neurologic deficit. Finally, skin pallor or necrosis may be present with vascular occlusion.

DIAGNOSIS AND DIFFERENTIAL

Laboratory Studies of Coagulation

The most common laboratory studies to be used by the emergency physician in the evaluation of a hypocoagulable patient are the complete blood count (CBC), prothrombin time with international normalized ratio (PT/INR), and the activated partial thromboplastin time (PTT). These tests screen for abnormalities of both primary and secondary hemostasis.

The CBC provides information regarding the quantity of platelets. However, it does not measure any aspect of platelet function. Consequently, a patient may have a normal number of platelets, but this does not ensure that those platelets are effective in primary hemostasis. The presence of thrombocytopenia alone does indicate that the potential for impaired platelet plug formation is present. Thrombocytopenia may be caused by disorders of platelet production (e.g., myeloproliferative disorders and alcoholism), sequestration (e.g., portal hypertension), or destruction (e.g., idiopathic thrombocytopenic purpura, thrombotic thrombocytopenic purpura, and disseminated intravascular coagulation). The CBC also includes a hemoglobin and hematocrit determination, which may be useful in determining the need for packed red blood cell (PRBC) transfusion.

The PT/INR and PTT are used to measure the function of secondary hemostasis. INR values are comparable between laboratories because the INR is a measure of the

PT adjusted to account for differences between varying reagents used to measure the PT in different laboratories. Common causes of PT prolongation include liver disease and therapy with vitamin K antagonists such as warfarin. Prolongation of the PTT can be caused by von Willebrand's disease, hemophilia, factor VIII or IX inhibitors, antiphospholipid antibodies, and therapy with heparin.

Tests of fibrinolytic activity include measurements of fibrinogen, fibrin degradation products (FDPs), and D-dimer. As more fibrinolysis occurs, the fibrinogen level falls, and the FDP and D-dimer levels rise. FDPs are created when plasmin acts on a fibrin clot to disassemble fibrinogen and fibrin monomers. D-Dimers are a product of cross-linked fibrin degradation by plasmin acting on a fibrin clot. A low fibrinogen level may indicate consumption by disseminated intravascular coagulation (DIC) or poor production secondary to liver disease. The FDP and D-dimer levels rise in DIC and also have been used as screening tests for occult thromboembolism such as deep venous thrombosis and pulmonary embolus. A number of other studies used to define coagulopathic disorders exist that are best left to the hematologist and are not generally useful to the emergency physician. Bleeding time as a measure of a qualitative platelet disorder is one example. Others are coagulation factor levels testing for hemophilias. A 1:1 of patient and normal serum is used as a screening test for the presence of a factor inhibitor. Antiphospholipid antibodies and heparin-induced thrombocytopenia antibodies also may be determined.

Hypocoagulability

Abnormal bleeding may be the result of deranged blood vessel architecture, ranging in severity from benign to life-threatening. Abnormal vascular proliferations such as hemangiomas and telangiectasias can bleed secondary to vascular fragility. Connective tissue disorders are implicated in other disease states. Senile purpura is the result of an age-dependent loss of subcutaneous tissue support for dermal blood vessels.[15] Vitamin C deficiency, chronic glucocorticoid therapy, and Ehlers-Danlos syndrome involve increased bleeding through poor blood vessel collagen support. Marfan syndrome is caused by abnormal fibrillin production and is associated with aortic dissection. Infiltrative diseases such as amyloidosis and inflammatory diseases such as the vasculitides also can result in bleeding.

Quantitative and qualitative platelet disorders impair primary hemostasis, resulting in bleeding complications. Thrombocytopenia of between 10,000 and 50,000 platelets/dL tends to result in prolonged bleeding times but does not result in spontaneous hemorrhage. Platelet counts of less than 10,000 platelets/dL are associated with spontaneous hemorrhage, including those involving the central nervous system. As mentioned previously, thrombocytopenia has multiple causes, including disorders of platelet production, sequestration, and destruction.

In the event that the platelet count, INR, and PTT are normal but the patient still has pathologic hemorrhage, a qualitative platelet disorder is the likely etiology. An accurate past medical history and medication history are the best means of determining if this might be the cause of the hemorrhage. Common causes of qualitative platelet disorders are iatrogenic. Aspirin permanently inhibits platelet cyclooxygenase-1 through acetylation. In turn, the affected platelets do not produce thromboxane, which promotes platelet aggregation. This effect is present for the life of the platelet. The more recent cyclooxygenase-2 inhibitors celecoxib and rofecoxib do not impair thromboxane production; therefore, platelet aggregation is unaffected. Platelet adenosine diphosphate (ADP) receptor blockers, ticlopidine and clopidogrel, also impair platelet aggregation. The final common pathway of platelet aggregation involves the glycoprotein IIb-IIIa receptor. Inhibitors of this receptor (e.g., abciximab, eptifibatide, and tirofiban) are often used in the emergency setting for treatment of acute coronary syndromes.

Platelet aggregation also may be impaired by endogenous substances associated with other disease states. The dysproteinemias (e.g., multiple myeloma and Waldenström's macroglobulinemia), hepatic failure, and uremia have been implicated in hemorrhage through this mechanism. Guanidinosuccinic acid, a by-product of urea synthesis, and other substances associated with uremia have been shown to inhibit platelets.[16,17] The interaction of vWF and platelets also seems to be negatively affected by uremia.[18]

Coagulation factor disorders also may result in a bleeding diathesis. These disorders cause a prolongation of the PT or PTT depending on the factors that are involved. Among the elderly population, the most clinically important of these are iatrogenic. Warfarin is the most commonly used vitamin K antagonist in the United States. It typically results in a prolonged INR but also can prolong the PTT in high doses. The risk of major hemorrhage is increased in elderly individuals taking warfarin compared with younger patients taking warfarin.[19,20] Hepatic failure also will result in coagulation factor deficiencies. The liver synthesizes all the coagulation factors, as well as proteins C and S, antithrombin, and plasminogen. A prolonged INR appears to correlate best with the level of hepatocellular damage and hemorrhage.[21] Hemophilia A (factor VIII deficiency) and hemophilia B (factor IX deficiency) will both prolong the PTT, although these diseases are almost universally identified in childhood. Factor inhibitors, antibodies to specific coagulation factors, most commonly present in hemophiliacs but also can arise spontaneously. Approximately half of those individuals with a spontaneous factor VIII inhibitor, the most common factor inhibitor, are otherwise healthy individuals over age 65.[22]

Some disorders involve both platelet and coagulation factor dysfunction. One such entity is von Willebrand's disease, in which a diminished quantity or abnormally structured vWF is produced. vWF plays a role in platelet aggregation to the vascular endothelium, as well as functioning as a carrier protein for factor VIII. Consequently, the patient's bleeding time and PTT will be prolonged. Another combined disorder is DIC. DIC is a syndrome associated with critically ill individuals in which tissue factor liberation results in the activation of secondary hemostasis and microthromboembolism. These, in turn, result in the depletion of coagulation factors and platelets, fibrinolysis, traumatic hemolysis, and ischemic tissue damage. This schema is depicted in Fig. 64-4. DIC is caused most commonly by overwhelming infection. Multiple other causes exist, including trauma, shock, carcinoma and leukemia, and acute respiratory distress syn-

drome. Laboratory studies in DIC demonstrate prolonged INR and PTT, elevated FDPs and D-dimer, diminished fibrinogen, anemia, and thrombocytopenia.

Thrombotic thrombocytopenic purpura (TTP) is a disorder that ultimately can result in hemorrhage, but it is believed to be caused by a prothrombotic mechanism related to a plasma protease deficiency that results in a highly platelet-aggregating form of vWF.[23] This leads to platelet consumption in the microvasculature, causing thrombocytopenia and placing the patient at risk of hemorrhagic complications. TTP typically presents with microangiopathic hemolytic anemia, thrombocytopenia, fever, renal insufficiency, and prominent neurologic abnormalities in the face of a normal INR and PTT.

Hypercoagulability

Unlike in the hypocoagulable states, the routine laboratory studies previously discussed are normal in the hypercoagulable states. Given that abnormal physical examination findings may be subtle or absent, the emergency physician has to rely on an accurate history of the chief complaint and a high clinical suspicion in order to diagnose a thromboembolic disease. Specific attention must be given to known acquired and inherited thromboembolic risk factors. Previously described acquired ve-

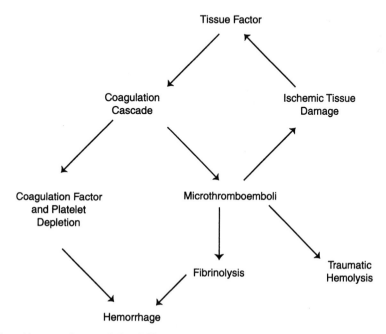

Fig. 64-4   Disseminated intravascular coagulation (DIC).

nous thromboembolic risk factors include advancing age, malignancy, immobilization, vascular trauma, HRT, and atherosclerosis. Multiple inherited disorders also predispose to venous thromboembolic disease.

Several inherited thrombophilias have been described in the literature. Although not usually diagnosed by the emergency physician, their presence should raise the clinical suspicion of thromboembolic disease states. Activated protein C (APC) resistance by factor V is one example. Most commonly, a gene mutation in factor V (e.g., factor V_{Leiden}) results in the inability of APC to inhibit factor V activity. Deficiencies of antithrombin, protein C, and protein S all have been implicated in predisposing to venous thromboembolism. The prothrombin 20210A mutation results in elevated prothrombin levels and an increased likelihood of venous thromboembolism. Finally, hyperhomocystinemia is a risk factor for arterial and venous thrombosis.[24,25] Special laboratory studies are required to diagnose these diseases and are best left to a hematologist. The presence of one or more of these factors, coupled with an asymmetrically swollen or painful extremity, should prompt a venous duplex study for confirmation of venous thrombosis.

Arterial thromboembolic disease is typically a function of atherosclerosis or cardiac pathology. At the time the fibrin cap of an atheroma ruptures, the prothrombotic lipid core is exposed, inducing thrombus formation, which may cause narrowing or occlusion of the affected vessel. Another means of arterial compromise involves cardiac mural thrombus formation with embolization into the peripheral arterial vasculature. Atrial fibrillation and ventricular wall motion abnormalities predispose to this type of disease. The site of arterial thromboembolism and degree of stenosis determine the clinical picture resulting in stroke, myocardial infarction, or peripheral artery occlusion, to name a few. Doppler studies and angiograms may be used to confirm the diagnosis of arterial occlusion.

EMERGENCY DEPARTMENT CARE AND DISPOSITION

Initial Management

Completing a rapid assessment of the patient for immediately life-threatening pathology and intervening on identification is a part of every emergency evaluation. Managing disorders of bleeding and coagulation is no different. Airway patency, the presence of protective airway reflexes, and adequate ventilation and oxygenation all should be confirmed prior to obtaining additional in-

formation. Tissue perfusion should then be assessed, and shock should be treated expeditiously. If hemorrhagic shock is present, then early transfusion of PRBCs is indicated to quickly increase oxygen-carrying capacity. This is especially important in the geriatric patient because underlying cardiovascular disease, which impairs physiologic reserve, is often present prior to the acute insult. Equally important is close monitoring of the patient's volume status, being careful to avoid volume overload. Once these issues have been addressed adequately, a rapid neurologic evaluation should be performed to search for signs of stroke or intracranial hemorrhage. If a focal neurologic deficit is identified in a patient with a known bleeding diathesis, then component-replacement therapy should be undertaken prior to diagnostic imaging. Only after all these issues have been addressed should the emergency physician proceed with the remainder of the evaluation and treatment.

Treatment of Hypocoagulable Disorders

Treatment of the vascular disorders that result in abnormal bleeding is directed toward treatment of the underlying disease process rather than the blood components involved in coagulation. Abnormal vascular proliferations may undergo chemical sclerosis. Vitamin C supplementation cures scurvy. Diminishing glucocorticoid doses may improve vascular fragility in those patients on chronic steroid therapy. Vasculitides often are treated with steroids to impair inflammatory reactions.

Platelet disorders may be treated by a variety of means. Platelet transfusions are used to raise the platelet count. Each unit of platelets transfused should raise the total platelet count by approximately 10,000 platelets/dL if continued platelet loss is not present. Platelet counts of between 10,000 and 50,000 platelets/dL indicate that bleeding times will be prolonged, but the risk of spontaneous hemorrhage is low. Platelet transfusion in a patient with this level of thrombocytopenia is only indicated if active bleeding is present. A platelet count of less than 10,000 platelets/dL requires emergent platelet transfusion, even in the absence of active bleeding, because thrombocytopenia this extreme is associated with spontaneous hemorrhage. Bleeding into the central nervous system may have catastrophic neurologic consequences. Platelet transfusions for thrombocytopenia associated with DIC and TTP should be avoided unless the platelet count falls below 10,000 platelets/dL. Platelet transfusions at higher levels in these diseases may contribute to the microangiopathic thrombus formation, exacerbating ischemic tissue damage.

Platelet transfusions also may be used to limit or stop bleeding associated with the platelet dysfunction caused by aspirin ingestion. More often, though, bleeding associated with platelet dysfunction from drug ingestion will only require discontinuation of the drug because the effects on platelet inhibition of most drugs are not as prolonged as that of aspirin. Aspirin is unique in that it creates a permanent platelet aggregation defect lasting the life of the platelet, which is approximately 10 days.

Platelet dysfunction caused by renal disease may be addressed by a variety of means. Dialysis reduces uremic retention products impairing platelet aggregation. Correction of the anemia of renal disease to a hemoglobin level of 8 to 10 g/dL is speculated to improve platelet distribution in the vasculature, allowing more efficient platelet and endothelial interactions.[16] Desmopressin (DDAVP) improves platelet aggregation in 50 to 75 percent of uremic patients.[16] DDAVP is usually administered in a dose of 0.3 µg/kg every 12 hours by the intravenous or subcutaneous route. DDAVP also may be administered intranasally in an amount of 150 to 300 µg every 12 hours. Conjugated estrogens also may be given intravenously in a dose of 0.6 mg/kg daily to improve bleeding times.

Platelet hypercoagulability associated with TTP is treated using plasma exchange with fresh-frozen plasma (FFP) in an attempt to replace the abnormal plasma protease with the properly functioning protease.[23]

The hallmark of treatment for disorders of coagulation factors is replacement of the deficient factors. Transfusion of FFP results in immediate replacement of all the coagulation factors. Cryoprecipitate is rich in vWF, factors VIII and XIII, and fibrinogen but lacks significant amounts of other coagulation proteins. Transmission of blood-borne pathogens is a rare, but still possible, problem with transfusions of FFPs or cryoprecipitate (as well as PRBCs and platelets). Another problem with transfusion therapy, especially in the elderly, in whom cardiac and renal disease is not uncommon, is the volume of fluid that must be infused, creating the possibility for volume overload. Specific recombinant factor replacement carries no risk of blood-borne pathogen transmission but is expensive. Finally, vitamin K supplementation in an oral or intravenous dose of 5 to 10 mg can be used to replenish factors II, VII, IX, and X by increasing hepatic synthesis; the effect of this therapy, however, is delayed a day or more.

Hemophiliacs suspected of having hemorrhage into the central nervous system, retroperitoneum, oropharynx, or neck should undergo immediate factor VIII or IX replacement for hemophilia A and B, respectively, in a dose of 50 units/kg intravenously. Factor replacement should be accomplished prior to any diagnostic testing. Patients with factor VIII inhibitors, both in hemophiliac and spontaneous cases, are more difficult to manage. Treatment strategies in this group include using recombinant factor VII, high-dose factor VIII with or without immunosuppressive agents, and porcine factor VIII.[26–29] Consultation with a hematologist is warranted under these circumstances.

Treatment of the combined platelet and coagulation factor disorders uses a combination of therapies. Von Willebrand's disease is treated most commonly with DDAVP (0.3 µg/kg intravenously or subcutaneously or 150–300 µg intranasal), which triples or quadruples the amount of circulating vWF.[30] Treatment with factor VIII replacement, using FFP, cryoprecipitate, or recombinant factor VIII, may be necessary in the minority of patients with the type II and III variants of this disease. The coagulopathy of DIC is treated with a combination of FFP, cryoprecipitate, and platelet transfusion for thrombocytopenia less than 10,000 platelets/dL. Recently, recombinant factor VII also has been used to treat DIC.[31] However, the most important treatment of DIC is addressing the underlying trigger for the syndrome. Treatment may include antibiotics for infection, volume expansion and vasopressors for shock, chemotherapy for carcinoma, and ventilatory support for acute respiratory distress syndrome. The use of heparin in low doses is controversial, and a hematologist should be consulted regarding this treatment.

Treatment of Hypercoagulable Disorders

The inherited thrombophilias are treated most commonly with a vitamin K antagonist such as warfarin to achieve an INR of two to three times normal. Because warfarin also inhibits the synthesis of proteins C and S, heparin or low-molecular-weight heparin (LMWH) should be administered concurrently at the start of therapy to diminish the likelihood of thrombus formation. Heparin is a catalyst for antithrombin, and LMWH inhibits factor Xa. Heparin or LMWH is withdrawn after a therapeutic INR is achieved. Heparin is not useful in the treatment of acute venous thromboembolic disease associated with antithrombin deficiency unless an antithrombin concentrate is administered concurrently.[32] In addition to heparin or LMWH and warfarin, individuals with hyperhomocystinemia are treated chronically with vitamin B_{12}, vitamin B_6, and folate to lower homocysteine levels in the blood.

Antiplatelet agents play a more significant role in the treatment of arterial as compared with venous thromboembolic disease. Aspirin, clopidogrel, and the glycoprotein IIb-IIIa inhibitors are used commonly in the treatment of acute coronary syndromes. Aspirin, clopidogrel, and warfarin can be used in the prevention of ischemic stroke. Acute ischemic stroke of less than 3 hours duration may be treated with intravenous tPA. Other thrombolytic agents that are available include reteplase and tenecteplase. which are used in the treatment of acute ST-segment-elevation myocardial infarction. Thrombolytics are also used in the treatment of massive pulmonary embolus with heart failure, peripheral arterial occlusion, and occasionally, deep venous thrombosis. Consultation with an appropriate specialist (e.g., neurology, pulmonology, or vascular surgery) is warranted when using thrombolytic therapy in these clinical settings.

REFERENCES

1. Fihn SC, McDonnel M, Martin D, et al: Risk factors for complications of chronic anticoagulation: A multicenter study. *Ann Intern Med* 118:511, 1993.
2. Stroke Prevention in Atrial Fibrillation Investigators: Warfarin versus aspirin for prevention of thromboembolism in atrial fibrillation: Stroke prevention in atrial fibrillation II study. *Lancet* 343:687, 1994.
3. Rodeghiero F, Castaman G, Dini E: Epidemiological investigation of the prevalence of von Willebrand's disease. *Blood* 69:454, 1987.
4. Green D, Lechner K: A survey of 215 non-hemophiliac patients with inhibitors to factor VIII. *Thromb Haemost* 45:2000, 1981.
5. Cortelazzo S, Finazzi G, Buelli M, et al: High risk of severe bleeding in aged patients with chronic idiopathic thrombocytopenic purpura. *Blood* 77:31, 1991.
6. Centers for Disease Control and Prevention: *National Vital Statistics Reports* 47(19), 1999.
7. Heit JA, Silverstein MD, Mohr DN, et al: The epidemiology of venous thromboembolism in the community. *Thromb Haemost* 86:252, 2001.
8. Anderson FA, Wheeler HB, Goldberg RJ, et al: A population based perspective of the hospital incidence and case fatality rates of deep venous thrombosis and pulmonary embolism. *Arch Intern Med* 151:933, 1991.
9. Goldhaber SZ, Visani L, DeRosa M: Acute pulmonary embolism: Clinical outcomes in the International Cooperative Pulmonary Embolism Registry (ICOPER). *Lancet* 353:1386, 1999.
10. Kearon C, Salzman EW, Hirsh J: Epidemiology, pathogenesis, and natural history of venous thrombosis, in Colman RW, Hirsh J, Marder VJ, et al (eds): *Hemostasis and Thrombosis: Basic Principles and Clinical Practice*, 4th ed.

Philadelphia, Lippincott, Williams, and Wilkins, 2001, p 1153.
11. Karpatkin S, Nierodzik ML, Klepfish A: Role of platelets and thrombin in cancer. *Vessels* 2:17, 1996.
12. Curatolo L, Colucci M, Cambini AL, et al: Evidence that cells from experimental tumors can activate coagulation factor X. *Br J Cancer* 40:228, 1979.
13. Stamatakis JD, Kakka VV, Sagar S, et al: Femoral vein thrombosis and total hip replacement. *Br Med J* 2:223, 1977.
14. Daly E, Vessey MP, Hawkins MM, et al: Risk of venous thromboembolism in users of hormone replacement therapy. *Lancet* 348:977, 1996.
15. Shiozawa S, Tanaka T, Miyahara T, et al: Age-related change in the reducible cross-link of human skin and aorta collagens. *Gerontology* 25:247, 1979.
16. Eberst ME, Berkowitz LR: Hemostasis in renal disease: Pathophysiology and management. *Am J Med* 96:168, 1994.
17. Horowitz HI, Stein IM, Cohen BD, et al: Further studies on the platelet-inhibitory effects of guanidinosuccinic acid and its role in uremic bleeding. *Am J Med* 49:336, 1970.
18. Escolar G, Cases A, Bastida E, et al: Uremic platelets have a functional defect affecting the interaction of von Willebrand factor with glycoprotein IIb-IIIa. *Blood* 76:1336, 1990.
19. Landefeld C, Goldman L: Major bleeding in outpatients treated with warfarin: Incidence and prediction by factors known at the start of outpatient therapy. Stroke Prevention in Reversible Ischemia (SPIRIT) Study Group. *Am J Med* 87:144, 1989.
20. Torn M, Algra A, Rosendaal FR: Oral anticoagulation for cerebral ischemia of arterial origin: High initial bleeding risk. *Neurology* 57:1993, 2001.
21. Lechner K, Niesser H, Thaler E: Coagulation abnormalities in liver disease. *Semin Thromb Hemost* 4:40, 1977.
22. Shapiro SS, Hultin M: Acquired inhibitors to the blood coagulation factors. *Semin Thromb Hemost* 1:336, 1975.
23. Elliott MA, Nichols WL: Thrombotic thrombocytopenic purpura and hemolytic uremic syndrome. *Mayo Clin Proc* 76:1154, 2001.
24. Nygard O, Nordrehaug JE, Refsum H, et al: Plasma homocysteine levels and mortality in patients with coronary artery disease. *New Engl J Med* 337:230, 1997.
25. den Heijer M, Rosendaal FR, Blom HJ, et al: Hyperhomocysteinemia and venous thrombosis: A meta-analysis. *Thromb Haemost* 80:874, 1998.
26. Hedner U, Glazer S, Falch J: Recombinant activated factor VII in the treatment of bleeding episodes in patients with inherited and acquired bleeding disorders. *Transfus Med Rev* 7:78, 1993.
27. Mariani G, Ghirardini A, Bellocco R: Immune tolerance in hemophilia: Principal results from the International Registry. Report of factor VIII and IX subcommittee. *Thromb Haemost* 72:155, 1994.
28. Hay C, Lozier JN: Porcine factor VIII therapy in patients with factor VIII inhibitor. *Adv Exp Med Biol* 386:143, 1995.
29. Kulkarni R, Aledort LM, Berntorp E, et al: Therapeutic

choices for patients with hemophilia and high-titer inhibitors. *Am J Hematol* 67:240, 2001.

30. Rodeghiero F, Castaman G, DiBona E, et al: Hyper-responsiveness to DDAVP for patients with type I von Willebrand disease and normal intra-platelet von Willebrand factor. *Eur J Haematol* 40:163, 1988.

31. Moscardo F, Perez F, De La Ruba J, et al: Successful treatment of severe intra-abdominal bleeding associated with disseminated intravascular coagulation using recombinant activated factor VII. *Br J Haematol* 113:174, 2001.

32. Lechner K, Kyrle P: Antithrombin III concentrates: Are they clinically useful? *Thromb Haemost* 73:340, 1995.

65

Anemia

Ryan Davis
Alex Garza

HIGH-YIELD FACTS

- The most common causes of anemia in the elderly are chronic disease and iron deficiency.
- The main indication for transfusion is a symptomatic patient with a hemoglobin level of less than 8 g/dL or a hematocrit of less than 25 percent.
- Care must be taken to avoid increased venous pressure and pulmonary congestion with blood transfusion in the elderly.

Although elderly patients experience the same causes of anemia as younger patients, the elderly respond differently. Elderly patients have decreased functional reserves in many organ systems and have a higher incidence of co-existing conditions, such as cognitive impairment, congestive heart failure, postural hypotension, and coronary artery disease.[1] Because of this, elderly patients require more aggressive intervention, and they respond differently to specific interventions than the younger population.

In the emergency department (ED), physicians commonly encounter anemic patients with either acute blood loss or chronic anemia. Making a firm diagnosis for the etiology of the anemia is not always achieved in the ED setting. It is important, however, to recognize that anemia may exacerbate many underlying medical conditions of the elderly.

EPIDEMIOLOGY

Anemia is the most common hematologic disorder encountered in the elderly, with an incidence that increases with age.[2] Anemia has a prevalence of approximately 10 to 20 percent in the elderly.[3] Anemia of chronic disease and iron-deficiency anemia are the two most common

causes of anemia in the elderly. Iron-deficiency anemia has a prevalence of 2 percent in the elderly population.[4]

Overall, elderly individuals have an increased incidence of anemia secondary to several coexisting conditions unrelated to age.[5] Several factors may contribute to the increased incidence of anemia in the elderly, such as decreased exercise activity and a leaner body mass. Reduced levels of testosterone and a decreased response to testosterone are hypothesized as contributing to anemia in men.

PATHOPHYSIOLOGY

Classification of Anemia

Anemia is defined by the World Health Organization (WHO) as a hemoglobin level below 12 g/dL in women and 13 g/dL in men.[6] Anemia can be classified either by morphology or etiology. Morphologic classifications include microcytic, macrocytic, and normocytic. Etiologic classification includes red blood cell (RBC) loss, excessive RBC destruction, and impaired RBC formation.[7]

Anemia Secondary to RBC Loss

Loss of RBCs can be either acute or chronic. Common causes of acute hemorrhage include gastrointestinal bleed, trauma, epistaxis, and ruptured abdominal aortic aneurysm. During acute hemorrhage states, bone marrow does not have the capacity to replace the loss of RBCs in a timely fashion. Chronic blood loss in the elderly sometimes is difficult to assess and usually is secondary to more serious etiologies. Common causes of chronic blood loss in the elderly include gastric erosion from non-steroidal anti-inflammatory drugs, bleeding colonic polyps, and angiodysplasia.[8–10]

Anemia Secondary to RBC Destruction

Hemolysis can be secondary to autoimmune hemolytic anemia or drug-related. Another cause of hemolysis in the elderly is traumatic hemolysis secondary to prosthetic heart valves. Hemolytic anemia is uncommon and usually is normocytic and normochromic.[11–14]

Anemia Secondary to Impaired Production of RBCs

Microcytic Anemia

The differential diagnosis for microcytic anemia includes iron-deficiency anemia, anemia of chronic disease, thalassemias, and sideroblastic anemia. Iron-deficiency anemia is rarely caused by dietary deficiencies. Anemia of chronic disease is more common in the elderly than younger individuals and is usually secondary to chronic inflammation, such as long-standing urinary tract infections, osteomyelitis, rheumatoid arthritis, or lupus. Anemia of chronic disease is also prominent in certain malignancies such as Hodgkin's disease. It is important to consider thalassemia trait as a cause of microcytic anemia.

Normocytic Anemia

Normocytic chronic anemia occurs from bone marrow stem cell failure. Common causes include chronic renal failure, endocrine disorders, liver disease, scurvy, infections, chemical exposure, myelodysplastic syndromes, radiation, and idiopathic causes.[15] Anemia in chronic renal failure occurs from decreased erythropoietin production. Many of these anemias are refractory and are treated by addressing the underlying disorder.

Macrocytic Anemia

Macrocytic anemia occurs from impaired DNA synthesis and usually is caused by a deficiency of folate or vitamin B_{12}. Folate deficiency is extremely common in the elderly; multiple factors contribute to it, which include mechanical reasons (loss of teeth) and socioeconomic reasons, such as alcoholism and diets consisting primarily of canned foods, which destroy the folic acid. Vitamin B_{12} deficiency usually results from decreased absorption rather than decreased dietary intake. Gastrectomies and gastric cancer can cause decreased absorption of vitamin B_{12}.[16]

CLINICAL FEATURES

The high prevalence of anemia in the elderly makes the signs and symptoms of anemia very common. However, physicians for several reasons frequently overlook diagnostic clues. First, elderly patients often attribute symptoms of anemia, such as fatigue, dyspnea, and weakness, to advancing age rather than to an underlying disorder. Second, symptom onset is usually insidious. Elderly individuals will adjust their activities and their bodies make physiologic adaptations to compensate for the decrease in RBCs. Finally, signs of anemia, such as pallor, can be difficult to detect in the elderly. One study demonstrated that physicians were able to detect conjunctival pallor at extremely low hematocrit levels but were less accurate as the hematocrit level increased.[14]

Although symptoms are sometimes difficult to discern in the elderly, patients will become symptomatic at higher hemoglobin concentrations than younger patients. Elderly patients frequently have more comorbid disease processes that can be aggravated by anemia, such as coronary artery disease, congestive heart failure, and postural hypotension. Therefore, anemia is an important diagnosis to consider in elderly patients who present with an exacerbation of an underlying medical condition.

DIAGNOSIS AND DIFFERENTIAL

The diagnosis of anemia in the elderly patient is established with decreased hemoglobin and hematocrit levels on evaluation of a complete blood cell count (CBC). It is important to remember that the clinical presentation of anemia can be varied in the elderly. Any patient with an exacerbation of existing medical condition or signs and symptoms consistent with anemia should be evaluated for anemia. It is essential to initially assess for acute causes of hemorrhage, such as trauma, epistaxis, or gastrointestinal bleeding. An occult gastrointestinal hemorrhage should be evaluated with rectal examination and stool Hemoccult in all patients suspected of being anemic. Laboratory studies should include CBC with indices, reticulocyte count, peripheral smear, coagulation studies, and type and cross-match if needed.

The mean corpuscular volume (MCV) is beneficial for determining whether the anemia is microcytic, macrocytic, or normocytic. Once the morphologic classification is determined, further studies are useful in determining etiologic classification. The reticulocyte count is used to determine the activity of the bone marrow. Peripheral blood smears are helpful in distinguishing the size of the RBCs, identifying abnormal RBC shapes, and examining for other cell lines, such as platelets and white blood cells. Coagulation studies and type and cross-match are important in the elderly patient who is anemic secondary to acute hemorrhage.

EMERGENCY DEPARTMENT CARE AND DISPOSITION

The initial ED evaluation of the elderly patient with signs and symptoms of anemia should start with assessment of the airway, breathing, and circulation. Correction of hypoventilation, hypoxia, and hypovolemia in the elderly anemic patient may stabilize an initially critically ill patient. Once the patient has been stabilized, the secondary survey can be initiated. At this point laboratory studies may be obtained, and a detailed physical examination should be conducted to investigate other less obvious causes of hemorrhage.

The initial management of acute hemorrhage should consist of crystalloid solution for volume replacement. Once the hemoglobin and hematocrit levels have been determined and the response to fluid resuscitation has been assessed, a decision can be made regarding transfusion of packed RBCs. When making this decision, it is important to consider underlying cardiovascular and cerebrovascular disease, as well as measures of tissue oxygenation.[17]

Concerns surrounding the risks and costs of blood products have led to many studies regarding the hemoglobin level for transfusion. Multiple studies have determined that packed RBC transfusion for hemoglobin levels of less than 7 g/dL is in general indicated.[18–20] An exception to this rule involves patients with myocardial infarction and unstable angina. A more liberal transfusion strategy of maintaining hemoglobin concentrations between 10 and 12 g/dL should be followed for these patients.[21,22]

Patients presenting to the ED with chronic anemia require a thorough evaluation. Laboratory studies should include a CBC with indices, reticulocyte count, peripheral smear, coagulation studies, and type and crossmatch, if needed. Discussion with the primary care physician is essential in determining further evaluation and disposition.

Any patient presenting with symptomatic anemia requiring transfusion should be admitted for observation and further evaluation. Patients with multiple comorbid diseases that are exacerbated by anemia also require admission. Patients with chronic anemia or newly diagnosed anemia not related to blood loss may not necessarily require admission if close follow-up can be arranged with their primary care physician.[23] Disposition ultimately is a clinical decision based on age, severity of anemia, treatment undertaken in the ED, comorbid medical conditions, and overall clinical picture.

ADDITIONAL ASPECTS

The following are pitfalls in the evaluation of elderly patients with anemia:

- Evaluation of anemia in the elderly is difficult because they may have multiple comorbid disease processes. One study of hospitalized patients found that 70 percent of the diagnoses contributed to anemia in the elderly.[24]

- Anemia of elderly patients is often overlooked because of a physician's belief that age is the primary reason for decreased hemoglobin levels. Only the hemoglobin levels in men decrease with age and by only 1 to 2 g/dL.

- Although low serum iron levels are present in both iron-deficiency anemia and anemia of chronic disease, anemia of chronic disease will not respond to iron supplementation.

- The mortality risk in healthy elderly patients with anemia is increased twofold, and the mortality risk from infectious and malignant diseases is higher in elderly patients with anemia.

REFERENCES

1. Izaks GJ, Westendorp RG, Knook DL: The definition of anemia in older persons. *JAMA* 281:1714, 1999.
2. Gautier M, Crawford J, Cohen HJ: Hematologic disorders, in Duthie EH (ed): *Practice of Geriatrics,* 3d ed. Philadelphia, Saunders, 1998, p 397.
3. Guyatt GH, Patterson C, Ali M, et al: Diagnosis of iron-deficiency anemia in the elderly. *Am J Med* 88:205, 1990.
4. Walsh JR: Hematologic problems, in Cassel CK, et al (eds): *Geriatric Medicine,* 3d ed. New York, Springer-Verlag, 1997, p 627.
5. Newland AC, Evans TG: Haematological disorders at the extremes of life. *Clin Rev* 314:1262, 1997.
6. Jolobe OMP: Does this elderly patient have iron deficiency anemia and what is the underlying cause? *Postgrad Med J* 76:195, 2000.
7. Looker AC, Dallman PR, Carroll MD, et al: Prevalence of iron deficiency in the United States. *JAMA* 277:973, 1997.
8. Freedman ML: Normal aging and patterns of hematologic disease. *Compr Ther* 22:304, 1996.
9. Lipschitz DA, Udupa KB, Milton KY, et al: Effect of age on hematopoiesis in man. *Blood* 63(3):502, 1984.
10. Scott RB: Common blood disorders: A primary care approach. *Geriatrics* 48(4):72, 1993.
11. Scott RB: Common blood disorders in the elderly. *Compr Ther* 20(10):575, 1994.
12. Rockey DC, Cello JP: Evaluation of the gastrointestinal tract in patients with iron deficiency anemia. *New Engl J Med* 329:1691, 1993.
13. Freedman ML, Sutin DG: Blood disorders and their management in old age, in Tallis R (ed): *Brocklehurst's Textbook of Geriatric Medicine and Gerontology,* 5th ed. New York, Churchill-Livingstone, 1998, p. 1247.
14. Hung OL, Kwon NS, Cole AE, et al: Evaluation of the physician's ability to recognize the presence or absence of anemia, fever, and jaundice. *Acad Emerg Med* 7:146, 2000.

15. Kruskall MS, Mintz PD, Bergin JJ, et al: Transfusion therapy in emergency medicine. *Ann Emerg Med* 17(4):327, 1988.
16. Eberst ME: Evaluation of anemia and the bleeding patient, in Tintinalli JE (ed): *Emergency Medicine: A Comprehensive Study Guide,* 5th ed. New York, McGraw-Hill, 2000, p 1365.
17. Chatta GS, Lipschitz DA: Anemia, in Hazzard WR (ed): *Principles of Geriatric Medicine and Gerontology,* 4d ed. New York, McGraw-Hill, 1999, p 899.
18. Hebert PC: Is a low transfusion threshold safe in critically ill patients with cardiovascular disease. *Crit Care Med* 29:227, 2001.
19. Welch HG: Prudent strategies for elective red blood cell transfusion. *Ann Intern Med* 116:393, 1992.
20. Hebert PC: Transfusion requirements in critical care. *JAMA* 273(18):1439, 1995.
21. Hebert PC: A multicenter, randomized, controlled clinical trial of transfusion requirements in critical care. *New Engl J Med* 340:409, 1999.
22. Goodenough LT: Transfusion medicine. *New Engl J Med* 340:438, 1999.
23. Damon LE: Anemias of chronic disease in the aged: Diagnosis and treatment. *Geriatrics* 47:47, 1992.
24. Smith DL: Anemia in the elderly. *Am Fam Phys* 62:1565, 2000.

66

Emergency Complications of Malignancy

John P. Sverha
O. John Ma

HIGH-YIELD FACTS

- For spinal cord compression secondary to metastatic disease, once weakness develops, further neurologic deterioration is rapid, with some patients progressing from weakness to complete paralysis in a matter of hours.

- Patients with confusion or seizures secondary to the syndrome of inappropriate antiuretic hormone (SIADH)–induced hyponatremia should be treated with hypertonic saline infusion.

- Adrenal crisis should be considered in all hypotensive cancer patients and, when suspected, should be treated immediately with hydrocortisone 100 mg intravenously.

- Hyperviscosity of the blood can cause central nervous system (CNS) dysfunction and respiratory distress. It usually occurs when the white blood cell count is greater than 100,000/mm³, the hematocrit is greater than 60 percent, or there are increased concentrations of serum proteins (e.g., Waldenström's macroglobulinemia and multiple myeloma).

- Cancer patients with fever and neutropenia require a meticulous physical examination to identify a source of infection and early administration of empirical antibiotics.

The majority of patients with cancer are over the age of 65 years. The treatment of patients with emergency complications of malignancy can be hindered by many factors. Patients may be uncomfortable or have insufficient knowledge to candidly discuss the extent of their malignancy in the emergency department (ED). The emergency physician may be unfamiliar with the large and frequently changing number of chemotherapeutic agents as well as the complex classification and staging of malignancies. Lastly, both patients and physicians may have the false impression that aggressive diagnostic and therapeutic interventions are futile in the presence of advanced malignancy.

Current trends in the management of cancer-related emergencies include an increasing number of older patients receiving chemotherapy, more aggressive chemotherapy regimens, broader use of chemotherapy (particularly with solid tumors), and an increasing use of bone marrow transplantation. These trends, coupled with an increasing prevalence of malignant disease and longer patient survival, require emergency physicians to recognize and treat a wide spectrum of oncologic emergencies. Myelosuppression from chemotherapy and radiotherapy can result in coagulopathies and infection. Tumor growth can produce signs and symptoms of local compression on the spinal cord or airway, and certain tumors are associated with unique complications, such as hyperviscosity syndromes from tumor-related gammopathies. Table 66-1 lists the most important life-threatening oncologic emergencies.

ACUTE SPINAL CORD COMPRESSION

Pathophysiology

Spinal cord compression is typically associated with metastatic breast, lung, or prostate cancer but also can be seen in patients with myeloma, renal cell carcinoma, and lymphoma.[1] There are four ways in which tumors typically compress the spinal cord. First and most commonly, a tumor that has metastasized to a vertebral body may extend outward into the spinal canal and compress the spinal cord. Second, a tumor metastasis may cause a pathologic compression fracture of the vertebral body, resulting in bony fragments being retropulsed into the cord. Third, tumor outside the spinal canal can invade posterolaterally through the neural foramina and compress the cord. Last and least commonly, pressure on the spinal cord can occur secondary to a metastasis that originates within the spinal cord (intramedullary metastasis).[2]

Clinical Features

It is estimated that 5 percent of patients with cancer will incur symptoms secondary to spinal cord compression.[3] In the

Table 66-1. Emergency Complications of Malignancy

Related to local tumor compression
    Acute spinal cord compression
    Upper airway obstruction
    Malignant pericardial effusion with tamponade
    Superior vena cava syndrome
Related to biochemical derangements and systemic collapse
    Hypercalcemia of malignancy
    Syndrome of inappropriate antidiuretic hormone (SIADH)
    Hyperviscosity syndrome
    Adrenocortical insufficiency with shock
Related to myelosuppression
    Granulocytopenia and sepsis
    Immunosuppression and opportunistic infections
    Thrombocytopenia and hemorrhage
    Anaphylaxis and transfusion reactions

majority of patients these symptoms will occur in the setting of previously diagnosed cancer; in perhaps 10 percent of patients these will be the first symptoms of malignancy.[4]

Approximately 95 percent of persons with spinal cord compression will have pain as their initial symptom.[5] The pain is typically continuous, progressive, and requires analgesics. It may precede the diagnosis by weeks or months. The pain may be localized to the involved vertebra or may be radicular, especially if the thoracic spine is involved.[1]

Weakness is typically the next symptom that occurs. Weakness almost always first develops in the legs, regardless of the site of spinal cord compression. Once weakness develops, further neurologic deterioration is rapid, with some patients progressing from weakness to complete paralysis in a matter of hours.[1] Sensory and autonomic deficits typically follow the development of weakness. Once neurologic deficits occur, they are difficult to reverse. Emergent treatment is then needed to enhance the likelihood of recovery and to prevent further progression of deficits.[2]

Diagnosis and Differential

Patients with a history of cancer and unexplained back pain without other neurologic symptoms should first have plain radiographs performed. Most patients will have abnormalities on plain radiographs if their symptoms are due to metastatic disease.[6] If the pain persists despite normal plain radiographs, magnetic resonance imaging (MRI) is required.

Patients with a history of cancer, back pain, and the acute onset of weakness, numbness, or autonomic dysfunction require an emergency MRI. The entire spine should be imaged due to the high incidence of asymptomatic multilevel disease.[2]

Emergency Department Care and Disposition

Once the diagnosis of spinal cord compression is made, treatment should begin immediately. All patients should first receive corticosteroids. The optimal dosing of corticosteroids in the setting of acute spinal cord compression is controversial. Authors typically recommend initial doses of dexamethasone between 10 and 100 mg intravenously.[7]

Additional treatments for acute spinal cord compression secondary to malignancy include radiation therapy, chemotherapy, and surgery. The treatment recommended is based on the tumor type, location, and response to previous treatment. Radiation therapy is the definitive treatment for most patients.[1] Surgical laminectomy and decompression are indicated if there is architectural instability, tissue confirmation of cancer is required, maximal radiation therapy has been given previously, or the tumor is particularly radioresistant.[2] The patient often will need to be assessed by physicians specializing in neurosurgery, oncology, and radiation oncology before an individualized treatment plan can be developed.

UPPER AIRWAY OBSTRUCTION

Acute upper airway obstruction is seen more commonly in patients with cancers of the base of the tongue, hypopharynx, larynx, and thyroid. It also can be caused by compression of the trachea in the mediastinum secondary to lymphoma or metastatic disease.[8]

Patients with upper airway obstruction typically will have stridor. Acute worsening of symptoms is often due to progressive edema, tumor growth, bleeding, or inspissated secretions. Initial stabilization should include attempts to clear the upper airway of secretions and foreign bodies. Helium-oxygen mixtures reduce respiratory work and may be administered as a temporizing measure.[8] Intravenous steroids may be given. If respiratory difficulty persists, direct control of the airway is required through orotracheal intubation or tracheostomy. Fiberoptic visualization of the upper airway may be necessary for successful orotracheal intubation. Once stabilized, the patient may benefit from surgical resection of the tumor, airway stent placement, radiation therapy, or photodynamic therapy.[9]

MALIGNANT PERICARDIAL EFFUSION WITH TAMPONADE

Pathophysiology

A pericardial effusion develops when fluid enters the pericardial sac more rapidly than it is reabsorbed. In cancer patients, failure to reabsorb pericardial fluid occurs when efferent lymphatic vessels are obstructed or when metastases to subcarinal lymph nodes prevent effective drainage. Fluid also may accumulate within the pericardium as a result of bleeding from tumor implants. Malignant pericardial effusions are associated most commonly with breast cancer, lung cancer, lymphoma, leukemia, and melanoma.[8] Cancer patients also may develop pericardial effusions in response to radiation or chemotherapy. Drugs associated with development of pericardial effusion include cyclophosphamide, granulocyte-macrophage colony-stimulating factor (GM-CSF), and cytarabine.[10]

Cardiac tamponade occurs when pressure from the effusion prevents adequate venous return to the heart. This can occur with both small and large effusions because the pericardial fluid pressure depends on both the rate of pericardial fluid accumulation and the distensibility of the pericardial sac. As little as 100 mL of pericardial fluid may cause symptoms in a patient with a scarred or infiltrated pericardium, whereas more than 1 L of fluid may cause minimal symptoms if it accumulates slowly in a patient with an elastic pericardium.[11]

Clinical Features

Patients with malignant pericardial effusions may present with dyspnea, cough, chest discomfort, or peripheral edema.[12] Patients with cardiac tamponade typically are hypotensive with a narrow pulse pressure. They exhibit jugular venous distension, diminished heart sounds, and a pulsus paradoxus greater than 10 mmHg. The electrocardiogram (ECG) may reveal electrical alternans, in which the QRS voltage becomes larger and smaller on alternate complexes.[11]

Diagnosis and Differential

The preferred method for diagnosing pericardial effusions is echocardiography.[13] The presence of an effusion may be suggested on chest radiograph if the size of the cardiac silhouette has increased compared with previous studies.

Emergency Department Care and Disposition

Patients with evidence of cardiac tamponade who are in extremis require emergency pericardiocentesis. The treatment of more stable patients should be discussed with an oncologist. The patient's tumor type, symptom severity, and prognosis are all considered in determining a treatment plan that may include systemic chemotherapy, intrapericardial chemotherapy, elective pericardiocentesis, creation of a pleuropericardial window, or other surgical techniques.[12]

SUPERIOR VENA CAVA SYNDROME

Pathophysiology

Superior vena cava (SVC) syndrome is caused by obstruction of blood flow through the SVC. This can be due to extrinsic compression by a mass, invasion by a tumor, or thrombosis. Cancers most often associated with SVC syndrome include lung cancer (typically small cell lung cancer), lymphoma (typically non-Hodgkin's lymphoma), and metastatic breast cancer.[14] Cancer patients also may develop SVC syndrome secondary to thrombosis around an indwelling vascular catheter.

Clinical Features

SVC syndrome typically has an insidious onset. The most common presenting symptom is dyspnea. Other common presenting symptoms include face or arm swelling, head fullness, cough, chest pain, and hoarseness.[14] Symptoms may worsen when bending forward. Elevated intracranial pressure can cause agitation, seizures, or syncope; however, theses are rare findings.[8] Physical examination may reveal venous distension of the neck and chest wall, facial edema, cyanosis, arm edema, and occasionally, papilledema.[14] Vocal cord paralysis or Horner's syndrome can occur. A palpable supraclavicular mass due to direct tumor extension occasionally can be noted with tumors of the superior mediastinum.[9]

Diagnosis and Differential

The chest radiograph in patients with SVC syndrome usually shows superior mediastinal widening. Other common findings on chest radiograph include pleural effusion and a right hilar mass. Contrast-enhanced chest computed tomographic (CT) scanning is the primary means of confirming the clinical suspicion of SVC syndrome. In addition to visualizing the SVC, chest CT scanning allows visualization of other mediastinal structures that may be compromised by tumor extension.

Emergency Department Care and Disposition

Most patients with SVC syndrome do not require emergency treatment. Exceptions include patients with neurologic symptoms or signs of airway compromise. Symptomatic patients may receive some relief by elevating the head of the bed and administering oxygen. Steroids such as dexamethasone (10 mg intravenously or orally) may help, although their efficacy for most patients has not been proven.[8] Diuretics such as furosemide (20–40 mg intravenously or orally) may reduce symptomatic edema.

More definitive treatment of SVC syndrome is provided by reducing the size of the tumor through radiation therapy or chemotherapy. Distinguishing the tumor type helps in determining which therapy would be most effective. A treatment option that provides immediate relief is percutaneous endovascular angioplasty with stent placement. This is becoming increasingly common and is used often in conjunction with radiation and chemotherapy. Surgery to bypass the occluded SVC is another option and may be indicated if the occlusion is due to an aortic aneurysm or retrosternal goiter.[14] Lastly, thrombolytic therapy is often effective in patients with SVC syndrome due to an indwelling vascular catheter.[8]

HYPERCALCEMIA OF MALIGNANCY

Pathophysiology

Hypercalcemia of malignancy is primarily due to increased osteoclastic bone resorption, although increased uptake of calcium through the renal tubules may contribute as well. The most common mediator of cancer-associated hypercalcemia appears to be parathyroid hormone–related protein (PTH-RP). Typically not present in the general circulation, it is found at high levels in patients with hypercalcemia from various solid tumors. Other potential mediators of malignancy-associated hypercalcemia include prostaglandins and cytokines, such as the transforming growth factors and interleukin-6.[15] The most common tumors associated with hypercalcemia include carcinoma of the breast and lung, myeloma, lym-

phoma, and the squamous cell cancers of the head and neck.[16]

Clinical Features

Hypercalcemia is the most common life-threatening metabolic disorder in patients with cancer, occurring in 10 to 20 percent of patients at some time during their disease course.[17] The severity of symptoms caused by hypercalcemia is not directly related to the degree of elevation in serum calcium. The rapidity of the onset of hypercalcemia is important as well, with severe symptoms manifesting at levels of 12 to 13 mg/dL if the elevation is acute, whereas some patients with chronic calcium levels of 16 mg/dL may have few, if any, symptoms.[15]

The most common presenting symptoms of hypercalcemia include nausea, weakness, constipation, and polyuria. Patients typically are dehydrated due to the nausea and an accompanying nephrogenic diabetes insipidus. Patients with long-standing hypercalcemia may develop kidney stones. More severe symptoms of hypercalcemia include confusion, seizures, and coma.

Diagnosis and Differential

Serum calcium is highly bound to albumin, and measurements of serum calcium levels change with serum protein concentrations. The serum calcium level can be adjusted for abnormal serum albumin levels using the formula

$$\text{Corrected calcium (mg/dL)} = \text{measured calcium (mg/dL)} - \text{albumin (g/dL)} + 4.0$$

Measurement of serum ionized calcium is also possible and is independent of the serum protein level. Measurement of a serum ionized calcium level is essential in patients with myeloma and hypercalcemia due to a large increase in serum calcium-binding proteins.

Emergency Department Care and Disposition

Therapies for malignancy-associated hypercalcemia aim to decrease serum calcium through either increasing renal excretion of calcium or decreasing bone resorption by inhibiting osteoclast function. Administration of normal saline intravenous fluids should be the first treatment provided because most patients with hypercalcemia are dehydrated. Assuming that renal and cardiac functions are adequate, infusion of intravenous normal saline at 300 to 400 mL/h over the first 3 to 4 hours will increase renal blood flow and promote calcium excretion. The addition of furosemide to promote calcium excretion is no longer routinely recommended.[15] Its use should be restricted to balancing fluid intake and urinary output once patients have been fully rehydrated.

Most patients with serum calcium levels greater than 12 mg/dL will not have adequate reductions in serum calcium with intravenous fluids only.[18] After rehydration and adequate urinary output have been achieved, these patients should be administered pamidronate (60 mg intravenously over 4 hours or 90 mg intravenously over 24 hours). Pamidronate is the most efficacious of the bisphosphonates, which reduce serum calcium levels by inhibiting the activity of osteoclasts.[16] Reductions in calcium levels occur 24 to 48 hours after initiation of the infusion.

Patients with serum calcium levels greater than 15 mg/dL or severe symptoms also may benefit from the early administration of calcitonin (6–8 IU/kg intramuscularly every 6 hours).[19] Calcitonin increases urinary excretion of calcium and helps prevent bone resorption. The onset of action is rapid, with decreases in calcium levels occurring within 2 to 4 hours.[20] However, the magnitude of the hypocalcemic response is small compared with pamidronate.

Other agents used to treat malignancy-associated hypercalcemia include gallium nitrate, phosphates, and plicamycin, although each has significant side effects. Administration of corticosteroids may be useful in some cancers such as lymphoma, leukemia, myeloma, and certain breast cancers.[16] Dialysis should be considered in patients with severe hypercalcemia and marked renal insufficiency.

SYNDROME OF INAPPROPRIATE ANTIDIURETIC HORMONE SECRETION

Pathophysiology

Common causes of the syndrome of inappropriate antidiuretic hormone (SIADH) secretion in cancer patients include ectopic ADH production by tumor cells and chemotherapy-induced excessive release of ADH from the pituitary gland. Tumors that are often associated with ectopic ADH production include small cell lung cancer, pancreatic cancer, prostate cancer, and bladder cancer.[21] Chemotherapeutic agents associated with SIADH include cyclophosphamide, vincristine, and vinblastine.[16] Patients with SIADH are impaired in their ability to excrete water, which results in euvolemic hyponatremia.

Clinical Features

The symptoms of SIADH are those of hyponatremia. The severity of symptoms is related to both the degree of hyponatremia and the rapidity of its onset. Symptoms may include nausea, weakness, headache, seizures, and coma. Seizures typically are associated with serum sodium levels of less than 120 meq/L.

Diagnosis and Differential

Patients with SIADH are clinically euvolemic. Laboratory studies reveal hyponatremia, decreased serum osmolality, concentrated urine, and excessive urine sodium excretion (U_{Na} > 30 meq/L). Other conditions that can cause similar findings include adrenal insufficiency and chronic diuretic use.

Emergency Department Care and Disposition

The mainstay of therapy in patients with SIADH is water restriction. Patients with a serum sodium level above 125 meq/L or mild symptoms generally can be managed through restricting water intake to approximately 500 mL/day. This should increase serum sodium concentrations by 2 to 3 meq/L/day.

Patients with severe confusion, seizures, or coma should be treated with hypertonic saline infusion. Patients should be infused with a 3% normal saline solution at a rate of 0.05 mL/kg/min.[21] This should increase serum sodium concentration by approximately 2 meq/L/h. Serum sodium measurements should be performed hourly. Hypertonic saline administration should be discontinued as soon as symptoms abate or the serum sodium level returns halfway back to normal, whichever comes first. Patients should never have their serum sodium corrected by more than 12 to 15 meq/L over a 24-hour period because this puts them at risk of developing osmotic demyelination syndrome.[21]

HYPERVISCOSITY SYNDROME

Pathophysiology

Hyperviscosity syndrome (HVS) is caused by severe elevations in serum paraproteins, white blood cells, or red blood cells. The end result is a marked increase in blood viscosity, causing decreased perfusion of the microcirculation and vascular stasis. The dysproteinemias most commonly associated with HVS are Waldenström's macroglobulinemia and multiple myeloma.[22] HVS due to leukocytosis typically occurs when white blood cell (WBC) counts exceed 100,000/mm^3. This is seen most often in the blastic phase of chronic myelogenous leukemia and chronic granulocytic leukemia and the blast cell crisis of acute lymphoblastic leukemia.[22] HVS due to erythrocytosis usually occurs at a hematocrit greater than 60 percent, which can be seen in polycythemia vera.

Clinical Features

Early symptoms of HVS include fatigue, anorexia, and visual disturbances. Patients also may develop confusion, seizures, dyspnea, or coma. Physical examination may reveal engorgement of retinal veins (e.g., boxcar or sausage-link segmentation) or papilledema.[23] Patients also may exhibit signs of congestive heart failure or renal insufficiency. The emergency physician should be aware that symptoms of HSV may be the first sign of an undiagnosed malignancy, especially many plasma cell dyscrasias.

Diagnosis and Differential

The diagnosis of HVS typically is made in the laboratory when a symptomatic patient is found to have a WBC greater than 100,000/mm^3, a hematocrit greater than 60 percent, or an abnormal serum electrophoresis. Since serum electrophoresis results often are not available immediately, a first clue to the presence of increased serum viscosity may be the inability of the laboratory to run chemistry tests because the blood is "too thick." Increased serum viscosity also should be considered in the setting of anemia with rouleaux formation on a peripheral smear.

Emergency Department Care and Disposition

Initial therapy is rehydration with normal saline followed by hematology consultation. Patients with frank coma may benefit from a 2-unit phlebotomy with concurrent replacement of fluids with normal saline.[22] Definitive treatment is provided by plasmapheresis, leukapheresis, or the initiation of chemotherapy.

ADRENAL INSUFFICIENCY AND SHOCK

Pathophysiology

Adrenal insufficiency in cancer patients can be due to destruction of the adrenal gland by metastases but more commonly is due to the withdrawal of chronic steroid therapy.[15] Cancers known to metastasize to the adrenal gland include lung and breast cancers, melanoma, and various retroperitoneal malignancies. Even if metastasis to the adrenal glands is evident by CT scan or MRI, most of these patients will not be adrenal insufficient.[24]

Clinical Features

Symptoms of adrenal insufficiency include weakness, dizziness, nausea, and skin hyperpigmentation. In cases of primary adrenal insufficiency, laboratory studies may reveal hyponatremia with hyperkalemia. Confirmation of adrenal insufficiency is best made through adrenocorticotropin hormone (ACTH) stimulation testing.

Adrenal crisis occurs when patients with underlying adrenal insufficiency encounter a major stress such as infection, trauma, or surgery. Patients may develop life-threatening hypotension that is minimally responsive to intravenous fluid administration and vasopressors. The diagnosis of adrenal crisis should be considered in all hypotensive cancer patients, and if suspected, it should result in immediate treatment. Serum levels of cortisol and ACTH should be drawn prior to treatment for later laboratory confirmation of the diagnosis.

Emergency Department Care and Disposition

Patients with adrenal insufficiency require daily supplementation with glucocorticoids (typically prednisone 7.5 mg/day or cortisol 30 mg/day) and mineralocorticoids (fludrocortisone 0.05–0.10 mg/day). Patients in adrenal crisis require immediate administration of hydrocortisone 100 mg intravenously, with repeat doses of 100 mg given every 6 hours. Mineralocorticoids are not needed when high doses of hydrocortisone are given because hydrocortisone itself has mineralocorticoid effects at these doses.

FEVER AND NEUTROPENIA

Clinical Features

Cancer patients can become neutropenic as a direct consequence of their malignancy or because of chemotherapy or radiation therapy. Neutropenia is usually defined as an absolute neutrophil count (ANC) of less than 500/mm^3 or an ANC of less than 1000/mm^3 with a predicted decrease to less than 500/mm^3. Patients who develop a fever while they are neutropenic are at high risk for bacteremia and sepsis. Fever in these neutropenic patients typically is defined as a single oral temperature greater than or equal to 38.3°C or an oral temperature greater than equal to 38.0°C for at least 1 hour.[25]

Diagnosis and Differential

The patient with fever and neutropenia requires a meticulous physical examination.[26] Special attention should be given to the oropharynx, skin, vascular catheter sites, and perineum. Signs and symptoms of inflammation may be minimal in these patients. For example, the only sign of a perirectal abscess may be local tenderness without any overlying erythema or warmth.

In looking for the source of the fever, these patients should have a chest radiograph, urinalysis, urine culture, and at least two sets of blood cultures ordered. If a vascular catheter is in place, at least one set of blood cultures should be obtained from each port.

Emergency Department Care and Disposition

If the source of infection is not apparent after the physical examination and initial diagnostic testing, empirical antibiotic therapy should be initiated promptly. According to the *2002 Guidelines for the Management of Fever and Neutropenia in Caner Patients* published by the Infectious Disease Society of America (IDSA), there are several acceptable empirical antibiotic regimens.[25] The regimen chosen should depend on whether the patient is at high or low risk for severe infection.

Patients are considered to be at low risk for severe infection if they have the following characteristics: ANC greater than 100/mm³, absolute monocyte count greater than 100/mm³, normal chest radiograph, no intravenous catheter infection, normal hepatic and renal tests, duration of neutropenia less than 7 days, expected resolution of neutropenia in less than 10 days, evidence of early bone marrow recovery, malignancy in remission, peak temperature less than 39.0°C, not ill-appearing or confused, and no hypotension or vomiting.

Adults determined to be at low risk by the preceding criteria are eligible for oral administration of antibiotics. The oral antibiotic regimen recommended is cipro-floxacin and amoxicillin-clavulanate. In at least two recent studies, this regimen has been shown to be as effective as intravenous antibiotic regimens in low-risk hospitalized patients.[27,28] However, discharge of these low-risk patients directly from the ED on oral antibiotic therapy is still controversial because home oral treatment has not yet been studied in prospective trials.[29,30]

There are multiple intravenous antibiotic regimens that have been shown to be effective in patients hospitalized with cancer-associated neutropenia and fever. Each regimen has a slightly different spectrum of antibacterial activity and a slightly different side-effect profile. Consideration should be given to local patterns of infection and antibiotic susceptibility when choosing one of these regimens. The efficacy of monotherapy with ceftazidime, cefepime, imipenem-cilastatin, or meropenem has been well established, although recently it has been shown that ceftazidime monotherapy may be inferior against *Streptococcus viridans* and pneumococci.[31–33] Two-drug therapy is also an option, with accepted regimens combining an aminoglycoside with an antipseudomonal penicillin, cefepime, ceftazidime, or a carbapenem. Vancomycin generally should not be part of an empirical antibiotic regimen in patients with neutropenia and cancer. However, it may reasonably be added to one of the preceding regimens in patients with a clinically suspected severe catheter infection, known colonization with penicillin- and cephalosporin-resistant pneumococci, or methicillin-resistant *Staphylococcus aureus,* severe sepsis with hypotension, or severe mucositis or in patients already on fluoroquinolone prophylaxis.[25]

GASTROINTESTINAL SYNDROMES

Acute upper gastrointestinal (UGI) hemorrhage is a common problem in both the general population and cancer patients. Clinicians should not presume that UGI bleeding in a cancer patient is directly related to the cancer because the most common causes of UGI bleeding in these patients are still hemorrhagic gastritis, peptic ulcer disease, variceal bleeding, and esophagitis.[8] Some cancer patients receiving chemotherapy and radiotherapy develop UGI bleeding due to Mallory-Weiss tears caused by severe vomiting.

Small bowel obstruction secondary to metastases is common in patients with ovarian, pancreatic, and gastric cancers. Large bowel obstruction is most commonly due to colorectal cancer.[34] Cancer patients are also at risk for large or small bowel ileus as a consequence of electrolyte abnormalities, narcotic use, and phenothiazine use.

Typhlitis is an inflammatory condition of the cecum most commonly seen in neutropenic cancer patients. It is a common cause of abdominal pain in patients with acute leukemia. The pathogenesis of this disorder is believed to be bacterial invasion of the bowel wall of the cecum.

Symptoms include fever, abdominal pain, and right lower quadrant pain and abdominal tenderness. Patients often improve with antibiotics alone. The role of surgery is controversial.[34]

UROLOGIC SYNDROMES

Urologic emergencies in the cancer patient include bladder hemorrhage, urinary tract obstruction, and priapism. Bladder hemorrhage in cancer patients may be secondary to chemotherapeutic agents or previous radiation therapy. Bladder hemorrhage is fairly common with the use of cyclophosphamide, occurring in almost 5 percent of patients on this agent.[35] Bleeding is due to the toxic effect on the bladder wall of acrolein, which is a by-product of cyclophosphamide metabolism. Bleeding typically occurs during or shortly after a chemotherapy treatment with intravenous cyclophosphamide, although delayed hemorrhage may occur when taking the oral form of this medication. Radiation therapy for various cancers can result in later bladder hemorrhage. This is usually due to the development of friable, telangiectatic blood vessels on the surface of the bladder mucosa. Bladder hemorrhage in both scenarios just described can be massive and life-threatening.[36] Initial treatment involves placement of a large-diameter and multiple-hole ureteral catheter to initiate saline lavage and clot evacuation. If bleeding continues, cystoscopic removal of clots with fulguration of bleeding sites may be indicated. Persistent bleeding despite these measures may require intravesical instillation of a hemostatic agent such formalin, alum, or prostaglandins.[35]

Urinary tract obstruction can occur at any level of the urinary tract. Ureteral obstruction in cancer patients can be secondary to direct tumor compression of the ureter, encasement of the ureter by retroperitoneal lymph nodes, or occasionally by direct metastases to the ureter. The most commonly associated malignancies are prostate, bladder, cervical, colon, and lymphoma. Ureteral obstruction also may occur as a consequence of radiation therapy. This is seen most commonly after radiation therapy for cervical cancer and can occur many months or years following the treatment.[37] Treatment of ureteral obstruction is most commonly through percutaneous nephrostomy or ureteral stent placement. Urinary retention at the level of the bladder is also seen in cancer patients. It can be caused by mechanical bladder outlet obstruction, brain or spinal cord metastases, or as a side effect of medications. Initial treatment is urethral catheter placement followed by urologic consultation.

Priapism in cancer patients may be caused by a primary hematologic malignancy (e.g., leukemia), metastases to the corporal bodies of the penis, or because venous outflow from the penis is obstructed by a pelvic tumor.[35] Treatment depends of the cause of the priapism but may include chemotherapy and radiation. Corporal shunting procedures used for idiopathic priapism usually are ineffective in priapism caused by malignancy.[36]

BONE MARROW TRANSPLANTS

Emergency physicians can expect to care for increasing numbers of bone marrow transplant patients due to the rising prevalence and survivability of this procedure. It is currently estimated that there are over 20,000 persons in the United States that have survived more than 5 years after bone marrow transplantation.[38] Bone marrow transplants currently are performed for malignant conditions such as leukemia, lymphoma, and selected solid tumors, as well as for nonmalignant conditions such as aplastic anemia, thalassemia, and sickle cell anemia.[39]

Emergency physicians are unlikely to encounter the acute complications of bone marrow transplantation because these patients often are kept in the hospital for several weeks following their transplant until engraftment occurs. However, emergency physicians should be aware of the long-term complications and consequences of bone marrow transplantation. Like solid-organ transplant recipients, bone marrow recipients are at increased risk of infection. This risk is not just confined to the period of granulocytopenia preceding engraftment. Even with a normal neutrophil count, bone marrow transplant patients have a residual cellular and humoral immunodeficiency that persists for 12 to 24 months after transplantation.[40] Bone marrow transplant patients are at particular risk of infection from encapsulated bacteria, *Pneumocystis carinii,* cytomegalovirus (CMV), varicella-zoster virus, *Candida,* and *Aspergillus.* CMV pneumonitis is the most common infectious cause of death after bone marrow transplantation and typically occurs 1 to 6 months following the transplant.[41] To decrease the risk of opportunistic infection, bone marrow transplant patients are often prophylactically administered penicillin, trimethoprim-sulfamethoxazole, and ganciclovir for the first 3 to 6 months following their transplant.[42] Fever or other signs of infection should be taken very seriously in a bone marrow transplant patient (even if the neutrophil count is normal), and a treatment plan should be developed in conjunction with the patient's hematologist.

A complication unique to bone marrow transplant patients is graft-versus-host disease (GVHD). This disorder occurs only in allogeneic transplant patients. It is caused by immunologically competent donor cells attacking target antigens in the recipient. Acute GVHD (within 100 days of transplantation) is a major life-threatening complication. Patients develop rash, diarrhea, liver dysfunction, and immune compromise of varying severity. The diagnosis is confirmed by biopsy. Treatment consists of immunosuppressive agents such as corticosteroids, tacrolimus, and cyclosporine. Chronic GVHD (occurring later than 100 days after transplantation) affects 30 to 60 percent of all bone marrow transplant recipients.[43] Findings include skin dryness and changes in pigmentation, mouth dryness, abnormal liver function tests, odynophagia, and joint contractures.[39] Chronic GVHD is not usually life-threatening, but it is a marker of persistent deficits in humoral and cellular immunity that can result in severe infections.[44] Treatment should be discussed with the transplant team but often involves long courses of immunosuppressive therapy.

REFERENCES

1. Fuller BG, Heiss JD, Oldfield EH: Spinal cord compression, in DeVita VT, Hellman S, Rosenberg SA (eds): *Cancer: Principles and Practice of Oncology*, 6th ed. Philadelphia, Lippincott Williams & Wilkins, 2001.

2. Quinn JA, DeAngelis LM: Neurologic emergencies in the cancer patient. *Semin Oncol* 27:311, 2000.

3. Byrne TN: Spinal cord compression from epideural metastases. *New Engl J Med* 327:614, 1992.

4. Boogerd W, van der Sande JJ: Treatment of complications: Diagnosis and treatment of spinal cord compression in malignant disease. *Cancer Treat Rep* 19:129, 1993.

5. Gilbert RW, Kim J-H, Posner JB: Epidural spinal cord compression from metastatic tumor: Diagnosis and treatment. *Ann Neurol* 3:40, 1978.

6. Sorensen S, Helweg-Larsen S, Mouridsen H et al: Effect of high-dose dexamethasone in carcinomatous metastatic spinal cord compression treated with radiotherapy: A randomized trial. *Eur J Cancer* 30A:22, 1994.

7. Loblaw DA, Laperriere NJ: Emergency treatment of malignant extradural spinal cord compression: An evidence-based guideline. *J Clin Oncol* 16:1613, 1998.

8. Morris JC, Holland JF: Oncologic emergencies, in Holland JF, Frei E III, Bast RC, et al (eds): *Cancer Medicine*, 4th ed. Baltimore: Williams & Wilkins, 1997.

9. Aurora R, Milite F, Vander Els NJ: Respiratory emergencies. *Semin Oncol* 27:256, 2000.

10. Sverha JJ, Borenstein M: Emergency complications of malignancy, in Tintinalli JE, Kelen GD, Stapczynski JS (eds): *Emergency Medicine: A Comprehensive Study Guide*, 5th ed. New York: McGraw-Hill, 2000.

11. Ewer MS, Benjamin RS: Cardiac complications, in Holland JF, Frei E III, Bast RC, et al (eds): *Cancer Medicine*, 4th ed. Baltimore: Williams & Wilkins, 1997.

12. Vaitkus PT, Herrmann HC, LeWinter MM: Treatment of malignant pericardial effusion. *JAMA* 272:59, 1994.

13. Keefe DL: Cardiovascular emergencies in the cancer patient. *Semin Oncol* 27:244, 2000.

14. Yahalom J: Superior vena cava syndrome, in DeVita VT, Hellman S, Rosenberg SA (eds): *Cancer: Principles and Practice of Oncology*, 6th ed. Philadelphia, Lippincott Williams & Wilkins, 2001.

15. Warrell RP: Metabolic emergencies, in DeVita VT, Hellman S, Rosenberg SA (eds): *Cancer: Principles and Practice of Oncology*, 6th ed. Philadelphia: Lippincott Williams & Wilkins, 2001.

16. Flombaum CD: Metabolic emergencies in the cancer patient. *Semin Oncol* 27:322, 2000.

17. Mundy GR, Guise TA: Hypercalcemia of malignancy. *Am J Med* 103:134, 1997.

18. Hosking DJ, Cowley A, Bucknall CA: Rehydration in the treatment of severe hypercalcemia. *Q J Med* 200:473, 1981.

19. Warrell RP Jr, Crown JP: Recovery from extreme hypercalcemia (letter). *Lancet* 342:375, 1993.

20. Warrell RP Jr, Israel R, Frisone M, et al: A randomized double-blind study of gallium nitrate versus calcitonin for acute treatment of cancer-related hypercalcemia. *Ann Intern Med* 108:669, 1988.

21. Robertson GL: Antidiuretic hormone: normal and disordered function. *Endocrinol Metab Clin North Am* 30:671, 2001.

22. Gertz MA, Kyle RA: Hyperviscosity syndrome. *J Intens Care Med* 10:128, 1995.

23. Blumenthal DT, Glenn MJ: Neurologic manifestations of hematologic disorders. *Neurol Clin* 20:265, 2002.

24. Redman DG, Pazdur R, Singas AP, et al: Prospective evaluation of adrenal insufficiency in patients with adrenal metastasis. *Cancer* 60:103, 1987.

25. Hughes WT, Armstrong D, Bodey GP et al: 2002 Guidelines for the use of antimicrobial agents in neutropenic patients with cancer. *Clin Infect Dis* 34:730, 2002.

26. Barber FD: Management of fever in neutropenic patients with cancer. *Nurs Clin North Am* 36:631, 2001.

27. Freifeld A, Marchigiani D, Walsh T, et al: A double-blind comparison of empirical oral and intravenous antibiotic therapy for low-risk febrile patients with neutropenia during cancer chemotherapy. *New Engl J Med* 341:305, 1999.

28. Kern WV, Cometta A, DeBock R, et al: Oral versus intravenous empirical antimicrobial therapy for fever in patients with granulocytopenia who are receiving cancer chemotherapy. *New Engl J Med* 341:312, 1999.

29. Finberg RW, Talcott JA: Fever and neutropenia: How to use a new treatment strategy. *New Engl J Med* 341:362, 1999.

30. Kern WV: Risk assessment and risk-based therapeutic strategies in febrile neutropenia. *Curr Opin Infect Dis* 14:415, 2001.

31. Feld R, DePauw B, Berman S, et al: Meropenem versus ceftazidime in the treatment of cancer patients with febrile neu-

tropenia: A randomized, double-blind trial. *J Clin Oncol* 18:3690, 2000.

32. Owens RC, Owens CA, Holloway WJ: Reduction in vancomycin consumption in patients with fever and neutropenia (abstract 458). *Clin Infect Dis* 31:291, 2000.

33. Vandercam B, Gerain J, Humblet Y, et al: Meropenem versus ceftazidime as empirical monotherapy for febrile neutropenic patients. *Ann Hematol* 79:152, 2000.

34. Schnoll-Sussman F, Kurtz RC: Gastrointestinal emergencies in the critically ill cancer patient. *Semin Oncol* 27:270, 2000.

35. Russo P: Urologic emergencies in the cancer patient. *Semin Oncol* 27:284, 2000.

36. Walther MM: Urologic emergencies, in DeVita VT, Hellman S, Rosenberg SA (eds): *Cancer: Principles and Practice of Oncology*, 6th ed. Philadelphia: Lippincott Williams & Wilkins, 2001.

37. Montana GS, Fowler WC: Carcinoma of the cervix: Analysis of bladder and rectal radiation dose and complications. *Int J Radiat Oncol Biol Phys* 16:95, 1989.

38. Horowitz M: Uses and growth of hematopoietic cell transplantation, in Thomas ED, Blume KG, Forman SJ (eds): *Hematopoietic cell transplantation*, 2d ed. Malden, MA, Blackwell Science, 1999.

39. Soutar RL, King DJ: Bone marrow transplantation. *Br Med J* 310:31, 1995.

40. Lum LG: The kinetics of immune reconstitution after bone marrow transplantation. *Blood* 69:369, 1987.

41. Rowe JM, Ciobanu N, Ascensao J et al: Recommended guidelines for the management of autologous and allogeneic bone marrow transplantation. *Ann Intern Med* 120:143, 1994.

42. Momin F, Chandrasekar PH: Antimicrobial prophylaxis in bone marrow transplantation. *Ann Intern Med* 123:205, 1995.

43. Cutler C, Giri S, Jeyapalan S et al: Acute and chronic graft-versus-host disease after allogeneic peripheral-blood, stem-cell, and bone marrow transplantation: A meta-analysis. *J Clin Oncol* 19:3685, 2001.

44. Antin J: Long-term care after hematopoietic-cell transplantation in adults. *New Engl J Med* 347:36, 2002.

67

Back Pain

Andrew D. Perron
Brian F. Erling

HIGH-YIELD FACTS

- Back pain is a frequent complaint in the geriatric patient population presenting to the emergency department (ED) or primary care office.

- A careful history and focused physical examination remain the cornerstones of clinical decision making in the geriatric patient with back pain. Laboratory and imaging studies are indicated in carefully defined circumstances.

- While the most frequent etiology of back pain in this patient population is mechanical in nature, the clinician needs to have a heightened suspicion for more sinister pathologic processes, such as metastatic disease, metabolic disease (e.g., Paget's disease), or compression fracture as a consequence of osteoporosis.

- Spinal degenerative disease is a very common radiologic finding in this patient population. The clinician should be cautious in ascribing symptoms to this finding until other pathologic entities have been ruled out.

- A great number of back pain "mimics" can occur in the elderly patient population, including abdominal aortic aneurysm, pancreatic tumors, and posterior duodenal ulcers.

- Medications routinely used in the treatment of back pain in a younger patient population (e.g., nonsteroidal anti-inflammatory drugs) can cause significant morbidity in the elderly patient population.

Low back pain is one of the most common human ailments and is a nearly universal phenomenon in modern Western society. As many as 85 percent of the Western world population will suffer from back pain at some time, yet as few as 20 percent can ever be given a precise pathoanatomic diagnosis.[1,2] The chief complaint of back pain accounts for nearly 1 percent of all emergency department (ED) visits.[3,4] ED evaluation of back pain in a younger patient population involves the search for certain "red flags" that raise the possibility of significant pathology as the etiologic mechanism. These red flags are well known and include a history of cancer, unexplained weight loss, rest pain, a history of intravenous drug use, presence of infection, and *age over 50 years*.[5,6] It is estimated that the presence of even a single one of these red flags can increase the chances of finding significant pathology to 10 percent.[1] Unfortunately, the entire patient population being discussed in this chapter falls under this last high-risk group, making the emergency physician's job all the more difficult.

In addition to the common benign causes of low back pain resulting from mechanical factors, elderly patients are at increased risk for spinal stenosis and other degenerative diseases, osteoporotic compression fracture, metastatic disease, infectious etiologies, and retroperitoneal processes that can mimic spinal disease. As with the younger patient population with this complaint in the ED, the clinician is charged with the job of determining who harbors routine mechanical low back pain and who has a more significant pathologic etiology. The clinician needs to develop a systematic approach to these patients that specifically addresses the various causes of back pain.

Fundamentally, evaluation of the elderly patient with back pain is not significantly different from that in the general ED population. However, the emergency physician must bear in mind that in the geriatric patient population the incidence of significant pathology is higher, the challenges to accurate diagnoses are greater, the threshold for diagnostic studies needs to be lower, and the potential for adverse drug reactions, once a diagnosis is made, is greater.

EPIDEMIOLOGY

The exact incidence and prevalence of back pain in the elderly are unknown. This has been attributed to a lack of standardized definition of illness, referral bias, and the wide variety of clinical practices where these patients are likely to present (ED, primary care office, orthopedist, neurosurgeon, and chiropractor).[7] It is known that the risk of serious disease processes that can present with back pain increases in the elderly, but correlation of these disease processes with ED presentation of back pain has not been done.

It is recognized that 60 to 80 percent of the adult population will be affected by an acute episode of back pain at some time.[8,9] One older study found a 20 percent annual incidence of back pain in a cohort of 3000 patients

in their sixties.[10] From this same study, approximately 5 percent of the patient population was reported to have been hospitalized because of their back pain, and 1 percent required surgery. A second study performed in this same time period found a 38 percent annual incidence of back pain in a cohort of septogenerians.[11] Both studies were limited by their design (self-reporting), and neither addressed final medical diagnoses.

PATHOPHYSIOLOGY

The pathophysiology of back pain is as widely varied as its etiology (Table 67-1). Virtually any innervated structure in the region may be the source of the patient's pain. The cause of the pain can be from structures within the back itself, such as the muscles, fascia, bones, periosteum, and joints. Pain also can be generated by pressure on nerves and meningeal structures. Additionally, pain may emanate from vascular structures or the retroperitoneum. Finally, visceral disorders that involve the pancreas, colon, duodenum, kidneys, and gallbladder all may generate painful sensations perceived in the back due to shared segmental innervation.[5]

Table 67-1. Differential Diagnosis of Back Pain in the Elderly

Mechanical	Gastrointestinal
Disc herniation	Pancreatitis
Spinal stenosis	Posterior penetrating ulcer
Osteoporotic compression fracture	Cholecystitis/biliary colic
Osteoarthritis/DJD	Diverticular disease
Spondylolisthesis	Rheumatologic
"Musculoskeletal"	Ankylosing spondylitis
Infectious	Polymyalgia rheumatica
Epidural abscess	Seronegative arthropathies
Discitis	Rheumatoid arthritis
Vertebral osteomyelitis	Genitourinary
Pyelonephritis	Renal colic
Malignant	Prostatitis
Metastatic disease (breast, lung, prostate, renal)	Pulmonary
Multiple myeloma	Pulmonary embolism
Lymphoma	Pneumonia
Vascular	Miscellaneous
AAA	Retroperitoneal mass/hemorrhage
Aortic dissection	Herpes zoster
Epidural hematoma	Pericarditis
	Transverse myelitis

CLINICAL FEATURES

A fundamental branch point in the evaluation of back pain in any patient population involves the division into traumatic versus nontraumatic etiologies. The clinician should keep in mind that even seemingly minor traumatic injuries may be significant in this patient population owing to the osteopenia and osteoporosis frequently associated with advancing age. Traumatic causes are addressed in Chap. 47.

The goal in the ED evaluation of these patients is twofold: to search for potentially serious pathologic etiologies of their back pain and, absent these, to identify, if possible, the source of the pain and suggest a rational course of treatment. While most patients are unlikely to harbor these serious pathologic entities, significant morbidity and even mortality can be avoided or minimized with a directed, efficient evaluation to exclude their presence. Most of these pathologic etiologies of back pain can be screened for with a careful history and physical examination.[12] Patients who harbor red flags evident on history or physical examination likely will need a more thorough evaluation that may include plain-film or advanced imaging, laboratory studies, and potential admission for further diagnostic workup.

History

As with any medical history, the onset and character of the pain should be identified. Similarly, aggravating and alleviating factors should be sought out to give a clue to the diagnosis. For example, the pain from a herniated disk typically is lessened with recumbancy, whereas pain from a tumor usually worsens in this position.

There are a number of historical features that are felt to be red flags for serious pathology in atraumatic back pain in the elderly (Table 67-2). A history of fever should raise the concern for an infectious etiology, specifically osteomyelitis, spinal epidural abscess, and discitis. A history of fever in association with night sweats and weight loss raises the concern for malignancy. The classic description of back pain in these patients is slowly progressive pain that is worse at night and with recumbancy. Most spinal malignancies are metastatic, particularly from primary cancers of the lung, breast, prostate, and kidney.[2,7,13] Progressive back pain in association with a history of these cancers should trigger an aggressive search for a metastatic lesion. Besides fever, complaints of systemic illness such as nausea or diaphoresis associated with the back pain should alert the examiner to the possibility of nonmechanical causes.

Other key historical issues that should be sought specifically include a detailed past medical history. The presence of diabetes or any other sort of immunosuppression (as from cancer, chemotherapy, or treatment of transplanted organs) can predispose the patient to infections etiologies for back pain. A history of collagen-vascular disease, spondyloarthropathies, recent spinal surgery, intravenous drug abuse, and known abdominal aortic aneurysm should raise suspicion. Recent treatment for infectious processes (e.g., urinary tract infection) should raise the possibility of an infectious etiology to the back pain.

A careful medication history also can help the examiner in the search for pathology. A history of steroid use (infection, compression fracture, peptic ulcer) and anticoagulants (retroperitoneal/intraspinal hemorrhage) should be determined. Nonsteroidal anti-inflammatory drugs (NSAIDs) and aspirin are both risk factors for peptic ulcer disease. Antihypertensive agents do not predispose to spinal disease but may blunt the patient's physiologic response to such diseases and should be noted if present.

Finally, historical features that are of concern for spinal cord compression should be sought out. Urinary and fecal retention or incontinence, focal weakness, and paresthesias can all be indicators of spinal cord impingement.

Table 67-2. Back Pain in the Elderly Patient: Pathologic Etiologies and Associated Historical Factors

Disease	Historical Factors
Cancer	Night sweats, fever, weight loss, pain increased with rest/recumbancy, progressive pain/motor weakness
Infection	Fever, recent infectious process, weight loss, immunosuppression
Vascular disorder	Previous peripheral vascular occlusive disease, hypertension, vascular claudication (Pain with ambulation, relieved with rest)
Spinal stenosis	Neurogenic claudication (Pain with walking erect, relieved by bending forward, not relieved with rest), leg numbness

Physical Examination

The ED physical examination should be focused yet broad enough to detect systemic illness. Vital signs should be assessed and reviewed, being sure to include a temperature determination. Needless to say, abnormal vital signs must be addressed and explained. Hypotension raises the possibility of aortic catastrophe, whereas fever should raise the possibility of an infectious etiology. In the geriatric population, the clinician should remember that it is not uncommon for elderly patients to be on beta-blocking agents that can blunt a pulse response. The determination of temperature is vitally important in these patients because fever can be one of the few clues to an infectious etiology. One recent study of spinal infections noted that in the presence back pain, fever increases the odds of spinal infection by a factor of 26.[14,15]

The general physical examination should include evaluation of the abdomen for a pulsatile mass, evidence of peritoneal irritation, gallbladder tenderness, or a focal intraabdominal source of the pain. Peripheral pulses should be assessed for pulse deficits. Evidence of acute ischemia (e.g., cool extremity) or chronic ischemia (e.g., loss of hair, nonhealing ulcer) should be sought. The back examination should include palpation for focal tenderness, scoliosis, and spasm. Neurologic examination includes an observation of gait as well as testing the motor and sensory systems. Hyper- or hyporeflexia, clonus, and an abnormal Babinski test all should be noted. If there is any concern over bowel or bladder impairment, as in the cauda equina syndrome, rectal tone and post-void residual bladder volume should be determined.

DIAGNOSIS AND DIFFERENTIAL

Laboratory Investigations

If a benign mechanical cause of back pain is thought to be the etiology of the patient's complaint, laboratory studies are of virtually no use. However, when a systemic cause of back pain is being considered, limited laboratory investigation may be warranted.

Complete Blood Count (CBC)

An elevated white blood cell (WBC) count increases odds of spinal infection by a factor of 7. Leukocytosis is present in 40 to 50 percent of patients with spinal infection and 6 percent of patients *without* infectious etiology.[14,16]

Erythrocyte Sedimentation Rate (ESR)

The ESR is a very nonspecific test that can be elevated in a wide variety of clinical processes. The sensitivity of the ESR, however, may make it a useful diagnostic adjunct when the pretest probability of tumor or vertebral osteomyelitis is increased.[15,17] In a study of cancer patients, it was shown that an ESR of more than 100 mm/hr was associated with a likelihood ratio of 55 for a serious etiology of back pain (metastases/infection).[14]

Urinalysis

Urinalysis is useful if urinary tract infection or stone is in the differential diagnosis. One caveat is that a small percentage of patients with an expanding or ruptured abdominal aortic aneurysm will demonstrate hematuria on urinalysis, which can cause confusion of that diagnosis with nephrolithiasis.[18,19]

Calcium/Alkaline Phosphatase/Phosphate

These may be elevated in patients with metabolic or tumor-related etiologies of back pain.

Radiographic Investigations

The Agency for Health Care Policy and Research (AHCPR) guidelines recommend plain radiographs in patients presenting with back pain who are at risk for fracture, malignancy, or infection.[120] When obtained, plain radiographs should be limited to anteroposterior and lateral views. Oblique views add little information and double the radiation exposure.[21,22] It should be noted, however, that by age 65, most of the population will demonstrate radiographic evidence of degenerative spine disease.[7] A number of studies, however, have demonstrated that this finding does not necessarily correlate with symptoms.[23,24] As a result, the clinician should be wary about ascribing symptoms to degenerative changes on the plain films. When evaluating plain films for the possibility of metastatic disease, it is important to note that 30 to 50 percent of a bone's mass must be demineralized in order to note an abnormality on a plain film unless the destruction occurs at a cortical margin.[7,14,25] (Fig. 67-1A) Computed tomographic (CT) imaging is best for bony pathology of the spine, such as spinal stenosis and fracture.[13,26,27] When used in combination with myelography, CT scanning can be effective at identifying neoplasms, epidural space infections, and herniated discs.[5,6,8] Magnetic resonance imaging (MRI) is the study of choice for

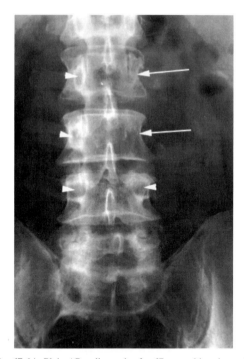

Fig. 67-1A Plain AP radiograph of a 67-year-old patient with newly diagnosed renal cell cancer, who presented with back pain. Plain x-ray demonstrates loss of pedicles at L2 and L3 (*arrows*). This is from tumor replacement of the bone in these regions. Normal pedicles are indicated by arrowheads.

patients with a continued concern for infection, spinal cord compression, or malignancy despite normal or nondiagnostic plain radiographs (Fig. 67-1B). It is the preferred study when the patient has an acute significant neurologic deficit referable to the spine, such as cauda equina syndrome. MRI also provides the most extensive ability to assess the soft tissue surrounding the spine.[28,29]

Differential Diagnosis

As is demonstrated in Table 67-1, the differential diagnosis of back pain in the elderly is vast. An exhaustive discussion of all causes of back pain is beyond the scope of this chapter. A more detailed description of the most common, as well as the more serious etiologies, follows.

Disk Herniation

While rupture of the nucleus pulposis is relatively common in patients 30 to 50 years of age, it is relatively uncommon in the elderly.[1,4,7,8] This is thought to be due to desiccation of the nucleus pulposis, rendering it more fibrotic and hence less likely to extrude.[1,4] Symptoms of disk herniation can be acute, subacute, or chronic. Symptoms in the elderly are the same as in a younger population, with pain exacerbated by sitting and Valsalva maneuvers and typically radiating in a radicular pattern. While rare, cauda equina syndrome is the most feared complication, heralded by the triad of bowel/bladder dysfunction, saddle anesthesia, and lower extremity weakness. MRI is the study of choice for evaluation. Cauda equina syndrome is a surgical emergency and warrants emergent consultation with a spine surgeon. A symptomatic herniated disk is treated conservatively unless there is evidence of a progressive neurologic deficit.

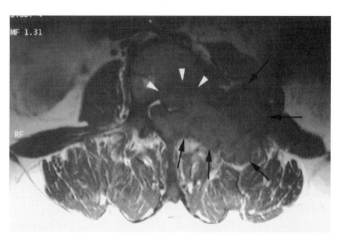

Fig. 67-1B MRI of same patient as in 1A. Black arrows indicate renal cell cancer in the paraspinal musculature, and white arrowheads indicate areas where the tumor has replaced the bone.

Spinal Stenosis

Decreased volume of the spinal canal is an extremely common condition in the aging spine. With degenerative changes affecting the spine, the body compensates by increasing spinal load bearing through pathologic hypertrophy of the ligamentum flavum and the facet joints. This process, with progression, results in compression of the nerve roots within the spinal column. The history is usually much more revealing than the physical examination in these patients. The syndrome of "pseudoclaudication" frequently is described by patients: bilateral leg pain or weakness of gradual onset aggravated by standing or walking and improved by flexion of the lumbar spine, sitting, or lying down.[30] The discomfort with walking frequently is described as a crampy or rubbery feeling in the legs. Walking downhill exacerbates the symptoms (due to spine extension), and walking uphill improves symptoms (due to forward spine flexion). Nerve tension signs (e.g., straight-leg raise) are rarely positive with this disease, and measurable weakness is seen in only one-third of patients.[7,30] Plain films are not helpful in making this diagnosis, and CT remains the diagnostic study of choice. Initial treatment is conservative unless there is demonstrable progressive neurologic compromise.

Tumor

Malignant tumors of the spine can be primary or metastatic. Overall, malignancy is responsible for less than 1 percent of back pain, with 80 percent of affected patients over age 50.[5,14] Most primary spinal tumors are found in patients younger than age 30. Metastatic disease generally is found in those older than age 50. Metastatic lesions are the most common neoplasm of the bone, and 70 percent of these will occur in the axial skeleton.[7] It has been reported that up to 30 percent of cancer patients ultimately will develop spinal metastases.[31,32] The vast majority of primary tumors responsible for spinal metastases are breast, lung, and prostate, and approximately half of all patients with these primary tumors will develop bony metastases.[7] Back pain in the context of known or suspected malignancy should be considered a red flag and prompt further diagnostic imaging in the ED. An elevated ESR is sensitive (but not specific) for malignancy. The incidence of primary skeletal malignancies is relatively small, with multiple myeloma being the most common. It is only rarely seen before age 40, and the incidence rises progressively into the eighth decade.[7]

Metabolic Disease

Osteoporosis is the metabolic bone disorder of greatest clinical and economic significance in the elderly.[7,33] It manifests in pathologic compression fractures at a rate estimated at half a million new cases per year (Fig. 67-2). By age 80, over half the white female population will have at least one compression fracture,[33] yet there is frequently no history of trauma to account for such fractures. Physical examination is of limited use, and neurologic problems are rare with compression fractures. The back pain associated with such a fracture generally resolves within 1 to 3 months with conservative treatment.[7,33]

Paget's disease, or osteitis deformans, is relatively common in the elderly. Occurring in approximately 3 percent of the elderly patient population, the exact etiology of the disease is unknown, but it is manifest with increased bone turnover, especially in the vertebrae. Paget's disease is frequently asymptomatic or manifests with mild chronic back pain. Radiographically, lesions initially appear lytic but later evolve into osteoblastic lesions, producing a homogeneously increased density.

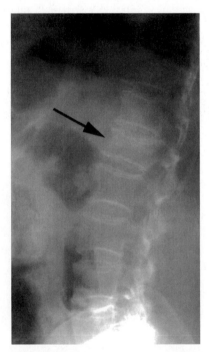

Fig. 67-2 L1 compression fracture (*black arrow*) from a minor fall in a 71-year-old female. Note loss of height in the L1 vertebra, with mild anterior wedging.

Spinal Epidural Abscess

Infectious processes are a relatively rare cause of back pain in the general population, accounting for approximately 0.01 percent of cases overall.[5] The at-risk population includes patients with diabetes, chronic renal insufficiency, intravenous drug abuse, alcoholism, cancer, recent spinal surgery, and recent systemic infection. Thoracic and lumbar sites are affected predominantly. Fever is variable, present in up to 50 percent.[34,35] The WBC count is elevated in 50 percent of patients, whereas the ESR is elevated in virtually all patients.[35,36] Localized bony tenderness along the spine is classic, and focal neurologic findings are late (<50 percent of patients). MRI is the study modality of choice. When spinal epidural abscess is identified, emergent consultation of a spine surgeon is required for decompression and debridement.

Vertebral Osteomyelitis

The at-risk group here is the same as for spinal epidural abscess. Onset may be insidious, with back pain and tenderness preceding neurologic involvement by a considerable amount of time. Many present with fever (50 percent demonstrate temperature elevation) and other constitutional symptoms. CBC and blood culture yields generally are low, with leukocytosis identified in approximately 40 to 50 percent of patients.[37] Plain films are diagnostic in 80 to 95 percent but only with prolonged disease. MRI is the definitive study. As with spinal epidural abscess, consultation with a spine surgeon should be sought when this diagnosis is made.

Abdominal Aortic Aneurysm (AAA)

AAA is found in 2 to 4 percent of the population over age 50, with an average age at diagnosis of 65 to 70 years.[38] Pain can be precipitated by ruptured or expanding aneurysm and usually is experienced in the back, flank, or abdomen (Fig. 67-3A,B). It is usually described as acute in onset and frequently radiates to the scrotum. Alternatively, the patient may present solely with syncope. Physical examination includes a search for a pulsatile ab-

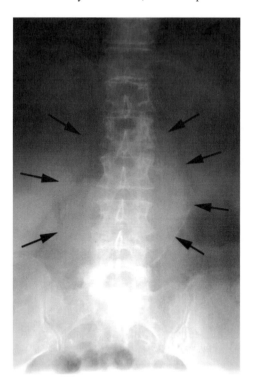

Fig. 67-3A AP radiograph of 66-year-old female presenting to the ED with low back pain. Arrows indicate outline of 13cm abdominal aortic aneurysm that at surgery was found to have a contained rupture in the retroperitoneum.

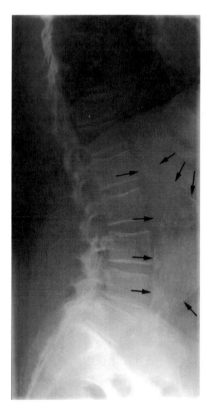

Fig. 67-3B Lateral lumbar spine film of the same patient as above. Arrows indicate outline of 13cm AAA.

dominal mass, diminished lower extremity pulses, and hypoperfusion. Bedside ultrasonography is used for the unstable patient. AAA can mimic renal colic, gastrointestinal bleeding, and diverticulitis. Studies report that from 10 to 30 percent of the time the patient is misdiagnosed initially, most commonly with ureteral colic.[39] Emergent consultation with a vascular surgeon should be obtained early in the evaluation process of patients with a possibility of this diagnosis.

EMERGENCY DEPARTMENT CARE AND DISPOSITION

Needless to say, patients with identified clear surgical emergencies require emergent consultation for definitive treatment. These include perforated viscus, spinal epidural abscess, cauda equina syndrome, ruptured AAA, and aortic dissection. Most patients, however, are not going to fall into this category. Studies in the general ED population report that an exact etiology of a patient's back pain can be identified only infrequently, with the great majority (>85 percent) of these patients leaving the ED without a precise pathoanatomic diagnosis of their pain.[1,2] The goal of the emergency clinician in these patients should to be to provide reassurance, treat the pain, establish a follow-up pathway, and avoid iatrogenic harm. The latter is a distinct possibility in the older patient population, frequently as a side effect of drug treatment.

In the elderly patient population, drug therapy should be monitored carefully and generally started at lower doses than in young adults. The American Geriatric Society has published *Clinical Practice Guidelines for the Management of Chronic Pain in Older Persons.*[40] It can be shown that there is little difference in outcome in a proper treatment setting between geriatric patients and those who are younger.[41] A recent meta-analysis has found NSAIDs to be effective in the treatment of acute low back pain, but not when the condition is chronic.[42] Older patients are at particular risk for adverse side effects, especially gastrointestinal bleeding and renal impairment.[43] Acetaminophen should be considered before NSAIDs because it demonstrates low toxicity compared with NSAIDs in this patient population.[44] Judicious use of narcotic analgesics is appropriate.

Follow-up instructions should be clear and time-specific (e.g., return *immediately* for bowel or bladder dysfunction, leg weakness, etc.). The instructions should be specific regarding any activity limitations, medication usage (including what side effects to watch for), and where to go for follow-up.

ADDITIONAL ASPECTS

As with younger patients, a probabilistic approach to clinical decision making in elderly patients presenting with back pain to the ED is the most prudent course. Understanding that, by definition, this patient population already has a red flag, the clinician must be vigilant for other clues that may indicate more sinister pathology. Most patients seen are unlikely to harbor significant disease despite their age and comorbidities. A careful history and physical examination, coupled with a low threshold to pursue limited diagnostic studies in the ED, will rule out significant pathology in most of this patient population.

REFERENCES

1. Wipf JE, Deyo RA: Low back pain, *Med Clin North Am* 79:231, 1995.
2. Deyo RA, Rainville J, Kent DL: What can the history and physical examination tell us about low back pain? *JAMA* 268:760, 1992.
3. Dvorak J: Epidemiology, physical examination, and neurodiagnostics. *Spine* 23:2663, 1998.
4. Brody M: Low back pain. *Ann Emerg Med* 27:454, 1996.
5. Rodgers KG, Jones JB: Back pain, in Marx JA, Hockberger RS, Walls RM (eds): *Rosen's Emergency Medicine*, 5th ed. St Louis, Mosby, 2001, p 223.
6. Tawney PJW, Siegel CB, LaBan MM: Thoracic and lumbar pain syndromes, in Tintinalli JE, Kelen GD, Stapczynski JS (eds): *Emergency Medicine: A Comprehensive Study Guide*, 5th ed. New York, McGraw-Hill, 2000, p 1866.
7. Svara CJ, Hadler NM: Back pain. *Clin Geriatr Med* 4:395, 1988.
8. Borenstein D: Epidemiology, etiology, diagnostic evaluation, and treatment of low back pain. *Curr Opin Rheumatol* 8:124, 1996.
9. Frymoyer JW, Cats-Baril WL: An overview of the incidences and cost of low back pain. *Orthop Clin North Am* 22:263, 1991.
10. Kavsky-Shulan M, Wallace RB, Kohout FJ, et al: Prevalence and functional correlates of low back pain in the elderly: The Iowa 65+ Rural Health Study. *J Am Geriatr Soc* 33:23, 1985.
11. Bergstrom G, Bjelle A, Sundh V, et al: Joint disorders at ages 70, 75 and 79 years: A cross-sectional comparison. *Br J Rheumatol* 25:333, 1986.
12. Deyo RA, Rainville J, Kent DL: What can the history and physical examination tell us about low back pain? *JAMA* 268:760, 1992.
13. Grobler LJ: Back and leg pain in older adults: Presentation, diagnosis, and treatment. *Clin Geriatr Med* 14:543, 1998.
14. Deyo RA, Diehl AK: Cancer as a cause of back pain: Fre-

quency, clinical presentation, and diagnostic strategies. *J Gen Intern Med* 3:230, 1988.

15. Lurie JD, Gerber PD, Sox HC: A pain in the back. *New Engl J Med* 343:723, 2000.

16. Deyo RA: Early diagnostic evaluation of low back pain. *J Gen Intern Med* 1:328, 1986.

17. Sox HC, Liang MH: The erythrocyte sedimentation rate: Guidelines for rational use. *Ann Intern Med* 104:515, 1986.

18. Akkersdijk GJ, van Bockle JH: Ruptured abdominal aortic aneurysm: Initial misdiagnosis and the effect on treatment. *Eur J Surg* 164:29, 1998.

19. Marston WA, Ahlquist R, Johnson G, et al: Misdiagnosis of ruptured abdominal aortic aneurysm. *J Vasc Surg* 16:17, 1992.

20. Bigos S, Bowyer O, Braen O, et al: *Clinical Practice Guidelines: Quick Reference Guide Number 14: Acute Low Back pain Problems in Adults.* AHCPR Publication No 95-0643. Rockville, MD, AHCPR, U.S. Dept. of Health and Human Services, 1994.

21. Scavone JG, Latshaw RF, Rohrer GV: Anterior posterior and lateral radiographs and adequate lumbar spine examination. *AJR* 136:715, 1997.

22. Suarez-Almazor ME, Belseck E, Russell AS, et al: Use of lumbar radiographs for the early diagnosis of low back pain. *JAMA* 277:1782, 1997.

23. Torgerson WR, Dotter WE: Comparative roentgenographic study of the asymptomatic and symptomatic lumbar spine. *J Bone Joint Surg* 58A:850, 1976.

24. Spengler DM: Degenerative stenosis of the lumbar spine. *J Bone Joint Surg* 69A:305, 1987.

25. McGowin PR, Borenstein D, Wiesel SW: The current approach to the medical diagnosis of low back pain. *Orthop Clin North Am* 22:315, 1991.

26. Bridwell KH: Lumbar spinal stenosis: Diagnosis, management, and treatment. *Clin Geriatr Med* 10:677, 1994

27. Kent DL, Haynor DR, Larson EB, et al: Diagnosis of lumbar spinal stenosis in adults: A meta-analysis of the accuracy of CT, MR, and myelography. *AJR* 158:1135, 1992.

28. An HS, Haughton VM: Non-discogenic lumbar radiculopathy: Imaging considerations. *Semin Ultrasound CT MR* 14:425, 1993.

29. Yu S, Haughton VM, Rosenbaum AE: Magnetic resonance imaging and anatomy of the spine. *Radiol Clin North Am* 29:691, 1991.

30. Hall S, Bartleson JD, Onofrio BM, et al: Spinal stenosis: Clinical features, diagnostic procedures, and results of surgical treatment in 68 patients. *Ann Intern Med* 103:271, 1985.

31. Wiegel B, Maghsudi M, Neumann C, et al: Surgical management of symptomatic spinal metastases. *Spine* 24:2240, 1999.

32. Clouston PD, DeAngelis LM, Posner JB: The spectrum of neurological disease in patients with systemic cancer. *Ann Neurol* 31:268, 1992.

33. Cummings SR, Kelsey JL, Nevitt MC, et al: Epidemiology of osteoporosis and osteoporotic fractures. *Epidemiol Rev* 7:178, 1985.

34. Hlavin ML, Kaminski HJ, Ross JS, et al: Spinal epidural abscess: A ten-year perspective. *Neurosurgery* 27:177, 1990.

35. Perron AD, Huff JS: Spinal cord disorders, in Marx JA, Hockberger RS, Walls RM (eds): *Rosen's Emergency Medicine*, 5th ed. St Louis, Mosby, 2001, p 1496.

36. Sampath P, Rigamonti D: Spinal epidural abscess: A review of epidemiology, diagnosis, and treatment. *J Spinal Disord* 12:89, 1999.

37. Babinchak AK, Riley DK, Rotheram EB: Pyogenic vertebral osteomyelitis of the posterior elements. *Clin Infect Dis* 25:221, 1997.

38. Bengtsson H, Bergqvist D, Sternby NH: Increasing prevalence of abdominal aortic aneurysms: A necropsy study. *Eur J Surg* 158:19, 1992.

39. Valentine RJ, Barth MJ, Myers SI, et al: Nonvascular emergencies presenting as ruptured abdominal aortic aneurysms. *Surgery* 113:286, 1993.

40. Management of chronic pain in older persons: Clinical practice guidelines. Written under the auspices of the American Geriatric Society (AGS) Panel on Chronic Pain in Older Persons. *J Am Geriatr Soc* 46:635, 1998.

41. Cutler RB, Fishbain DA, Steele-Rosomoff R, et al: Outcome in treatment of pain in geriatric and younger age groups. *Arch Phys Med* 75:457, 1994.

42. VanTulder MW, Koes BW, Bouter LM: Low back pain, in *Primary Care: Effectiveness of Diagnostic and Therapeutic Interventions.* Amsterdam, EMGO Institute, Vrije University, 1996.

43. Deyo RA: Drug therapy for back pain: Which drugs help which patients? *Spine* 21:2840, 1996.

44. Saag KG, Cowedry JS,: Spine update: nonsteroidal anti-inflammatory drugs: Balancing benefits AND Risks. *Spine* 19:1530, 1994.

68

Acute Arthritis

Harriet Young

HIGH-YIELD FACTS

- Absence of fever and leukocytosis in an elderly patient complaining of joint pain does not rule out infection; joint aspiration and cultures must be done.
- Patients with rheumatoid arthritis or osteoarthritis have a high risk of developing septic arthritis.
- Never start uric acid-lowering agents such as allopurinol during a gout exacerbation because it will worsen the attack.
- Take a careful drug history in the elderly; this is especially helpful for diagnosing drug-induced lupus, gout exacerbation in a patient on diuretics, hemarthrosis in a patient on warfarin, and septic arthritis in a patient on immunosuppressive agents.
- There is a high incidence of malignancy in those diagnosed with polymyositis and dermatomyositis.

Older patients commonly present to the emergency department (ED) with complaints of acute arthritis. Although the many arthritides are similar to those in younger populations, the elderly more often experience atypical presentations. As the population ages, it is important to be aware of the differences between the older-age-onset and younger-age-onset manifestations of rheumatic disease. Many causes of acute arthritis exist in the elderly[1]. Etiologies to consider include septic, crystal-induced arthritis, osteoarthritis (OA), remitting seronegative symmetric synovitis with pitting edema (RS$_3$ PE) syndrome, malignancy, and systemic diseases such as rheumatoid arthritis (RA), systemic lupus erythematosus (SLE), drug-induced lupus, polymyalgia rheumatica (PMR), and giant cell arthritis (GCA) (see Chap. 69). A useful classification characterizing the number of joints involved and the possible diagnostic considerations is given in Table 68-1.

Table 68-1. Classification of Arthritis by Number of Affected Joints

No. Affected Joints	Differential Considerations
1 = Monoarthritis	Trauma-induced arthritis
	Infection/septic arthritis
	Crystal-induced (gout, pseudogout)
	Osteoarthritis (acute)
	Lyme disease
	Avascular necrosis
	Tumor
2–3 = Oligoarthritis	Lyme disease
	Reiter's syndrome
	Ankylosing spondylitis
	Gonococcal arthritis
	Rheumatic fever
>3 = Polyarthritis	Rheumatoid arthritis
	Systemic lupus erythematosus
	Viral arthritis
	Osteoarthritis (chronic)

SEPTIC ARTHRITIS

There are four types of septic arthritis: bacterial and viral, which are usually acute, and mycobacterial and fungal, which are usually indolent. Given its relative prevalence and clinical importance, bacterial septic arthritis will be the focus of this section.

Most joint infections are caused by *Staphylococcus aureus,* followed by *Streptococcus* and gram-negative bacilli. In polyarticular septic arthritis, *S. aureus* accounts for at least half the cases, followed by *Neisseria gonorrhea, Bacteroides fragilis, Streptococcus pneumoniae,* group G *Streptococcus, Hemophilus influenzae,* and mixed aerobic with anaerobic organisms.[2]

Acute pain, tenderness, swelling, or redness in a single joint out of proportion to the other joints should lead to a suspicion of a septic joint, even in elderly patients with chronic arthritis, such as rheumatoid arthritis or osteoarthritis. Septic arthritis involving the shoulder may be more common in the elderly and may be misdiagnosed as frozen shoulder or tendinitis. It is important to distinguish any acute arthritis from a more focal periarticular inflammatory process, such as cellulitis, tendinitis, or bursitis. True articular inflammation results in pain with both passive and active range of motion. Septic sternoclavicular arthritis has been reported in those with rheumatoid arthritis and presents with complaints of localized anterior chest discomfort, fever, gross swelling over the joint, and a decreased range of motion of the shoulder. Be aware that patients with rheumatoid arthritis are prone to develop polyarticular septic arthritis as well.[2]

In a retrospective study of polyarticular septic arthritis compared with monoarticular septic arthritis, the following traits were noted: male predominance; knee involvement most common, followed by elbow, shoulder, and hip; and an average of four joints were affected. *S. aureus* was the most common etiology (80 percent) and was blood culture-positive in a significant majority. However, fever and leukocytosis were not present in 40 percent of patients. A history of rheumatoid arthritis also was present in 40 percent. Overall mortality was 30 percent, compared with 4 percent in those with monoarticular infections.[3]

Many elders with septic arthritis are afebrile and have a normal white blood cell count. Useful ancillary tests include an erythrocyte sedimentation rate (ESR) or a C-reactive protein (CRP) determination. Both these tests are commonly elevated but lack sensitivity and specificity for septic arthritis.

Arthrocentesis is the most important diagnostic test for evaluation of a septic joint (or any acute arthritis).[4] Synovial fluid cultures and Gram stain should be obtained, and synovial fluid should be inspected for crystals and cell count (Table 68-2). Treatment consists of admission for immediate intravenous antibiotics and joint irrigation. A second- or third-generation cephalosporin or nafcillin with an aminoglycoside is indicated empirically, pending culture results, and treatment should be continued for 2 to 4 weeks.

Acute arthritis is worrisome in patients with prosthetic joints because of the devastating possibility of infection involving the protheses. The most frequent source is seeding from infected skin lesions.[4] Staphylococci cause 70 to 80 percent of prosthetic joint infections; *S. epidermidis* is found most frequently in perioperative infections, whereas *S. aureus* is from later postoperative infections. Other frequently found bacteria from prosthetic joints are gram-negative bacilli, non-group A streptococci, and anaerobes. Infections usually present within the first few months after surgery with pain, swelling, fever, and drainage.[2]

Late prosthetic joint infections usually manifest as gradual onset of increasing joint pain; often it is hard to differentiate between septic and aseptic joint loosening. Fever may occur in less than half of late prosthetic joint infections, and only 10 percent of patients have an elevated white blood cell count. ESR and CRP usually are increased but are nonspecific. Radiographs may show loosening of the prosthesis but cannot ascertain whether the cause is bacterial or mechanical. Scintigraphy also may be used but, again, is not definitive. If there is a suspicion of prosthetic joint infection, joint fluid and tissue must be analyzed; hip aspirations are done with computed tomographic (CT) guidance. If CT-guided joint aspiration is unsuccessful, open surgical aspiration and biopsy of the synovium and periprosthetic tissue must be done, and the specimen must be sent off for aerobic and anaerobic cultures. Treatment requires admission for a protracted course of antibiotics and urgent surgical consultation for debridement. Unfortunately, less than 10 percent of pros-

Table 68-2. Examination of Synovial Fluid

	Normal	Noninflammatory	Inflammatory	Septic
Clarity	Transparent	Transparent	Cloudy	Cloudy
Color	Clear	Yellow	Yellow	Yellow
WBC/mL	<200	<200–2000	200–50,000	>50,000
PMNs, %	<25	<25	>50	>50
Culture	Negative	Negative	Negative	>50% positive
Crystals	None	None	Multiple or none	None
Associated conditions		Osteoarthritis, trauma, rheumatic fever	Gout, pseudogout, spondylo-arthropathies, rheumatoid, Lyme disease, SLE	Nongonococcal or gono-coccal septic arthritis

Note: The white blood cell count (WBC) and percent polymorphonuclear leucocytes (%PMNs) are affected by a number of factors, including disease progression, affecting organism, and host immune status. The joint aspirate WBC and %PMNs should be considered part of a continuum for each disease, particularly septic arthritis, and should be correlated with other clinical information. SLE, systemic lupus erythematosus.

thetic hip infections can be treated successfully without prothesis removal. Mortality rates have been reported to be 5 to 20 percent in those with prosthetic joint infections.[2]

CRYSTAL-INDUCED ARTHRITIS

Gout

Acute gouty arthritis is due to deposition of uric acid crystals in joints from supersaturated extracellular fluids. Gout is predominantly a disorder affecting middle-aged men; however, the frequency of gout among the elderly is increasing. With patients having new onset of gout after age 60, the ratio of men to women has equalized; after age 80, women outnumber men. Associated factors of younger-onset gout include alcohol consumption, obesity, hypertension, and hypertriglyceridemia; in elderly-onset gout, associated features include renal insufficiency and diuretic use.[5] Interestingly, gout is seen rarely in patients with systemic lupus erythematosus, rheumatoid arthritis, or ankylosing spondylitis.[2]

Typically, the initial gout exacerbation presents as an acute monoarticular atrthritis. As a rule, the affected joint is red, swollen, and very painful. Sixty percent of initial exacerbations involve the first metatarsophalangeal joint. Duration of attacks may be from a few days to a few weeks. If gout remains untreated, it may become polyarticular, increase in frequency, and present with fever and constitutional symptoms. Long-standing gout may produce tophaceous deposits on elbows or fingers.

There are several differences between elder-onset and younger-onset gout. Elders are more likely than their younger cohorts to have polyarticular symptoms. The mean age of polyarticular gout is 60 to 64 years. In such patients, gout and rheumatoid arthritis bear a striking resemblance; it may be difficult to differentiate between the two. Second, females outnumber their male counterparts in elderly-onset gout, whereas in younger-onset gout, middle-aged men are the most afflicted group. Up to 85 percent of women are afflicted with gout after menopause. Women constitute more than half the subjects with new-onset gout over age 60; over age 80, almost all patients are female. Third, small joints of the fingers are affected more often in the elderly, whereas in younger-onset gout, lower extremity involvement (podagra) is more common. Last, tophi formation occurs earlier in the course and in unusual places such as the fingers in elderly-onset gout, whereas in younger-onset gout, tophi occur after long-standing disease and typically are present in the elbow.[5]

The definitive diagnosis of gout is made by arthrocentesis and crystal analysis. Needle-shaped, negatively birefringent urate crystals are easily demonstrated using a polarizing microscope. Since patients with gout may present with fever, a thorough workup to rule out acute bacterial arthritis is recommended.

Acute gout is treated with colchicine, nonsteroidal anti-inflammatory drugs (NSAIDs), corticotropin (ACTH), and corticosteroids. Colchicine should be used with care in the elderly because it can cause nausea, vomiting, and abdominal cramping with diarrhea; patients with renal and hepatic insufficiency should avoid colchicine. In the el-derly, it is not usually recommended for gout treatment.[5,6] NSAIDs also should be avoided in the elderly because of their gastrointestinal GI and renal toxicity. Currently, ACTH and corticosteroids have been used more frequently and with less toxic effects, especially in elders with comorbidities. Intraarticular steroid injection after arthrocentesis and aspiration of large joint effusions can be very effective. For small joints such as the hands or feet, 5 to 10 mg triamcinolone is used, whereas for larger joints, such as the knee, 40 to 60 mg is sufficient. Systemic corticosteroids may be indicated in patients with polyarticular involvement or in those in whom colchicine or NSAIDs should be avoided. Prednisone, 40 to 60 mg by mouth, and a single intramuscular injection of 40 units ACTH or 40 to 60 mg triamcinolone are treatment options. These steroid treatments have been shown to be as effective as NSAIDs for acute gout. Low-dose cholchicine (0.6 mg once or twice a day) or allopurinol may be used for prophylaxis. However, long-term therapy to lower serum uric acid levels should not be initiated during an acute attack because these agents will worsen symptoms.

Pseudogout

Pseudogout is a disorder involving deposition of calcium pyrophosphate dihydrate in articular cartilage and is especially common in the elderly. Osteoarthritis often coexists with pseudogout. Pseudogout may be asymptomatic, result in acute exacerbations of mono- or polyarticular arthritis, or present as a chronic arthropathy coupled with osteoarthritis. Joints affected most often are the hip, knee, shoulder, and wrist. Knee involvement is characteristic of pseudogout. Patients may have joint stiffness, pain, and high ESRs. Fever and mental status changes also have been reported. For patients with these dramatic presentations, rheumatoid arthritis and bacterial meningitis are additional considerations.[5]

Radiographs of the affected joint may show calcification in joints, tendon insertions, ligaments, and bursa. Bilateral meniscal calcification in the knees or in the triangular ligament at the radioulnar joint of the wrist is typical of pseudogout. There are no erosive bony changes as in rheumatoid arthritis. Definitive diagnosis can be made following arthrocentesis. Crystal analysis will demonstrate weakly positive birefringence with yellow, rhomboid crystals under polarized microscopy.[5] The synovial fluid may show leukocyte counts of 10,000 to 20,000/mm3 due to inflammation.

Treatment of pseudogout is similar to that for acute gout: rest, NSAIDs, or intraarticular corticosteroid injection in the affected joint. Colchicine should be avoided in the elderly because of its toxicity. Intramuscular or subcutaneous ACTH (40 units) or intramuscular triamcinolone (60 mg) can control the acute exacerbation. For chronic pseudogout, hydroxychloroquine 200 to 400 mg/d can be helpful.[5]

OSTEOARTHRITIS

Osteoarthritis involves chronic, localized loss of hyaline articular cartilage with formation of osteophytes and bony sclerosis; surrounding joint structures are affected due to inflammatory changes in the synovium and preexisting weak ligaments and muscles. Osteoarthritis is encountered frequently in the elderly because prevalence increases with age. Before age 50, men are affected more than women; however, after age 50, more women are affected than men. Osteoarthritis frequently affects the knee and hip and less often the hands. This section will focus only on joints of the knee, hip, and hands.

In the pathogenesis of osteoarthritis, several systemic and local biomechanical factors, especially of weight-bearing joints, affect osteoarthritis development. Systemic factors include advancing age, female gender, ethnic characteristics, bone density, lack of estrogen-replacement therapy in postmenopausal women, and genetics. Local biomechanical factors include obesity; joint injury with knee laxity and lack of proprioception; joint deformity; occupational factors, such as those involving repetitive tasks that can affect hands, knee, and hip joints; sports participation; and muscle weakness. The combination of these systemic and local biomechanical factors and a susceptibility to osteoarthritis result in osteoarthritis of varying severity at the affected sites.[7]

Factors associated with osteoarthritis and patient disability include psychosocial factors such as pain severity and depression, decreased aerobic capacity, muscle weakness, and radiographic arthritic severity.[7]

History and clinical presentations are often typical. Morning stiffness lasting 10 to 25 minutes is common; inactivity worsens symptoms. Patients will report loss of movement or instability of a joint. Physical examination often reveals bony swelling around the joint and crepitus. Heberden's and Bouchard's nodes are found on the hands. Effusions may be seen in osteoarthritis involving the knee. Radiographic imaging typically shows loss of joint space, marginal osteophytes, subchondral sclerosis, cysts, tibial spiking in the knees, and loss of alignment.

Although truly effective treatment of osteoarthritis is lacking, mild to moderate joint pain can be relieved with acetaminophen. For moderate to severe pain, tramadol, a synthetic opioid agonist that prevents reuptake of norepinephrine and serotonin, can be used when acetaminophen fails or if NSAIDs are contraindicated. Efficacy of tramadol is similar to ibuprofen in patients with both knee and hip osteoarthritis. Nausea, drowsiness, constipation, and rarely, seizures have been reported in patients taking tramadol. If tramadol is not effective, consider NSAIDs or cyclooxygenase 2 (COX-2) inhibitors such as celecoxib and rofecoxib. For patients who have pain that is resistant to or who cannot tolerate tramadol and NSAIDs, consider opioid analgesics.[8]

Use of glucosamine and chondroitin is common but of unproven efficacy. The rationale for their use is that they increase proteoglycan synthesis in articular cartilage; chondroitin sulfate also hinders leukocyte elastase and decreases the breakdown of cartilage collagen and proteoglycans.[8] Currently, a National Institutes of Health-funded multicenter randomized, double-blind, placebo-controlled study of subjects taking glucosamine alone, chondroitin sulfate alone, both glucosamine and chondroitin sulfate, or placebo is underway, and results are expected in 2004.

For those with osteoarthritis of the hand or knee and mild to moderate pain, topical analgesics, such as capsaicin cream, can be used as a single agent or with combination therapy. Side effects may include a local burning sensation.[8]

There are several adjunctive therapies for osteoarthritis. Exercise involving muscle conditioning and aerobic exercise have been shown to decrease symptoms in knee osteoarthritis. Bracing and corrective footwear have been employed for treatment of knee osteoarthritis. Acupuncture use is controversial but promising. The premise is that it relieves pain through stimulation of the gate-control system where large nerve fibers are activated and small fibers that conduct signals in the dorsal horn of the spinal cord are hindered or through discharge of neurochemicals in the central nervous system (CNS). Behavioral interventions such as individualized telephone-based interventions and group programs also have been used with success.[8]

Surgical approaches are considered after failure of medical treatment and include osteotomy, arthroscopy, arthrodesis, and arthroplasty. Osteotomies are done in patients with early osteoarthritis and may relieve symptoms. Arthroscopic debridement and lavage may help with degenerative meniscal tears. Arthrodesis by fusion is often performed in the spine and in small joints of the hand and foot. Total-joint arthroplasty is the basis of surgical treatment of the hip, knee, and glenohumeral joints. For the elderly, this total-joint replacement probably will endure their lifetime.[8]

In the future, biologic repair of articular cartilage may be done routinely. Two different approaches exist: First, host hyaline cartilage is induced to repair the defects by mechanical means (osteotomy) or by biologic stimulation of bone marrow progenitor cells or growth factors, and second, cartilage transplantation takes articular cartilage and supplants it with adult tissue. The three types of cartilage transplantation are osteochondral autografting, osteochondral allografting, and tissue engineering. The latter places committed differentiated chondrocytes or undifferentiated chondroprogenitor cells in a carrier to restore osteochondral defects. Although grafting does not seem to be suitable for most joints with osteoarthritis because of the large articular cartilage defects present, tissue engineering appears promising.[8]

REMITTING SERONEGATIVE SYMMETRIC SYNOVITIS WITH PITTING EDEMA (RS₃ PE) SYNDROME

This syndrome, involving an acute synovitis and edema, was described only recently (in 1985) and occurs mostly in the elderly.[9] Men are afflicted twice as frequently as women, and the average age of onset is 75 years. Patients typically report a sudden onset of redness, warmth, and symmetric soft tissue swelling of the wrists, dorsal surfaces of forearms, feet, and pretibial areas. Carpal tunnel syndrome may be noted. Protracted morning stiffness, lasting up to 6 hours, may be reported, and patients may be debilitated by their symptoms. The ESR is frequently elevated as high as 93 mm/hr. Rheumatoid factor is negative, and low anti-nuclear antibody (ANA) titers may be observed. HLA typing reveals large number of patients having HLA-B7. Low-dose prednisone usually yields good clinical results. Other treatments such as NSAIDs, hydroxychloroquine, and gold have been tried. Most patients experience remission within 1 year

but may still have a slight decrease in range of motion in the hands and wrists.[10]

MALIGNANCY

When an elderly patient presents with new-onset polyarthritis or oligoarthritis, suspicion of secondary malignancy should be considered. Secondary malignancy is usually observed more frequently than primary malignancy. Usually the lower extremities, such as the hip or knee, are affected more often than upper extremities. The most commonly associated malignancies are breast and prostate cancer. Plain radiographs of affected joints will demonstrate pathologic lesions and are indicated in the initial evaluation.

SYSTEMIC DISEASES

Rheumatoid Arthritis (RA)

RA is a chronic systemic inflammatory disease involving hyperplasia, expanding vascularity, and infiltration of CD4+ T cells into the synovial fluid. RA is linked to the major histocompatibility complex class II antigens HLA-DRB1*0404 and DRB1*0401, which present antigenic peptides to CD4+ T cells. Once the antigen-activated CD4+ T cells influence monocytes, macrophages, and synovial fibroblasts to create cytokines interleukin 1 (IL-1), IL-6, and tumor necrosis factor (TNF), the inflammatory cascade in RA is initiated.[11]

The highest incidence of RA occurs in women from 30 to 50 years of age; average onset is 55 years. Elderly-onset RA is defined by distinctly different symptoms that develop after age 60 and makes up one-third of all patients who develop RA.[12] About 10 to 20 percent of patients with RA develop Sjögren's syndrome.[1]

In elderly-onset RA, the following are distinct from the younger-onset RA:

1. Ratio of women to men affected is 1:1; in younger-onset RA, it is 3:1.

2. Acute onset and "infectious-like"; in younger-onset RA, gradual onset is common.

3. More involvement of large, proximal joints (oligoarticular) such as the shoulder; in younger-onset RA, small joints of the hands and feet (polyarticular) are affected.

4. More diffuse systemic symptoms and higher ESR at presentation; although both subsets may have weight

loss, weakness, and elevated ESRs, these findings are more pronounced in the elderly.

5. Decrease in prevalence of positive rheumatoid factor (RF) (66 percent compared with 80 percent in younger-onset RA).[12]

Poorer prognosis occurs in elders with other comorbidities. Life expectancy is decreased for the elderly with functional decline, drug toxicities from RA treatment, and other significant medical conditions. Death usually results from infection, coronary heart disease, or RA itself.[12]

Treatment of RA is not different for the elderly patient. NSAID medications can be started but must be used with care due to renal, gastrointestinal, and CNS side effects. Proton-pump inhibitors, misoprostol, or H2 blockers also should be combined with NSAIDs. COX-2 inhibitors also may be used instead of NSAIDs to lessen gastrointestinal and platelet side effects.[12]

Patients with persistent synovitis and radiographic erosions are often started on either methotrexate or the new disease-modifying antirheumatic drugs (DMARDs) leflunomide and etanercept. Both leflunomide and etanercept are effective when used as monotherapy, but infliximab, which is a foreign protein and another DMARD, must be given with methotrexate to avoid an immune response. In acute RA, leflunomide has been noted to produce a clinical response equal or inferior to methotrexate. Even though etanercept has been compared directly with methotrexate for early RA, studies of patients with chronic RA are complicated because most of these patients are already on methotrexate. In addition, infliximab plus methotrexate has been found to be better than methotrexate alone in stopping radiographic progression of disease. Studies are still underway about the long-term safety and efficacy of these new DMARDs.[13]

Since methotrexate can cause hepatic, pulmonary, and renal toxicity, supplemental folate is given, and a baseline chest radiograph as well as hepatic and renal functional assessments is paramount. If the patient does not have a good response to oral methotrexate and folic acid, parenteral methotrexate is started. If parenteral methotrexate does not work, sulfasalazine and hydroxychloroquine can be added as triple therapy. This combination has been found to have marked clinical response with less toxicity than methotrexate alone. Side effects of hydroxychloroquine include pigmentary retinitis, neuropathies, and myopathies. Side effects of sulfasalazine include neutropenia, thrombocytopenia, and hemolysis in patients with glucose-6-phosphate dehydrogenase deficiency.[13]

Leflunomide is a pyrimidine synthesis inhibitor; side effects include diarrhea, rash, reversible alopecia, and hepatotoxicity. Etanercept and infliximab are both inhibitors of TNF. They work by targeting TNF and preventing activation of lymphocytes and leukocytes, which are increased in the synovial fluid of patients with RA.[13] Side effects of etanercept may include minor irritation at injection site, upper respiratory tract infections, headache, and diarrhea. About 5 to 9 percent of patients develop autoantibodies to double-stranded DNA (dsDNA). In infliximab, reported side effects include upper respiratory tract infections, headache, diarrhea, and abdominal pain. Antibodies to dsDNA were found in about 16 percent of people taking infliximab.

Systemic Lupus Erythematosus (SLE)

SLE is an autoimmune disorder afflicting mostly women during the reproductive age; however, late-onset SLE, defined as onset of symptoms at 50 to 55 years or later, has been observed.[14]

The presentation of younger versus older cohorts is different. The ratio of female predominance is 7:1 in late-onset SLE, lower than the 9:1 ratio in younger cohorts; there is a longer mean interval from symptom onset to diagnosis (32.5 months) in older cohorts; and a white predominance, instead of African-American, is noted in late-onset SLE. However, 5-year survival rates for both younger and older patients are similar.[14]

The diagnosis is difficult to make in late-onset SLE, which explains the longer time it requires for diagnosis of this condition in the elderly. The following classic findings are more common in early-onset or classic SLE: oral and nasal ulcers, alopecia, malar rash, photosensitivity, glomerulonephritis, and lymphadenopathy. Both younger and older patients may experience arthritis, arthralgia, and rash. However, late-onset SLE often presents atypically, and interstitial pneumonitis, serositis, hematocytopenias, peripheral neuropathy, and symptoms suggestive of Sjögren's syndrome are more common in late-onset SLE. Late-onset SLE is usually less severe; patients often die from unrelated causes, such as infections, coronary heart disease, perforated peptic ulcers, or other causes.[14]

Diagnosis of late-onset SLE is elusive given some of its nonspecific symptoms: ill health, muscular aches and pains, weight loss, and behavioral and mood changes. Since infections and endocrine disorders are more common in the elderly, workup must be complete before considering late-onset SLE. Another difficulty is that the

ANA titer is nonspecific, with 36 percent of healthy elderly having low-titer ANAs. Since autoantibodies to dsDNA and Sm are characteristic of SLE and occur in 60 and 8 percent of patients, respectively, in late-onset SLE, they can help with the diagnosis.[14]

Management is directed toward the severity of the disease. Since most elderly patients experience mild symptoms, use of corticosteroids and immunosuppressive agents is not warranted. Arthritis and serositis are treated with anti-inflammatory analgesics. Treatment failure may warrant a short course of corticosteroids with analgesics such as acetaminophen or a narcotic-acetaminophen combination. Antimalarial agents such as chloroquine, hydroxychloroquine, and quinacrine are reserved for dermatologic and arthritis complications. Side effects of these medications include myopathy, retinopathy, heart block, cardiomyopathy, and dyskinesias.[14]

Corticosteroid use is indicated for lupus pneumonitis, thrombocytopenia, and hemolytic anemia. Complications of steroid use include sepsis, aseptic necrosis, osteoporotic vertebral compression fractures, steroid atrophy, electrolyte abnormalities, purpura, fluid retention, glaucoma, hypertension, and adrenal insufficiency. Although glomerulonephritis is not seen as commonly in late-onset SLE, it is managed similarly as in younger patients, with corticosteroids and intravenous pulse cyclophosphamide. Side effects of cyclophosphamide include dehydration from persistent nausea and vomiting, myelosuppression, hemorrhagic cystitis, and superinfection, including herpes zoster.[14]

Neurologic symptoms of late-onset SLE are less common than in early-onset SLE. In an elderly lupus patient with neurologic symptoms, antiphospholipid antibody syndrome and stroke or neurologic complications of hypertension also must be considered. Consultation with both a neurologist and a hematologist may be needed to determine whether anticoagulation should be initiated.[14]

Drug-induced Lupus

The incidence of drug-induced lupus increases with age. About 10 percent of all cases of lupus are drug-related. Medications with a definite association with drug-induced lupus are hydralazine, procainamide, phenytoin, quinidine, isoniazid, methyldopa, and chlorpromazine. Hydralazine, seen mostly in females, and procainamide, noted mostly in males, are the most frequent culprits. Common symptoms include polyarthritis, fever, myalgias, and polyserositis. Rarely, the CNS and kidneys are involved.[15] Antihistone antibodies are distinctive for drug-induced lupus but are not specific. Antibodies to native dsDNA are not seen in procainamide- or hydralazine-induced lupus. Patients also may have antiphospholipid antibody and its thromboembolic tendencies. Drug-induced lupus usually resolves within 4 to 6 weeks after treatment with the offending agent is terminated; however, ANA titers can remain positive for 6 to 12 months.[16] Recently, etanercept and infliximab, two TNF inhibitors used to treat rheumatoid arthritis, have been demonstrated to increase the incidence of drug-induced lupus and resulting positive ANA titers.

Polymyalgia Rheumatica (PMR) and Giant Cell Arteritis (GCA)

Both polymyalgia rheumatica and giant cell arteritis are common conditions in the elderly and are interrelated. Half of all patients with GCA have PMR, whereas 4 to 40 percent of patients with PMR have GCA as well. Both these conditions are discussed in Chap. 69.

DIFFERENTIAL DIAGNOSIS

Avascular Necrosis

Avascular necrosis (AVN) is often the by-product of corticosteroid treatment, and when it is compounded by osteoporosis in the elderly, the results can be devastating. AVN can present as hip pain and often mimics osteoarthritis. A suspicion of avascular necrosis should be considered in elderly patients who have a history of persistent hip pain despite use of pain medication.

Myopathies

Myopathies can mimic some of the symptoms of arthritis suffered by the elderly. Both polymyositis (PM) and dermatomyositis (DM) cause chronic progressive muscle weakness symmetrically affecting the proximal extremities. Other symptoms include polyarthralgias, polyarthritis, and constitutional symptoms. Increases in serum muscle enzyme levels, typical inflammatory changes on electromyography, and abnormal inflammatory changes around myocytes and vessels are noted on muscle biopsy. Be aware that these two conditions have a high association with malignancy, especially in the elderly. Myopathy of hypothyroidism usually involves weakness, pain, cramping, and stiffness of the proximal muscle groups that may simulate fibromyalgia or polymyalgia rheumatica. Drug-induced myopathies also should be considered in the differential. Offending agents include corticosteroids (proximal hip girdle muscles), alcohol, colchicine, and lipid-lowering agents such as HMG-CoA reductase inhibitors, clofibrate, gemfibrozil, and nicotinic acid.

Trauma

When trauma to a joint results in an intraarticular deformity, hemarthrosis, or fracture, it can be mistaken for acute arthritis. A history of warfarin use or a clotting deficiency may result in hemarthrosis following minor trauma. Penetrating injuries from wood fragments, thorns, or other foreign bodies may lead to an acute synovitis either acutely or months later.[4]

Bursitis and Tendinitis

Chronic friction, crystal deposition, trauma, infection, and systemic diseases such as RA and gout can inflame bursae and tendons. In all cases, patients usually present with pain in periarticular structures, which should be distinguished from a true arthritis. Tenderness is usually elicited by palpation around the joint. Most of these soft tissue inflammations are treated conservatively with rest, ice initially and later warm packs, and NSAIDs (if there are no contraindications). Olecranon and prepatellar bursitis can be difficult to distinguish from septic bursitis, which also affects these areas. If there is a suspicion of infection, these bursae should be aspirated and the fluid sent for Gram stain and culture. Patients should be given antibiotics effective against *S. aureus*. Steroid injections are strongly discouraged because they can increase the risk for spontaneous rupture, and worsening infection.

ADDITIONAL ASPECTS

In elderly patients with chronic arthritis, including rheumatoid arthritis or osteoarthritis, any acute pain, tenderness, swelling, or redness in a single joint out of proportion to the other joints should lead not only to a suspicion of gout but also to consideration of a septic joint.

Although treatment for many of rheumatologic diseases typically is not started in the ED, knowledge of the presentation, treatment, and treatment side effects of these diseases is essential.

REFERENCES

1. Calkins E, Vladutiu AO: Musculoskeletal Disorders in Duthie EH, Katz PR (eds): *Practice of Geriatrics,* 3d ed. Philadelphia, Saunders, 1998; p. 421.
2. Goldenberg DL: Bacterial arthritis in Ruddy S (eds): *Kelley's Textbook of Rheumatology,* 6th ed. Philadelphia, Saunders, 2001; p. 469.
3. Dubost J, Fis I, Denis P, et al: Polyarticular Septic Arthritis. *Medicine* 72: 296, 1993.
4. Baker DG, Schumacher HR: Acute monoarthritis. *New Engl J Med* 329:1013, 1993.
5. Aguedo CA, Wise CM: Crystal associated arthritis in the elderly. *Rheum Dis Clin North Am* 26(3):527, 2000
6. Emmerson BT: The management of gout. *New Engl J Med* 334:445, 1996.
7. Jordan JM, Kington RS, Lane NE, et al: Systemic risk factors for osteoarthritis, in Felson DT (conference chair): Osteoarthritis: New insights: 1. The disease and its risk factors. *Ann Intern Med* 133:637, 2000.
8. Hochberg MC, McAlindon T, Felson DT: Systemic and topical treatments, in Felson DT (conference chair): Osteoarthritis: New insights: 2. Treatment approaches. *Ann Intern Med* 133:726, 2000.
9. McCarty DJ, O'Duffy JD, Person L, et al: Remitting seronegative symmetrical synovitis with pitting edema. RS3PE Syndrome. *JAMA* 254:2763, 1985.
10. Oliveri I, Salvarani C, Cantini F: RS3PE Syndrome: an overview. *Clin Exp Rheumatol* 18:S53, 2000.
11. Choy EHS, Panayi GS: Cytokine pathways and joint inflammation in rheumatoid arthritis. *New Engl J Med* 334:907, 2001.
12. Yazici Y, Paget SA:. Elderly onset rheumatoid arthritis. *Rheum Dis Clin North Am* 26(3):517, 2000.
13. Kremer JM: Rational use of new and existing disease-modifying agents in rheumatoid arthritis. *Ann Intern Med* 134:695, 2001.
14. Kammer GM, Mishra N: Systemic lupus erythematosus in the elderly. *Rheum Dis Clin North Am* 26(3):475, 2000
15. Pinals RS: Polyarthritis and fever. *New Engl J Med* 330:769, 1994.
16. Mills JA: Systemic lupus erythematosus. *New Engl J Med* 330:1871, 1994.

69

Giant Cell Arteritis (Temporal Arteritis) and Polymyalgia Rheumatica

Mark Levine

HIGH-YIELD FACTS

- Giant cell arteritis (GCA) and polymyalgia rheumatica (PMR) are found almost exclusively in patients over age 50.

- Approximately 40 percent of patients do not present with classic signs and symptoms.

- Laboratory evaluation typically reveals an elevated erythrocyte sedimentation rate (ESR) for both disease processes.

- New headache, abnormal temporal artery biopsy, jaw or tongue claudication, and visual abnormalities are cardinal features of GCA.

- Immediate treatment with steroids, even prior to confirmatory testing, has been shown to improve long-term outcome.

There are historical references to giant cell arteritis (GCA) and polymyalgia rheumatica (PMR) in the tombs of Egypt, in writings of Mesopotamia, and on Italian and Dutch art murals from the fifteenth century.[1] The symptoms of PMR were first described in 1888 as "senile rheumatic gout," and the term *polymyalgia rheumatica* was first used in 1957 to describe a syndrome of myalgias and stiffness of the shoulder and muscle girdles along with an increased erythrocyte sedimentation rate (ESR) in patients over age 50.[2,3] The first modern description of GCA was given in 1890 and includes "a peculiar form of thrombotic arteritis of the aged . . . whose superficial temporal arteries were so swollen and painful that he was unable to wear a hat." The clinical and microscopic profiles of GCA were elucidated in 1932.[1] PMR and GCA are found primarily in the geriatric population, and sometimes both can be present in the same patient in rates of 20 to 60 percent of the time.[3] Both diseases have constitutional complaints associated with

them, including malaise, fatigue, weight loss, anemia, and an elevation of acute-phase reactants. In addition, both show a rapid response to the use of corticosteroids. The major complication of GCA is visual loss and permanent blindness when not treated promptly. Patients with GCA or PMR do not have any higher increased rate of mortality compared with controls. The diagnoses of these diseases are sometimes obscured by nonspecific constitutional complaints and other confounding illnesses that may lead the practitioner away from making the appropriate diagnosis. Since the mean age of onset for these diseases is 70 years, there may be difficulties obtaining a history from patients because problems with of cognitive impairment and communication. In addition, the diagnosis may be obscured by variations in laboratory results and biopsy results.

EPIDEMIOLOGY

These are relatively common diseases in the elderly population and mainly afflict white individuals of northern European and Scandinavian background. The annual incidence of PMR ranges from 0.49 to 27.3 cases per 100,000 in adults over age 50,[3] whereas the incidence of GCA is approximately 18 cases per 100,000 persons.[4] Approximately 50 percent of patients with GCA also may have symptoms of classic PMR. Biopsy-proven GCA has been reported in approximately 20 percent of patients with PMR.[5] GCA is rarely seen in the African-American, Asian, and Latino populations.[3,6] Giant cell arteritis is twice as common in women as in men, and the prevalence of GCA increases from southern to northern latitudes.[3] Other risk factors for GCA and PMR are smoking (in women only), sun exposure (secondary to solar radiation–induced degradation of the internal elastic lamina of superficial arteries), and nulliparity (due to hyperestrogenic effects on the arterial wall).[7]

PATHOPHYSIOLOGY

There are multiple hypotheses as to the causes of GCA and PMR. PMR and GCA were believed initially to have an infectious etiology such as adenovirus, respiratory syncitial virus, *Mycoplasma pneumoniae,* or parainfluenza virus, but this has never been proven.[4,7] Since biopsies of the temporal and other large arteries show a T-lymphocyte proliferation in the arterial walls, another hypothesis is that GCA and PMR have an immune-based etiology. In this hypothesis, an insult to the arterial wall provokes an autoimmune response, and the subsequent reparative process leads to an increase in immune cell and smooth muscle infiltration in the lumen, forming a hyperplastic intima that occludes the lumen.[8,9] This infiltration of the vasculature affects the arterial walls in a patchy pattern. The degree of luminal compromise varies throughout the course of the vessel wall. Lymphocytes, histiocytes, epithelioid cells, and multinucleated giant cells are also found within the cellular mix in the lumina. These giant cells form calcifications by the fusion of modified smooth muscle cells. Other giant cells attack these calcifications, attracting lymphocytes and causing activation of mononuclear cells that cause further destruction and dilatation of the arterial wall.[8] The aorta and the subclavian and axillary arteries and their subsequent branches are the most commonly involved vessels in GCA and are affected in a centripetal fashion.[2,10] Intracranial arteries are less often involved, possibly due to a lesser amount of internal elastic lamina.[2,10] The immune response that is seen in PMR appears to be a more systemic and mild reaction, whereas in GCA it is a more intense and localized.[4] In PMR, the vasculature is not affected, but lymphocytic inflammation and synovitis have been found in the joints of patients with PMR. Muscle biopsies in PMR are normal or show minimal atrophy.

The increased risk of visual loss in patients with GCA may be related to cytokine production in the affected vessels. Interferon gamma is produced in cranial arteritis, in contrast to subjects with PMR, where the T cells produce IL-2. Interferon gamma stimulates macrophages to produce local growth factors, leading to intimal hyperplasia and arterial wall destruction, whereas IL-2 does not have the same effects on platelet growth factors and stimulation of the wall hyperplasia and thus does not result in as severe of disease. It is still unclear whether anticoagulation or platelet inhibitors would be helpful in the treatment or prevention of these diseases.[11]

CLINICAL FEATURES

The onset of PMR and GCA usually occurs at about 70 years of age and has a female-to-male predilection of 2:1. Frequently, the onset of these diseases is insidious. Patients with PMR frequently complain of pain and stiffness of the proximal muscle girdles of the pelvis and neck. The proximal extremities also may be involved. Frequently, the pain is so intense that the patient cannot get out of bed in the morning; however, strength is usually not compromised. Other generalized complaints in PMR include night sweats, anorexia, weight loss, and

vomiting.[4] Active motion is painful, whereas passive motion is relatively pain-free. Synovitis is present in about 15 percent of patients. Virtually all patients with PMR have subacromial or subdeltoid bursitis, and there is also some aspect of mild to moderate proximal joint synovitis.[5] Patients with PMR also may develop distal arthritis and may manifest with distal extremity swelling and pitting edema, neither of which is seen with GCA.[5,12,13]

Symptoms of GCA are related to the vasculature involved. Headache and scalp tenderness described as "boring" or lancinating is typical when the temporal artery is involved. The headache is usually new onset and may be generalized; however, it is usually unilateral and found in the area of the affected temporal artery.[3] The temporal artery itself is usually pulseless and swollen. Jaw claudication is a frequent complaint and has high specificity for GCA.[14] In addition, odynophagia, hoarseness, cough, otalgia, and sudden loss of hearing or visual changes are described frequently. Approximately one-half of patients may be febrile with temperatures of up to 39.5°C.[15]

Importantly, however, up to 40 percent of patients with GCA present in an occult fashion with either systemic or local symptoms resulting from involvement of the large arteries. At times, GCA may present as anorexia, weight loss, depression, or failure to thrive.[10]

Ocular involvement is the most common and most severe complications of GCA. Headaches usually precede the onset of visual symptoms, although this time frame may vary significantly and has been reported to be from 4 to 240 days. Decreased visual acuity, diplopia, ptosis, hemianopsia, and a monocular vision loss are all manifestations of the disease process.[16] Amaurosis fugax also may occur, but it is a rare initial finding. Blindness and visual symptoms are relatively rare in biopsy-negative cases.[17] Involvement of the lingual artery can cause pain and blanching of the tongue, infrequently leading to gangrene. Involvement of the arteries in the otic region can cause hearing loss, tinnitus, and vertigo.[4]

Larger vessel disease may occur in up to 15 percent of patients and include aortic valve incompetence, dissecting aneurysms, claudication, Raynaud's phenomenon, paresthesias, bruits (found in approximately 30–80 percent of patients with GCA),[10,14] decreased pulses, myocardial infarction, or neurologic symptoms secondary to vertebral arteritis. Aneurysms, both dissecting and nondissecting, occur approximately 17 times more often than in unaffected subjects.[10] Large-vessel GCA does not represent a more advanced disease process but instead appears to be a different pattern of arterial involvement.

Neurologic manifestations may include ataxia, lateral medullary syndrome, hemianopsia, hearing loss, and dementia. Peripheral neuropathies occur in approximately 7 percent of patients with GCA due to vasculitis of the adjacent arteries that supply the affected nerves. Involvement of the vertebrobasilar system is common in patients with GCA. However, transient ischemic attacks and stroke are relatively uncommon and are noted only in 6 and 3 percent of biopsy-proven cases, respectively.[16,17] Some patients report cognitive and memory disorders, delirium, depression, or psychotic features, including visual hallucinations.

DIAGNOSIS AND DIFFERENTIAL

PMR and GCA are clinical diagnoses in the emergency department (ED) setting based on patient age, presentation, and the presence of an elevated ESR. PMR and GCA are both associated with moderately to significantly elevated ESR. Sedimentation rates of approximately 40 to 60 mm/h are noted in PMR. In GCA, more marked elevations, often approximating 100 mm/h, are seen. It is important to remember that the ESR is usually abnormal in these disease states, although the elevation may be anywhere from the 40 to 100+ mm/h range.[3] In one study, only 5 percent of GCA patients had a normal (<40 mm/h) ESR at the time of diagnosis; in this same study, 20 percent of patients with PMR were reported to have a normal ESR at the time of diagnosis.[18] Other acute-phase reactants such as CRP, fibrinogen, platelet count, and complement level also can be elevated. Of these, CRP is most useful as a diagnostic aid. The white blood cell count is usually normal, and a normochromic, normocytic anemia is found frequently. It is not uncommon to have a lower ESR elevation or other laboratory value in a patient who is unable to mount an acute-phase serologic response or a patient who has a very localized arteritis.[18]

The criterion standard for confirmation of GCA is superficial temporal artery biopsy. Because of the patchy nature of the disease process,[3] the biopsy area should be 3 to 5 cm long and at the area of the greatest tenderness. Although this is considered to be the criterion standard for the diagnosis of GCA, the sensitivity of a single biopsy has been reported to be as low as 60 to 80 percent.[4] Biopsy-proven cases tend to appear more severe at the time of diagnosis, possibly because the disease process has progressed to such a point that the diagnosis is clear and other differentials have been exhausted.[17] False-negative rates of 5 percent, usually caused by skip lesions at the biopsy site, are probably more typical.[19] If temporal artery biopsy is normal and clinical suspicion remains high, then a repeat biopsy should be performed and/or empirical therapy should be given. If both biopsies are negative, alternative etiologies of the elevated ESR should be considered. If the ESR is normal and a unilateral biopsy is negative, there is a lesser chance of the patient having GCA. If suspicion is high, an alternate side biopsy may be performed.

The diagnosis of GCA can be made regardless of biopsy results if three of five of the following American College of Rheumatology criteria are met: (1) patient is older than age 50, (2) presents with a new-onset headache, (3) has a temporal artery abnormality (tenderness on palpation or decreased temporal artery pulse unrelated to arteriosclerosis of the cervical arteries), (4) has an elevated ESR, and (5) has an abnormal arterial biopsy (vasculitis characterized by a predominance of mononuclear cell infiltration or granulomatous inflammation, usually with multinucleated giant cells).

Patients with a clinical picture of PMR usually have a lower ESR, resolution of symptomatology with low-dose steroids, a male predominance, a lower frequency of anemia, elevated CRP, and lower frequency of abnormal protein electrophoresis. In addition, they are younger, have a longer duration of symptoms prior to final diagnosis, have a lower incidence of fever, a lower frequency of weight loss, and do not respond well to NSAIDs.

Diagnostic imaging is useful occasionally for GCA and PMR. Ultrasonography, computed tomography, angiography, and magnetic resonance imaging all have been used to confirm the diagnosis of these conditions.

Color duplex ultrasonography can determine areas of vascular stenosis and occlusion consistent with GCA. A hypoechoic halo secondary to edema of the artery wall is found in 73 percent of patients diagnosed with GCA. The halo, when displayed in two planes, is always circumferential. Skip lesions also are seen on ultrasound. Normal temporal arteries show a fully perfused lumen and a bright vessel wall. Although ultrasound can diagnose vasculitis with a high degree of sensitivity and specificity and detect changes in velocity that indicate the degree of stenosis and wall thickness, there can be false-negative results because the hypoechoic area is not noted in all patients.[20,21] Vascular ultrasound also can be used to follow remission in patients with GCA because edema of the vessel wall will disappear within 2 to 3 weeks of the initiation of steroids.[4] In patients with PMR, inflammation of the subacromial and subdeltoid bursae of the shoulders and iliopectineal bursae can be determined with the use of ultrasound as well. Peripheral synovitis is observed in 31 to 38 percent of patients with PMR, and hip synovitis is also seen very frequently.

Magnetic resonance imaging (MRI) reveals musculotendinous and articular structures well, and fluid accumulation in bursae, joints, and tendon sheaths can be noted. MRI has a higher sensitivity than ultrasound in the diagnosis of peripheral synovitis and distal swelling of the extremities, although it is much more expensive. MRI, however, is less sensitive diagnosing fluid in large joints.[22,23]

Intravenous angiography will show a pattern of arteriographic stenoses and/or occlusions with a smooth, tapered appearance in the subclavian, axillary, and proximal brachial arteries. Lesions in the femoral regions are found infrequently. Stenotic lesions are the dominant feature with angiography proven GCA. Angiographic studies may be done if there is a concern of aortic arch syndrome or other related large-artery arteritis. Angiography may show alternating dilatation and constriction of affected large arteries and a lack of irregular plaques and ulcerations consistent with the skip lesions found on biopsy. Aortic involvement is more common in the later stages of GCA. Importantly, inflammation of the arterial wall cannot be detected by angiography. MRI, computed tomographic (CT) scanning, and ultrasonography are better suited for that purpose.

CT scanning and MRI are also most appropriate for evaluation of aneurysms secondary to GCA. One of the limitations of CT scanning is related to the orientation of the acquired images. Vessels that are oriented horizontal to the plane of the section are not seen well enough for diagnostic purposes; those imaged in cross section or in the long axis are better able to be evaluated.[21] Last, CT scanning and MRI are relatively good choices for evaluation of the end stages of vasculitic and ischemic changes, lymphadenopathy, and effusions that may occur with large-vessel vasculitis. [24]

The differential of GCA and PMR includes other inflammatory and noninflammatory rheumatic diseases, malignancies, and infections. Arthritis is one of the most common peripheral manifestations of GCA. The elevated ESR is helpful in differentiating several other diseases such as fibromyositis, tendinitis, and capsulitis, as well as seronegative and seropositive rheumatoid arthritis.[13] Polymyositis should be considered in the differential of PMR. Characteristic findings of muscular weakness, elevated muscle enzymes [creatine phosphokinase (CPK)], and abnormal electromyography are found in polymyositis, which distinguish it from PMR. Hypothyroidism and hyperparathyroidism also may have symptoms that can be confused with PMR. Additional diagnostic considerations include infections, malignancy, depression, osteoarthritis, and rheumatoid arthritis.

EMERGENCY DEPARTMENT CARE AND DISPOSITION

PMR is treated with 10 to 15 mg prednisone orally each morning. Usually dramatic relief occurs within a few days, which helps confirm the diagnosis. Steroid therapy is also effective in PMR associated bursitis and synovitis. After a decrease in symptoms, the dosage is tapered to a maintenance level that provides symptomatic relief and maintains a lower ESR. PMR may be self-limiting or may require low maintenance dose of prednisone over the course of many years. Too rapid taper of the prednisone dose usually causes a relapse. GCA also responds dramatically to initial high doses of prednisone (60–80 mg orally daily) or methylpredinisolone sodium succinate (Solu-Medrol; 125–250 mg parenterally every 6 hours). Symptoms should resolve in 24 to 48 hours. If there is a recurrence of symptoms, an increase in the prednisone dose should be given until symptoms clear, followed by a more gradual reduction of the taper.[3] If there is no improvement in the symptoms within 4 days, another diagnosis should be considered.[3] Ocular involvement is the most common and most severe complications of GCA. Partial or complete visual loss occurs in 8 to 20 percent of patients.[11] Transient visual symptoms and an elevated platelet count are reported risk factors for permanent visual loss. Once visual loss occurs, it is not reversible. However, a lower incidence of permanent visual changes occurs with early recognition of GCA and treatment with glucocorticoids.[11] Since changes in arterial wall inflammation can be recognized even after initiation of steroids, it is imperative to begin steroid treatment immediately, even if a biopsy cannot be performed imminently. Pathologic findings on biopsy can be noted for up to 2 weeks after therapy.[3] The route of steroid administration is probably not critical. In patients with GCA and vision loss, intravenous steroids have demonstrated a difference in subjective improvement of vision but not a statistically significant increase in visual acuity compared with those treated with oral steroids. In a study of patients with biopsy-proven GCA, there was no difference in oral versus intravenous steroid administration.[25] Evidence of neurologic improvement is also noted in the majority (74 percent) of GCA patients treated with steroids.[16] Steroid therapy may worsen GCA-associated psychiatric symptoms, and patients with psychosis may need to be treated with antipsychotic medication.[16] Tapering of the steroid doses in GCA should be done in 10 percent increments over the course of at least 2 years. However, this should not be started until the ESR has normalized.

Proper follow-up with neurology and ophthalmology

is of utmost importance for the patient whom the clinician believes is afflicted with GCA or PMR. Hospitalization is rarely emergently required but may be discussed with consulting services. Prompt initiation of corticosteroid therapy should begin prior to discharge or admission.

ADDITIONAL ASPECTS

When interpreting ESR results, it should be noted that mild elevations, typically less than 40 mm/h, are common in older patients. The formula (age + 10)/2 is a useful rule of thumb in determining appropriate age-related upper limits for the ESR.

Although GCA and PMR can be chronic vasculitic conditions, there appears to be no correlation with an increased risk of death from cardiovascular disease in these patients. Several studies have shown similar mortality rates without respect to disease and controls.[26]

High doses of steroids interfere with the hypothalamic-pituitary-adrenal axis and may result in life-threatening adrenal insufficiency. In addition, the long-term use of corticosteroids increases the risk of osteoporosis, hyperglycemia, susceptibility to infection, hypertension, cataracts, glaucoma, and the incidence of fracture and decreases wound healing. Long-term steroid treatment regimens should balance the benefits and risks of steroid therapy and involve the patient in treatment decisions.

REFERENCES

1. Portioli I: The history of polymyalgia rheumatic/giant cell arteritis. *Clin Exp Rheumatol* 18(4 suppl 20):S1, 2000.
2. Cassel CK, Cohen HJ, Larson EB (eds): *Geriatric Medicine*, 34th ed. New York, Springer, 1997.
3. Meskimen S, Cook TD, Blake RL: Management of giant cell arteritis and polymyalgia rheumatica. 61(7):2061, 1991.
4. Epperly TD, Moore KE, Harrover JD: Polymyalgia rheumatica and temporal arteritis. *Am Fam Physician* 62(4):789, 2001.
5. Gonzalez-Gay MA, Garcia-Porrua C, Salvarani C: Diagnostic approach in a patient presenting with polymyalgial. *Clin Exp Rheumatol* 17(3):276, 1999.
6. Liu NH, LaBree LD, Feldon SE, et al: The epidemiology of giant cell arteritis: A 12-year retrospective study. *Ophthalmology* 108(6):1145, 2001.
7. Cimmino MA, Zaccaria A: Epidemiology of polymyalgia rheumatica. *Clin Exp Rheumatol* 18(4 suppl 20):S9, 2000.
8. Nordborg C, Nordborg E, Petursdottir V: The pathogenesis

of giant cell arteritis: Morphological aspects. *Clin Exp Rheumatol* 18(4 suppl 20):S18, 2000.
9. Weyand CM: The Dunlop-Dottridge Lecture: The pathogenesis of giant cell arteritis. *J Rheumatol* 27(2):517, 2000.
10. Kelly J, Rudd AG: Giant cell arteritis presenting with arm claudication. *Age Ageing* 30:167, 2001.
11. Liozon E, Herrmann F, Ly K, et al: Risk factors for visual loss in giant cell (temporal) arteritis: A prospective study of 174 patients. *Am J Med* 111(3):211, 2001.
12. Narvaez J, Nolla-Sole JM, Clavaguera MT, et al: Musculoskeletal manifestations in polymyalgia rheumatica and temporal arteritis. *Ann Rheum Dis* 60(11):1060, 2001.
13. Salvarani C, Hunder GG: Musculoskeletal manifestations in a population-based cohort of patients with giant cell arteritis. *Arthritis Rheum* 42(6):1259, 1999.
14. Brack A, Martinez-Taboada V, Stanson A, et al: Disease pattern in cranial and large-vessel giant cell arteritis. *Arthritis Rheum* 42(2):311, 1999.
15. Hu Z, Yang Q, Zheng S, et al: Temporal arteritis and fever: Report of a case and clinical reanalysis of 360 cases. *Angiology* 51(11):953, 2000.
16. Nesher G: Neurologic manifestations of giant cell arteritis. *Clin Exp Rheumatol* 18(4 suppl 20):S24, 2000.
17. Duhaut P, Pinede L, Bornet H, et al: Biopsy proven and biopsy negative temporal arteritis: Differences in clinical spectrum at the onset of the disease. *Ann Rheum Dis* 58(6):335, 1999.
18. Salvarani C, Hunder GG: Giant cell arteritis with low erythrocyte sedimentaion rate: Frequency of occurrence in a population-bsred study. *Arthritis Rheum* 45(2):140, 2001.
19. Lee AG, Brazis PW: Temporal arteritis: A clinical approach. *J Am Geriatr Soc* 47(11):1364, 1999.
20. Schmidt WA: Doppler ultrasonography in the diagnosis of giant cell arteritis. *Clin Exp Rheumatol* 18(4 suppl 20):S40, 2000.
21. Stanson AW: Imaging findings in extracranial (giant cell) temporal arteritis. *Clin Exp Rheumatol* 18(4 suppl 20):S43, 2000.
22. Martinez-Taboada VM, Blanco R, Rodriguez-Valverde V: Polymyalgia rheumatica with normal erythrocyte sedimentation rate: clinical aspects. *Clin Exp Rheumatol* 18(4 suppl 20):S34, 2000.
23. Pavlica P, Barozzi L, Salvarani C, et al: Magnetic resonance imaging in the diagnosis of PMR. *Clin Exp Rheumatol* 18(4 suppl 20):S38, 2000.
24. Atalay MK, Bluemke DA: Magnetic resonance imaging of large vessel vasculitis. *Curr Opin Rheumatol* 13(1):41, 2001.
25. Chan CC, Paine M, O'Day J: Steroid management in giant cell arteritis. *Br J Ophthalmol* 85(9):1061, 2001.
26. Gran JT, Myklebust G, Wilsgaard T, et al: Survival in polymyalgia rheumatica and temporal arteritis: A study of 398 cases and matched population controls. *Rheumatology* 40(100):1238, 2001.

70

Ankylosing Spondylitis

John R. Lindbergh
Andrew D. Perron

HIGH-YIELD FACTS

- Ankylosing spondylitis is a seronegative arthritis; it is one of the inflammatory arthropathies that lacks serum rheumatoid factor and is closely linked with the HLA-B27 haplotype.

- While ankylosing spondylitis should be considered in younger patients with back pain and associated morning stiffness persisting for more than 3 months, sequelae are often seen in older persons with advanced disease.

- Sacroiliitis is a common early complaint, and long-term sequelae include eventual fusing of the spinal column and the pathognomonic "bamboo spine" on radiographs.

- Extraskeletal manifestations include uveitis, aortitis, cardiac conduction disturbance, pulmonary disease, renal disease, and the cauda equina syndrome.

- Emergency department (ED) management can be complicated by airway issues related to cervical spine ankylosis.

- Patients with ankylosing spondylitis can have significant spinal injuries such as fracture, atlantoaxial or atlanto-occipital subluxation, or spinal epidural hematoma secondary to minor trauma.

Ankylosing spondylitis ranks among the more common of the seronegative spondyloarthropathies. The term *seronegative* refers to the absence of rheumatoid factor in the patient's serum. These are a group of related disorders that lead to inflammation and sometimes to fusion of the axial skeleton. In addition to ankylosing spondylitis, the spectrum of these disorders includes Reiter's syndrome, psoriatic arthritis, and the arthropathy of inflammatory bowel disease. Additionally, there are peripheral arthridities and extraskeletal manifestations that may precede the skeletal symptoms or may occur concurrently.

Ankylosing spondylitis puts the geriatric patients at risk for chronic back pain and immobility in the mildest of cases and atlantoaxial subluxation, aortitis, cardiac conduction disturbances, pulmonary fibrosis, and renal impairment in the more severe cases. With emphasis on the geriatric population, the extraskeletal manifestations are much more likely to occur in the later stages of the disease and usually are expressed in the second to third decade of symptomatic disease. With respect to emergency medicine, some of the more pertinent sequelae of ankylosing spondylitis occur in the later stages of the disease, when the cervical spine becomes fused, brittle, and deformed. This can lead to airway management difficulties, as well as significant injuries that occur as a result of relatively minor trauma.

EPIDEMIOLOGY

Ankylosing spondylitis occurs more commonly in men than in women, with a 2:1 to 3:1 ratio.[1] The reasons for this are unclear; it is possible that the disease occurs equally among the sexes but is more severe in men and therefore diagnosed more frequently.

HLA-B27 is the only gene thus far identified that is unambiguously associated with spondyloarthropathy. The frequency of HLA-B27 in a given population closely parallels that of the prevalence of ankylosing spondylitis. HLA-B27 also has been found to be linked to Reiter's syndrome, which, in turn, is associated with bacterial pathogens such as *Chlamydia* and *Yersinia*. This linkage has suggested the role of infectious pathogens in ankylosing spondylitis as well.[2]

HLA-B27 can be identified in 80 to 95 percent of Caucasians with ankylosing spondylitis.[3] It is not, however, the sole contributor to the disease. Family, twin, and genetic studies suggest a model involving multiple genes and environmental factors interacting together. In the general population, ankylosing spondylitis is likely to develop in 1 to 2 percent of HLA-B27-positive adults. Among Caucasians, the estimated prevalence of ankylosing spondylitis ranges from 67 per 100,000 people over the age of 20 in the Netherlands to 197 per 100,000 in the United States.[4]

PATHOPHYSIOLOGY

The term *ankylosing spondylitis* is derived from the Greek roots *ankylos* meaning "fused" and *spondylos* meaning "vertebrae," combined with *-itis*, which implies inflammation. The pathophysiology underlying ankylosing spondylitis remains unclear. It is thought that the disease is due to an immune response that is genetically determined but also is modulated by environmental factors. Some hypothesize a role for gram-negative bacteria, such as *Klebsiella pneumoniae*.[2,5] It is thought that these bacteria have antigens that resemble HLA-B27 and cause an immune response that gives rise to autoantibodies.

The site of insertion of tendons and ligaments into bone is known as the *enthesis*, and *enthesitis* refers to inflammation at these sites. Enthesitis is the primary progenitor of the skeletal manifestations of ankylosing spondylitis. As the disease progresses, calcification and reduced range of motion of affected joints ensue. This ultimately leads to the radiologic finding of squaring of the vertebral bodies, vertebral end plate destruction, and the eventual functional fusion of the vertebrae. The precise pathophysiology of the extraskeletal manifestations is unclear but likely also stems from a similar immunopathology.

CLINICAL FEATURES

Back pain is an extremely common symptom, especially among the elderly. Fortunately, there are some special features of ankylosing spondylitis that may distinguish it from the more ordinary causes of persistent back pain. The presence of ankylosing spondylitis is heralded by the insidious onset of back discomfort, usually before age 40, persistence of this pain for more than 3 months, and the presence of morning stiffness. Ankylosing spondylitis is unlikely to present after age 40; however, there is a subset of patients who present later than the typical patient. Thus the diagnosis should not be excluded based solely on the age of onset.[6]

The discomfort is described initially as a deep-seated pain in the gluteal region, which may occur unilaterally or bilaterally and which at this stage is difficult to characterize or to localize. The pain then most commonly settles in the sacroiliac joints but may radiate in a sciatic distribution. The morning stiffness may last up to 3 hours and, as in rheumatoid arthritis, may abate with a hot shower or range-of-motion exercises. Eventually, ankylosing spondylitis can progress to involve the entire spinal column, which results in deformities, including fixed flexion of the cervical spine, thoracic kyphosis, and loss of the lumbar spine lordosis.[7]

Extra-axial Manifestations

Generalized systemic symptoms, such as weight loss, fever, and fatigue, may occur commonly. Other more localized extraarticular manifestations may include anterior uveitis, aortitis, cardiac conduction disturbances, pulmonary fibrosis, amyloidosis, and renal disease.

The shoulders and the hip are the most frequently involved extraaxial joints, and pain in these joints may be the presenting complaint in up to 15 percent of patients.[4] Hip involvement seems to correlate with earlier age of onset. Enthesitis also can commonly cause tenderness at other sites, such as the vertebral spinous processes, iliac crests, greater trochanters, ischial tuberosities, tibial tubercles, plantar fascia, and Achilles tendon insertion.

Many patients complain of chest pain, which is secondary to enthesitis of the costovertebral and sternocostal insertions. A mild to moderate reduction in chest expansion due to fibrosis of these areas is often detectable in the early stages of this disease. Interestingly, pulmonary volume capacities usually are not greatly affected due to increased diaphragmatic compensation for thoracic immobility.

Acute anterior uveitis is the most common extraarticular manifestation.[1] It can occur in up to 25 to 30 percent of patients at some time in the course of their disease.[4] The symptoms are typically acute in onset, with unilateral eye inflammation and pain progressing to glaucoma and loss of vision in untreated cases.

Neurologic sequelae of ankylosing spondylitis are quite common and can result from fractures, spinal compression, spinal instability, and spinal stenosis. Atlantoaxial and atlanto-occipital subluxation can occur due to trauma or can occur spontaneously and cause spinal cord compression. Involvement of the lumbrosacral nerve roots can bring about the cauda equina syndrome, with resulting saddle anesthesia, urinary and fecal incontinence, and loss of lower extremity reflexes.

Cardiac involvement can include ascending aortitis, aortic valve disease, and progressive conduction disturbance. Pulmonary disease is usually a late feature of ankylosing spondylitis, involving the upper lobes of the lungs with slowly progressive fibrosis. Renal disease often is secondary to IgA nephropathy or amyloid deposition and can produce a variably progressive renal failure. A more complete listing of the skeletal and extraskeletal manifestations of ankylosing spondylitis can be found in Table 70-1.

Table 70-1. Manifestations of Ankylosing Spondylitis

Articular/skeletal
    Axial arthritis
        Sacroiliitis
        Spondylitis
        Spinal fracture
        Atlantoaxial subluxation
        Atlanto-occipital subluxation
    Extraaxial arthritis
        Hip
        Shoulder
        Peripheral arthritis
        Enthesopathy
            Achilles tendonitis
            Costochondritis
    Osteoporosis
Extraskeletal
    Anterior uveitis
    Iritis
    Aortitis
    Cardiac conduction abnormalities
    Pulmonary fibrosis
    Amyloidosis
    IgA nephropathy
    Neurologic complications
        Spinal cord compression
        Spinal stenosis
        Cauda-equina syndrome
        Spinal epidural hematoma

Table 70-2. Differential Diagnosis of Ankylosing Spondylitis

Seronegative arthridities
    Reiter's syndrome
    Psoriatic arthritis
    Arthropathy of inflammatory bowel disease
    Undifferentiated spondyloarthropathies
Noninflammatory arthridities
    Osteoarthritis
    Gout
    Pseudogout
Seropositive arthridities
    Rheumatoid arthritis
    Lupus arthritis
Tuberculous spondylitis
Paget's disease
Parathyroid disease
Septic discitis

too nonspecific, and testing for the HLA-B27 allele in the ED is not feasible. Therefore, if the diagnosis has not been made already or the patient is unaware or unable to give a history of the disease, the emergency physician must rely on a high suspicion for the disease and recognition of radiographic clues in the appropriate clinical milieu.

DIAGNOSIS AND DIFFERENTIAL

Typically, ankylosing spondylitis presents with low back pain, which is also one of the most common presenting complaints to the emergency department (ED). This makes de novo diagnosis in the ED unlikely. However, the occasional undiagnosed patient may present with the typical clinical course, sacroiliitis, or the pathognomonic bamboo spine on radiographs. Thus it is important for the emergency physician to be able to identify this clinical constellation because it may have important implications for management of the patient. The differential diagnosis for ankylosing spondylitis is listed in Table 70-2.

There are no laboratory tests that are helpful in the acute setting for the diagnosis of ankylosing spondylitis. The erythrocyte sedimentation rate (ESR) and the C-reactive protein test, although readily available, are much

Radiographic Investigations

The sacral spine is typically the earliest involved region of the spine and the area where initial radiographic investigation is likely to provide a diagnosis. Sacroiliitis is usually symmetric and consists radiographically of blurring of the subchondral bone surface with erosions and sclerosis of adjacent bone. Usually these changes are more prominent on the iliac side of the joint (Fig. 70-1). In later stages of the disease, the vertebral column becomes almost completely fused, resulting in the pathognomonic bamboo spine. This consists of gradual ossification of the annulus fibrosis and eventual bridging of the vertebrae by syndesmophytes. This brings about the eventual squaring of the vertebral bodies and calcification of the intervertebral spaces with an undulating contour, leading to the characteristic bamboo appearance on lumbar spine radiographs (Fig. 70-2).

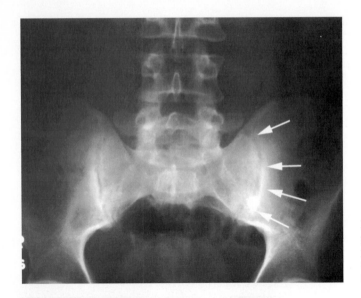

Fig. 70-1 Anteroposterior (AP) pelvis view of a patient with ankylosing spondylitis. Sacroiliitis is present bilaterally, as manifest by sclerosis of both sacroiliac joints with notable osseous erosions of adjacent bone (*arrows*).

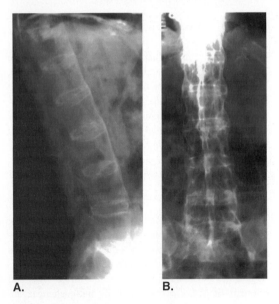

A.   **B.**

Fig. 70-2*A*. Lateral radiograph of the lumbar spine in a patient with ankylosing spondylitis. Note marked calcification of the intervertebral spaces and the undulating anterior contour of the spine classic for bamboo spine. *B*. AP radiograph of the lumbar spine in a patient with ankylosing spondylitis. There is marked calcification of the intervertebral spaces and an undulating contour characteristic of bamboo spine.

EMERGENCY DEPARTMENT CARE AND DISPOSITION

Patients with the advanced stages of ankylosing spondylitis, characterized by fusion and inflexibility of the cervical spine, can present special challenges to the emergency physician. The inflexibility of the cervical spine becomes particularly important when the patient is in respiratory distress or respiratory failure and in need of an artificial airway. Additionally, fusion of the spine eventually leads to immobility and subsequently osteoporosis. This can al-

low relatively minor trauma to cause significant injuries and disability.

Emergent airway management of a patient with an inflexible spine can prove to be exceedingly difficult. Historically, the anesthesia literature suggests awake fiberoptic-assisted intubation.[8] However, in the emergency setting, this modality is not always feasible or readily available. Until recently, the only reliable alternatives available to the emergency physician would have been cricothyrotomy, which is an invasive procedure with a potential for significant complications. Several reports in the recent literature have advocated the use of the Laryngeal Mask Airway or the LMA-Fastrach (LMA North America, Inc., San Diego, CA).[9–11] The Laryngeal Mask Airway, when used alone, is not a substitute for endotracheal intubation because it does not reliably protect the airway from the effects of regurgitation and aspiration. It is therefore relatively contraindicated in patients in whom fasting cannot be confirmed, as in most ED patients. The LMA-Fastrach, on the other hand, is a device designed to facilitate tracheal intubation with an endotracheal tube without requiring special positioning of the head or neck. With this device, the Laryngeal Mask Airway is placed, and then a specially adapted endotracheal tube is placed through the device into the trachea. The LMA is then removed while the endotracheal tube is left in place. It is a simple procedure to learn, is noninvasive, and has a high degree of success.

When patients with ankylosing spondylitis present to the ED with trauma, the physician should have a higher suspicion for spinal injury and a lower threshold for further workup of these patients. The immobilization brought about by ankylosis eventually results in osteoporosis and spinal fragility. Spinal fractures from minor traffic accidents are not uncommon. The C5 to C7 levels are the most commonly involved locations for traumatic fractures; therefore, adequate radiographs of this area are of the utmost importance.

Spinal epidural hematoma is a rare entity in the general population, but its incidence is much higher in patients with ankylosing spondylitis. In one series of 300 patients with spinal cord injury, 8 had ankylosing spondylitis, and of these, 4 had a spinal epidural hematoma. No spinal epidural hematoma was seen in any of the other 292 patients without ankylosing spondylitis.[12] Clinically, it manifests as an incomplete spinal cord injury with a subsequent deterioration in neurologic function. The deterioration is due to external spinal cord compression from a rapidly expanding epidural hematoma. Early detection and rapid surgical decompression are critical if neurologic function is to be preserved.

Atlanto-axial and atlanto-occipital subluxations are seen in patients with ankylosing spondylitis but not as commonly as seen in patients with rheumatoid arthritis. Subluxation can result from relatively inconsequential trauma, or it can occur spontaneously. Clinically, these injuries are characterized by symptoms of cord compression, and they carry a risk of sudden death. Again, the emergency physician must have a high degree of suspicion for injury in patients with ankylosing spondylitis who present with any neurologic complaints, regardless of the degree of trauma.

ADDITIONAL ASPECTS

The seronegative spondyloarthropathies, in particular ankylosing spondylitis, can present unique challenges to the emergency physician. In addition to being a cause of chronic sacral and back pain, its later stages, characterized by spinal ankylosis and fragility, can give rise to unexpected injuries and difficulties in airway management. Knowledge of the chronic sequelae of the disease and a high degree of suspicion for these complications can significantly alter ED management.

REFERENCES

1. Kerr H, Sturrock R: Clinical aspects, outcome assessment, disease course, and extra-articular features of spondyloarthropathies. *Curr Opin Rheumatol* 11:235, 1999.
2. Hyrich K, Inman R: Infectious agents in chronic rheumatic diseases. *Curr Opin Rheumatol* 13:300, 2001.
3. Reveille J, Ball E, Khan M: HLA-B27 and genetic predisposing factors in spondyloarthropathies. *Curr Opin Rheumatol* 13:265, 2001.
4. van der Linden S, van der Heijde D: Clinical aspects outcome assessment and management of ankylosing spondylitis and postenteric reactive arthritis. *Curr Opin Rheumatol* 12:263, 2000.
5. Yu D, Wiesenhutter C: HLA-B27 and the pathogenesis of Reiter's syndrome and ankylosing spondylitis. *Up to Date* 8(1), 2000.
6. Olivieri I, Salvarani C, Cantini F, et al: Ankylosing spondylitis and undifferentiated spondyloarthropathies: A clinical review and description of a disease subset with older age at onset. *Curr Opin Rheumatol* 13:280, 2001.
7. Gladman D: Clinical aspects of the spondyloarthropathies. *Am J Med Sci* 316:234, 1998.
8. Roberts K, Solgonick R: A modification of retrograde wire-guided, fiberoptic-assisted endotracheal intubation in a patient with ankylosing spondylitis. *Anesth Analg* 82:1290, 1996.
9. Hsin S, Chen C, Juan CH, et al: A modified method for intubation of a patient with ankylosing spondylitis using intubating Laryngeal Mask Airway (LMA-Fastrach): A case report. *Acta Anaesthesiol Sinica* 39:179, 2001.
10. Lu P, Brimacombe J, Ho A, et al: The intubating laryngeal mask airway in severe ankylosing spondylitis. *Can J Anaesth* 48:1015, 2001.
11. Defalque R, Hyder M: Laryngeal mask airway in severe cervical ankylosis. *Can J Anaesth* 44:305, 1997.
12. Wu C, Lee S: Spinal epidural hematoma and ankylosing spondylitis: Case report and review of the literature. *J Trauma* 44:558, 1998.

71

Depression and Suicide

Stephen W. Meldon
Sarah Delaney-Rowland

HIGH-YIELD FACTS

- Depression is the most common psychiatric disorder in community-dwelling older adults, with a prevalence of 2 to 10 percent for major depressive disorder and 15 to 30 percent for depressive symptoms.

- The prevalence of depression in older emergency department (ED) patients is approximately 30 percent.

- Risks for depression include female gender, single marital status, and lack of social support.

- Suicide rates are highest for older white males (five times the national average).

- Risk factors for suicide include depression, male gender, alcohol use, and recent death of a loved one.

- Pharmacotherapy, such as selective serotonin reuptake inhibitors (SSRIs), is an effective treatment for depression in this age group, with response rates of 60 to 80 percent.

Depression is the most common psychiatric disorder among elderly persons, yet it often remains unrecognized.[1] Depression contributes significantly to increased morbidity and mortality, diminished quality of life, and increased health care use and costs. Depression causes a decrease in functional well-being that is comparable to other chronic major medical problems[2] and results in increased health care use and an increased overall mortality compared with nondepressed persons.[3,4] Despite increased public awareness of depression and effective treatments for this disorder, depression in older adults remains underrecognized and undertreated. Furthermore, older adults are less likely to receive specialty mental health services and more likely to present to their primary care physicians and emergency department (ED). Studies involving older ED patients show that depression is very prevalent yet is generally unrecognized.[5–7]

An understanding of the prevalence and presentation of this common psychiatric disorder will enable emergency physicians to recognize and refer patients appropriately.

EPIDEMIOLOGY

The prevalence of major depressive disorder in community-dwelling older persons varies from approximately 2 to 10 percent.[8] However, estimation of the prevalence of late-life depression varies according to the criteria used and the characteristics of study population. In community-dwelling elderly adults, the prevalence of major depression is approximately 2 percent, and the prevalence of depressive symptoms is 15 to 30 percent.[9] Approximately 5 to 10 percent of older patients visiting primary care clinics have major depressive disorders or depressive symptoms.[10] Patients hospitalized for medical reasons experience depressive symptoms at a rate of 10 to 30 percent. In nursing home residents, the prevalence of major depression is approximately 10 percent, and the rate of depressive symptoms approaches 30 percent.[11] Studies using brief screening tools to evaluate geriatric ED patients have found fairly consistent prevalence rates of between 27 and 32 percent when ED patients over age 65 were screened for depression.[5–7] Depression has a significant impact on all-cause mortality. Older patients with depression have odds of dying 4 times greater than those of their nondepressed peers.[4]

Important social and demographic risk factors for major depression include female gender, divorced or separated status, low socioeconomic status, poor social support, comorbid medical illnesses, cognitive impairment, and adverse life stressors.

Suicide is the eighth leading cause of death in the United States. Older white males are among those at highest risk, with the rate of 67.6 per 100,000, which is five times higher than the national average.[12] Major social demographic risk factors for suicides among the elderly are old age, male gender, white race, and unmarried status. Often these suicidal patients are suffering from their first episode of major depression, which is moderately severe yet which has been unrecognized and untreated.[10] Importantly, most elderly persons who commit suicide communicate their suicidal ideation to either family or friends prior to killing themselves. Additionally, more than three-fourths of these individuals have visited a primary care physician for general medical problems or somatic complaints in the 1 month preceding their suicide.[13]

PATHOPHYSIOLOGY

Depression is thought to result from disruption of the normal brain neurochemistry. Current therapies are focusing on regulatory proteins that activate specific target genes including brain-derived neurotrophic factor (BDNF), a neuroprotective factor that results in hippocampal nerve growth. It is now known that psychological stress, important in the pathogenesis of depression, can decrease the production of BDNF and result in hippocampal neuronal atrophy. In addition, a series of brain imaging studies has consistently shown that there is reduced neuronal activity in the prefrontal cortex that varies with the severity of depression. It appears that stress-induced vulnerability in genetically susceptible people may induce a cascade of neuronal mechanisms that increases or decreases specific neurotrophic factors influencing the development of specific brain neurons and resulting in clinical depression.[14] Specific neurotransmitters that are thought to be involved in the pathogenesis of depression include seratonin, norepinephrine, and glucocorticoid levels.

Depression also appears to affect other organ systems and disease courses. Depressive illnesses have been shown to be associated with increased rates of death and disability from cardiovascular disease, independent of other major risk factors, including age, ventricular ejection fraction, and the presence of diabetes.[15,16] Current mechanistic hypotheses include impaired platelet functioning, decreased heart rate variability and immune system activation, and increased cortisol levels as stressor responses to depression.[17]

CLINICAL FEATURES

Depressed mood is the typical feature of depression. However, in older persons this may be less prominent than other depressive symptoms, such as loss of appetite, sleeplessness, and anhedonia (loss of interests in activities). Older depressed persons are more likely to express somatic complaints, have less feelings of guilt, and minimize the presence of depressed mood than younger depressed adults.

In addition, elder depressed persons are more likely than younger persons to have psychotic or delusional depression. Typical themes of delusional depression are guilt, hypochondriasis, nihilism, persecution, and jealousy.

Specific symptoms that would warrant assessment for depression include psychological symptoms of sadness, anhedonia, worthlessness, somatic complaints (nonspecific aches, changes in appetite and weight, sleep disturbances), and cognitive symptoms (slow thinking, poor concentration, and impaired memory). However, many of these symptoms overlap with comorbid medical illnesses and cognitive impairment syndromes (such as Alzheimer's), which can make the assessment of depression difficult.

Symptoms of major depression are shown in Table 71-1. Symptoms of depressed mood (dysthymia) are similar but generally less severe and lack suicidal ideation. An increased incidence of nonspecific complaints and the presence of underlying chronic illnesses, such as chronic obstructive pulmonary disease (COPD) or chronic pain syndromes, have been correlated with depression.[18,19] In a study of geriatric ED patients, nonspecific complaints were more common in depressed patients, but the difference was not statistically significant. In addition, the prevalence of depression did not vary significantly when analyzed by specific chronic illnesses.[20] Another study of older ED patients found that depressed patients were

Table 71-1. Symptoms of Major Depression

Depressed mood
Loss of interest (anhedonia)
Appetite change or weight loss
Changes in sleep patterns
Psychomotor agitation and retardation
Loss of energy and fatigue
Feelings of worthlessness or guilt
Difficulty with concentration
Suicidal ideation or thoughts of death

---

more likely to report lower income, lower educational level, more medical conditions, less independence, living in assisted living, and poor overall health status than non-depressed patients.[21] Similar results were found in an earlier study that reported a strong association between self-reported "poor health" status and depression.[5]

DIAGNOSIS AND DIFFERENTIAL

Despite intensive research on the biologic and structural correlates of depression, there are no specific diagnostic tests that can be used to diagnose depression in clinical practice. The current criterion standard for diagnosis is the diagnostic criteria from the *Diagnostic and Statistical Manual of Mental Disorders,* 4th edition (DSM-IV). Criteria for major depressive disorder include depressed mood or loss of interest or pleasure most of the time for 2 or more weeks, plus symptoms affecting four of the following categories: sleep, interest, guilt, energy, concentration, appetite, psychomotor, and suicide. Symptoms must cause clinically significant distress or impairment in important areas of functioning, not be due to direct physiologic effects of substances such as drugs or medications and should not be secondary to bereavement. Structured psychiatric interviews using DSM-IV criteria, however, are of limited utility in a primary care or ED setting. For this reason, a number of short questionnaires have been developed to help providers identify depression in these settings. Commonly used screening tools include the Geriatric Depression Scale Short Form[22] and a similarly brief (11-item) depression scale developed for medically ill patients.[23] Many of these scales are simple yes/no questionnaires with standardized cutoff values to detect depressive symptoms and major depression. However, even 11- to 15-item questionnaires can be difficult to use in the ED.

Additional studies have looked at even briefer depression screens. One study examined a 2-item depression screen that consisted of the following questions: (1) During the past month have you often been bothered by feeling down, depressed, or hopeless? and (2) During the past month have you often been bothered by little interest or pleasure in doing things?[24] In a separate validation and case-finding study, this instrument was found to have a sensitivity of 96 percent and a specificity of 57 percent in detecting depression.[25] However, this validation study was not confined to a geriatric population.

A recent study[7] examined a very brief screening tool to detect depression in elderly ED patients using the following three questions:

1. Do you often feel sad or depressed?
2. Do you often feel helpless?
3. Do you often feel downhearted and blue?

An affirmative response to any of these three questions was considered a positive screen. This brief screen was compared with the Geriatric Depression Scale and found to have a sensitivity of 79 percent, a specificity of 66 percent, and a negative predictive value of 87 percent for detecting depression. Sensitivity (89 percent), specificity (73 percent), and negative predictive value (94 percent) all increased when cognitively impaired patients were excluded.[7]

These brief depression screens should be considered useful screening tools for the ED setting that can alert providers to patients with depressive symptoms and major depression and allow for additional in-depth evaluation.

It is important to remember that many signs and symptoms of depressive syndromes overlap with manifestations of other medical and neurologic diseases. Medical conditions that may mimic depression include hypothyroidism and apathetic thyrotoxicosis (see Chap. 51) and neurologic conditions that have significant frontal lobe involvement (frontal lobe syndrome). In addition, there are a number of neurologic diseases that result in major depressive symptoms. In older persons, depression occurs in approximately 20 to 25 percent of patients suffering a stroke.[26] Basal ganglia and left hemispheric lesions, especially those close to the frontal pole, are more frequently associated with poststroke depression. Prevalence of depression in Parkinson's disease is estimated to be 40 percent.[27] In addition, depressive symptoms occur in approximately half of patients with cognitive impairment. Major depression occurs in 15 to 20 percent of patients with Alzheimer's disease.[27]

It is common for depression to adversely affect memory and cognition. Some depressed elderly patients develop a dementia syndrome, referred to as *pseudodementia,* that resolves either completely or partially after remission of depression. Pseuodementia is a cognitive impairment associated with depression and is characterized by decreased mental performance. It also can present as extreme general apathy, which also simulates dementia. One distinguishing feature between the two is cognitive performance during a mini-mental status examination; persons with dementia will make an effort to perform the tasks but often fail, whereas those who are depressed will make little effort but with persistent coaxing will perform the task successfully.[28] Interestingly, depression accompanied by reversal of dementia may be predictive of subsequent irreversible dementia. Distinguishing between these two disorders may be difficult. Patients reporting a history of a mood disturbance prior to cognitive impairment are much more likely to have pseudodementia; in addition, pseudodementia associated with depression has a much more rapid onset than other dementias.

EMERGENCY DEPARTMENT CARE AND DISPOSITION

The first management priority, if one suspects depression in older patients, is to assess suicide risk. Suicide is the most serious consequence of depression. Careful evaluation for suicidal ideation risk factors should be part of any evaluation when depression is suspected. Risk factors for suicide in older patients include a history of previous suicide attempts, hopelessness, comorbid physical illnesses, alcohol use, and lack of treatment for depression.[29] Suicide assessment also should include whether the patient has a well-formed plan, has access to firearms, has hoarded medications, has given away possessions, or has talked about death. Questions should be direct and supportive, such as "During the past month, have you felt sad and hopeless?" or "Have you felt that life is not worth living or wanted to end it all?"[30] Affirmative response to these questions should mandate a further psychiatric evaluation.

Treatment of depression in older adults can reduce excessive levels of disability and result in improved levels of functioning. Psychotherapy, drug therapy, and electroconvulsive therapy (ECT) used alone or in combination have been shown to be effective in geriatric depression.[10,27] Therapy with an antidepressant agent is the preferred treatment in cases of moderate to severe depression. Although antidepressive therapy typically is not initiated in the ED, antidepressant medications, including the selective serotonin reuptake inhibitors (SSRIs), will be reviewed briefly. The rate of response to an antidepressant is approximately 60 percent and improves to 80 percent if a second medication is tried after an initial antidepressant drug failure.[31,32] The SSRIs are a common, preferred treatment for acute episodes of depression in the elderly because of their favorable side-effect profile, relative safety, ease of use, and smaller dose adjustments. Unlike tricyclic antidepressants, SSRIs have minimal cardiovascular effects and, because of less anticholinergic toxicity, do not worsen cognition.

Common side effects of SSRIs include nausea, diarrhea, insomnia, sedation, headache, agitation, and anxiety. Less common adverse effects include SSRI-induced syndrome of inappropriate antidiuretic hormone secretion (SIADH), extrapyramidal symptoms, and bradycardia.[13] In trials that directly compared SSRIs with tricyclic antidepressants (TCAs), the SSRIs fluoxetine, sertraline, and paroxetine were roughly equivalent to TCAs, with a response to treatment of about 60 to 80 percent.[13] Sertaline was found to have a significant advantage among patients age 70 and over with respect to response time and duration of remission. As with all medications in this age group, recommendations are to "start low and go slow" (i.e., use low initial doses and increase them gradually). Recommendations for length of maintenance treatment are at least for 6 months of treatment after recovery for those with first-onset late-life depression and at least 12 months for those with recurrent depression.

Older adults who suffer from depression are also likely to benefit from psychotherapeutic interventions. Cognitive-behavioral and interpersonal psychotherapies seem to be the most effective psychological interventions for late-life depression.[13]

Patients with significant depressive symptoms or suicidality or those with significant potential for suicide risk require an emergency psychiatric evaluation or admission. Patients with less severe depressive symptoms may be discharged home with family once outpatient follow-up has been arranged.

ADDITIONAL ASPECTS

There is some controversy regarding routine screening of older ED patients for depression. The report by the Society for Academic Emergency Medicine Public Health and Education Task Force Preventative Services Work Group noted that there was insufficient evidence to recommend either for or against instituting routine depression screens in the ED.[33] However, given the impact of geriatric depression, the risk of suicide, and the lack of recognition of geriatric depression by emergency physicians,[5,6] screening with brief instruments such as the three-item depression screening instrument may be indicated.

REFERENCES

1. Holt J, Alexopoulos G: Depression and the aged, in Robinson R, Rabins P (eds): *Depression and Coexisting Disease.* New York: Igaku-Shoin Medical, 1989, p 10.
2. Wells KB Steward A, Hay RD, et al: The functioning and well-being of depressed patients: Results from the Medical Outcomes Study. *JAMA* 262:914, 1989.

3. Hoeper EW, Nycz GR, Regier DA, et al: Diagnosis of mental disorders in adults and increased use of health services in four outpatient settings. *Am J Psychiatry* 137:207, 1980.

4. Bruce ML, Leaf PJ: Psychiatric disorders and 15-month mortality in a community sample of older adults. *Am J Public Health* 79:727, 1989.

5. Meldon SW, Emerman CL, Schubert DS, et al: Depression in geriatric ED patients: Prevalence and recognition. *Ann Emerg Med* 30:141, 1997.

6. Meldon SW, Emerman CL, Schubert DS: Recognition of depression in geriatric ED patients by emergency physicians. *Ann Emerg Med* 30:442, 1997.

7. Fabacher DA, Raccio-Robak N, McErlean MA: Validation of a brief screening tool to detect depression in elderly ED patients. *Am J Emerg Med* 20:99, 2002.

8. Unutzer J, Katon W, Sullivan M, et al: Treating depressed older adults in primary care: Narrowing the gap between efficacy and effectiveness. *Milbank Q* 77:225, 1999.

9. Montgomery SA, Beekman AFT, Sadavoy J, et al: Consensus statement on depression in the elderly: Primary care companion. *J Clin Psychiatry* 2:46, 2000.

10. NIH Consensus Conference: NIH Consensus Development Panel on Depression in Late Life: Diagnosis and treatment of depression in late life. *JAMA* 268:1018, 1992.

11. Blazer DG: Depression in the elderly: Myths and misconceptions. *Psychiatr Clin North Am* 20:111, 1997.

12. Jacobs DG: A 52-year old suicidal man. *JAMA* 283:2693, 2000.

13. Lebowitz BD, Person JL, Schneider LS, et al: Diagnosis and treatment of depression in late life: Consensus statement update. *JAMA* 278:1186, 1997.

14. Remick RA: Diagnosis and management of depression in primary care: A clinical update and review. *Can Med Assoc J* 167:1253, 2000.

15. Frasure-Smith N, Lespearance F, Talajic M: Depression and 19-month prognosis after myocardial infarction. *Circulation* 91:999, 1995.

16. Bush DE, Ziegelstein RC, Tayback M, et al: Even minimal symptoms of depression increase mortality risk after acute myocardial infarction. *Am J Cardiol* 88:337, 2001.

17. Musselman DL, Evans DL, Nemeroff CB: The relationship of depression to cardiovascular disease. *Arch Gen Psychiatry* 55:580, 1998.

18. Gerber PD, Barret JE, Barret JA: The relationship of presenting physical complaints to depressive symptoms in primary care patients. *J Gen Intern Med* 7:170, 1992.

19. Wilson DR, Widmer RB, Cadoret RJ, et al: Somatic symptoms: A major feature of depression in a family practice. *J Affect Disord* 5:199, 1983.

20. Meldon SW, Emerman CL, Moffa DA, et al: Utility of clinical characteristics in identifying depression in geriatric ED patients. *Am J Emerg Med* 17:522, 1999.

21. Raccio-Robak N, McErlean MA, Fabacher DA, et al: Socioeconomic and health status differences between depressed and nondepressed ED elders. *Am J Emerg Med* 20:71, 2002.

22. Sheikh JI, Yesavage JA: Geriatric depression scale: Recent evidence and development of a shorter version. *Clin Gerontol* 5:165, 1986.

23. Koenig HG, Cohen HJ, Blazer DG, et al: A brief depression scale for use in the medically ill. *Int J Psychiatr Med* 22:183, 1992.

24. Spitzer RL, Williams JB, Kroenke K, et al: Utility of a new procedure for diagnosing mental disorders in primary care. The PRIME-MD 1000 study. *JAMA* 272:1749, 1994.

25. Whooley MA, Avins AL, Miranda J, et al: Case-finding instruments for depression. *J Gen Intern Med* 12:439, 1997.

26. Rao R: Cerebrovascular disease and late life depression: An age old association revisited. *Int J Geriatr Psychiatry* 15:419, 2000.

27. Alexopoulos GS: Depression and other mood disorders. *Clin Geriatr* 8:69, 2000.

28. Evers MM, Marin DB: Effective management of major depressive disorder in the geriatric patient. *Geriatrics* 57:36, 2002.

29. Sable JA, Dunn LB, Zisook S: Late life depression: How to identify its symptoms and provide effective treatment. *Geriatrics* 57:18, 2002.

30. Lantz MS: Suicide in late life: Identifying and managing at-risk older patients. *Geriatrics* 56:47, 2001.

31. Joffe R, Sokolov S, Streiner D: Antidepressant treatment of depression: A meta-analysis. *Can J Psychiatry* 41:613, 1996.

32. Moller HJ, Fuger J, Kasper S: Efficacy of new generation antidepressant: Meta-analysis of imipramine-controlled studies. *Pharmacopsychiatry* 27:215, 1994.

33. Irvin B, Wyer PC, Gerson LW: Preventive care in the emergency department: II. Clinical preventive services—An emergency medicine evidence-based review. Society for Academic Emergency Medicine Public Health and Education Task Force Preventive Services Work Group. *Acad Emerg Med* 7:1042, 2000.

72

Psychosis

Stephen W. Meldon
Sarah Delaney-Rowland

HIGH-YIELD FACTS

- Psychosis may be functional or due to a number of organic etiologies.
- Psychotic symptoms are present in about 15 percent of depressed patients.
- Neurologic diseases, such as Alzheimer's and Parkinson's, often present with psychotic features.
- The newer atypical antipsychotics are the treatment of choice for severe symptoms or agitation.
- Psychosis should be considered to be organic (nonpsychiatric) until proven otherwise.

Psychoses are defined as disturbances in thought processing and behavior leading to a loss of contact with reality. *Acute psychosis* is a general term that refers to any major mental disorder of a psychiatric or emotional etiology that results in thought disturbances and personality derangement. New-onset psychoses are relatively uncommon in older persons. The most common functional causes in the elderly are psychotic depression, delusional disorders, and late-onset schizophrenia (LOS). A more recent nomenclature has been introduced that refers to LOS occurring after age 60 as *very-late-onset schizophrenia-like psychosis.*[1]

EPIDEMIOLOGY

Estimates of the incidence and prevalence of schizophrenia in geriatric persons are difficult to obtain because some diagnostic criteria exclude late-onset cases and many prevalence studies did not include patients older than 60 years of age. For individuals over age 65, the community prevalence of schizophrenia ranges from 0.1 to 0.5

percent.[2,3] The prevalence of paranoid ideation in the general elderly population is estimated to be around 5 percent, with the majority of these patients having dementia.[4]

PATHOPHYSIOLOGY

Etiologies and distinctive pathophysiologies of schizophrenia are at present unknown. There is no evidence that a progressive dementing disorder is associated with LOS or very-late-onset schizophrenia-like psychosis. Female gender is associated with LOS. Very-late-onset cases may arise in the context of sensory impairment and social isolation.[5]

Psychotic depression and delusional disorders also may cause acute psychoses in older persons. *Delusional disorder* is defined as persistent delusions without evidence of schizophrenia or mood disorders and without prominent hallucinations or evidence of organic dysfunction.[6] Delusional disorders are more common in the elderly population, especially women. Psychotic symptoms occur in about 15 percent of all depressed patients. Psychotic depression also appears to be slightly more prevalent in the geriatric population when compared with younger adults and results in more cognitive impairment than nonpsychotic depression.[7]

Risk factors for psychotic symptoms in the elderly include cognitive impairment, female gender, chronic bed rest, sensory impairment, and social isolation.

CLINICAL FEATURES

Psychosis in older persons must be differentiated from other causes of altered mental status, such as coma, dementia, and delirium (see Chap. 39).

Important historical information includes the onset and course of the episode, the presence of hallucinations and delusions, and whether there is a prior psychiatric history. The onset may be variable, but the course over days is often stable. Cognition may be selectively impaired, and attention may be abnormally high or low. In contrast to delirium, attention is not invariably disordered. Hallucinations are predominantly auditory, and delusions are often sustained, complex, and systematized. Psychomotor activity may be variably affected, and agitation is frequent. Speech is typically coherent. Early and LOS are similar in terms of symptomatology. However, extreme old age onset is associated with less evidence of a formal thought disorder and a higher prevalence of visual hallucinations.[8]

The physical examination should focus on assessment of vital signs, general appearance, and neurologic examination. A cardiovascular assessment should consider congestive heart failure and myocardial infarction. Evidence should be sought for infectious processes; fluid, electrolyte, and metabolic derangements; and central nervous system disorders (subdural hematomas, CNS infections). Environmental etiology (heat stroke) and intoxication/withdrawal syndromes should be additional areas of focus.

DIAGNOSIS AND DIFFERENTIAL

The diagnosis of psychosis should be one of exclusion, especially in the older age group. There are no specific tests that can be used to diagnose psychosis in the clinical setting. Furthermore, neuropsychiatric disorders such as psychosis may occur alone or in combination with other neurologic or medical illness.[9,10] For example, psychotic symptoms, such as paranoid delusions and hallucinations (which are more commonly visual), occur in up to one-third of patients with Alzheimer's dementia. The differential diagnosis is fairly extensive and includes both functional and medical etiologies (Table 72-1).

Altered mental status should be characterized as a decreased *level* of consciousness or disturbed *content* of consciousness. Disturbed content of consciousness includes delirium, dementia, and psychosis.[11]

Initial emergency department (ED) diagnostic tests that should be considered in all older patients with mental status changes include serum electrolytes and glucose, blood urea nitrogen (BUN) and creatinine, calcium, urinalysis, arterial blood gases and pulse oximetry, a chest radiograph, and an electrocardiogram. Additional tests should be based on patient presentation and clinical picture. Considerations for selected patients include neuroimaging (computed tomography and magnetic resonance imaging), lumbar puncture, toxicologic screens (including alcohol and serum ammonia levels), and thyroid function tests.[11]

EMERGENCY DEPARTMENT CARE AND DISPOSITION

Immediate management priorities are to diagnose and address serious medical etiologies that might present as psychosis. Rapid determination of blood glucose concentration should be performed in all patients with mental status alterations. Thiamine also should be considered depending on the history and presentation. After rapid assessment and stabilization, altered mental status should be characterized as a decreased *level* of consciousness or disturbed *content* of consciousness. Disturbed content of consciousness should then be further delineated into delirium, dementia, and psychosis.[11]

This distinction between and diagnosis of an underlying etiology may be difficult. Frequent reevaluation is essential. In this age group it is wise to assume that changes in behavior and mental status are nonpsychiatric until a comprehensive workup has been completed.

General management principles are to discover and treat underlying etiologies and address identifiable psychosocial triggers.[12] Management of severe psychotic symptoms, such as severe agitation and threatening behavior, may require the use of antipsychotic agents. Use of the newer atypical antipsychotics, such as olanzapine and risperidone, is recommended because of efficacy and a safer side-effect profile.[13–15] Use of conventional neuroleptics in older patients is associated with high rates of tardive dyskinesia, especially in the setting of alcohol abuse and preexisting movement disorders.[16]

The management and disposition of the acutely psy-

Table 72-1. Differential Diagnosis of Psychosis

Psychiatric	Major depression, schizophrenia, delusional disorder
Neurologic	Dementia, Parkinson's, stroke, tumor, temporal lobe seizure
Medical	Hypo- and hyperglycemia, hypo- and hyperthyroidism, electrolyte imbalance, Cushing's syndrome, B_{12} deficiency
Drugs	Anticholinergic agents, antiparkinsonian agents, benzodiazepines and alcohol (including withdrawal), opiates, corticosteroids, stimulants
Delirium	
Pain	

Source: Adapted from Reuben DB, Herr K, Pacala JT, et al: *Geriatrics at Your Fingertips,* 2002 ed. Malden, MA: Blackwell Sciences, Inc., for the American Geriatrics Society, 2002, p 128.

chotic older patient will depend on patient presentation and the diagnosis, as well as existing patient social support systems. Psychiatric consultation in the ED setting may be warranted. Episodes that are severe enough to present to the ED generally warrant an admission to the hospital for observation and further evaluation and management.

ADDITIONAL ASPECTS

The number of elderly persons with psychosis likely will increase as the geriatric population increases. Psychosis in this population will represent early-onset (as younger patients with schizophrenia age), late-onset, and very-late-onset schizophrenia-like psychosis. Likewise, the prevalence of neurologic diseases, such as Alzheimer's dementia and Parkinson's disease, which can present with psychosis, also will increase.

Psychiatric disposition prior to a thorough medical and neurologic evaluation in older persons with psychosis should be discouraged.

REFERENCES

1. Howard R, Rabins PV, Seeman MV: Late-onset schizophrenia and very-late-onset schizophrenia-like psychosis: An international consensus. *Am J Psychiatry* 57:172, 2000.
2. Copeland JRM, Dewey ME, Scott A, et al: Schizophrenia and delusional disorder in older age: Community prevalence, incidence, comorbidity and outcome. *Schizophr Bull* 24:153, 1998.
3. Castle DJ, Murray RM: The epidemiology of late-onset schizophrenia. *Schizophr Bull* 19:691, 1993.
4. Forsell Y, Henderson AS: Epidemiology of paranoid symptoms in an elderly population. *Br J Psychiatry* 172:429, 1998.
5. Kay DWK, Roth M: Environmental and hereditary factors in the schizophrenias of old age ("late paraphrenia") and their bearing on the general problem of causation in schizophrenia. *J Ment Sci* 107:649, 1961.
6. Lacro JP, Jeste DV: Geriatric psychosis. *Psychiatr Q* 68:247, 1997.
7. Jests DV, Heaton SC, Paulsen JS, et al: Clinical and neuropsychological comparison of psychotic depression with nonpsychotic depression and schizophrenia. *Am J Psychiatry* 153:490, 1996.
8. Howard R, Castle D, Wessely S, et al: A comparative study of 470 cases of early- and late-onset schizophrenia. *Br J Psychiatry* 163:352, 1993.
9. Jenike MA: Psychiatric illnesses in the elderly: A review. *J Geriatr Psychiatry Neurol* 9:57, 1996.
10. Factor SA, Molho ES: Emergency department presentations of patients with Parkinson's disease. *Am J Emerg Med* 18:209, 2000.
11. Kalbfleisch N: Altered mental status, in Sanders AB (ED): *Emergency Care of the Elder Person.* St louis, Beverly Cracom Publications, 1996, p 119.
12. Reuben DB, Herr K, Pacala JT, et al: *Geriatrics at Your Fingertips,* 2002 ed. Malden, MA: Blackwell Sciences, for the American Geriatrics Society, 2002, p 128.
13. Madhusoodanan S, Sinha S, Brenner R, et al: Use of olanzapine for elderly patients with psychotic disorders: A review. *Ann Clin Psychiatry* 3:201, 2001.
14. Daniel DG: Antipsychotic treatment of psychosis and agitation in the elderly. *J Clin Psychiatry* 61:49, 2000.
15. Bhana N, Spencer CM: Risperidone: A review of its use in the management of the behavioural and psychological symptoms of dementia. *Drugs Aging* 16:451, 2000.
16. Jests DV, Caligiuri MP, Paulsen JS: Risk of tardive dyskinesia in older patients: A prospective longitudinal study of 266 outpatients. *Arch Gen Psychiatry* 52:756, 1995.

73

Alcoholism in the Elderly

James W. Campbell

HIGH-YIELD FACTS

- Older patients presenting to the emergency department (ED) should be screened for alcoholism.

- Pharmacokinetic changes and increased ratio of body fat to body water make alcohol more potent in older persons.

- No laboratory tests or physical examination findings perform as well as screening tools. Most detect late-stage disease or have very low specificity.

- Short, consequence-based questionnaires are the best screening tools. Quantity and frequency inquiries perform poorly as screening for alcohol problems.

- Heavy alcohol use and alcohol abuse are associated with falls, osteoporosis, and hip fractures.

- Alcohol-induced dementia (which is often mistaken for progressive degenerative dementia of the Alzheimer's type) improves significantly with sobriety.

Alcoholism is a high-prevalence illness in older populations. Fourteen percent of elders presenting to an emergency department (ED) have diagnosable alcoholism.[1] Alcoholism is appropriately screened for with short, consequence-based questionnaires. More in-depth reviews can confirm the diagnosis. Alcoholism is a serious cause of morbidity and mortality among seniors. Alcoholism is treated successfully at all ages, and success rates are actually greater in older populations. The ED is a very likely location for the diagnosis to first be suspected. Brief intervention is an effective tool to initiate treatment and is practical in the ED setting.

EPIDEMIOLOGY

Alcoholism is present in 6 to 11 percent of older persons admitted to the hospital.[1] Alcohol use significant enough to impair health is present in up to 20 percent of patients hospitalized on medical-surgical units. Alcoholism is the third most common psychiatric disorder among older persons. Up to 16 percent of men and 8 percent of women have alcohol use disorders.[2] Despite screening tools with good sensitivity and specificity being available, screening is often ignored. Older women represent the most underdiagnosed population. Twelve percent of older women regularly drink in excess, and older women have a swifter progression to alcohol-related illnesses.[3] The rates of use of nonprescribed "illicit" drugs are thought to be low; a national comorbidity study suggests that illicit drug use declines with age.[4] As the baby boomers age, this picture may change.

Substance-related disorders of all types remain overlooked in geriatric patients. Smoking is still one of the most medically damaging substances. The Center for Medicare and Medicaid Studies is of the opinion that smoking is the single most preventable cause of illness. Over 10 percent of the population aged 65 years and over are smokers, specifically 12.9 percent of persons aged 65 to 74 smoke, and 6.1 percent of persons over age 75 smoke. Smokers over age 65 are identified as the most likely to benefit from smoking cessation. Treatment based on brief intervention and 12-step programs is effective in all substance abuse disorders.

Nomenclature is complicated in this field, but a simple method of approaching any alcohol use that is deleterious to health in a broad biopsychosocial format is appropriate. Alcoholism may be subcategorized as chronic or late-onset depending on the presentation of first symptoms before or after age 65. These two groups do not perform significantly differently on screening tests or in treatment. The language used regarding leukemia is useful to emphasize the medical model. Alcoholism can be considered to be active or in remission, with activities such as relapse prevention groups functioning as mechanisms to prolong a remission.

PATHOPHYSIOLOGY

The elderly patient's metabolism of various substances is unique based on the altered pharmacokinetics present in older individuals. A decrease in gastric acid secretion impairs absorption, but slowed gastric motility increases absorption. Clearance of many toxins is decreased as a result of decreased liver and kidney mass as well as decreased flow rates through both these organs. This results in a high-risk situation with drug concentrations often higher than expected. Serum creatinine can be deceiving; the decreased creatinine source pool in a thin, older patient can mean that a "normal" serum creatinine level may represent a patient with significant impairment in clearance. Drug receptor sensitivity changes lead to inconsistent drug activity. The volume of distribution of water-soluble agents is altered as the body-fat-to-body-water ratio changes with age. A standard dose of alcohol (1.5 oz of liquor, 4 oz of wine, or 12 oz of beer) produces a much higher blood alcohol concentration in an older person than a younger person of the same weight. Alcoholism is a heritable disease. Genetic predisposition is estimated to account for 40 to 60 percent of the etiology of the disease of alcoholism.[5]

CLINICAL FEATURES

Classic clinical clues of alcoholism are often mistakenly attributed to age-related changes or diseases common in old age (Table 73-1). The negative consequences that cause a younger person to seek help—job loss, divorce, or legal pressures—are less likely to occur in older persons. The use of other substances, particularly nicotine, should serve as a red flag to increase your suspicion that an older person may have a drinking problem. Seventy percent of alcoholics smoke more than 20 cigarettes a day compared with 10 percent of the general population.[5] Alcohol abuse should be investigated in patients with anxiety and depression. Hip fractures should trigger screening for alcoholism because research has shown a 2.6 times increased risk of hip fracture over 5 years in pa-

tients with a history of admission for alcohol-related disorders.[6] Physical examination finding consistent with alcoholism occur late in the disease process.

DIAGNOSIS AND DIFFERENTIAL

The best definition of harmful use of any substance is *use resulting in a negative consequence followed by continued use.* Negative consequences can be in the arenas of medical, legal, family, occupational, social, psychological, and/or economic. In older persons, social, family and health consequences are most prevalent. Older persons can have negative effects despite lower quantity and frequency of use. Older persons presenting to the ED for congestive heart failure, dementia, depression, delirium, falls, fractures, hypertension, incontinence, insomnia, malnutrition, sexual dysfunction, gastrointestinal complaints, and many other conditions actually may have underlying alcoholism.

Alcohol abuse in older persons also can exacerbate virtually any chronic illness, even if the condition is not caused primarily by alcohol.

No laboratory screening test with reasonable sensitivity and specificity exists. Elevations in mean corpuscular volume (MCV) and Gamma Glutamyl Transpeptidase (γGT) are reasonably sensitive but very nonspecific. Aspartate Amino-transferase (AST) and Alanine Amino-transferase (ALT) elevations most often represent late-stage disease. Carbohydrate-deficient transferrin (CDT currently available at specialized centers) is analogous to Hemoglobin Alc (glycosylated hemoglobin) in diabetes because a permanently altered protein possibly gives a measure of alcohol intake over time. CDT offers more promise as a monitor of treatment as opposed to a screening tool.

Table 73-1. Emergency Presentations of Alcoholism Misattributed to Diseases Common in Old Age

Clue	Disease	Alcohol
Cognitive impairment	Alzheimer's type dementia	Alcohol direct cause of dementia, Wernicke-Korsakoff syndrome, and delirium
Congestive heart failure	Ischemic heart disease	Alcohol-induced cardiomyopathy
Elevated blood pressure	Essential hypertension	Alcohol direct cause of secondary BP elevation
Delirium	Dementia	Alcohol directly causes DTs and confusion
Fall	Gait instability ± osteoarthritis	Alcohol increases risk of falls directly
Fracture	Osteoporosis	Alcohol directly induces falls and osteoporosis
Incontinence	Urinary tract infection	Alcohol-induced diuresis
Pneumonia	Community-acquired pneumonia	Alcohol-induced aspiration

A brief questionnaire is an appropriate screen for all elders presenting to the ED. The CAGE questionnaire exhibits excellent sensitivity, especially with the geriatric corrected positive score of one positive answer (91 percent sensitive, 48 percent specific).[7] This tool has four simple questions based on the CAGE mnemonic:

1. Have you ever felt you should *c*ut down on your drinking?

2. Have people *a*nnoyed you by criticizing your drinking?

3. Have you ever felt bad or *g*uilty about your drinking?

4. Have you ever had a drink first thing in the morning to steady your nerves or get rid of a hangover (i.e., as an *e*ye opener)?

The interview process is important because the CAGE becomes less sensitive if preceded by questions on quantity and frequency. The CAGE often can indicate the diagnosis even in a patient with significant denial. The patient may offer as evidence of his or her control his or her ability to cut down. The simple fact that he or she is working to limit his or her intake helps make the diagnosis of alcoholism. Another more recently developed tool, the Alcohol-Related Problems Survey (short version; ARPS), also exhibits 92 percent sensitivity and 51 percent specificity.[8]

Standardized diagnostic interviews are the current "gold standard" for diagnosis. Many of these diagnostic interviews are hours in length; however, the geriatric version of the Michigan Alcoholism Screening Test (G-MAST short version) is one of the best practical-length tools available (Fig. 73-1). This brief screening tool has been shown to have 94 percent sensitivity and 78 percent specificity when compared with a longitudinal evaluation done by an expert employing all available data.[9] Its brevity makes it useful in the ED setting.

Alcoholism is in the differential diagnosis as an etiology or exacerbating factor in almost all the geriatric syndromes: cognitive impairment, delirium, depression, falls, functional decline, osteoporosis, polypharmacy, and urinary incontinence. Likewise, alcohol abuse, heavy alcohol use, or alcoholism can be a direct etiologic factor or a clear cause of worsening of diseases prevalent in old age. As many as 10 percent of demented elders are suffering from an alcohol-induced dementia. This dementia is one of the most responsive to treatment. Alcoholic dementia remains very underdiagnosed. Another important consideration is the differentiation of aging from substance abuse disorders. Table 73-2 lists examples of presentations symptomatic of pathologic alcohol use often incorrectly attributed to aging.

Table 73-2. Clinical Clues to the Diagnosis of Alcoholism Misattributed to "Normal" Aging

Decreased social support
Frequent ED visits
Functional decline
Gait instability
Impaired driving
Increased use of analgesics
Increased use of OTC drugs
Motor vehicle accidents
Peripheral neuropathy
Poor dentition
Poor nutrition
Self-neglect
Trauma
Slow postanesthetic recovery

EMERGENCY DEPARTMENT CARE AND DISPOSITION

In the ED an organized approach to screening, diagnosis, management, and disposition of substance abuse in elders is essential. An approach for seniors is summarized in Fig. 73-2. Substance abuse treatment centers on Alcoholics Anonymous (AA) and similar long-term programs. Brief intervention done in an ED setting is often effective to initiate recovery.[10] Family involvement is key to success in any treatment. The standard sobriety prescription includes (1) discontinue all substance use, (2) attend 90 meetings in the first 90 days, and (3) become active in a long-term program and attend meetings regularly. AA is readily available and can be applied for any substance abuse disorder. Formal research on AA is by definition difficult, however; studies have shown attendance at 90 meetings in the first 90 days to be the most powerful predictor of long-term sobriety. AA is senior-appropriate, and a third of all calls to AA are from persons over age 55. In contrast to classic theory, a nonjudgmental approach without "labeling" appears to be more effective in older persons. Elders often are strongly averse to accepting the label *alcoholic* and are able to enter into treatment more readily by accepting their drinking as unhealthy. Presenting sobriety in the framework of hope is a far more successful strategy for behavior change than fear or shame.

1. After drinking have you ever noticed an increase in your heart rate or beating in your chest?

2. When talking with others, do you ever underestimate how much you actually drink?

3. Does alcohol make you sleepy so that you often fall asleep in your chair?

4. After a few drinks, have you sometimes not eaten or been able to skip a meal because you don't feel hungry?

5. Does having a few drinks help decrease your shakiness or tremors?

6. Does alcohol sometimes make it hard for you to remember parts of the day or night?

7. Do you have rules for yourself that you won't drink before a certain time of day?

8. Have you lost interest in hobbies or activities you used to enjoy?

9. When you wake up in the morning do you have trouble remembering part of the night before?

10. Does having a drink help you sleep?

11. Do you hide your alcohol bottles from family members?

12. After a social gathering, have you ever felt embarrassed because you drank too much?

13. Have you ever been concerned that drinking might be harmful to your health?

14. Do you like to end an evening with a night cap?

15. Did you find your drinking increased after someone close to you died?

16. In general, would you prefer to have a few drinks at home rather than go out to social events?

17. Are you drinking more now than in the past?

18. Do you usually take a drink to relax or calm your nerves?

19. Do you drink to take your mind off your problems?

20. Have you ever increased your drinking after experiencing a loss in your life?

21. Do you sometimes drive when you have had too much to drink?

22. Has a doctor or nurse ever said they were worried or concerned about your drinking?

23. Have you ever made rules to mange your drinking?

24. When you feel lonely does having a drink help?

QUESTIONS SHOULD BE ANSWERED "YES" OR "NO". SCORING 5 OR MORE "YES' RESPONSES IS INDICATIVE OF AN ALCOHOL PROBLEM.

Fig. 73-1 Michigan Alcoholism Screening Test Geriatric Version (MAST-G).

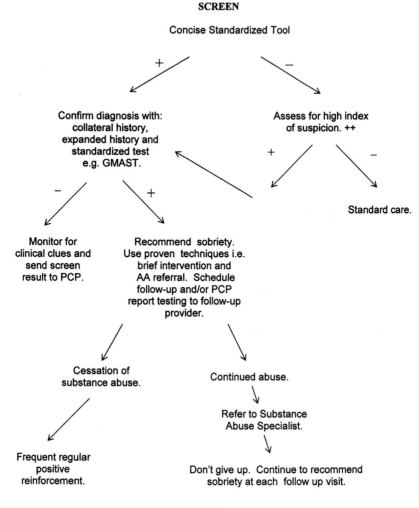

Fig. 73-2 Clinical approach to alcoholism in elders.

Alcohol detoxification needs to be closely managed. The older patient is more susceptible to medical complications of withdrawal. Similarly, drugs such as Antabuse are of limited utility in older persons because an Antabuse reaction may have major medical consequences or be potentially fatal. Naltrexone, a pharmacologic adjunct to treatment, although well grounded in appropriate physiology, prevents the "high" from substance use, and therefore should lessen risk of relapse. However, it is of limited utility because of cost.

A key fact to remember is that treatment is actually more likely to be successful in older persons. Initiation of treatment for substance abuse disorders through brief intervention has been found to be effective in older patients. Brief intervention including education of patients regarding risks and benefits of continued use, combined with one follow-up resulted in a significant success rate on the order of 10 to 15 percent. This rate is low in absolute terms but extremely high compared with the success of treatment of other chronic diseases in two visits. Older patients completing treatment showed significant change in most areas targeted, including motivation, cognition, and interpersonal support, showing improvement.[11] The improved prognosis compared with younger individuals may be due to the fact that the older cohort has single-substance abuse.

ADDITIONAL ASPECTS

There is debate regarding the beneficial effects of low-dose drinking. In younger persons, low-dose controlled alcohol use may improve cardiovascular risk factors. No clear evidence exists of benefits from drinking for elders. On the contrary, many diseases and medications used by the elderly have contraindications to alcohol use.

Interactions between alcohol and prescription and over-the-counter (OTC) medications are potentially serious problems, especially in older persons.[12] Two-thirds of older persons use OTC medications, and two-thirds of the OTC use is analgesics, including aspirin, nonsteroidal anti-inflammatory drugs (NSAIDs), and acetaminophen products. Acetaminophen specifically interacts with alcohol and can form a dangerous drug-drug interaction with toxin formation. This phenomenon is exacerbated by heavy alcohol use. Acetaminophen highlights another concern; this ingredient is found in many OTC and prescription combination agents and therefore can be ingested accidentally in toxic doses.

REFERENCES

1. National Institute on Alcohol Abuse and Alcoholism: *Alcohol Alert No. 40: Alcohol and Aging.* Bethesda, MD, NIAAA, April 1998.
2. Menninger JA: Assessment and treatment of alcoholism and substance related disorders in the elderly. *Bull Menninger Clin* 66(2):166, 2002.
3. Blow FC: Treatment of older women with alcohol problems: Meeting the challenge for a special population. *Alcohol Clin Exp Res* 24(8):1257, 2000.
4. Hinkin CH, Castellon SA, Dickson-Fuhrman E: Screening for drug and alcohol abuse among older adults using a modified version of the CAGE. *Am J Addict* 10:319, 2001.
5. Enoch M, Goldman D: Problem drinking and alcoholism: Diagnosis and treatment. *Am Fam Phys* 65:441, 2002.
6. Yuan Z, Dawson N, Cooper G, et al: Effects of alcohol-related disease on hip fracture and mortality: A retrospective cohort study of hospitalized Medicare beneficiaries. *Am J Public Health* 91:1089, 2001.
7. Buchsbaum DG, Buchanan BA, Welsh MA, et al. Screening for drinking in the elderly using the CAGE questionnaire. *J Am Geriatr Soc* 40:662, 1992.
8. Moore AA, Beck JC, Babor TF, et al: Beyond alcoholism: Identifying older, at risk drinkers in primary care. *J Stud Alcohol* 63:316, 2002.
9. Widlitz M, Marin DB. Substance abuse in older adults: An Overview. *Geriatrics*. 57:29, 2002.
10. Arndt S, Schultz SK, Turvey C, et al: Screening for alcoholism in the primary care setting: Are we talking to the right people? *J Fam Pract* 51(1):41, 2002.
11. Lemke S, Moos RH: Prognosis of older patients in mixed-age alcoholism treatment programs. *J Subst Abuse Treat* 22(1):2, 2002.
12. Rigler SK: Alcoholism in the elderly. *Am Fam Phys* 15(61):1710, 2000.

RELEVANT WORLD WIDE WEB SITES

www.cms.hhs.gov/healthyaging/1b.asp: Issues related to tobacco use.

www.niaaa.nih.gov: Many government reports on alcoholism.

www.surgeongeneral.gov/library/mentalhealth/chapter4/sec5.html#service_substance: Alcohol and substance use disorders in older adults," "Older adults and mental health," "Mental health: A report of the Surgeon General" (1999).

http://silk.nih.gov/silk/niaaa1/publication/agepage.htm:. "Age and alcohol abuse," Age Page, National Institute on Aging.

http://silk.nih.gov/silk/niaaa1/publication/aa40.htm: "Alcohol alert: Alcohol and aging," National Institute on Alcohol Abuse and Alcoholism.

http://silk.nih.gov/silk/niaaa1/publication/handout.htm: "How to cut down on your drinking," National Institute on Alcohol Abuse and Alcoholism.

INDEX

Note: Page numbers followed by "t" indicate tables, page numbers followed by "f" indicate figures, page numbers followed by "b" indicate boxes.

A

AA (Alcoholics Anonymous), 555
AAA (abdominal aortic aneurysm), 173, 174
  atypical presentations of, 272t
  back pain and, 523–524
  classic triad in, 268
  complications of, 273
  CT scan for, 270
  diagnosis of, 269
  ED care/disposition of, 271
  epidemiology of, 267–268
  facts related to, 267
  findings in symptomatic, 269t
  males v. females and, 267
  MRI for, 270–271
  pathophysiology of, 268
  physical examinations for, 269
  plain abdominal radiography for, 269
  risk factors for, 268t
  risk-management "pearls" for, 273t
  rupture, risk of, with, 267–268
  symptomatic unruptured, 268
  ultrasound for, 269–270, 270f
AACG (acute-angle-closure glaucoma), 308
ABCDEF approach, for ventricular tachycardia, 103
Abdomen, anatomic zones of, 351
Abdominal aorta, branches of, 227–228
Abdominal aortic aneurysm. See AAA
Abdominal pain
  ACS with, 175
  analgesia for, 177
  antibiotic coverage for, 177
  appendicitis and, 220, 221
  biliary tract disease with, 215
  bowel obstruction with, 177, 198
  clinical features of, 174–175
  constipation and, 210
  CT scan for, 176
  differential diagnosis of, 175, 175t
  ED care/disposition of, 176–177
  epidemiology of, 173

  facts related, 173b
  history taking for, 174
  hospitalization for, 177
  laboratory evaluation for, 175
  outpatient therapy for, 177
  pathophysiology of, 173–174
  physical examination for, 174–175
  pitfalls managing, 177–178
  radiographs, plain, for, 175–176
  types of, 173–174
  ultrasonography for, 176
Abdominal trauma, 350–351
  DPL for, 355
  emergent laparotomy for, 355
  FAST for, 355
  Kehr's sign in, 350–351
  pitfalls managing, 356
ABG (arterial blood gas)
  dyspnea and, 142
  PE and, 167
ABI (ankle-brachial index), arterial insufficiency's use of, 282
Abuse/Neglect
  agencies investigating, 32
  approaching patients/victims of, 38t
  clinical features of, 33
  decubiti as, 37
  differential diagnosis for, 36
  ED care/disposition of, 36–38
  epidemiology of, 33
  examples of, 32
  facts related to, 32b
  findings, typical, of, 36t
  forms of, 32
  intervention, case management of, 34f, 39f
  interviews to uncover, 33, 35t
  mnemonic for identification of, 37t
  orthopedic injuries from, 359
  physical examination for, 35–36, 35t
  predisposition for, 33
  resources for physicians on, 38t

Abuse/Neglect *(contd.)*
  restraining orders for, 38
  signs of, 37t
  social services called for, 37
  warning signs pointing to, 33–34, 36
ACE (angiotensin-converting enzyme) inhibitors, 18
  ARF and, 239–240
  for heart failure, 94
  underused with elderly, 94
Acetabulum fractures, 362
Achalasia, 186
ACS (acute coronary syndrome), 71
  abdominal pain with, 175
  difficulty diagnosing, 73–74
  drug therapies for, 75
  ED care of, 74
  pitfalls in diagnosis/management of, 76
  thrombus formation in, 72
  vasospasm in, 72
  younger patients v. older patients with, 74–75, 76
Activated partial thromboplastin time. *See* APTT
Activities of daily living. *See* ADL
Acute coronary syndrome. *See* ACS
Acute decompensated heart failure, 92–93
Acute left ventricular failure, 125–126
  blood pressure and, 125–126
  pharmacologic agents for, 126
Acute myocardial infarction. *See* AMI
Acute otitis media, 481
Acute pulmonary edema, 88
  heart failure and, 92
  HOCM and, 92
Acute renal failure. *See* ARF
Acute subdural hematomas, 343–344, 344t
  GCS and, 347
  mortality rates with, 347
Acute-angle-closure glaucoma. *See* AACG
ADE (adverse drug events), definition of, 13
Adhesive bands, bowel obstruction from, 198
ADL (activities of daily living), 22, 23–24
  assessment of, 25
  dehydration and, 371
  hierarchy in loss of, 24
  Katz scale for measurement of, 23t
Admission rates, for older v. younger patients, 2
ADR (adverse drug reactions), definition of, 13
Adrenal insufficiency
  clinical features of, 511
  ED care/disposition of, 511
  pathophysiology of, 511
ADREs (adverse drug related event)

  definition of, 13
  etiology of, 14
  herbal remedies, cause of, 14
  mimic other conditions, 20
Advance directives, 44
Advanced life support. *See* ALS
Adverse drug event. *See* ADE
Adverse drug reactions. *See* ADR
Adverse drug related events. *See* ADREs
Afebrile bacteremia, infections, cause of, 56
African-Americans, type 2 diabetes and
Age structure, factors contributing to, 1
Aging
  characteristics of, 4
  chemical/biological changes with, 58, 60
  clinical significance of, 5
  definition of, 4
  emergency physicians and, 5
  facts regarding, 4b
  physiologic changes of, 5–11
  physiology of, 6t-7t
  types of, 4
Aging population, demographics of, 1
AICDs (automatic internal cardiac defibrillators), for dysrhythmia, 109
Alcoholics Anonymous. *See* AA
Alcoholism
  AA and, 555
  clinical approach to, 557f
  clinical features of, 554
  clues in diagnosing, 555t
  detoxification and, 557
  differential diagnosis of, 554–555
  ED care/disposition of, 555
  epidemiology of, 553
  facts related to, 553b
  G-MAST short version for, 555, 556f
  misattribution of, 554t
  OTC medications and, 558
  pathophysiology of, 553–554
  screening questionnaire for, 555
Allis maneuver, 365f
ALS (advanced life support), nursing home transfers and, 51
Alzheimer's disease
  language impairment in, 293
  pathophysiology of, 293
  psychiatric symptoms of, 293
AMI (acute myocardial infarction)
  CAD and, 71, 72
  ECG and, 73

painless presentation of, 73
ST-segment elevation, 74
Anemia
 classification of, 502
 clinical features of, 503
 differential diagnosis of, 503
 ED care/disposition of, 503–504
 epidemiology of, 502
 facts related to, 502b
 macrocytic, 503
 microcytic, 502–503
 nomocytic, 503
 pitfalls evaluating, 504
 RBC destruction and, 502
 RBC impaired production and, 502–503
 RBC loss and, 502
Anergy, rates relating to, 57
Aneurysms
 ruptured, 268–269
 unruptured, 268
Angiodysplasia, 180
Angiography, for mesenteric ischemia, 232
Angiotensin-converting enzyme inhibitors. *See* ACE
 inhibitors
Angiotensin-receptor blockers. *See* ARBs
Ankle-brachial index. *See* ABI
Ankylosing spondylitis
 airway management and, 542
 challenges of, 543
 clinical features of, 540
 differential diagnosis of, 541, 541t
 ED care/disposition of, 542–543
 epidemiology of, 539
 extra-axial manifestations of, 540, 541t
 facts related to, 539b
 pathophysiology of, 540
 radiographic investigations for, 541, 542t
Anoscopy, for constipation, 211
Antibodies/autoantibodies, immune deficiencies and, 60
Antimicrobials, for pneumonia, 149
Aortic dissection
 aortic intima weakening in, 276
 aortic regurgitation with, 277
 aortography for, 277
 blood pressure with, 276
 classification systems for, 275
 clinical features of, 276–277
 differential diagnosis of, 277, 277t
 ED care/disposition of, 278
 epidemiology/etiology of, 275
 facts related to, 275b

hypertension and, 125
medications for, 278
mortality rates for, 275
neurological symptoms with, 276
pain, nature of, with, 276
pathophysiology for, 276
pharmacologic agents for, 125
preexisting conditions with, 275
presentation of, 125
surgery for, 278
syncope with, 276
TEE for, 277
Aortic regurgitation
 acute, 114
 chronic, 114
 clinical features of, 114
 ED care/disposition of, 114
 pathophysiology of, 114
Aortic stenosis
 aortic valve calcification in, 111, 113
 cardiac catheterization for, 113
 clinical features of, 112
 echocardiography for, 113
 ED care/disposition of, 113–114
 epidemiology of, 111
 etiologies responsible for, 112
 life expectancy with, 112
 pathophysiology of, 111–112
 signs of, 113t
 sudden cardiac death from, 112
 symptoms of, 112
 syncope and, 112t, 113f
Aortic valve, calcification of, 111, 113
Aortography, aortic dissection's use of, 277
Appendicitis
 abdominal pain and, 221
 clinical features of, 221–222
 constipation with, 222
 CRP and, 223
 CT scan for, 223–224
 differential diagnosis for, 222–223
 difficulties diagnosing, 220
 disorders confused with, 224
 ED care/disposition of, 224, 225t
 epidemiology of, 221
 events responsible for, 221, 222
 facts related to, 220b
 laboratory investigations for, 223
 management algorithm for, 225t
 pathophysiology of, 221
 reevaluation for, 226

Appendicitis *(contd.)*
    ultrasound for, 224
    younger v. older patients with, 222t
APTT (activated partial thromboplastin time) levels,
        DVT and, 228
ARBs (angiotensin-receptor blockers), hypertension
        managed with, 94
ARF (acute renal failure). *See also* Renal failure
    ACE inhibitors and, 239–240
    anuric failure in, 238–239
    clinical features of, 241
    contrast material-induced, 240–241
    COX-2 inhibitors and, 239
    ED care/disposition of, 242–243
    embolic, 241
    epidemiology of, 237
    facts related, 237b
    history taking for, 241
    hospital acquired, 237
    hyperkalemia and, 238
    intrinsic renal failure in, 240
    laboratory test for, 242t
    medications causing, 243
    multiple myeloma, 241
    obstructive, 241
    oliguric failure in, 239
    pathophysiology of, 237–238
    prerenal failure and, 239
    prerenal failure in, 239
    survival rate from, 237
    ultrasonography for, 243
    vasomotor disorders in, 239
Arterial blood gas. *See* ABG
Arterial insufficiency. *See also* Atherosclerosis;
        Diabetic microangiopathy
    ABI used in, 282
    arteriography for, 282
    claudification with, 281
    clinical features of, 281
    diagnosis of, 282
    ED care/disposition of, 282
    facts related, 280
    Fontaine classification for chronic, 281
    invasive therapy for, 283
    lifestyle changes with, 282
    MRA for, 282
    pathophysiology of, 280–281
    peripheral vascular disease, same as, 280
    pharmacotherapy for, 282–283
    smoking cessation for, 282
Arterial intima, 7

Arteriosclerosis. *See* Atherosclerosis
Arthritis
    acute, 527
    bursitis, tendonitis and, 533
    classification by affected joints, 526t
    crystal-induced, 528
    differential diagnosis of, 532–533
    malignancy with, 530
    myopathies of, 532
    osteo, 529–530
    septic, 526–528
    trauma and, 533
Aspirin therapy, for mitral regurgitation, 117
ASSENT-2 trial, 75
Asymptomatic bacteriuria, 264
Atheroma. *See* Atherosclerosis
Atherosclerosis
    arterial intima in, 7
    coronary, 71
    hypertension complicated by, 123
    pathophysiology of, 281
Atrial fibrillation, 99, 101, 101f
    embolic stroke concurrent with, 116
    mitral stenosis and, 115
Atrial flutter, 101f
Atrial tachycardias, types of, 101
Atrophic vaginitis, 255
Automatic internal cardiac defibrillators. *See* AICDs
AV (atrioventricular) junction level, of supraventricular
        dysrhythmia, 101, 102f
AVN (avascular necrosis), 532

B
Back pain
    AAA and, 523
    calcium/alkaline phosphatase/phosphate and, 520
    causes of, 517
    CBC for, 520
    clinical features of, 519
    differential diagnosis of, 518t, 520
    disk herniation and, 521
    ED care/disposition of, 524
    epidemiology of, 518
    ESR for, 520
    etiologies of, 519t
    facts related to, 517b
    historical factors of, 519, 519t
    metabolic diseases and, 522
    osteoporosis and, 522
    pathophysiology of, 518
    physical examination for, 520

probabilistic approach to, 524
radiographic investigations of, 520–521, 521f
spinal epidural abscess and, 523
spinal stenosis and, 522
tumors and, 522
urinalysis for, 520
vertebral osteomyelitis and, 523
Bacteremia
UTI and, 64
white blood cell count in predicting, 63–64
Bacteriuria
asymptomatic, 264
catheter-associated, 264, 264t
Bacteroides fragilis, 526
"Bad news," guidelines for delivering, 46t
Balantis/Posthitis, 248
Baltimore Longitudinal Study of Aging, 75
Barium-/Gastrografin-contrasted swallow studies, for
esophageal disease, 188
Barret's esophagus, from GERD, 187, 189
Basal metabolic rate. *See* BMR
B-cell activity, 60
Benign positional vertigo. *See* BPV
benign prostatic hypertrophy, urinary retention and, 247
Beta blockers, for heart failure, 95
Biliary stones, types of, 214
Biliary tract disease. *See also* Cholecystitis
abdominal pain with, 215
antibiotic regimens for, 218t
biliary stones, types of, in, 214
cholecystitis and, 215
clinical features of, 215–216
CT scan for, 216
differential diagnosis of, 216–217
ED care/disposition of, 217–218
epidemiology of, 214
facts related to, 214b
gallstones in, 214, 216, 217f
geriatric v. younger patients with, 215
laboratory studies for, 216
opiates for, 218
pathophysiology of, 214–215
pitfalls managing, 218–219
ultrasonography for, 216
Bleeding disorders
acquired, 492
clinical features of, 494–495
coagulopathies, synonym for, 491
differential diagnosis of, 495–498
ED care/disposition of, 498
epidemiology of, 491–492

facts related to, 491b
fibrinolysis and, 492, 494, 494f
hemostasis and, 492, 493f
hypocoagulability and, 494–495
pathophysiology of, 492, 494
thromboembolic diseases as, 492
treatment of, 498–500
Blocks
diagnosis of, 106
types of, 105–106
Blood pressure
acute elevations in, 122
aging's effect on, 5
Blood urea nitrogen. *See* BUN
Bloom-Singer voice prosthesis, 486
Blunt trauma, 354–355
cardiac contusion in, 355
Blunted fever response, 55–56
BMI (body mass index), malnutrition and, 421
BMR (basal metabolic rate), temperature, body, and, 11
BNP (brain natriuretic peptide) test, heart failure and,
90
Body mass index. *See* BMI
Body water, three compartments of, 369
Bone marrow transplants, GVHD and, 513
Bowel obstruction
abdominal pain with, 198
from adhesive bands, 198
air-fluid levels in, 199
clinical features of, 199
differential diagnosis of, 199–200
ED care/disposition of, 200
epidemiology of, 198
facts related to, 198b
ileocecal valve competence and, 189–199, 200
large v. small, 199
medications for, 200
pathophysiology of, 198–199
pitfalls managing, 200
strangulated groin hernia and, 198
volvulus and, 202
BP (bullous pemphigoid)
clinical features of, 435
differential diagnosis of, 435–436
ED care/disposition of, 435–436
epidemiology of, 435
pathophysiology of, 435
BPV (benign positional vertigo), 334–335
Bradydysrhythmias
pacemakers and, 108
SCD and, 132

Brain abscess
    antibiotics for, 307
    clinical features of, 307
    ED care/disposition of, 307
Brain natriuretic peptide. *See* BNP
Bronchitis, COPD and, 157
Bronchodilators, 160t
    classes of, 160
    methods of delivering, 161
Bullous myringitis, 481
Bullous pemphigoid. *See* BP
BUN (blood urea nitrogen)
    dehydration and, 126
    diabetes mellitus and, 396
    renal deterioration and, 126
Burns, 339, 446
    prevention of, 448
    treatment of, 448
Bursitis, 533

C

CAD (coronary artery disease)
    ACS as, 71
    AMI as, 71
    clinical features of, 72–73
    clinical presentations of, 71
    epidemiology of, 71–72
    facts related, 71b
    Glycoprotein IIb/IIIa platelet inhibitors for, 76
    pathophysiology of, 72
Calcium, 379
    conditions precipitating, 245
    deficiency of, 420–421
Calcium channel blockers. *See* CCBs
CAM (Confusion Assessment Method), delirium
    screening using, 297, 298f
Cancer
    cervical, 251
    ovarian, 251
    vaginal, 255–256
Candida, 254
Carbon monoxide poisoning, headaches, dizziness with,
    309
Cardiac contusion, blunt trauma and, 355
Cardiac output, exercise with, 7
Cardiac syncope, 78
    causes of, 80
Cardiac tamponade, 355
Cardiac valves, normal function of, 111
Cardiogenic shock, 113
    etiology of, 88

heart failure as, 92
    pathophysiology of, 88
Cardiology consult, urgent, 91t
Cardiopulmonary resuscitation. *See* CPR
Cardiovascular system, 5, 7
    blood pressure of, 5
    cardiac output of, 5, 7
Catheterization, urethral, 264
Catheters, ballon-tipped pacer, pacemakers and,
    108–109
CBC (complete blood count), for hypocoagulability,
    495
CCBs (calcium channel blockers), DDIs from, 18
Central nervous system. *See* CNS
Cephalosporins, for pneumonia, 149
Cervical cancer, 251
Cervical hypertrophic osteoarthropathy, 186
Cervicogenic headache, cervical spondylosis as, 312
CH (cluster headache)
    clinical features of, 311
    ED care/disposition of, 311
    epidemiology of, 311
    oxygen, high-flow, for, 311
Chest pain, differential diagnosis of, 74t
Chest radiograph. *See* CXR
Chest trauma, 350
    hemothorax as, 354
    management principles for, 353–354
    PEA and, 354
    pitfalls managing, 356
CHF (congestive heart failure)
    dyspnea and, 138
    ischemia in, 73
Chicken pox, HZ, cause of, 438
Cholecystitis
    factors leading to, 215
    medication for, 218
    pathogens involved in, 215
    presentation of, 215
    surgery for, 218
    ultrasonography for, 217f
Cholesteatoma, 482
Chronic obstructive pulmonary disease. *See* COPD
Chronic otitis media, 481
Chronic subdural hematoma. *See* CSH
Chronic venous insufficiency. *See* CVI
Chronologic aging, 4
Cincinnati Prehospital Stroke Scale, 320t
Circadian rhythms, SCD and, 131
CK-MB, 74
Cluster headache. *See* CH

CNS (central nervous system)
   dysrhythmia and, 99
   hypothermia and, 387
Coagulation, laboratory studies of, 495–496
Communication
   and ED care provider, 53
   end of life, 45, 45t
   with families following death, 46
Complete blood count. *See* CBC
Computed tomographic scan. *See* CT scan
Confusion Assessment Method. *See* CAM
Congestive heart failure. *See* CHF
Conjunctivitis, 469, 472
   clinical features of, 470
   differential diagnosis of, 470–471
   ED care/disposition of, 471–472
Constipation
   abdominal pain in, 210
   anoscopy for, 211
   appendicitis and, 222
   chronic, 211
   clinical features of, 210–211
   complications of, 212
   diet/fluid intake and, 210
   differential diagnosis of, 211
   ED care/disposition of, 212
   epidemiology of, 208–209
   etiology of, 209–210, 209t
   facts regarding, 208
   GI bleeding, lower, and, 181
   irritable bowel syndrome and, 211
   laxative use for, 212
   mechanisms involved in, 208
   medication for, 212
   medications causing, 209
   pathophysiology of, 209
   pitfalls managing, 212
   radiologic investigation with, 211
   rectal examination in, 210–211
   subjective nature of, 208
Conversations, documenting of, 43
COPD (chronic obstructive pulmonary disease), 138
   antibiotics for, 161–162
   bacterial infections exacerbating, 157
   bronchitis and, 157
   bronchodilators for, 160–161, 160t
   causes of, 154
   clinical features of, 157
   corticosteroids for, 161
   differential diagnosis of, 157–158, 159t
   dyspnea and, 155, 158, 162

ECG for, 157–158
   ED care/disposition of, 158
   emphysema and, 156, 157
   environmental pollution's effect on, 155–156
   epidemiology, natural history, prognosis for, 155
   exacerbations of, 154, 157
   facts related to, 154b
   genetics and, 156
   hallmarks of, 155
   hospital mortality rates for, 154
   management principles for, 162
   methylxanthines for, 161
   oxygen therapy for, 159–160
   pathophysiology of, 155–156
   pharmacologic intervention for, 159
   pitfalls managing, 163
   prevention of, 162–163
   progression of, 156
   smoking, cause of/effect on, 154, 155, 155f, 156
   ventilatory support for, 162
Corneal blindness, HSV-1 and, 469
Coronary artery disease. *See* CAD
Coronary atherosclerosis, 71
Coronary ischemia, nitroglycerin for, 113
Coronary syndrome, acute, hypertension and, 124
Corticosteroids, for COPD, 161
COX-2 (cyclooxygenase 2) inhibitors, ARF and, 239
CPR (cardiopulmonary resuscitation)
   nursing home patients and, 52
   withholding of, 44
Creatine clearance, formula for correction of, 16
Cricoarytenoiditis, 483
CRP (C-reactive protein), appendicitis and, 223
Crystal-induced arthritis, gout as, 528
CSH (chronic subdural hematoma)
   CT scan for, 305
   headache with, 305
   MRI for, 305
CT (computed tomographic) scan
   for abdominal pain, 176
   for appendicitis, 223–224
   for biliary tract disease, 216
   for diverticular disease, 194
   for mesenteric ischemia, 231–232
   for PE, 168–169
   for renal calculus, 246
CVI (chronic venous insufficiency), 285
   epidemiology of, 285
   pathophysiology of, 285
   presenting symptoms of, 286
CXR (chest radiograph), pneumonia and, 64

D

DDIs (drug-drug interactions)
CCBs, cause of, 18
definition of, 13
Deceased patients, procedures on, 46
Decision-making capacity
Code of Ethics of the American College of
Emergency Physicians on, 41
coercion and, 41
definition of, 41
determination of, 40, 41, 41t
documentation of, 43
impediments to, 41–42
Mini-Mental Status Examination for, 42t
QCS for, 42t
surrogates and, 43
Decubiti, as abuse/neglect, 37
Deep venous thrombophlebitis. *See* DVT
Defecation, events involved in, 209
Dehydration
blood pressure and, 371
BUN and, 372
clinical features of, 371–372
diagnosing difficulties with, 372
diagnosis of, 372
ED care of, 372
epidemiology/impact of, 370–371
facts related to, 369b
risk factors for, 371
triggers of, 371t
types of, 370
Delirium, 291–292
causes of, 292
diagnosis of, 296
pathophysiology of, 292
precipitants of, 293t
v. dementia, 292, 295
Delusional disorder, 550
Dementia
Alzheimer's disease, 293
characteristics of, 295t
degenerative brain disorders and, 292
etiologies of, 292–293
FTD as, 294
hypoactive-hyperactive psychomotor pattern in, 295
hypothyroidism in, 294
Parkinson's disease, 293–294
pitfalls unique to, 297
reversible causes of, 294
v. delirium, 292, 295
vascular, 293

Depression
clinical features of, 546–547
dementia and, 547
detecting, 547
differential diagnosis of, 547–548
ED care/disposition of, 548
epidemiology of, 545–546
facts related to, 545b
Koenig Scale for, 297, 300f
pathophysiology of, 546
SSRIs for, 548
symptoms of major, 546t
treatment of, 548
Diabetes insipidus, causes of, 375t
Diabetes mellitus
clinical features of, 395
commonly used insulin preparations for, 399t
complications associated with, 400
diabetic microangiopathy and, 280–281
diagnosis of, 396
disposition of, 400
ED care/disposition of, 396–397
epidemiology of, 394–395
facts related to, 394b
hyperglycemia and, 395
hypertension therapy with, 398
immunizations and, 399
insulin for, 398, 399t
long-term therapy for, 397–399
oral antidiabetic agents for, 399t
pathophysiology of, 395
personalized treatment for, 398
smoking and, 399
Diabetic ketoacidosis. *See* DKA
Diabetic microangiopathy, diabetes and, 280–281
Diabetic ulcers, treatment of, 450
Diagnostic peritoneal lavage. *See* DPL
Diarrhea, bloody, 181
Diastolic dysfunction, 5, 87
DIC (disseminated intravascular coagulation)
causes of, 497f
fibrinogen levels and, 496
Digitalis toxicity, junctional tachycardia and, 102
Digoxin, for heart failure, 94–95
Disease prevalence, differences in, 57
Disseminated intravascular coagulation. *See* DIC
Disseminated varicella, 440
Distal radius fractures
clinical features of, 366–367
differential diagnosis of, 367
ED care/disposition of, 367

Diuretics, heart failure and, 93
Diverticular abscesses, grading system for, 196t
Diverticular disease
  abdominal radiograph for, 194
  analgesia for, 195
  antibiotic coverage for, 195
  collagen-vascular disorders and, 191
  colonoscopy for, 194
  CT scan for, 194
  diet and, 191
  differential diagnosis of, 193, 193t
  diverticulitis as, 192
  ED care/disposition of, 195–196
  epidemiology of, 191
  ethnicity and, 191
  hospitalization for, 195
  MRI for, 195
  outpatient therapy for, 195–196
  pathophysiology of, 191–192
  ultrasonography for, 194
  urinalysis for, 194
Diverticulitis
  in diverticulosis, 192
  leukocytosis in, 193
  symptoms of, 192–193
Diverticulosis, 191
  diverticular hemorrhage with, 193
  high-fiber diet for, 196
Dizziness
  postural hypotension, cause of, 334
  symptoms of, 333
DKA (diabetic ketoacidosis), 395, 396
  principles of therapy for, 397
  v. HHNS, 396t
DNR (do not resuscitate)
  document, 45
  dyspnea and, 142
  SCD and, 133
Documentation, importance of, 43
DPL (diagnostic peritoneal lavage), thoracoabdominal
  trauma and, 352
Drug interactions/side effects, 67t
Drug metabolism
  factors affecting, 17
  metabolic changes from, 16
Drug-drug interactions. *See* DDIs
Drug-induced fevers, sources of, 63t
Durable power of attorney, 44
DVT (deep venous thrombophlebitis), 286
  APTT (Activated Partial Thromboplastin Time)
    levels and, 288

D-dimer levels with, 287–288
differential diagnosis for, 286–287, 288
diseases mimicking, 288
duplex ultrasound for, 287
ED care/disposition of, 288
embolism, risk of, with, 286
laboratory investigations of, 287–288
LMWH for, 288
predicting pretest probability of, 287t
presenting symptoms of, 286
radiologic investigations of, 287
risk factors for, 286, 286t
younger patients v. older patients with, 286
Dysphagia. *See also* Esophageal disease; GERD
  (gastroesophageal reflux disease)
  causes of, 187
  diffuse esophageal spasm in, 186
  ED care/disposition of, 188–189
  epidemiology of, 185
  esophageal, 185
  oropharyngeal, 185
  pathophysiology of, 185–186
  radiographic studies for, 188
Dyspnea
  ABG determination for, 142
  acute v. subacute onset of, 139
  causes of, 139–140
  CHF, symptom of, 138
  clinical features of, 139–140
  COPD and, 156, 158, 162
  descriptors for, 137, 140t
  differential diagnosis of, 140, 141t, 142
  drugs for, 142–143
  ECG for, 140
  ED care/disposition of, 142
  end-of-life care for, 142
  epidemiology of, 138
  facts related to, 137b
  neural circuit of, 139t
  pathophysiology of, 138–139
  quantifying-scales, 137
Dysrhythmia(s)
  AICDs for, 109
  blocks, 105–106
  clinical features of, 99–100
  CNS and, 99
  ED care/disposition of, 108–109
  epidemiology of, 99
  facts related to, 99b
  hypotension and, 100
  pathophysiology of, 99

Dysrhythmia(s) *(contd.)*
    SA node, source of, 100
    supraventricular, 100–102, 100f
    ventricular, 102–103, 105
    vital signs with, 100

E
Ear, nose, throat infections. *See* ENT infection(s)
ECG (electrocardiogram)
    in AMI, 73
    in aortic stenosis, 112
    for dyspnea, 140
    heart failure and, 89
    for PE, 167
    tachycardia and, 103
Echocardiogram
    aortic stenosis and, 113
    heart failure and, 90–91
ED (emergency department) (use)
    admission rates, older v. younger patients for, 2
    ADREs and, 13, 14
    approach to febrile elderly, 65f
    characteristics of elder visits to, 1
    environment, ideal, of, 3
    facts regarding, 1b
    geriatric care model for, 2–3
    overcrowding of, 2
    role in abuse/neglect, 37
    syncope and, 78
    usage, demographics of, 2
Elderly populations, studies of, age and, 57
Electricity, for tachydysrhythmias, 108
Electrolyte disorders
    facts related to, 369b
    sodium in, 373
ELISA (enzyme-linked immunosorbent assay), for PE,
    168
Embolic stroke, atrial fibrillation concurrent with, 116
Emergency department care, 51–52
    SAEM and, 52
Emergency physicians, aging and, 5
Emphysema, COPD and, 156
Encephalitis
    clinical features of, 307
    HSV-1 causes herpetic, 306
End of life
    communication at, 45, 45t
    ethical issues at, 43–44
    physician's role at, 45
    rituals at, 45

Endocarditis
    antibiotics for, 118
    prosthetic valve, 119
Endocrine disease, heart failure and, 87
Endocrine system
    glucose regulation in, 9
    sexual function in, 9
    thyroid function in, 9
Endometrial carcinoma, postmenopausal bleeding and,
    255
Endotracheal intubation. *See* ET
ENT infection(s)
    acute otitis media as, 481
    cholesteatoma as, 482
    chronic otitis media as, 481
    cricoarytenoiditis as, 483
    epidemiology of, 479
    epiglottitis and, 483
    furunculosis as, 481
    Ludwig's angina as, 482–483
    malignant otitis externa as, 480
    nasopharyngitis as, 482
    otitis externa as, 480
    otomycosis as, 480–481
    pathophysiology of, 479–480
    peritonsillar abscess as, 483
    serious otitis externa as, 480
    sinusitis as, 482
    younger v. older patients with, 479
Environmental pollution, COPD and, 155–156
Enzyme-linked immunosorbent assay. *See* ELISA
Epididymitis
    clinical features of, 249
    diagnostic studies of, 249
    differential diagnosis of, 249
    ED care of, 249
    epidemiology of, 248–249
Epistaxis
    anterior, 477
    bleeding with, 476
    causes of, 475
    clinical features of, 476
    differential diagnosis of, 477
    ED care/disposition of, 477–478
    epidemiology of, 475
    facts related to, 475b
    pathophysiology of, 475–476
    posterior, 477–478
Erythrocyte sedimentation rate. *See* ESR
Esmolol, for hypertensive emergencies, 128

Esophageal disease
    Barium-/Gastrografin-contrasted swallow studies for, 188
    clinical features of, 186–187
    differential diagnosis of, 187–188
    pitfalls managing, 189
    symptoms of, 186
Esophageal injuries, 355
ESR (erythrocyte sedimentation rate)
    back pain and, 520, 536
    changes with age and, 538
Estrogen, intact uterus and, 252
ET (endotracheal intubation), for COPD, 162
Ethical issue(s)
    end of life, 43–44
    facts related to, 40b
    general principles regarding, 40
    resuscitation as, 43–44
Euthyroid sick syndrome, 412
Exercise, cardiac output with, 7
Eye infection(s)
    conjunctivitis as, 469
    herpes infections and, 469
    preseptal, orbital cellulitis as, 469–470
Eyelids, 455

F

Falls, 338
    clinical features of, 29
    consequences of, 28
    diagnosis regarding, 30
    epidemiology of, 28–29
    facts related, 28b
    injuries resulting from, 30
    institutionalized adults and, 28–29
    orthopedic injuries from, 359
    pathophysiology of, 29
    pitfalls, avoidance of, in treatment of, 31
    prehospital considerations for, 29
    prevention of, 30–31
    risk factors for, 29t
    syncope and, 30
    treatment of, 30
Family violence, high-risk history for, 35t
FAST (focused assessment with sonography for trauma)
    thoracoabdominal trauma and, 353
FDP (fibrin degradation products), fibrinolytic activity and, 496
Fecal impaction, 212

Femoral
    head fractures, 363
    neck fractures, 363
Fenoldopam, for hypertensive emergencies, 129
Fever
    blunted fever response as, 55–56
    causes of, 59f
    common etiologies of, 61t
    differential diagnosis/relative frequencies of, 62t
    ESR/PPD to evaluate, 63
    facts related, 55b
    infections and, 5
    lowering threshold for, 56
    medications for drug-induced, 63t
    sources of drug-induced, 63t
    thermometer's relevance with, 56
    treatments for, 66t
    young patients v. old patients with, 57
Fever of unknown origin. *See* FUO
Fibrin degradation products. *See* FDP
Fibrinolysis, 492, 494f
Fluoroquinolones, for pneumonia, 148–149
Focused assessment with sonography for trauma. *See* FAST
Folate deficiency, 419–420
Foley catheter
    hematuria and, 247
    urinary retention and, 247
Fontaine classification, for chronic peripheral arterial disease, 281
Fournier's gangrene, 248
FTD (frontotemporal dementia), 294
Functional assessment/decline
    epidemiology of, 22–23
    facts related, 22b
    measures of, 23–26
Functional screening, 25
FUO (fever of unknown origin), 61–62
    younger patients v. older patients and, 61
Furunculosis, 481
Fusion beats, 106f
Futility
    concept of, 44–45
    determination of, 44

G

Gallstones, ultrasonography for, 217f
Gastroesophageal reflux disease. *See* GERD
Gastrointestinal system, 10–11
    constipation in, 10

Gastrointestinal tract, 209
GCA (giant cell arteritis)
   clinical features of, 305–306
   ED care/disposition of, 306
   PMR and, 532
   temporal arteritis, synonym for, 305
GCA/PMR
   clinical features of, 535–536
   differential diagnosis of, 536–537
   ED care/disposition of, 537–538
   epidemiology of, 534
   facts related to, 534b
   historical references to, 534
   pathophysiology of, 534–535
   steroid administration for, 537, 538
GCS (Glasgow Coma Scale), 346t
   geriatric trauma and, 341
   head trauma and, 345
GERD (gastroesophageal reflux disease), 186
   Barret's esophagus from, 187, 189
   H. pylori and, 189
   H_2 blockers for, 188
   Maalox, viscous lidocaine cocktail for, 188
Geriatric trauma
   blood pressure and, 340
   burns as, 339
   comorbid conditions and, 341
   differential diagnosis of, 340
   ED care/disposition of, 340–341
   epidemiology of, 337–338
   facts related to, 337b
   falls as, 338
   GCS and, 341
   history taking for, 339
   ICU for, 340
   medication and, 341
   mortality rate and, 341
   motor vehicle crashes as, 338
   pedestrian-automobile accidents as, 338
   pitfalls in management of, 341–342
   prehospital considerations and, 339
   violence as, 339
   vital signs and, 339–340
GI (gastrointestinal) bleeding. *See also* Peptic ulcer
   disease
   aspirin/NSAIDs and, 180
   ED care/disposition of, 182–183
   epidemiology of, 179
   H_2 antagonist for, 183
   hypovolemic shock from, 183

laboratory evaluation for, 182
   mortality from, 179
   nitroglycerin (intravenous) for, 183
   peptic ulcers and, 180
   pitfalls in management of, 183
   somatostatin for, 183
   vasopressin (intravenous) for, 183
GI bleeding, lower, 180–181
   colonic diverticula and, 180
   constipation and, 181
   diarrhea, bloody, and, 181
   hematochezia and, 182
   hemorrhoids present in, 181
   v. GI bleeding, upper, 180
GI bleeding, upper, 180
   men and, 180
   NSAIDs and, 180
   peptic ulcers and, 180
Giant cell arteritis. *See* GCA
Glasgow Coma Scale. *See* GCS
Glasgow Outcome Scale. *See* GOS
Glaucoma
   AACG as, 308–309
   Caucasian patients with, 308
   clinical features of, 309, 463
   ED care/disposition of, 309, 463
   epidemiology of, 462
   IOP and, 462
   medications, side-effects for, 464t
   osmotic diuretics for, 464
   pathophysiology of, 462–463
   types of, 462
   women v. men with, 308
Glycoprotein IIb/IIIa platelet inhibitors, CAD and, 76
Glycyrrhizic acid, hypokalemia, caused by, 376–377
G-MAST short version (Michigan Alcoholism
   Screening Test), 555
GOS (Glascow Outcome Scale), 347t
   acute subdural hematoma and, 347
Gout
   elder-onset v. younger onset, 528
   pseudo, 528–529
   treatment of, 528
Graft-v.-host disease. *See* GVHD
GVHD (graft-v.-host disease), bone marrow transplants
   and, 513–514
Gynecologic emergencies
   clinical features of, 252
   ED care/disposition of, 257–258
   facts related, 251b

history taking in, 252
pathophysiology of, 251–252
Gynecologic examination, 252–254
steps in, 253
Gynecologic malignancies, epidemiology of, 251

H

H. pylori
GERD and, 189
peptic ulcer disease and, 179, 181
H$_2$ antagonist for, for GI bleeding, 183
H$_2$ blockers, for GERD, 188
Head trauma
acceleration-deceleration force and, 343
acute subdural hematomas as, 343–344
analgesics, short-acting, for, 347
clinical features of, 344
differential diagnosis for, 345–346
ED care/disposition of, 346–347
epidemiology of, 343
ET in, 346
facts related to, 343b
financial impact of, 347
history taking with, 345
morbidity/mortality from, 347
neurologic examination for, 345
neurosurgical intervention for, 346
out-of-hospital considerations with, 344–345
pathophysiology of, 343–344
physical examination for, 345
subdural hygroma as, 344, 344t
syncope, cause of, 346
Headache(s). *See also* Brain abscesses; Cervicogenic
headache; CH; CSH; Encephalitis; GCA;
Glaucoma; Meningitis; Migraine; MIH; SAH;
Stroke; Trigeminal neuralgia; TTH; Tumor
facts related to, 304
MSG, cause of, 309
neuroimaging in, 307t
SAH as, 304–305
serious, 304t
sodium nitrate, cause of, 309
subarachnoid hemorrhage as, 304–305
toxic, metabolic, 309–310
Heart failure
ACE inhibitors for, 94
acute decompensated, 92–93
acute pulmonary edema with, 88, 92
beta blockers for, 95
BNP test for, 90

cardiogenic shock as, 88, 92
chest radiograph for, 90
clinical features of, 89
clinical presentations of, 88t
comorbidity with, 91
concomitant diseases with, 86
diastolic, 87–88
differential diagnosis of, 91t
digoxin for, 94–95
diuretics for, 93
ECG for, 89
echocardiogram and, 90–91
ED care/disposition of, 91
endocrine disease in, 87
epidemiology of, 86
facts related, 86b
laboratory studies for, 90
natriuretic peptides and, 87
New York Heart Association (NYHA) class IV, 86,
86t
90 day readmission rates for, 95t
observation unit discharge guidelines for, 96t
observation unit treatment for, 96t
pathophysiology of, 86–87
prognosis of, 86
readmission for, 91
spironolactone for, 95
symptoms of, 89
Heart failure, acute decompensated, 92–93
nesiritide for, 93
Heartburn, 186
Heat stroke, 389, 390
ED care/disposition of, 391
tachycardia in, 390
Hematochezia, GI bleeding and, 182
Hematuria
clinical features of, 249–250
ED care of, 250
epidemiology of, 249
false, 249
Foley catheter use in, 250
microscopic/gross, 262–263
Hemophilus influenzae, 526
Hemothorax, 354
Heparin, 75
PE and, 169
Hepatic function, 16–17
drugs related to, 17t
Herbal remedies, ADREs exacerbated by, 14
Herniated disk, 521

Herpes ocular infection, ED care/disposition of, 472

Herpes Opthalmicus, 440, 441f

Herpes simplex keratitis, 471, 472–473

Herpes zoster. *See* HZ

HHNS (hyperglycemic, hyperosmolar, nonketoic syndrome), 395
 principles of therapy for, 397
 v. DKA, 396t

Hiatal hernia, 186

Hip dislocations
 Allis maneuver for, 365f
 clinical features of, 364
 differential diagnosis of, 364, 365f
 ED care/disposition of, 364
 Stimson maneuver for, 365f

Hip fractures
 clinical features of, 363
 differential diagnosis of, 363
 ED care/disposition of, 363–364
 femoral head fractures as, 363
 femoral neck fractures as, 363
 functional decline from, 66
 intertrochanteric fractures as, 363–364
 subtrochanteric fractures as, 364

Hispanic/Mexican-Americans, type 2 diabetes and, 394

HOCM (hypertrophic obstructive cardiomyopathy), acute pulmonary edema and, 92

Homeostatis/homeostatic mechanisms, 4

HRT (hormone-replacement therapy), 252
 breakthrough bleeding in, 254

HSV-1 (herpes simplex virus)
 corneal blindness and, 469
 encephalitis and, 306
 ocular, 469, 470

Humerus fractures
 clinical features of, 364
 differential diagnosis of, 365
 ED care/disposition of, 365–366
 Neer classification system for proximal, 366f
 types of, 366

HVS (hyperviscosity syndrome)
 clinical features of, 511
 differential diagnosis of, 511
 ED care/disposition of, 511
 pathophysiology of, 510–511

Hydralazine-isosorbide dinitrate, 94

Hypercalcemia
 causes of, 380, 381t
 clinical features of, 379
 ED treatment for, 381
 effects of, 380t, 381t

Hypercalcemia of malignancy
 clinical features of, 509
 differential diagnosis of, 509
 ED care/disposition of, 509–510
 pathophysiology of, 509

Hypercholesterolemia, aortic stenosis in, 111

Hypercoagulability, 495
 differential diagnosis of, 497–498
 treatment of, 499–500

Hyperglycemia, diabetes mellitus and, 395

Hyperglycemic, hyperosmolar, nonketoic syndrome. *See* HHNS

Hyperkalemia
 ARF and, 238, 242
 causes of, 377–378, 378t
 clinical features of, 378
 ED treatment for, 378–379
 medications associated with, 378t
 potassium and, 377–378

Hypermagnesemia
 causes of, 383t
 clinical features of, 383
 ED treatment for, 383
 underlying process in, 383

Hypernatremia
 clinical features of, 375
 ED treatment for, 375
 types of, 374–375

Hyperphosphatemia
 causes of, 385
 clinical features of, 385
 ED treatment of, 385
 mesenteric ischemia and, 231

Hypertension
 acute coronary syndromes and, 124–125
 ARBs management of, 94
 atherosclerosis' complication of, 123
 autoregulation in, 122
 Caucasians v. African-Americans with, 122
 diabetes mellitus and, 398
 history taking for, 123
 MAP, higher, with, 122
 physical examination for, 123–124
 prevalence of, 121
 renal failure and, 126
 stroke syndromes and, 126–127
 symptoms of, 123
 transient, 123

Hypertensive emergencies
  chronic hypertension and, 121
  definition of, 121, 123
  differential diagnosis for, 127
  ED care/disposition of, 127
  epidemiology of, 121–122
  facts related to, 121b
  hypertensive urgencies v., 121
  intensive care unit admission for, 127
Hypertensive encephalopathy
  nitroprusside for, 124
  presentation of, 124
Hypertensive urgency, 121, 123
Hyperthermia
  clinical features of, 390–391
  CNS dysfunction in, 390
  cooling techniques for, 391–392
  CT scan for, 391
  differential diagnosis of, 391
  drugs and, 390
  ED care/disposition of, 391–392
  epidemiology of, 389
  heat stroke as, 389, 390
  pathophysiology of, 390
Hyperthyroidism
  clinical features of, 407–409
  diagnosis of, 409
  epidemiology of, 407
  pathophysiology of, 407
  subclinical, 413
  thyrotoxicosis as, 407, 408
Hypertrophic obstructive cardiomyopathy. *See*
    HOCM
Hyperviscosity syndrome. *See* HVS
Hypocalcemia
  causes of, 379, 380t
  clinical features of, 379
  ED treatment for, 379
  effects of, 380
Hypocoagulability, 494–495
  causes of, 496
  CBC for, 495
  differential diagnosis of, 496–497
  PT/INR for, 495
  PTT and, 495
  treatment of, 498–499
Hypoglycemia, therapy for, 397
Hypokalemia
  causes of, 376, 376t
  clinical features of, 377

ED treatment for, 377
  glycyrrhizic acid, cause of, 376–377
  potassium and, 376
Hypomagnesemia
  categories of, 381–382
  causes of, 382t
  clinical features of, 382
  ED treatment for, 382–383
Hyponatremia
  clinical features of, 374
  ED treatment of, 374
  hypotonic, 373, 374t
  SIADH and, 373
  types of, 373
Hypophosphatemia
  causes of, 384, 384t
  clinical features of, 384
  ED treatment for, 384
  mechanisms of, 384
Hypotension
  dysrhythmia and, 100
  mesenteric ischemia and, 230
  nesiritide, cause of, 93
  orthostatic, 80–81
  postural, 334
Hypothermia
  accidental, 386, 388
  behavioral changes for, 387
  causes of, 387
  clinical features of, 387
  definition of, 386
  differential diagnosis of, 388
  drug therapy for, 389
  ED care/disposition of, 388–389
  epidemiology of, 386
  pathophysiology of, 386–387
  respiratory system and, 387
  rewarming techniques for, 388–389
Hypothyroidism
  clinical features of, 403
  dementia and, 294, 295
  diagnosis of, 403–404
  epidemiology of, 402
  myxedema coma and, 404–405
  pathophysiology of, 402
  precipitating events for, 404t
  signs, symptoms of, 403t
  subclinical, 412–413
  thyroid storm as, 403, 403t
  TSH and, 402, 409

Hypovitaminosis
  definition of, 416
  studies of, 417
Hypovolemic shock, from GI bleeding, 183
Hypoxia/hypercapnia, 309
HZ (herpes zoster)
  antiviral medications for, 439
  bacterial superinfection and, 442
  chicken pox caused by, 438
  clinical features of, 438–439, 439t
  CNS involvement in, 441–442
  differential diagnosis of, 439
  disseminated varicella and, 440
  ED care/disposition of, 439–440
  epidemiology of, 438
  facts related to, 438b
  herpes opthalmicus and, 440, 441f
  Hutchinson's Sign and, 442
  pathophysiology of, 438
  postherpetic neuralgia and, 440
  prednisone for, 440
  prevention of, 442
  prognosis for, 442
  Ramsey Hunt syndrome and, 442
  zoster sine herpete and, 442

I

IADLs (instrumental activities of daily living)
  assessment of, 25
  Lawton and Brody scale of, 24t
  mortality predicted by, 24
ICD (implantable cardioverter-defibrillator), SCD
  prevention by, 133
ICP (intracranial pressure), headaches and, 306
ICU (intensive care unit)
  admission indications for, 95t
  for elderly trauma patients, 340
  for severe pneumonia, 151
  severe pneumonia and, 151
Identifications of Seniors at Risk. *See* ISAR
IL-2 (interleukin 2) synthesis, T-cell function and, 58
Ileocecal valve competence, bowel obstruction from,
  189–199, 200
Iliac wing fractures, 362
Immune function/system, 55
  altered, causes of, 59f
  antibodies/autoantibodies and, 60
  cellular components of, 60
Immunization, age's effect on, 57
Implantable cardioverter-defibrillator. *See* ICD
Inappropriate antidiuretic hormone secretion. *See* SIADH

Infections
  afebrile bacteremia from, 56
  malnutrition and, 58
  pathophysiology of, 58
  presentation of patients with, 56–57
  risks/manifestations of, 55
  younger patients v. older patients and, 56–57
Injury Severity Score. *See* ISS
Institutionalized adults, falls and, 28–29
Instrumental activities of daily living. *See* IADLs
Insulin, diabetes mellitus and, 398
Integumentary system, physical examination includes,
  63
Intensive care unit. *See* ICU
Intertrochanteric fractures, 363
Interviewing, for abuse/neglect, 35t
Intestinal angina, mesenteric ischemia and, 229
Intraabdominal pathology, lack of pain with, 62
Intracranial hemorrhage, 321f
Intracranial pressure. *See* ICP
ION (ischemic optic neuropathy)
  clinical features of, 467–468
  ED care/disposition of, 468
  epidemiology of, 467
  pathophysiology of, 467
IOP (intraocular pressure), 462, 463
Irritable bowel syndrome, constipation and, 211
ISAR (Identifications of Seniors at Risk), 25t
Ischemia, cell death from, 318f
Ischemic heart disease, men and, 72
Ischemic optic neuropathy. *See* ION
Ischemic stroke, treatment of, 322
Isolated bony fractures, 362
ISS (Injury Severity Score), mortality and, 341

J

Joint infections
  causes of, 526
  prosthetic, 527
  treatment of, 527
Junctional escape rhythm, 102f
Junctional tachycardia, digitalis toxicity and, 102

K

Katz Activities of Daily Living, 22
Kehr's sign, 350–351

L

Labetalol, for hypertensive emergencies, 128
Labrynthitis, 335
Lacrimal system, 455–456

β-lactams, for pneumonia, 149
LAFB (left anterior fascicular block), 106
Laryngeal Mask Airway. *See* LMA
Lawson and Brody Instrumental Activities of Daily Living, 22
Laxative use, constipation and, 212
LBBB (left bundle-branch block), 106
Leukocytosis, in diverticulitis, 193
Living will, 44
LMA (Laryngeal Mask Airway), ankylosing spondylitis, use of, 543
LMWH (low-molecular-weight heparin)
    for DVT, 286
    for PE, 170
    varieties of, 170
LP (lumbar puncture), SAH and, 322
LPFB (left posterior fascicular block), 106, 108f
Ludwig's angina, 482–483
Lumbar puncture, *See* LP
Lung compliance, age-related increase in, 7–8
Lupus, drug-induced, 532

M

Maalox/viscous lidocaine cocktail, for GERD, 188
Macrocytic anemia, 503
Macrolides, for pneumonia, 149
Magnesium, 381
Magnetic resonance angiography. *See* MRA
Malignancy(ies)
    adrenal insufficiency and, 511
    bone marrow transplants and, 513–514
    facts related to, 506b
    HVS and, 510–511
    hypercalcemia of, 509–510
    malignant pericardial effusion with tamponade and, 508
    neutropenia and, 511–512
    SIADH as, 510
    spinal cord compression and, 506–507
    SVC and, 508–509
    UGI hemorrhage and, 512–513
    upper airway obstruction and, 507
    urologic syndromes and, 513
Malignant otitis externa, 480
Malignant pericardial effusion with tamponade
    clinical features of, 508
    differential diagnosis of, 508
    ED care/disposition of, 508
    malignancy and, 508
    pathophysiology of, 508
Malnutrition. *See also* individual vitamins
    BMI calculation in, 421
    clinical features of, 421–422
    definition of, 416
    differential diagnosis of, 422–423
    epidemiology of, 417
    facts related to, 416b
    multivitamin supplementation for, 423
    physical findings of, 422t
    prevention of, 423
    prognosis for, 423
    protein-calorie deficiencies as, 417
Malnutrition, infections and, 58
MAP (mean arterial pressure), hypertension and, 122
Medication-induced headache. *See* MIH
Meningitis
    bacterial, 308
    clinical features of, 308
    ED care/disposition of, 308
    nosocomial v. community acquired, 308
    younger v. older patients with, 307–308
Mental status impairment. *See also* Alzheimer's disease; Delirium; Dementia
    CAM screening in, 297
    clinical features of, 294
    delirium as, 291–292
    ED care/disposition of, 296–297
    ED cognitive assessment tools for, 297
    epidemiology of, 291–292
    etiologies of, 292
    facts related to, 291b
    medications, cause of, 300
    nonrecognition of, 297
    OMC screening in, 297
    restraint for, 297
    societal impact of, 291
    types of, 292
Mesenteric ischemia
    abdominal aorta anatomy and, 227–228
    abdominal examination in, 230
    angiography for, 232
    cardiac examination in, 230
    chronic, 235
    clinical features of, 229–230
    comorbid diseases with, 229
    confounding features of, 230
    CT scans for, 231–232
    diagnostic laparascopy for, 233
    differential diagnosis of, 230–233
    ED care/disposition of, 233, 234f
    epidemiology of, 227
    etiologies of, 228

Mesenteric ischemia *(contd.)*
   facts related to, 227b
   heart rate and, 230
   hyperphosphatemia and, 231
   hypotension and, 230
   intestinal angina with, 229
   laboratory studies for, 231
   mesenteric venous thrombosis and, 235
   mortality rate for, 230
   MRA for, 232
   MRI for, 232
   nonocclusive, 228, 233, 235
   pathophysiology of, 227–228
   pitfalls in management of, 235
   rectal examination in, 230
   respiratory rate and, 230
   risk factors for, 227, 228–229, 229t
   serological factors identifying, 231
   SMA embolism and, 233
   SMA thrombosis and, 235
   triad for, 229
Mesenteric venous thrombosis, mesenteric ischemia
      and, 235
Metabolic changes, drug metabolism as cause of, 16
Methylxanthines, for COPD, 161
MI (myocardial infarction), syncope and, 82
Michigan Alcoholism Screening Test. *See* G-MAST
      short version
Microlytic anemia, 502–503
Migraine
   clinical features of, 310
   ED care/disposition of, 310
   pathophysiology of, 310
   pharmacologic treatment for, 310
MIH (medication-induced headache)
   ED care/disposition of, 312–313
   medication withdrawal headache as, 312
Mini-Mental Status Examination, 42t
Mitral regurgitation
   acute, 116–117
   acute v. chronic, 117t
   aspirin therapy for, 117
   chronic, 117
   ED care/disposition of, 117
   epidemiology of, 116
   nitroglycerin for, 117
   pathophysiology of, 116
   surgery for, 117
Mitral stenosis
   atrial fibrillation in, 115
   clinical features of, 115

   ED care/disposition of, 115–116
   epidemiology of, 115
   pathophysiology of, 115
   signs of, 115
   TEE for, 115
Mitral valve prolapse
   clinical features of, 118
   ED care/disposition of, 118
   epidemiology of, 118
   pathophysiology of, 118
Monokines, decreased in elderly, 60
Mortality, IADLs prediction of, 24
MRA (magnetic resonance angiography), for
      mesenteric ischemia, 232
MRI (magnetic resonance imaging), for mesenteric
      ischemia, 232
Multiple sclerosis, vertigo and, 335
Muscular system, lean body mass in, 8
MVCs (motor vehicle crashes), 338
   orthopedic injuries from, 359
Myocardial infarction. *See* MI
Myxedema coma
   clinical features of, 404–405, 405t
   diagnosis of, 405
   ED care/disposition of, 405–406, 406t
   precipitating events for, 404
   treatment recommendations in, 406–407

N

Nasogastric suction, for bowel obstruction, 177
Nasopharyngitis, 482
National Institute of Neurological Disorders and Stroke.
      See NINDS
National Institutes of Health Stroke Scale, 319t
Neer classification system, humerus fractures and,
      366f
Neisseria gonorrhoea, 526
Nesiritide
   for acutely decompensated heart failure, 93
   contraindications for, 94
   hypotension caused by, 93
Neurologic system, physical examination includes, 63
Neutropenia
   clinical features of, 511–512
   differential diagnosis of, 512
   ED care/disposition of, 512
Niacin deficiency, 420
NINDS (National Institute of Neurological Disorders
      and Stroke)
   thrombolytic therapy and, 322
   timeline for evaluation of stroke by, 318t

Nitroglycerin
  for coronary ischemia, 113
  for GI bleeding, 183
  for hypertensive emergencies, 128–129
  for mitral regurgitation, 117
NOMI (nonocclusive mesenteric ischemia), risk factors
    for, 228
Nomocytic anemia, 503
Nonparoxysmal atrial tachycardia. *See* PAT
NPPV (noninvasive positive-pressure ventilation), for
    COPD, 162
NSAIDs (non steroidal anti-inflammatory drugs), 18
  ARF and, 239
  GI bleeding from, 180
Nursing home transfers
  ALS and, 51
  approach for, 53
  ED interventions with, 52
  epidemiology of, 51
  facts related, 51b
  forms for, 52
Nursing homes, increased infections in, 57–58
Nutritional issues
  benchmarks for, 416
  RDAs and, 416

O

Ocular complaints
  anterior chamber in, 456
  conjunctiva in, 456
  cornea in, 456
  epidemiology/pathophysiology of, 455
  eyelids in, 455
  facts related to, 455b
  iris in, 456
  lacrimal system in, 455–456
  lens in, 456
  physical examination for, 457–460
  prevention, prognosis, outcome of, 460
  retina in, 456
  vitreous in, 456
Ocular examination, components of, 457–460
Odynophagia, 186
OMC (Orientation Memory Concentration Test),
    delirium screening using, 297, 299f
Opiates, for biliary tract disease, 218
Orthopedic injuries
  clinical features of, 359
  comorbid diseases with, 358–359
  epidemiology of, 358
  facts related to, 358b

  mechanisms of, 359
  osteoporosis as, 358
  pathologic fractures as, 358
  pathophysiology of, 358–359
  pitfalls in management of, 368
Orthostatic hypotension, 80–81
Osmolality, 369
Osmotic diuretics, for glaucoma, 464
Osteoarthritis
  factors associated with, 529
  pathogenesis of, 529
  treatment of, 529–530
Osteoporosis, 522
  compression fractures and, 522f
  male, 358
  menopause and, 358
  primary, types of, 9
OTC (over-the-counter) medications, 13
  effect on metabolism, 15t
Otitis externa, 480
Otomycosis, 480–481
Ovarian cancer, 251
  symptoms of, 256
Oxygen therapy, for COPD, 159–160

P

Pacemakers, 105
  balloon-tipped pacer catheters and, 108–109
  bradydysrhythmias and, 108
  electronic interrogation of, 106f, 107f
PADI (potential adverse drug interaction), 13
PAMI (Primary Angioplasty in Myocardial Infarction),
    75
PaO$_2$ respiratory system's decline of, 8
Paraneoplastic pemphigus. *See* PNP
Paraphimosis, 248
Paroxysmal supraventricular tachycardia. PSVT
Partial thromboplastin time. *See* PTT
PAT (nonparoxysmal atrial tachycardia), 101
  with block, 102f
Patient disposition, 52–53
PCP (primary care provider), 14
PDAs (personal digital assistants), pharmaceutical
    databases for, 20
PE (pulmonary embolism), 165. *See also* VTE (venous
    thromboembolism)
  ABG and, 167
  anticoagulation initiated for, 169
  care, subsequent, for, 170
  clinical features of, 166–167
  CT scan for, 168–169

PE (pulmonary embolism) *(contd.)*
  D-Dimer test for, 168
  differential diagnosis of, 167–168, 167t
  disposition of, 170
  ECG and, 167
  echocardiogram for, 169
  ED care/disposition of, 169
  ELISA for, 168
  epidemiology of, 165
  evaluation for, 167
  facts related to, 165b
  heparin therapy for, 169
  LMWH for, 170
  pathophysiology of, 165–166
  pitfalls regarding, 171
  pretest probability for, 167t
  pulmonary angiogram for, 167
  venous ultrasonography for, 168
  ventilation-perfusion scan for, 168
  and VTE, 165
  warfarin for, 170
PEA (pulseless electrical activity), chest trauma and, 354
Pedestrian-automobile accidents, 338
Pelvic floor disorders, 251
Pelvic injury(ies)
  acetabulum fractures as, 362
  classification of, 359–360, 360t
  complex pelvic fractures as, 362
  differential diagnosis of, 362
  ED care/disposition of, 362
  iliac wing fractures as, 362
  isolated bony fractures, avulsions as, 361–362
  pelvic ring fracture as, 360–361, 360f-361f
  pubic ramus fractures as, 362
  specific, 360–362
Pelvic mass(es), 256
  causes of, 257t
  large, 258
  ovarian cysts as, 256
  ovarian masses as, 256
Pelvic organ prolapse, 256–257
  examination for, 253
  non-surgical therapy for, 258
  pessaries, cause of, 257
  presenting symptoms of, 257t
  urinary catheterization for, 258
Pelvic ring fractures, 362
Pemphigus vulgaris. *See* PV
Penile conditions
  balantis, posthitis as, 248

paraphimosis as, 248
penile swelling as, 248
phimosis as, 248
Peptic ulcer disease
  clinical features of, 181
  differential diagnosis of, 181–182
  ED care/disposition of, 182
  endoscopy/upper GI series for, 181
  facts related to, 179b
  GI bleeding and, 180
  H. pylori and, 179, 181
  pathophysiology of, 179–180
  pitfalls in management of, 183
Peripheral vascular disease, arterial insufficiency, same as, 280
Peritonsillar abscess, 483
Personal digital assistants. *See* PDAs
Pharmacodynamics, in elders, 16
Pharmacokinetics
  in elders, 16
  renal function and, 64
Pharmacotherapy
  facts regarding, 13b
  successful, steps for, 20
Phimosos, 248
Phosphorus, 383–384
  loss of, 384t
Physical examination, 62–63
  for abuse/neglect, 35
  components of, 62
Physician, emergency
  aging and, 5
  elder's decision making capacity and, 40
Physiologic age
  v. biologic age, 1
  v. chronologic age, 337
Physiologic aging, 4
Physiologic reserve, 337
PMR (polymyalgia rheumatica), GCA and, 532
Pneumonia
  antibiotic therapy for, 147–148, 148t
  antimicrobials, other, for, 149
  blood cultures for, 147
  cephalosporins for, 149
  chest examination for, 145, 146
  clinical features of, 145–146
  complications of, 146
  CXR and, 64
  differential diagnosis of, 147
  epidemiology of, 144
  facts related to, 144b

fluoroquinolones for, 148–149
functional decline from, 66
ICU for severe, 151
β-lactams for, 149
macrolides for, 149
microbial etiology of, 145
microbial testing for, 146
mortality rates of, 144
nonpharmacologic management of, 147
nursing home-acquired, 151
outpatient management of, 149, 150
pathogens causing, 145
pathophysiology of, 144–145
PORT for assessing, 149, 150t
prevention of, 151
radiographic appearance of, 146
sputum gram stain and culture for, 146–147
"typical" v. "atypical," 145
vital signs with, 145
PNP (paraneoplastic pemphigus)
    clinical features of, 433–434
    differential diagnosis of, 434
    ED care/disposition of, 434–435
    epidemiology of, 432
    pathophysiology of, 433
Polymyalgia rheumatica. *See* PMR
Polypharmacy, 14
PORT (Pneumonia Severity Index), assessing
    pneumonia via, 149, 150t
Positive predictive value. *See* PPV
Postherpetic neuralgia
    capsaicin for, 440
    tricyclic antidepressants for, 440
Postmenopausal bleeding
    causes of, 254t
    endometrial carcinoma and, 255
Potassium, 375–376
    excretion routes of, 376
    hyperkalemia and, 377–378
    hypokalemia and, 376
Potential adverse drug interaction. *See* PADI
PPV (positive predictive value), of pyuria, 262
Prednisone, for HZ, 440
Premature ventricular contraction. *See* PVC
Prerenal failure, ARF and, 239
Preseptal, orbital cellulitis, 469–470, 473
    clinical features of, 470
    differential diagnosis of, 471
    ED care/disposition of, 472
Pressure ulcers, treatment, prevention of, 449–450
Presyncope, causes of, 333t

Primary Angioplasty in Myocardial Infarction. *See*
    PAMI
Primary care provider. *See* PCP
Prolonged QT-interval syndrome, associated with
    SCD, 132
Prostatitis
    clinical features and, 262
    treatment options and, 263
Prosthetic valve
    complications/management of, 119
    endocarditis, 119
Protein-calorie deficiencies, 417
Prothrombin time with international normalized
    ration. *See* PT/INR
Pseudogout, 528–529
PSVT (paroxysmal supraventricular tachycardia),
    101
Psychological aging, 4
Psychosis
    brain disease, underlying, and, 294
    clinical features of, 550–551
    delusional disorder as, 550
    differential diagnosis of, 551, 551t
    ED care/disposition of, 551
    epidemiology of, 550
    evaluation, challenges of, 295
    facts related to, 550b
    late life, 292
    pathophysiology of, 550
PT/INR (prothrombin time with international
    normalized ratio), hypocoagulability and, 495
PTT (partial thromboplastin time), hypocoagulability
    and, 495
Pubic ramus fractures, 362
Pulmonary angiogram, for PE, 167
Pulmonary embolism. *See* PE
Pulseless electrical activity. *See* PEA
PV (pemphigus vulgaris)
    clinical features of, 433
    differential diagnosis of, 434
    ED care/disposition of, 434
    epidemiology of, 432
    pathophysiology of, 433
    variants of, 432
PVC (premature ventricular contraction), 102
    interpolated, 104f
Pyrosis (heartburn), 186
Pyuria, 263

Q
QCS (Quick Confusion Scale), 42

R

RA (rheumatoid arthritis)
  description of, 530
  elderly onset v. younger onset of, 530–531
  treatment of, 531
  women and, 530
Radiographs, plain, for abdominal pain, 175–176
RBC (red blood cells), anemia and, 502–503
RDAs (recommended dietary allowances), 416
Referred pain, 173
Remitting seronegative symmetric synovitis with
    pitting edema (RS₃ PE) syndrome. *See* RS₃ PE
    syndrome
Renal calculus
  clinical features of, 245–246
  differential diagnosis of, 245
  ED care for, 246
  epidemiology of, 245
  helical CT scanning for, 246
  hospital admission for, 246
  NSAIDs for, 246
  waxing/waning flank pain in, 245
Renal failure
  fenoldopam for, 126
  hypertension and, 126
Renal function, 16
  age-related decrease in, 16
  drugs related to, 17t
  pharmacokinetics altered by, 64
Renal system, 8
  renal blood flow decrease in, 8
  renal mass loss in, 8
Respiratory physiology, changes, age-related, in, 138
Respiratory system, 7–8
  chest wall changes in, 8
  lung compliance in, 7–8
  PaO₂ decline in, 8
Restraining orders, for abuse/neglect, 38
Resuscitation
  as ethical issue, 43
  family presence during, 45
Retinal vascular occlusions
  clinical features of, 466–467
  ED care/disposition of, 467
  epidemiology of, 466
  facts related to, 466b
  pathophysiology of, 466
Rheumatic endocarditis, scarring from, 115
Rheumatoid arthritis. *See* RA
RS₃ PE (remitting seronegative symmetric synovitis
    with pitting edema) syndrome, 530

S

S. aureus, 526
SA node, dysrhythmia and, 100
SAEM (Society of Academic Emergency Medicine),
    emergency department care and, 52
SAH (subarachnoid hemorrhage)
  cause of, 318
  clinical features of, 305
  ED care/disposition of, 305
  epidemiology of, 304–305
  LP for, 322
  medications and, 323
  misdiagnosis of, 304, 305
  stroke and, 317
  symptoms of, 305
  treatment of, 323–324
  "worst headache of life" as, 304
SCD (sudden cardiac death)
  aortic stenosis and, 112
  cardiac diseases related to, 131
  circadian rhythms and, 131
  epidemiology of, 131
  facts related to, 131b
  ICD prevents, 133
  interventions for, 133
  pathophysiology of, 131–132
  prevention of, 133
  prolonged QT-interval syndrome associated with, 132
  recovery from, 133–134
  resuscitation after, 134
  survival and, 132–133
  ventricular tachyarrhythmia and, 132
Scrotal pain, Fournier's gangrene as, 248
Seizures/status epilepticus
  anticonvulsants, standard, for, 331t
  aura symptoms with, 328
  causes of, 326, 327
  clinical features of, 327–328
  differential diagnosis of, 329
  drugs causing, 327
  ED care/disposition of, 329–330
  EEG for, 328–329
  epidemiology of, 326–327
  facts related to, 326b
  first, 330
  history taking for, 328
  home services with, 330

LP for, 328
   medications for, 329, 330
   neuroimaging for, 328
   pathophysiology of, 327
   physical examination for, 328
   types of, 327
   younger v. older patients with, 326
Selective serotonin reuptake inhibitors. *See* SSRIs
Sensory systems
   hearing in, 10
   vision in, 10
Septic arthritis
   arthrocentesis for, 527
   causes of, 526
Serious otitis externa, 482
Serotonin syndrome, 14
Sexual activity, geriatric women and, 252
SIADH (syndrome of inappropriate antidiuretic
    hormone secretion)
   clinical features of, 510
   differential diagnosis of, 510
   ED care/disposition of, 510
   hyponatremia and, 373–374
   pathophysiology of, 510
Side effects/drug interactions, 67t
SIGNET (Systematic Intervention for a Geriatric
    Network of Evaluation and Treatment), 25, 26t
   TRST of, 25, 26t
Sinoatrial node. *See* SA node
Sinusitis, 482
SJS-TEN (Stevens-Johnson syndrome-toxic epidermal
    necrolysis)
   clinical features of, 429–430
   comorbidities and, 429
   components of, 429
   differential diagnosis of, 429–430, 430t
   ED care/disposition of, 430
   epidemiology of, 427–428
   facts related to, 427b
   laboratory tests for, 430
   medications, cause of, 428, 429
   organs susceptible to, 428–429
   pathophysiology of, 428–429
   priorities with, 430
   therapies for, 430
Skeletal system, 8–9
   primary osteoporosis and, 9
Skin tears, 445
   Payne-Martin classification system for, 446t
   prevention strategies for, 446
   treatment of, 446, 447f, 448f

SLE (systemic lupus erythematosus). *See also* Lupus,
    drug-induced, 532
   diagnosis of late-onset, 531–532
   management of, 532
   younger v. older cohorts with, 531
SMA (superior mesenteric artery) embolism
   mesenteric ischemia and, 233
   thrombosis, 233
Smoking
   arterial insufficiency and, 283
   COPD and, 154, 155
   effects of, 155f
Social services, called for abuse/neglect, 37
Society of Academic Emergency Medicine. *See* SAEM
Sodium, electrolyte disorders and, 373
Sodium nitroprusside
   for hypertensive emergencies, 128
   for hypertensive encephalopathy, 124
Somatic pain, 173
Somatostatin, for GI bleeding, 183
Spinal cord compression, acute
   clinical features of, 406–407
   differential diagnosis of, 507
   ED care/disposition of, 507
   pathophysiology of, 406
Spinal epidural abscess, 523
Spinal stenosis, 522
Spine fractures
   clinical features of, 367
   differential diagnosis of, 367
   ED care/disposition of, 367
Spironolactone, for heart failure, 95
SSRIs (selective serotonin uptake inhibitors), for
    depression, 548
Staphylococcus autereus, 526
Status epilepticus. *See* Seizures/status epilepticus
Stevens-Johnson syndrome-toxic epidermal necrolysis.
    See SJS-TEN
Stimson maneuver, 365f
Strangulated groin hernia, bowel obstruction from, 198
Streptococcus, 526
   group G, 526
Streptococcus pneumoniae, 526
Stroke
   causes of, 316
   clinical features of, 318–319
   cranial nerve examination for, 320
   CT scan for, 321–322
   diagnostic tests for, 321–322, 321t
   differential diagnosis of, 317t, 321
   ED care/disposition of, 321–324

Stroke *(contd.)*
facts related to, 316
hemorrhagic, 323–324
history taking for, 318
hypertension and, 322
initial assessment for, 319
intracranial hemorrhage and, 321
ischemic, 322
mental status examination for, 319–320
National Institutes of Health scale for, 319
neurologic examination for, 319
pathophysiology of, 316
premonitory headache preceding, 306
SAH and, 317
seizures with, 323
sensory, motor examination for, 320
speech difficulties from, 320
symptoms of, 316–317
syndromes, 317t
team treatment of, 324
thrombolytic therapy for, 322, 323t
TIA, similarities with, 317
visual loss from, 320
Stroke syndromes, hypertension and, 126–127
ST-segment elevation, AMI, 74
Subarachnoid hemorrhage. *See* SAH
Subdural hygroma, 344, 344t
Subtrochanteric fractures, 363
Sudden cardiac death. *See* SCD
Superficial thrombophlebitis, 285–286
Superior mesenteric artery. *See* SMA
Superior vena cava syndrome. *See* SVC
Supraventricular dysrhythmias, 100–102, 100f
AV junction level of, 101
Surrogates, for decision-making, 43
SVC (superior vena cava syndrome)
clinical features of, 508
differential diagnosis of, 508–509
ED care/disposition of, 509
pathophysiology of, 508
Swallowing, phases of, 185–186
Syncope
ancillary testing for, 83–84
aortic dissection with, 276
aortic stenosis and, 112t, 113f
autonomic nervous system/endocrine system and, 79
cardiac, 78, 79–80, 82
cardiovascular presentations with, 333–334
causes, other, of, 81
definition of, 78, 333
differential diagnosis of, 83

ED care/disposition of, 84
epidemiology of, 78
etiology of, 79t
facts related, 78b
fall resulting in, 30
head trauma from, 346
laboratory testing for, 83
medications associated with, 81, 81t
MI and, 82
monitoring for, 113
neurologic causes of, 81, 82
orthostatic hypotension and, 80
pathophysiologic mechanism of, 78
physical examination for, 82
pitfalls in management of, 84
position at time of, 82
reflex-mediated, 80
situational, 80
vasovagal/neurocardiogenic, 80, 333–334
vital signs evaluated with, 83
Syndrome of inappropriate antidiuretic hormone
secretion. *See* SIADH
Synovial fluid, examination of, 527t
Systemic lupus erythematosus. *See* SLE

T
Tachycardia, heat stroke and, 390
Tachydysrhythmias, electricity for, 108
T-cell/thalamic function, 58, 60
aging's effect on, 58
TEE (transesophageal echocardiogram)
for aortic dissection, 277
for mitral stenosis, 115
Temperature, body, BMR (basal metabolic rate) and, 11
Temporal arteritis. *See* GCA
Tendonitis, 533
Tension-type headache. *See* TTH
Tetanus, prophylaxis for, 452
Thirst, 370
Thoracoabdominal trauma
cardiac output and, 350
causes of, 349
clinical features of, 350
comorbid diseases with, 350
CT scan for, 351–352
differential diagnosis of, 351
DPL for, 352
ED care/disposition of, 353
epidemiology of, 349
facts related to, 349b
FAST and, 353

laboratory testing for, 353
pathophysiology of, 349–350
radiographs for, 351
ultrasonography for, 353
Thrombolytic therapy
inclusion/exclusion criteria for, 323t
stroke and, 322
Thyroid disease, facts related to, 402b
Thyroid releasing hormone. *See* TRH
Thyroid stimulating hormone. *See* TSH
Thyroid storm, 403
adjunctive therapies for, 412t
diagnosis of, 410, 410t
ED care/disposition of, 410–411
hyperthyroidism and, 409
precipitants of, 409, 409t
treatment of, 411, 411t
Thyroid surgery, 413
Thyrotoxicosis, 407
apathetic, 408–409
TIA (transient ischemic attack)
crescendo, 317
stroke, similarities with, 317
Timed "up and go" test, 24–25
TPP (thyrotoxic periodic paralysis), 412
Tracheobronchial injuries, 354
Tracheostomy(ies)
bleeding, complication of, 488
care, suctioning of, 486–487
clinical features of, 485
facts related to, 485b
history of, 485
infection, complication of, 488
obstruction, complication of, 487–488
pathophysiology of, 485
speech and, 486
tracheal, stomal stenosis, complication of, 488
tracheoesophageal fistula, complication of, 488–489
tubes, 485–486, 486f, 487
Transient ischemic stroke. *See* TIA
TRH (thyroid releasing hormone)
TSH stimulated by, 402
Tricyclic antidepressants, postherpetic neuralgia and, 440
Trigeminal neuralgia
clinical features of, 312
ED care/disposition of, 312
TRST (Triage Risk Screening Tool), 25, 26t
cost of, 26
TSH (thyroid stimulating hormone)
hypothyroidism and, 402
TRH stimulation of, 402

TTH (tension-type headache)
clinical features of, 311
ED care/disposition of, 311–312
Tuberculosis, 151–152
Tumor
"brain tumor headache" and, 306
clinical features of, 306
ICP and, 306

U
UGI (upper gastrointestinal) hemorrhage, 512–513
Ulcers
diabetic, 449
pressure, 449
vascular, 449–450
Unruptured aneurysms, ED care/disposition of, 271
Upper airway obstruction, malignancy and, 507
Upper gastrointestinal hemorrhage. *See* UGI hemorrhage
Ureteral obstruction, conditions causing, 245
Urinary incontinence, 264
Urinary retention
benign prostatic hypertrophy and, 247
ED care of, 247
epidemiology of, 246–247
Foley catheter used in, 247
hospital admission for, 247
older males and, 246
penile causes of, 246–247
radiographs for, 247
ultrasound for, 247
Urinary tract infection. *See* UTI
Urologic emergencies
facts related, 245b
renal calculus as, 245
urinary retention as, 246–247
Urologic syndromes, 513
Uterine procidentia, 253f
UTI (urinary tract infection). *See also* Bacteriuria
antibiotic therapy in, 263–264
bacteremia and, 64
causes of, 261
chronic incontinence and, 264
clinical features of, 262
cost, morbidity, mortality of, 260
definitions of terms for, 259t
ED care/disposition of, 262–264
epidemiology of, 260–261
facts related to, 259
laboratory tests for, 263

UTI (urinary tract infection) *(contd.)*
  organisms causing bacterial, 261t
  pathophysiology of, 261–262
  prevalence of, 260
  prostatic disease and, 261
  risk factors of, 260–261
  symptomatic, 263
  treatment options for, 263t
  urine, foul smelling, in, 262
  younger patients v. older patients with, 262

V

Vaginal
  candidiasis, 255
  carcinoma, 255–256
  prolapse, 254
Vaginal bleeding
  differential diagnosis for, 254–255
  rectal bleeding, excluded with, 257
  treatment for, 257
  vulvar sources of, 255
Vaginitis, atrophic, 254
Valvular heart disease. *See also* Aortic stenosis
  facts related to, 111b
  prophylaxis for, 118–119
  right-sided, 118
Vascular ulcers, 450–451
Vasopressin (intravenous), for GI bleeding, 183
Vasospasm, ACS and, 72
Vasovagal/neurocardiogenic syncope, 80
VBI (vertebrobasilar insufficiency), vertigo as, 335
Venous disorder(s)
  CVI as, 285
  facts related, 285b
Venous thromboembolism, complications of, 285
Ventricular dysrhythmias, 102–103, 105
Ventricular tachyarrhythmia, SCD and, 132
Ventricular tachycardia, 102, 104f
  ABCDEF approach to, 103
  concordance as evidence for, 105f
  ECG for, 103
  left, 104f, 105f
Vertebral osteomyelitis, 523
Vertebrovascular insufficiency. *See* VBI
Vertigo. *See also* BPV
  causes of, 334–335, 334t
  central, 335
  CT scan for, 336
  definition of, 334
  ECG for, 335

ED care/disposition of, 335–336
  eighth cervical vertebra and, 335
  medication for, 336
  medications causing, 334t
  physical examination for, 335
  Ramsey Hunt syndrome and, 335
  VBI and, 335
VF (ventricular fibrillation), defibrillation for, 132
Viagra, death/hypotension from, 76
Violence, 339
Visceral pain, 173
Vitamin A deficiency, 417–418
Vitamin B$_1$/Thiamin deficiency, 418
Vitamin B$_6$/Pyridoxine deficiency, 419
Vitamin B$_{12}$/Cyanocobalamin deficiency, 419
Vitamin C/Ascorbic acid deficiency, 420
Vitamin D deficiency, 420–421
Vitamin E/α-Tocopherol deficiency, 421
Vitamin K deficiency, 421
Volvulus
  atypical presentation of, 204
  barium enema for, 206
  bowel obstruction and, 202
  cecal, 203, 204
  ED care/disposition of, 206
  epidemiology of, 202
  facts related to, 202b
  imaging studies for, 204, 205f, 206
  laboratory findings for, 204
  mortality from, 202
  nonoperative treatment for, 206
  pathophysiology of, 202–203
  pitfalls in the management of, 206
  presenting symptoms of, 203–204
  sigmoid, 202–203, 206
  surgical interventions for, 206
VTE (venous thromboembolism)
  DVT as, 165
  heparin v. LMWH for, 171
  PE as, 165
  prophylaxis of, 171
  risks for, 166t
Vulvar skin conditions, 257–258
Vulvovaginal disorder
  atrophic vaginitis as, 255
  vaginal candidiasis as, 255

W

Warfarin
  ADREs/DDIs from, 18
  for PE, 170

Water
  excretion of, 370
  loss of, 370
Wide-complex tachycardias, 103
"Worst headache of life" , SAH as, 304
Wounds
  acute, 445
  assessment of, 445, 451
  burns as, 446, 448
  chronic, 448–449, 451–452
  diabetic ulcers as, 450
  epidemiology of, 444
  facts related to, 444b
  medications inhibiting healing of, 445t
  pathophysiology of, 444–445
  pressure ulcers as, 449, 449t
  skin tears as, 445, 446t
  treatment of, 445–446, 451
  vascular ulcers as, 450–451

Z
Zenker's diverticulum, 186